TNM
Staging Atlas
with Oncoanatomy

TNM Staging Atlas
with Oncoanatomy

Second Edition

Philip Rubin, MD, FASTRO

Professor and Chair Emeritus of Department of Radiation Oncology
Former Associate Director, James P. Wilmot Cancer Center
Senior Associate in Surgery and Medicine, University of Rochester School of Medicine and Dentistry
University of Rochester Medical Center, Rochester, New York

John T. Hansen, PhD

Professor of Neurobiology and Anatomy, and Associate Dean
University of Rochester School of Medicine and Dentistry, Rochester, New York

Wolters Kluwer | Lippincott Williams & Wilkins
Health

Philadelphia · Baltimore · New York · London
Buenos Aires · Hong Kong · Sydney · Tokyo

Senior Executive Editor: Jonathan W. Pine, Jr.
Senior Product Manager: Emilie Moyer
Vendor Manager: Alicia Jackson
Senior Manufacturing Manager: Benjamin Rivera
Senior Marketing Manager: Angela Panetta
Designer: Teresa Mallon
Production Service: Aptara, Inc.

Printed in China

Library of Congress Cataloging-in-Publication Data

Rubin, Philip, 1927-
    TNM staging atlas with oncoanatomy / Philip Rubin, John T. Hansen.—2nd ed.
        p. ; cm.
    Includes bibliographical references and index.
    ISBN 978-1-60913-144-9 (hardback : alk.paper)
    1. Tumors—Classification—Atlases. 2.
Cancer—Classification—Atlases.   I. Hansen, John T.   II. Title.
    [DNLM: 1. Neoplasm Staging—methods—Atlases.   2. Neoplasms—Atlases.
QZ 17]
    RC258.R83 2011
    616.99′4—dc23
                                                                2011024780

Care has been taken to confirm the accuracy of the information presented and to describe generally accepted practices. However, the authors, editors, and publisher are not responsible for errors or omissions or for any consequences from application of the information in this book and make no warranty, expressed or implied, with respect to the currency, completeness, or accuracy of the contents of the publication. Application of the information in a particular situation remains the professional responsibility of the practitioner.

The authors, editors, and publisher have exerted every effort to ensure that drug selection and dosage set forth in this text are in accordance with current recommendations and practice at the time of publication. However, in view of ongoing research, changes in government regulations, and the constant flow of information relating to drug therapy and drug reactions, the reader is urged to check the package insert for each drug for any change in indications and dosage and for added warnings and precautions. This is particularly important when the recommended agent is a new or infrequently employed drug.

Some drugs and medical devices presented in the publication have Food and Drug Administration (FDA) clearance for limited use in restricted research settings. It is the responsibility of the health care provider to ascertain the FDA status of each drug or device planned for use in their clinical practice.

To purchase additional copies of this book, call our customer service department at (800) 638-3030 or fax orders to (301) 223-2320. International customers should call (301) 223-2300.

Visit Lippincott Williams & Wilkins on the Internet: at LWW.com. Lippincott Williams & Wilkins customer service representatives are available from 8:30 am to 6 pm, EST.

10 9 8 7 6 5 4 3 2 1

Advisory and Section Editors

Joy Anderson, MD
Assistant Professor
Department of Radiation Oncology
James P. Wilmot Cancer Center
University of Rochester Medical Center
Rochester, New York
Section Editor of the Gynecologic Section

Ralph A. Brasacchio, MD
Associate Professor
Department of Radiation Oncology
James P. Wilmot Cancer Center
University of Rochester Medical Center
Rochester, New York
Section Editor of the Male Genitourinary Section

Yuhchyau Chen, MD, PhD
Professor and Chair
Director of Clinical Investigation
Department of Radiation Oncology
James P. Wilmot Cancer Center
University of Rochester Medical Center
Rochester, New York
Senior Advisory Editor and Section Editor of the Head and Neck and Thorax Sections

Louis S. Constine, MD, FASTRO
Professor of Radiation Oncology and Pediatrics
Vice Chair, Department of Radiation Oncology
James P. Wilmot Cancer Center
University of Rochester Medical Center
Rochester, New York
Section Editor of Generalized Sites, Eye, and CNS Sections

Alan W. Katz, MD, MPH
Associate Professor
Clinical Director
Department of Radiation Oncology
James P. Wilmot Cancer Center
University of Rochester Medical Center
Rochester, New York
Associate Editor and Section Editor of the Abdomen Section

Marilyn N. Ling, MD
Associate Professor
Department of Radiation Oncology
James P. Wilmot Cancer Center
University of Rochester Medical Center
Rochester, New York
Section Editor of the Breast Chapter

Michael T. Milano, MD, PhD
Associate Professor
Department of Radiation Oncology
James P. Wilmot Cancer Center
University of Rochester Medical Center
Rochester, New York
Associate Editor and Section Editor of Generalized Sites Section

George M. Uschold, RTT, EdD
Associate Professor
Department of Radiation Oncology
James P. Wilmot Cancer Center
University of Rochester Medical Center
Rochester, New York
Advisory Editor for Education and Training Applications

Sisi Lisa Chen
Information Analyst and Editorial Assistant
Department of Radiation Oncology
James P. Wilmot Cancer Center
University of Rochester Medical Center
Rochester, New York
Managing Editor

Contents

Foreword

TNM Staging Atlas with Oncoanatomy is a masterful attempt to bring order and understanding to the tumor staging systems. Staging systems play a critical role in describing the local/regional/distant extent of tumor spread for any given patient. Such systems enable clinicians to better communicate with each other, to sort patients into reasonably well-defined subgroups, and thus facilitate comparisons between like patients. Accurate staging is widely considered to be a prerequisite to optimal treatment. Nevertheless, staging systems are often simply *memorized* by practioners, rather than *understood*. In order to increase understanding, Rubin and Hansen summarize the patterns of spread for most solid tumors, and successfully relate these patterns to the normal anatomy of the affected organs. All of this information is presented in the context of the TNM staging system and is complemented by numerous clear colorful and instructive illustrations. A clear understanding of these anatomic principles and staging systems are needed for the safe practice of oncology.

Oncology is the word used to describe what we know about one of humanity's most-dreaded diseases. Anatomy is the term used to describe the very essence of our physical being. Students of anatomy are often struck by the beautiful complexity that lurks just beneath our skins. How could such complexities arise? And how is it that such complexities are recreated over and over again? I have always been struck by these two concepts: complexity yet inter-patient consistency. Cancer is such a vicious disease it almost seems to purposefully exploit the underlying anatomy.

Oncoanatomy is the fusion of these two words, (oncology and anatomy), and oncoanatomy is the paradigm for TNM oncotaxonomy. Philip Rubin has always had a flair for creating words and acronyms. The fusion of these two words is not just a convenience. For decades, Dr. Rubin has recognized the symbiotic relationship between understanding both anatomy and oncology. Knowledge of the anatomy helps to understand the behavior of cancer. Through our observations on the patterns of spread of cancer, we can gain greater insights into the underlying anatomy. Indeed, Dr. Rubin taught a course for the University of Rochester medical students and residents called "Oncoanatomy" (1) with Dr. John Hansen, the Senior Advisory Editor, who is one of the most gifted teachers of anatomy. While at Duke, we formed a similar course geared more towards residents in oncology-related disciplines (2, 3, 4, 5).

These educational initiatives, and this book, are recognitions of the inextricable link between cancer and anatomy. Indeed, given these linkages, oncologists (and radiation oncologists in particular) can play an important role in anatomy instruction for medical students. This book can serve as a tool to help to facilitate such instruction and establish electives in radiation oncology in medical schools.

The field of radiation oncology (and cancer care in general) is embracing more and more-complex technologies to care for our patients; e.g. better imaging with PET (positron emission tomography), better dose distributions with IMRT (intensity-modulated radiation therapy), and better localization with IGRT (image-guided radiation therapy). However, it is critical that we not lose sight of the underlying anatomic principles that help to explain how and why tumors spread. These underlying anatomic realities are not negated by these advanced technologies. For example, nasopharyngeal cancers will *still* tend to spread into the adjacent skull foramina, and such spread can be seen on imaging. Ideally, target volumes should be created with a firm understanding of these underlying anatomic principles rather than arbitrary 1 cm to 2 cm margins for planning volumes. Failure to do so will likely lead to marginal tumor misses.

This book is an outstanding resource for oncologists who need to continually consider these anatomic principles in their daily practice, as well as medical students who can better visualize three-planar anatomy through the window of cancer spread patterns and staging. It is the latest in a several-decades-long series of "Onco-Philip's" contributions to help us, as a medical specialty, better understand the apparent complexities of cancer and the anatomy sciences.

Lawrence B. Marks, MD

References

1. Hansen, J.T. and P. Rubin. Clinical anatomy in the oncology patient: a preclinical elective that reinforces cross-sectional anatomy using examples of cancer spread. *Clinical Anatomy* 1998;11:95–99.
2. Alvin R. Cabrera, MD, W. Robert Lee, MD, MS, MEd, Richard Madden, PhD, Ershela Sims, PhD, Jenny K. Hoang, MBBS, Leonard E. White, PhD, Lawrence B. Marks, MD, Junzo P. Chino, MD. Incorporating Gross Anatomy Education Into Radiation Oncology Residency: A 2-Year Curriculum With Evaluation of Resident Satisfaction. *J Am Coll Radiol* 2011;8:335–340.

3. Kelsey CR, Marks LB. Oncologic imaging/oncologic anatomy. In: Halperin EC, Perez CA, Brady LW, eds. *Perez and Brady's Principles and Practice of Radiation Oncology*, 5th edition. Philadelphia: Lippincott Williams & Wilkins; 2008:620–636.

4. Zumwalt AC, Marks L, Halperin EC. Integrating gross anatomy into a clinical oncology curriculum: the oncoanatomy course at Duke University School of Medicine. *Acad Med* 2007;82:469–474.

5. Chino JP, Lee WR, Madden R, et al. Teaching the anatomy of oncology: evaluating the impact of a dedicated oncoanatomy course. *Int J Radiat Oncol Biol Phys* 2011;79:853–859.

Preface

Since its inception, the TNM system has embraced the concept of determining the true anatomic extent of a cancer at the time of its initial diagnosis. The surgeon Pierre Denoix introduced the cancer language. The alphabet was simple: T, local tumor spread, N, regional lymph node involvement, and M, distant hematogenous seeding or metastases. The subscripts 1, 2, 3, and 4 delineated cancer advancement. The addition of stage grouping different TNM combinations allowed for simplification to four stages: I, II, III, and IV. Once cancer staging and classification became universally adopted by multidisciplinary oncologists, it resulted in a more uniform design of clinical trial target groups for their randomization. Prognosis has become more accurate and, most important, end-results reporting of survival and outcomes following treatment has allowed for comparisons between cancer centers for the sake of therapeutic improvements and gains.

The first edition of the *Cancer Staging Manual* (CSM) of the American Joint Committee on Cancer (AJCC) arrived in 1976, following a national conference devoted to the concept of cancer staging. By the third edition in the 1980s, all major cancer sites were included, and both the AJCC and International Union Against Cancer/Union Internationale Contre le Cancer (UICC) agreed to a joint publication, leading to its international use. In the 1990s, a number of revisions of the TNM staging system began and were made to adopt the staging systems of major surgical and medical oncology cooperative investigative groups, including the International Federation of Gynecology and Obstetrics (FIGO), among others.

The sixth edition of the CSM, published in 2002, and especially the seventh edition, published in October 2009, have numerous revisions, which raises the issue of consistency versus change and its impact on assessing the oncology literature. The first dilemma is use of the same TNM designations, whereby the stage has been redefined and assigned to different degrees of tumor advancement. Second, improvements in diagnostic techniques such as computed tomography (CT), magnetic resonance imaging (MRI), and positron emission tomography (PET) can lead to more accurate staging and, with it, stage migration. Finally, the oncology literature, which spans the last five decades, has constantly shown improvements in survival rates at different anatomic sites, but this may reflect both revisions and modifications in staging rather than true therapeutic gains.

A picture is worth a thousand words; a well-designed illustration is worth even more. This *TNM Staging Atlas* is intended to be a companion volume to major multidisciplinary oncology textbooks providing a visual reference with clear, full-color diagrams of TNM stages by organ site and their TNM anatomy to augment the detailed verbal anatomic descriptions at the beginning of each chapter of the CSM. It is designed to enable practicing oncologists and physicians to access the data they need in oncologic diagnostic, prognostic, and treatment decision making. For consistency, chapters are arranged in the same sequence, and when possible related figures, tables, and text appear together on the same two-page spread to minimize the need to flip back and forth. For medical students and residents, the volume is central to understanding three-dimensional (3D) human anatomy by cancer spread patterns. The primary site oncoanatomy is presented in 3D/three-planar fashion to correlate with CT/MR images generated clinically. The regional nodal anatomy illustrates the sentinel lymph node and the first station of regional nodes. The draining veins and vascular spread patterns leading to distant metastases are also presented together.

Our continued interest in the staging and classification of cancers dates back to the first edition (1977) of the *AJCC Cancer Staging Manual*, which was the first compilation of all primary sites staged to that time. At that time, one of the present authors (P. R.) was privileged to be one of the editors along with Ollie Beahrs (Surgery) and David Carr (Medicine) of the Mayo Clinic to organize and establish this important endeavor. In *Clinical Oncology and Oncoimaging Multidisciplinary Approach for Physicians and Students* (first through eighth editions) and *Oncologic Imaging* (first and second editions), we have illustrated cancer staging. The medical illustrations of cancer staging were introduced into our oncology textbook, *Clinical Oncology: A Multidisciplinary Approach Medical Students and Physicians*, sponsored and printed by the American Cancer Society, and reprinted in color in *Oncologic Imaging* as well as in the numerous editions of *Principles and Practice of Radiation Oncology* by C. A. Perez, L. W. Brady, and E. C. Halperin.

Philip Rubin

John T. Hansen

Acknowledgments

Every book places high demands on the creative processes of many individuals to produce a unique and singular volume. *The seminal concept of providing oncoanatomy as the paradigm for understanding the basis for the TNM oncotaxonomy staging of cancer* was germinated with John Hansen as a learning elective for medical students and residents.

We are grateful to our publisher, Lippincott Williams & Wilkins, for their encouragement and support to produce this endeavor. Specifically, Jonathan Pine provided a generous grant for the artwork essential to foster the initial and revised phases of the project. Emilie Moyer, senior product manager, was responsible for coordinating the editorial and illustrative aspects to produce the book. We are most appreciative to Lippincott Williams & Wilkins for allowing us to integrate illustration assets from other publications into the TNM Staging Atlas.

The editing of the *TNM Staging Atlas* is a demanding task, which includes meticulous detailed attention to page design. In the present edition, my Managing Editor Sisi Lisa Chen, in coordination with Emilie Moyer of LWW, edited the page proofs. Chris Miller of Aptara has been steadfast through the creation and printing of the page layouts, as was Donna Kessler of Aptara for the first edition.

The initiation and development of the concept of using cancer spread patterns to provide a scaffold for appreciating 3D anatomy are in large part due to the enthusiastic response of medical students and radiation oncology residents. The term **oncoanatomy** embodies the idea of the cancer crab's six basic directions of invasion and was endorsed by our faculty in our teaching seminars. Of special note are Alvin Ureles, George Uschold, and Pat Fultz, together with the department of radiation oncology faculty and colleagues who have reviewed this text as section editors and offered their encouragement to pursue this venture. The electronic version has been assembled and updated by Seth Rubin, our webmaster, who created a website to allow for multiple section editors to participate in the final review for this second edition.

The medical illustrator Margaret Pence, of the Rochester Institute of Technology (RIT) faculty, has been untiring, imaginative, and most reliable in updating the TNM Stage Group figures illustrating the advancement of primary and lymph nodes as were the medical illustrators, Tiffany Gagnon and Kristen Johnson of RIT, who rallied in the summer of 2008 to actualize this demanding assignment for the first edition.

The major burden of assembling the text, figures, and tables of the first edition, which became a Sisyphean chore, was carried by Heike Kross, my editorial and research assistant, with dedication and devotion. Also, Frank Stock, a gifted artist undertook the final task of refining the art to meet publication requirements for high-resolution illustrations in the first edition.

Finally, my beautiful granddaughters to whom this book is dedicated have all participated actively in numerous draft versions of this volume. Of particular note are Sara, Amanda, Madelyn, as well as Rebecca and Lisa, who actively participated in formulating and configurating the three-planar anatomy during college breaks and holidays and over past summers.

Special Recognition

The *AJCC Cancer Staging Manual* has undergone seven editions since its origin in the 1960s by the American Joint Committee for Cancer (AJCC) in coordination with the International Union Contra Cancer (UICC). As one of the authors of the first *AJCC Cancer Staging Manual* edition with Ollie Bears (surgeon) and David Carr (internist) of the Mayo Clinic, I appreciate the arduous task of creating new staging systems and modification of an existing TNM system. The number of TNM cancer site specific systems has doubled from 30 to more than 70 over the past 5 decades. The multidisciplinary interaction of the American College of Physicians, Surgeons, and Radiologists and Pathologists in addition to numerous sponsoring and liaison organizations is the essential element to widespread acceptance and use by the world's onocologists on all six continents. There are 13 task forces with 180 members of key cancer committees. We are most appreciative for their permission to enable us to illustrate the cancer progression as presented in the 7th Edition *AJCC Cancer Staging Manual*. To assure accuracy in verbal and numeric categories, we have added a group of section editors from our faculty who are actively practicing oncologists specializing in the cancer region/sites using the current staging systems on a daily basis.

Medical Book of the Year Award 2008

TNM Staging Atlas by Philip Rubin and John T. Hansen won the celebrated British Medical Association (BMA) Medical Book of the Year Award 2008, and also secured First Prize in the oncology class. The BMA Medical Book Competition has been held annually since 1994 by the BMA's Board of Science and administered by the BMA Library. It aims to encourage and reward excellence in medical publishing and patient information. A total of 640 books were entered in this international competition.

How to Use the Atlas
The Concept of TNM Oncoanatomy

- The oncoanatomy is the paradigm for the oncotaxonomy, that is, the anatomic extent of cancer spread is the basis for cancer classification and staging.
- The oncoanatomy refers to the normal tissue organization of a specific anatomic site that determines the clinical behavior of the cancer that originates there and its pattern of spread.
- The cancer crab invades the anatomic site of origin in six basic directions: superior-inferior, medial-lateral, anterior-posterior (SIMLAP). Although cancer can infiltrate in a myriad of directions, it usually follows the path of least resistance around these six vectors. The tumor infiltrates along fascial and muscle planes, invading fatty areolar spaces, and enters low pressure lymphatics and venous channels.
- The three-dimensional anatomic aspects and construct of a region is readily appreciated by utilizing the model of cancer spread patterns. That is, each manifestation of the cancer clinically is based upon a specific vector of tumor involvement, providing a geographic, anatomic-physiologic basis as its explanation.
- The most important decision in cancer treatment is the first decision once the neoplasm is definitely diagnosed as to its histopathologic type and grade.
- Knowing the anatomic extent of the cancer or its stage is most often the key determinant in achieving a successful outcome and selection of treatment.
- The oncoanatomy is presented as Regional Sections (7), which then are divided into Primary Cancer Sites (61). Then each regional section is presented first as an orientation diagram in an anterior and lateral projection, with surface anatomy landmarks and a radiographic osseous feature, the vertebral level.
- Each anatomic region is presented in 3D/3-planar sections; a coronal, a sagittal, and a transverse axial section of anatomy. There are seven anatomic regions, each with several primary cancer sites, which are ordered from cephalad to caudad.
- This "companion volume" to major multidisciplinary, multiauthored oncology textbooks is designed for the oncologist to have a visual illustrated reference to TNM staging to complement the associated verbal descriptive anatomy that begins each chapter in all editions of the AJCC and UICC (seventh edition).
- Each cancer site is introduced by a diagram of anatomic features identifiable on physical or radiographic examination.
- The derivative normal cellular and histologic features of each site provide a basis for the WHO histopathologic classification of cancers at each anatomic site.
- The patterns of cancer spread at the primary site (T), to regional nodes (N), and to a distant target organ of first metastases (M), often based on venous drainage, are concisely presented as the logic built into the TNM system of tumor progression.
- The 3D/3-planar oncoanatomy of the primary site and the regional nodes along with its venous drainage are presented in succession.
- The first-station lymph nodes (N) are shown for each primary site, with emphasis on the sentinel lymph node and tabulation of regional lymph nodes.
- Hematogenous spread via draining venous channels (M) will often determine the target metastatic organ.
- The clinical imaging criteria for staging with onco-imaging annotations are emphasized in the rules for TNM classification.
- The cancer survival results over the past 5 decades are presented as Surveillance Epidemiology and End Results (SEER) 5-year survival data (1950–2000).
- In reviewing the staging systems that have been designed, adopted, and modified over time, we have utilized the international anatomical terminology (*Terminologia Anatomica*) to improve the accuracy of reporting by oncologic disciplines to supplement the numbering of lymph node stations in a region.

Chapter Organization

The Design of Individual Cancer Site Chapters follows a similar page layout to minimize page turning.

- *One topic* is assigned to each set of facing pages: text on left page, figures on right page, tables on either side.
1. **Histopathology** of the dominant cancer is illustrated in microsections from *Rubin's Pathology* and is accompanied by WHO Histopathology Table. (Table 1 and Figure 1).
2. **Pathology and Patterns of Cancer Spread** is illustrated in two views of the anatomy (Figures 2A and 2B).
   A. Coronal B. Sagittal, whenever possible. Six patterns of cancer spread are presented: Superior, Inferior, Medial, Lateral, Anterior, and Posterior. (SIMLAP Tables accompany Patterns of Spread figures; Table 2 and Figure 2).
3. **TNM Staging Criteria and Changes** summarized according to the 7th Edition of American Joint Committee of Cancer/UICC Cancer Staging Manual

(published in 2010). Two additional features are a **Stage Summary Matrix** and a concise overview summarizing 6th and 7th edition changes of each staging system.

- **TNM Stage Groups** are presented diagrammatically in five color-coded lanes with portrayal of T progression and N advancement. Definitions are on the left side and Stage Groups are on the right side. (Figure 3).
- **TNM Stage Summary Matrix** allows ease in identifying Stage Group once T and N stages are defined. (Table 3).

4. **T-Oncoanatomy** consists of phantom figures to orient the three-planar anatomy in coronal, sagittal, and axial sections at the anatomic isocenter of the cancer site (Nexus).
   - **T-Oncoanatomy** is identified by coronal/sagittal crosshair diagrams based on trigeminal landmarks (Figure 4).
   - **T-Oncoanatomy** is displayed in three dissection planes based mainly on *Grant's Atlas of Anatomy*. (Figure 5).

5. **N-Oncoanatomy** describes the sentinel lymph node and regional lymph nodes, which are tabulated and displayed in Table 4, and Figure 6.
   M-Oncoanatomy describes the venous drainage pattern and target metastatic organ.
   - **N and M-Oncoanatomy** of lymph nodes and veins are illustrated based on *Grant's Atlas of Anatomy* (Figure 6A for N-Oncoanatomy, and Figure 6B for M-Oncoanatomy orientation).
   - **Incidence and Distribution** of Lymph Node and Distant Metastases by Stage are tabulated and diagrammed when available in literature.

6. **Rules and Staging Work-up** emphasize imaging with CT/MRI/PET/US with "Oncoimaging Annotations" based on *Oncologic Imaging* by Bragg, Rubin, and Hricak, 2nd Edition, Elsevier, 2002, Table 5. A normal transverse axial CT/MRI is presented to allow correlation with axial anatomy section. (Table 5).
   - **CT and MR imaging** in axial plane is offered as a correlate to T-oncoanatomy three planar (Figure 7).
   - **Prognostic Factors and Survival Statistics** are summarized (Table 6) based on 7th Edition AJCC data in the form of bar graphs, by stage and five year survival rates. (Figure 8).

When the TNM oncoanatomy is the same, multiple histopathologies, each with its own staging system, are added as separate TNM staging figures. Examples are in Head and Neck: Ethmoid Sinus Cancer/Mucosal Melanoma, Thorax: Esophagus vs. Esophagogastric Junction, Abdomen: Stromal Cancer and Stromal Tumor, Liver and Intrahepatic Bile Ducts, Gynecologic: Fundus Cancer vs. Sarcomas, GAS: Basal/Squamous Cell Cancers vs. Merkel Cell Carcinoma, Eye: Choroid Melanomas.

In a similar fashion, **multiple anatomic sites** with identical anatomies are consolidated into one chapter: the Glottis and Subglottis in the Head and Neck, Liver and Intrahepatic Bile Ducts, Distal and Proximal Bile Ducts in the Abdomen, Penis and Urethra in the Male Genital Site, and the Ovary and Fallopian Tube in the Gynecologic site.

Special Features: Color Code

A unifying feature of this atlas is a color code that portrays the spectrum of cancer progression at primary sites (T) and lymph node regions (N), and of stage grouping. The head and neck oropharynx cancer site illustrates the color code.

- **The unifying feature is the Color Code for Cancer Progression of primary tumors and lymph nodes. The Head and Neck Oropharynx cancer illustrates the design of figures.**

T0 or TIs	Yellow
T1	Green
T2	Blue
T3	Purple
T4a	Red
T4b	Black

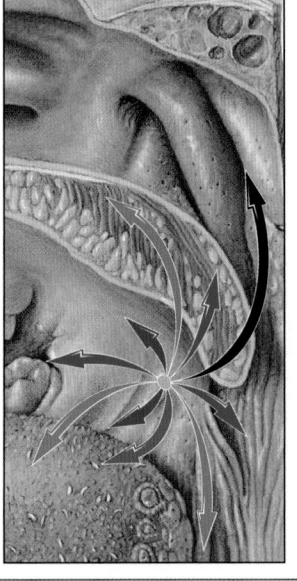

Coronal

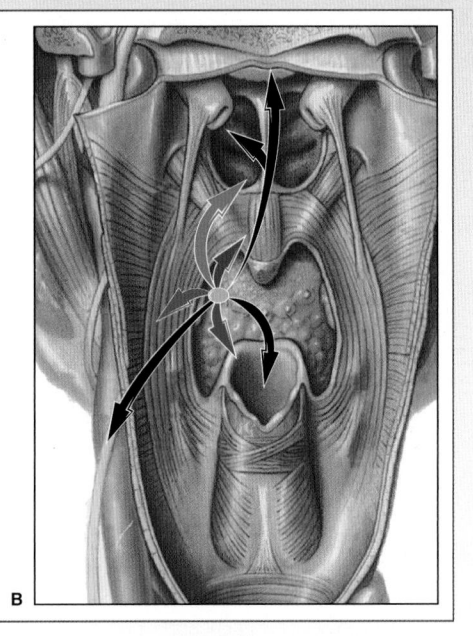

Sagittal

TABLE 7.2 SIMLAP*

Oropharynx (Tonsil)		
S	Nasopharynx	• T4b
	Skull base	• T4b
I	Hypopharynx, larynx	• T4b
M	Medial pterygoid muscle	• T4b
L	Mandible	• T4a
	Lateral pterygoid muscle	• T4b
	Encases carotid	• T4b
A	Hard palate	• T4a
P	Prevertebral space	• T4b

There are six basic directions or vectors (arrows): The six vectors of invasion are <u>S</u>uperior, <u>I</u>nferior, <u>M</u>edial, <u>L</u>ateral, <u>A</u>nterior, and <u>P</u>osterior. The color-coded dots correlate the T stage with specific anatomic structure involved.

- **For the primary (T)**, color-coded arrows on the cancer crab spread patterns allow the reader to immediately appreciate cancer progression and advancement. Each arrow points to specific structures that advance the stage when invaded. Arrow color changes and length increases as stage advances.
- **SIMLAP Tables** act as legends for Figure 1 **Patterns of Spread** by identifying the anatomy invaded and its impact on stage. There are six vectors of cancer infiltrations: <u>S</u>uperior, <u>I</u>nferior, <u>M</u>edical, <u>L</u>ateral, <u>A</u>nterior, and <u>P</u>osterior. The T stage advancement assigns the color-code dot next to specific structures provides the T stage if involved by cancer.
- For primary and regional nodes, the designation of nodal progression N1, N2, N3 is colored the same as T1, T2, and T3. Beyond, T4a,b and N3 refers to second station or echelon of nodes. We are suggesting M_N for such regional lymph nodes, which are considered truly juxtaregional but not placed in M1. Such metatastic juxtaregional nodes are quite distant and rarely curable.
- For TNM Stage Grouping (the third figure in each chapter), the color code remains the same. Horizontal color bars encompass T and N categories, which vary in each stage group. Variations in cancer staging, A and B, when applied to stages III and IV, in effect creates five or six stages. In such situations, color coding may vary but is designed to show progression of a more advanced stage.
- The vertical arrangement of TNM is to allow the reader to read across the page to check T and N.
- **Definitions on left** with pictorial display and **stage groupings on right**. When stage group is not shown in diagram, an asterisk alerts the reader and is annotated in the legend.

T0 or TIs	Yellow	N0
T1	Green	N1
T2	Blue	N2
T3	Purple	N3
T4a	Red	N4 N_m
T4b	Black	N4 M_1

DEFINITION OF TNM

T1
Tumor ≤2 cm in greatest dimension

N0
No regional lymph node metastasis

T2
Tumor >2 cm but not more than 4 cm in greatest dimension

N0
No regional lymph node metastasis

T3
Tumor >4 cm in greatest dimension

N1
Metastasis in a single ipsilateral lymph node, ≤3 cm in greatest dimension

T4a
Tumor invades the larynx, deep/extrinsic muscle of tongue, medial pterygoid, hard palate, or mandible

N2
(N2a) Metastasis in a single ipsilateral lymph node, >3 cm but ≤6;
(N2b) Metastasis in multiple ipsilateral lymph nodes, none >6 cm;
(N2c) Metastasis in bilateral or contralateral lymph nodes, none >6 cm

T4b
IVB
T4b Tumor invades lateral pterygoid muscle, pterygoid plates, lateral nasopharynx, or skull base or encases carotid artery

N3
Metastasis in a lymph node >6 cm in greatest dimension

STAGE GROUPINGS

Stage I
T1 N0 M0

Stage II
T2 N0 M0

Stage III
T3 N0 M0
T1 N1 M0
T2 N1 M0
T3 N1 M0

Stage IVA
T4a N0 M0
T4a N1 M0
T1 N2 M0
T2 N2 M0
T3 N2 M0
T4a N2 M0

Stage IVB
T4b Any N M0
Any T N3 M0

Stage IVC
Any T Any N M1

TABLE 7.3	Stage Summary Matrix				
	Stage T1	**Stage T2**	**Stage T3**	**Stage T4a**	**Stage T4b**
N0	I	II	III	IVA	IVB
N1	III	III	III	IVA	IVB
N2	IVA	IVA	IVA	IVA	IVB
N3	IVB	IVB	IVB	IVB	IVB
M1	IVC	IVC	IVC	IVC	IVC

* *T stage* determines stage group
  * T1 = I, T2 + II, T3 = III, T4 = IV
* *N stage* N1 = T3 and then progresses as T stage progresses
  * N1 = T3, N2 = T4a, N3 = T4b
* *M stage* is a separate stage
  * M1 = Stage IVC

- **Stage Summary Matrix figures** are designed in color code as in Stage Groups for ease in determining exact stage group to complement Stage Group figures.
- **Orientation of T-oncoanatomy:** The crosshair diagrams provide landmarks for the anatomic isocenter, which is the nexus for three-planar anatomy. Trigeminal landmarks are readily identified in surface (ectoderm), skeletal (mesoderm), and visceral (endoderm).

- The anatomic isocenter is at the axial level, in this case, at level C3. Figure A shows the coronal view. Figure B shows the Sagittal view.

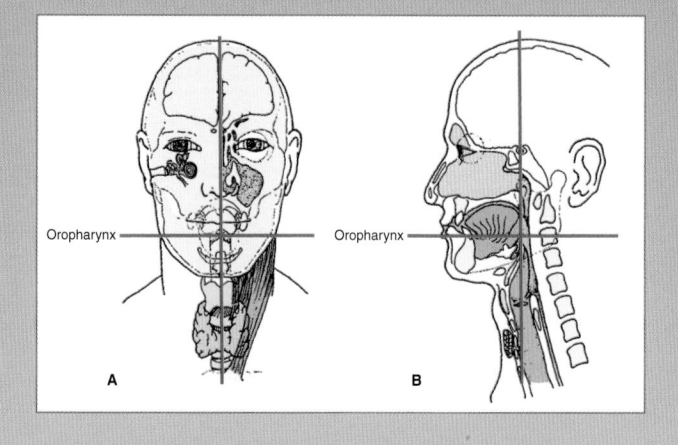

- **T-Oncoanatomy legend of Three-Planar Views** have been the anatomy leadlines and labels, also with color-code dots assigned to cancer progression by stage.
- Connecting the dots via color code allows for integrating the oncoanatomy into the TNM oncotaxonomy.
- *Three-planar anatomy has similar color code dots identifying specific structures invaded as cancer invasion progresses.

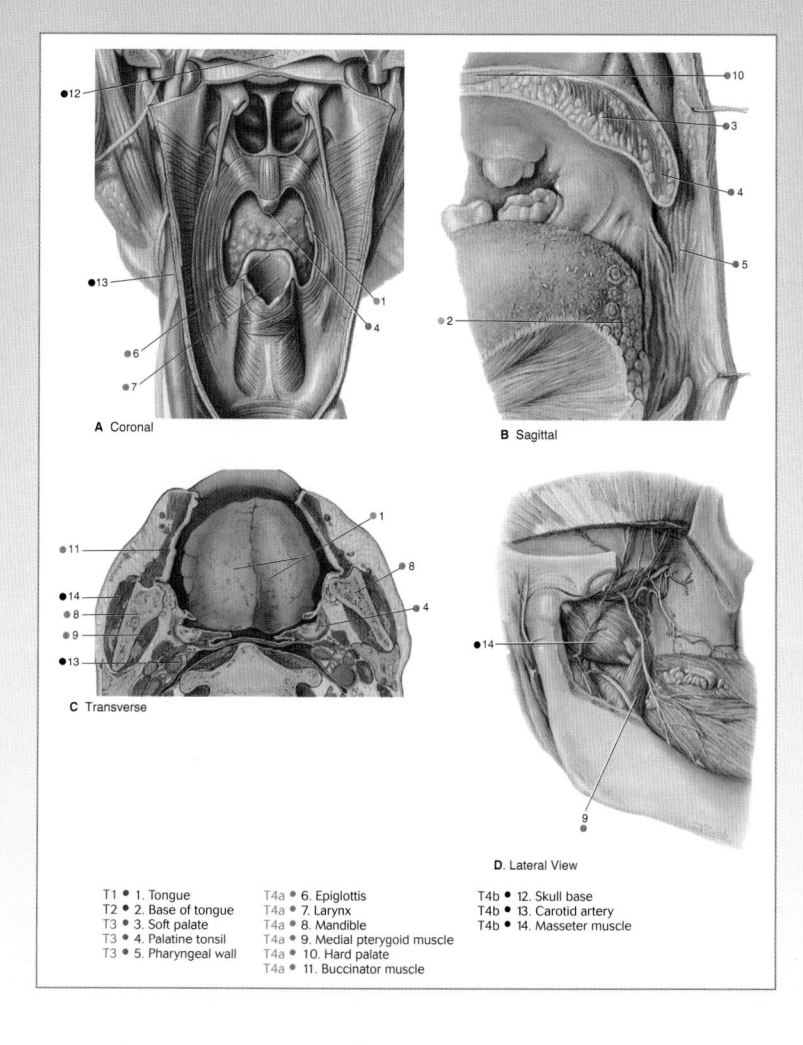

A Coronal

B Sagittal

C Transverse

D. Lateral View

T1 • 1. Tongue	T4a • 6. Epiglottis	T4b • 12. Skull base
T2 • 2. Base of tongue	T4a • 7. Larynx	T4b • 13. Carotid artery
T3 • 3. Soft palate	T4a • 8. Mandible	T4b • 14. Masseter muscle
T3 • 4. Palatine tonsil	T4a • 9. Medial pterygoid muscle	
T3 • 5. Pharyngeal wall	T4a • 10. Hard palate	
	T4a • 11. Buccinator muscle	

Concept of the Cancer Staging Process: Connecting the Dots

Oncoanatomy is the paradigm of TNM Oncotaxonomy. The clinical oncologist most often will rely on some form of cross-sectional imaging: CT/MRI/PET to determine anatomic extent of the cancer, its stage.

Thus, by "Connecting the Dots" in anatomy, it alerts the clinical oncologist what anatomy details he or she needs to discern for T staging.

- **The Gross Tumor Volume (GTV)** will be defined by size and details as to normal anatomy structures invaded by the cancer.
- **The Gross Nodal Volume (GNV)** is determined by sentinel and regional lymph node involvement and is defined by size, number, and geographic location of nodes in relation to primary site. Such aspects as mobility, matting, and ulceration are assessed on clinical examination.
- **Connecting the Dots** is a new feature in which the Patterns of Spread figures are color coded for cancer advancement in SIMLAP (Table 2).
- **T-Oncoanatomy** legends are color coded for cancer invasion stage.

*Connecting the Dots assists and abets the Staging Process (Figure 5).

SECTION 1
Head and Neck Primary Sites

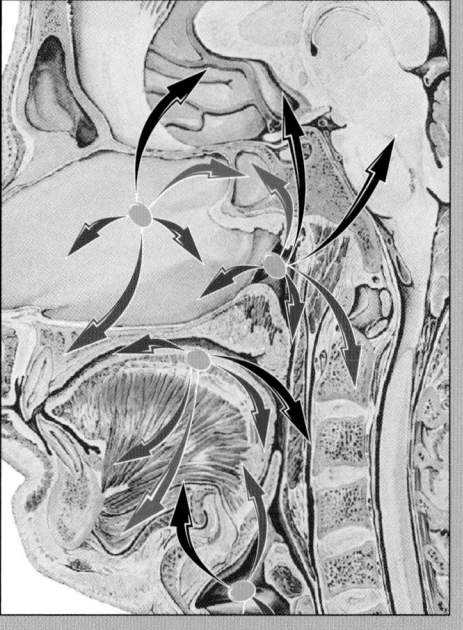

Introduction and Orientation

PERSPECTIVE AND PATTERNS OF SPREAD

The study of the patterns of tumor spread and their invasive behavior provides a unique spyglass through which one can view and understand this regional anatomy three dimensionally.

PERSPECTIVE AND PATTERNS OF SPREAD

The head and neck area is a very complex region consisting of a series of mazes and channels that constitute the upper aerodigestive passages. A large variety of tumors arise from the different tissues that constitute the various structures of the head and neck sites. This section focuses on malignancies arising from the surface epithelium, which are the most frequently encountered cancers. They are very destructive if allowed to progress, and because of the resultant functional disabilities, their impact on social presentation, particularly with regard to self-image, speech, and communication, can be extremely

detrimental. The challenge is not only to be able to control these cancers, but also to maintain normal anatomic relationships and structure. The TNM staging reflects the patterns of spread and the oncologic anatomy (Fig. 1.1). The common cancers arising in the upper aerodigestive passages are mainly in the pharyngeal and laryngeal tubes (Table 1.1).

Although head and neck cancers are clustered together, they comprise a very diverse group of tumors. If facial and scalp skin cancers and melanomas were included with extracranial head and neck tumors, this would be the most common anatomic site for malignancy. When typically limited to mucosal cancers of the upper aerodigestive tract, it accounts for 3% of all cancers and ranks 6th worldwide—7th for men and 11th for women. The classic patient population presenting with head and neck cancers consists of those with excessive smoking and alcohol habits. Essential to success are programs designed for posttreatment abstinence to avoid a recurrence of malignant tumors.

Cancers in the head and neck region are similar in terms of their biologic behavior; it is the differences in primary site anatomy that define the uniqueness of their clinical

TABLE 1.1	SIMLAP*	
Oral Cavity (Oral Tongue)		
S	Hard Palate	• T4a
	Maxillary Sinus	• T4a
	Skull Base	• T4b
I	Floor of Mouth, Deep Extrinsic Muscles (Genioglossus, hyoglossus, palatoglossus and Styloglossus)	• T4a
M		
L	Mandible Cortical Bone	• T4a
	Skin of Face	• T4a
A	Skin of Face	• T4a
P	Masticator Space	• T4b
	Pterygoid Plates	• T4b
	Carotid Artery	• T4b

*There are six basic directions or vectors (*arrows*): The six vectors of invasion are Superior, Inferior, Medial, Lateral, Anterior, and Posterior. The colored dots correlate the T stage with specific anatomic structure involved.

manifestations. The conceptualization of three-dimensional anatomy of the head and neck region is therefore appreciated through cancer spread (Fig. 1.1). The cancer crab can spread in six basic directions: superiorly–inferiorly, medially–laterally, and anteriorly–posteriorly (SIMLAP). There are an infinite number of possible patterns around these six basic vectors; however, these are predetermined by the arrangement of muscle and fascial planes. Cancers of the head and neck tend to follow the path of least resistance, invading fatty areolar spaces, which are particularly vulnerable; along nerves through perineural invasion; and entering bony ostia and foramina. Lymphatics and vessels also provide low-pressure flow channels of minimal resistance.

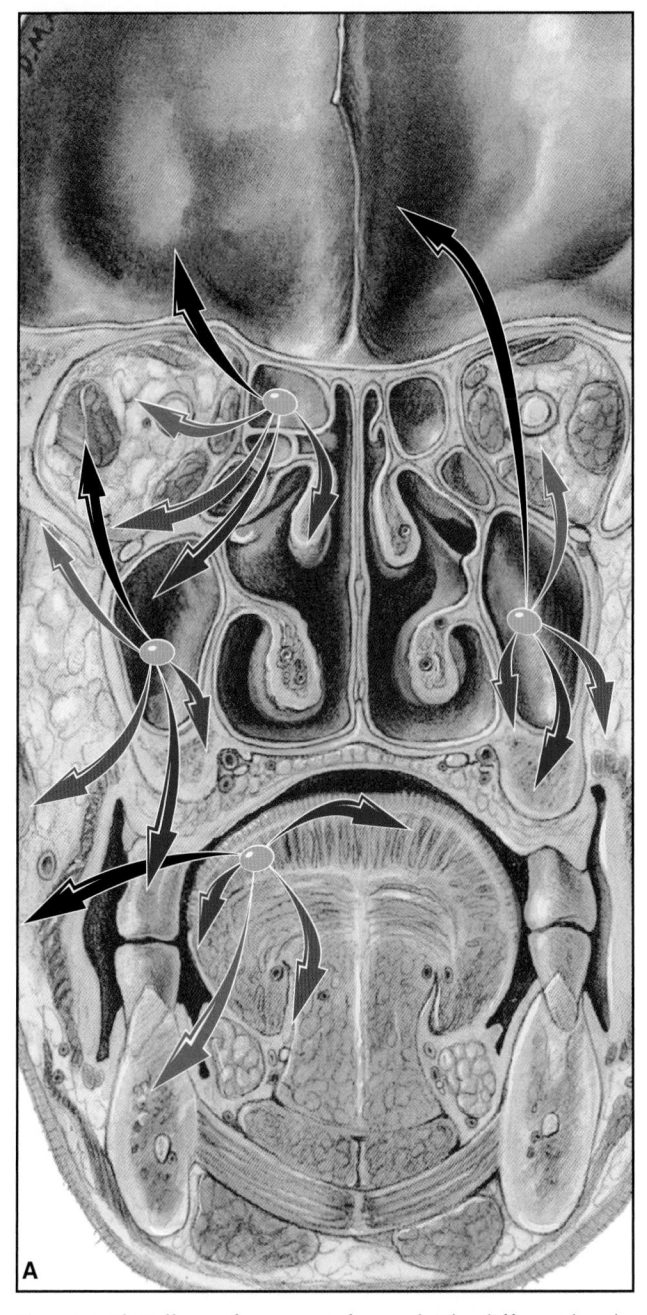
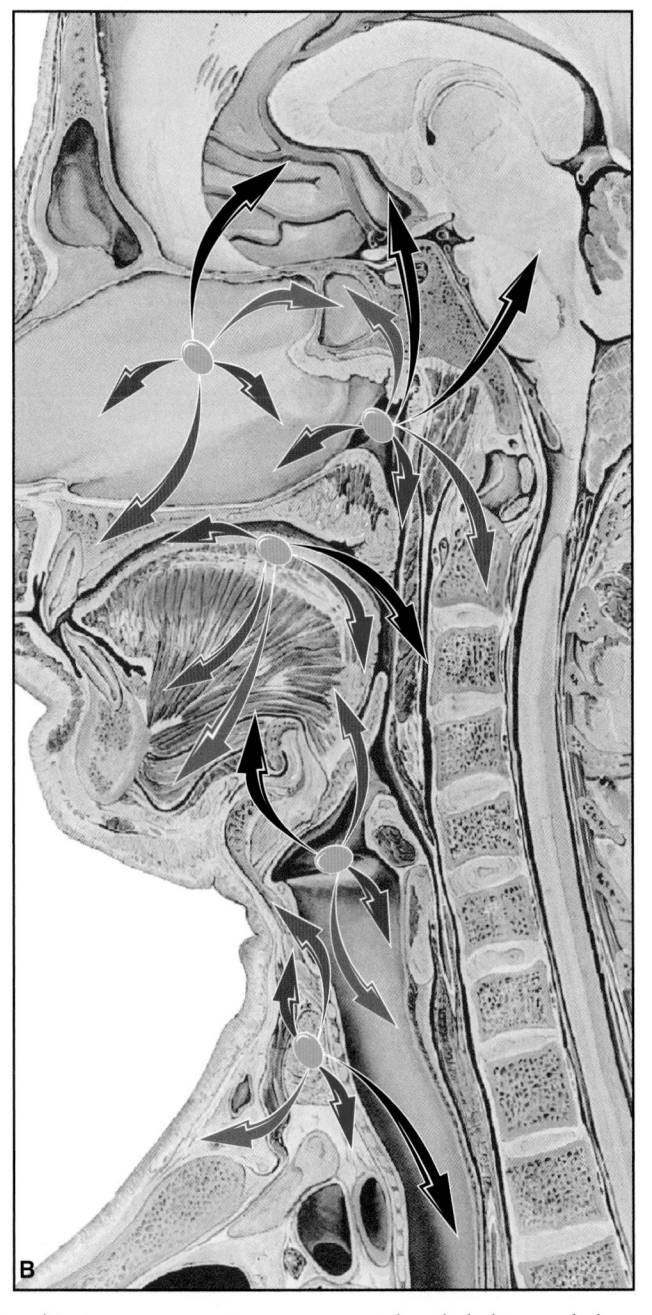

Figure 1.1 | Collage of patterns of spread. The different head and neck primary cancer sites are presented cephalad to caudad. **A.** Coronal: Ethmoid, maxillary antrum, and oral cavity. **B.** Sagittal: maxillary antral, nasopharynx, oral cavity, larynx, and thyroid. There are six basic directions or vectors (*arrows*): anterior–posterior, medial–lateral, superior–inferior. The *arrows* are color-coded for T stage category: T is yellow, T1 green, T2 blue, T3 purple, T4a red, T4b black. The concept of visualizing patterns of spread to appreciate the surrounding anatomy is well demonstrated by the six directional pattern i.e. SIMLAP Table 1.1.

OVERVIEW OF HISTOGENESIS

The mucosal surfaces of the two major sectors differ (Fig. 1.2; Table 1.2). The respiratory passage is a ciliated columnar or pseudostratified columnar epithelium (Fig. 1.2B–D), and the digestive passage is a stratified squamous epithelium (Fig. 1.2E,F). Both give rise mainly to squamous cell cancers. Most cancers are epithelial in origin, arising from the surface and evolving into four general patterns of invasion; shallow, mucosal, premalignant leukoplakia-like warty lesions often become submucosal (Fig. 1.3A).

- *Verrucous growths:* Wartlike, spreading on the surface rather than in depth;
- *Exophytic and exuberant growth:* An polyploid mushroom in appearance that undergoes;
- *Fungation, necrosis of growth:* This type of tumor usually, but not always, undergoes ulceration; and
- *Endophytic invasive growth:* Infiltration into muscle or erosion of bone and cartilage, and invasion perineurally of the cranial nerves and their branches.

Adenocarcinomas arise from the endocrine thyroid gland and the exocrine salivary glands (Figs. 1.2C–G and 1.3B).

Because most of the sites consist of different tissue layers (an epithelial surface, underlying muscle, and/or bone with an air-containing cavity), the study of primary tumor sites, where neoplasms commonly arise, requires an appreciation of the surrounding structures. Fat collections in specific pockets in and about the face, pharynx and larynx, and the areolar spaces, which are normally collapsed, are preestablished planes for cancer spread and infection. These spaces allow for mobility and the sliding of muscles during deglutition and speech. The various foramina are particularly vulnerable to spread. Because nerves pass through these openings in their course, perineural infiltration is often a problem.

TABLE 1.2	**Overview of the Histogenesis at Primary Cancer Sites**		
Primary Site Structure	**Derivative Normal Cell**	**Cancer Histopathology**	**Axial Level**
Ethmoid sinus, nasal cavity	Ciliated pseudostratified columnar epithelial	Adenocarcinoma	Sphenoid sinus
	Olfactory bipolar neurons	Esthesioneuroblastoma	
Maxillary sinus	Ciliated pseudostratified columnar epithelial	Squamous cell cancer, undifferentiated	Clivus
Nasopharynx	Ciliated pseudostratified columnar epithelial	Lymphoepithelioma	C1
	Waldeyer's lymphoid cells		
Oral cavity	Stratified squamous epithelial	Squamous cell cancer	C2/3
	Minor salivary gland epithelial	Adenocarcinoma	
Parotid gland	Serous acini cuboidal epithelial	Acini adenocarcinoma	Clivus–C3
		Adenoid cystic cancer	
Oropharynx	Stratified squamous epithelial	Squamous cell cancer	C3
Hypopharynx	Stratified squamous epithelial	Squamous cell cancer, more differentiated	C4
Supraglottis	Ciliated pseudostratified columnar epithelial	Squamous cell cancer Less differentiated	C4
Glottis	Stratified squamous epithelial	Squamous cell cancer Very differentiated	C5
Subglottis	Ciliated columnar and pseudostratified columnar epithelium	Squamous cell cancer Less differentiated	C6
Thyroid	Lining cuboidal epithelium of follicles	Adenocarcinomas Follicular, papillary, medullary	C5–T1

No major changes have been made in nodal classification staging; N2 is stage IVA, N3 is stage IVB, and for a notation as to an upper and lower neck node.

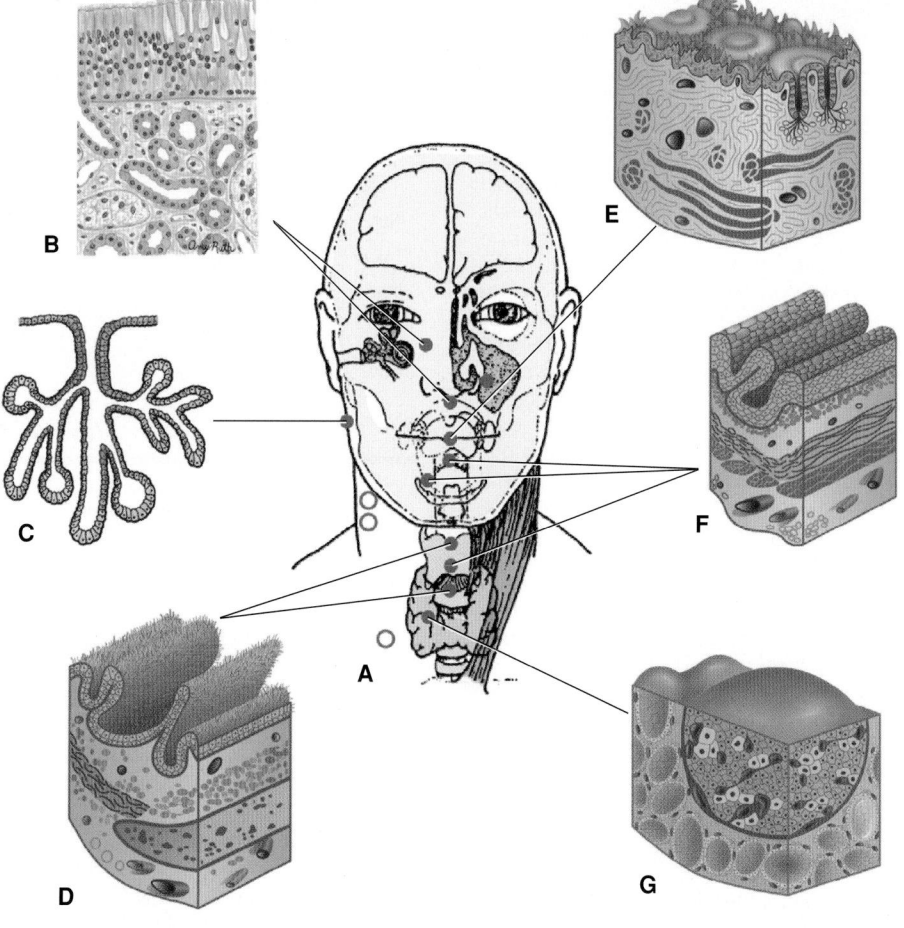

Figure 1.2 | Overview of Histogenesis. A. Primary cancer site isocenters. **B.** Paranasal sinus and nasopharynx. **C.** Salivary gland. **D.** Supraglottic and subglottic larynx. **E.** Oral cavity and tongue. **F.** Oropharynx and hypopharynx. **G.** Thyroid.

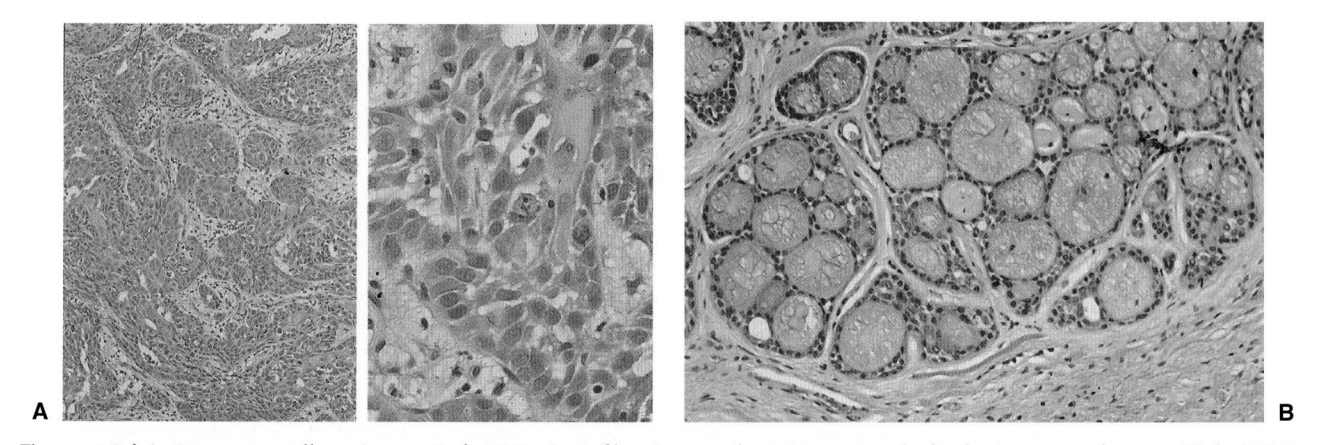

Figure 1.3 | A. Squamous cell carcinoma. Left (LM): An infiltrative neoplasm is composed of cohesive nests of tumor. **Right (HM):** A less differentiated tumor displays cells with pleomorphic nuclei, prominent nucleoli, brightly eosinophilic cytoplasm indicating keratinization, and intercellular bridges connecting adjacent cells. **B: Adenoid cystic carcinoma** showing cribriform growth in which cystlike spaces are filled with basophilic material. The cyst spaces are really pseudocysts surrounded by myoepithelial cells.

TNM STAGING CRITERIA

TNM STAGING CRITERIA

The head and neck area is generally considered one anatomic and physiologic unit because their boundaries are not well defined. Cancers arising in the different sites of the upper aerodigestive passages spread into the neck nodes as first station nodes. The specific site of the first node to be affected varies according to the origin of the primary tumor. In fact, every primary site drains into the cervical nodes as noted, but each site has a preference for a specific sentinel node. This is often the first evidence of cancer somewhere in the head, of an unknown primary. Because many midline areas drain bilaterally, both sides of the neck are vulnerable to cancer spread. Bilateral and contralateral lymphatic involvement also are common. Once one node is affected, the entire complex of lymph nodes in the neck is at risk because of altered flow into collateral channels.

The classification and staging of head and neck cancers are excellent prototypes for the classification and staging of cancer in general. There has always been a guiding principle to maintain uniform criteria across all anatomic primary sites. Two major modifications of T and N categories and stage grouping have been made based on survival data of clinical trials. Major changes in nodal criteria occurred with the third edition (1987) when criteria as N2 mobility versus N3 fixation of lymph nodes were changed to size. Size of nodes was adopted as the criterion to be more objective. A fixed node to the carotid artery was replaced by >6 cm in greatest diameter, and the N definitions N1 ≤3 cm, N2 3 to 6 cm, and N3 >6 cm have been uniformly applied across all head and neck sites except for the nasopharynx. In the sixth edition (2002), a major change in all sites was dividing the primary cancer into stage IVA T4a resectable, stage IVB T4b N2 unresectable, and stage IVC is for distant metastases.

In general, every effort has been made to bring the stage groupings of the head and neck to a relatively uniform combination of TNM criteria for all sites. This useful attribute would be beneficial to adopt at other anatomic cancer sites.

SUMMARY OF CHANGES SEVENTH EDITION AMERICAN JOINT COMMITTEE ON CANCER (AJCC)

- The terms "resectable" and "unresectable" are replaced with "moderately advanced" and "very advanced"

- No major changes have been made in the N staging for any sites except that a descriptor has been added. Extracapsular spread (ECS) of disease is added as ECS + or ECS − as a descriptor. These descriptors will not influence staging system.

- The T stage determines the stage grouping with modifications by N stage. Size implying depth of invasion is the key criterion for primary tumors: T1 is <2 cm, T2 is 2 to 4 cm, and T3 > 4 cm. A uniform description of advanced tumors has been recommended: T4 lesions are divided into T4a resectable, T4b unresectable, and assignment to stage IVA and stage IVB, respectively. Stage IVC is metastatic disease.

TABLE 1.3 Stage Summary Matrix

	Stage T1	Stage T2	Stage T3	Stage T4a	Stage T4b
N0	I	II	III	IVA	IVB
N1	III	III	III	IVA	IVB
N2	IVA	IVA	IVA	IVA	IVB
N3	IVB	IVB	IVB	IVB	IVB
M1	IVC	IVC	IVC	IVC	IVC

- *T stage* determines stage group
  - T1 = I, T2 + II, T3 = III, T4 = IV
- *N stage* N1 = T3 *and then progresses as T stage progresses*
  - N1 = T3, N2 = T4a, N3 = T4b
- *M stage* is separate stage
  - M1 = Stage IVC

- In the 7th Edition there have been moderate changes 2+ in Nasopharynx, and minor changes 1+ in the Thyroid.

- A new cancer site staging system for Muscosal Melanoma, which is illustrated in the Ethmoid Sinus chapter (Chapter 2).

Linguistically the T stage determines the stage group with modification by N stage. A major modification occurred when stage IV in fifth edition was divided into IVA, IVB, and IVC based on nodal extent (i.e., N1, N2, N3). In the sixth edition, T4 was divided into T4a and T4b and stage IVA and stage IVB, respectively. Size of primary tumor (<2, <4, >4 cm) and size of regional lymph nodes (<3, <6, >6 cm) remain the most important staging criteria. Figure 1.4 shows the TNM staging criteria for four key sites in the Head and Neck.

Genesis and Evolution of TNM Stages: First to Seventh Editions

The head and neck TNM staging system has remained relatively consistent over five decades with an important guiding principle; that is to maintain uniform definitions of T and N across all sites. Modifications of T and N categories in stage grouping are based on survival data of clinical trials in the literature using the American Joint Committee on Cancer/ International Union Against Cancer (AJCC/UICC) systems. Benchmark survival curves are presented for major primary sites by stage.

Roman Numerals = Edition of AJCC/UICC
Scoring:
No change = yellow 0
Minor = green 1+
Moderate = blue 2+
Marked = purple 3+
Major = red 4+
New = black 5+

I	0
II	0
III	3+
IV	0
V	2+
VI	3+
VII	1+

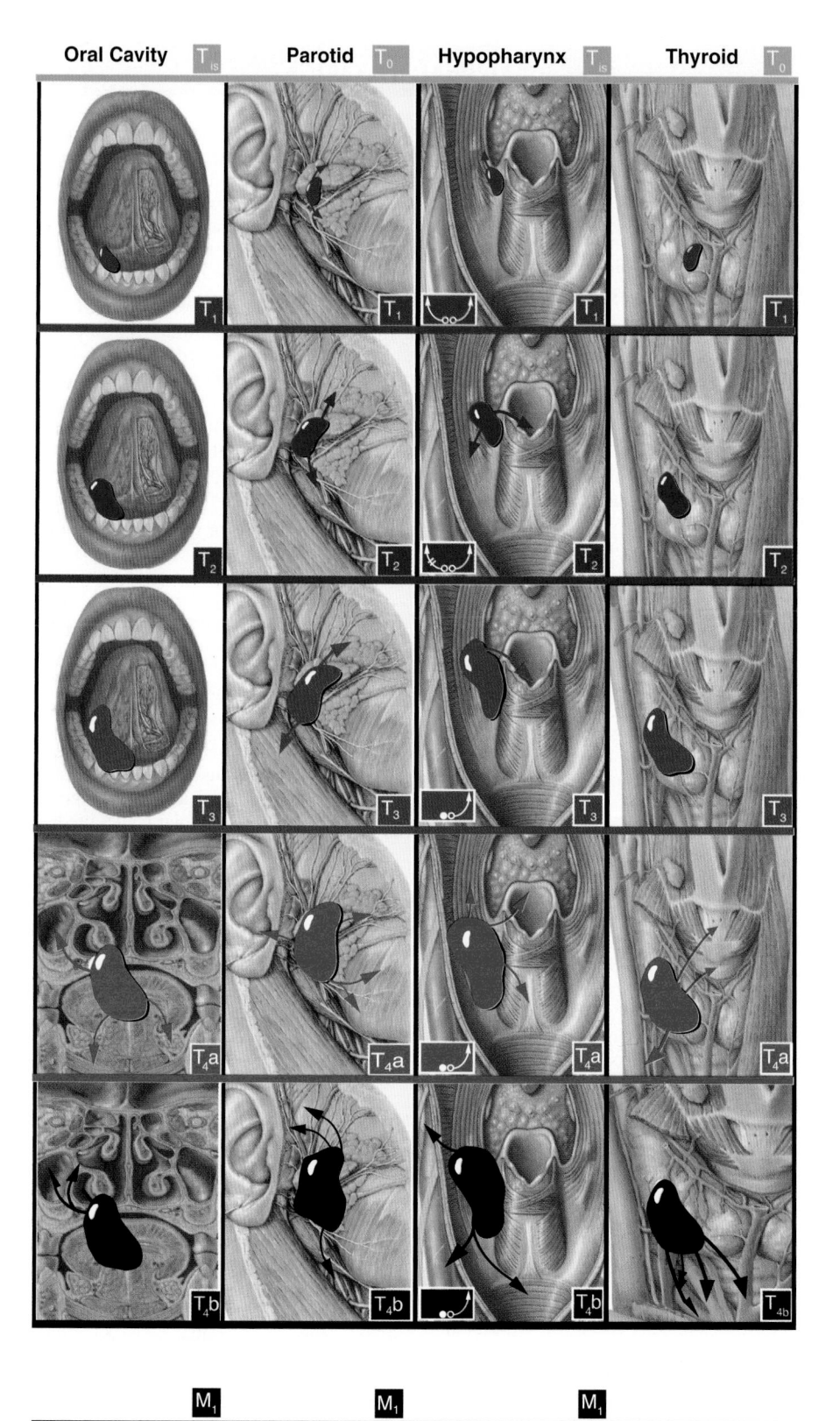

Figure 1.4 | **T stage grouping.** Vertical presentations of stage groupings for Oral Cavity, Parotid, Hypopharynx, and Thyroid, which follow same color code for cancer stage advancement are organized in horizontal lanes: Stage 0, yellow; I, green; II, blue; III, purple; IVA, red; and IVB, black. Definitions of TN on left and stage grouping on right.

T-ONCOANATOMY

ORIENTATION OF T-ONCOANATOMY: ODYSSEY OF PRIMARY SITES

The anatomic isocenter of a primary cancer site is the intersection of the three planar T-oncoanatomy views: coronal, sagittal, and transverse, taken from *Grant's Atlas of Human Anatomy*. The axial orientation of the vertebral level is an important imaging reference point. Surface anatomy can vary from patient to patient; however, it is presented as a guide for the localization of the cancer in both accessible and internal anatomic sites that cannot be assessed on routine physical examination. The red bullets in our multilayered coronal (Fig. 1.5A) and sagittal (Fig. 1.5B) planes are a combination of both superficial and deep landmarks to identify primary sites. The tabulation of oncologic anatomy in the head and neck region starts at the base of the skull, and primary sites of head and neck cancers are noted in an axial fashion from cephalad to caudad and are arranged along planes anterior to the entire cervical spine from C1 to C7. There are two major anatomic sectors with 11 distinct cancer primary sites currently staged (Fig. 1.5C; Table 1.4). These sectors are the upper aerorespiratory passage consisting of the nasal cavity, paranasal sinuses, the nasopharynx and the larynx; and the upper digestive passage, which contains the oral cavity, lips, oropharynx, and hypopharynx. Taken together, the anatomic physiologic complexity lies in the oropharynx, which is common to both systems.

Cervical fascial planes are important for compartmentalizing the neck and have a major impact on staging. To appreciate the neck compartments, axial and sagittal views are required. The anterior compartment is defined by an investing fascia that envelopes the sternocleidomastoid muscle, and superficial muscles, which are usually considered resectable (Stage IVA), and houses the pharynx, larynx, and thyroid gland. Therefore, when pharyngeal cancer spread is anterior and inferior, it is more often amenable to surgical removal. With posterior and superior invasion patterns, pharyngeal cancers penetrate the prevertebral fascia into the prevertebral space, which is not resectable (Stage IVB). Lateral spread into the carotid sheath is also an ominous sign; fixation of lymph nodes to the carotid artery renders the cancer unresectable. Clinically, it is difficult to diagnose cancer fixation to arteries; therefore, cancer node size >6 cm makes the evaluation more objective and has been shown to correlate with carotid artery involvement. The retropharyngeal space is ideal for pharyngeal cancer (Fig. 1.3C) spread vertically, but once the prevertebral fascia has been invaded, the cancer is no longer resectable. A concise overview (odyssey) of the 11 primary sites follows:

1. Cancers of the ethmoid sinus are the most superior in the head and neck region, whereas frontal sinuses and the sphenoid sinus tumefaction are rare and secondary to other neoplastic processes. Esthesioneuroblastoma can arise in the roof of the nasal cavity and involve the cribriform plate. Paranasal sinus cancer spread into other sinuses and orbital invasion are common.

2. Cancers of the nasopharynx can be insidious in onset and highly metastatic to lymph nodes. Cranial nerve involvement is due to cancer entry of the cavernous sinus via the foramen lacerum involving cranial nerves III, IV, V, and VI. In contrast, enlarging cervical metastatic lymph nodes, the highest in the deep cervical chain (Rouviere's node), can compress cranial nerves IX, X, XI, and XII.

3. Cancers of the maxillary antra can masquerade as unilateral sinusitis and only become evident as the paper-thin bones (lamina papyracea) erode, loosening of molar teeth occurs, erosion into the cheek, destroying the zygomatic arch, occurs, and most catastrophically erosion into the orbit. The sentinel node tends to be submaxillary and therefore misleading.

4. Cancer of the lips and oral cavity can arise at numerous subsites that initiate the upper digestive passage. The common sites of malignancies are the food gutters, namely the floor of mouth and lateral border of the tongue. The sentinel nodes are often a function of the exact anatomic location of the primary cancer. With 10 different oral cavity subsites, anterior cancers lead to submental and submaxillary nodal invasion, whereas posterior neoplasms result in jugulodigastric nodes.

5. Neoplasms of the parotid gland are highly varied, and even benign mixed pleomorphic adenomas tend to recur, as can low-grade mixed mucoepidermoid cancers. Perineural invasion of cranial nerves VII, V, or both is a characteristic of cylindromas. The parotid gland lymph nodes are both the regional and sentinel nodes in this location. Prolonged survival even in the face of pulmonary metastasis is a peculiarity of some salivary gland cancers.

6. Cancer of the oropharynx arises at the isocenter of the upper aerodigestive passage, which houses Waldeyer's ring, a favored site for malignant transformation. The underlying muscular planes predetermine spread patterns. The sentinel node is the jugulodigastric. Odynophagia referred to the middle ear is due to Jacobson's branch of cranial nerve IX.

7. Cancers of the hypopharynx may surround the larynx and block the food bolus, leading to aspiration into the larynx. Dysphagia can be caused by local invasion as well as cranial nerve involvement. The jugulo-omohyoid is often the sentinel node and can be invaded in contiguity with a primary.

8–10. Cancers of the larynx are divided into three parts: the supraglottis, glottis, and subglottis. Vocal cord involvement can be an early sign of malignancy. The malignant gradient varies with true glottic cancers being most readily detected in the earlier stages and therefore highly curable, whereas both the supraglottic and especially the subglottic cancers can be silent and more egregious in onset. Transglottic cancers advance as the cancer crosses the vocal cords. Paratracheal or paralaryngeal nodes can be the sentinel nodes. Odynophagia referred to the outer external ear is due to Arnold's nerve, a branch of the vagus (cranial nerve X), which supplies sensation to the larynx.

11. Thyroid cancers, although considered part of head and neck tumors, are unique because they arise from an endocrine gland and not an epithelial surface. The cancers can be well-differentiated colloid or papillary adenocarcinomas compatible with long survival despite lymph node invasion. Although the Delphic lymph node located above the isthmus can be the sentinel node, more often the inferior deep jugulo-omohyoid nodes are at risk. Anaplastic cancers can be highly lethal and metastasize early to the lungs.

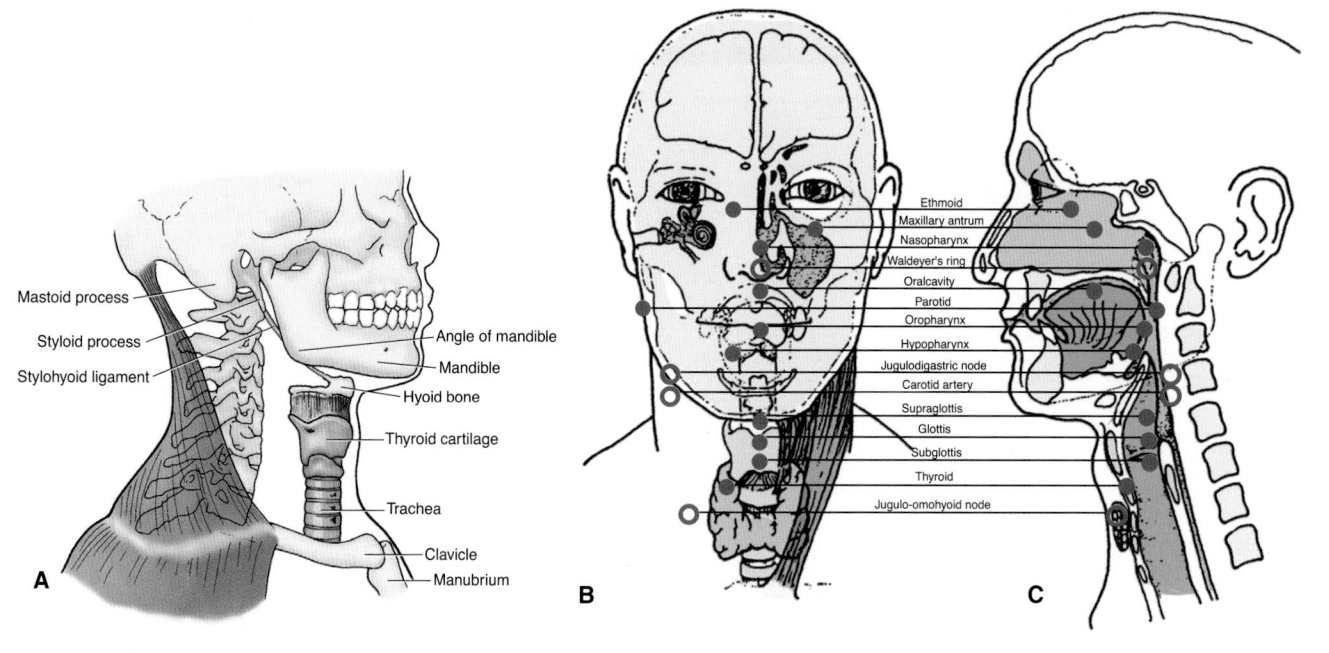

Figure 1.5 | Orientation of T-oncoanatomy. The locations of 11 primary cancer sites are indicated at their anatomic isocenters with red bullets. Open circles are important lymph nodes. **A.** Bone and cartilage frame for head and neck primary sites. **B.** Coronal. **C.** Sagittal.

TABLE 1.4	Orientation and Overview of T-oncoanatomy: Odyssey of T Sites and Landmarks		
Primary Site Structure	**Coronal**	**Sagittal**	**Transverse**
Ethmoid sinus, nasal cavity	Right/left of midline, orbit	Zygomatic arch	Sphenoid sinus
Maxillary sinus	Right/left bridge of nose	Zygomatic arch	Clivus
Nasopharynx	Hard palate	External auditory meatus	C1
Oral cavity	Lips	Teeth	C2/3
Parotid gland	Ramus mandible	Angle of mandible	Clivus–C3
Oropharynx	Lips/teeth	Angle of mandible	C3
Hypopharynx	Hyoid	Greater horn of hyoid bone	C4
Supraglottis	Thyroid cartilage notch	Horn of thyroid cartilage	C4
Glottis	Below thyroid cartilage notch	Horn of thyroid cartilage	C5
Subglottis	Cricoid cartilage	Cricoid cartilage	C6
Thyroid	Right/left paratracheal	Paratracheal	C5–T1

N-ONCOANATOMY

ORIENTATION OF REGIONAL LYMPH NODES: N-ONCOANATOMY

Understanding the complex anatomy of the neck is essential to appreciate the many nuances and evolution of changes. Most important is an appreciation that the major regional nodal areas are divided into superficial and deep cervical node chains; the latter includes the high retropharyngeal and parapharyngeal nodes. Each of the major head and neck cancer sites drain into a specific region of neck nodes—sentinel nodes (Fig. 1.6; Table 1.5). Some have unilateral drainage, others bilateral. The most commonly involved lymph nodes are those along the internal jugular vein, which are subdivided into superior, mid, and inferior deep cervical node chains. They include the jugulodigastric and jugulo-omohyoid, and the scalene nodes in the anterior aspect of the supraclavicular fossae. A series of two planar orientation diagrams of regional lymph nodes and their lymphatics are shown in anterior and lateral views (Fig. 1.6A–C). Each primary anatomic site or subsite has a sentinel node or favored nodes to which it drains preferentially. This can be determined clinically by injecting a radiocolloid such as Tc^{99m} or methylene blue dye at the primary site and dissecting the node that concentrates the most radioactivity. It is equally important to be aware of all the lymph nodes at risk. The clinician needs to locate first station nodes in three planes to determine if they are accessible for physical examination.

Traditionally, the triangles of the neck are used to define the topographic anatomy that consists of anterior and posterior triangles (Fig. 1.6D). *The sternocleidomastoid muscle divides the neck into these two major triangles; many other small triangles exist.* The external jugular vein and the platysma muscle are superficial to the sternocleidomastoid muscle. Deep to the sternocleidomastoid are the carotid artery, internal jugular vein, and some cranial nerves. Deep cervical lymph nodes also surround the carotid sheath. The lymphatic channels and lymph nodes are located more anteriorly as they follow the sternocleidomastoid muscle inferiorly. The nodes in the neck make up one of the most important sections of oncologic anatomy. The lymphatics of the head are, in essence, the lymphatic channels in the neck and their lymph nodes. Regional nodes are not always the closest anatomically to the primary site nor are the sentinel nodes solely involved with cancers of the head and neck. Distant primary sites both above and below the diaphragm can spread to neck nodes, especially supraclavicular nodes (Virchow's node).

The nomenclature we use is that of *The International Anatomical Terminology,* and this correlates with various staging systems and terms proposed by the AJCC. The AJCC has grouped regional lymph nodes in the neck into seven levels and subdivided specific anatomic subsites (Fig. 1.6D). Each level is designated by a roman numeral (I–VII). *Lymph node-bearing region* is promulgated by Hodgkin's lymphoma staging rather than anatomic physiologic considerations and deserves to be reconsidered in terms of cancer spread. According to AJCC/UICC clinical staging for Hodgkin's lymphoma, each side of the neck is one lymph node–bearing region (Fig. 1.6E). The lymphoid tissue of Waldeyer's ring is an extranodal lymphoid collection that forms the palatine tonsils. The lymphoid tissue extends superiorly into the pharyngeal wall and the roof of the nasopharynx and inferiorly into the base of the tongue. Midline anatomic sites such as Waldeyer's ring drain bilaterally, whereas paired or parallel structures drain unilaterally to their respective deep jugular nodes, right or left.

TABLE 1.5	Sentinel Nodes			
			Level/Location of Node(s)*	
Primary Site Structure	**Sentinel Node(s)**		**Axial Level**	**AJCC Level**
Ethmoid sinus, nasal cavity	Retropharyngeal		Sphenoid sinus	nl
Maxillary sinus	Submandibular		Clivus	I
Nasopharynx	Retropharyngeal		C1	nl
Oral cavity	Submandibular Jugulodigastric		C2/3	I II
Parotid gland	Parotid nodes		Clivus–C3	I
Oropharynx	Jugulodigastric, superior deep cervical		C3	II
Hypopharynx	Mid deep cervical		C4	III
Supraglottis	Jugulodigastric, superior/mid deep cervical		C4	II
Glottis	Prelaryngeal		C5	VI
Subglottis	Jugulo-omohyoid, inferior deep cervical		C6	IV
Thyroid	Jugulo-omohyoid Inferior/mid/superior deep cervical		C5–T1	IV III/II

*Sentinel nodes transfer axial level; they may not be at the same level as the primary site.
nl, not listed.

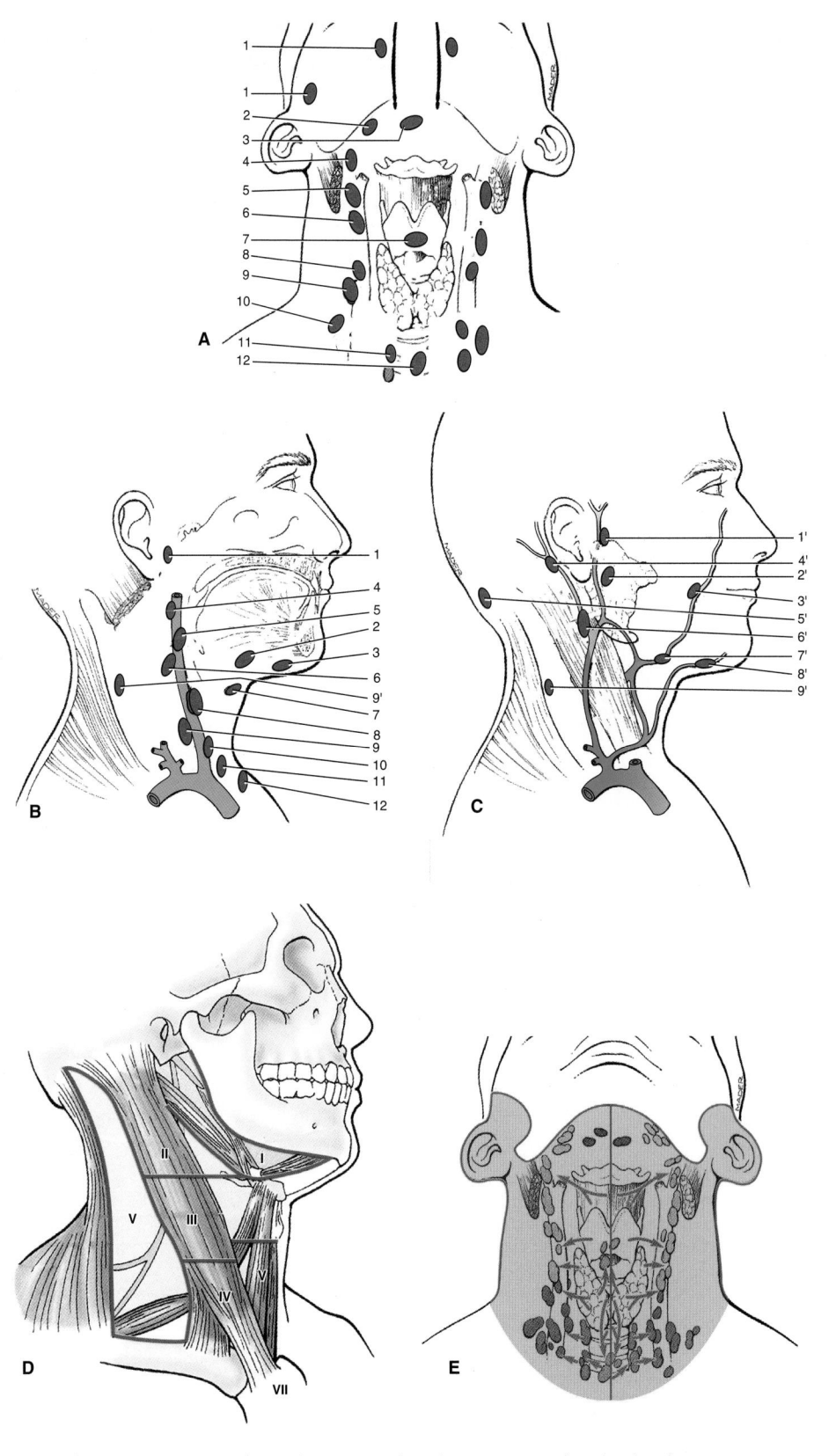

Figure 1.6 | Orientation of N-oncoanatomy. The neck or cervical nodes are regional nodes for the 11 primary cancer sites. Any cluster can be a sentinel node that drains a specific site (A, B, C). These are assigned using the international anatomical terminology and are identified by number to note clusters of regional nodes that could be sentinel nodes. **A.** Anterior view of deep jugular nodes. **B.** Lateral view of deep nodes with the sternocleidomastoid muscle removed. Anterior deep jugular (A) and lateral (no sternocleidomastoid muscle, (B) lymph nodes: (1) retropharyngeal; (2) submandibular; (3) submental; (4) superior deep cervical; (5) jugulodigastric; (6) mid deep jugular; (7) prelaryngeal; (8) jugulo-omohyoid; (9) inferior deep cervical (jugular); (10) supraclavicular; (11) paratracheal; and (12) pretracheal. (C) Lateral view of superficial nodes: (1′) preauricular; (2′) parotid; (3′) facial; (4′) mastoid; (5′) superficial cervical; (7′) submandibular; (8′) submental; and (9′) spinal accessory. **D.** AJCC nomenclature of seven levels of cervical lymph nodes. **E.** Node-bearing region according to staging in Hodgkin's lymphoma.

M-ONCOANATOMY

M-ONCOANATOMY OF REGIONAL VEINS AND THE NEUROVASCULAR BUNDLE

The head and neck are generally considered an anatomic and physiologic unit; all sites share a common regional arterial blood supply and venous drainage (Fig. 1.7A). Most of the upper aerodigestive passages are supplied by the branches of the carotid artery. Their venous drainage is through the pterygoid venous plexus deep to the masseter muscle and is retropharyngeal, next to the posterior aspect of the parotid gland and then by way of the jugular veins. Cancer can disseminate hematogenously through vascular routing most often to the superior vena cava to the right side of the heart and lung via the pulmonary circulation and then to other organs sys-

temically. Lung is the target organ for the first signs of distant metastases for the majority of head and neck cancers.

The cranial nerves become peripheral as they exit the skull to innervate the head and neck region. Cranial nerves IX, X, XI, and XII descend in the neck with the carotid artery and internal jugular vein and constitute the major neurovascular bundle in the head and neck region (Fig. 1.7B). Metastatic cancer to the deep chain of jugular lymph nodes can produce cranial neuropathy. Rouviere's node is the highest cervical node; it is clinically inaccessible and retropharyngeal in location (Fig. 1.7C,D).

Jugular foramen syndrome is characterized by loss of the gag reflex (cranial nerve IX), vocal cord paralysis (cranial nerve X), atrophy of the trapezius muscle (cranial nerve XI), and deviation of the uvula (cranial nerve X) and tongue on protrusion (cranial nerve XII).

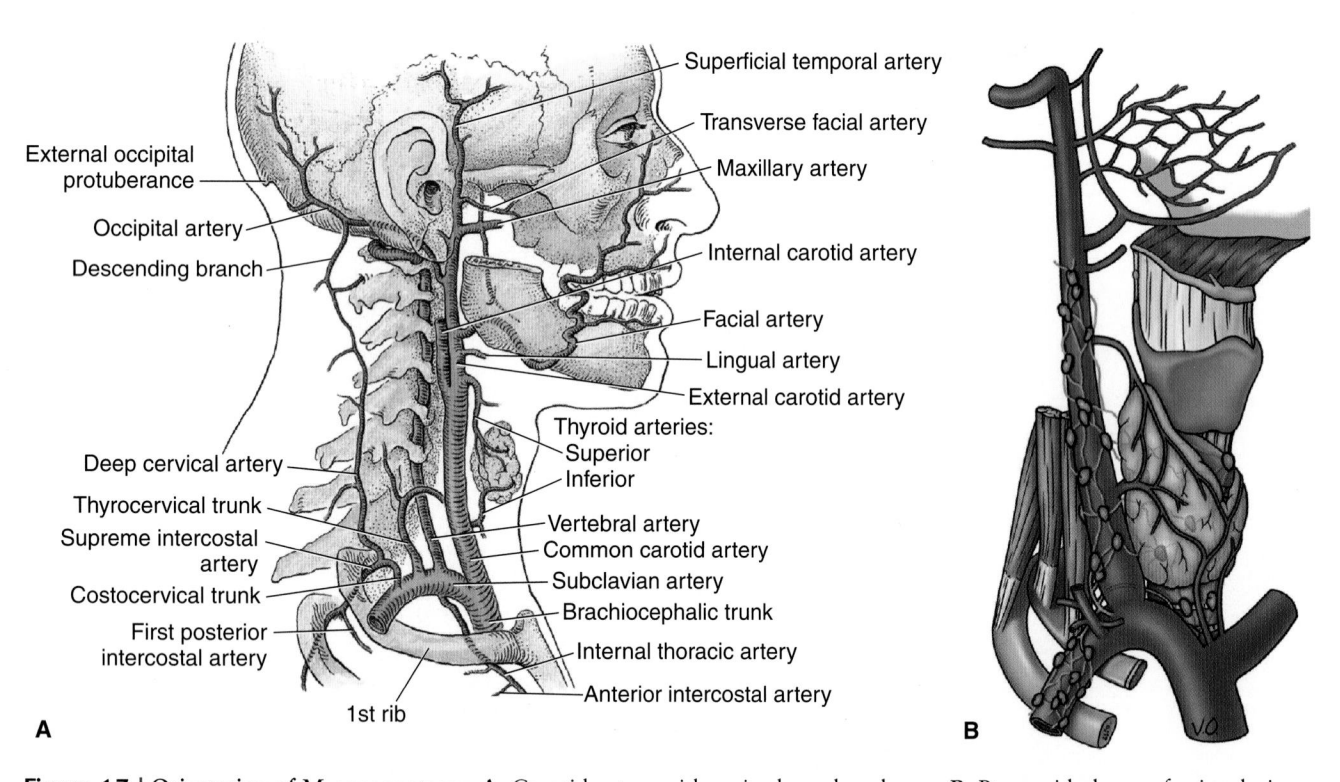

Figure 1.7 | Orientation of M-oncoanatomy. A. Carotid artery with major branches shown. **B.** Pterygoid plexus of veins drains most of head and neck sites into internal deep jugular. Note green small normal lymph nodes are juxtaposed. The jugular vein drains into the superior vena cava and then into the right heart, making lung the target organ.

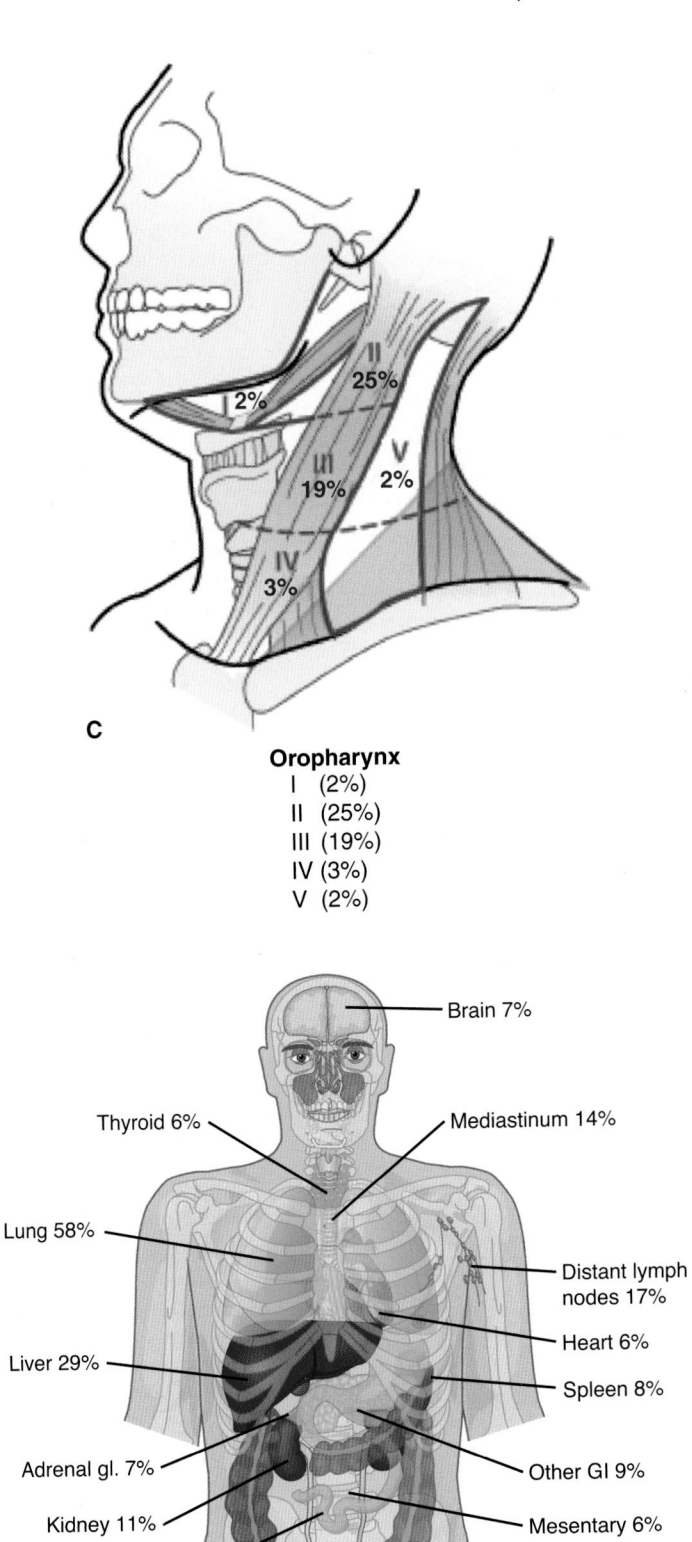

Oropharynx
I   (2%)
II (25%)
III (19%)
IV (3%)
V   (2%)

Figure 1.7 C&D| C. Percent of positive nodes in clinically negative (N0) neck in Oropharyngeal cancer according to AJCC levels. D. The Incidence and Distribution of Distant Metastases of Oropharyngeal Cancers. The oropharyngeal cancers can serve as a prototype for head and neck cancers. Lung (58%) is the target organ with liver metastases next (29%) and bone metastases third (22%) followed by distant lymph nodes (17%), mediastinum (14%). The remainder of sites are 11% (kidney) or less than 10%.

CRANIAL NERVES AND NEUROVASCULAR BUNDLE

The importance of appreciating the complex anatomy of cranial nerves lies in the patterns of cancer spread at the primary cancer site as well as nodal spread patterns. Perineural invasion or compression by metastatic lymph nodes often is manifested by specific neurologic symptoms and signs. The overview of cranial nerves provides an intricate roadmap as to points of vulnerability (Figure 1.8).

Cranial nerve invasion can produce specific syndromes and neurologic evaluation is a vital part of physical diagnosis in all head and neck cancers.

A tabulation of potential neurologic syndromes either due to perineural invasion at the primary site or nodal compression will alert the astute clinician to extent of cancer advancement anatomically (Table 1.6).

1. *Ethmoid sinus cancers* are midline and invade the nasal cavity at the crista galli and the penetrating branches of the olfactory nerve. The *esthesioneuroblastoma* arises from the ganglion organ of Jacobson. Cancers pick off the V_2, resulting in hypesthesia of upper lip, then invade the orbit, can compress III, IV, VI, and optic nerve II.

   Nodal drainage to retropharyngeal nodes (Rouviere's node) can lead to compression of IX, X, XI, or XII as they exit along the carotid artery and jugular vein.

2. *Maxillary antrum* cancers tend to invade lamina papyrea, then bone walls (i.e., superiorly the infraorbital nerve will result in a circle of anesthesia below the lower eyelid and then invasion of the orbit resulting extraocular invasion of III, IV, VI and eventually II posteriorly).

3. *Nasopharynx cancers* enter the parapharyngeal space and then invade through the foramen lacerum, enter the cavernous sinus and pick off CN V, IV, and III in that order causing diplopia. As it extends laterally, the Gasserian ganglion is encountered. V_1 eyelid anesthesia, V_2 upper lip and nasal anesthesia, and V_3 lower face anesthesia can occur when Retropharyngeal (Rouviere's) node compresses the neurovascular bundle of CN IX, X, XI, and XII, exiting the skull alongside the carotid artery and jugular vein.

4. *Oropharynx* cancers invade the CN IX first and refer pain on swallowing along the vagus nerve to the middle ear (Jacobson's nerve). The sytlopharyngeal muscle as well as palate is paralyzed and there is absence of gag reflex. Taste is affected on the posterior third of the tongue. Retropharyngeal nodes can entrap (CN IX, X, XI, and XII) in the neurovascular bundle.

5. *Salivary gland* or *parotid gland* cancers tend to invade the facial nerve CN VII as it exists from the stylohyoid foramen and result in impairment of facial musculature depending on its invasion of branches versus the main nerve. Sensory taste in the anterior two thirds of the tongue and soft palate can be altered. Cylindromas are notorious for perineural invasion and if branches of V_3 mandibular nerve are involved, it can penetrate into the Gasserian ganglion into the middle fossa.

   Retroparotidean nodes can compress IX, X, XI, and XII, especially if the primary involves the deep lobe.

6. *Oral cavity cancers* can invade the floor of the mouth and the hypoglossus CN XII leads to unilateral paralysis with tongue on protrusion pointing to the paralytic side. Invasion of V_3 mandibular branch results in sensory loss of lower third of face. Muscle impairment of mastication muscles can result in drooling. Submandibular nodes rarely lead to neurologic events.

7. *Hypopharyngeal cancers* tend to invade the CN X vagus nerve, causing vocal cord paresis and pain on swallowing is referred to external ear (Arnold's nerve).

   Deep cervical nodes on the right side can extend into the supraclavicular nodes and entrap the recurrent laryngeal nerve on that side. Massive extranodal invasion could involve the spinal accessory nerve CN XI and lead to paresis of sternocleidomastoid muscle and trapezius.

8. *Larynx cancers* directly invade into vocal cord, and hoarseness results rather than nerve invasion. Supraglottic cancers can lead to referred pain and swallowing along CN X Arnold's nerve to outer ear.

   Deep cervical nodes in advanced stages can entrap the recurrent laryngeal nerve on the right side.

9. *Ear tumors* vary depending on location:

   Acoustic neuromas lead to deafness and can compress the intermediate branch of CN VII, altering taste in the anterior two thirds of the tongue.

   Jugular foramen chemodectomas can compress the neurovascular bundle and mimic retropharyngeal node, impairing CN IX, X, XI, and, by eypansion, XII.

   External auditory canal cancers can invade and involve the facial nerve CN VII and lead to unilateral facial muscular paresis.

TABLE 1.6	Potential Neurologic Syndromes Due to Invasion of Cranial Nerves	
	T Site*	**N Site***
Ethmoid sinus	I, (II), V_2 (III, IV, VI)	IX, X, XI, XII
Maxillary sinus	V_2 (III, IV, VI)	—
Nasopharynx	VI, IV, III ($V_{1,2,3}$)	IX, X, XI, XII
Oral Cavity	XII	—
Oropharynx	IX, X_A	IX, X, XI, XII
Parotid Gland	VII, V_3	IX, X, XI, XII
Hypopharynx	X_J	XX_{RL} (XI)
Larynx	X_J	—
Thyroid	X	(XI)
Ear	VIII, VII IX, X, XI, XII	—

*Those within parentheses indicate extensive invasion T4.

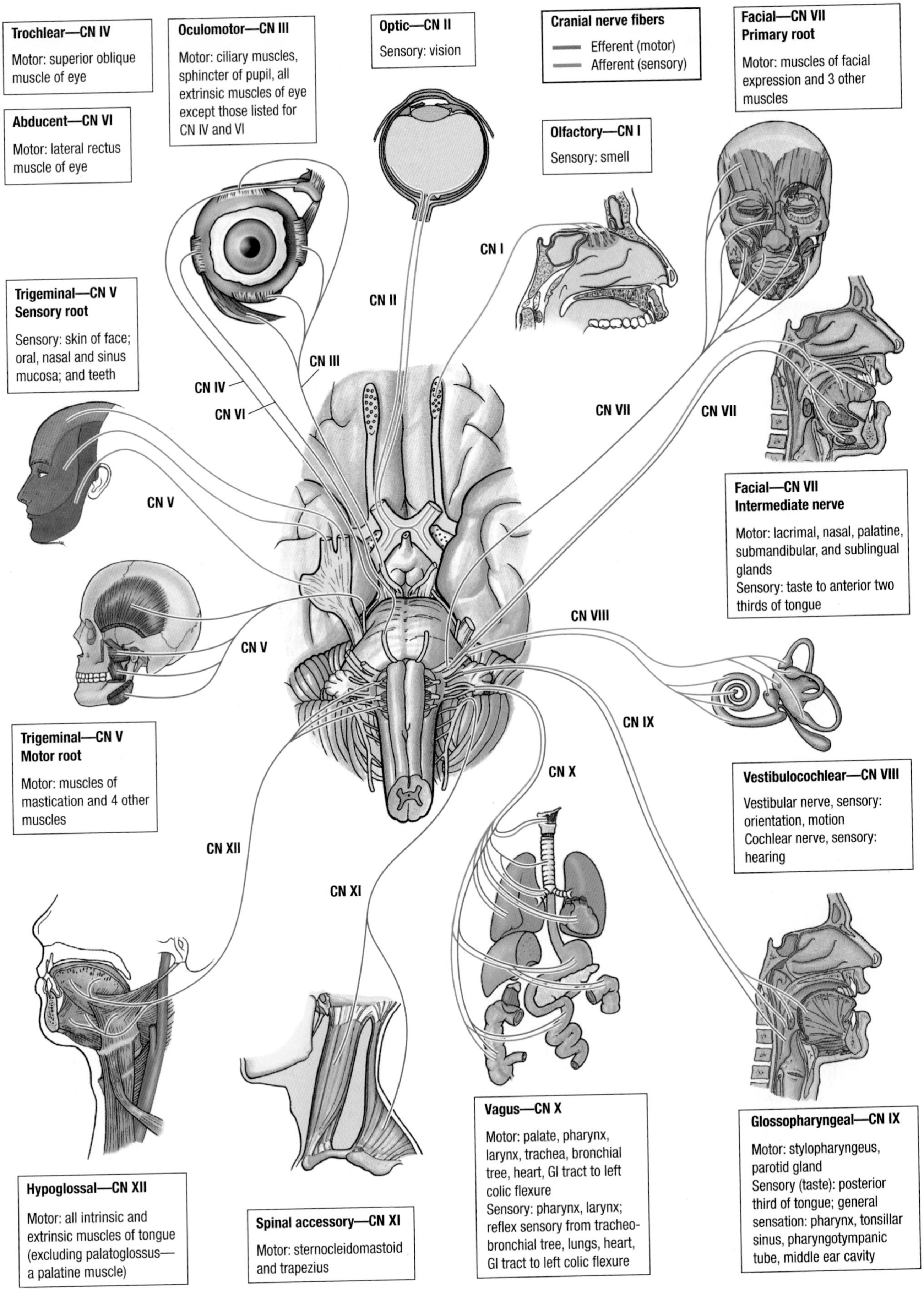

Trochlear—CN IV

Motor: superior oblique muscle of eye

Abducent—CN VI

Motor: lateral rectus muscle of eye

Oculomotor—CN III

Motor: ciliary muscles, sphincter of pupil, all extrinsic muscles of eye except those listed for CN IV and VI

Optic—CN II

Sensory: vision

Cranial nerve fibers

━━━ Efferent (motor)
━━━ Afferent (sensory)

Facial—CN VII Primary root

Motor: muscles of facial expression and 3 other muscles

Olfactory—CN I

Sensory: smell

CN I

CN II

CN III

CN IV

CN VI

CN VII

CN VII

Trigeminal—CN V Sensory root

Sensory: skin of face; oral, nasal and sinus mucosa; and teeth

CN V

Facial—CN VII Intermediate nerve

Motor: lacrimal, nasal, palatine, submandibular, and sublingual glands
Sensory: taste to anterior two thirds of tongue

CN VIII

CN V

CN IX

Trigeminal—CN V Motor root

Motor: muscles of mastication and 4 other muscles

CN X

Vestibulocochlear—CN VIII

Vestibular nerve, sensory: orientation, motion
Cochlear nerve, sensory: hearing

CN XII

CN XI

Hypoglossal—CN XII

Motor: all intrinsic and extrinsic muscles of tongue (excluding palatoglossus—a palatine muscle)

Spinal accessory—CN XI

Motor: sternocleidomastoid and trapezius

Vagus—CN X

Motor: palate, pharynx, larynx, trachea, bronchial tree, heart, GI tract to left colic flexure
Sensory: pharynx, larynx; reflex sensory from tracheo-bronchial tree, lungs, heart, GI tract to left colic flexure

Glossopharyngeal—CN IX

Motor: stylopharyngeus, parotid gland
Sensory (taste): posterior third of tongue; general sensation: pharynx, tonsillar sinus, pharyngotympanic tube, middle ear cavity

Figure 1.8 | Cranial nerves

STAGING WORKUP

RULES FOR CLASSIFICATION AND STAGING

Clinical Staging and Imaging

Clinical staging is an essential step in establishing meaningful data. Physical examination includes visualization of upper aerodigestive passage whenever possible and is often combined with mirror or direct endoscopy. Palpation is critical to define endophytic induration whenever feasible. Imaging is important, particularly spiral computed tomography (CT) and magnetic resonance imaging (MRI), which can provide superb visualization of the three-planar anatomy. MRI provides better visualization of soft tissue cancer infiltration; CT better detects bone destruction. The difference in density of tissue planes allows for viewing fat as black on CT and white on MRI, in contrast to the gray of muscles and viscera in contrasting these diagnostic modes (Fig. 1.9). Cancer can be enhanced by contrast administration owing to a greater degree of tumor neovascularization versus normal tissue vascularity. However, MRI is better than CT in that tumorous infiltrates appear intensely white. Identification of enlarged lymph nodes (>1 cm^2) requires contrast visualization of arteries and veins (white) on CT; blood flow allows for a black image of the neck vessels on MRI. Each anatomic site is discussed for nuances, imaging highlights, and notations. Suspicious neck nodes need fine needle aspiration for confirmation (Table 1.7). An excellent reference from which oncoimaging notations highlight important aspects of cancer spread and staging at each primary site is by Bragg, Rubin, and Hricak (2002).

Pathologic Staging

Gross specimen should be evaluated for margins. Unresected gross residual tumor must be reported and marked with clips. All resected lymph node specimens should describe size, number, and level of involved nodes and whether there is extracapsular spread. Specimens postradiation and/or chemotherapy need to be so noted. Specimen shrinkages may occur up to 30% after resection itself. Designations pT and pN should be used after histopathologic evaluation. Perineural invasion deserves special notation.

Histogenesis

The histopathology grading of squamous cell cancers are recommended to be defined in a four-grade system generally is defined as:

Gx Grade cannot be assessed

G1 Well differentiated

G2 Moderately differentiated

G3 Poorly differentiated

G4 Undifferentiated

Lymph node dissections are defined as:

Selective when six nodes are removed, if there is a lesser number they should still be pathologically assessed.

TABLE 1.7	Imaging Modalities and Strategies for Diagnosis and Staging for Head and Neck	
Modality	**Strategy**	**Recommended**
Primary Tumor and Nodes		
Computed tomography	Excellent for defining extent of primary depth of invasion and enlargement of involved nodes. Preferred for bone invasion.	Yes—3–5 mm cuts, 3 mm for primary site, 5 mm for neck
Magnetic resonance imaging	Offers best 3D or 3-planar views of primary and nodes, especially soft tissue extensions. Gadolinium contrast for extensions and perineuronal spread.	Yes—≤4 cm slices Gd—for intracranial and perineuronal spread
Magnetic resonance spectroscopy	Provides metabolic and biochemical analysis of tumor, choline/creatinine ratio elevated in tumor vs. normal tissues.	No.
Positron emission tomography	Functional and metabolic imaging of ^{18}FDG is based on 2-deoxy modification inhibits the molecule from subsequent enzymatic conversion and is "metabolically trapped" in tumor cells.	No—potential exists for distinguishing Recurrence from tissue necrosis
Single photon emission computed tomography	^{201}Thallium used to detect tumor recurrence vs. normal tissue imaging, especially central nervous system.	No—high uptake normally in salivary and thyroid glands
Metastases		
Chest film	Search for metastases.	Yes
Radionuclide scan	^{99m}Tc for bone metastases	Yes—if symptomatic

3D, three-dimensional; FDG, fluorodeoxyglucose.

scan level

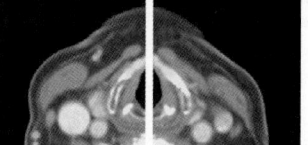

scan level

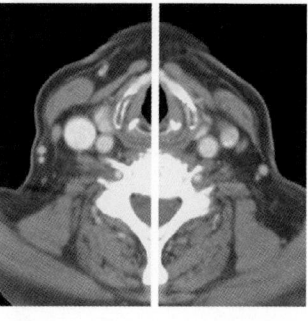

1. pharynx
2. epiglottis
3. aryepiglottic fold
4. hyoid bone
5. false vocal cord
6. laryngeal ventricle
7. true vocal cord
8. tracheal lumen
9. thyroid gland
10. carotid art
11. internal jugular vein

1. mandible
2. base of tongue
3. hyoid bone
4. epiglottis
5. preepiglottic space
6. vallecula
7. false vocal cord
8. laryngeal ventricle
9. true vocal cord
10. cricoid cartilage
11. tracheal lumen
12. esophagus
13. spinal canal
14. manubrium

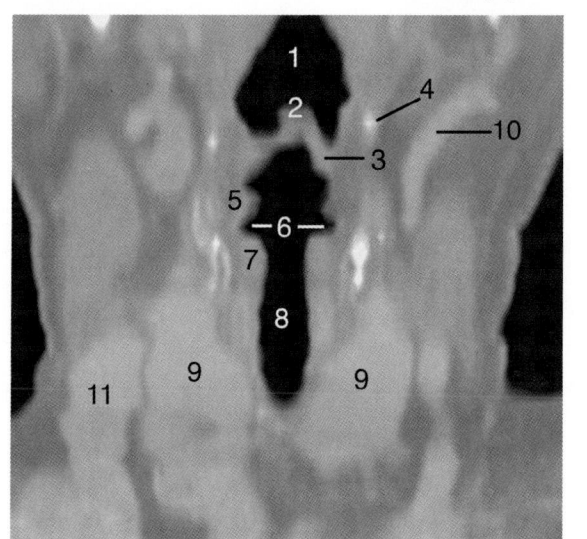

Figure 1.9 | CT scans of head and neck. Another new feature is the addition of CT or MR images to correlate with the axial level in each site specific chapter.

Radical or modified radical requires at least 10 or more nodes are removed.

Imaging criteria for nodal involvement in addition to size are noted for extracapsular spread (ECS) (i.e., speculated margins, loss of intranodal fat, and change in shape from oval to round).

General performance can impact survival. The Performance Scale (ZuGrod, European Cooperative Oncology Group [ECOG]) should be used:

0. Fully active, able to carry on all predisease activities without restriction (Karnofsky 90–100)

1. Restricted in physically strenuous activity but ambulatory and able to carry work of a light or sedentary nature. For example, light housework, office work (Karnofsky 70–80).

2. Ambulatory and capable of all self-care but unable to carry out any work activities. Up and about more than 50% of waking hours (Karnofsky 50–60).

3. Capable of only limited self-care, confined to bed or chair 50% or more of waking hours (Karnofsky 30–40).

4. Completely disabled. Cannot carry on self-care. Totally confined to bed (Karnofsky 10–20).

5. Death (Karnofsky 0).

- *Comorbidities* are advised to be included in medical record such as depression and diabetes; infection such as human papilloma virus (HPV) or AIDS/HIV.

- *Lifestyle* habits as tobacco use in past years and alcohol use as drinks/day/week/month, etc.

- *Weight loss* of more than 10%.

Head and Neck Glossary

(U) Upper

(L) Lower

(ESC) Extracapsular Spread (E) Evident and on clinical/imaging work up

(En) No Extranodal Extension **Applies to ECS**

(Em) Microscopic **Applies to ECS**

(Eg) Gross **Applies to ECS**

(NMSC) Non melanoma skin cancer

(PPS) Prestyloid space

(CS) Carotid space

(RPS) Retropharyngeal space

(PVS) Prevertebral space

pN Selective neck dissection 6 nodes

PROGNOSIS AND CANCER SURVIVAL

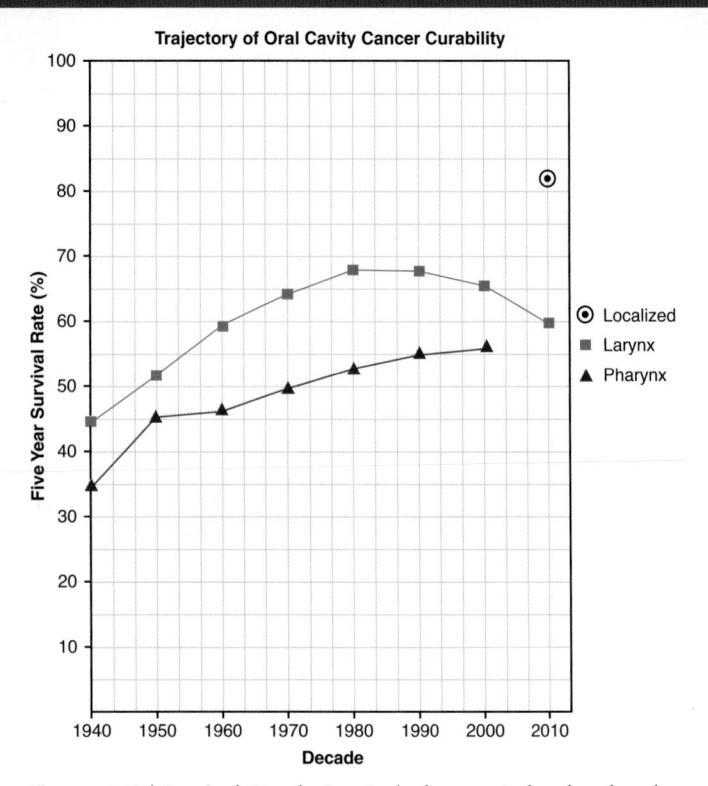

Figure 1.10 | Survival Graph. Survival of cancer in head and neck over seven decades: 1940 through 2010 based on ACS SEER data.

PROGNOSIS AND SURVIVAL

Prognostic Factors

Prognostic factors related to the host are variously cited throughout the head and neck sites.

Specific Tabulation of prognostic factors that are Site Specific Factors recommended for collection is a new feature and varies in its details.

Clinically significant:

- Size of lymph nodes
- Extracapsular extension from lymph nodes for head and neck
- Head and neck lymph nodes levels I-III
- Head and neck lymph nodes levels IV-V
- Head and neck lymph nodes levels VI-VII
- Other lymph node group
- Clinical location of cervical nodes
- Extracapsular spread (ECS) clinical
- Extracapsular spread (ECS) pathologic
- Human papillomavirus (HPV) status
- Tumor thickness*

CANCER STATISTICS AND SURVIVAL

Cancers of the oral cavity and pharynx—the upper digestive passage—account for 36,540 new cases per year. In addition,

*The foregoing passage is from Edge SB, Byrd DR, and Compton CC, et al, *AJCC Cancer Staging Manual, 7th edition*. New York, Springer, 2010, p. 38.

cancers of the larynx provide another 12,720 patients and thyroid cancers, 44,670. Approximately 25% of head and neck cancer patients die annually, often from other causes. For long-term survival, thyroid cancers, with only 1,500 deaths (5%), are the exception. The improvement in oral cavity and pharyngeal tumors from 1950 to 2000 was modest (14%) and matches larynx (15%). A multidisciplinary approach is vital and normal tissue conservation and reconstructive techniques have added greatly to quality of life. Unfortunately, this patient population comprises ethanol and nicotine abusers and it is difficult to change their habits. Persistence of smoking and drinking contributes to their demise, often from second malignant tumors in adjacent sites (Fig. 1.10).

Remarkably, >55% of patients are alive at 5 years; the majority live to 10 years. When treatment fails, death is within 2 years in 90% of patients and is often painful and disfiguring. African Americans in particular tend to die at a higher rate (75%). Another source for assessing the gains in survival in head and neck cancers is based on the multidisciplinary approach to management in national cooperative groups. The large database accumulated by the Radiation Therapy Oncology Group allows for 5-year survival analysis by major anatomic sites and their subsites as a function of stage. Stage I patients survive at the 60% to 80% level, stage II at 40% to 60%, stage III at 30% to 60%, and stage IV at 15% to 30%. With combined modality treatment, chemoradiation and surgery yields complete response rates of 45% to 95% depending on stage and often allows for preservation of normal structures (e.g., larynx).

In reviewing, the AJCC 7th Edition data confirms the importance of early diagnosis in head and neck cancers where survival is better than 50% prior to development of lymph node metastases (Fig. 1.11).

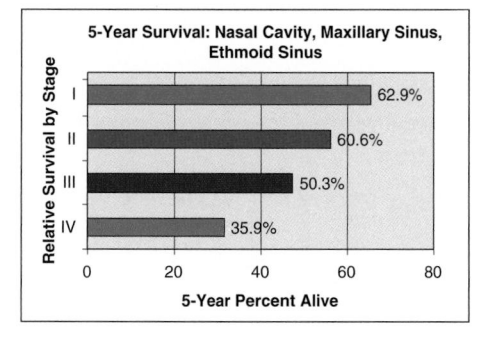

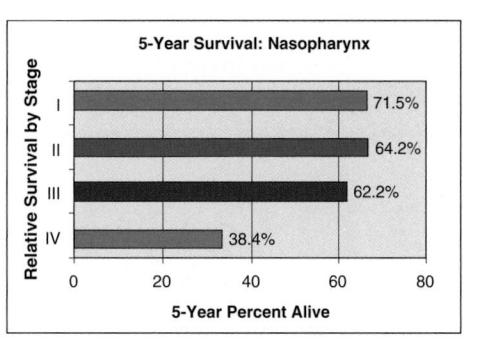

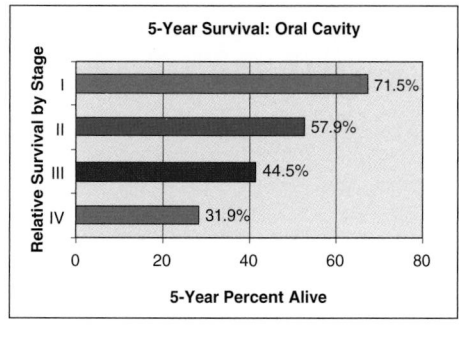

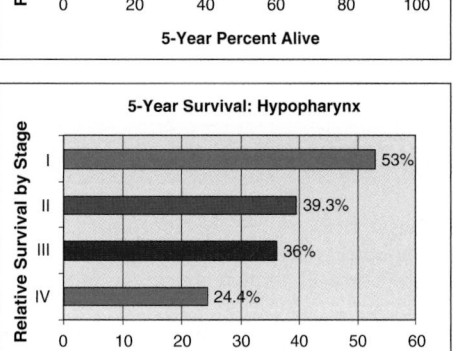

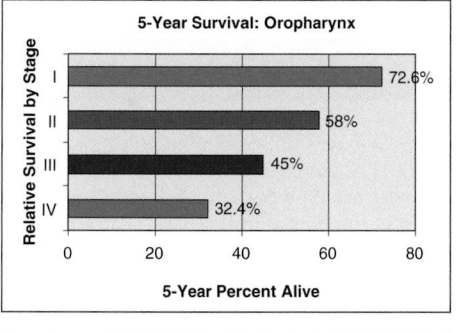

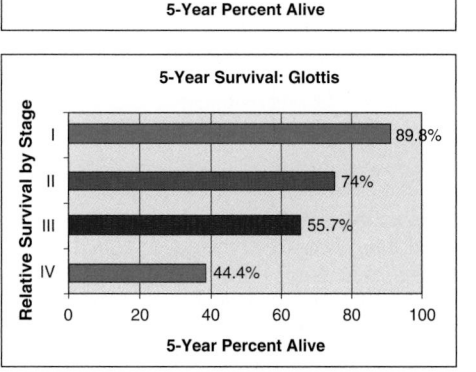

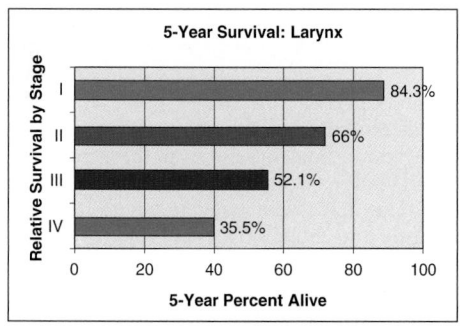

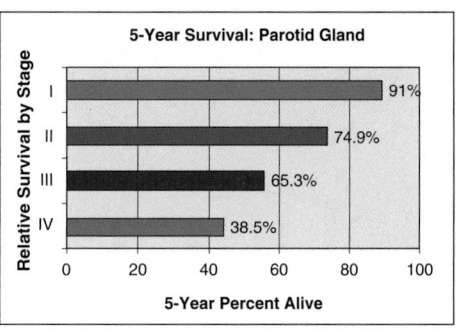

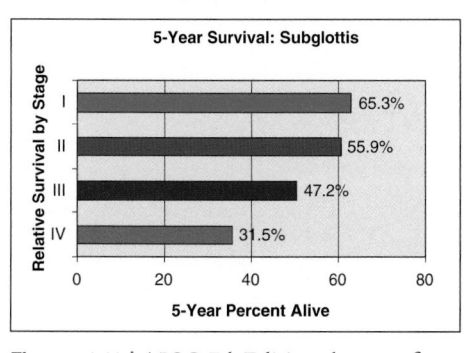

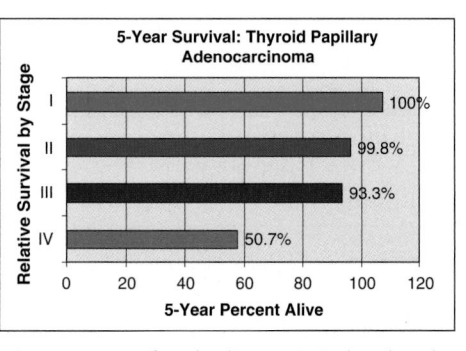

Figure 1.11 | AJCC 7th Edition data confirms the importance of early diagnosis in head and neck cancers where survival is better than 50% prior to development of lymph node metastases. Once cervical lymph node metastases occurs, the survival decreases to 30–40% but varies with larynx cancer still yielding 50–55% survival in advanced Stage III due to effective chemoradiation regimens. Exception to the rule is thyroid papillary/follicular adenocarcinomas that have 90–100% survival for stage I–III. (Data from Edge SB, Byrd DR, and Compton CC, et al, *AJCC Cancer Staging Manual, 7th edition*. New York, Springer, 2010.)

Paranasal Ethmoid Sinus and Mucosal Melanomas

PERSPECTIVE, PATTERNS OF SPREAD, AND PATHOLOGY

The ethmoid sinuses and nasal passages are the appropriate introduction to the upper respiratory tract oncoanatomy since the malignant gradient of the ethmoid sinus is its access and invasion into all of the other paranasal sinuses.

Also included in this chapter is a new site, mucosal melanoma of the head and neck, and its staging criteria. It has been included in this chapter because of the similarity in histopathology of these sites.

PERSPECTIVE AND PATTERNS OF SPREAD

Ethmoid sinus cancer, although rare, is more common than cancers of the sphenoid or frontal sinus. Because of their deep-seated location, these neoplasms are even more difficult to diagnose than maxillary antral cancers. The cancer is insidious in onset, but each manifestation is explicable by the pattern of invasion of the surrounding anatomy. A deep-seated headache around or posterior to the eyes suggests invasion into the surrounding sinuses—the frontal anteriorly, the sphenoid posteriorly, or the contralateral ethmoid or the maxillary sinus inferiorly (Fig. 2.2).

TABLE 2.1	Histopathologic Type: Common Cancers of the Paranasal Ethmoid Sinus
Squamous Cell Carcinoma Microscopic Variants	
Keratinizing; well differentiated; moderately well differentiated; poorly differentiated	
Nonkeratinizing; anaplastic squamous carcinoma	
Transitional cell carcinoma	
Spindle cell squamous carcinoma	

With lateral extension, orbital invasion and globe displacement can occur. The clinical triad of symptoms and signs of ethmoid sinus cancer are diplopia, a bloody nasal discharge, and loss of sensation in the upper lip (Fig. 2.2). Patterns of Spread are presented as a cancer crab that can invade in six basic directions Superior-Inferior, Medial-Lateral, Anterior-Posterior (SIMLAP) of adjacent anatomic sites (Fig. 2.2; Table 2.2).

PATHOLOGY

These mucoperiosteum spaces have ciliated, thin pseudo-stratified columnar epithelium that sweeps mucus to the nasal cavity. Ethmoid cancers arise from these mucosal linings of the sinus and tend to be adenocarcinomas as well as squamous cell cancers. They have been associated with the shavings and dust of furniture and cabinetmakers (Table 2.1; Fig. 2.1).

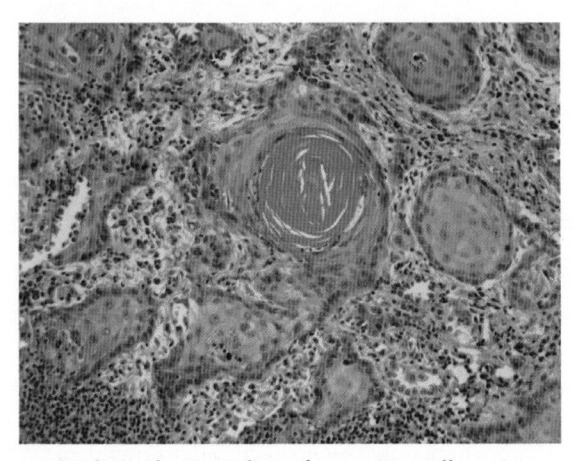

Figure 2.1 | Cytologic grading of squamous cell carcinoma. Well-differentiated (grade 1) squamous cell carcinoma. The tumor cells bear a strong resemblance to normal squamous cells and synthesize keratin, as evidenced by epithelial pearls.

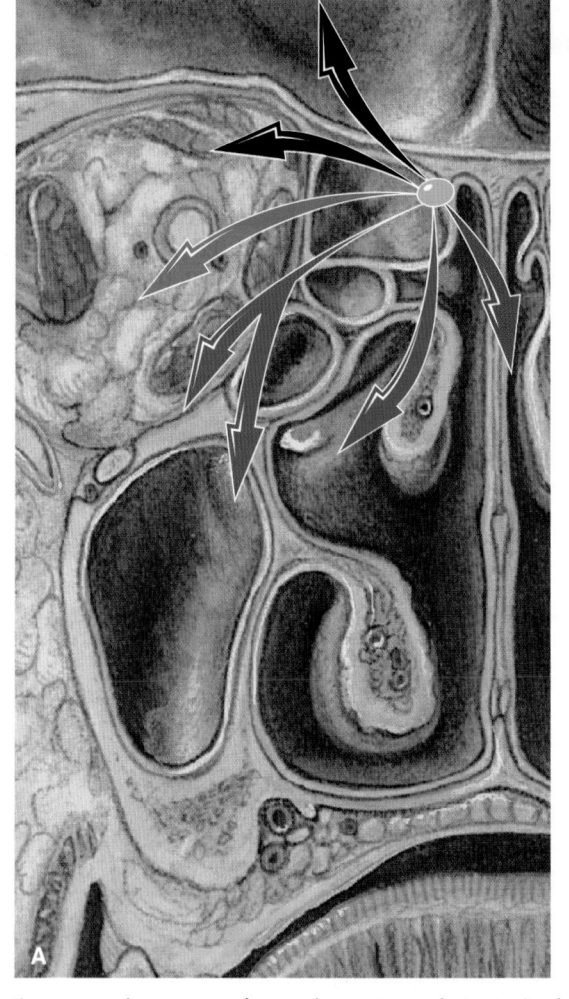
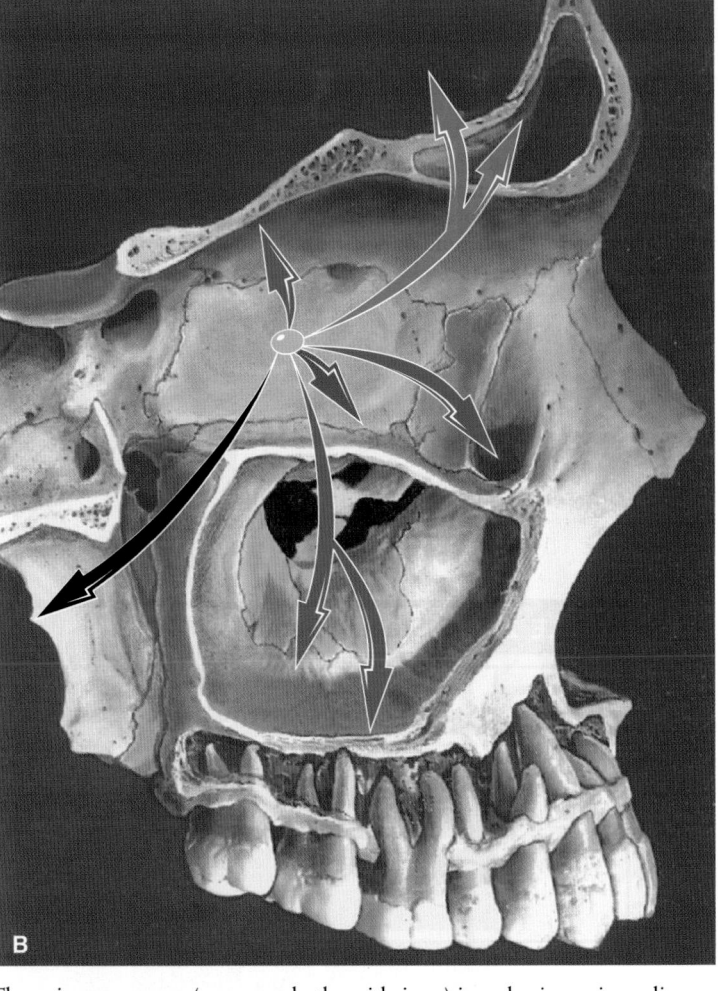

Figure 2.2 | Patterns of spread. A. Coronal. B. Sagittal. The primary cancer (paranasal ethmoid sinus) invades in various directions, which are color-coded vectors (*arrows*) representing stage of progression: Tis, yellow; T1, green; T2, blue; T3, purple; T4a, red; T4b, black. Three vectors of invasion are into orbit, into nasal passage, and paranasal sinuses and intracranially. The concept of visualizing patterns of spread to appreciate the surrounding anatomy is well demonstrated by the six directional patterns, i.e. SIMLAP Table 2.2.

TABLE 2.2	SIMLAP*	
Ethmoid Sinus (T1)		
S	Cribriform plate	• T3
I	Nasal cavity	• T2
M	Contralateral sinus	• T2
L	Orbit medial wall	• T2
	Orbit floor	• T3
A	Maxillary sinus, palate	• T3
	Ant. orbit, frontal sinus	• T4a
	Ant. cranial fossa	• T4a
P	Pterygoid plates	• T4b
	Orbital apex, dura, brain, midcranial fossa, CN nasopharynx, clivus	• T4b

There are six basic directions or vectors (arrows): The six vectors of invasion are S̲uperior, I̲nferior, M̲edial, L̲ateral, A̲nterior, and P̲osterior. The color-coded dots correlate the T stage with specific anatomic structure involved.

TNM STAGING CRITERIA

MUCOSAL MELANOMAS

Mucosal melanomas of the head and neck are highly malignant tumors and fortunately are rare. Of the different categories, the mucosal melanomas that occur in the sinuses are the most lethal, followed in the oral cavity, pharynx, and intranasal lesions. These mucosal melanomas represent a small percentage of all melanomas (i.e., 1% to 2% in most large series as compared to cutaneous melanomas) (Fig. 2.3B).

- *Mucosal melanomas* are derived from mucosa of neuroectodermal origin–derived mucosa whereas nonectodermally derived mucosa such as mucosa of nasopharynx, larynx, and tracheobronchial, which are of endodermal origin, are therefore more free of mucosal melanomas.

- *Sinonasal mucosal melanomas,* primarily a disease of adults and the elderly, have an onset characteristically two decades later than skin melanomas; 60% are older than 55 years of age.

- *Most common sites* are palate (34%) and paranasal sinuses (20%) then oral cavity; floor of mouth and tongue constitute only 2% to 10%.

- *Advanced stage* presentation is common, thus the current TNM system starts at T3, T4a, T4b, since often the exact site of origin can be obscured. Unilateral nasal or sinus obstruction and epistaxis accounted for 85% to 90% of symptoms encountered, often persisting for months. In the oral cavity approximately 35% have preexisting benign mucosal melanotosis because the primary is obscured; they more often present as a metastatic neck node clinically (Fig. 2.3C).

- *Pathologic diagnosis* requires identification of intracellular melanin, which occurs in 50% to 70% of cases. Enzyme immunochemistry improves accuracy as does the finding of premelanosomes.

- *Histologic cellular composition* is composed of three types of cells: spindle cell, polygonal cell, and mixed cell.

- *Depth of invasion* is a key prognostic factor (i.e., <0.5 cm survival is 30%, 0.6 cm to 1 cm is 18%, and >1 cm is only 10%). Size of lesion is less useful for prognosis.

- *Angioinvasiveness* is another feature and it predicts for early metastatic spread.

- *Staging of mucosal melanomas* in the literature generally indicates 75% are localized, 18% have regional nodes, and 6% to 10% present as metastases.

- *Local failure* despite treatment is common and salvage is approximately 25% or less. Distant metastases increase over-time: 51% after treatment but rises to 75% with local failure.

- *Survival* from pooled series (approximately 1,000 patients), mean survival is 39%, at 5 years 17%; 10 years mean survival drops to 5%, and over 10 years survival is 1% to 2%.

- *Treatment* is mostly surgical, survival is better for nasal (31%) or oral cavity (12%) and poorest for paranasal sinus (0%).

- *Radiation,* when used as the primary treatment, is given in a hypofractionation schedule, and local control has been reported to vary from 44% to 61%. Neutron therapy has also had some success.

- *Chemotherapy* and immunotherapy (BCG) has been used as an adjuvant with little success.

TABLE 2.3B	**Staging Summary Matrix**		

	Stage T3	**Stage T4a**	**Stage T4b**
N0	III	IVA	IVB
N1	III	IVA	IVB
N2	IVA	IVA	IVB
N3	IVB	IVB	IVB
M1	IVC	IVC	IVC

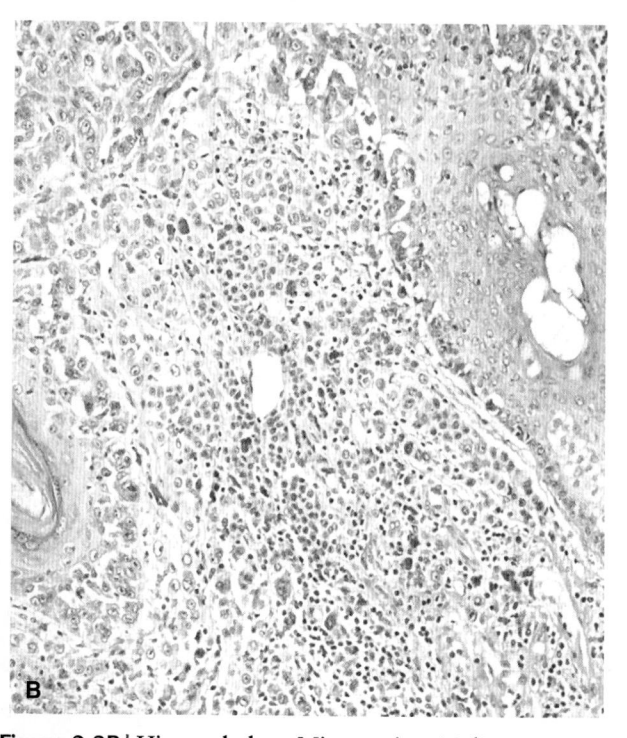

Figure 2.3B I Histopathology Microsection. Malignant melanoma, vertical growth phase. The host response consists of lymphocytes infiltrating amid the melanocytes ("tumor-infiltrating lymphocytes").

MUCOSAL MELANOMAS

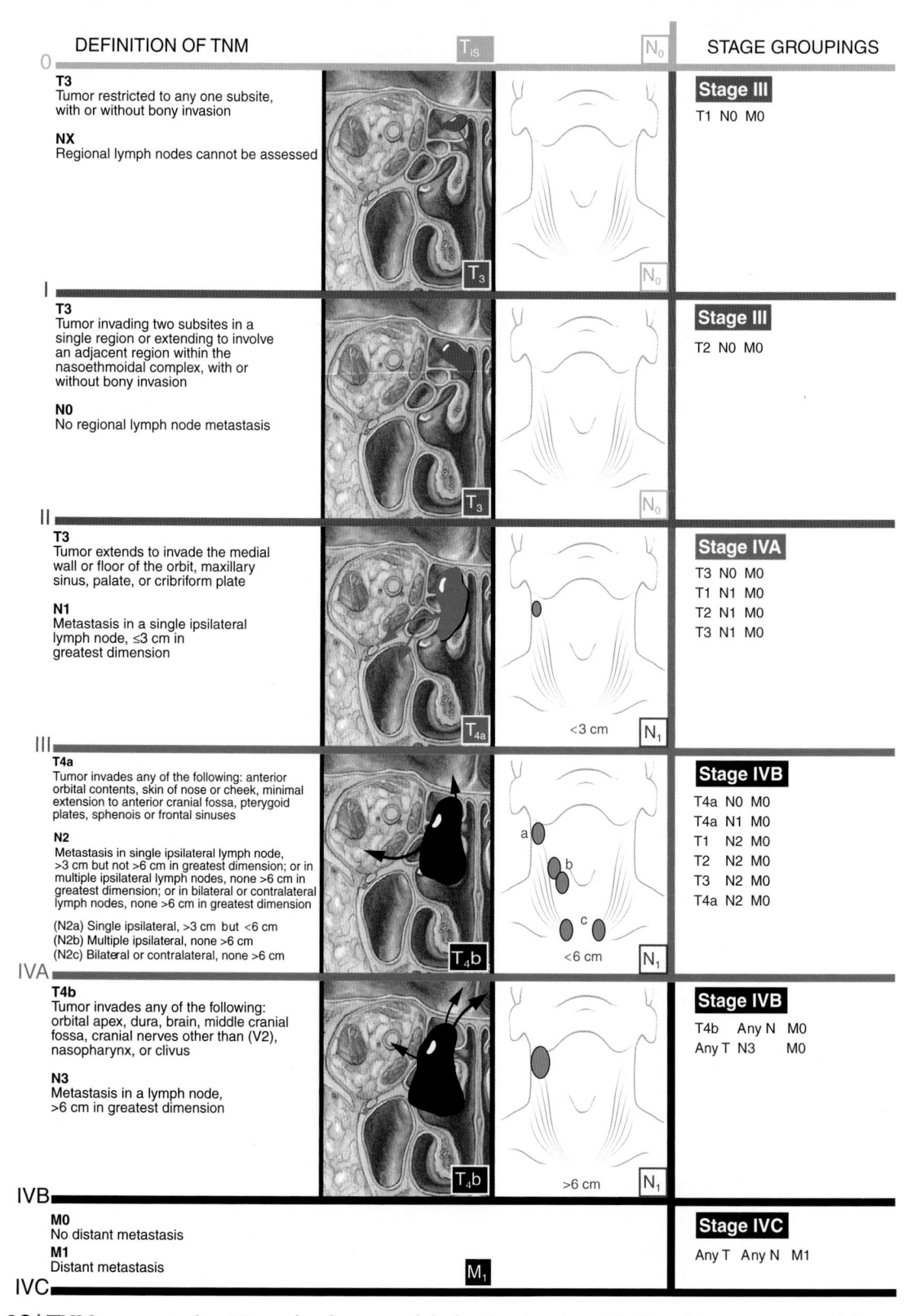

Figure 2.3C | TNM stage grouping. Mucosal melanomas of the head and neck are highly malignant tumors and fortunately are rare. Of the different categories, the mucosal melanomas that occur in the sinuses are the most lethal, followed in the oral cavity, pharynx, and intranasal lesions. These mucosal melanomas represent a small percentage of all melanomas i.e. 1%–2% in most large series as compared to cutaneous melanomas. Vertical presentations of stage groupings, which follow the same color code for cancer stage advancement, are organized in horizontal lanes: stage 0, yellow; I, green; II, blue; III, purple; IVA, red; IVB, black. Definitions of TN on left and stage grouping on right.

T-ONCOANATOMY

ORIENTATION OF THREE-PLANAR T-ONCOANATOMY

The ethmoid sinus is the anatomic isocenter of all paranasal sinuses. The anatomic isocenter is at the level of the floor of the orbit and extends to the sphenoid at the skull base. The anterior surface bullet enters to the right or left of the midsagittal plane at or below the medial canthus of the eye (Fig. 2.4A). The lateral bullet is at or below the lateral canthus of the eye (Fig. 2.4B).

T-oncoanatomy

The ethmoid sinuses and nasal passages are the appropriate introduction to the upper respiratory tract. The four paired sinuses are the maxillary, ethmoid, frontal sinuses, and the sphenoid. Although the sphenoid appears as a single midline sinus, it is a paired sinus. A three-dimensional reconstruction, focusing on bony anatomy, allows for an understanding of the interrelationships. The anatomy may be divided by drawing three parallel lines across the frontal view of the skull, one line passing above and another below the orbits, the third passing through the floor of the antra or hard palate. The two vertical lines separate the ethmoid and nasal fossa from the maxillary antra. The nasal septum separates the ethmoid and nasal fossa into right and left sides. In a comparison with anteroposterior and lateral projections or coronal and sagittal sections, three important planes become evident: (i) The floor of the anterior fossa of the skull is the roof of the nasal cavity and ethmoid; (ii) The hard palate is the floor of the maxillary antra; and (iii) An imaginary plane below the orbits divides the paranasal sinuses into a suprastructure and an infrastructure. The suprastructure contains the ethmoids, superomedial to which is the apex of the nasal cavity and cribriform (olfactory region). Posterior to this are the sphenoid sinuses, lateral are the orbits, and inferior are the nasal fossa and turbinates. The infrastructure contains the maxillary antra and the major portion of the nasal cavity or vestibule. These planes are helpful in relating the surface anatomy to the radiographic anatomy. The three-dimensional planar views are crucial to understanding the malignant gradient:

- *Coronal plane* (Fig. 2.5A): In the coronal view, the lateral anterior wall separates the ethmoid sinus from the orbit and inferiorly drains into the nasal cavity.

- *Sagittal plane* (Fig. 2.5B): The relationship to the maxillary antrum is readily seen as well as to the sphenoid sinus. Superior to the ethmoid is the cribriform plate and cranial nerve I (olfactory).

- *Axial plane* (Fig. 2.5C): The orbit and its relation to the ethmoid sinus is shown and illustrates the fineness of the walls separating the two cavities. The sphenoid sinus has the most complex anatomic location in contrast to the frontal sinus, which has the simplest. To understand cranial nerve anatomy, one must relate the course of the first six nerves to the walls of the sphenoid sinuses. The various divisions and branches of the cranial nerve V and its trigeminal ganglion are in its vicinity. This is detailed when studying the nasopharynx, which is directly below the sphenoid sinuses and cavernous sinus.

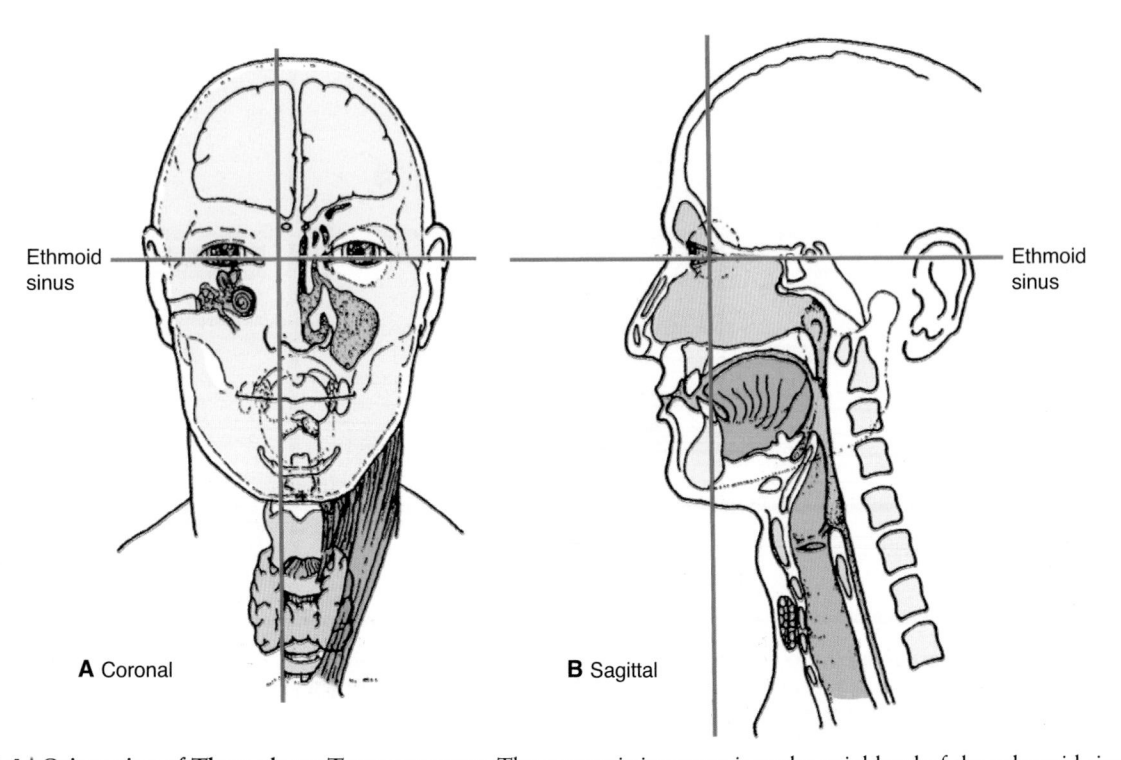

A Coronal   **B** Sagittal

Figure 2.4 | Orientation of Three-planar T-oncoanatomy. The anatomic isocenter is at the axial level of the sphenoid sinus. **A.** Coronal. **B.** Sagittal. Landmarks: Coronal, Right/Left of midline orbit; Sagittal, Zygomatic arch; Transverse, Sphenoid Sinus.

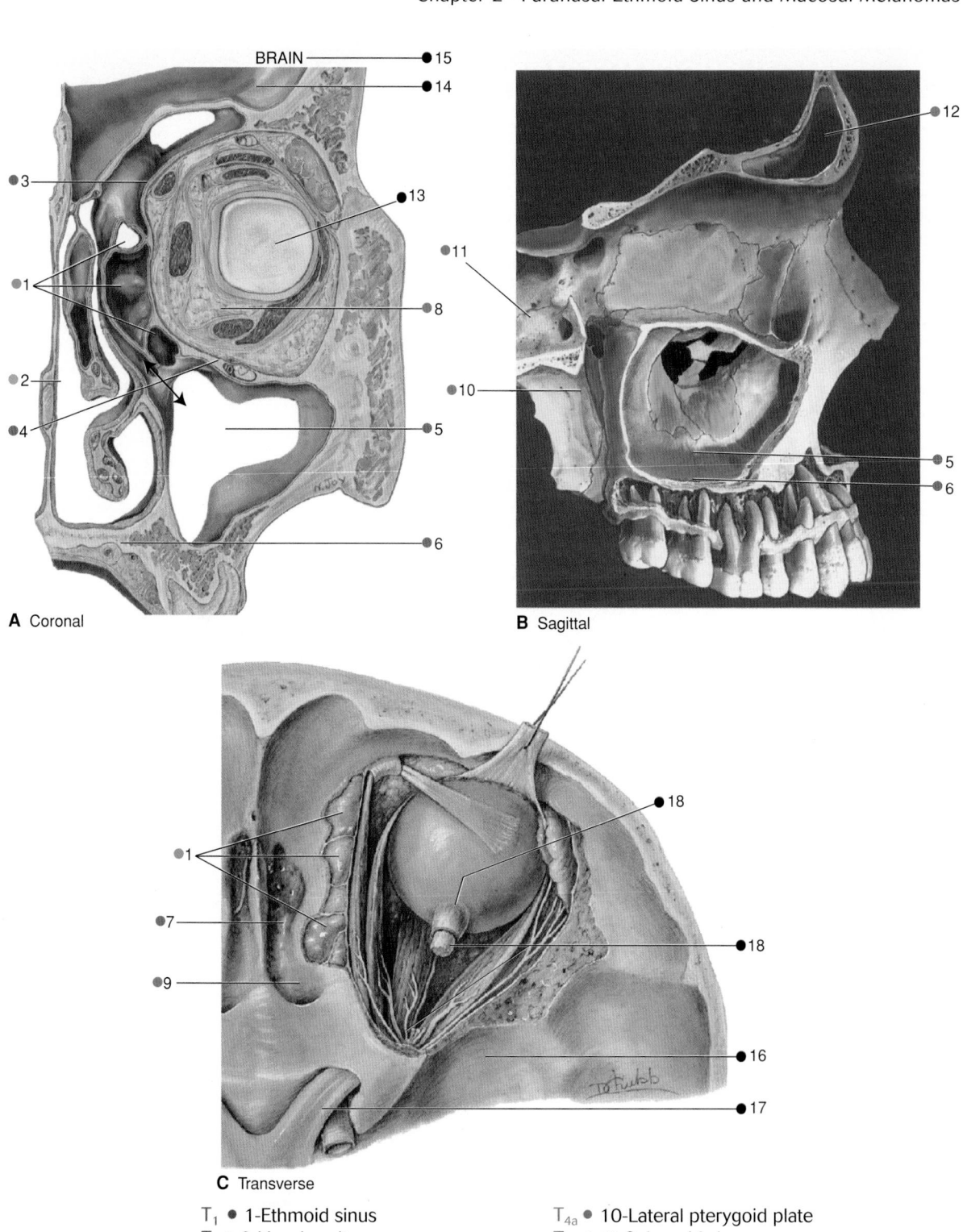

A Coronal

B Sagittal

C Transverse

T₁ ● 1-Ethmoid sinus	T₄ₐ ● 10-Lateral pterygoid plate
T₂ ● 2-Nasal cavity	T₄ₐ ● 11-Sphenoid sinus
T₃ ● 3-Orbit, medical wall	T₄ₐ ● 12-Frontal sinus
T₃ ● 4-Orbit, floor	T₄ᵦ ● 13-Orbit (eyeball)
T₃ ● 5-Maxillary sinus	T₄ᵦ ● 14-Dura
T₃ ● 6-Palate	T₄ᵦ ● 15-Brain
T₃ ● 7-Cribriform plate	T₄ᵦ ● 16-Middle cranial fossa
T₄ₐ ● 8-Anterior orbit	T₄ᵦ ● 17-Optic nerve
T₄ₐ ● 9-Anterior (phasal fossa minimal)	T₄ᵦ ● 18-Apex of orbit (optic nerve)

Figure 2.5 | T-oncoanatomy. The Color Code for the anatomic sites correlates with the color code for the stage group (Figure 2.3) and patterns of spread (Figure 2.2) and SIMLAP table (Table 2.2). Connecting the dots in similar colors will provide an appreciation for the 3D Oncoanatomy.

N-ONCOANATOMY AND M-ONCOANATOMY

N-ONCOANATOMY

The sentinel nodes are the high retroparapharyngeal and para-pharyngeal nodes along the carotid sheath. When they are involved and extend into the retrostyloid compartment (Fig. 2.6), this leads to entrapment of the cranial nerves emerging alongside the jugular foramen. The nodes in this region are named after Rouviere, famous for his treatise on lymphoid anatomy. Again, numerous neurologic syndromes can occur. Retroparotidian syndrome, or the jugular foramen syndrome, is characterized by loss of the gag reflex (cranial nerve IX), vocal cord paralysis (cranial nerve X), atrophy of the trapezius muscle (cranial nerve XI), and

deviation of the uvula (cranial nerve X) and tongue on protrusion (cranial nerve XII) (Table 2.4).

M-ONCOANATOMY

The lateral pterygoid buccal venous plexus drains into the jugular vein and then into the brachiocephalic veins and to the superior vena cava. Hematogenous spread, although uncommon, can include lung and bone as favored sites of involvement; distant metastases occur infrequently (Fig. 2.7A,B).

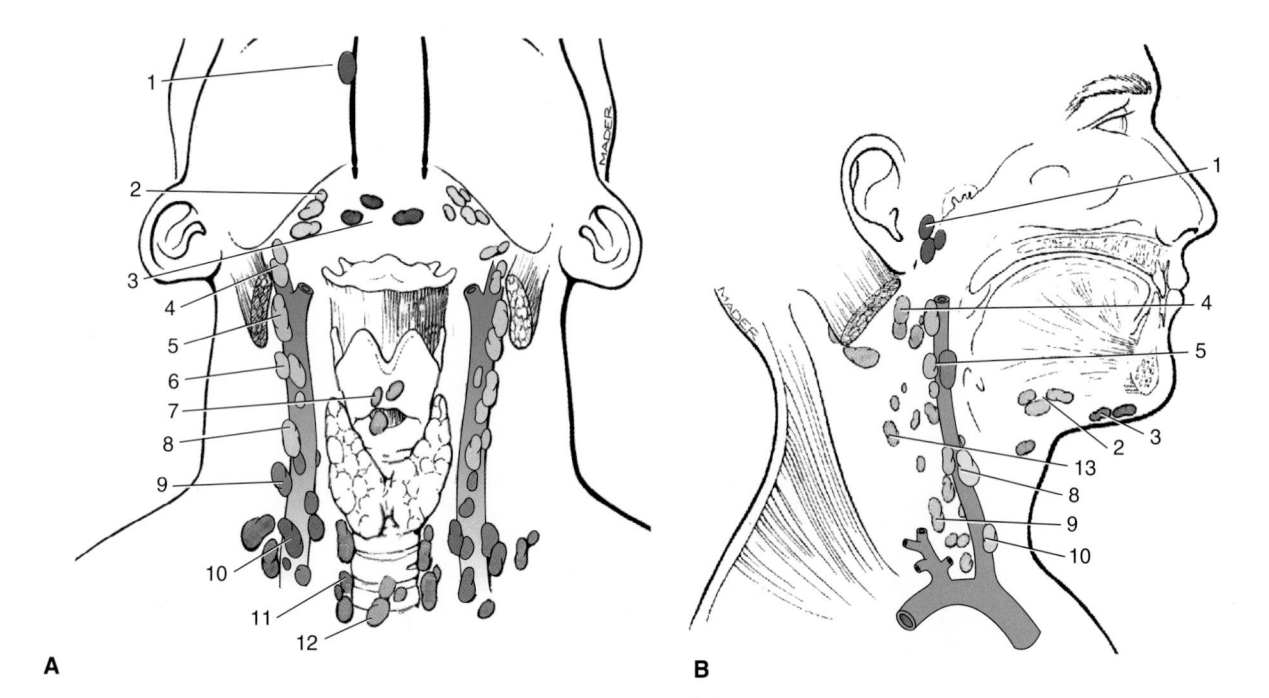

A   **B**

Figure 2.6 | N-oncoanatomy. The red node highlights the sentinel node, which is the highest retropharyngeal node. **A.** Anterior view. **B.** Lateral view. Once the sentinel node is involved, all of the neck nodes are at risk for metastases. The regional nodes include: (1) retropharyngeal; (2) submandibular; (3) submental; (4) superior deep cervical; (5) jugulodigastric; and (6) midjugular. The juxtaregional nodes are: (7) prelaryngeal; (8) jugulo-omohyoid; (9) inferior deep cervical; (10) supraclavicular; (11) paratracheal; (12) pretracheal; and (13) spinal accessory. **M-oncoanatomy** is determined by the jugular vein, which joins with the subclavian vein to form the right brachiocephalic vein on the right, and the left brachiocephalic vein on the left; both brachiocephalic veins form the superior vena cava, which drains into the right side of the heart and then into lung.

TABLE 2.4	Sentinel and Regional Nodes: Ethmoid Sinus (Bilateral)		
		Level/Location of Node(s)	
S Sentinel Node		**Axial Level**	**AJCC Level**
S1 Retropharyngeal Rouviere's Node		C1	nI
R Regional Nodes			
R1 Jugulodigastric, superior deep cervical		C3/4	II
R2 Mid deep cervical		C4	III
R3 Jugulodigastric, superior/mid deep cervical		C3/4	II
R4 Jugulo-omohyoid, inferior deep cervical		C7	IV

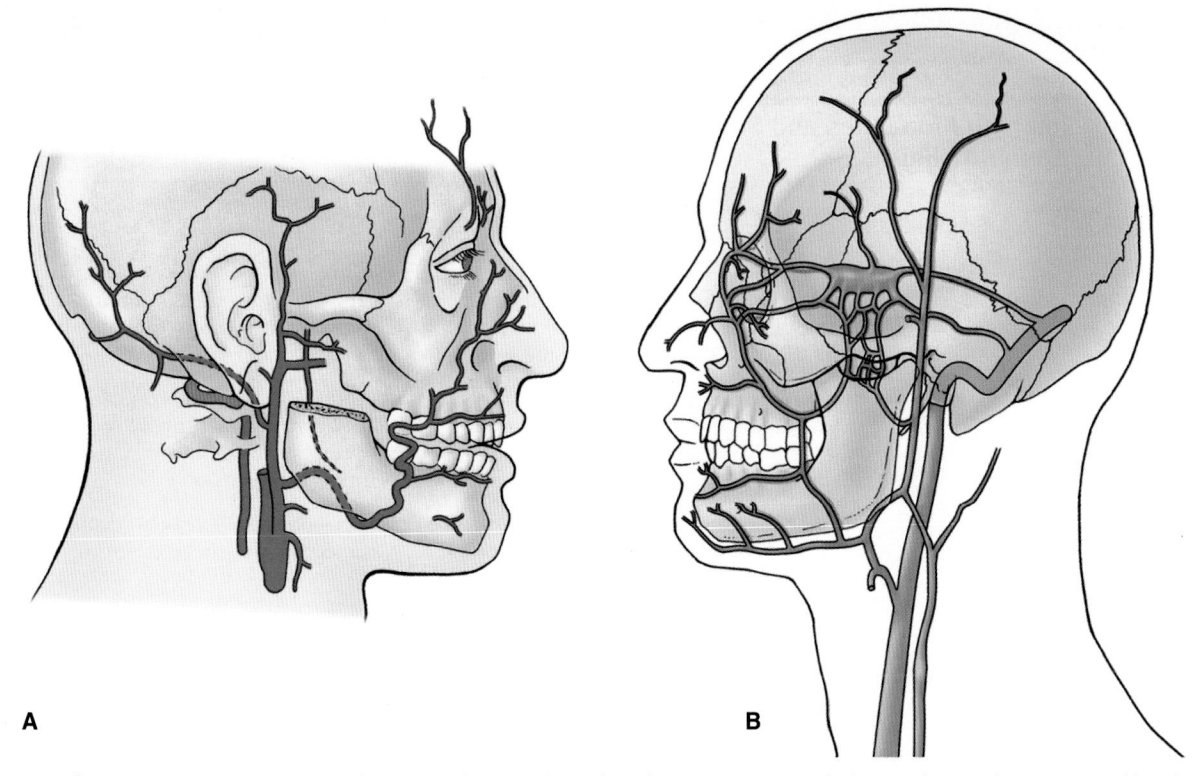

Figure 2.7 | M-oncoanatomy. **A.** Carotid artery with major branches shown. **B.** Pterygoid plexus of veins drains most of head and neck sites into internal deep jugular. The jugular vein drains into the superior vena cava and then into the right heart, making jung the target organ.

Perineural invasion and compression of Ethmoid Cancers is V_2 external nasal branch as the cancer invades into Nasal Cavity. The infraorbital perineural invasion occurs with ero-sion of the lateral wall and floor of the orbit resulting in a round spot of hypoesthesia below the lower eyelid (Fig. 2.7C).

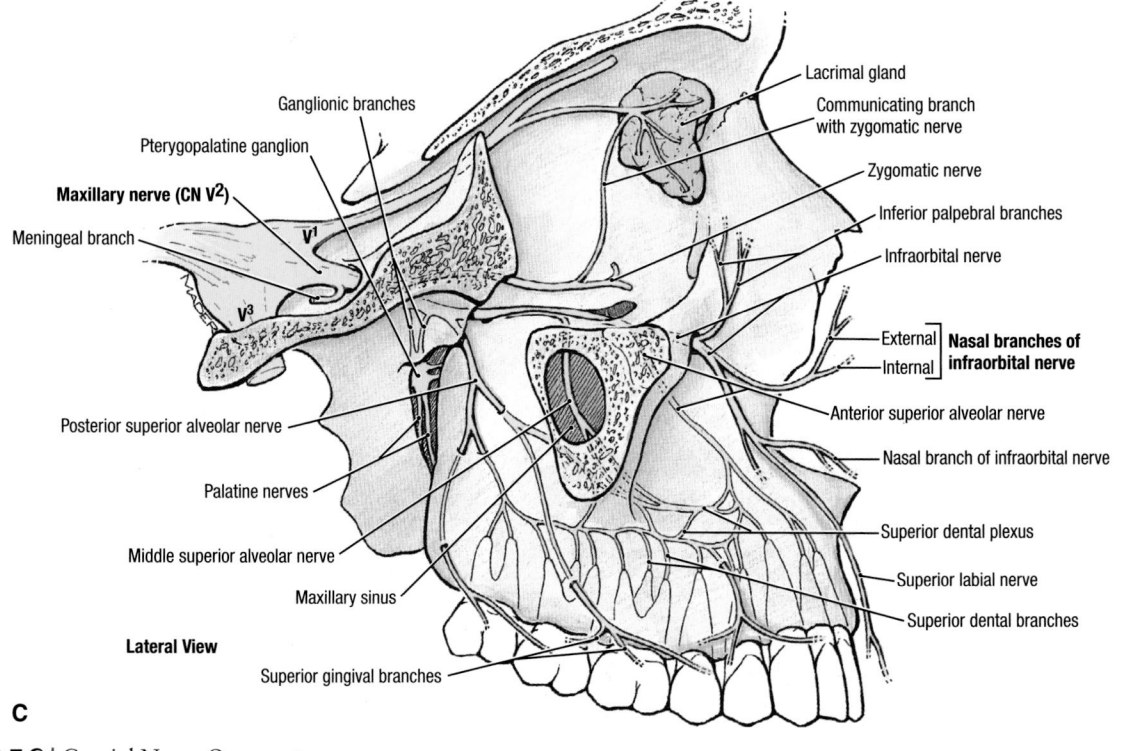

Figure 2.7 C | Cranial Nerve Oncoanatomy.

STAGING WORKUP

TABLE 2.5	Imaging Modalities and Strategies for Diagnosis and Staging for Head and Neck: Ethmoid Sinus	
Modality	**Strategy**	**Recommended**
Primary Tumor and Nodes		
Computed tomography	Excellent for defining extent of primary depth of invasion enlargement of involved nodes. (Preferred for bone invasion.)	Yes—3–5 mm cuts, 3 mm for primary sites, 5 mm for neck. Bone sclerosis rare
Magnetic resonance imaging	Offers best 3D and 3-planar views of primary and nodes, especially soft tissue extensions. Gadolinium contrast for extensions and perineuronal spread.	Yes—≤4 cm slices Gd for intracranial and perineuronal spread. T1 & T2. Orbital invasion DDx. (Cancer vs. sinusitis/secretions?)**
Positron emission spectroscopy	Functional and metabolic imaging of ^{18}FDG is based on 2-deoxy modification, which inhibits the molecule from subsequent enzymatic conversion and is "metabolically trapped" in tumor cells.	Yes—potential exists for distinguishing cancer vs. sinusitis/secretions.
Metastases		
Chest film	Search for metastases.	Yes.
Radionuclide scan	^{99m}Tc for bone metastases.	No/Yes—If symptomatic

3D, three-dimensional; FDG, fluorodeoxyglucose.

RULES OF CLASSIFICATION AND STAGING

Clinical Staging and Imaging

Inspection and palpation of paranasal sinuses is limited in early localized stages. For ethmoid cancers, orbital invasion may displace the globe and trap the anterior ethmoid branch of cranial nerve V_1, leading to altered sensation in the upper lip. Maxillary antral cancers, when advanced, fill the gingival buccal gutter, loosen molar teeth, and invade the cheek and hard palate. Infection and inflammatory sinusitis obscures cancers. Both magnetic resonance imaging (MRI) and computed tomography enhancement (CT_e) are recommended to distinguish tumor from fluid. CT_e is best for determining bone erosion of the paper-thin lamina bones of sinus walls. For evaluation of retropharyngeal nodes imaging is essential (Table 2.5 and Figure 2.8).

Pathologic Staging

The gross specimen should be evaluated for margins. Unresected gross residual tumor must be included and marked with clips. All resected lymph node specimens should describe the size, number, and level of involved nodes and whether there is extracapsular spread. Specimens taken after radiation or chemotherapy need to be noted as such; specimen shrinkages may occur up to 30% after resection itself. Designations pT and pN should be used after histopathologic evaluation. Perineural invasion deserves special notation.

Oncoimaging Annotations

- MRI and CT play complementary roles in the assessment and staging process for these tumors.

- MRI is best at detecting tumor extension outside the sinonasal cavity. CT is most sensitive in assessing anatomy and bone invasion with these tumors. The hallmark of sinonasal malignancy is bone destruction, seen in approximately 80% of all CT scans in these patients.

- MRI aids in separating complex sinonasal secretions/infections from tumor. Combined T1- and T2-weighted, contrast medium-enhanced images are needed for this evaluation.

- Orbital extension is manifest on CT and MRI by bone erosion and changes in the orbital fat. MRI tends to underestimate orbital invasions.

- Sinonasal bony sclerosis caused by tumor is rare; its presence is normally related to coexistent chronic inflammatory changes.

PROGNOSIS AND CANCER SURVIVAL

PROGNOSTIC FACTORS

The seventh edition of the AJCC Cancer Staging Manual lists the following prognostic factors for nasal ethmoid sinus cancers:

- Size of lymph nodes
- Extracapsular extension from lymph nodes for head and neck
- Head and neck lymph nodes levels I-III
- Head and neck lymph nodes levels IV-V
- Head and neck lymph nodes levels VI-VII
- Other lymph node group
- Clinical location of cervical nodes
- Extracapsular spread (ECS) clinical
- Extracapsular spread (ECS) pathologic
- Human papillomavirus (HPV) status
- Tumor thickness*

*The foregoing passage is from Edge SB, Byrd DR, and Compton CC, et al, *AJCC Cancer Staging Manual, 7th edition.* New York, Springer, 2010, p. 99.

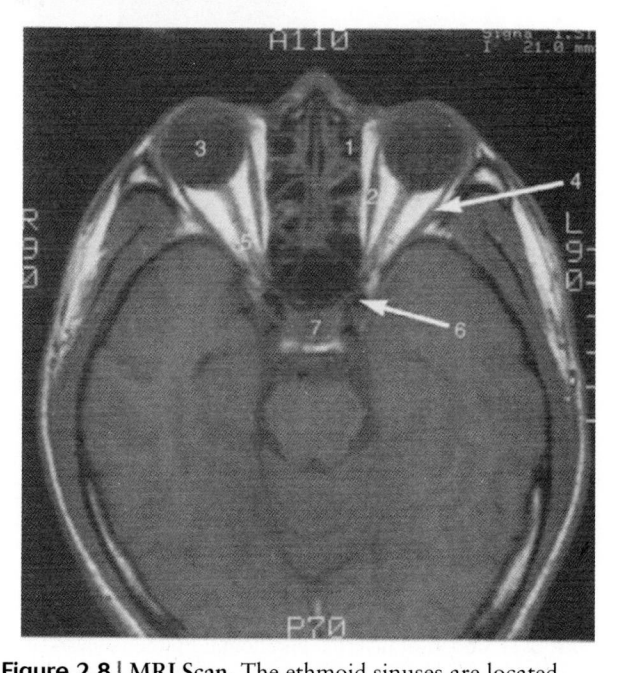

1. ethmoid sinus
2. medial rectus muscle
3. globe
4. lateral rectus muscle
5. optic nerve
6. carotid artery
7. pituitary fossa

Figure 2.8 | MRI Scan. The ethmoid sinuses are located between or orbits and demonstrates why lateral invasion into orbit is a common pattern of invasion. The CT/MRI transverse section can be correlated with the anatomy in Fig. 2.5C as an assist to staging.

CANCER STATISTICS AND SURVIVAL

Generally, cancers of the oral cavity and pharynx (the upper digestive passage) account for 36,540 new cases. In addition, cancer of the larynx affects another 12,720 patients and thyroid cancers, 44,670. Approximately 25% of head and neck cancer patients die annually, often owing to other causes. Long-term survival rates in patients with thyroid cancer, with only 1,500 deaths (5%), is the exception. The improvement in survival rates in patients with oral cavity and pharyngeal tumors from 1950 to 2000 was modest at 14% and matches that for patients with tumors of the larynx at 15%. A multidisciplinary approach is vital, and normal tissue conservation and reconstructive techniques have both added greatly to quality of life. Unfortunately, this patient population contains ethanol and nicotine abusers, and it is difficult to change these habits. Persistence of smoking and drinking contributes to their demise, often from second malignant tumors in adjacent sites.

Specifically, paranasal sinus cancers are detected late due to being mistaken for sinusitis. Both ethmoid and maxillary central cancers remain well below 50% 5-year survival. If diagnosed early survival rates are above 50% 5-year survival (Fig. 2.9).

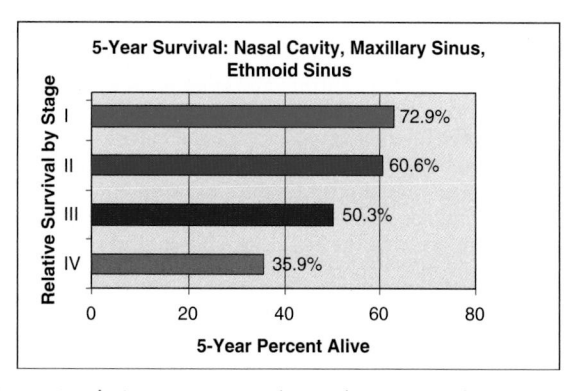

Figure 2.9 | Five-year survival rates by stage at diagnosis. (Data from Edge SB, Byrd DR, and Compton CC, et al., *AJCC Cancer Staging Manual, 7th edition.* New York, Springer, 2010.)

Maxillary Sinus Antrum

PERSPECTIVE, PATTERNS OF SPREAD, AND PATHOLOGY

The use of Ohngren's plane provides the malignant gradient of the maxillary antrum, dividing the sinus into an anterior-inferior compartment and a posterior-superior pocket.

PERSPECTIVE AND PATTERNS OF SPREAD

Tumors arising in the paranasal sinuses can be both very destructive and deforming. Fortunately, they are uncommon. Cancers of the maxillary antrum and ethmoid are among those more frequently encountered. The unique anatomic feature at these sites is the direct juxtaposition of the mucous membrane with very thin bony walls. Unfortunately, the manifestations of localized cancers are similar to sinusitis. Consequently, most cancers masquerade as infections and go unrecognized. It is no surprise, therefore, that the first detectable clinical signs of cancer are of advanced spread, most often owing to invasion through bony walls (Fig. 3.2). To the astute clinician, a persistent unilateral sinusitis may be a clue to an underlying cancer.

As for most sites, the cancer infiltrates the surrounding structures, which depends on its site of origin. Pathways of least resistance are at the foramina or where the bone is thinnest and are manifested by displaying a number of typical signs. The infrastructure of the maxillary sinus is the most common site of cancer origin, and the medial wall is easy to penetrate because of the normal ostia. Bloody nasal discharge appears before erosion of this paper-thin wall. As the mass extends medially into the nose, nasal obstruction can occur. The floor of the maxillary

TABLE 3.1	Histopathologic Type: Common Cancers of the Maxillary Antrum
Squamous Cell Carcinoma Microscopic Variants	
Keratinizing; well differentiated; moderately well differentiated; poorly differentiated	
Nonkeratinizing; anaplastic squamous carcinoma	
Transitional cell carcinoma	
Spindle cell squamous carcinoma	

sinus is in close contact with molar dental roots and their nerves. Consequently, as the bone is destroyed with inferior spread, there is filling of the gingivobuccal gutter, loosening of teeth, and finally an ulcerating lesion and loss of the alveolar bone with extension into the hard palate (Fig. 3.2A,B).

Cancers of the suprastructure usually occur at the summit of the sinusoidal pyramid. They extend into the malar bone and the outer half of the floor of the orbit into the temporal fossa. The skin of the cheek rapidly expands, often as a result of infection, and the zygomatic arch can be destroyed. The eye can be displaced and become proptotic when there is superior invasion. A posterior location and spread of cancer is less common, but in advanced states, the tumor, particularly when it is aggressive, can explode the sinus cavity and move in all directions via the associated infection. Under these circumstances, the cancer invades the pterygoid

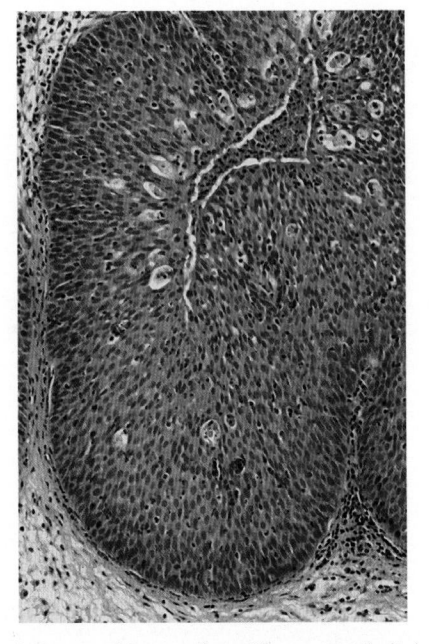

Figure 3.1 | Sinonasal inverted papilloma. Epithelial nests are growing downward (inverted) into the submucosa. They are composed of a uniform cellular proliferation, which displays an inflammatory cell infiltrate and scattered microcysts.

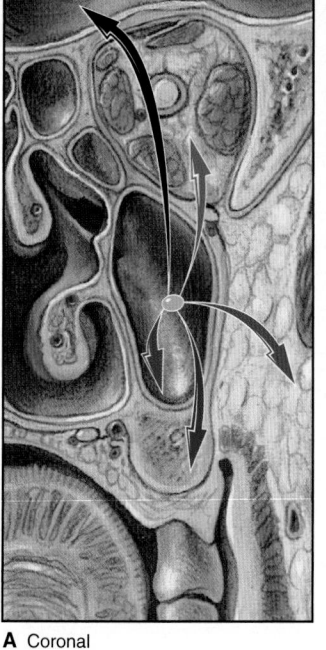
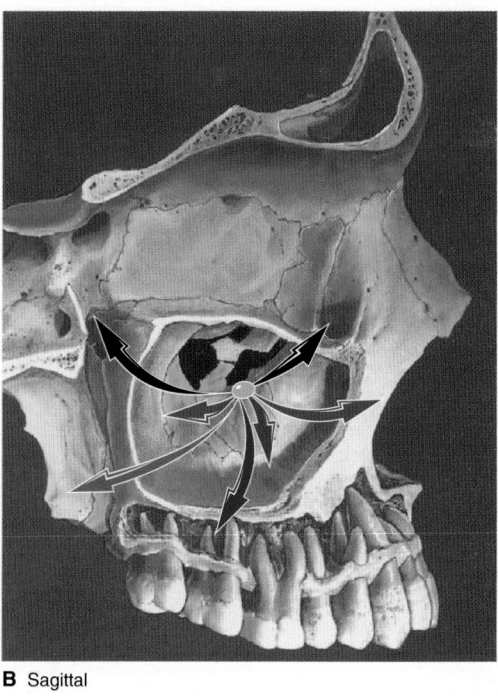

A Coronal   **B** Sagittal

Figure 3.2 | Patterns of spread. A. Coronal. Patterns of Spread into orbit superiorly, check laterally, and palate inferiorly. **B. Sagittal.** Pattern of Spread into palate inferiorly and pterygoid fossa posteriorly. The primary cancer (maxillary sinus antrum) invades in various directions, which are color-coded vectors (*arrows*) representing stage of progression. Tis, yellow; T1, green; T2, blue; T3, purple; T4a, red; and T4b, black. The concept of visualizing patterns of spread to appreciate the surrounding anatomy is well demonstrated by the six directional pattern, i.e. SIMLAP Table 3.2.

plates and muscles, leading to trismus (Fig. 3.2B). Patterns of Spread are presented as a cancer crab that can invade in six basic directions Superior-Inferior, Medial-Lateral, Anterior-Posterior (SIMLAP) of adjacent anatomic sites (Fig. 3.2; Table 3.2).

PATHOLOGY

Papillomas of the nasal cavities and paranasal sinuses show inversion patterns of surface epithelia that are in the underly-

ing stroma (Figure 3.1). Often HPV have been associated. In a small percentage (≤5%) become squamous cell cancers. Most maxillary antral cancers are squamous cell cancers (Table 3.1). Ethmoid cancers can be either squamous cell or adenocarcinomas. In contrast, tumors of the nose are highly varied, although again, they are most often squamous cell cancers.

TABLE 3.2	SIMLAP*	
Maxillary Antrum		
S	Floor and medial wall orbit	• T3
	Ethmoid sinus	• T3
I	Hard palate	• T2
	Loosen 1st and 2nd molar teeth	• T2
M	Middle meatus	• T2
L	Pterygoid fossa	• T3
A	Subcutaneous	• T3
	Skin of cheek	• T4a
P	Posterior wall	• T3
	Pterygoid plates	• T4a
	Infratemporal fossa	• T4a
	Nasopharynx	• T4b
	Clivus, C$_1$	• T4b

*There are six basic directions or vectors (arrows): The six vectors of invasion are Superior, Inferior, Medial, Lateral, Anterior, and Posterior. The color-coded dots correlate the T stage with specific anatomic structure involved.

TNM STAGING CRITERIA

TNM STAGING CRITERIA

The TNM criteria for the maxillary antrum was initiated in the first edition of the American Joint Committee on Cancer/International Union Against Cancer (AJCC/UICC) and are based on patterns of spread into subsites rather than size. The subsite criteria were introduced with the fourth edition of the AJCC/ UICC (1992) and are based on patterns of spread rather than size (Fig. 3.3). The use of Ohngren's plane provides the malignant gradient of the maxillary antrum, dividing the sinus into an anterior-inferior compartment and a posterior-superior pocket. With massive invasion, cancer of the maxillary sinus can invade other paranasal sinuses, enter into the cranial fossa, and even reach the lateral pterygoid space. Lymph node progression from N1, N2, to N3 is the same as most head and neck cancer sites and is based on size, laterality, and number of nodes.

SUMMARY OF CHANGES SEVENTH EDITION AJCC

The TNM stages according to the 7th Edition of AJCC are illustrated in color code of advancement (Fig. 3.3). T4 lesions have been divided into T4a (moderately advanced local disease) and T4b (very advanced local disease), leading to the stratification of Stage IV into Stage IVA (moderately advanced local/regional disease), Stage IVB (very advanced local/regional disease), and Stage IVC (distant metastatic disease). The TNM Staging Matrix is color coded for identification of Stage Group once T and N stages are determined (Table 3.3).

TABLE 3.3 | **Stage Summary Matrix**

	Stage T1	Stage T2	Stage T3	Stage T4a	Stage T4b
N0	I	II	III	IVA	IVB
N1	III	III	III	IVA	IVB
N2	IVA	IVA	IVA	IVA	IVB
N3	IVB	IVB	IVB	IVB	IVB
M1	IVC	IVC	IVC	IVC	IVC

Head and Neck: All Sites
- *T stage* determines stage group
  - T1 = I, T2 + II, T3 = III, T4 = IV
- *N stage* N1 = T3 and then progresses as T stage progresses
  - N1 = T3, N2 = T4a, N3 = T4b
- *M stage* is a separate stage
  - M1 = Stage IVC

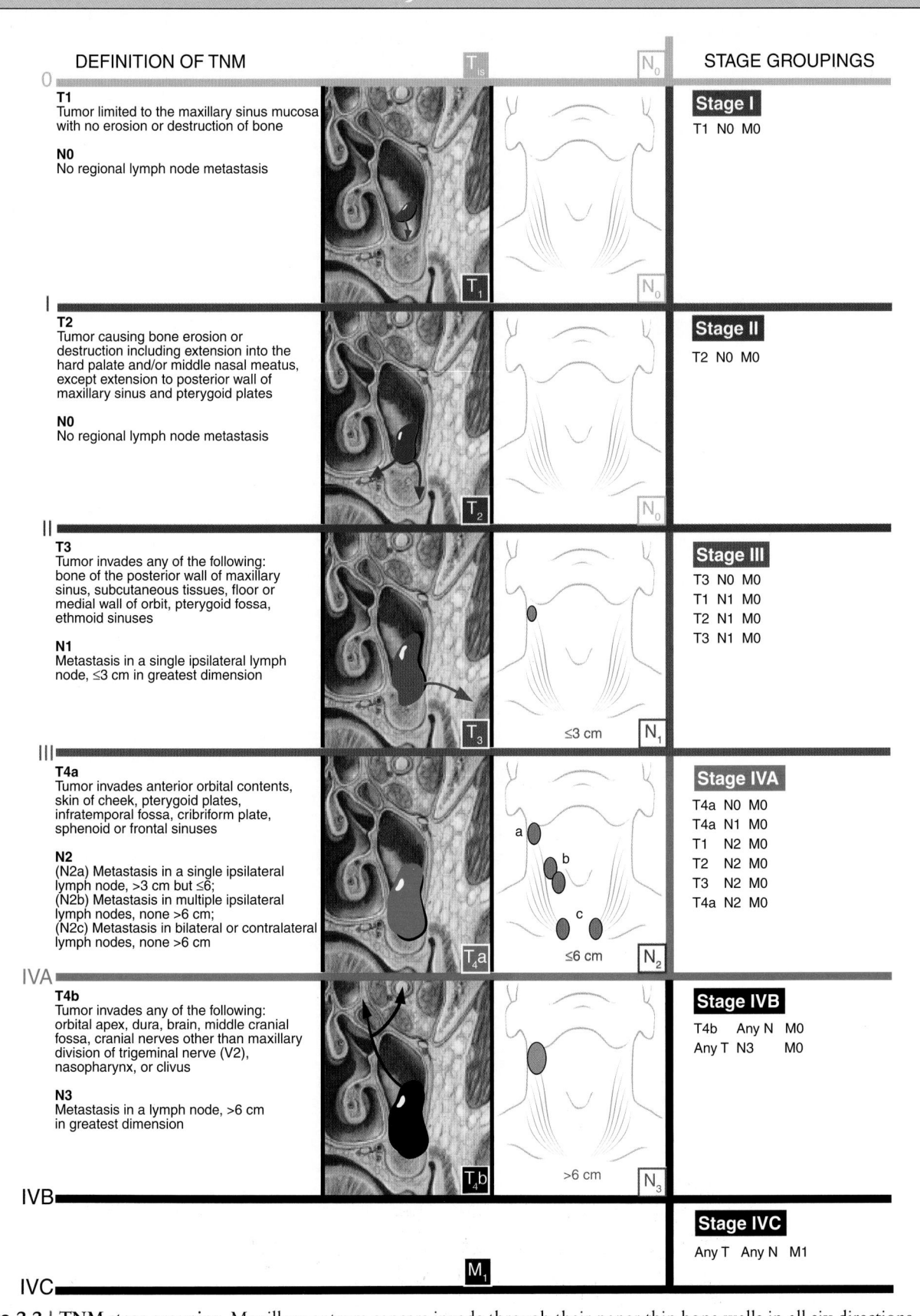

MAXILLARY SINUS ANTRUM

DEFINITION OF TNM

T1
Tumor limited to the maxillary sinus mucosa with no erosion or destruction of bone

N0
No regional lymph node metastasis

T2
Tumor causing bone erosion or destruction including extension into the hard palate and/or middle nasal meatus, except extension to posterior wall of maxillary sinus and pterygoid plates

N0
No regional lymph node metastasis

T3
Tumor invades any of the following: bone of the posterior wall of maxillary sinus, subcutaneous tissues, floor or medial wall of orbit, pterygoid fossa, ethmoid sinuses

N1
Metastasis in a single ipsilateral lymph node, ≤3 cm in greatest dimension

T4a
Tumor invades anterior orbital contents, skin of cheek, pterygoid plates, infratemporal fossa, cribriform plate, sphenoid or frontal sinuses

N2
(N2a) Metastasis in a single ipsilateral lymph node, >3 cm but ≤6;
(N2b) Metastasis in multiple ipsilateral lymph nodes, none >6 cm;
(N2c) Metastasis in bilateral or contralateral lymph nodes, none >6 cm

T4b
Tumor invades any of the following: orbital apex, dura, brain, middle cranial fossa, cranial nerves other than maxillary division of trigeminal nerve (V2), nasopharynx, or clivus

N3
Metastasis in a lymph node, >6 cm in greatest dimension

STAGE GROUPINGS

Stage I
T1 N0 M0

Stage II
T2 N0 M0

Stage III
T3 N0 M0
T1 N1 M0
T2 N1 M0
T3 N1 M0

Stage IVA
T4a N0 M0
T4a N1 M0
T1 N2 M0
T2 N2 M0
T3 N2 M0
T4a N2 M0

Stage IVB
T4b Any N M0
Any T N3 M0

Stage IVC
Any T Any N M1

Figure 3.3 | TNM stage grouping. Maxillary antrum cancers invade through their paper-thin bone walls in all six directions. Vertical presentations of stage groupings, which follow the same color code for cancer stage advancement, are organized in horizontal lanes. Stage 0, yellow; I, green; II, blue; III, purple; IVA, red; IVB and IVC, black. Definitions of TN on left and stage grouping on right.

T-ONCOANATOMY

ORIENTATION OF THREE-PLANAR ONCOANATOMY

For the maxillary antrum the anatomic isocenter is at the level of the clivus. The anterior surface bullet is at the level of or slightly inferior to the bridge of the nose to the right and left of the midline (Fig. 3.4A). Centered inferior to the pupil of the eye (Fig 3.4B), the lateral bullet is at the level of the external auditory canal and inferior to a line connecting the lateral canthus of the eye and the external auditory canal.

T-oncoanatomy

To appreciate the manifestation of cancer of the paranasal sinus, a thorough knowledge of the three-dimensional aspects of paranasal sinus anatomy is essential. The eight major sinuses in the face and skull are in direct continuity. The four paired sinuses are the maxillary, the ethmoid, frontal sinuses, and the sphenoid. Although the sphenoid appears as a single midline sinus, it is also a paired sinus. A three-dimensional reconstruction, focusing on bony anatomy, allows for an understanding of the interrelationships. The anatomy may be divided by drawing three parallel lines across the frontal view of the skull, one line passing above and another below the orbits, the third passing through the floor of the antra or hard palate. The two vertical lines separate the ethmoid and nasal fossa from the maxillary antra. The nasal septum separates the ethmoid and nasal fossa into the right and left sides.

- *Coronal plane* (Fig. 3.5A): In a comparison of anteroposterior and lateral projections or coronal and sagittal sections, three important planes become evident: (i) The floor of the anterior fossa of the skull (in the roof of the nasal cavity and ethmoid); (ii) The hard palate, in the floor of the maxillary antra; and (iii) An imaginary plane below the orbits that divides the paranasal sinuses into a suprastructure and an infrastructure. The suprastructure contains the ethmoids, anterior to which is the apex of the nasal cavity and cribriform (olfactory region). The sphenoid sinus is poste-

rior, the orbits are medial, and the nasal fossa and turbinates are inferior to the suprastructure. The infrastructure contains the maxillary antra and the major portion of the nasal cavity or vestibule. These planes are helpful in relating the external anatomy of physical diagnosis to the radiographic anatomy.

- *Sagittal plane* (Fig. 3.5B): The relationship of the teeth in the superior alveolus determines which teeth are affected as tumor invasion of the floor occurs. First, the second premolar or bicuspid and the first and second molars are in the floor itself and become loosened. The upper canine may become involved when there is more anterior invasion. Rarely, however, are the incisors affected. The third molar can be loosened when there is posterior extension. The ethmoid sinuses are the central paranasal space in the suprastructure with communication to the frontal sphenoid sinuses and the nasal cavity. The ethmoid bone also constitutes the cribriform plate and the superior and medial concha. The important nerves in its walls are (i) the anterior ethmoidal branch of the ophthalmic division of the cranial nerve V (anterior at the junction with the frontal sinus); (ii) the olfactory nerve and bulb in and above the cribriform plate; and (iii) the nasociliary nerve inside the orbit that branches into the posterior and anterior ethmoidal nerves, infratrochlear, and the internal nasal branches.

- *Transverse plane* (Fig. 3.5C): The maxillary antrum is the essential paranasal sinus to study in the infrastructure. It is pyramidal with its apex at the malar arch and base at the nasal cavity. It projects as a triangulated space from virtually every view. The bony walls consist of the maxillary bone in its entirety laterally, anteriorly, and inferiorly. The medial wall is constituted inferiorly by the concha and palatine bone, superiorly and laterally by the zygomatic bone, and posteriorly by the pterygoid plates of the sphenoid. The important nerves to identify in these walls are those in the infraorbital branch of the maxillary division of cranial nerve V through the canal in the perpendicular plate of the palatine posteriorly. The posterior aspect and its relationship to the pterygoid plates and muscle with its access to major vessels and retropharyngeal nodes should be noted.

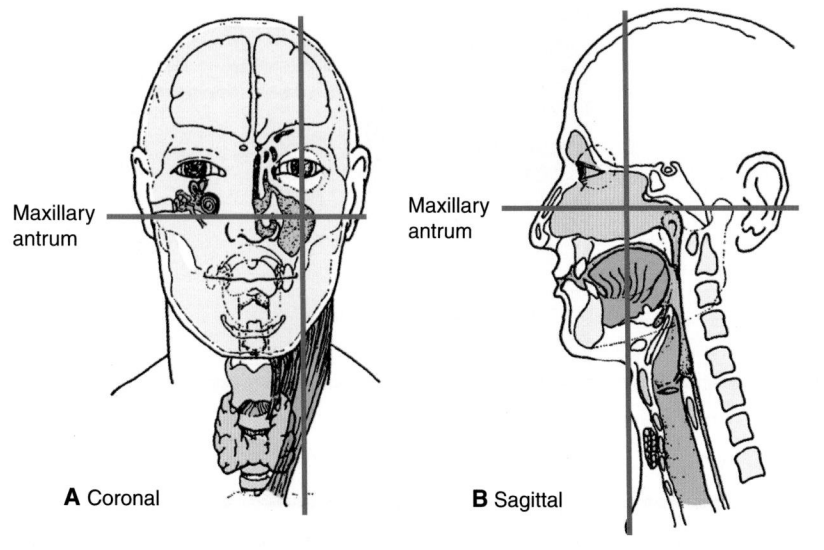

Maxillary antrum

Maxillary antrum

A Coronal   **B** Sagittal

Figure 3.4 | Orientation of three-planar T-oncoanatomy. The anatomic isocenter is at the axial level of the clivus. **A.** Coronal. **B.** Sagittal.

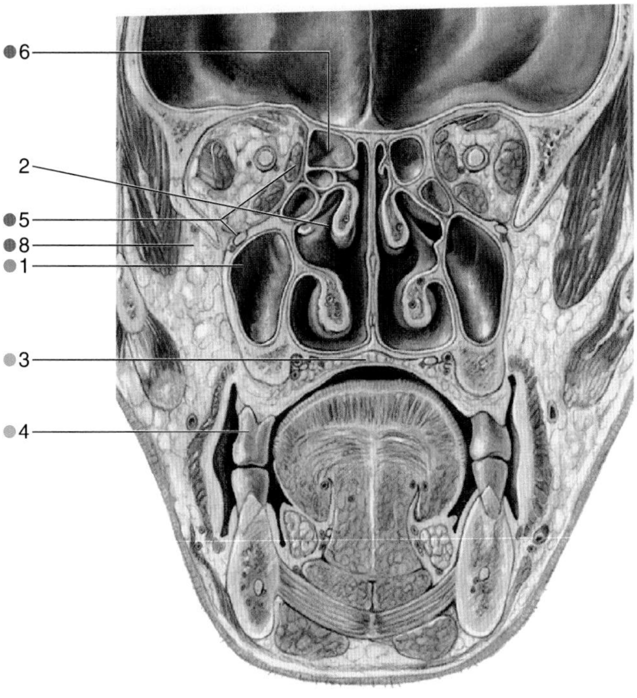

A Coronal

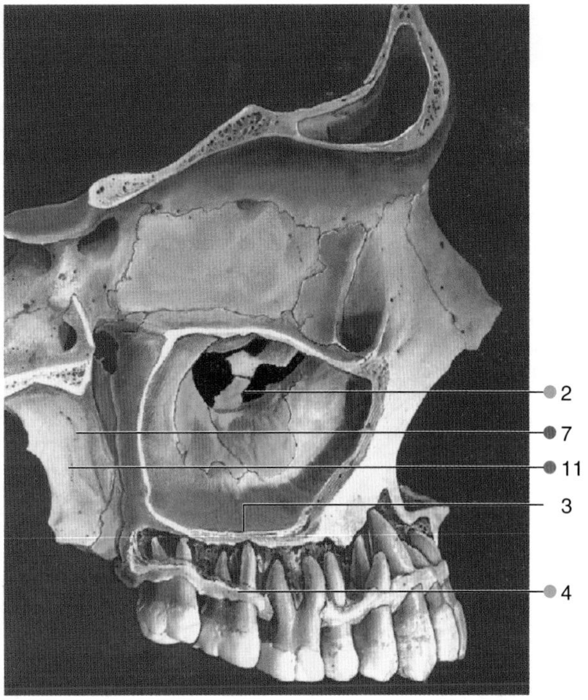

B Sagittal

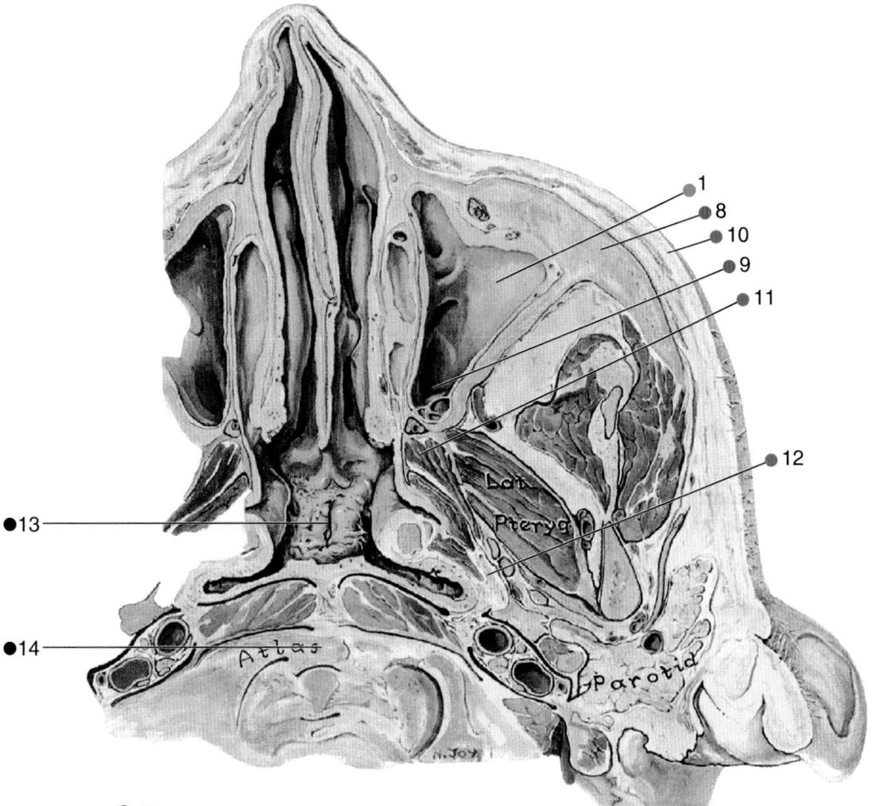

C Transverse

T1 ●	1. Maxillary antrum	T3 ●	5. Floor and medial orbital wall	T4a ●	10. Skin of cheek
T2 ●	2. Middle meatus	T3 ●	6. Ethmoid sinus	T4a ●	11. Lateral Pterygoid Plate
T2 ●	3. Hard Palate	T3 ●	7. Pterygoid fossa	T4a ●	12. Infratemporal fossa
T2 ●	4. Loosen 1st 1 2nd molar teeth	T3 ●	8. Subcutaneous fat (buccal fat pad)	T4b ●	13. Nasopharynx
		T3 ●	9. Posterior wall	T4b ●	14. Atlas, C1

Figure 3.5 | **T-oncoanatomy.** The Color Code for the anatomic sites correlates with the color code for the stage group (Fig. 3.3) and patterns of spread (Fig. 3.2) and SIMLAP table (Table 3.2). Connecting the dots in similar colors will provide an appreciation for the 3D Oncoanatomy.

4

Nasopharynx

PERSPECTIVE, PATTERNS OF SPREAD, AND PATHOLOGY

To understand the malignant gradient of the nasopharynx in terms of the oncoanatomy of the head and face, it is essential to understand both its superior aspect and its relationship to the cavernous sinus in the skull.

PERSPECTIVE AND PATTERNS OF SPREAD

Nasopharyngeal cancer is uncommon in white populations and accounts for only 2% of all head and neck cancers in the United States. The nasopharynx can be a harbinger of malignant disease, particularly common among the Chinese population. This is true for specific provinces and subpopulations; the risk is maintained even after migrating to the United States and applies to second-generation Chinese. Its etiology is being investigated from the point of view of viral induction, immunologic response, environmental pollutants, and ingestion of nitrates in food. The Epstein-Barr virus is commonly identified in elevated antibody titers, but it also has been associated with other malignances and is not truly specific for this site.

Cancer of the nasopharynx has two major spread patterns, depending on whether the primary tumor extends locally or metastasizes to parapharyngeal nodes (Fig. 4.2A). The juxtaposi-

tion of the mucosa to the base of the skull allows for immediate access to the cranial fossa. The foramen lacerum is accessible and is the only foramen medial to the pharyngeal tube and its fascia. Once the base of the skull is invaded, the tumor enters into the cavernous sinus and can involve a number of cranial nerves. There are numerous clinical syndromes, depending on which combination of nerves is involved. Invasion of cranial nerves, inferiorly to superiorly, are cranial nerves III, IV, and VI, which can cause diplopia or ophthalmoplegia because of the resultant partial paralysis of one eye (Fig. 4.2B). Deafness is caused by local obstruction of the eustachian tube leading to tympanic membrane fixation, and not caused by involvement of cranial nerve VIII. The acoustic nerve is well encased in the mastoid bone of the inner ear with its meatus in the posterior fossa. Despite the fact that the eustachian tube is open, cancer rarely invades along this pathway into the middle ear, probably because of the cartilaginous wall of the tube and the absence of a good vascular bed. Proptosis, periorbital edema, and orbital invasion are a result of extensive invasion along the base of the skull and/or thrombosis of the cavernous sinuses. Patterns of Spread are presented as a cancer crab that can invade in six basic directions Superior-Inferior, Medial-Lateral, Anterior-Posterior (SIMLAP) of adjacent anatomic sites (Fig. 4.2 and Table 4.2).

PATHOLOGY

The epithelium of the nasopharynx varies from a stratified squamous in its lower part to a pseudostratified ciliated

TABLE 4.1 Histopathologic Type: Common Cancers of the Nasopharyngeal Carcinoma

WHO Classification	Former Terminology
Type 1	
Squamous cell carcinoma	Squamous cell carcinoma
Type 2	
Nonkeratinizing carcinoma	Transitional cell carcinoma
Without lymphoid stroma	Intermediate cell carcinoma
With lymphoid stroma	Lymphoepithelial carcinoma (Regaud)
Type 3	
Undifferentiated carcinoma	Anaplastic carcinoma
Without lymphoid stroma	Clear cell carcinoma
With lymphoid stroma	Lymphoepithelial carcinoma (Schmincke)

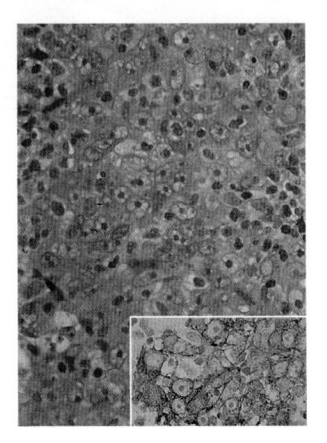

Figure 4.1 | Nasopharyngeal nonkeratinizing carcinoma, undifferentiated type. The cells have large nuclei and prominent eosinophilic nucleoli. The cells are cytokeratin-positive (by immunohistochemistry; *inset*) indicating an epithelial cell proliferation.

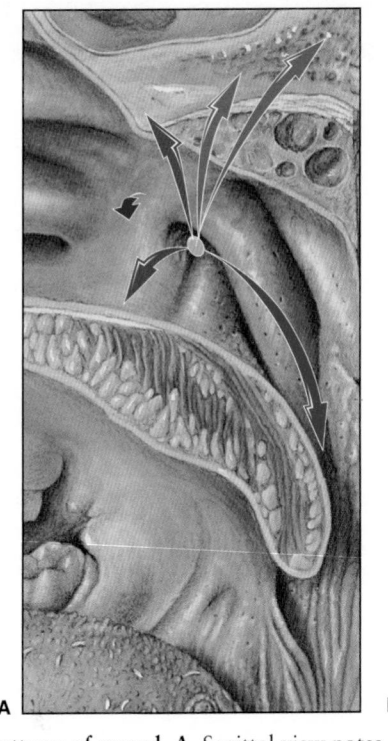
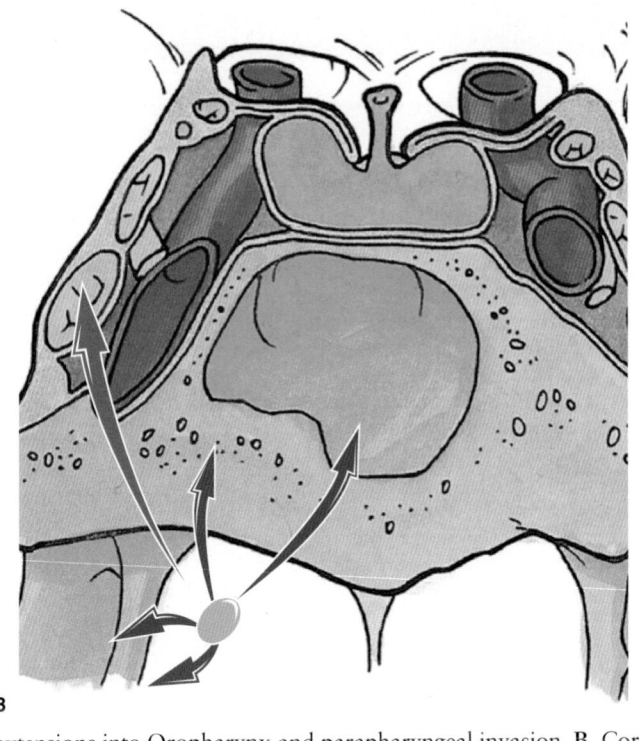

Figure 4.2 | Patterns of spread. A. Sagittal view notes extensions into Oropharynx and parapharyngeal invasion. **B.** Coronal view notes invasion of skull base, cavernous sinus and cranial nerves. The primary cancer (nasopharynx) invades in various directions which are color-coded vectors (*arrows*) representing stage of progression: Tis, yellow; T1, green; T2, blue; T3, purple; T4, red; and T4, black. The concept of visualizing patterns of spread to appreciate the surrounding anatomy is well demonstrated by the six directional pattern i.e. SIMLAP Table 4.2.

columnar epithelium along its walls and roof. Because of Waldeyer's lymphatic ring, many different tumors can arise in this site—lymphoepitheliomas and lymphosarcomas in addition to carcinomas (Table 4.1). The most common, however, are carcinomas, which are locally invasive and destructive to the bony structures of the skull (Fig. 4.1). Lymphoepitheliomas tend to spread bilaterally to nodes in the neck and may present in this fashion. Lymphosarcomas are bulky lesions that tend to interfere with breathing but tend to be less destructive.

TABLE 4.2	**SIMLAP***	
Nasopharynx (Fossa Rosenmüller)		
S	Intracranial, cranial nerves	• T4
	Sphenoid sinus	• T3
	Cavernous sinus	• T4
	Pituitary gland	• T4
I	Oropharynx	• T2a
	Hypopharynx	• T4
M	Eustachian tube	• **T1**
L	Parapharyngeal wall	• T2b
	Infratemporal fossa	• T4
	Masticator space	
A	Nasal cavity	• T2a
	Maxillary sinus, ethmoid sinus	• T3
	Orbit	• T4
P	Clivus	• T3
	Foramen lacerum, F. ovale, F. rotundum	• T3

*There are six basic directions or vectors (arrows): The six vectors of invasion are <u>S</u>uperior, <u>I</u>nferior, <u>M</u>edial, <u>L</u>ateral, <u>A</u>nterior, and <u>P</u>osterior. The color-coded dots correlate the T stage with specific anatomic structure involved.

TMN STAGING CRITERIA

TNM STAGING CRITERIA

The classification and staging of nasopharyngeal cancers, both for primary (T) and nodes (N) criteria, are unique to this site and do not follow the majority of head and neck cancer sites. The major variable has been assessment of the suprastructure involvement of the base of the skull and contents of cavernous sinus, cranial nerves III, IV, and VI. Essentially, the T progression is into subsites of the nasopharyngeal region; however, T4 has been, since the first edition of American Joint Committee on Cancer/International Union Against Cancer (AJCC/UICC), an invasion of suprastructure bone and cranial nerves. Nodal progression was similar to other head and neck sites until the fifth and sixth editions of AJCC/UICC.

Nasopharyngeal cancer is different from other cancers of the head and neck, but has remained relatively unchanged since its introduction in the third edition of the AJCC/UICC classifications (1988). The vectors of invasion vary with the biologic behavior of these different malignancies.

SUMMARY OF CHANGES SEVENTH EDITION AJCC

The TNM stages according to the 7th Edition of AJCC are illustrated in color code of advancement (Fig. 4.3). For Nasopharynx, T2a lesions will now be designated T1. Stage IIA will therefore be Stage I. Lesions previously staged T2b will be T2 and therefore Stage IIB will now be designated Stage II. Retropharyngeal lymph node(s), regardless of unilateral or bilateral location, is considered N1. T2a lesions are T1 confined to nasopharynx with extension to oropharynx or nasal cavity. T2b lesions are T2 parapharyngeal extension. The TNM Staging Matrix is color coded for identification of Stage Group once T and N stages are determined (Table 4.3).

| TABLE 4.3 | Stage Summary Matrix |

	N0	N1	N2	N3	M1
T1	I	II	III	IVB	IVC
T2	II	II	III	IVB	IVC
T2	IIB	IIB	III	IVB	IVC
T3	III	III	III	IVB	IVC
T4	IVA	IVA	IVA	IVB	IVC

Unlike the majority of head and neck cancer sites, nasopharynx stage groups in Rule III where in both T and N progression determine stage group.

- *T Stage* progression determines Stage Group
- *N Stage* progression also determines Stage Group

NASOPHARYNX

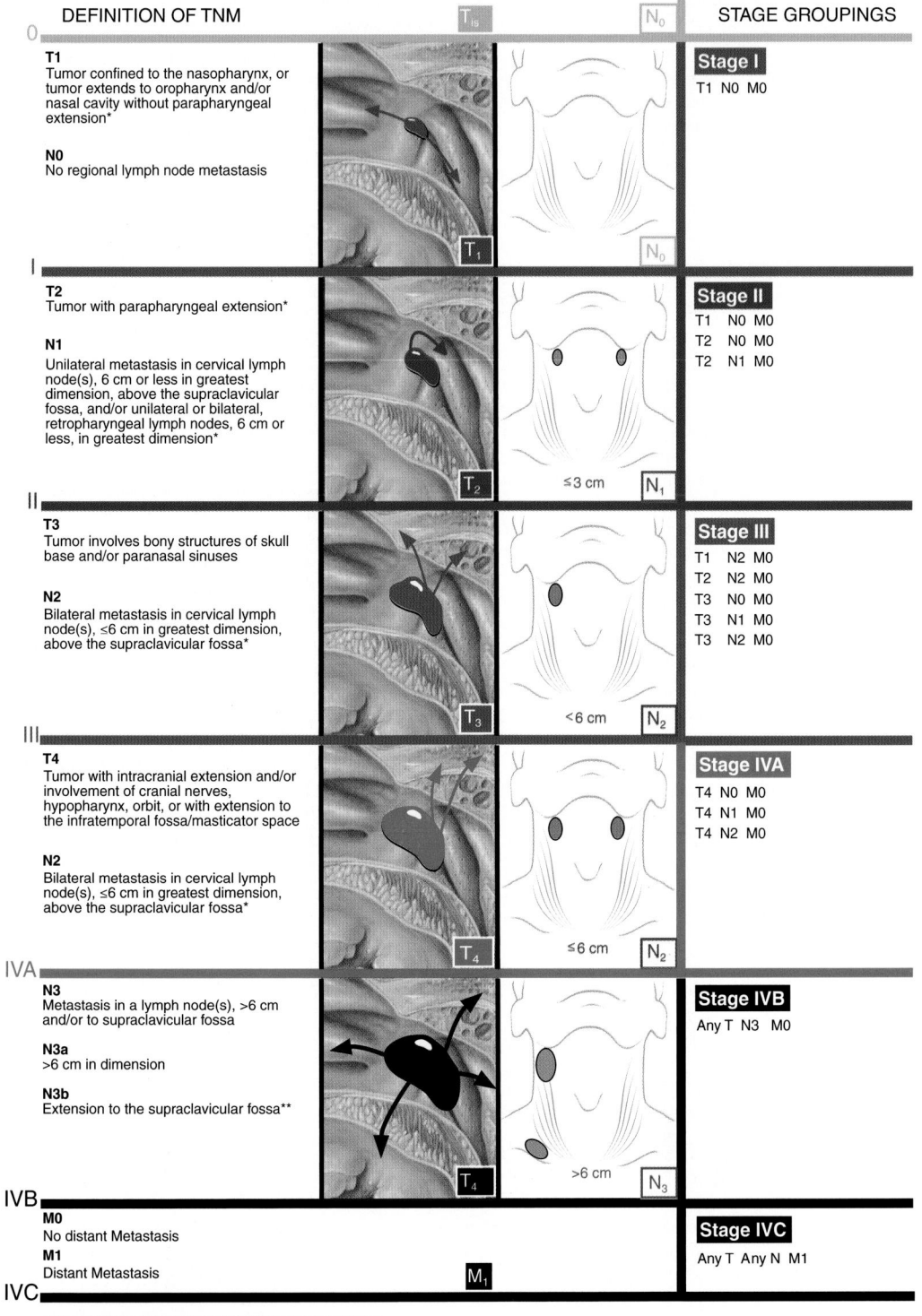

DEFINITION OF TNM

T1
Tumor confined to the nasopharynx, or tumor extends to oropharynx and/or nasal cavity without parapharyngeal extension*

N0
No regional lymph node metastasis

T2
Tumor with parapharyngeal extension*

N1
Unilateral metastasis in cervical lymph node(s), 6 cm or less in greatest dimension, above the supraclavicular fossa, and/or unilateral or bilateral, retropharyngeal lymph nodes, 6 cm or less, in greatest dimension*

T3
Tumor involves bony structures of skull base and/or paranasal sinuses

N2
Bilateral metastasis in cervical lymph node(s), ≤6 cm in greatest dimension, above the supraclavicular fossa*

T4
Tumor with intracranial extension and/or involvement of cranial nerves, hypopharynx, orbit, or with extension to the infratemporal fossa/masticator space

N2
Bilateral metastasis in cervical lymph node(s), ≤6 cm in greatest dimension, above the supraclavicular fossa*

N3
Metastasis in a lymph node(s), >6 cm and/or to supraclavicular fossa

N3a
>6 cm in dimension

N3b
Extension to the supraclavicular fossa**

M0
No distant Metastasis
M1
Distant Metastasis

STAGE GROUPINGS

Stage I
T1　N0　M0

Stage II
T1　N0　M0
T2　N0　M0
T2　N1　M0

Stage III
T1　N2　M0
T2　N2　M0
T3　N0　M0
T3　N1　M0
T3　N2　M0

Stage IVA
T4　N0　M0
T4　N1　M0
T4　N2　M0

Stage IVB
Any T　N3　M0

Stage IVC
Any T　Any N　M1

*Note: Midline nodes are considered ipsilateral nodes.

**Note: Supraclavicular zone or fossa is relevant to the staging of nasopharyngeal carcinoma and is the triangular region originally described by Ho. It is defined by three points:
(1) the superior margin of the sternal end of the clavicle,
(2) the superior margin of the lateral end of the clavicle,
(3) the point where the neck meets the shoulder (Figure 4.2).
Note that this would include caudal portions of levels IV and VB. All cases with lymph nodes (whole or part) in the fossa are considered N3b.

Figure 4.3 | TNM stage grouping. Nasopharyngeal cancers are not resectable and staging categories differ from other head and neck sites as to T/N definitions. Vertical presentations of stage groupings, which follow the same color code for cancer stage advancement, are organized in horizontal lanes: Stage 0, yellow; I, green; II, blue; III, purple; IVA, red; and IVB, black. Definitions of TN on left and stage grouping on right.

T-ONCOANATOMY

ORIENTATION OF THREE-PLANAR ONCOANATOMY

For the nasopharynx, the anatomic isocenter is at the level of C1, the atlas. The anterior surface bullet enters through the tip of the nose (Fig. 4.4A) and the lateral bullet is at the temporal mandibular joint, just below the level of the external auditory canal (Fig. 4.4B).

T-oncoanatomy

The nasopharynx is a small, box-like space in the center of the head, posterior to the nasal cavity and superior to the pharyngeal tube. The anterior limit of the nasopharynx is the chona, through which it is continuous with the nasal cavity. Its roof is attached to the base of the skull, and slopes downward to become continuous with the posterior pharyngeal wall. The lateral wall is composed of the torus tubarius, the eustachian tube orifice, and that posterior portion of the mucosa, the fossa of Rosenmüller, extending up to its apex and junction with the roof. The inferior limit of the nasopharynx is level with the plane of the hard palate.

To understand the importance of the nasopharynx in terms of the anatomy of the head and face, it is essential to understand both its superior aspect and its relationship to the skull and lateral walls. The pharyngeal fascia is attached to the base of the skull. This can be diagrammed in relationship to those foramina, which may be invaded and destroyed by carcinomas. The superior attachment of the pharyngobasilar fascia starts from the midline pharyngeal tubercle on the basiocciput, extending across the petrous portion of the temporal bone to a point in front of the carotid canal. From there, it passes posteromedially to the petrotympanic fissure in the region where the eustachian tube attaches and the levator palati originates, and then attaches to the medial pterygoid lamina. The fascia inferiorly is continuous over the superior pharyngeal constrictor muscle.

- *Coronal section* (Fig. 4.5A) provides a view from the retropharyngeal space. The roof of the nasopharynx is occupied by the sphenoid sinus, alongside of which are the cavernous sinuses. Within its contents are three cranial nerves responsible for extraocular motion (III, IV, and VI), laterally lies the Gasserian (trigeminal) ganglion (cranial nerve V) and its major branches as they exit through different foramina along the base of the skull into the parapharyngeal space, paranasal sinuses, and orbit.

- *Sagittal plane* (Fig. 4.5B) shows the lateral walls of the nasopharynx, which consist of the eustachian tube and its two related muscles, the tensor veli palatini and the levator veli palati, the latter of which is more important functionally for tubal patency. The muscles are continuous with the palatopharyngeus muscles and superior constrictor, forming the pharyngeal muscular tube.

- *Transverse plane* (Fig. 4.5C) shows the parapharyngeal space divided into three compartments by the styloid process, its muscles, and the related fascial expansions from the carotid sheath and prevertebral fascia. A neoplastic process may extend into and follow these preformed spaces but, unlike an inflammatory process, also may extend through these barriers and invade nerves.

The *retropharyngeal compartment* houses Rouviere's node, which is a major focus of metastatic spread. As these parapharyngeal nodes enlarge, they compress the neurovascular bundle in the carotid sheath. The retrostyloid compartment contains the internal carotid artery, the last four cranial nerves, and cervical sympathetics. The prestyloid is formed by the tensor palatini muscle and the pterygoid muscles. It contains the maxillary artery and important nerves. Once this latter space is invaded, access is gained laterally into the deep portion of the parotid gland and inferiorly to the submaxillary gland.

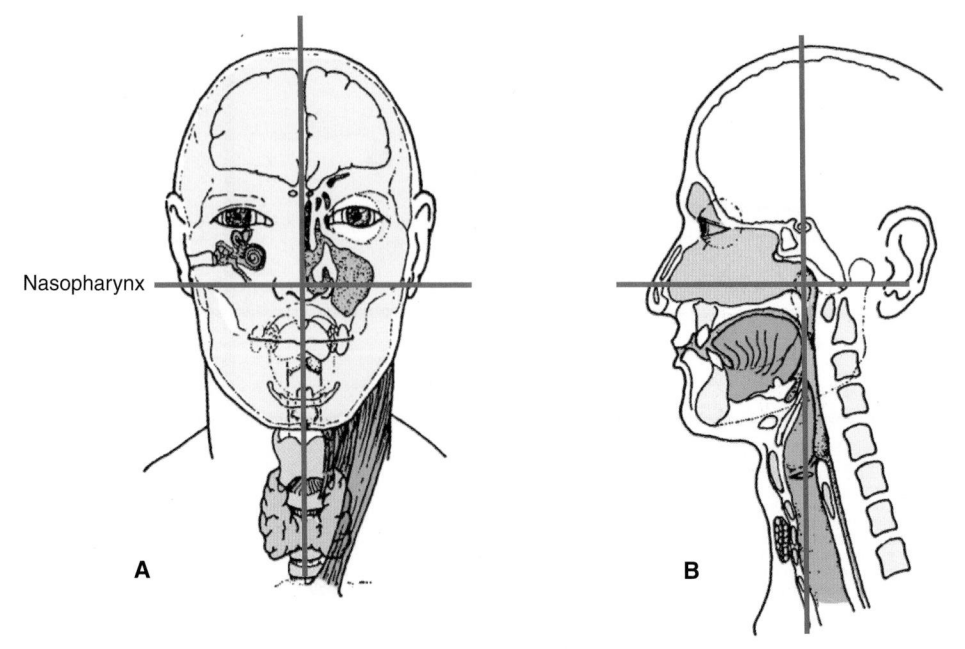

Nasopharynx

A   B

Figure 4.4 | Orientation of three-planar T-oncoanatomy. The anatomic isocenter is at the axial level at clivus/C1. **A.** Coronal. **B.** Sagittal.

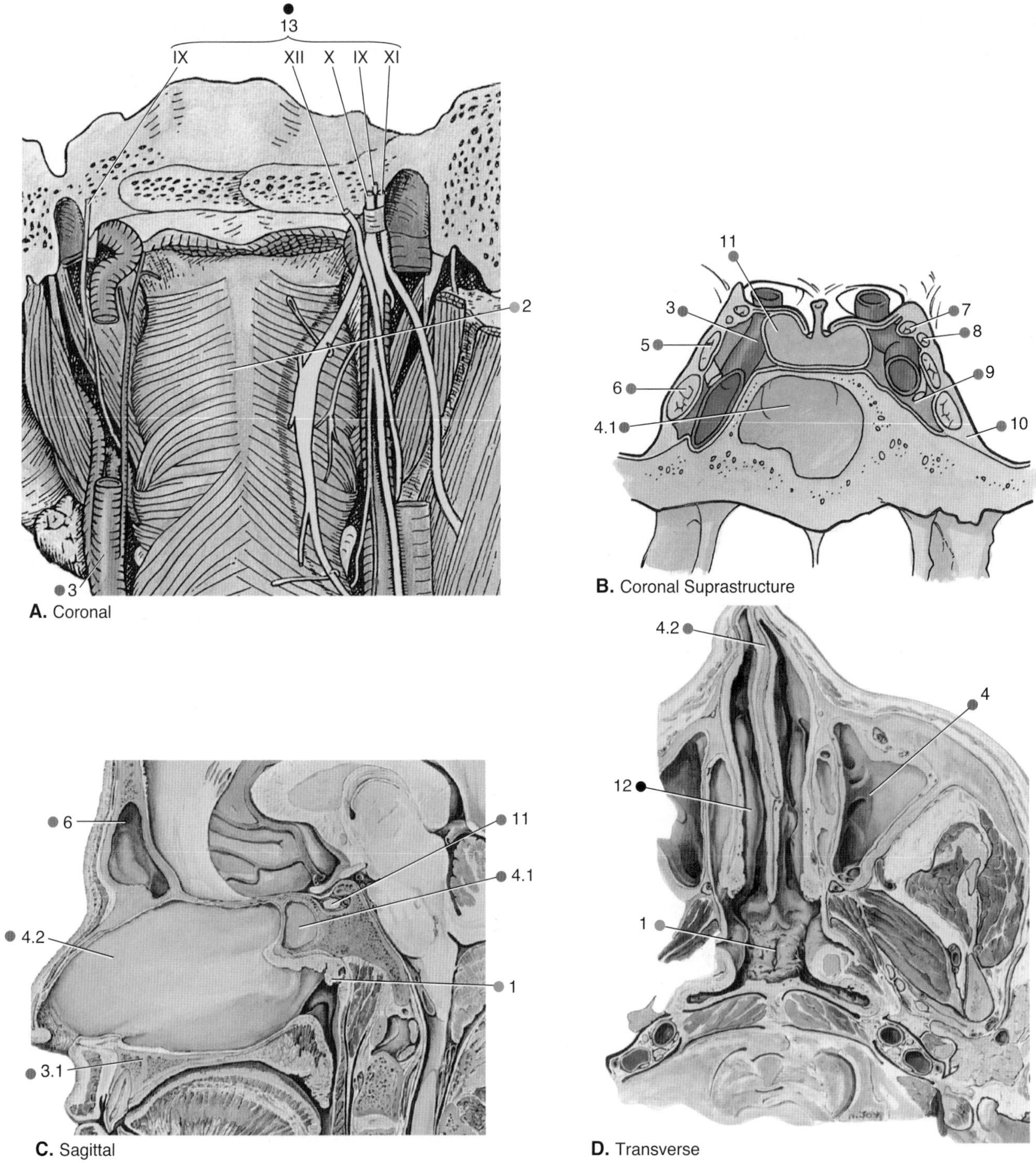

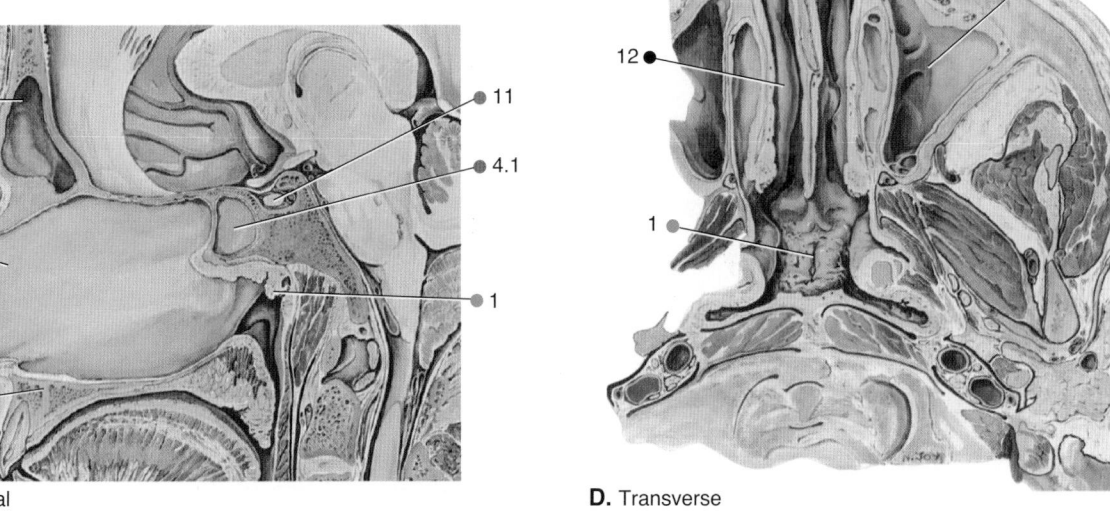

13
IX
XII X IX XI
2
3
A. Coronal
11
3
7
8
5
9
6
4.1
10
B. Coronal Suprastructure
4.2
4
12
1
6
11
4.1
4.2
1
3.1
C. Sagittal
D. Transverse

T1 • 1. Nasopharyngeal tonsil
T2 • 2. Muscle wall superior constrictor
T3 • 3. Internal carotid artery
T3 • 3.1. Hard palate
T3 • 4. Sphenoid sinus
T3 • 4.1′. Maxillary sinus
T3 • 4.2″. Nasal septum
T4a • 5. Ophthalmic nerve
T4a • 6. Maxillary nerve
T4a • 7. Oculomotor nerve
T4a • 8. Trochlear nerve
T4a • 9. Abducent nerve
T4a • 10. Dura
T4a • 11. Hypophysis
N1,2,3 • 12. Middle conclia
N1,2,3 • 13. Cranial nerves IX,X,XI,XII

Figure 4.5 | **T-oncoanatomy.** The Color Code for the anatomic sites correlates with the color code for the stage group (Fig. 4.3) and patterns of spread (Fig. 4.2) and SIMLAP table (Table 4.2). Connecting the dots in similar colors will provide an appreciation for the 3D Oncoanatomy.

N-ONCOANATOMY AND M-ONCOANATOMY

N-ONCOANATOMY

With nodal dissemination, the high parapharyngeal nodes along the carotid sheath are involved and extend into the retrostyloid compartment (Fig. 4.6). This leads to entrapment of the cranial nerves emerging alongside the jugular foramen. The nodes in this region are named after Rouviere—famous for his treatise on lymphoid anatomy. Again, numerous neurologic syndromes can occur. The retroparotidian syndrome, or the jugular foramen syndrome, is characterized by loss of the gag reflex (cranial nerve IX), vocal cord paralysis (cranial nerve X), atrophy of the trapezius muscle (cranial nerve XI),

and deviation of the uvula (cranial nerve X) and tongue on protrusion (cranial nerve XII).

In addition to retropharyngeal and parapharyngeal nodes, the main routes of lymphatic spread of the nasopharynx are into the first station nodes, that is, the jugulodigastric, jugulo-omohyoid, upper deep cervical, lower deep cervical, and submaxillary and submental lymph nodes. Bilateral node spread is common (Table 4.4). Mediastinal lymph node metastases are considered distant metastases. Distant spread to the lungs is common in this type of cancer. Incidence and distribution of neck node metastases in a clinically negative (N0) neck are presented in Figure 4.7A.

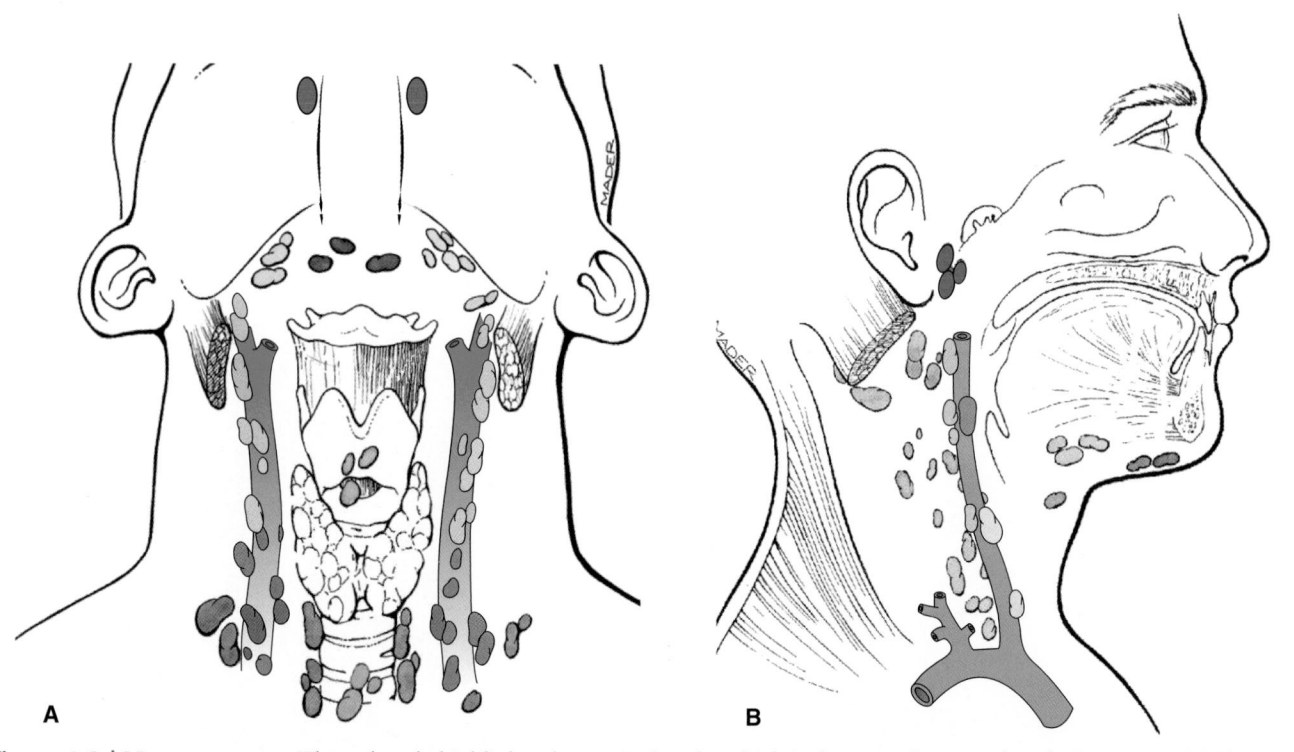

Figure 4.6 | N-oncoanatomy. The red node highlights the sentinel node, which is the retropharyngeal node (Rouviere's Node). **A.** Anterior view. **B.** Lateral view. **M-oncoanatomy** is determined by the jugular vein, which joins with the subclavian vein to form the superior vena cava on the right, and the innominate vein, which drains into the right side of the heart and then into lung.

TABLE 4.4	Sentinel and Regional Nodes: Nasopharynx (Bilateral)		
		Level/Location of Node(s)	
S Sentinel Node		**Axial Level**	**AJCC Level**
S1 Retropharyngeal Rouviere's node		C1	nI
R Regional Nodes			
R1 Mastoid (postcervical)		C3	I
R2 Jugulodigastric, superior deep cervical		C3/4	II
R3 Mid deep cervical		C4	III
R4 Jugulo-omohyoid, inferior deep cervical		C7	IV
R5 Jugulo-omohyoid		C3-T1, T2	
Inferior/mid/superior deep cervical			

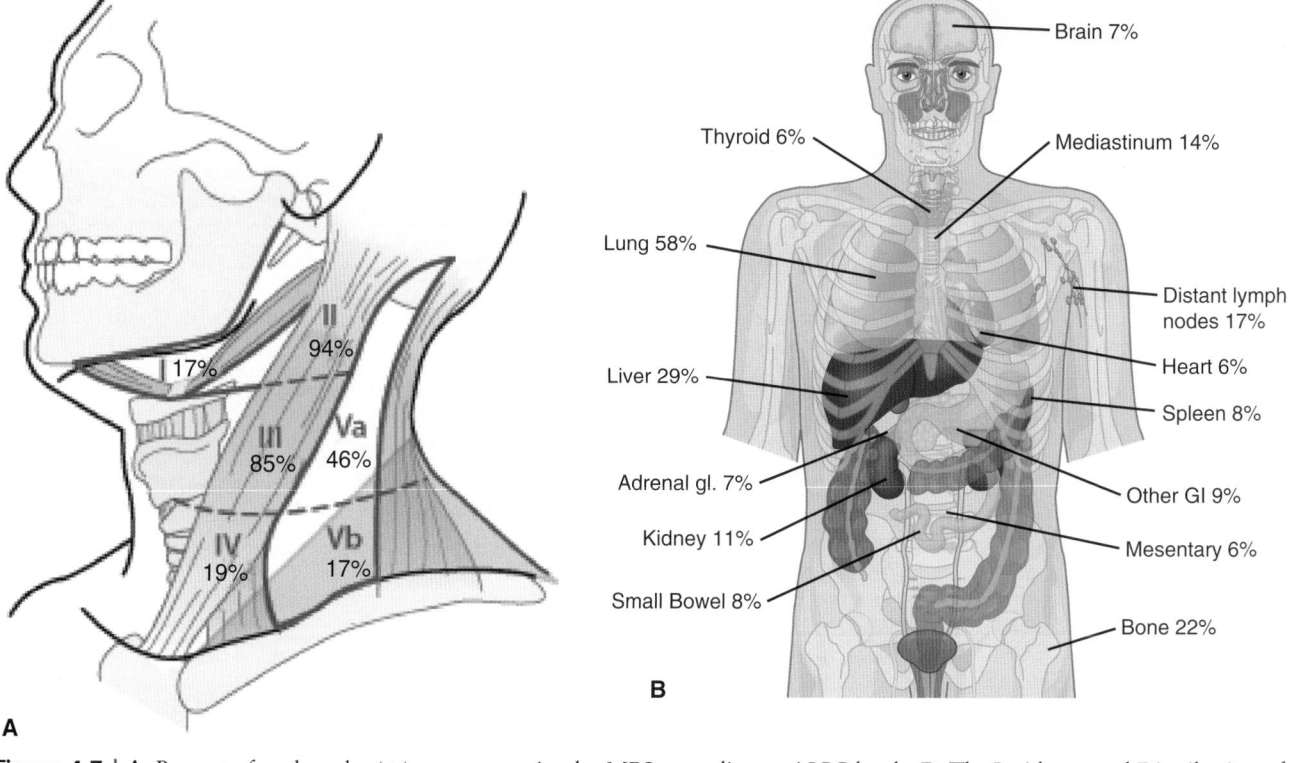

Figure 4.7 | **A.** Percent of neck nodes (+) on presentation by MRI according to AJCC levels. **B.** The Incidence and Distribution of Distant Metastases. The Oropharyngeal Cancers can serve as a prototype for head and neck cancers. Lung (58%) is the target organ with liver metastases next (29%) and bone metastases third (22%) followed by distant lymph nodes (17%), mediastinum (14%). The remainder of sites are 11% (kidney) or less than 10%.

M-ONCOANATOMY

The cavernous sinus and lateral pterygoid buccal venous plexus drains into the jugular vein, brachiocephalic vein, and then into the subclavian vein and right superior vena cava. Hematogenous spread, although uncommon, can include lung and bone as favored sites of involvement. Skeletal and other distant metastases occur infrequently (see Fig. 4.7B; Table 4.5).

CRANIAL NERVES AND NEUROVASCULAR BUNDLE

Nasopharynx cancers first invade parapharyngeal space and then invade through the foramen, lacerum, and then enter the

cavernous sinus and pack off CN VI, IV, and III in that order causing diplopia. As it extends laterally, the Gasserian ganglion is encountered and as each branch of cranial nerve veins become involved, each produces a specific neurologic defect: V_1 eyelid anesthesia, V_2 upper lip and nasal anesthesia, and V_3 lower face anesthesia. Retropharyngeal (Rouviere's) Node compresses the neurovascular bundle of CN IX, X, XI, XII exiting the skull along side the carotid artery and jugular vein (Table 4.5).

The importance of appreciating the complex anatomy of cranial nerves lies in the patterns of cancer spread at the primary cancer site as well as nodal spread patterns. Perineural invasion or compression by metastatic lymph nodes often is manifested by specific neurologic symptoms and signs. The overview of cranial nerves provides an intricate roadmap as to points of vulnerability.

Cranial nerve invasion can produce specific syndromes and neurologic evaluation is a vital part of physical diagnosis in all head and neck cancers.

A tabulation of potential neurologic syndromes either due to perineural invasion at the primary site or nodal compression will alert the astute clinician to extent of cancer advancement anatomically.

TABLE 4.5	Potential Neurologic Syndromes Due to Invasion of Cranial Nerves I–XII	
Nasopharynx	T Site VI, IV, III ($V_{1,2,3}$)	N Site IX, X, XI, XII

STAGING WORKUP

TABLE 4.6	Imaging Modalities and Strategies for Diagnosis and Staging for Head and Neck Nasopharynx	
Modality	Strategy	Recommended
Primary Tumor and Nodes		
Computed tomography	Excellent for defining extent of primary depth of invasion enlargement of involved nodes. (Preferred for bone invasion.)	Yes—3–5 mm cuts, 3 mm for primary sites, 5 mm for neck.
Magnetic resonance imaging	Offers best 3D and 3-planar views of primary and nodes, especially soft tissue extensions. Gadolinium contrast for extensions and perineuronal spread.	Yes—≤4 cm slices Gd for intracranial and perineuronal spread.
Positron emission tomography	Functional and metabolic imaging of ^{18}FDG is based on 2-deoxy modification, which inhibits the molecule from subsequent enzymatic conversion and is "metabolically trapped" in tumor cells.	Yes—potential exists for distinguishing from tissue necrosis.
Metastases		
Chest film	Search for metastases.	Yes.
Radionuclide scan	^{99m}Tc for bone metastases.	No/Yes—if symptomatic.

3D, three-dimensional; FDG, fluorodeoxyglucose.

RULES OF CLASSIFICATION AND STAGING

Clinical Staging and Imaging

For nasopharyngeal cancers, careful history taking and inspection and palpations of the face and neck are essential. Testing all cranial nerves is critical. Both direct and indirect endoscopy are useful. Despite patient cooperation, pharyngeal cancers are inaccessible and imaging is important. To determine the true extent of primary nasopharyngeal cancers, imaging is essential. Magnetic resonance imaging (MRI) is superior to computed tomography (CT) in demonstrating soft tissue extension, skull base bone changes, and perineural invasion (see Table 4.6 and Figure 4.8).

Pathologic Staging

Histopathologic verification of primary and nodes is performed by needle aspiration or biopsy. Nasopharyngeal cancers are not resectable.

Oncoimaging Annotations

- Most nasopharyngeal tumors arise in the fossa of Rosenmüller and tend to spread deeply, often obstructing the eustachian tube.

- The vast majority (75%) of nasopharyngeal cancer patients have cervical node metastases at presentation. Bilateral involvement occurs in up to 80%.

- MRI is superior to CT in demonstrating the soft tissue extent of the tumor and skull base changes. CT often underestimates the frequency and extent of skull base involvement.

- After successful radiation therapy, there is usually complete tumor resolution on images within 3 months. A baseline, posttreatment scan should be obtained at approximately 6 months. Differentiating tumor recurrence from fibrosis can be a formidable task.

- Positron emission tomography (PET) with fluorine-18–labeled deoxy-D-glucose (FDG) enhancement may be useful in evaluating tumor recurrence. Both PET and thallium 201 single-photon emission computed tomography (SPECT) may be used to differentiate tumor from radiation-induced necrosis.

- CT and MRI can identify Rouviere's node opposite C1 transverse process.

PROGNOSIS AND CANCER SURVIVAL

PROGNOSTIC FACTORS

The seventh edition of the AJCC Cancer Staging Manual lists the following prognostic factors for nasal ethmoid sinus cancers:

- Size of lymph nodes
- Extracapsular extension from lymph nodes for head and neck
- Head and neck lymph nodes levels I-III
- Head and neck lymph nodes levels IV-V
- Head and neck lymph nodes levels VI-VII
- Other lymph node group
- Clinical location of cervical nodes
- Extracapsular spread (ECS) clinical
- Extracapsular spread (ECS) pathologic
- Human papillomavirus (HPV) status
- Tumor thickness*

*The foregoing passage is from Edge SB, Byrd DR, and Compton CC, et al, *AJCC Cancer Staging Manual, 7th edition*. New York, Springer, 2010, p. 99.

CANCER STATISTICS AND SURVIVAL

Generally, cancers of the oral cavity and pharynx, the upper digestive passage, account for 36,540 new cases per year. In addition, cancer of the larynx affects another 12,720 patients and thyroid cancers, 44,670. Approximately 25% of head and neck cancer patients die annually, often due to other causes. Long-term survival in thyroid cancer is the exception, with only 1,500 deaths (5%). The improvement in oral cavity and pharyngeal tumors from 1950 to 2000 was modest at 14% and matches larynx at 15%. A multidisciplinary approach is vital.

Specifically, nasopharyngeal cancers are difficult to detect and metastasize to bilateral neck nodes with generally poor overall survival for all stages. When encountered in early stages in high-risk Chinese populations, 5-year survival is at the 90% level. Combined chemoradiation regimens (Cis-platinum and 5-fluoracil with radiation) have dramatically improved response rates and survival. Recent AJCC survival data indicated improved survival rates for all stages as compared to other head and neck sites (Fig. 4.9).

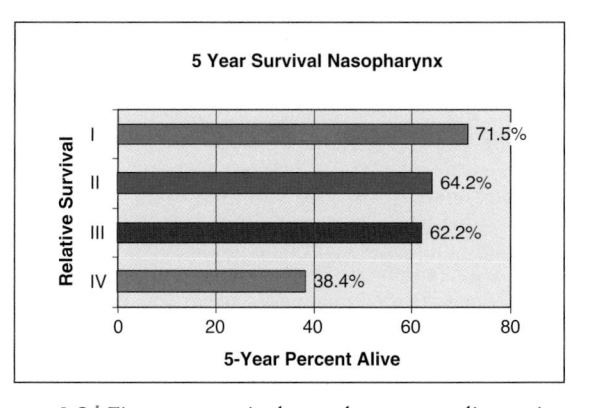

Figure 4.9 | Five-year survival rates by stage at diagnosis. (Data from Edge SB, Byrd DR, and Compton CC, et al., *AJCC Cancer Staging Manual, 7th edition*. New York, Springer, 2010.)

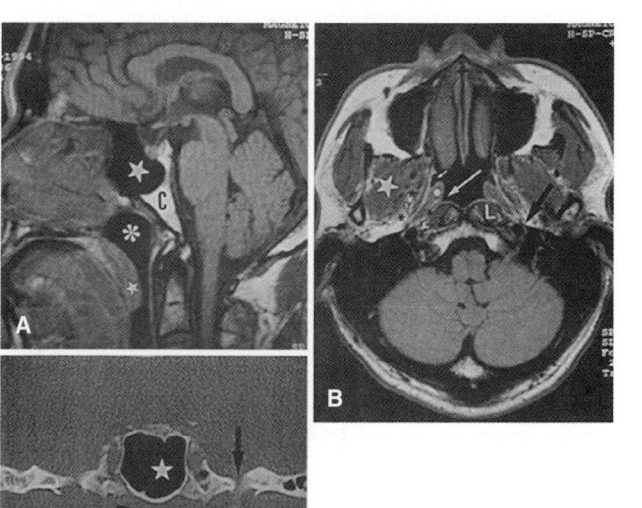

Figure 4.8 | MRI of nasal cavity and nasopharynx—Transverse (axial) inferior view. Normal anatomy of the nasopharynx. **A:** Sagittal contrast-enhanced magnetic resonance (*MR*) image shows the nasopharynx (*asterick*), sphenoid sinus (*large star*), clivus (*C*), and soft palate (*small star*). **B:** Axial T1-weighted MR image shows the right Eustachian tube opening (*small arrow*), torus tubarius (small arrow), torus tubaris (*small white asterisk*), fossa of Rosenmuller (*large white arrow*), parapharyngeal space (*black asterick*), masticator space (*star*), left carotid space (*black arrow*), and left longus colli muscle (L). **C:** Coronal CT shows the sphenoid sinus (*star*), left torus tubarius (*asterick*), fossa of Rosenmüller (*thick white arrow*), eustachian tube opening (*thin white arrow*), and foramen ovale (*black arrow*). The CT/MRI transverse section can be correlated with the anatomy in Fig. 4.5C. (Bragg DG, Rubin P, Hricak H. *Oncologic Imaging, 2nd edition*. Philadelphia, W.B. Saunders, 2002.)

Oral Cavity

PERSPECTIVE, PATTERNS OF SPREAD, AND PATHOLOGY

In the oral cavity, the location of the cancer is a powerful prognosticator of its malignant gradient; a shift of a few centimeters alters the prognosis of the cancer significantly.

PERSPECTIVE AND PATTERNS OF SPREAD

Each specific cancer subsite in the oral cavity has the potential to give rise to different manifestations. Each requires individualized management, dictated by local anatomy and patterns of spread (Fig. 5.2). Thus, lip cancers appear as superficial ulcerations that grow slowly. They rarely enter lymphatic channels or have metastases to lymph nodes, unless there is a deep invasion of the orbicularis oris muscle. By contrast, cancers of the tongue tend to arise along the lateral borders due to irritation of broken teeth and the microtrauma of swallowing foods, alcohol, and smoking tobacco. The underlying musculature is readily invaded and, because of its rich lymphatic network, leads to rapid infiltration and lymph node involvement.

Oral cavity cancers are the most common upper aerodigestive cancers and are predominantly male oriented (88%); lip followed by tongue is the most common site. The malignant gradient in the oral cavity increases from anterior to posterior and from lateral to medial loci. Cancers arising in the posterior portion of the floor of the mouth tend to carry a poor prognosis because the mylohyoid muscle is shorter in its anterior–posterior diameter and is deficient in its posterior part, no longer providing a muscular floor to the oral cavity. Invasion at this particular junction allows the tumor to extend directly into a gap and enter into direct contact with the submandibular salivary gland and tissues of the neck. This leads to the retromylohyoid space and permits the easy propagation of both an infectious and/or neoplastic process directly from the mouth to the neck. The buccal mucosa gives rise to superficial lesions, much as the lip; they tend to be ulcerating, and also arise from irritation due to broken teeth. Deep invasion into the buccinator muscle can lead to swelling of the cheek and access to the deep pterygoid plexus of veins. Unrecognized advancement can become rapidly debilitating, interfering with speech and swallowing and producing a malodorous halitosis. Patterns of Spread are presented as a cancer crab that can invade in six basic directions Superior-Inferior, Medial-Lateral, Anterior-Posterior (SIMLAP) of adjacent anatomic sites (Fig. 5.2; Table 5.2).

PATHOLOGY

There are a large variety of carcinomas (Table 5.1), but the most common are squamous cell cancers (Fig 5.1); adenocarcinomas are less common.

TABLE 5.1	Histopathologic Type: Common Cancers of the Oral Cavity	
Squamous Cell Carcinoma Microscopic Variants	**Adenocarcinoma Major or Minor Salivary Gland**
Keratinizing; well differentiated; moderately well differentiated; poorly differentiated	Low-grade adenocarcinoma Adenoid cystic carcinoma
Nonkeratinizing; anaplastic squamous carcinoma	Mucoepidermoid (low or high grade)
Lymphoepithelioma	With lymphoid stroma
Transitional cell carcinoma	Carcinoma expleomorphic adenoma
Spindle cell squamous carcinoma	Poorly differentiated adenocarcinoma

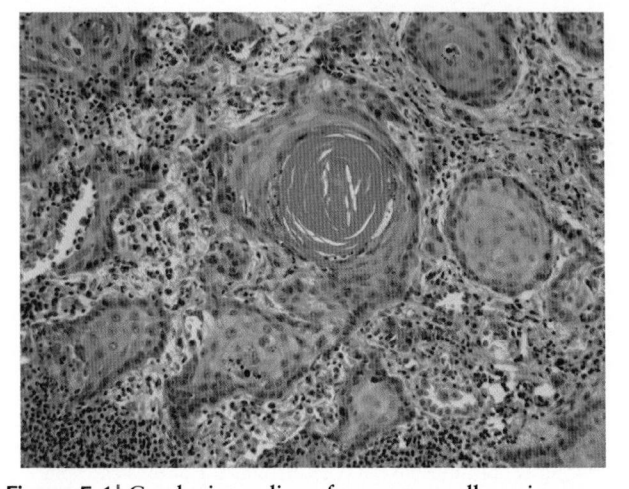

Figure 5.1| Cytologic grading of squamous cell carcinoma. Well-differentiated (grade 1) squamous cell carcinoma. The tumor cells bear a strong resemblance to normal squamous cells and synthesize keratin, as evidenced by epithelial pearls.

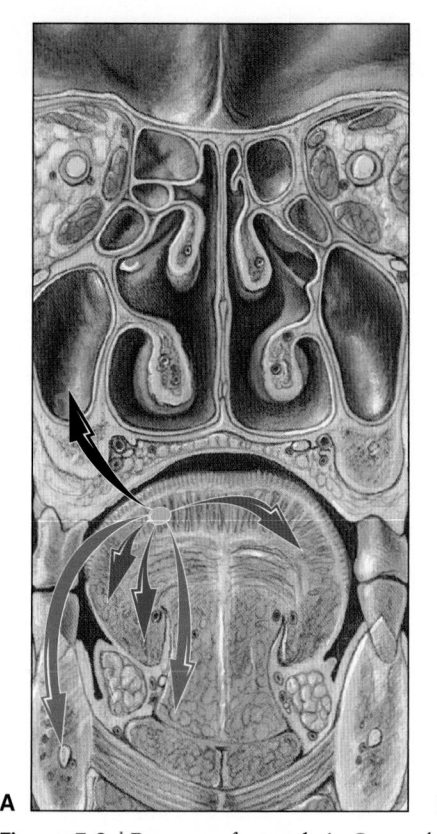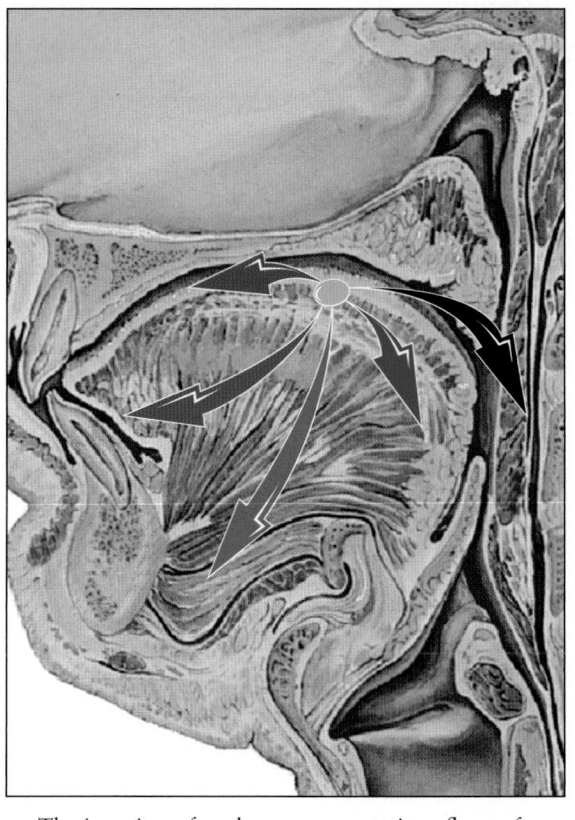

Figure 5.2 | Patterns of spread. A. Coronal view: The invasion of oral tongue cancer into floor of mouth and alveolar ridges. **B.** Sagittal view: The invasion of oral tongue into extrinsic floor of mouth musculature and posterior tongue. The primary cancer (oral cavity) invades in various directions, which are color-coded vectors (*arrows*) representing stage of progression: Tis, yellow; T1, green; T2, blue; T3, purple; T4A, red; and T4B, black. The concept of visualizing patterns of spread to appreciate the surrounding anatomy is well demonstrated by the six directional pattern i.e. SIMLAP Table 2.2.

TABLE 5.2	SIMLAP*	
Oral Cavity (Oral Tongue)		
S	Hard palate	• T4a
	Maxillary sinus	• T4a
	Skull base	**• T4b**
I	Floor of mouth, deep extrinsic muscles (genioglossus, hyoglossus, palatoglossus, and styloglossus)	• T4a
M		
L	Mandible cortical bone	• T4a
	Skin of face	• T4a
A	Skin of face	• T4a
P	Masticator space	**• T4b**
	Pterygoid plates	**• T4b**
	Carotid artery	**• T4b**

There are six basic directions or vectors (arrows): The six vectors of invasion are Superior, Inferior, Medial, Lateral, Anterior, and Posterior. The color-coded dots correlate the T stage with specific anatomic structure involved.

TNM STAGING CRITERIA

TNM STAGING CRITERIA

These lesions tend to be either exophytic or endophytic, with the greatest concern being cancer of the tongue that, because of the interdigitations of its intrinsic and extrinsic muscles, leads to invasion of the floor of the mouth. Cancers arising in the floor of the mouth tend to be shallow ulcerations, usually in the gutters, and invade into the muscles of the tongue. They can readily attach and destroy the mandible. The lateral angles of the floor are important and precise landmarks for cancer spread in the mouth, because they merge into the alveololingual sulcus of the oropharynx.

In the oral cavity, the location of the cancer is a powerful prognosticator. As noted, a shift of a few centimeters alters the prognosis of the cancer significantly. Buccal cancers, alveolar ridges, and retromolar cancers are more unilaterally localized and are likely to spread into ipsilateral lymph nodes. Structures in the midline, such as the tongue, floor of the mouth, and palate, tend to drain bilaterally and have a poorer prognosis.

SUMMARY OF CHANGES SEVENTH EDITION AMERICAN JOINT COMMITTEE ON CANCER (AJCC)

The TNM stages according to the 7th Edition of AJCC are illustrated in color code of advancement (Fig. 5.3). T4 lesions have been divided into T4a (moderately advanced local disease) and T4b (very advanced local disease), leading to the stratification of Stage IV into Stage IVA (moderately advanced local/regional disease), Stage IVB (very advanced local/regional disease), and Stage IVC (distant metastatic disease). The TNM Staging Matrix is color coded for identification of Stage Group once T and N stages are determined (Table 5.3).

TABLE 5.3 Stage Summary Matrix

	Stage T1	Stage T2	Stage T3	Stage T4a	Stage T4b
N0	I	II	III	IVA	IVB
N1	III	III	III	IVA	IVB
N2	IVA	IVA	IVA	IVA	IVB
N3	IVB	IVB	IVB	IVB	IVB
M1	IVC	IVC	IVC	IVC	IVC

- *T stage* determines stage group
  - T1 = I, T2 + II, T3 = III, T4 = IV
- *N stage* N1 = T3 and then progresses as T stage progresses
  - N1 = T3, N2 = T4a, N3 = T4b
- *M stage* is a separate stage
  - M1 = Stage IVC

ORAL CAVITY

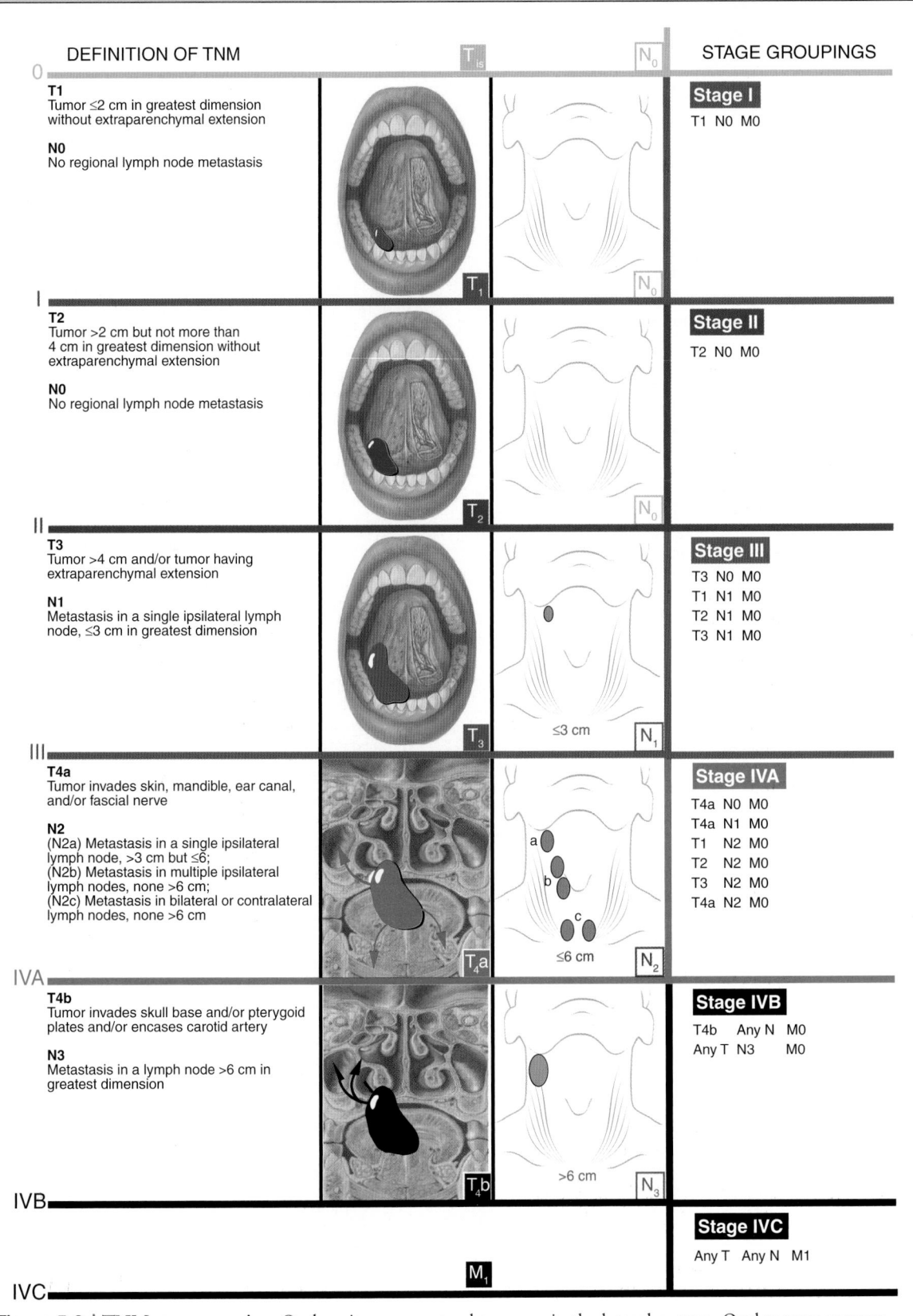

DEFINITION OF TNM

0

T1
Tumor ≤2 cm in greatest dimension
without extraparenchymal extension

N0
No regional lymph node metastasis

I

T2
Tumor >2 cm but not more than
4 cm in greatest dimension without
extraparenchymal extension

N0
No regional lymph node metastasis

II

T3
Tumor >4 cm and/or tumor having
extraparenchymal extension

N1
Metastasis in a single ipsilateral lymph
node, ≤3 cm in greatest dimension

III

T4a
Tumor invades skin, mandible, ear canal,
and/or fascial nerve

N2
(N2a) Metastasis in a single ipsilateral
lymph node, >3 cm but ≤6;
(N2b) Metastasis in multiple ipsilateral
lymph nodes, none >6 cm;
(N2c) Metastasis in bilateral or contralateral
lymph nodes, none >6 cm

IVA

T4b
Tumor invades skull base and/or pterygoid
plates and/or encases carotid artery

N3
Metastasis in a lymph node >6 cm in
greatest dimension

IVB

IVC

STAGE GROUPINGS

Stage I
T1 N0 M0

Stage II
T2 N0 M0

Stage III
T3 N0 M0
T1 N1 M0
T2 N1 M0
T3 N1 M0

Stage IVA
T4a N0 M0
T4a N1 M0
T1 N2 M0
T2 N2 M0
T3 N2 M0
T4a N2 M0

Stage IVB
T4b   Any N   M0
Any T N3   M0

Stage IVC
Any T Any N M1

Figure 5.3 | TNM stage grouping. Oral cavity cancers tend to occur in the lateral gutters. Oral tongue cancers invade the floor of the mouth because of interdigitation of intrinsic and extrinsic musculature. Vertical presentations of stage groupings, which follow the same color code for cancer stage advancement, are organized in horizontal lanes: Stage 0, yellow; I, green; II, blue; III, purple; IVA, red; and IVB, black. Definitions of TN on left and stage grouping on right.

T-ONCOANATOMY

ORIENTATION OF THREE-PLANAR ONCOANATOMY

The anatomic isocenter of the oral cavity is the C2/C3 level. The anterior bullet enters in the midline at the upper lip (Fig. 5.4A) and the lateral bullet is posterior to the lateral commissure of the lips (Fig. 5.4B).

T-oncoanatomy

The oral cavity extends from the skin–vermillion junction of the lips to the junction of the hard and soft palate anteriorly and the anterior pillar (palatoglossal of the oropharynx) and to the line of the circumvallate papillae inferiorly, which divides the tongue into the anterior two-thirds and posterior one-third of the tongue. The various subsites of the oral cavity are noted. The major structures are the tongue, floor of the mouth, alveolar ridges, gingival, and hard palate within the oral cavity proper; the mandible separates the buccal mucosa and lips.

The deeper and more complex anatomy requires knowledge of the underlying musculature, which suspends the upper aerodigestive tract from the mandible and hyoid bone to the vertebral column and base of the skull. Swallowing, mastication, and the initiation of digestion through salivary gland secretion occur in the oral cavity. The tongue aids in food consumption and the sensation of taste is principally located here. The tongue is vital to social intercourse for verbalization, articulation, conversation, and osculation. All of these complex functions relate to the musculature, namely, the muscles of the lips and cheek, including the orbicularis oris and the deeper muscles of the face, the levator anguli oris, the mentalis, and the buccinator muscle of the cheek. The muscles of the tongue and floor of the mouth include the intrinsic muscles of the tongue (longitudinal, transverse, and vertical), the extrinsic tongue muscles (genioglossus, styloglossus, and hyoglossus), and the geniohyoid and mylohyoid muscles, which are the muscles of the floor of the mouth.

The retromolar trigone, when viewed from its superficial mucosa to its deeper underlying structure, shows the complexity of the oral cavity particularly as it relates to the oropharynx. Beneath the retromolar trigone mucosa lies the pterygomandibular raphe, which forms the boundary between the vestibule of the oral cavity and the anterior pillar of the fauces,

containing the palatoglossal muscle in its free border. The fibers of the superior pharyngeal constrictor muscle attach laterally and the buccinator anteriorly to the pterygomandibular raphe. When these muscles and the superior constrictor muscle are removed, the various spaces around the tonsillar fossa and the mandible are readily identified with the important underlying nerves. The lingual nerve and buccal nerve are identified, as is the glossopharyngeal nerve and the inferior alveolar nerve. The various spaces are the parapharyngeal space, which lies medial to the lateral pterygoid muscle; the pterygomandibular space, which is occupied by buccal fat and lies lateral to the medial pterygoid muscle; the buccal space, which is lateral to the mandible; and the masseter muscle.

Perhaps no area illustrates the complexity of the underlying anatomy of the oral cavity better than the retromolar trigone. This site is of particular interest to radiation oncologists because cancers in this area tend to be more radiosensitive and carry a better prognosis than cancers of the oropharynx. The retromolar trigone is formed by the posterior boundary of the retromolar space, posterior to the opening of Stensen's (parotid) duct, and extends posteriorly to the anterior surface of the mandible. With the mouth open, the retromolar trigone comes into prominence and assumes a triangular form with a pale mucous membrane. The base of the retromolar trigone is situated superiorly behind the third upper molar tooth, and the apex lies inferiorly behind the third lower molar tooth. The stretching of the mucous membrane in this region results in the lengthening and projection of the underlying elevator muscles. The medial boundary of the trigone forms the border between the oral cavity and the oropharynx.

- *Coronal plane* (Fig. 5.5A): The coronal plane stratifies the oral tongue and floor of mouth as a set of interdigitating muscles constituted by the intrinsic and extrinsic muscles of the oral cavity.

- *Sagittal plane* (Fig. 5.5B): This view presents the tongue as a contiguous structure of both the oral cavity and tongue attached to the mandible and hyoid bone, respectively.

- *Transverse plane* (Fig. 5.5C): Note the pterygomandibular raphe, which defines the retromolar trigone as the buccal mucosa anterior to the anterior tonsillar pillar. The buccinator muscle and medial pterygoid meet at the raphe. The parapharyngeal space and the pterygomandibular space are avenues into lymph nodes, carotid artery encasement, and perineural invasion of the lingual and glossal pharyngeal nerves.

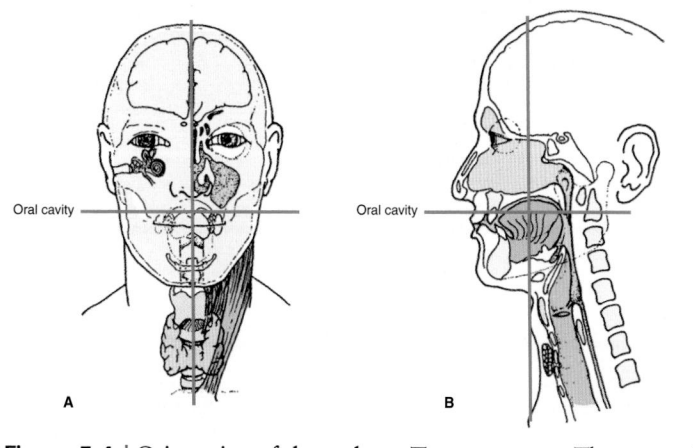

A   B

Figure 5.4 | Orientation of three-planar T-oncoanatomy. The anatomic isocenter is at the axial level at C2/C3. **A.** Coronal. **B.** Sagittal.

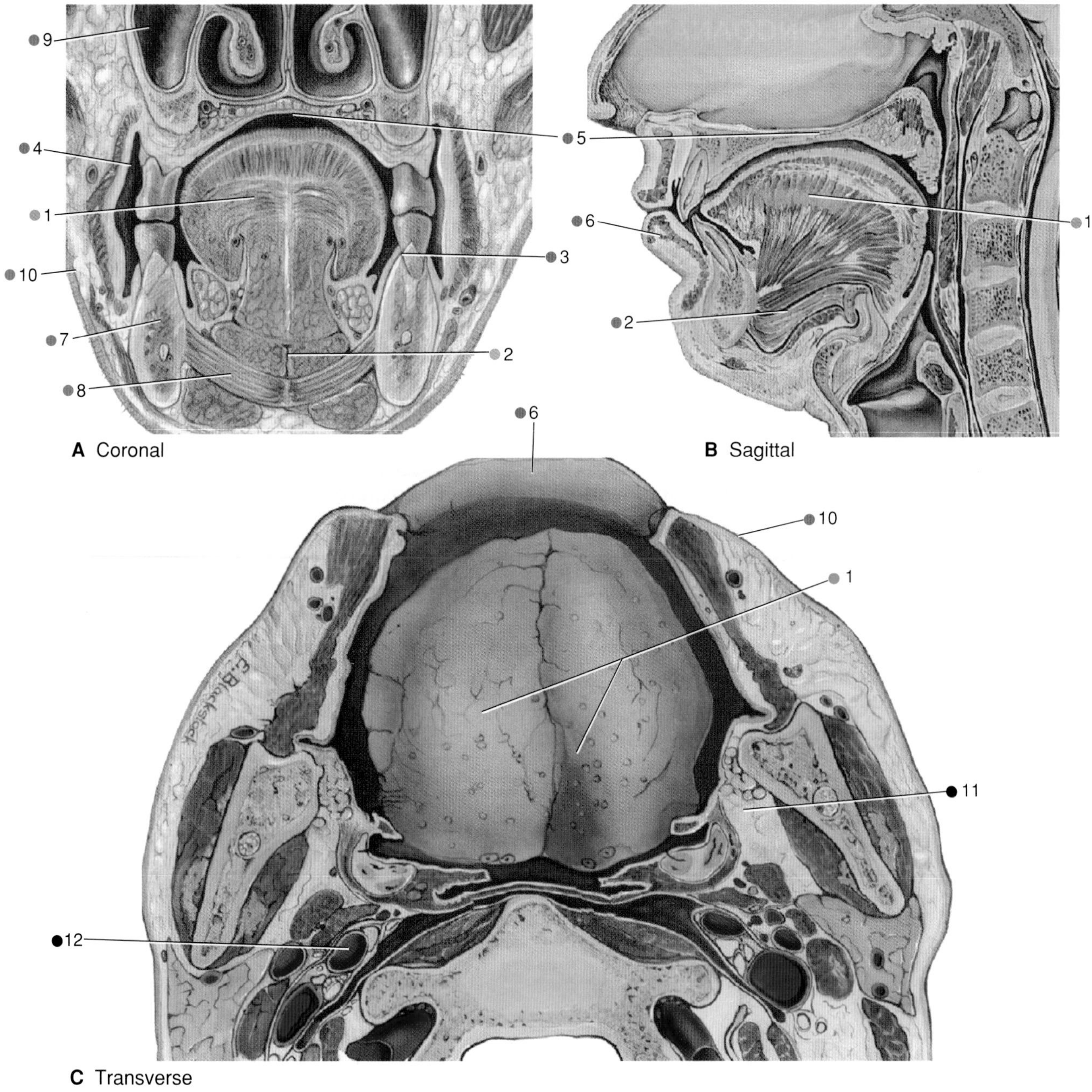
9
4
1
10
7
8
5
3
2
6
1
6
2
A Coronal
B Sagittal
10
1
11
12
E.Blackstock
C Transverse

T_1 • 1. Tongue
T_2 • 2. Geniohyoid muscle
T_3 • 3. Alveolar ridge (gum)
T_3 • 4. Buccal mucosa
T_3 • 5. Hard palate
T_3 • 6. Lip
T_{4a} • 7. Mandible
T_{4a} • 8. Mylohyoid muscle
T_{4a} • 9. Maxillary sinus
T_{4a} • 10. Skin of face
T_{4b} • 11. Masticular space
T_{4b} • 12. Internal carotid artery

Figure 5.5 | T-oncoanatomy. The Color Code for the anatomic sites correlates with the color code for the stage group (Fig. 5.3) and patterns of spread (Fig. 5.2) and SIMLAP table (Table 5.2). Connecting the dots in similar colors will provide an appreciation for the 3D Oncoanatomy.

TNM STAGING CRITERIA

TNM STAGING CRITERIA

The staging system for salivary glands appeared in the fourth edition of the American Joint Committee on Cancer/ International Union Against Cancer (AJCC/UICC) guidelines (1992), and was based on an extensive retrospective study of malignant tumors of the major salivary glands collected from 11 participating American and Canadian institutions. Although statistical analysis of the data revealed that numerous factors affected patient survival, the classification proposed involved only four clinical variables: Tumor size, local extension of the tumor, palpability and suspicion of nodes, and presence or absence of distant metastasis. The anatomic configuration and location predetermines the staging features of the parotid gland. Involvement of the pterygoid plates or skull base renders tumors unresectable (T4b).

SUMMARY OF CHANGES SEVENTH EDITION AJCC

The TNM stages according to the 7th Edition of AJCC are illustrated in color code of advancement (Fig. 6.3). T4 lesions have been divided into T4a (moderately advanced local disease) and T4b (very advanced local disease), leading to the stratification of Stage IV into Stage IVA (moderately advanced local/regional disease), Stage IVB (very advanced local/ regional disease), and Stage IVC (distant metastatic disease). The TNM Staging Matrix is color coded for identification of Stage Group once T and N stages are determined (Table 6.3).

TABLE 6.3 | Stage Summary Matrix

	Stage T1	Stage T2	Stage T3	Stage T4a	Stage T4b
N0	I	II	III	IVA	IVB
N1	III	III	III	IVA	IVB
N2	IVA	IVA	IVA	IVA	IVB
N3	IVB	IVB	IVB	IVB	IVB
M1	IVC	IVC	IVC	IVC	IVC

- *T stage* determines stage group
  - T1 = I, T2 + II, T3 = III, T4 = IV
- *N stage* N1 = T3 and then progresses as T stage progresses
  - N1 = T3, N2 = T4a, N3 = T4b
- *M stage* is a separate stage
  - M1 = Stage IVC

PAROTID GLAND

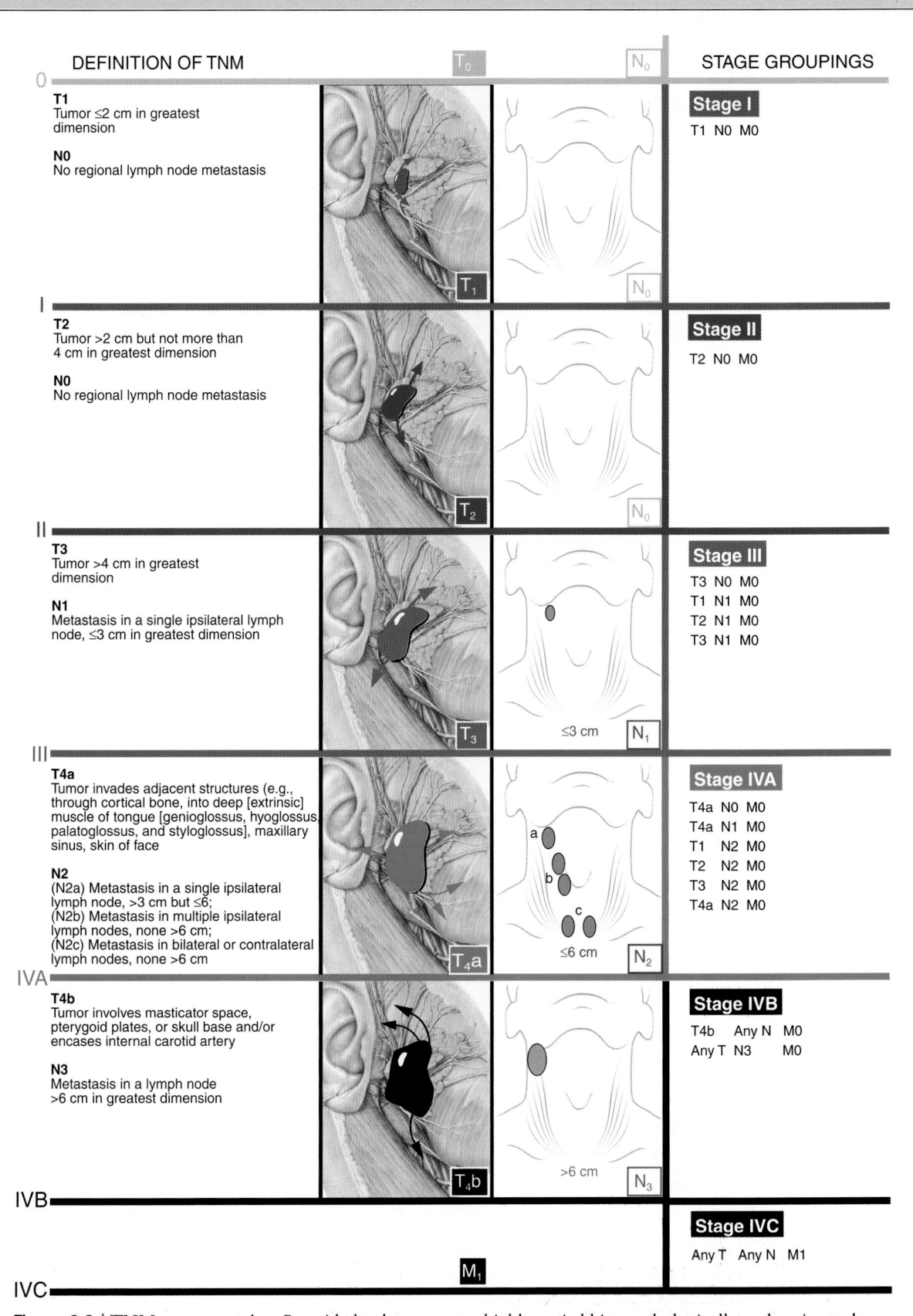

DEFINITION OF TNM

T1
Tumor ≤2 cm in greatest dimension

N0
No regional lymph node metastasis

T2
Tumor >2 cm but not more than 4 cm in greatest dimension

N0
No regional lymph node metastasis

T3
Tumor >4 cm in greatest dimension

N1
Metastasis in a single ipsilateral lymph node, ≤3 cm in greatest dimension

T4a
Tumor invades adjacent structures (e.g., through cortical bone, into deep [extrinsic] muscle of tongue [genioglossus, hyoglossus, palatoglossus, and styloglossus], maxillary sinus, skin of face

N2
(N2a) Metastasis in a single ipsilateral lymph node, >3 cm but ≤6;
(N2b) Metastasis in multiple ipsilateral lymph nodes, none >6 cm;
(N2c) Metastasis in bilateral or contralateral lymph nodes, none >6 cm

T4b
Tumor involves masticator space, pterygoid plates, or skull base and/or encases internal carotid artery

N3
Metastasis in a lymph node >6 cm in greatest dimension

STAGE GROUPINGS

Stage I
T1 N0 M0

Stage II
T2 N0 M0

Stage III
T3 N0 M0
T1 N1 M0
T2 N1 M0
T3 N1 M0

Stage IVA
T4a N0 M0
T4a N1 M0
T1   N2 M0
T2   N2 M0
T3   N2 M0
T4a N2 M0

Stage IVB
T4b Any N M0
Any T N3   M0

Stage IVC
Any T Any N M1

Figure 6.3 | TNM stage grouping. Parotid gland cancers are highly varied histopathologically and perineural invasion of the VIIth and Vth cranial nerves are the major concern. Vertical presentations of stage groupings, which follow the same color code for cancer stage advancement, are organized in horizontal lanes: Stage 0, yellow; I, green; II, blue; III, purple; IVA, red; and IVB, black. Definitions of TN on left and stage grouping on right.

T-ONCOANATOMY

ORIENTATION OF THREE-PLANAR ONCOANATOMY

The parotid is a superficial gland above the angle of the mandible and wraps around the ramus. The anatomic isocenter is axially at the level of the bodies of C2 and C3. The anterior bullet skims the cheek at the level of the lobule of the external ear (Fig. 6.4A) and the lateral bullet is through the body of the ramus of the mandible superior to the angle of the jaw (Fig. 6.4B).

T-oncoanatomy

The parotid, submaxillary, and sublingual glands are the major salivary glands in contradistinction to the many minor salivary glands, each and all providing digestive enzymes, lubrication, or both for the lumen of the upper digestive passage. The major salivary glands are best oriented (Fig. 6.4AB) to the oral cavity because their major ducts empty into this region. Stensen's duct opens into the buccal cavity opposite the

2nd maxillary molar and Wharton's duct empties into the floor of mouth along the frenulum of the tongue. The three-dimensional planar views (Fig. 6.5A–C) are essential to appreciate the oncoanatomy.

- *Sagittal plane* (Fig. 6.5A): The sagittal view is the most informative; the cranial nerve VII (facial nerve) enters and exits through the parotid gland between the superficial lobe and the mandible, innervating multiple muscles of the face. Equally important are branches of cranial nerve V3 and the lingual nerve, both of which can be involved with deep lobe cancers. Perineural invasion can occur, particularly with cylindromas. Such cancers can travel retrograde along the nerve and penetrate into the middle fossa of the skull and the Gasserian ganglion of cranial nerve V.

- *Coronal plane* (Fig. 6.5B): The coronal view demonstrates the relationship of the parotid and submaxillary gland to the mandible.

- *Transverse plane* (Fig. 6.5C): This view is essential to define the retroparotidian space through which the carotid artery, jugular vein, parapharyngeal nodes, and cranial nerves IX, X, XI, and XII pass along the posterior pharyngeal wall.

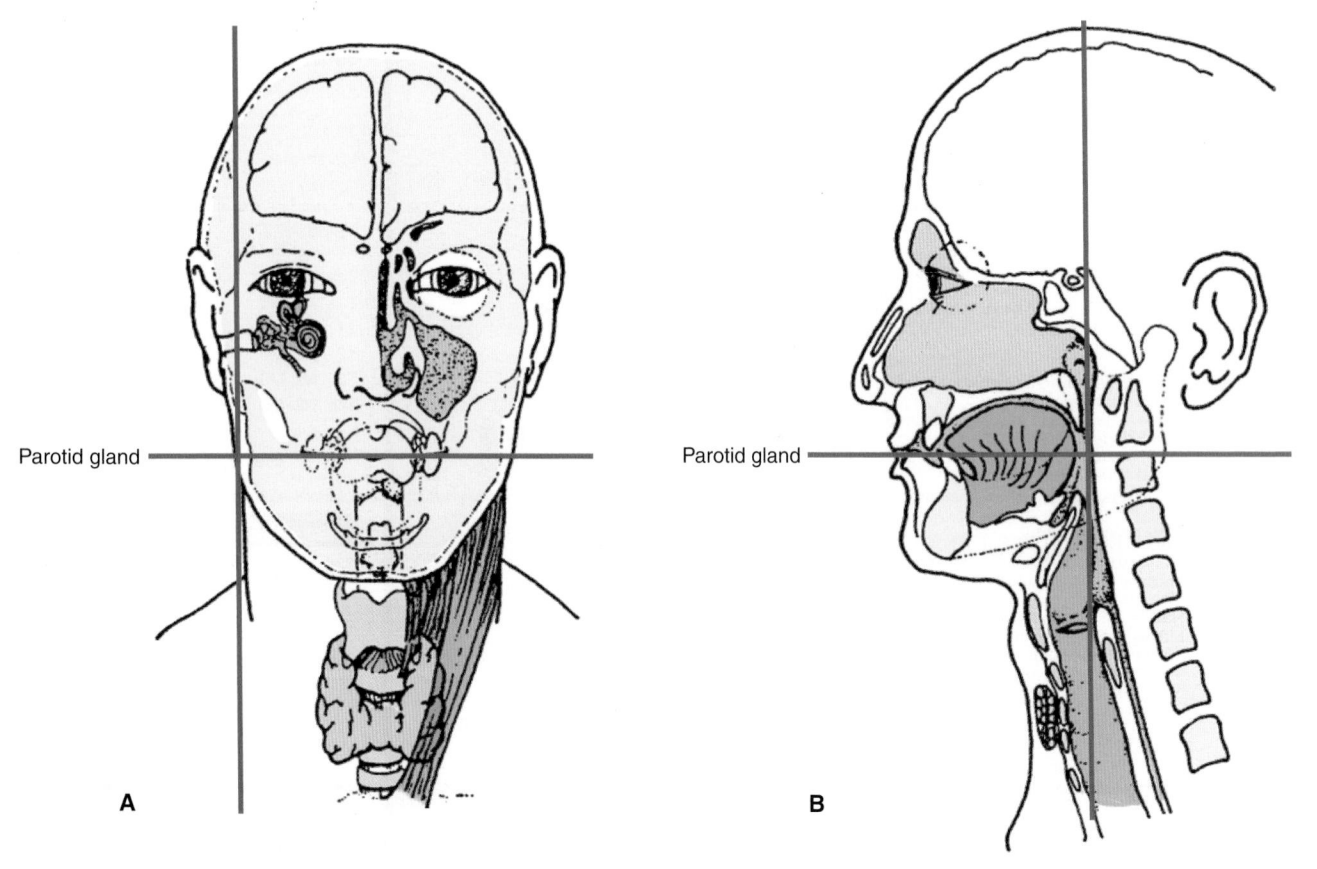

Parotid gland

A

Parotid gland

B

Figure 6.4 | Orientation of three-planar T-oncoanatomy. The anatomic isocenter is at the axial level at C2/C3. **A.** Coronal. **B.** Sagittal.

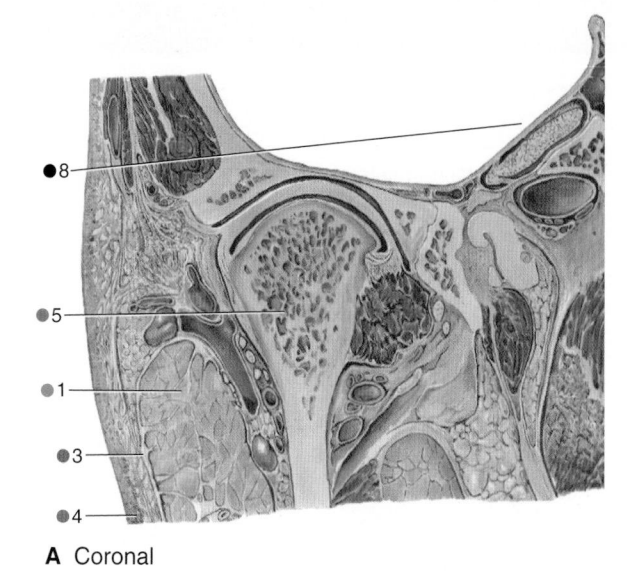

A Coronal

B Sagittal

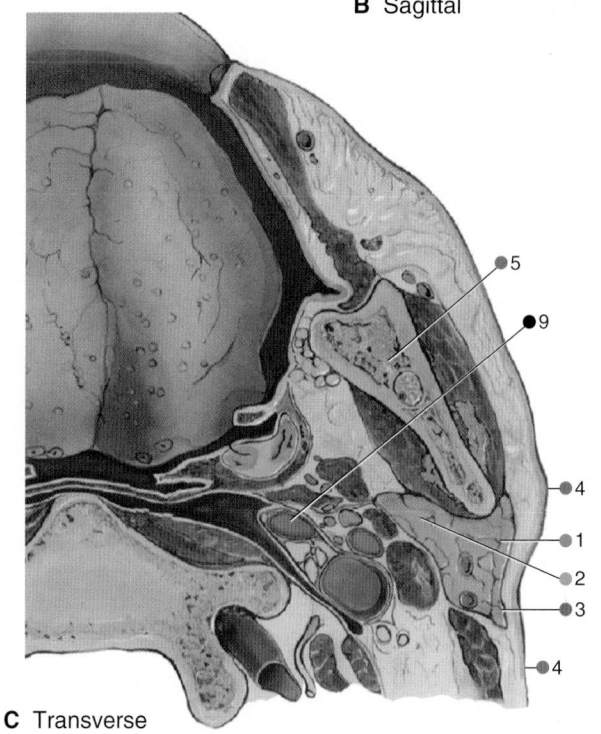

C Transverse

T1 ● 1. Superficial lobe		T4a ● 4. Skin		T4b ● 8. Skull base	
T2 ● 2. Deep lobe		T4a ● 5. Mandible		T4b ● 9. Carotid artery	
T3 ● 3. Capsule (extraparenchymal extension)		T4a ● 6. External ear canal			
		T4a ● 7. Facial nerve			

Figure 6.5 | **T-oncoanatomy.** The Color Code for the anatomic sites correlates with the color code for the stage group (Fig. 6.3) and patterns of spread (Fig. 6.2) and SIMLAP table (Table 6.2). Connecting the dots in similar colors will provide an appreciation for the 3D Oncoanatomy.

N-ONCOANATOMY AND M-ONCOANATOMY

N-ONCOANATOMY

The rich network of superficial lymphatics of the face, including the scalp and eyelids, drains into the preauricular and parotid lymph nodes (Fig. 6.6; Table 6.4). The jugulodigastric lymph node is just inferior to the parotid gland. The deep lobe of the parotid drains into the retropharyngeal lymph nodes. The submaxillary gland drains into submandibular nodes (Fig. 6.6). The risk estimation for percent positive neck nodes is based on T score/stage and histopathology (Table 6.5A).

M-ONCOANATOMY

The parotid gland drains to the pterygoid venous plexus, facial vein, internal jugular vein, brachiocephalic vein and superior vena cava, and into the right side of the heart. The target metastatic organ is lung, but the pulmonary vascular bed acts as a sanctuary housing metastases that often do not produce any severe or life-threatening loss of pulmonary function (see Fig. 6.7A).

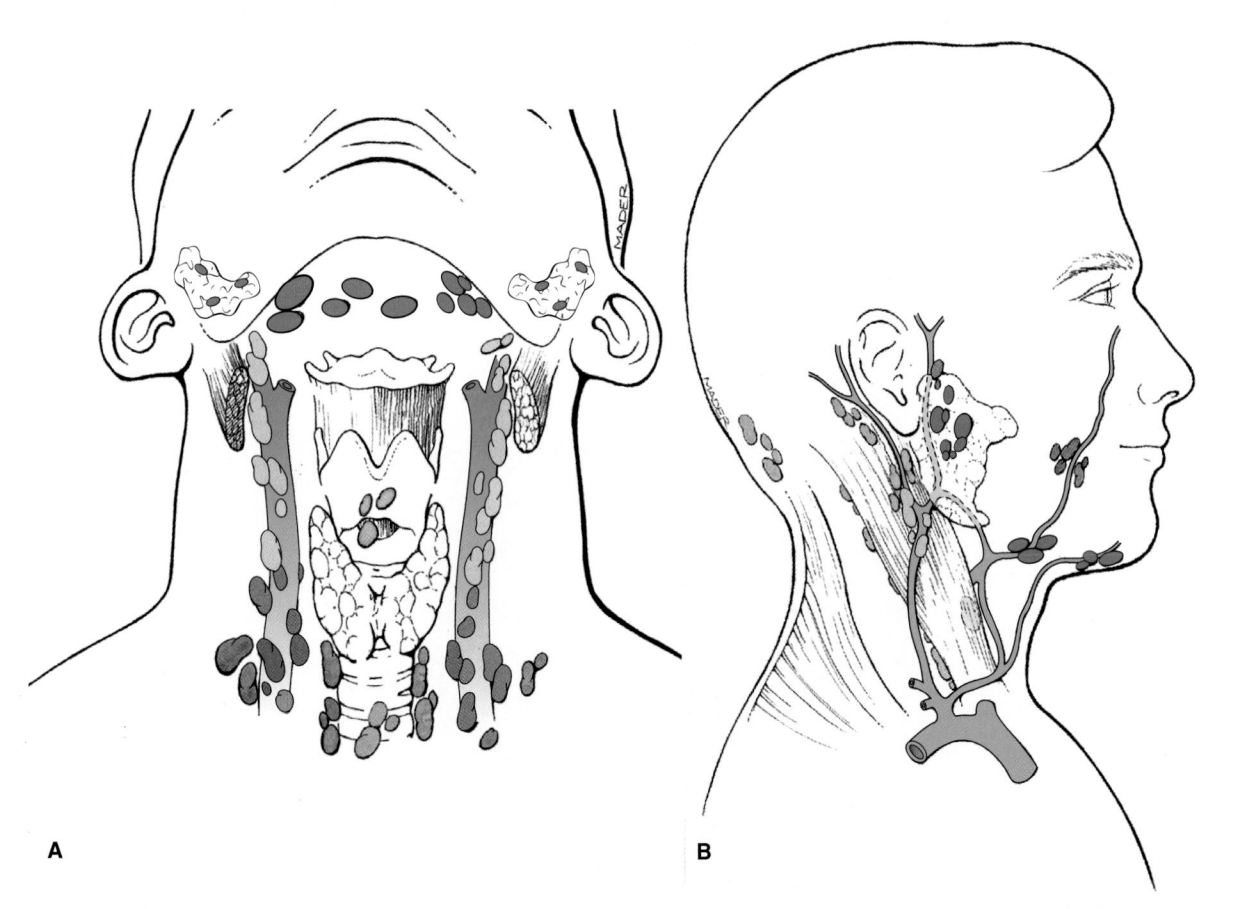

A   B

Figure 6.6 | **N-oncoanatomy.** The red node highlights the sentinel node, which are the parotid node and submandibular node. **A.** Anterior view. **B.** Lateral view. **M-oncoanatomy** is determined by the jugular vein, which joins with the subclavian vein to form the superior vena cava on the right, and the innominate vein, which drains into the right side of the heart and then into lung.

TABLE 6.4	Sentinel and Regional Nodes: Parotid Gland (Ipsilateral)	
	Level/Location of Node(s)	
S Sentinel Node	**Axial Level**	**AJCC Level**
S1 Parotid nodes	C2/C3	I
R Regional Nodes		
R1 Submandibular	C3	I
R2 Jugulodigastric, superior deep cervical	C3	II
R3 Mid deep cervical	C4	III
R4 Jugulo-omohyoid, inferior deep cervical	C7	IV

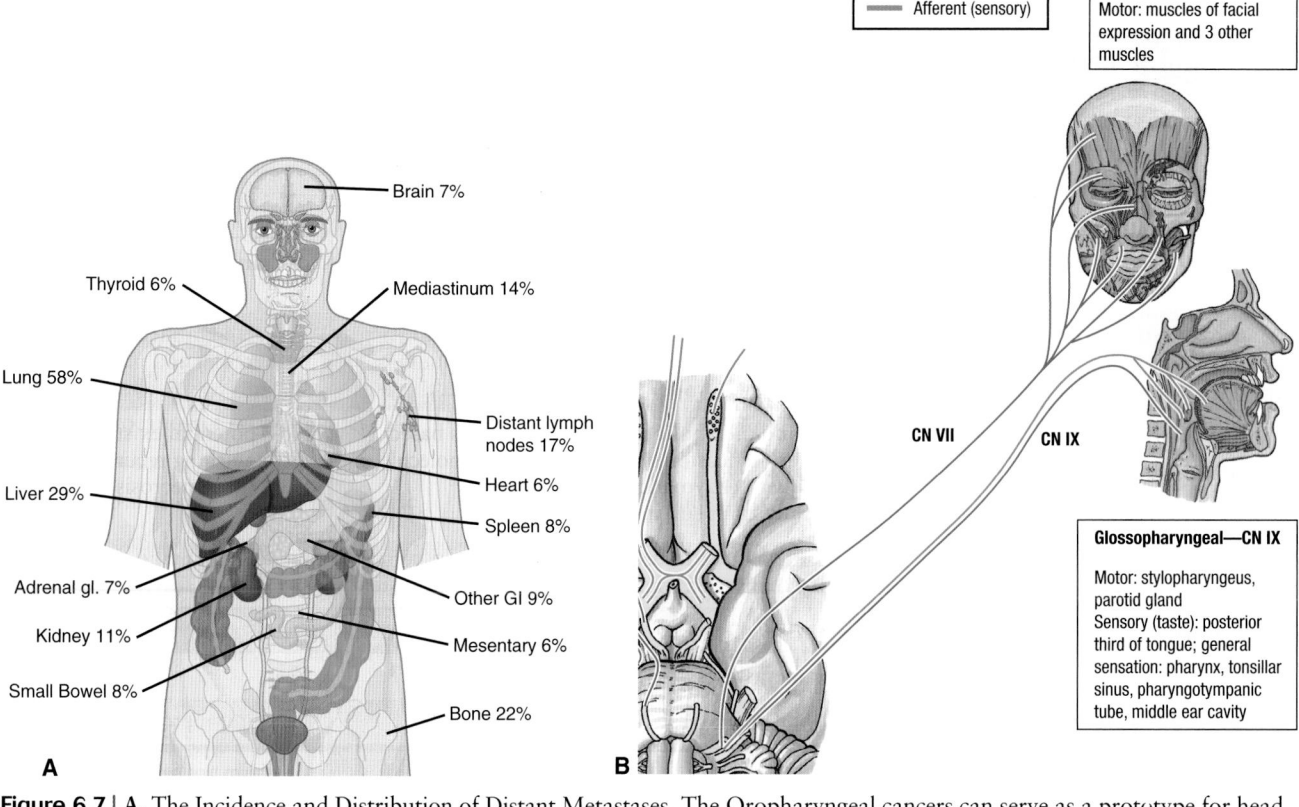

Figure 6.7 | A. The Incidence and Distribution of Distant Metastases. The Oropharyngeal cancers can serve as a prototype for head and neck cancers. Lung (58%) is the target organ with liver metastases next (29%) and bone metastases third (22%) followed by distant lymph nodes (17%), mediastinum (14%). The remainder of sites are 11% (kidney) or less than 10%. **B.** Cranial nerve for Parotid Gland CN IX.

CRANIAL NERVES AND NEUROVASCULAR BUNDLE

The importance of appreciating the complex anatomy of cranial nerves lies in the patterns of cancer spread at the primary cancer site as well as nodal spread patterns. Perineural invasion or compression by metastatic lymph nodes often is manifested by specific neurologic symptoms and signs. The overview of cranial nerves provides an intricate roadmap as to points of vulnerability (Fig. 6.7B; Table 6.5B).

Cranial nerve invasion can produce specific syndromes and neurologic evaluation is a vital part of physical diagnosis in all head and neck cancers.

A tabulation of potential neurologic syndromes either due to perineural invasion at the primary site or nodal compression will alert the astute clinician to extent of cancer advancement anatomically.

Salivary gland or parotid gland cancers tend to invade the facial nerve CN VII as it exists from the stylohyoid foramen and result in impairment of facial musculature depending on its invasion of branches vs. the main nerve. Sensory taste in the anterior 2/3 of tongue and soft palate can be altered. Cylindromas are notorious for perineural invasion and if branches of V_3 mandibular nerve are involved, it can penetrate into the bassercan ganglion into the middle fossa.

Retroparotidean nodes can compress IX, X, XI, XII, especially if the primary involves the deep lobe.

TABLE 6.5A	Risk Estimation (%) for Positive Neck Nodes
Summation: T Score + Histologic Type Score	Parotid Gland
2	4
3	12
4	25
5	33
6	38

T1 = 1, T2 = 2, T3-4 = 3; acinic/adenoid cystic/carcinoma ex pleomorphic adenoma = 1, mucoepidermoid = 2, squamous/undifferentiated = 3.

TABLE 6.5B	Potential Neurologic Syndromes Due to Invasion of Cranial Nerves I-XII	
	T Site	N Site
Parotid Gland	VII, V_3	IX, X, XI, XII

Oropharynx

PERSPECTIVE, PATTERNS OF SPREAD, AND PATHOLOGY

The TNM patterns of spread and the malignant gradient are predetermined by the underlying musculature anatomy of the tonsillar pillars.

PERSPECTIVE AND PATTERNS OF SPREAD

The oropharynx is the isocenter of the upper aerodigestive tract and is composed of a series of large sphincters, which receives the bolus of food and initiates the act of swallowing. The need for sphincteric mechanisms arises because the physiology of deglutition ensures that the contents of tubular structures move in one direction to ensure their proper digestion. Once the bolus is swallowed, a series of involuntary muscular movements of the tube propel the food onward. The chief sphincter of the upper aerodigestive tract is the muscular pharynx (Fig. 7.2).

Cancers of the anterior pillar follow the palatoglossal muscle, which either encircle the soft palate and uvula or, alternately, follow the fascial plane inferiorly and infiltrate the tongue. Cancers of the pharyngonasal sphincter (Passavant's fold) consist of palatal neoplasms that act as a nasopharyngeal neoplasm. This sphincter prevents nasal regurgitation and, in effect, ensures closure and separation of the nasal passage from the oral cavity and pharynx while swallowing. Cancers

of the posterior pillar (palatopharyngeal muscle) of the tonsil invade the posterior wall of the pharynx (Fig. 7.2). The contraction of the superior constrictor muscle of the pharynx during swallowing forms a prominence known as Passavant's fold on the posterior wall of the nasopharynx, which acts as a protective barrier. Cancers in this area tend to appear as irregular surface lesions, spreading circumferentially on the oral and pharyngeal surface. Odynophagia (pain on swallowing) may be ignored and attributed to the common cold. To the astute clinician, dysphagia-producing pain referred to the middle ear is attributed to the referral of pain to the nerve of Jacobson, a branch of the glossopharyngeal nerve (cranial nerve IX). Patterns of Spread are presented as a cancer crab that can invade in six basic directions Superior-Inferior, Medial-Lateral, Anterior-Posterior (SIMLAP) of adjacent anatomic sites (Fig. 7.2; Table 7.2).

PATHOLOGY

Tumors of the oropharynx arise from the mucosal lining and are similar to those of the nasopharynx; the tonsil and base of the tongue are a continuation of Waldeyer's ring. The most common neoplasms are squamous cell cancers exhibiting

TABLE 7.1	Histopathologic Type: Common Cancers of the Oropharynx	
Squamous Cell Carcinoma Microscopic Variants	**Adenocarcinoma Major or Minor Salivary Gland**
Keratinizing; well differentiated; moderately well differentiated; poorly differentiated	Low-grade adenocarcinoma
Nonkeratinizing; anaplastic squamous carcinoma	Adenoid cystic carcinoma
Lymphoepithelioma	Mucoepidermoid (low or high grade)
Transitional cell carcinoma	Carcinoma expleomorphic adenoma
Spindle cell squamous carcinoma	Poorly differentiated adenocarcinoma

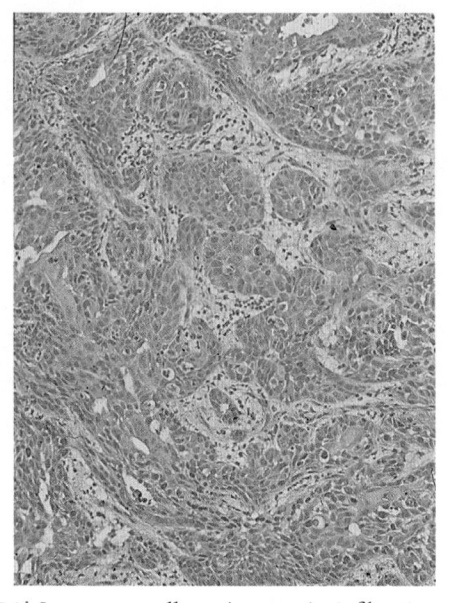

Figure 7.1 | Squamous cell carcinoma. An infiltrative neoplasm is composed of cohesive nests of tumor.

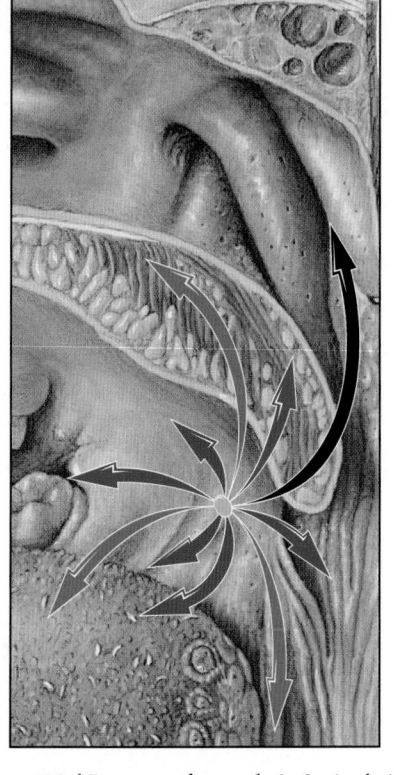
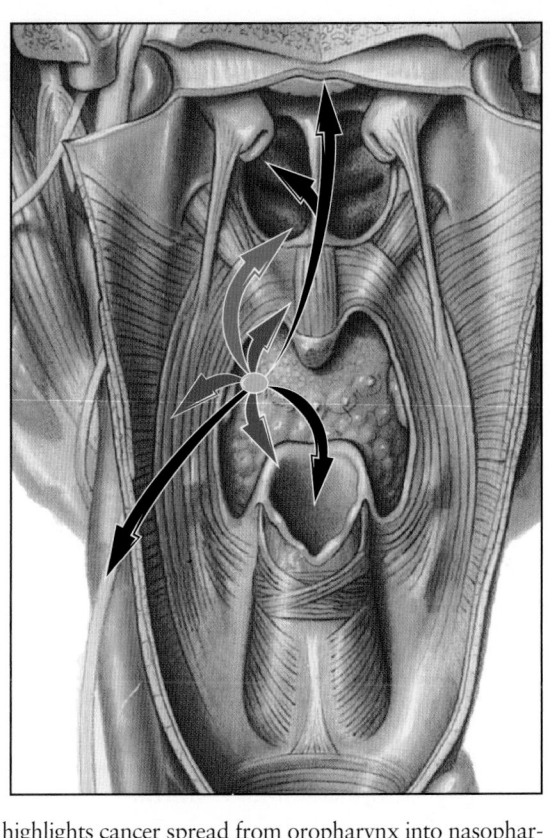

Figure 7.2 | Patterns of spread. A. Sagittal view: highlights cancer spread from oropharynx into nasopharynx and hypopharynx. **B.** Coronial view: indicates the sphincter muscular of the pharynx: middle constrictor between superior constrictor of nasopharynx and inferior constrictor of the hypopharynx as to invasive pathways of pharyngeal tube. The primary cancer (oropharynx) invades in various directions, which are color-coded vectors (*arrows*) representing stage of progression: Tis, yellow; T1, green; T2, blue; T3, purple; T4a; red; and T4b, black. The concept of visualizing patterns of spread to appreciate the surrounding anatomy is well demonstrated by the six directional pattern i.e. SIMLAP Table 7.2.

varying degrees of differentiation and anaplasia; most of the discussion surrounding these neoplasms refers to their pattern of spread (Table 7.1; Fig. 7.1). Lymphomas tend to be bulky exophytic lesions. They enlarge the palatine tonsils and/or lingual tonsils without deep infiltration. Although cancers can be exophytic, they invariably have a significant endophytic component. Lymphoepitheliomas have both epithelial and lymphatic cells and behave in a fashion consistent with both of these two components. Large primaries with bilateral adenopathy are frequently present at their onset.

TABLE 7.2	SIMLAP*	
Oropharynx (Tonsil)		
S	Nasopharynx	• T4b
	Skull base	• T4b
I	Hypopharynx, larynx	• T4b
M	Medial pterygoid muscle	• T4b
L	Mandible	• T4a
	Lateral pterygoid muscle	• T4b
	Encases carotid	• T4b
A	Hard palate	• T4a
P	Prevertebral space	• T4b

There are six basic directions or vectors (arrows): The six vectors of invasion are S̲uperior, I̲nferior, M̲edial, L̲ateral, A̲nterior, and P̲osterior. The color-coded dots correlate the T stage with specific anatomic structure involved.

TNM STAGING CRITERIA

TNM STAGING CRITERIA

The TNM patterns of spread are predetermined by the underlying musculature anatomy. The two pillars of the tonsillar fossa, which need to be distinguished from true tonsil remnants, are readily appreciated on surface anatomy. The two sphincters of the oropharynx are the pharyngonasal and buccopharyngeal sphincters.

Cancers can arise in the posterior pharyngeal wall in the area of the mucous membrane between the posterior pillars on the posterior pharyngeal wall over the bodies of C2 and C3. More frequently, the base of the tongue, which seals off regurgitation by pressing against the oropharyngeal bar, is a favored site for malignancy. The malignant gradient increases as the cancer arises in an anteromedial location versus a posterolateral site. Again, the intimate relationship of the tongue and tonsillar region is reflected in their anatomic structure and muscular arrangements. Deeply penetrating cancers from either site usually extend into and invade the other region. Unlike the oral tongue, the base of tongue contains some fat and lymphoid tissue in between the fibers, as well as a less distinct midline septum, making invasion across to the opposite side a more likely clinical occurrence.

SUMMARY OF CHANGES SEVENTH EDITION AMERICAN COMMITTEE ON CANCER (AJCC)

The TNM stages according to the 7th Edition of AJCC are illustrated in color code of advancement (Fig. 7.3). T4 lesions have been divided into T4a (moderately advanced local disease) and T4b (very advanced local disease), leading to the stratification of Stage IV into Stage IVA (moderately advanced local/regional disease), Stage IVB (very advanced local/regional disease), and Stage IVC (distant metastatic disease). The TNM Staging Matrix is color coded for identification of Stage Group once T and N stages are determined (Table 7.3).

TABLE 7.3 | **Stage Summary Matrix**

	Stage T1	Stage T2	Stage T3	Stage T4a	Stage T4b
N0	I	II	III	IVA	IVB
N1	III	III	III	IVA	IVB
N2	IVA	IVA	IVA	IVA	IVB
N3	IVB	IVB	IVB	IVB	IVB
M1	IVC	IVC	IVC	IVC	IVC

- *T stage* determines stage group
  - T1 = I, T2 + II, T3 = III, T4 = IV
- *N stage* N1 = T3 and then progresses as T stage progresses
  - N1 = T3, N2 = T4a, N3 = T4b
- *M stage* is a separate stage
  - M1 = Stage IVC

OROPHARYNX

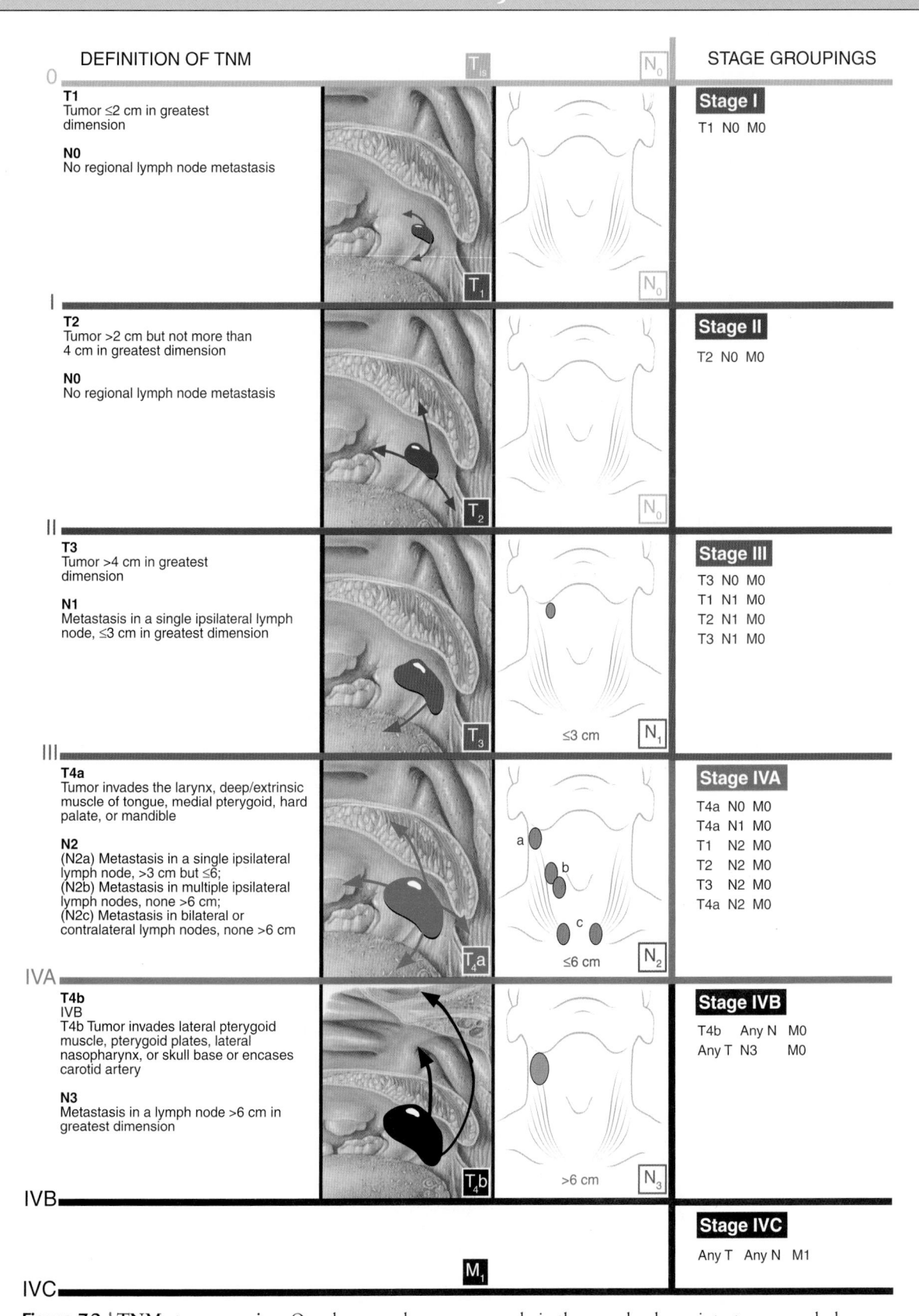

DEFINITION OF TNM

T1
Tumor ≤2 cm in greatest dimension

N0
No regional lymph node metastasis

T2
Tumor >2 cm but not more than 4 cm in greatest dimension

N0
No regional lymph node metastasis

T3
Tumor >4 cm in greatest dimension

N1
Metastasis in a single ipsilateral lymph node, ≤3 cm in greatest dimension

T4a
Tumor invades the larynx, deep/extrinsic muscle of tongue, medial pterygoid, hard palate, or mandible

N2
(N2a) Metastasis in a single ipsilateral lymph node, >3 cm but ≤6;
(N2b) Metastasis in multiple ipsilateral lymph nodes, none >6 cm;
(N2c) Metastasis in bilateral or contralateral lymph nodes, none >6 cm

T4b
IVB
T4b Tumor invades lateral pterygoid muscle, pterygoid plates, lateral nasopharynx, or skull base or encases carotid artery

N3
Metastasis in a lymph node >6 cm in greatest dimension

≤3 cm

≤6 cm

>6 cm

STAGE GROUPINGS

Stage I
T1 N0 M0

Stage II
T2 N0 M0

Stage III
T3 N0 M0
T1 N1 M0
T2 N1 M0
T3 N1 M0

Stage IVA
T4a N0 M0
T4a N1 M0
T1 N2 M0
T2 N2 M0
T3 N2 M0
T4a N2 M0

Stage IVB
T4b Any N M0
Any T N3 M0

Stage IVC
Any T Any N M1

Figure 7.3 | TNM stage grouping. Oropharyngeal cancers spread via the muscle planes into tongue and pharynx from palate in a circumferential fashion. Vertical presentations of stage groupings, which follow the same color code for cancer stage advancement, are organized in horizontal lanes: Stage 0, yellow; I, green; II, blue; III, purple; IVA, red; and IVB, black. Definitions of TN on left and stage grouping on right.

T-ONCOANATOMY

ORIENTATION OF THREE-PLANAR ONCOANATOMY

The anatomic isocenter is located at the C2-3 level and located along the anterior border of the ramus of the mandible and medial to it. A vertical line from the center of the ramus runs through the center of the pharyngeal tube. The anterior surface bullet is at the level of the lips in the midline (Fig. 7.4A) and the lateral bullet penetrates at the angle of the mandible (Fig. 7.4B).

T-oncoanatomy

The pharynx is a fibromuscular tube extending from the base of the skull to the esophagus, regulating the flow of food and air in the upper aerodigestive passage. The pharynx is composed of three sections: (i) the nasal, (ii) the oral, and (iii) the laryngeal pharynx.

● *Coronal plane* (Fig. 7.5A): There are four major sphincters in the pharynx that regulate the passage of air and food to their ultimate destinations. The sphincters, at the point of the entry, are the buccopharyngeal sphincters guarding the communication between the mouth and the pharynx (fauces). They are formed by the base of the tongue and the oropharyngeal bar, which is produced by a synchronized peristaltic contraction of the posterior oropharyngeal muscular wall. The upper or pharyngonasal opening between the nasopharynx and the oropharynx is protected by a sphincter formed by the soft palate and Passavant's fold. The lower or esophageal opening is protected by the cricopharyngeal sphincter formed by the cricopharyngeal bar and the back of the cricoid cartilage. Cancers invade posteriorly to the pterygoid plate and superiorly into the nasopharynx to the skull.

  The fibrous coat (pharyngobasilar fascia) is strong and anchors the pharynx to the base of the skull and the medial pterygoid plate. In a dissection of mucous membranes and tonsils from the lateral oropharyngeal wall, the following muscles may be identified: palatopharyngeus, superior constrictor, styloglossus, stylopharyngeus, and middle constrictor. As in all peristaltic activity in the digestive tract, there are constrictor muscles and longitudinal muscles. This pattern is seen in the pharyngeal wall. There are three inner constrictor muscles: (i) superior, (ii) middle, and (iii) inferior—and an outer, more longitudinal coat—the stylopharyngeus, stylohyoid, and palatopharyngeus muscles. The constrictor muscles are strategically attached to the mandible, the hyoid bone, and the thyroid and cricoid cartilages. They provide the form and structure of the pharyngeal tube.

  It is in the coronal plane that the prestyloid compartment can be identified by the fatty or areolar content from the lateral pharyngeal space with the stylopharyngeus and styloglossus muscles. The posterior belly of the digastric muscle arises posteriorly and spreads inferiorly in this space, as does the stylohyoid. Using these same muscles and the styloid process as landmarks, the lateral pharyngeal space is better appreciated with its contents. Posterior to the styloid process is the neurovascular bundle, identified previously in the nasopharyngeal wall.

● *Sagittal plane* (Fig. 7.5B): The palatopharyngeus muscle is shown, innervation by cranial nerve IX into the base of the tongue. On deep dissection of the tonsillar fossa, the palatopharyngeal and the stylopharyngeus muscles form the longitudinal coat. The constrictor muscles, superior and mainly middle, are the circular inner coat that controls swallowing. The glossopharyngeal nerve supplies one muscle, the stylopharyngeus, and provides special taste to the posterior third of the tongue and sensation to an entire half of the pharyngeal wall; absent gag reflex result when the nerve is lost.

● *Transverse plane* (Fig. 7.5C): At C2, it demonstrates the medial and lateral pterygoid muscles, than posteriorly the retropharyngeal nodes alongside the carotid and jugular vessels in the retroparotidian space laterally. Deep invasion of the posterior glossopharyngeal muscle along the posterior pillar into retropharyngeal nodes leads to neurologic loss, namely, cranial nerves IX, X, XI, and XII.

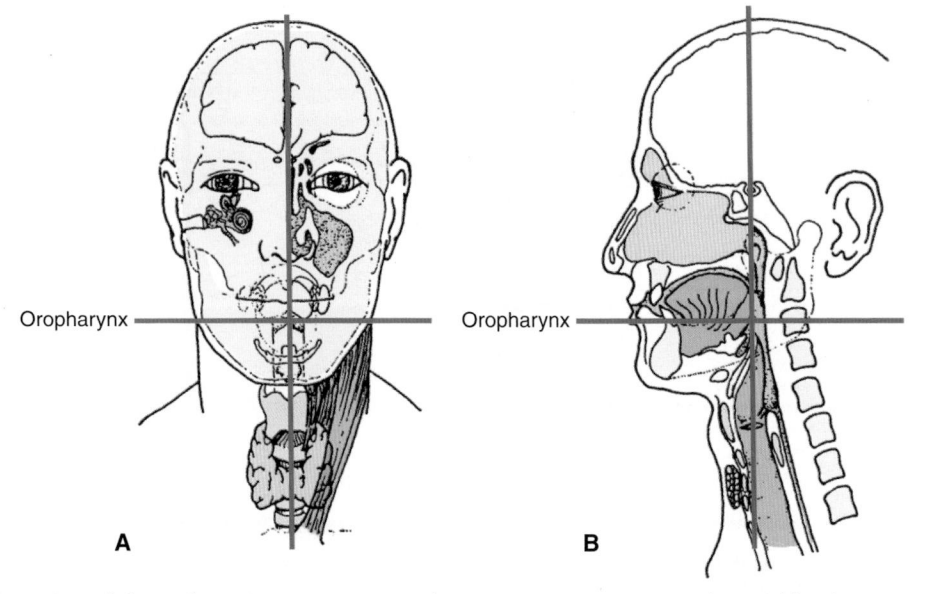

Oropharynx

Oropharynx

A

B

Figure 7.4 | **Orientation of three-planar T-oncoanatomy.** The anatomic isocenter is at the axial level at C3. **A.** Coronal. **B.** Sagittal.

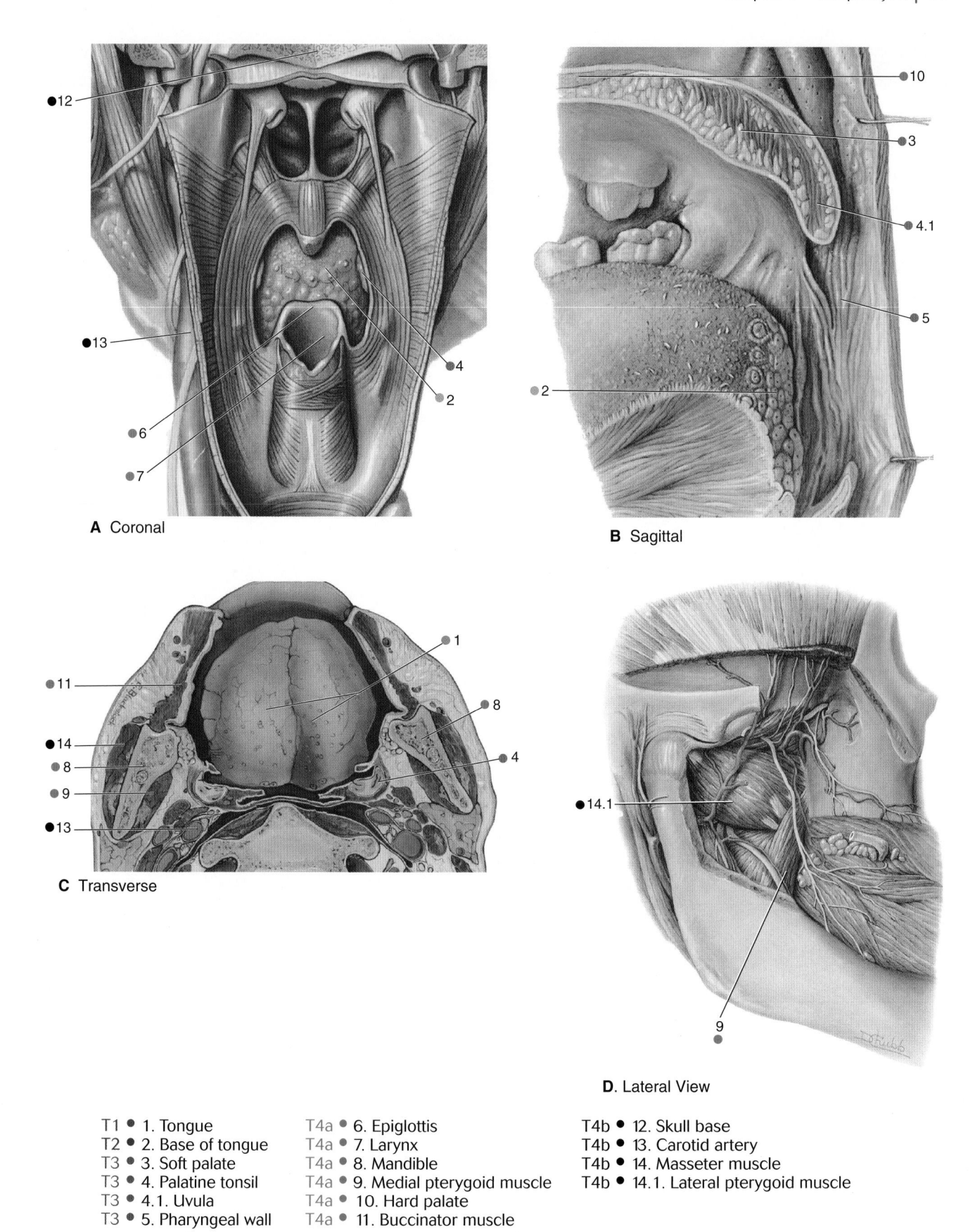

A Coronal

B Sagittal

C Transverse

D. Lateral View

T1 ● 1. Tongue	T4a ● 6. Epiglottis	T4b ● 12. Skull base
T2 ● 2. Base of tongue	T4a ● 7. Larynx	T4b ● 13. Carotid artery
T3 ● 3. Soft palate	T4a ● 8. Mandible	T4b ● 14. Masseter muscle
T3 ● 4. Palatine tonsil	T4a ● 9. Medial pterygoid muscle	T4b ● 14.1. Lateral pterygoid muscle
T3 ● 4.1. Uvula	T4a ● 10. Hard palate	
T3 ● 5. Pharyngeal wall	T4a ● 11. Buccinator muscle	

Figure 7.5 | **T-oncoanatomy.** The Color Code for the anatomic sites correlates with the color code for the stage group (Fig. 7.3) and patterns of spread (Fig. 7.2) and SIMLAP table (Table 7.2). Connecting the dots in similar colors will provide an appreciation for the 3D Oncoanatomy.

N-ONCOANATOMY AND M-ONCOANATOMY

N-ONCOANATOMY

There are three major collecting lymphatic trunks in the oropharynx: (i) the middle collecting, (ii) the palatine tonsil, and (iii) the posterior lingual. These drain into the parapharyngeal or retropharyngeal nodes (Fig. 7.6; Table 7.4). The jugulodigastric and jugulo-omohyoid are the most common draining nodes, although upper and lower deep cervical nodes also are first-station nodes. Because of the location of palatine tonsillar lymphoid tissue between the anterior and posterior pillars and the location of lingual tonsils in the base of the tongue, lymphomas commonly arise at these sites. Occasionally, all of Waldeyer's ring can be involved with lymphomatous infiltration, obstructing the oropharynx and nasopharynx. These tumors can become large, growing rapidly and remaining submucosal. Both lymphomas and carcinomas often spread into the jugulodigastric and omodigastric

nodes. Rapid spread into other cervical nodes and bilateral involvement is common, reflecting the bilateral drainage of the base of the tongue (Tables 7.5A and 7.5B; Fig. 7.7A). The incidence of neck node metastasis in clinical negative (N0) neck as presented in Figure 7.7A and Table 7.7A compared to a clinical positive neck (Table 7.5B).

M-ONCOANATOMY

Distant metastases are also possible because of the plexus of pharyngeal veins that drain into the jugular vein, and then into the superior vena cava, the right heart, and finally the lungs. The vascular supply of the pharynx arises from the external carotid. The carotid body and sinus located at the bifurcation of the common carotid are arterial chemoreceptor and baroreceptor areas, respectively (see Fig. 7.7B).

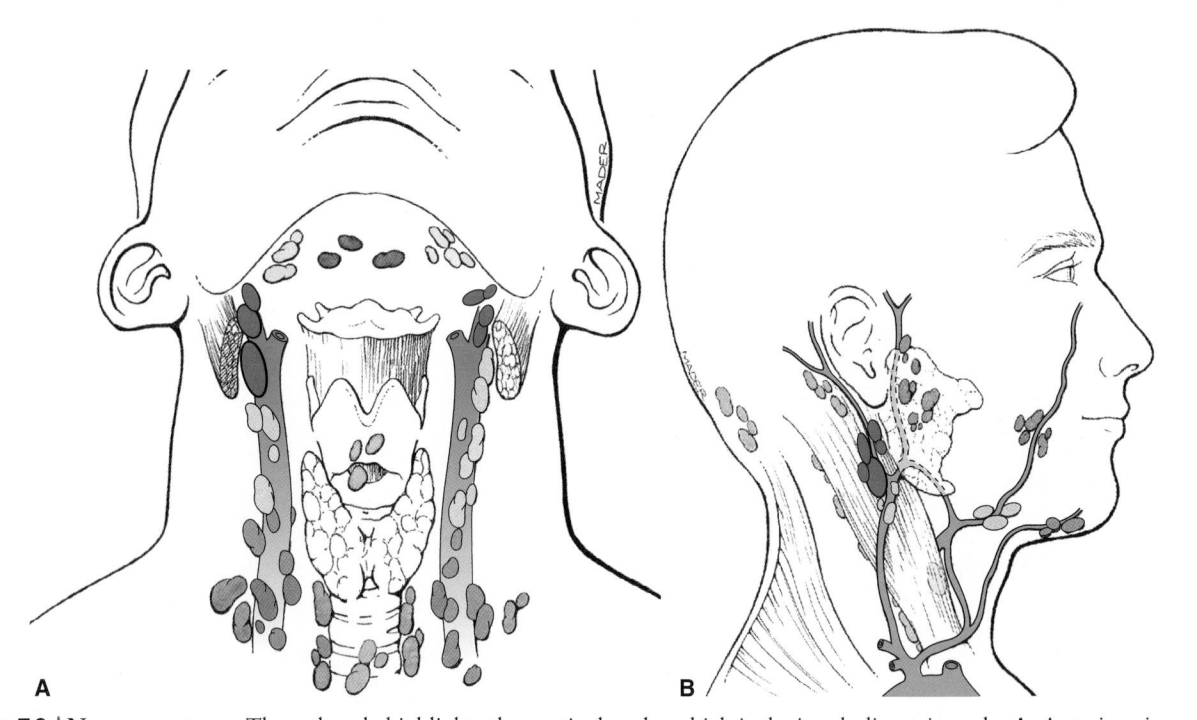

Figure 7.6 | N-oncoanatomy: The red node highlights the sentinel node, which is the jugulodigastric node. **A.** Anterior view. **B.** Lateral view. **M-oncoanatomy** is determined by the jugular vein, which joins with the subclavian vein to form the superior vena cava on the right, and the innominate vein, which drains into the right side of the heart and then into lung.

TABLE 7.4	Sentinel and Regional Nodes: Oropharynx (Uni and Bilateral)	
	Level/Location of Node(s)	
S Sentinel Node	**Axial Level**	**AJCC Level**
S1 Jugulodigastric	C3	II
R Regional Nodes		
R1 Retropharyngeal	C1	nI
R2 Jugulodigastric, superior deep cervical	C3	II
R3 Mid deep cervical	C4	III
R4 Jugulo-omohyoid, inferior deep cervical	C7	IV

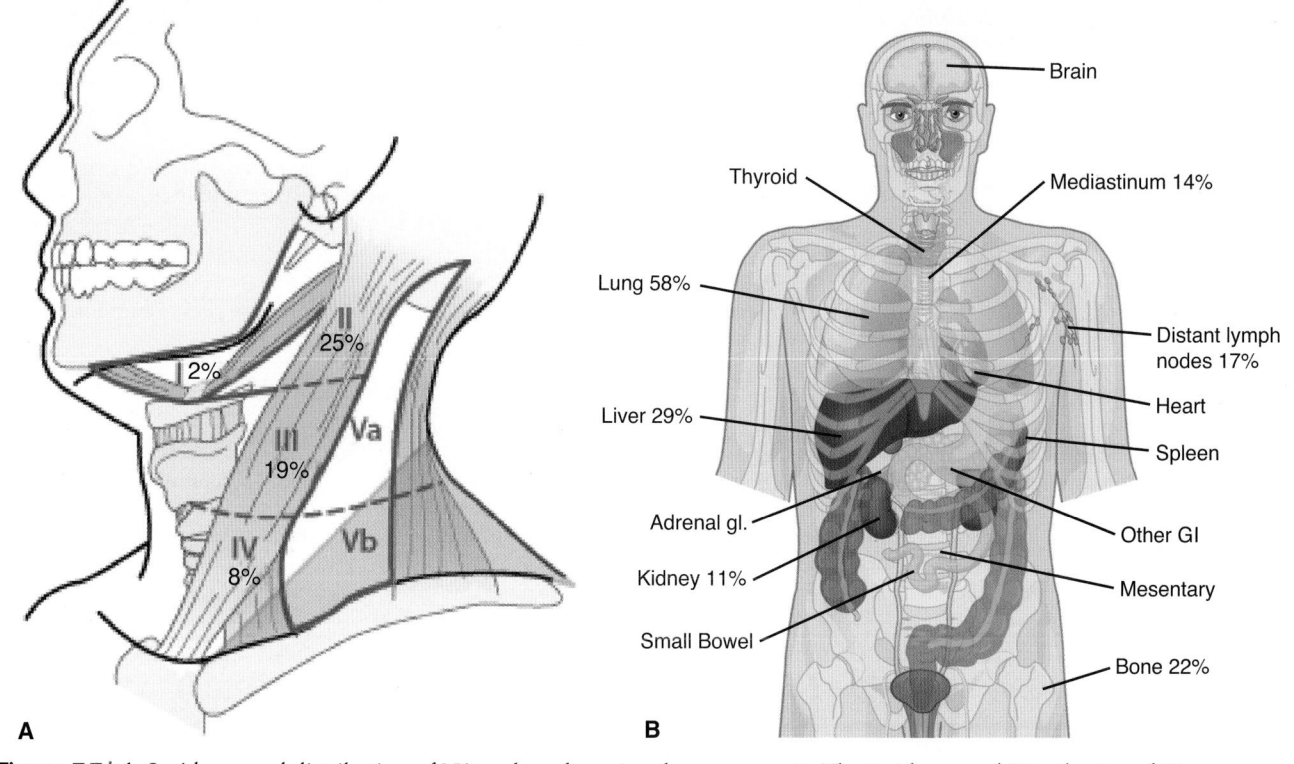

Figure 7.7 | A. Incidence and distribution of N0 neck node regional metastases. **B.** The Incidence and Distribution of Distant Metastases of Oropharynx Cancers. The Oropharyngeal Cancers can serve as a prototype for head and neck cancers. Lung (58%) is the target organ with liver metastases next (29%) and bone metastases third (22%) followed by distant lymph nodes (17%), mediastinum (14%). The remainder of sites are 11% (kidney) or less than 10%.

TABLE 7.5A	Incidence and Distribution of N0 Neck Node Regional Metastases

The sentinel node of oropharyngeal neck node metastases is the jugulodigastric node. This varies according to the stage of the primary cancer.

- Stage T1 = 2%
- Stage T2 = 25%
- Stage T3 = 19%
- Stage T4 = 8%

TABLE 7.5B	Incidence and Distribution of N+ Neck According to AJCC Neck Regions

Once the sentinel node is involved, the patterns of spread to the rest of the neck nodes at difference levels is due to collateralization of drainage both prograde and retrograde as well as contralateral spread. The neck node levels (%) involved:

Level I = 15%

Level II = 21%

Level III = 42%

Level IV = 27%

Level V = 9%

Incidence and Distribution of Distant Metastases

STAGING WORKUP

TABLE 7.6 Imaging Modalities and Strategies for Diagnosis and Staging for Head and Neck: Oropharynx

Modality	Strategy	Recommended
Primary Tumor and Nodes		
Computed tomography	Excellent for defining extent of primary depth of invasion enlargement of involved nodes. (Preferred for bone invasion.)	Yes—3–5 mm cuts, 3 mm for primary sites, 5 mm for neck.
Magnetic resonance imaging	Offers best 3D and 3-planar views of primary and nodes, especially soft tissue extensions. Gadolinium contrast for extensions and perineuronal spread.	Yes—$\leq$4 cm slices Gd for intracranial and perineuronal spread.
Positron emission tomography	Functional and metabolic imaging of ^{18}FDG is based on 2-deoxy modification, which inhibits the molecule from subsequent enzymatic conversion and is "metabolically trapped" in tumor cells.	No—potential exists for distinguishing recurrence from tissue necrosis.
Metastases		
Chest film	Search for metastases.	Yes.
Radionuclide scan	^{99m}Tc for bone metastases.	Yes—if symptomatic.

3D, three-dimensional; FDG, fluorodeoxyglucose.

RULES OF CLASSIFICATION AND STAGING

Clinical Staging and Imaging

For oropharyngeal cancers, careful history taking, inspection, and palpation of the face and neck are essential. Testing of all cranial nerves is critical. Both direct and indirect endoscopy are useful. Despite cooperation of the patient, pharyngeal cancers may be inaccessible and imaging is important. To determine the true extent of primary oropharyngeal cancers, imaging is essential. Magnetic resonance imaging (MRI) is superior to computed tomography (CT) in demonstrating soft tissue extension, skull base changes, and perineural invasion (see Table 7.6 and Fig. 7.8 Axial CT).

Pathologic Staging

The gross specimen should be evaluated for margins. Unresected gross residual tumor must be included and marked with clips. All resected lymph node specimens should describe size, number, and level of involved nodes and whether there is extracapsular spread. Specimens taken after radiation, chemotherapy, or both need to be so noted; specimen shrinkages may occur up to 30% after resection itself. Designations pT and pN should be used after histopathologic evaluation. Perineural invasion deserves special notation.

Oncoimaging Annotations

- Staging systems for oropharyngeal carcinomas are based mainly on tumor size criteria and deep extensions.

- All CT studies should be performed after contrast enhancement administered by using a bolus technique.

- Thirty percent of patients with squamous cell carcinoma of the base of the tongue have bilateral metastatic nodes at the time of initial clinical presentation. Many of these nodes are clinically silent and are detected on imaging studies.

- Evaluation of tonsillar and soft palate carcinomas is best done with MRI to determine soft tissue invasion.

PROGNOSIS AND CANCER SURVIVAL

PROGNOSTIC FACTORS

The seventh edition of the AJCC Cancer Staging Manual lists the following prognostic factors for nasal ethmoid sinus cancers:

- Size of lymph nodes
- Extracapsular extension from lymph nodes for head and neck
- Head and neck lymph nodes levels I-III
- Head and neck lymph nodes levels IV-V
- Head and neck lymph nodes levels VI-VII
- Other lymph node group
- Clinical location of cervical nodes
- Extracapsular spread (ECS) clinical
- Extracapsular spread (ECS) pathologic
- Human papillomavirus (HPV) status
- Tumor thickness*

*The foregoing passage is from Edge SB, Byrd DR, and Compton CC, et al, *AJCC Cancer Staging Manual, 7th edition.* New York, Springer, 2010, p. 99.

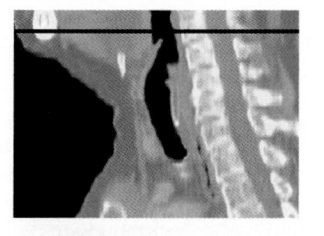

1. mandible
2. base of tongue
3. pharynx
4. internal jugular vein
5. common carotid art
6. sternocleidomastoid muscle
7. external jugular vein
8. vertebral art
9. vertebral body
10. posterior lamina

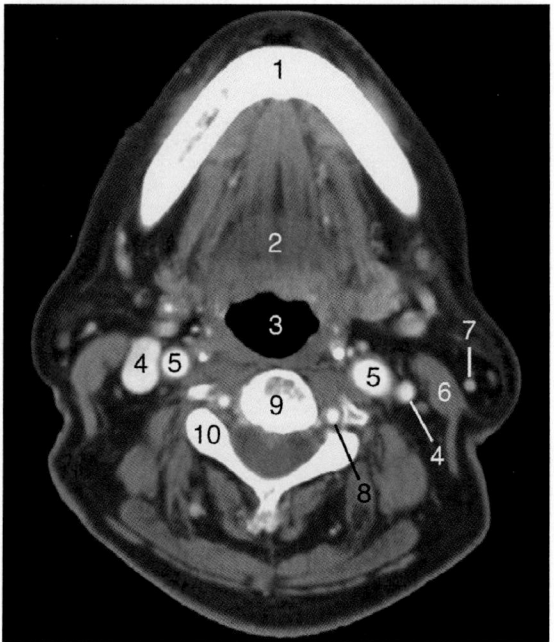

Figure 7.8 | Neck and Larynx—Axial CT view. The axial view at C3 provides relationships of oropharynx to oral cavity, and the parapharyngeal space with major blood vessels: carotid artery, jugular vein, and lymph nodes.

CANCER STATISTICS AND SURVIVAL

Generally, cancers of the oral cavity, pharynx, and the upper digestive passage account for 36,540 new cases per year. In addition, cancer of the larynx affects another 12,720 patients and thyroid cancers 44,670. Approximately 25% of head and neck cancer patients die annually, often due to other causes (Table 7.2). Long-term survival for patients with thyroid cancers is an exception, with only 1,500 deaths (5%). The improvement in oral cavity and pharyngeal tumors from 1950 to 2000 was modest at 14% and matches larynx at 15% (see Fig. 1.10). A multidisciplinary approach is vital and both normal tissue conservation and reconstructive techniques have added greatly to quality of life. Unfortunately, this patient population abuses ethanol and nicotine and it is difficult to change these habits. Persistence of smoking and drinking contributes to their demise often from second malignant tumors in adjacent sites.

Specifically, oropharyngeal cancer is often advanced stage II or III when detected and overall survival is only 30% to 40%. The best outcome is with early stage I tonsillar cancers and soft palate as compared to base of tongue and pharyngeal wall, that is, 85% to 90% versus 50% to 60%, respectively. The recent AJCC Survival data indicate T1 and T2 cancers without nodes yields a 5 year survival above 50%, where as nodal involvement stage decreases survival to less then 50%.

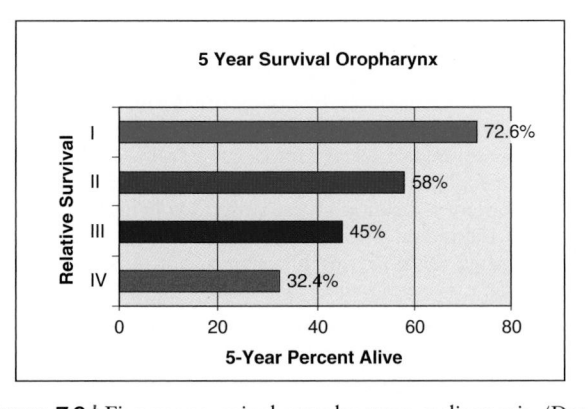

Figure 7.9 | Five-year survival rates by stage at diagnosis. (Data from Edge SB, Byrd DR, and Compton CC, et al, *AJCC Cancer Staging Manual, 7th edition.* New York, Springer, 2010.)

8

Hypopharynx

PERSPECTIVE, PATTERNS OF SPREAD, AND PATHOLOGY

The malignant gradient is an oblique plane following the hypopharyngeal circle. The circle begins with the valleculae at the base of the tongue and worsens as it extends to the piriform recesses laterally. The poorest prognosis is posteriorly at the postcricoid region above the esophageal inlet with the completion of the circle.

PERSPECTIVE AND PATTERNS OF SPREAD

Although the hypopharynx (laryngopharynx) and larynx are anatomically distinct, they require presentation together. In hunting animals such as the wolf and fox, the larynx projects into the nasopharynx, providing continuity for airways. There is no oropharynx when the epiglottis overrides the uvula and soft palate, providing a continuous air column. With evolution the two-part pharynx arose; as in bipedal man, the food bypasses the larynx laterally in the piriform recess. In this anatomic arrangement, food and fluids can be aspirated and is a common complaint when tumors arise in the hypopharynx. There is a malignant gradient of cancers arising in this site, with the anterior location at the valleculae being more favorable than the lateral piriform fossae, with the least desirable location being the posterior pharyngeal and postcricoid. The

common epithelial cancer is squamous cell, with other varieties occurring less often.

The major sites of malignancy in the hypopharynx occur in the zones of food traffic. The hypopharynx can be viewed as a circular gutter designed to allow the food bolus to circumvent the larynx, which is closed during deglutition. The circle, starting anteriorly, begins with the valleculae at the base of the tongue, extends to the piriform recesses laterally, and is completed posteriorly at the postcricoid region above the esophageal inlet. The epithelial cancers of the piriform recess are by far the most common. Superiorly, they extend into the lateral pharyngeal wall and the base of the tongue, and inferiorly into the cricopharyngeal area. Medially, they can spill into the larynx by infiltrating over the aryepiglottic fold. Very often they invade laterally directly into the soft tissues of the neck. An obscure piriform sinus cancer can present as aspiration pneumonitis. A majority of patients complain of difficulty in swallowing with referral of pain to the external ear, which is attributed to Arnold's nerve, a branch of the vagus nerve (cranial nerve X). This neurologic sign indicates invasion of the larynx. Other signs of cancer progression are fetor oris, difficulty swallowing saliva, and dyspnea. Hoarseness also indicates laryngeal invasion. Patterns of Spread are presented as a cancer crab that can invade in six basic directions Superior-Inferior, Medial-Lateral, Anterior-Posterior (SIMLAP) of adjacent anatomic sites (Fig. 8.2; Table 8.2).

TABLE 8.1	Histopathologic Type: Common Cancers of the Hypopharynx	
Squamous Cell Carcinoma Microscopic Variants	**Adenocarcinoma Major or Minor Salivary Gland**
Keratinizing; well differentiated; moderately well differentiated; poorly differentiated	Low-grade adenocarcinoma
Nonkeratinizing; anaplastic squamous carcinoma	Adenoid cystic carcinoma
Lymphoepithelioma	Mucoepidermoid (low or high grade)
Transitional cell carcinoma	Carcinoma expleomorphic adenoma
Spindle cell squamous carcinoma	Poorly differentiated adenocarcinoma

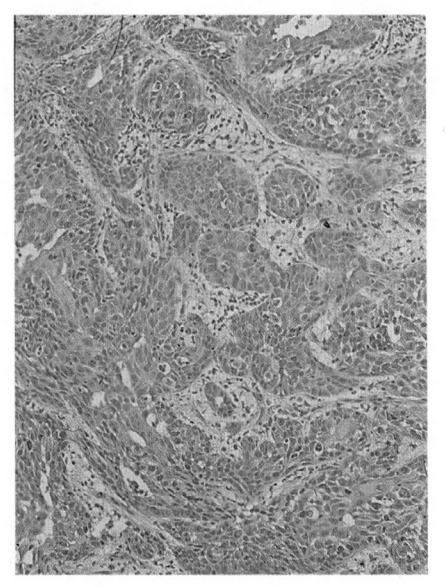

Figure 8.1 | Squamous cell carcinoma. An infiltrative neoplasm is composed of cohesive nests of tumor.

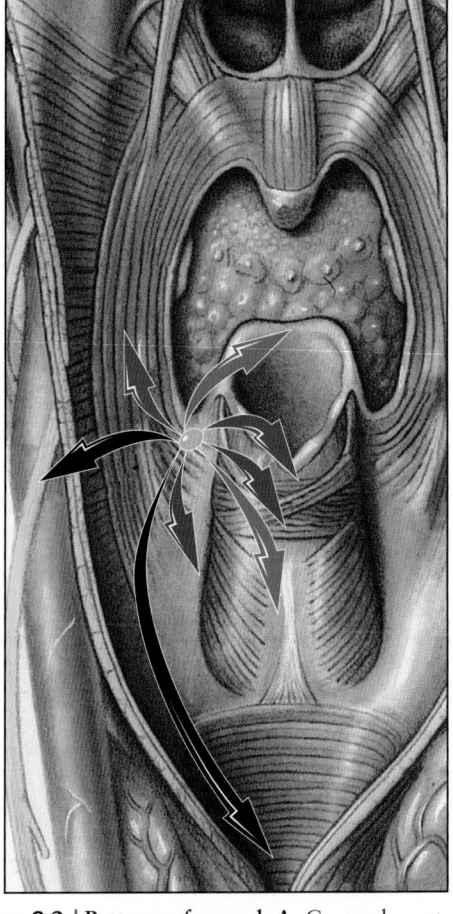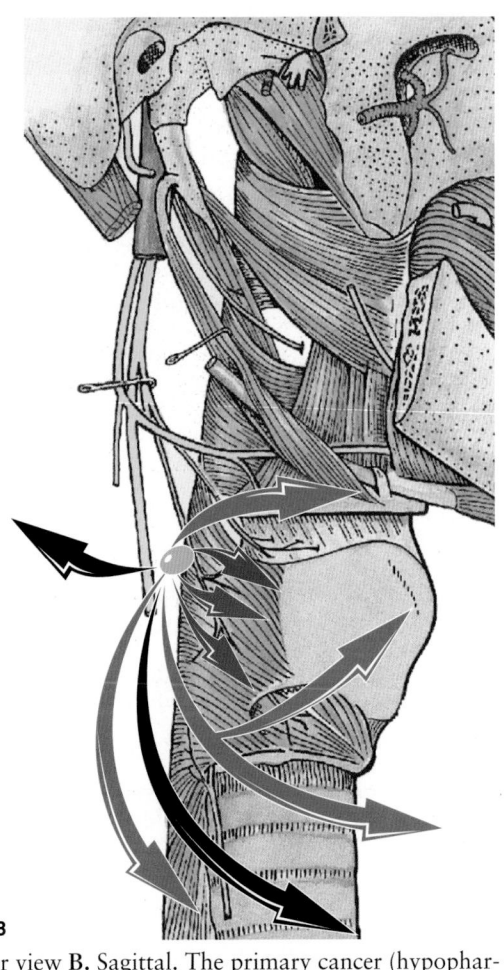

Figure 8.2 | Patterns of spread. A. Coronal, posterior view **B.** Sagittal. The primary cancer (hypopharynx) invades in various directions, which are color-coded vectors (*arrows*) representing stage of progression: Tis, yellow; T1, green; T2, blue; T3, purple; T4a, red; and T4b, black. The concept of visualizing patterns of spread to appreciate the surrounding anatomy is well demonstrated by the six directional pattern i.e. SIMLAP Table 8.2.

PATHOLOGY

Cancers of the piriform recess are usually squamous cell carcinomas, most often undifferentiated and advanced, spreading in all directions. The pharyngeal mucosa tends to be nonkeratinized stratified squamous epithelium, giving rise to squamous cell cancers predominantly with varying degrees of differentiation (Table 8.1 and Fig. 8.1).

TABLE 8.2	SIMLAP*	
Hypopharynx (Pyriform Sinus)		
S	Hyoid bone	• T4a
I	Esophagus	• T4a
M	Aryepiglottic fold (impaired cord)	• T2
	Mediastinal structures	• T4b
	Glottis (fixed cord)	• T3
L	Thyroid gland	• T4a
	Central soft tissues (strap muscles) neck	• T4a
A	Thyroid cartilage, cricoid cartilage	• T4a
P	Prevertebral space, encases caroid artery	• T4b

There are six basic directions or vectors (arrows): The six vectors of invasion are Superior, Inferior, Medial, Lateral, Anterior, and Posterior. The color-coded dots correlate the T stage with specific anatomic structure involved.

TNM STAGING CRITERIA

TNM STAGING CRITERIA

True postcricoid tumors are often difficult to distinguish from cancer of the cervical esophagus (Fig. 8.3). There are three definite groups of tumors: (i) cricopharyngeal, (ii) pharyngoesophageal, and (iii) cervical esophageal. There are certain peculiarities in these tumors. For example, they seem to be more common in women and are associated with difficulty in swallowing. The cricopharyngeus muscle, a muscular band formed by the lower part of the inferior constrictor, usually directs the tumor in an encircling fashion, where it tends to remain with extension superiorly. Involvement of the true larynx with invasion into the arytenoids and into the glottis is possible, but much less likely than inferior spread into the esophagus or superior spread into the posterior pharyngeal wall in the direction of peristalsis.

The most difficult cancers to recognize are those in the valleculae, which tend to burrow into the base of the tongue and destroy the epiglottis. Necrosis is common, and deep sinuses may develop in the tongue. Cartilage erosion and disfiguration of the epiglottis are frequently noted. Invasion of the pre-epiglottic, fat-filled space is common; it offers no resistance to cancer spread.

As stated, the malignant gradient of the hypopharynx is less anteriorly in the valleculae where the prognosis is better than posteriorly and laterally in the piriform recess and postcricoid regions. However, direct invasion into the soft tissues of the neck and even the jugular vein often lead to distant metastases.

SUMMARY OF CHANGES SEVENTH EDITION AMERICAN JOINT COMMITTEE ON CANCER (AJCC)

The TNM stages according to the 7th Edition of AJCC are illustrated in color code of advancement (Fig. 8.3). T4 lesions have been divided into T4a (moderately advanced local disease) and T4b (very advanced local disease), leading to the stratification of Stage IV into Stage IVA (moderately advanced local/regional disease), Stage IVB (very advanced local/regional disease), and Stage IVC (distant metastatic disease). The TNM Staging Matrix is color coded for identification of Stage Group once T and N stages are determined (Table 8.3).

TABLE 8.3	**Stage Summary Matrix**				
	Stage T1	**Stage T2**	**Stage T3**	**Stage T4a**	**Stage T4b**
N0	I	II	III	IVA	IVB
N1	III	III	III	IVA	IVB
N2	IVA	IVA	IVA	IVA	IVB
N3	IVB	IVB	IVB	IVB	IVB
M1	IVC	IVC	IVC	IVC	IVC

- *T stage* determines stage group
  - T1 = I, T2 + II, T3 = III, T4 = IV
- *N stage* N1 = T3 and then progresses as T stage progresses
  - N1 = T3, N2 = T4a, N3 = T4b
- *M stage* is a separate stage
  - M1 = Stage IVC

HYPOPHARYNX

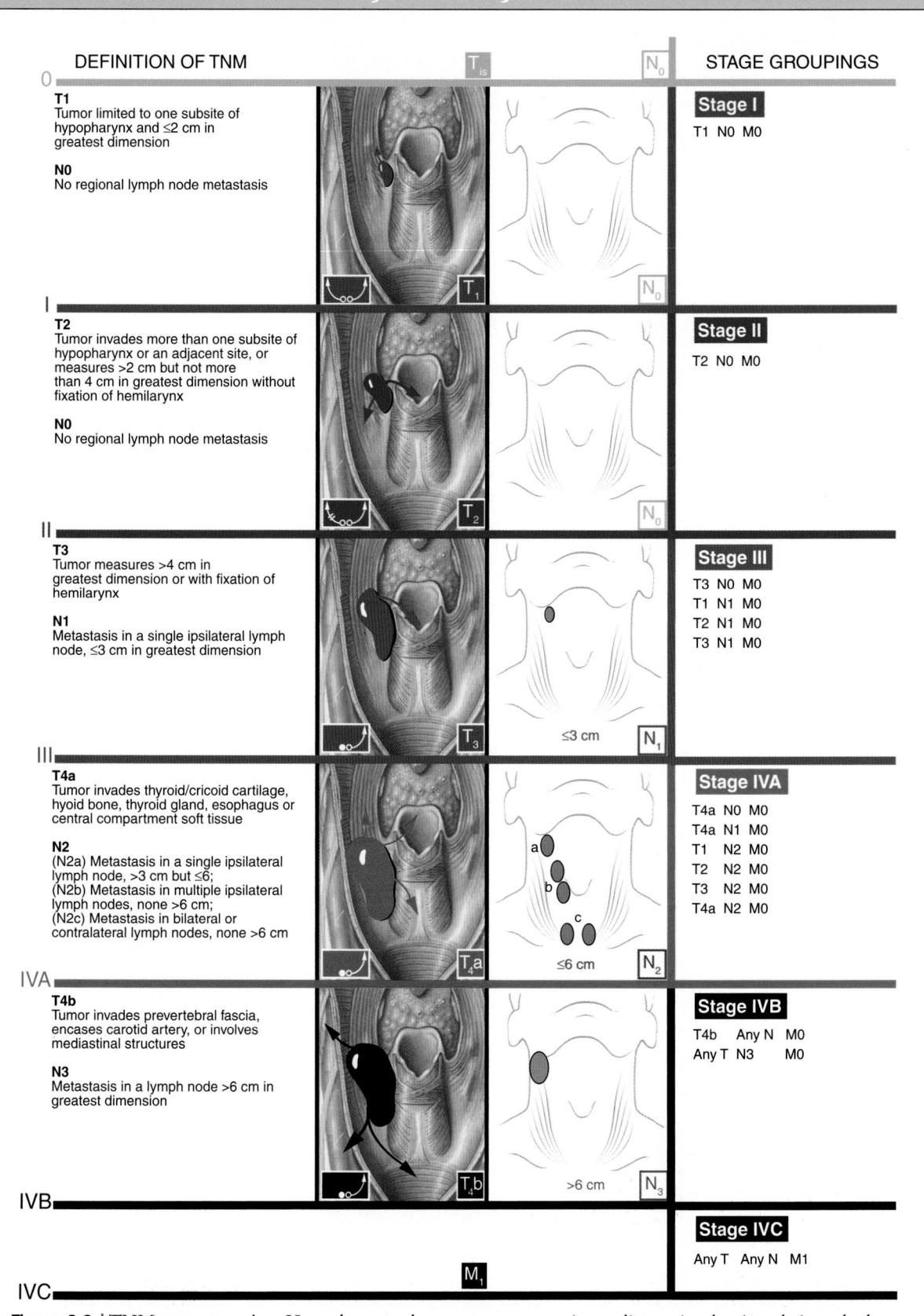

DEFINITION OF TNM

T1
Tumor limited to one subsite of hypopharynx and ≤2 cm in greatest dimension

N0
No regional lymph node metastasis

T2
Tumor invades more than one subsite of hypopharynx or an adjacent site, or measures >2 cm but not more than 4 cm in greatest dimension without fixation of hemilarynx

N0
No regional lymph node metastasis

T3
Tumor measures >4 cm in greatest dimension or with fixation of hemilarynx

N1
Metastasis in a single ipsilateral lymph node, ≤3 cm in greatest dimension

T4a
Tumor invades thyroid/cricoid cartilage, hyoid bone, thyroid gland, esophagus or central compartment soft tissue

N2
(N2a) Metastasis in a single ipsilateral lymph node, >3 cm but ≤6;
(N2b) Metastasis in multiple ipsilateral lymph nodes, none >6 cm;
(N2c) Metastasis in bilateral or contralateral lymph nodes, none >6 cm

T4b
Tumor invades prevertebral fascia, encases carotid artery, or involves mediastinal structures

N3
Metastasis in a lymph node >6 cm in greatest dimension

STAGE GROUPINGS

Stage I
T1 N0 M0

Stage II
T2 N0 M0

Stage III
T3 N0 M0
T1 N1 M0
T2 N1 M0
T3 N1 M0

Stage IVA
T4a N0 M0
T4a N1 M0
T1   N2 M0
T2   N2 M0
T3   N2 M0
T4a N2 M0

Stage IVB
T4b   Any N M0
Any T N3   M0

Stage IVC
Any T Any N M1

Figure 8.3 | TNM stage grouping. Hypopharyngeal cancers are aggressive malignancies that invade into the larynx and/or directly into cervical neck nodes. Vertical presentations of stage groupings, which follow same color code for cancer stage advancement, are organized in horizontal lanes: Stage 0, yellow; I, green; II, blue; III, purple; IVA, red; IVB, black. Definitions of TN on left and stage grouping on right.

T-ONCOANATOMY

ORIENTATION OF THREE-PLANAR ONCOANATOMY

The anatomic isocenter of the hypopharynx is at the C4–5 level. It is vertically in line with the anterior border of the ramus of the mandible and its inferior border anteriorly begins at level of the hyoid bone. The anterior bullet is the level of the hyoid bone to the left and right of midline (Fig. 8.4A) and the lateral bullet is just below the greater horns of the hyoid bone (Fig. 8.4B).

T-oncoanatomy

The hypopharynx is the lower continuation of the pharyngeal tube and is anatomically defined laterally and posteriorly by the middle and inferior constrictor muscles and anteriorly by the hyoid bone, thyroid, and cricoid cartilage (Fig. 8.5). If the larynx were postnasal, anatomy would be less complex and the oropharynx and hypopharynx functionally and structurally would be one. The descent of the larynx transforms the tube into a series of symmetrical gutters surrounding the larynx (Fig. 8.5).

- *Coronal view* (Fig. 8.5A): The hypopharynx is best understood anatomically from a posterior coronal view, obtained by separating the inferior constrictor muscles at the midline. The hypopharyngeal sphincters and the piriform recesses circumvent the larynx to lead food into the esophagus. The superior laryngeal nerve enters the larynx and can be trapped by piriform sinus cancers.

- *Sagittal plane* (Fig. 8.5B) allows identification of the postcricoid region and establishes the relationship to the larynx of the beginning of the trachea and the beginning of the esophagus.

- *Transverse plane* and a cross-section at C4–5 (Fig. 8.5C) basically identifies the intimate relationship of the pharyngeal tube to the cartilages, bones, and muscles in the neck. The carotid artery and its branches, as well as the jugular vein in the retropharyngeal space, has only cranial nerve X and the cervical sympathetics. Most of the neck volume is posterior to the prevertebral fascia, which contains the spinal cord and nerve trunks to form the brachial plexus.

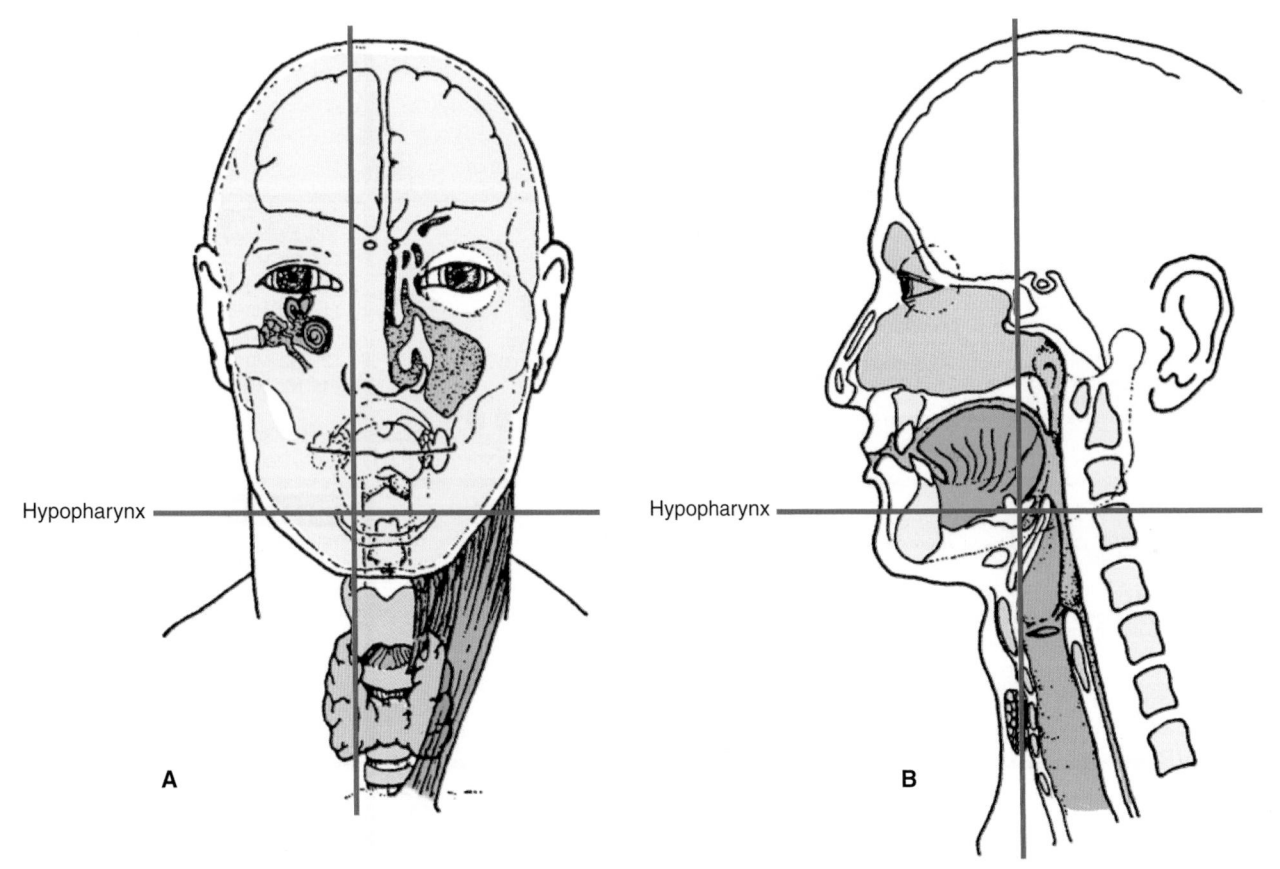

Hypopharynx

A

Hypopharynx

B

Figure 8.4 | Orientation of three-planar T-oncoanatomy. The anatomic isocenter is at the axial level at C4/C5. **A.** Coronal. **B.** Sagittal

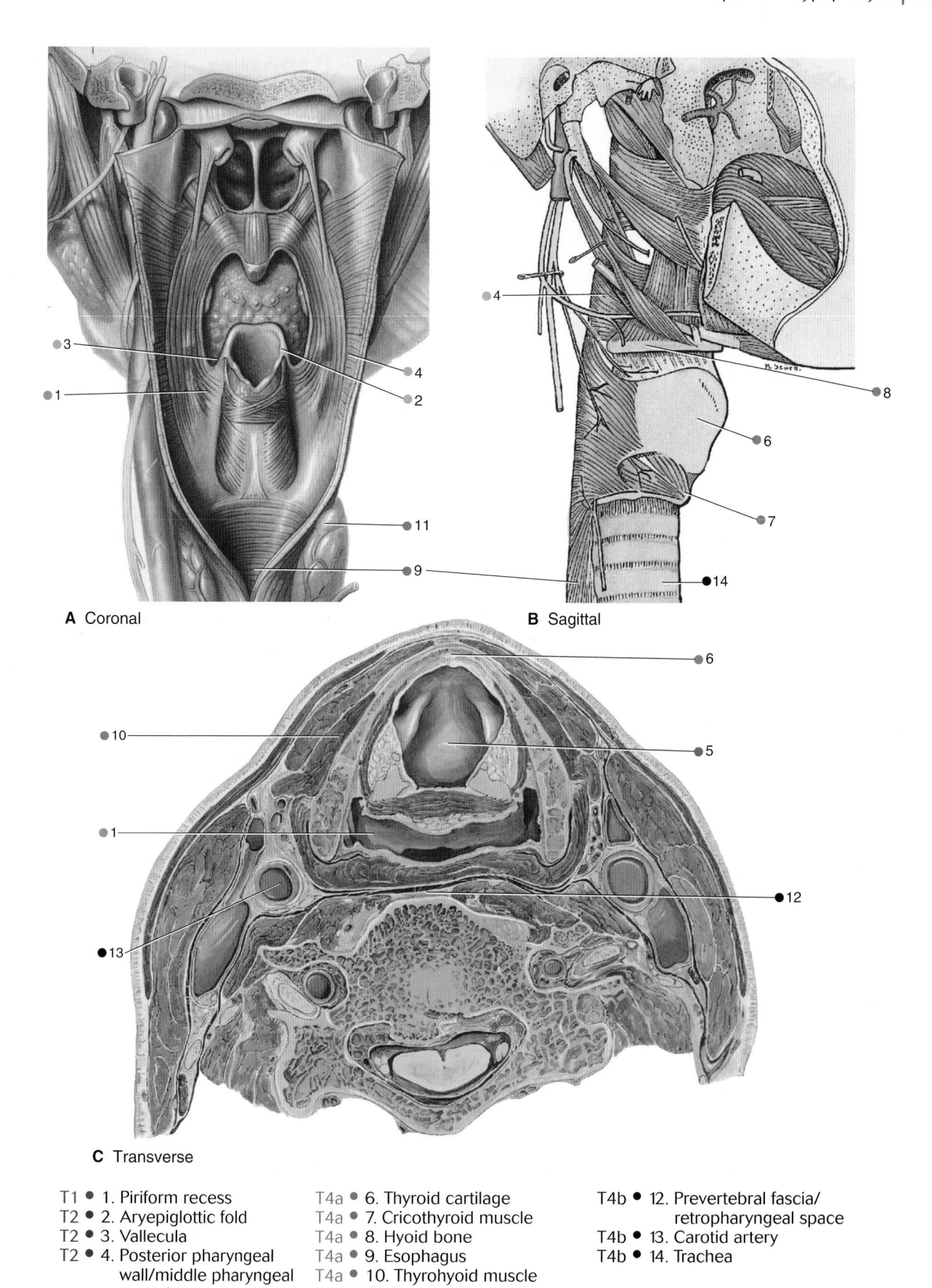

A Coronal

B Sagittal

C Transverse

T1 ● 1. Piriform recess
T2 ● 2. Aryepiglottic fold
T2 ● 3. Vallecula
T2 ● 4. Posterior pharyngeal
     wall/middle pharyngeal
     constrictor
T3 ● 5. Glottis

T4a ● 6. Thyroid cartilage
T4a ● 7. Cricothyroid muscle
T4a ● 8. Hyoid bone
T4a ● 9. Esophagus
T4a ● 10. Thyrohyoid muscle
T4a ● 11. Thyroid gland

T4b ● 12. Prevertebral fascia/
      retropharyngeal space
T4b ● 13. Carotid artery
T4b ● 14. Trachea

Figure 8.5 | T-oncoanatomy. The Color Code for the anatomic sites correlates with the color code for the stage group (Fig. 8.3) and patterns of spread (Fig. 8.2) and SIMLAP table (Table 8.2). Connecting the dots in similar colors will provide an appreciation for the 3D Oncoanatomy.

N-ONCOANATOMY AND M-ONCOANATOMY

N-ONCOANATOMY

The major lymph node drainage is into the jugular chain of nodes (Fig. 8.6; Table 8.4). The deep cervical node and posterior triangle nodes are also readily related to the hypopharynx. The vagus nerve (cranial nerve X) plays an important role in sensation and muscular innervation of the hypopharynx and larynx. Note that only the vagus nerve is left in the lower neck as the other cranial nerves terminate in the head with the exception of the spinal accessory XI nerve. The jugulo-omohyoid node is often the sentinel node for hypopharyngeal cancers. There is a high degree of lymph node involvement including the parapharyngeal and retropharyngeal nodes, as well as the jugulodigastric and jugulo-omohyoid nodes. The incidence and distribution of clinically negative

neck node (N0) Table 8.5A and clinically positive (N+) Table 8.5B according to AJCC levels (Fig. 8.7A,B).

M-ONCOANATOMY

Distant metastases are also possible because of the plexus of pharyngeal veins that drain into the jugular vein, and then into the superior vena cava, the right heart, and finally the lungs. The vascular supply of the pharynx arises from the external carotid. The carotid body and sinus located at the bifurcation of the common carotid is an arterial chemoreceptor and baroreceptor area, respectively (see Fig. 8.6).

The target organ for hypopharyngeal spread is classically the lung.

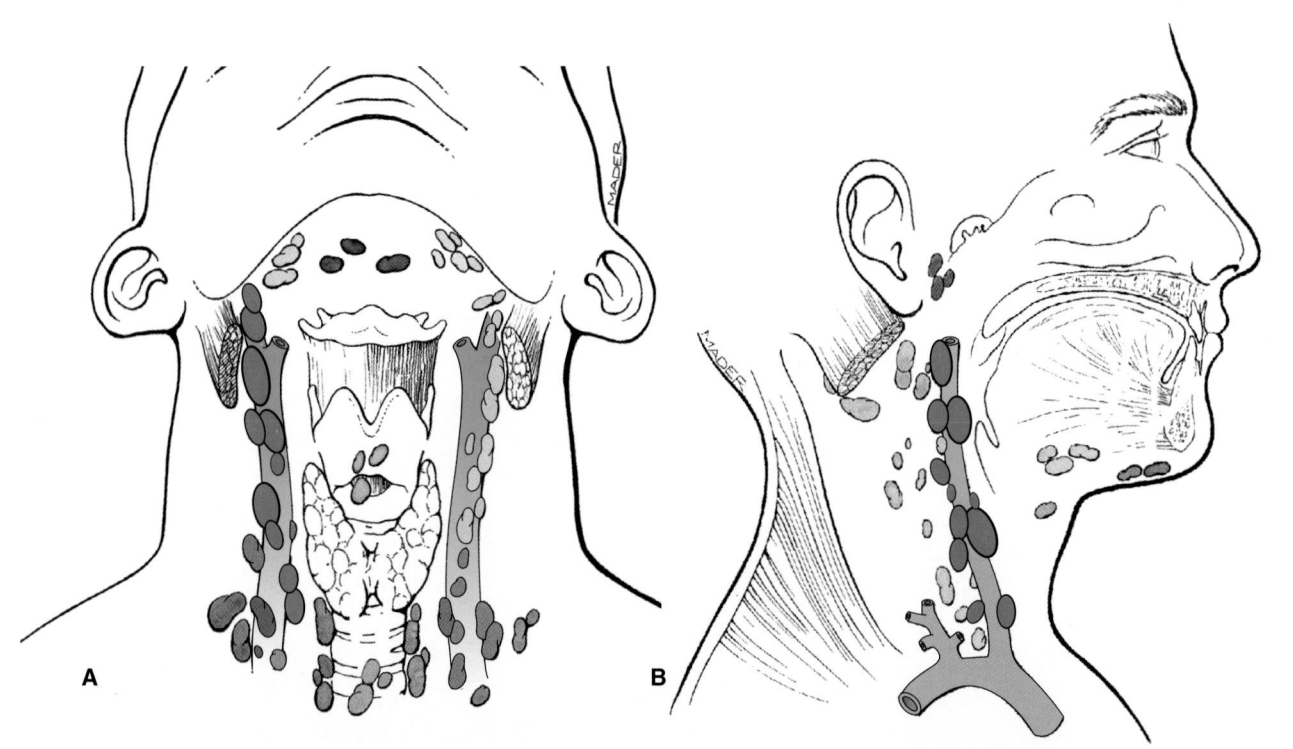

Figure 8.6 | N-oncoanatomy. The red node highlights the sentinel node, which is the jugulo-omohyoid node. **A.** Anterior view. **B.** Lateral view. **M-oncoanatomy** is determined by the right internal jugular vein, which joins with the right subclavian vein to form the right brachiocephalic vein, which drains into the superior vena cava on the right, and the left brachiocephalic vein, which drains into the superior vena cava and then the right side of the heart and then into the lung.

TABLE 8.4	Sentinel and Regional Nodes: Hypopharynx (Unilateral and Bilateral)	
	Level/Location of Node(s)	
S Sentinel Node	**Axial Level**	**AJCC Level**
S1 Jugulodigastric, superior/mid deep cervical	C4–5	II
R Regional Nodes		
R1 Jugulo-omohyoid, inferior deep cervical	C7	IV
R2 Retropharyngeal	C1	nI*
R3 Parotid nodes, retroparotidian space	C2–3	I

nl = not listed

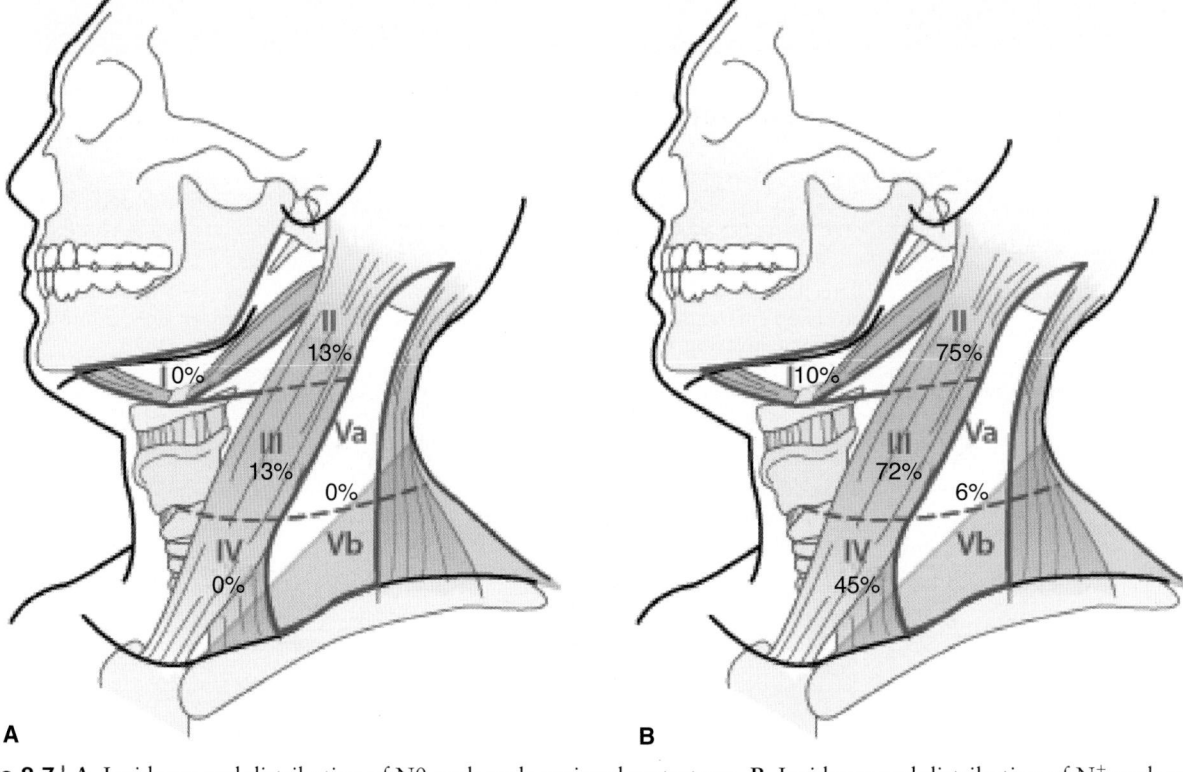

A

B

Figure 8.7 | A. Incidence and distribution of N0 neck node regional matastases. **B.** Incidence and distribution of N⁺ neck according to AJCC neck regions. Fig. 8.7A correlates with Table 8.5A. Fig. 8.7B correlates with Table 8.5B.

TABLE 8.5A	Incidence and Distribution of N0 Neck Node Regional Metastases

If neck nodes is N0 clinically then the incidence & distribution is as follows.

- I = 0%
- II = 13%
- III = 13%
- IV = 0%
- V = 0%

TABLE 8.5B	Incidence and Distribution of N⁺ Neck According to AJCC Neck Regions

Once the sentinel node is involved N+, the patterns of spread to the rest of the neck nodes at difference levels is due to collateralization of drainage both prograde and retrograde as well as contralateral spread. The neck node levels (%) involved:

Level I = 10%

Level II = 75%

Level III = 72%

Level IV = 45%

Level V = 6%

Incidence and Distribution of Distant Metastases

STAGING WORKUP

TABLE 8.6	Imaging Modalities and Strategies for Diagnosis and Staging for Head and Neck: Hypopharynx	
Modality	**Strategy**	**Recommended**
Primary Tumor and Nodes		
Computed tomography	Excellent for defining extent of primary depth of invasion enlargement of involved nodes. (Preferred for bone invasion.)	Yes—3–5 mm cuts, 3 mm for primary sites, 5 mm for neck.
Magnetic resonance imaging	Offers best 3D and 3-planar views of primary and nodes, especially soft tissue extensions. Gadolinium contrast for extensions and perineuronal spread.	Yes—≤4 cm slices Gd for intracranial and perineuronal spread.
Magnetic resonance spectroscopy	Provides metabolic and biochemical analysis of tumor, choline/creatinine ratio elevated in tumor vs. normal tissues.	No.
Positron emission tomography	Functional and metabolic imaging of ^{18}FDG is based on 2-deoxy modification, which inhibits the molecule from subsequent enzymatic conversion and is "metabolically trapped" in tumor cells.	No—potential exists for distinguishing recurrence from tissue necrosis.
Metastases		
Chest film	Search for metastases.	Yes.
Radionuclide scan	^{99m}Tc for bone metastases.	Yes—if symptomatic.

3D, three-dimensional; FDG, fluorodeoxyglucose.

RULES OF CLASSIFICATION AND STAGING

Clinical Staging and Imaging

For hypopharyngeal cancers, careful history taking, inspection, and palpations of the face and neck are essential. Testing all cranial nerves is critical. Both direct and indirect endoscopy are useful. Despite patient cooperation, pharyngeal cancers are inaccessible and imaging is important. To determine the true extent of primary hypopharyngeal cancers, imaging is essential. Magnetic resonance imaging (MRI) is superior to computed tomography (CT) in demonstrating soft tissue extension, skull base changes, and perineural invasion (see Table 8.6 and Fig. 8.8).

Pathologic Staging

The gross specimen should be evaluated for margins. Unresected gross residual tumor must be included and marked with clips. All resected lymph node specimens should describe size, number, and level of involved nodes and whether there is extracapsular spread. Specimens taken after radiation, chemotherapy, or both need to be so noted, but specimen shrinkages may occur up to 30% after resection itself. Designations pT and pN should be used after histopathologic evaluation. Perineural invasion deserves special notation.

Oncoimaging Annotations

- With hypopharyngeal carcinomas, cartilage invasion is often clinically occult and is therefore best detected by imaging. Submucosal extension is also better detected with imaging.

- All CT studies should be performed after contrast enhancement is administered by using a bolus technique.

- A collapsed (paralyzed) piriform sinus may mimic a tumor on both CT and MRI studies.

PROGNOSIS AND CANCER SURVIVAL

PROGNOSTIC FACTORS

The seventh edition of the AJCC Cancer Staging Manual lists the following prognostic factors for nasal ethmoid sinus cancers:

- Size of lymph nodes
- Extracapsular extension from lymph nodes for head and neck
- Head and neck lymph nodes levels I-III
- Head and neck lymph nodes levels IV-V
- Head and neck lymph nodes levels VI-VII
- Other lymph node group
- Clinical location of cervical nodes
- Extracapsular spread (ECS) clinical
- Extracapsular spread (ECS) pathologic
- Human papillomavirus (HPV) status
- Tumor thickness*

*The foregoing passage is from Edge SB, Byrd DR, and Compton CC, et al, *AJCC Cancer Staging Manual, 7th edition.* New York, Springer, 2010, p. 99.

CANCER STATISTICS AND SURVIVAL

Generally, cancers of the oral cavity, pharynx, and upper digestive passage account for 36,540 new cases per year. In addition, cancer of the larynx affects another 12,720 patients and thyroid cancers, 44,670.

Approximately 25% of head and neck cancer patients die annually, often due to other causes (Table 8.2). Long-term survival is exceptional in thyroid cancers, with only 1,500 deaths (5%). The improvement in oral cavity and pharyngeal tumors from 1950 to 2000 was modest at 14% and matches larynx at 15%. A multidisciplinary approach is vital, and normal tissue conservation and reconstructive techniques have both added greatly to quality of life. Unfortunately, this patient population abuses ethanol and nicotine, and it is difficult to change these habits. Persistence of smoking and drinking contributes to their demise, often from second malignant tumors in adjacent sites.

Specifically, hypopharyngeal cancers are found in advanced stages, particularly pyriform sinus and postcricoid cancers, with the poorest survival in head and neck sites at 20% to 25% at 5 years. Localized early cancers have a 5-year survival rate of 50% (Fig 8.9A and Fig 8.9B), whereas advanced malignancies hover in the 25% range.

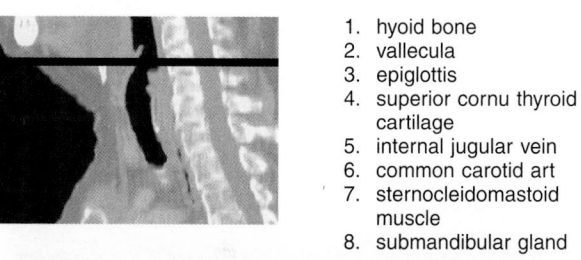

1. hyoid bone
2. vallecula
3. epiglottis
4. superior cornu thyroid cartilage
5. internal jugular vein
6. common carotid art
7. sternocleidomastoid muscle
8. submandibular gland

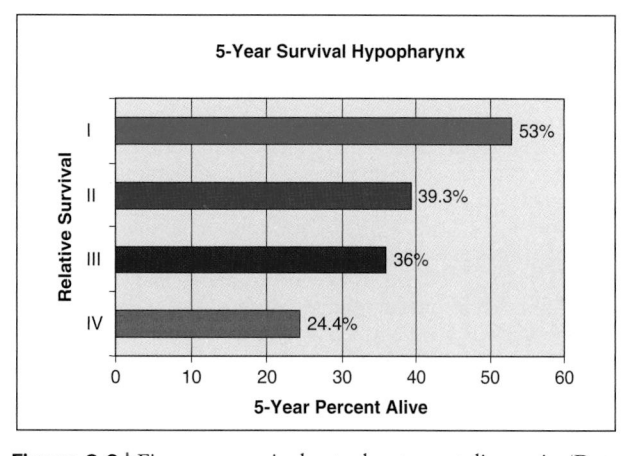

Figure 8.9 | Five-year survival rates by stage at diagnosis. (Data from Edge SB, Byrd DR, and Compton CC, et al, *AJCC Cancer Staging Manual, 7th edition.* New York, Springer, 2010.)

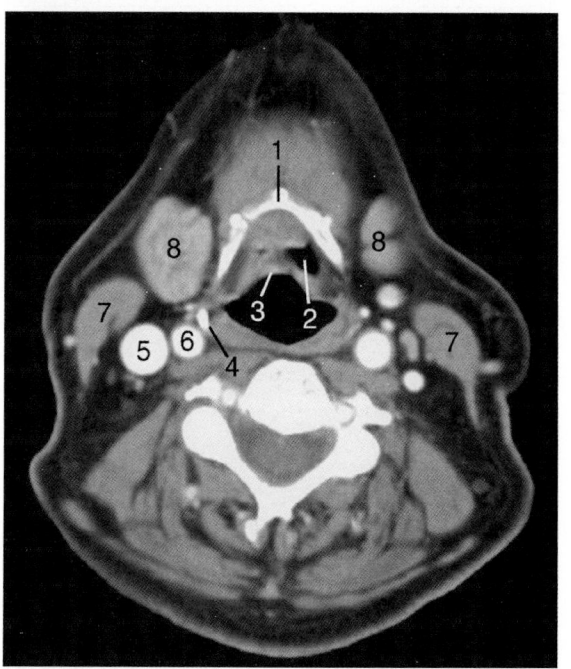

Figure 8.8 | Neck and Larynx—Axial CT scan. The CT/MRI transverse section can be correlated with the anatomy in Figure 8.5C as an assist to staging.

CHAPTER

9

Supraglottic Larynx

PERSPECTIVE, PATTERNS OF SPREAD, AND PATHOLOGY

The malignant gradient is in reference to the horizontal midplane through the true glottis. Cancers above have a better outcome and cancers below have a poorer prognosis.

PERSPECTIVE AND PATTERNS OF SPREAD

Cancers of the larynx are among the commonly occurring cancers in the upper respiratory passage and present the challenge of preservation of phonation. The larynx is a critical structure in the respiratory tract and is the major sphincter through which air enters and exits from the lung. It performs the essential function of closure to the airway entrance during deglutition. Once involved, laryngeal cancer can be an isolated nodule, but is often part of a field cancerization process due to habitual smoking. The likelihood of a recurrence or second primary in lung is inevitable if the host is either unwilling or unable to give up tobacco. Persistent hoarseness demands an otologic examination. The larynx is lined by pseudostratified ciliated columnar epithelium except on the superior surface of the epiglottis and vocal cords, which are covered by stratified squamous nonkeratinized epithelium. The malignant gradient is greater from anterior to posterior, from superior to inferior, and from medial to lateral. Most important is sparing of the vocal cords and voice preservation. A number of randomized studies have confirmed that chemoradiation regimens are able to yield comparable survival with laryngeal preservation versus radical laryngectomy.

Cancers arising in the different subsites of the larynx have patterns of spread that reflect the anatomy of a larynx in its development and function. The malignant gradient is in reference to the horizontal midplane through the true glottis. Cancers above have a less favorable outcome and cancers below have a better prognosis for readily apparent reasons relating to the ease of detection of supraglottic compared with subglottic cancers obscured by the vocal cords. Cancers of the true vocal cord are detected early because they alter voice quality and lead to hoarseness. They tend to arise from the free margin, but frequently cross to the opposite cord via the anterior commissure. The vocal cords are relatively avascular and are poor in lymphatics. Consequently, lymph node involvement and distant metastases are rare. Patterns of Spread are presented as a cancer crab that can invade in six basic directions Superior-Inferior, Medial-Lateral, Anterior-Posterior (SIMLAP) of adjacent anatomic sites (Fig. 9.2; Table 9.2).

PATHOLOGY

Most cancers are squamous cell cancer (Fig. 9.1), but a variety of malignancies can occur (Table 9.1). Vocal cord cancers tend to be well differentiated, and supraglottic and subglottic cancers tend to be more undifferentiated.

TABLE 9.1	Histopathologic Type: Common Cancers of the Glottic Larynx

Squamous Cell Carcinoma Microscopic Variants

Keratinizing; well differentiated; moderately well differentiated; poorly differentiated

Nonkeratinizing; anaplastic squamous carcinoma

Transitional cell carcinoma

Spindle cell squamous carcinoma

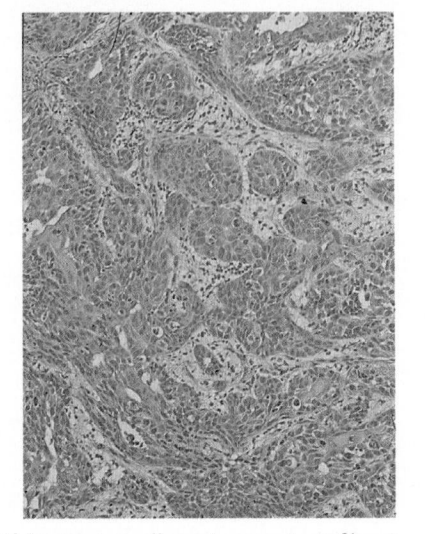

Figure 9.1 | Squamous cell carcinoma. An infiltrative neoplasm is composed of cohesive nests of tumor.

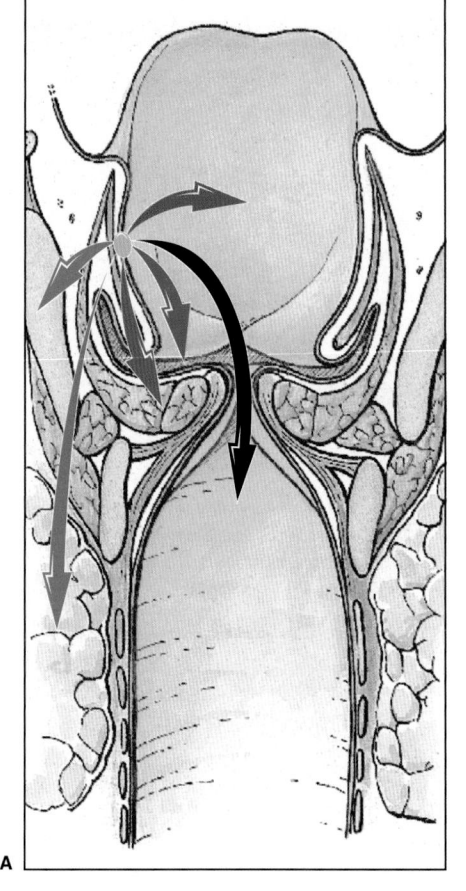 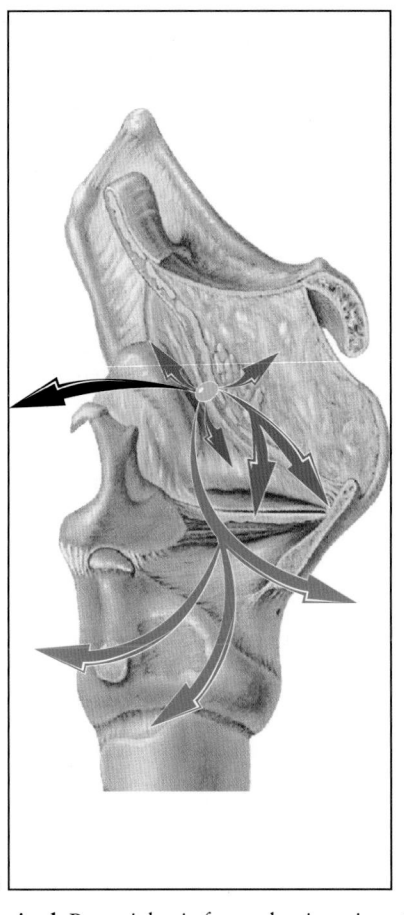

Figure 9.2 | Patterns of spread. A. Coronal. Transglottic invasion **B. Sagittal.** Pre-epiglottic fat pocket invasion allows for paralaryngeal spread. The primary cancer (supraglottic larynx) invades in various directions, which are color-coded vectors (*arrows*) representing stage of progression: Tis, yellow; T1, green; T2, blue; T3, purple; T4a, red; and T4b, black. The concept of visualizing patterns of spread to appreciate the surrounding anatomy is well demonstrated by the six directional pattern i.e. SIMLAP Table 9.2.

TABLE 9.2	SIMLAP*	
Supraglottis (False Cord)		
S	Deep, extrinsic muscles of the tongue	• T4a
I	True cord, glottis partial	• T2
	Fixed	• T3
	Trachea	• T4a
	Esophagus	• T4a
	Mediastinum	• T4b
M	Subsite without cord fixation	• T2
L	Thyroid gland	• T4a
A	Pre-epiglottic space	• T3
	Thyroid cartilage erosion	• T3
	Through thyroid cartilage	• T4a
	Soft tissues of the neck	• T4a
	Strap muscles	• T4a
P	Postcricoid area	• T3
	Prevertebral space	• T4b
	Carotid artery	• T4b

There are six basic directions or vectors (arrows): The six vectors of invasion are Superior, Inferior, Medial, Lateral, Anterior, and Posterior. The color-coded dots correlate the T stage with specific anatomic structure involved.

TNM STAGING CRITERIA

TNM STAGING CRITERIA

Supraglottic cancers can arise from a variety of different locations and tend to cause few symptoms until advanced (Fig. 9.3). The free surface of the epiglottis, false cords, and ventricles can all be involved. Transglottic cancers are usually advanced cancers that extend from the supraglottic area and invade the vocal cords and impair their function. These tumors spread rapidly because of the rich lymphatic network of this region. Bilateral neck nodes are often encountered. Another favored area of spread is the pre-epiglottic fat space.

Epilaryngeal cancers arise from the free border of the larynx where they come into contact with the pharynx. Cancers of the tip of the epiglottis can spill into the valleculae and can appear like a golf ball on a tee. Another common point of origin is the aryepiglottic fold, from which the cancer can spread into the supraglottic larynx or into the piriform sinus. Arytenoids cancers are unusual and obscure the normal double-beaded appearance of the posterior cartilages of the larynx.

Subglottic cancers, in terms of prognosis, are worse than other types. This is probably due to their tendency to invade the trachea and to reach a more advanced state before detection.

The larynx was initially staged with the development of the TNM system and appeared in the joint first edition of the American Joint Committee on Cancer/International Union Against Cancer guidelines (AJCC/UICC) (1978). The basis of progression of laryngeal cancers is related to their spread patterns to subsites (T2) as well as advancement from any one major site: glottic, supraglottic, subglottic to another, T2 if cord mobility is preserved. Loss of cord mobility indicates T3.

SUMMARY OF CHANGES SEVENTH EDITION AJCC

The TNM stages according to the 7th Edition of AJCC are illustrated in color code of advancement (Fig. 9.3). T4 lesions have been divided into T4a (moderately advanced local disease) and T4b (very advanced local disease), leading to the stratification of Stage IV into Stage IVA (moderately advanced local/regional disease), Stage IVB (very advanced local/regional disease), and Stage IVC (distant metastatic disease).

The TNM Staging Matrix is color coded for identification of Stage Group once T and N stages are determined (Table 9.3).

TABLE 9.3	Stage Summary Matrix				
	Stage T1	Stage T2	Stage T3	Stage T4a	Stage T4b
N0	I	II	III	IVA	IVB
N1	III	III	III	IVA	IVB
N2	IVA	IVA	IVA	IVA	IVB
N3	IVB	IVB	IVB	IVB	IVB
M1	IVC	IVC	IVC	IVC	IVC

- *T stage* determines stage group
  - T1 = I, T2 + II, T3 = III, T4 = IV
- *N stage* N1 = T3 and then progresses as T stage progresses
  - N1 = T3, N2 = T4a, N3 = T4b
- *M stage* is a separate stage
  - M1 = Stage IVC

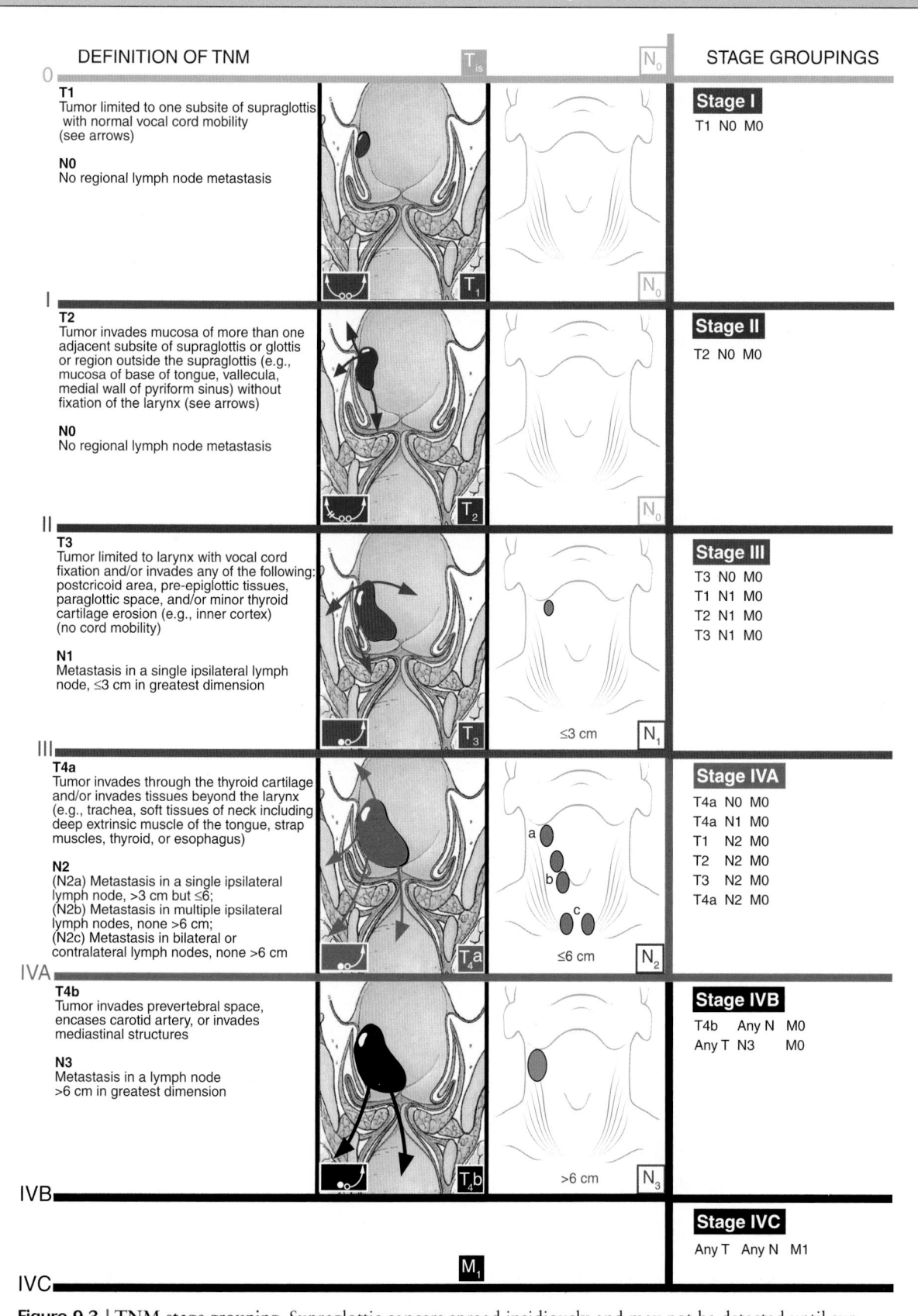

Figure 9.3 | TNM stage grouping. Supraglottic cancers spread insidiously and may not be detected until surrounding structures are invaded as vocal cords or spill into piriform fossa. Vertical presentations of stage groupings, which follow the same color code for cancer stage advancement, are organized in horizontal lanes: Stage 0, yellow; I, green; II, blue; III, purple; IVA, red; and IVB, black. Definitions of TN on left and stage grouping on right. Note inferior box on T-oncoanatomy provides a key to vocal cord mobility.

T-ONCOANATOMY

ORIENTATION OF THREE-PLANAR ONCOANATOMY

The anatomic isocenter of the supraglottic larynx is at the C5 level. The anterior surface bullet is at the level of the thyroid cartilage notch (Fig. 9.4A) and the lateral surface bullet is at the same level anterior to the greater horn of the thyroid cartilage (Fig. 9.4B).

T-oncoanatomy

The introduction to three-dimensional planar view of the larynx is best appreciated from the posterior coronal view with the constrictor musculature split.

- *Coronal plane* (Fig. 9.5A): The larynx is divided into three parts: (i) supraglottis, (ii) glottis, and (iii) subglottis; these three parts are known as the vestibule, ventricle (glottis), and infraglottic cavity, respectively. The epiglottis is readily visualized at its vestibule. The opening of the larynx, referred to as the aditus or the superior laryngeal aperture, can be traced from the epiglottis to the arytenoids. The aryepiglottic folds start at the free edge of the epiglottis and terminate at the corniculate and arytenoid cartilages. The

false cords and the true cords are separated by the ventricle. The true cords act as a sphincter that closes off the airway.

- *Sagittal plane* (Fig. 9.5B): The cartilaginous skeleton of the larynx consists of the epiglottis, thyroid, cricoid, arytenoids, cuneiform and corniculate cartilages and hyoid bone. A set of fine membranes and muscles hold this cartilage together, forming a rigid structure that is not easily destroyed by cancer invasion. The crieothyroid muscle tenses the vocal cords. The intrinsic muscles include the posterior and lateral cricoarytenoid, thyroarytenoids, vocalis, thyroepiglottis, and aryepiglottis. The essential function of these muscles is to open and close the glottis during breathing and to regulate cord tension during speaking. The true cords and the false cords are separated by a ventricle. The pre-epiglottic fat-filled space can be readily infiltrated from a cancer in the supraglottic region at its base because the epiglottic cartilage sits as an upside-down paddle. These features are best appreciated in the coronal and sagittal views.

- *Transverse view* (Fig. 9.5C): The axial view illustrates the paralaryngeal space between the thyroid and epiglottal cartilage and the position of the larynx to the pharynx. The prevertebral space is separated from the larynx by the hypopharynx and the prevertebral fascia is rarely invaded by true laryngeal malignancies.

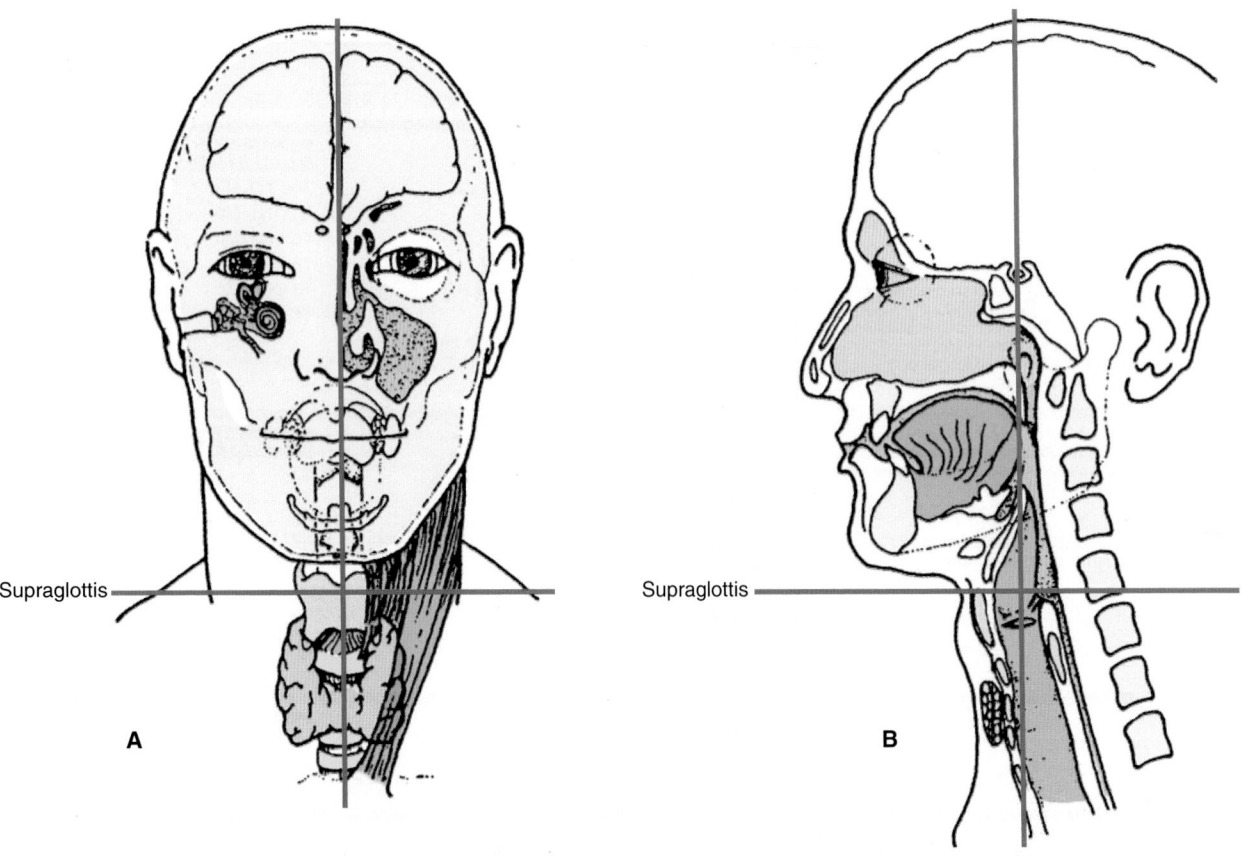

Figure 9.4 | Orientation of three-planar T-oncoanatomy. The anatomic isocenter is at the axial level at C5. **A.** Coronal. **B.** Sagittal.

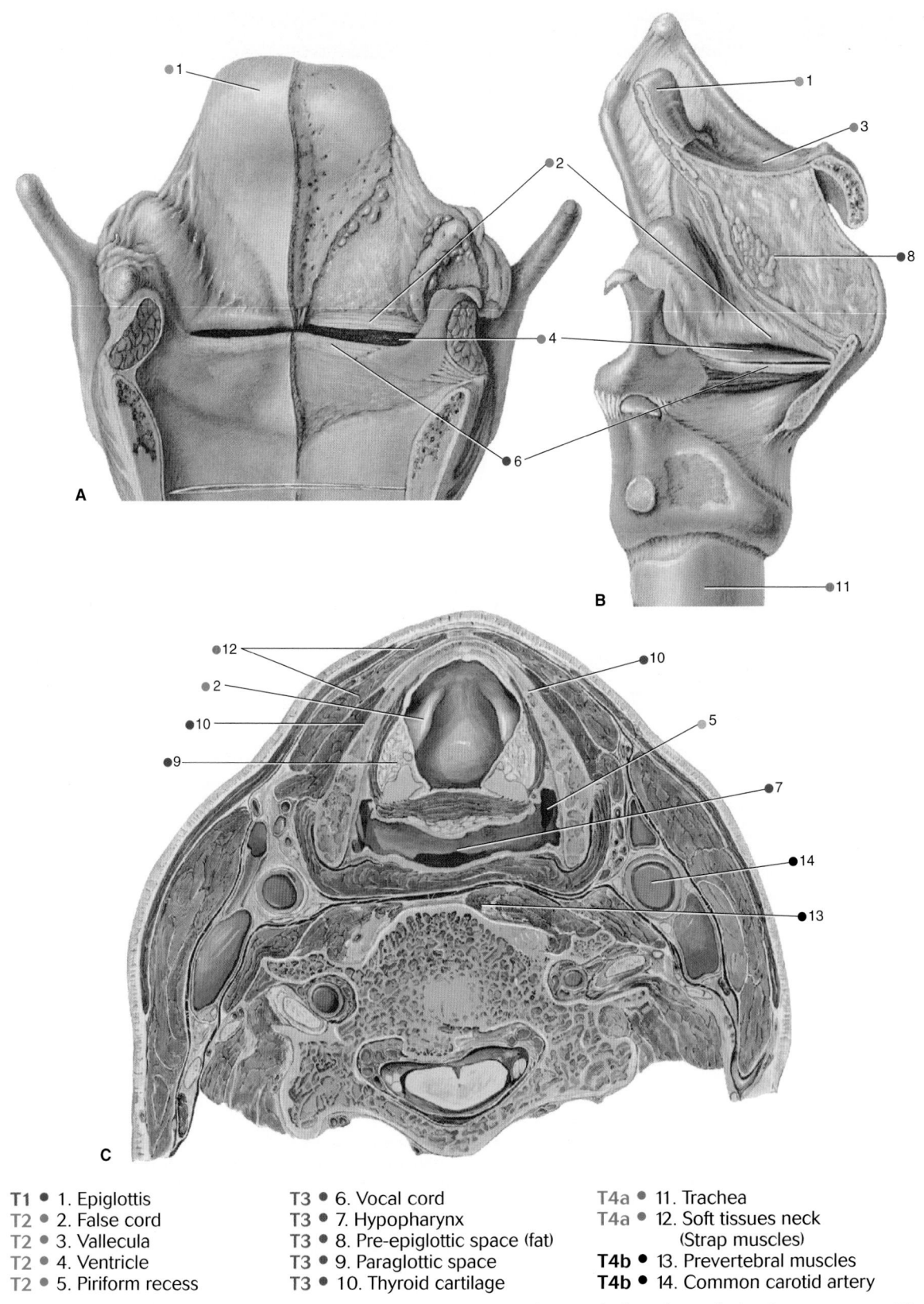

Figure 9.5 | T-oncoanatomy. The Color Code for the anatomic sites correlates with the color code for the stage group (Fig. 9.3) and patterns of spread (Fig. 9.2) and SIMLAP tables (Table 9.2). Connecting the dots in similar colors will provide an appreciation for the 3D Oncoanatomy.

T1	1. Epiglottis	T3	6. Vocal cord	T4a	11. Trachea
T2	2. False cord	T3	7. Hypopharynx	T4a	12. Soft tissues neck
T2	3. Vallecula	T3	8. Pre-epiglottic space (fat)		(Strap muscles)
T2	4. Ventricle	T3	9. Paraglottic space	T4b	13. Prevertebral muscles
T2	5. Piriform recess	T3	10. Thyroid cartilage	T4b	14. Common carotid artery

N-ONCOANATOMY AND M-ONCOANATOMY

N-ONCOANATOMY

Each segment of the larynx drains to a different sentinel node (Fig. 9.6; Table 9.4). The glottis or true vocal cords are not rich in lymphatics and drain to pretracheal or paralaryngeal lymph nodes. The supraglottis is richer in lymphatics and vascularization, with drainage favoring midjugular and jugulodigastric nodes. Infraglottic cancers drain to deeper cervical nodes, the jugulo-omohyoid, and even the scalene nodes. The incidence and distribution of clinically negative neck nodes (N0) Table 9.5A and clinically positive (N+) Table 9.5B according to AJCC levels (Fig. 8.7A,B).

M-ONCOANATOMY

The venous drainage of the larynx is by way of laryngeal veins into the internal jugular vein and ultimately into the superior vena cava. Metastases are most likely to target the lung.

The target organ for supraglottic spread is classically the lung (Fig. 9.7B).

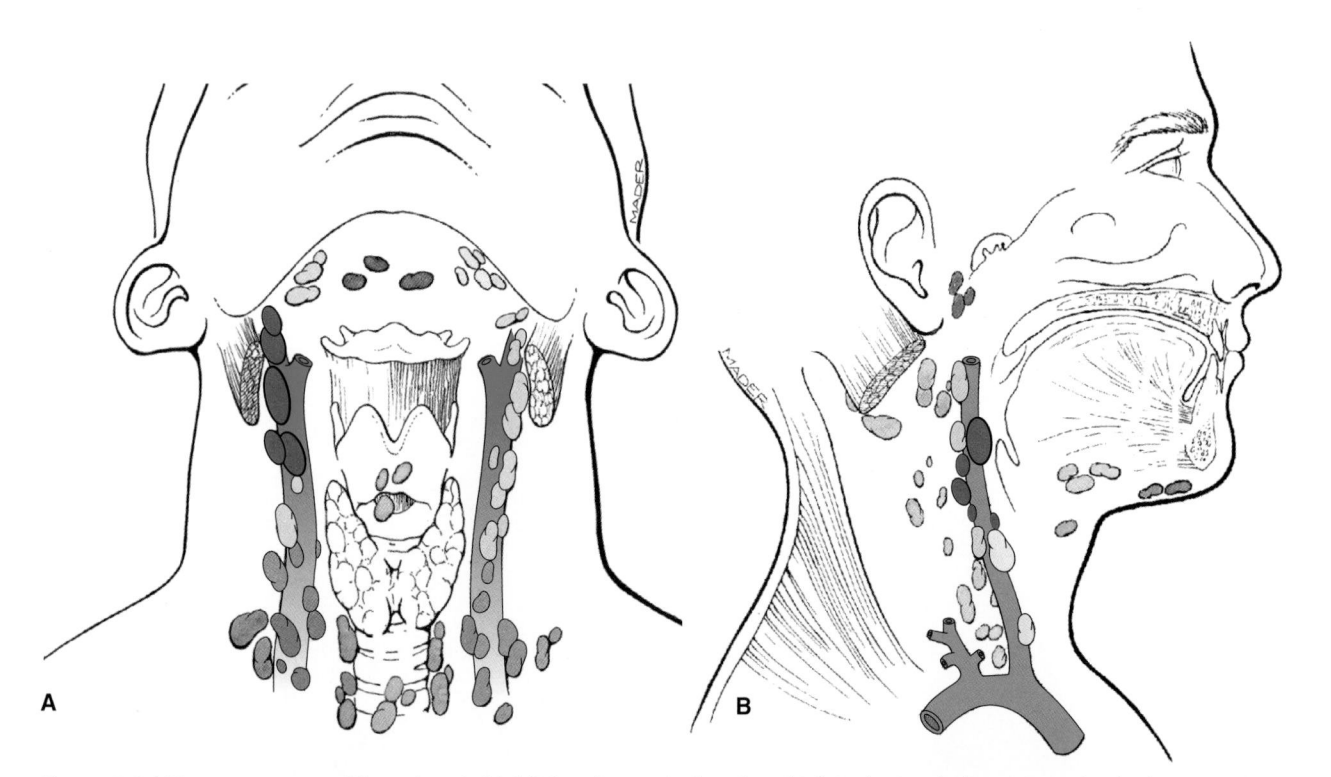

Figure 9.6 | N-oncoanatomy. The red node highlights the sentinel node, which is the jugulodigastric node. **A.** Anterior view. **B.** Lateral view. **M-oncoanatomy** is determined by the right internal jugular vein which joins with the right subclavian vein to form the right brachiocephalic vein, which drains into the superior vena cava on the right, and the left brachiocephalic vein, which drains into the superior vena cava and then the right side of the heart and then into lung.

TABLE 9.4	Sentinel and Regional Nodes: Supraglottic Larynx (Unilateral and Bilateral)		
		Level/Location of Node(s)	
S Sentinel Node		**Axial Level**	**AJCC Level**
S1 Jugulogastric, superior/mid deep cervical		C4–5	II
R Regional Nodes			
R1 Prelaryngeal		C5	VI
R2 Jugulo-omohyoid, inferior deep cervical		C7	IV
R3 Retropharyngeal		C1	nI*

*not listed

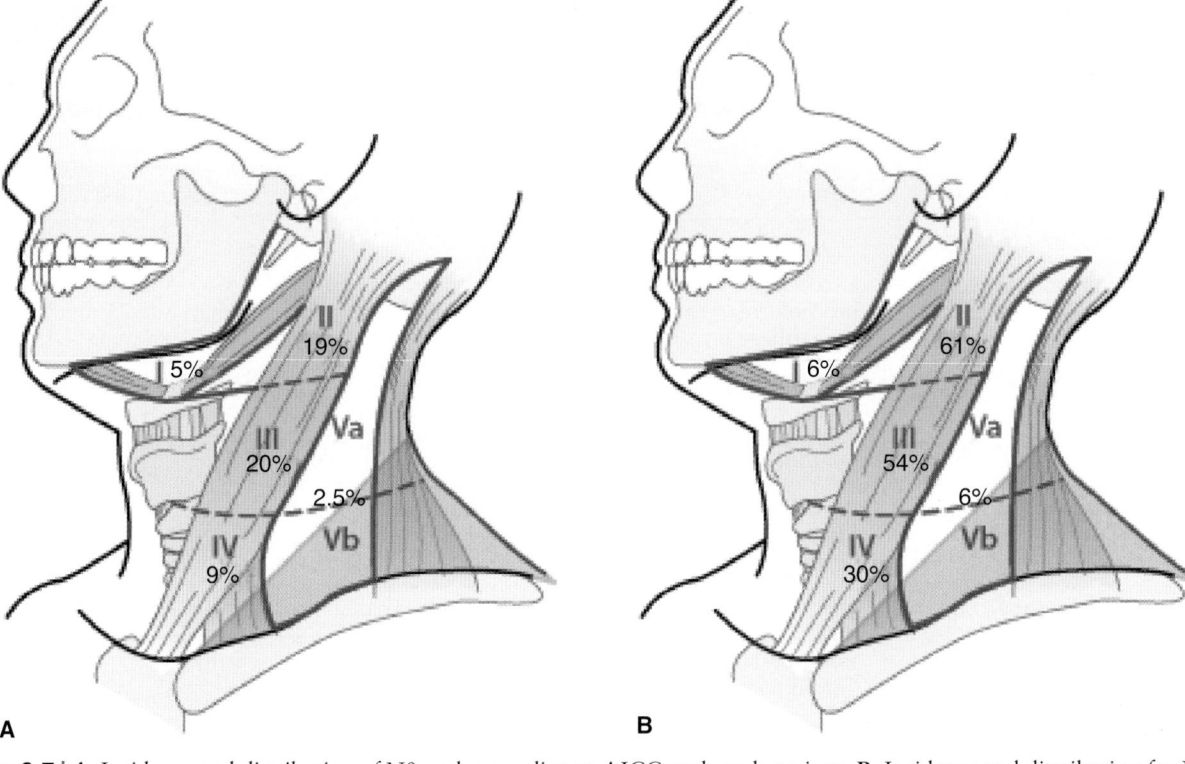

Figure 9.7 | **A.** Incidence and distribution of N0 neck according to AJCC neck node regions. **B.** Incidence and distribution for N⁺ neck according to AJCC neck regions.

TABLE 9.5A	Incidence and Distribution for N0 Neck According to AJCC Neck Node Regions

- I = 5%
- II = 19%
- III = 20%
- IV = 9%
- V = 2.5%

TABLE 9.5B	Incidence and Distribution for N+ Neck According to AJCC Neck Regions

Once the sentinel node is involved, the patterns of spread to the rest of the neck nodes at difference levels is due to collateralization of drainage both prograde and retrograde as well as to contralateral spread. The neck node levels (%) involved:

Level I = 6%

Level II = 61%

Level III = 54%

Level IV = 30%

Level V = 6%

Incidence and Distribution of Distant Metastases

STAGING WORKUP

TABLE 9.6	Imaging Modalities and Strategies for Diagnosis and Staging for Head and Neck: Supraglottic Larynx	
Modality	**Strategy**	**Recommended**
Primary Tumor and Nodes		
Computed tomography	Excellent for defining extent of primary depth of invasion enlargement of involved nodes. (Preferred for cartilage invasion.)	Yes—3–5 mm cuts, 3 mm for primary sites, 5 mm for neck.
Magnetic resonance imaging	Offers best 3D and 3-planar views of primary and nodes, especially soft tissue extensions. Gadolinium contrast for extensions and perineuronal spread. (Not for cartilage invasion.)	Yes—$\leq$4 cm slices Gd for intracranial and perineuronal spread.
Magnetic resonance spectroscopy	Provides metabolic and biochemical analysis of tumor, choline/creatinine ratio elevated in tumor vs. normal tissues.	No.
Positron emission tomography	Functional and metabolic imaging of ^{18}FDG is based on 2-deoxy modification, which inhibits the molecule from subsequent enzymatic conversion and is "metabolically trapped" in tumor cells.	No—potential exists for distinguishing cancer and its extensions.
Single photon emission computed tomography	Thallium-201 is used to detect tumor recurrence vs. normal tissue imaging, especially central nervous system.	No—high uptake normally in salivary and thyroid glands.
Metastases		
Chest film	Search for metastases.	Yes.
Radionuclide scan	^{99m}Tc for bone metastases.	Yes—if symptomatic.

3D, three-dimensional; FDG, fluorodeoxyglucose.

RULES OF CLASSIFICATION AND STAGING

Clinical Staging and Imaging

Assessment of the larynx in its three compartments—supraglottis, glottis, and infraglottis—is optimally performed with fiberoptic laryngoscope and often requires general anesthesia, which is advised often after completion of diagnostic imaging studies. Determining vocal cord motion, either partial or complete paralysis, is difficult; the normal cord can cross over to meet the involved cord. Imaging studies do not supplant endoscopy and are viewed as complementary. Distinction between the three compartments is essential to staging. Computed tomography (CT) (Fig. 9.8) and magnetic resonance imaging (MRI) are often complementary (see Table 9.6).

Pathologic Staging

The gross specimen should be evaluated for margins. Unresected gross residual tumor must be included and marked with clips. All resected lymph node specimens should describe size, number, and level of involved nodes and whether there is extracapsular spread. Specimens taken after radiation, chemotherapy, or both need to be noted; specimen shrinkages may occur up to 30% after resection itself. Designations pT and pN should be used after histopathologic evaluation. Perineural invasion deserves special notation.

Oncoimaging Annotations

- After contrast administration, cross-section CT studies of the larynx should be performed, extending from C1 to the thoracic inlet.

- MRI should be performed before and after gadolinium enhancement.

- Extralaryngeal tumor spread can cause cartilage sclerosis, erosion, and lysis, suggestive of cartilaginous cancer invasion on CT.

- A positive diagnosis of cartilage invasion on MRI should be made with caution because the positive predictive value of the altered signal behavior as a sign of invasion is low.

- Pretreatment CT imaging is predictive of local tumor control in patients treated with definitive radiation therapy. Tumor diameters of less than 2 cm have a high likelihood of local control, whereas tumor diameters greater than 2 cm have only a 50% chance of control.

- Both positron emission tomography with fluorine-18-labeled-deoxy-glucose and thallium-201 single photon emission computed tomography have useful potential in differentiating posttreatment radiation changes from recurrent tumor.

PROGNOSIS AND CANCER SURVIVAL

PROGNOSTIC FACTORS

The seventh edition of the AJCC Cancer Staging Manual lists the following prognostic factors for nasal ethmoid sinus cancers:

- Size of lymph nodes
- Extracapsular extension from lymph nodes for head and neck
- Head and neck lymph nodes levels I-III
- Head and neck lymph nodes levels IV-V
- Head and neck lymph nodes levels VI-VII
- Other lymph node group
- Clinical location of cervical nodes
- Extracapsular spread (ECS) clinical
- Extracapsular spread (ECS) pathologic
- Human papillomavirus (HPV) status
- Tumor thickness*

*The foregoing passage is from Edge SB, Byrd DR, and Compton CC, et al, *AJCC Cancer Staging Manual, 7th edition.* New York, Springer, 2010, p. 99.

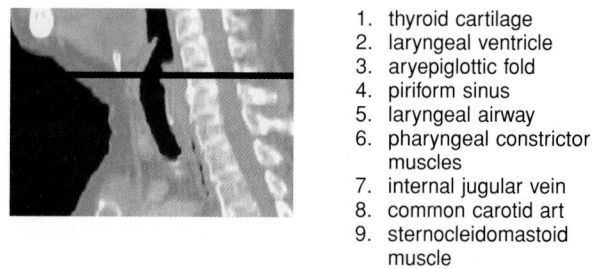

1. thyroid cartilage
2. laryngeal ventricle
3. aryepiglottic fold
4. piriform sinus
5. laryngeal airway
6. pharyngeal constrictor muscles
7. internal jugular vein
8. common carotid art
9. sternocleidomastoid muscle
10. external jugular vein
11. vertebral body
12. vertebral art

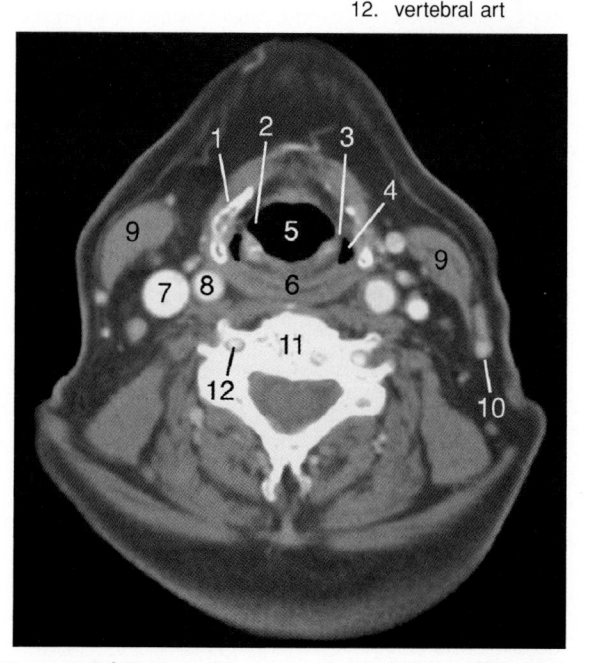

Figure 9.8 | Neck and Larynx—Axial CT scan. The CT/MRI transverse section can be correlated with the anatomy in Figure 9.5C as an assist to staging.

CANCER STATISTICS AND SURVIVAL

Generally, cancers of the oral cavity, pharynx, and upper digestive passage account for 36,540 new cases each year. In addition, cancer of the larynx affects another 12,720 patients and thyroid cancers, 44,670.

Approximately 25% of head and neck cancer patients die annually, often due to other causes. Long-term survival in thyroid cancers is exceptional, with only 1,500 deaths (5%). The improvement in oral cavity and pharyngeal tumors from 1950 to 2000 was modest at 14% and matches larynx at 15%. A multidisciplinary approach is vital, and normal tissue conservation and reconstructive techniques have both added greatly to quality of life. Unfortunately, this patient population abuses ethanol and nicotine and it is difficult to change these habits. Persistence of smoking and drinking contributes to their demise, often from second malignant tumors in adjacent sites.

Specifically, laryngeal cancers are a more favorable site in head and neck cancers because hoarseness allows for early detection. With early detection, stage I glottic cancers have 95% survival at 5 years and overall stages at 85%. Success in advanced stages in both survival and preservation of voice is due to chemoradiation regimens, which yield high complete response rates (i.e. 50% 5 years survival and somewhat better for stages I and II).

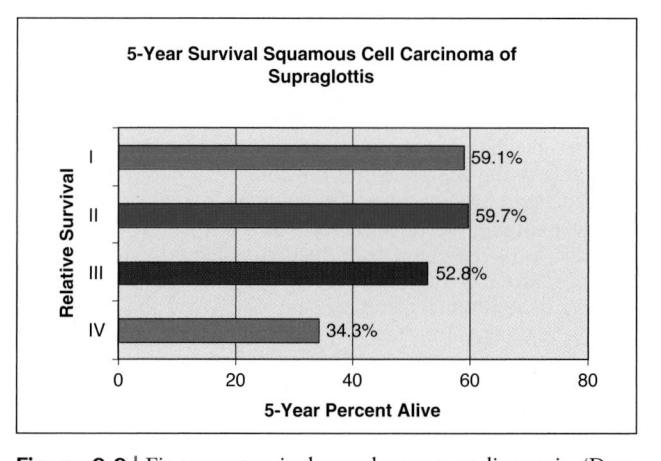

Figure 9.9 | Five-year survival rates by stage at diagnosis. (Data from Edge SB, Byrd DR, and Compton CC, et al, *AJCC Cancer Staging Manual, 7th edition.* New York, Springer, 2010.)

Glottic and Subglottic Larynx

PERSPECTIVE, PATTERNS OF SPREAD, AND PATHOLOGY

The malignant gradient is vertical in reference to the horizontal midplane through the true glottis; it is greater above and below the vocal cords.

PERSPECTIVE AND PATTERNS OF SPREAD

Cancers of the larynx are among the most commonly occurring cancers in the upper respiratory passage and present the challenge of preservation of phonation. The larynx is a critical structure in the respiratory tract and is the major sphincter through which air enters and exits from the lung. It performs the essential function of closure to the airway entrance during deglutition. Once involved the laryngeal cancer can be an isolated nodule, but is often part of a field cancerization process due to habitual smoking. The likelihood of a recurrence or second primary in lung is inevitable if the host is either unwilling or unable to give up tobacco. Persistent hoarseness demands an otologic examination.

The malignant gradient is from anterior to posterior, from superior to inferior, and from medial to lateral. Most important is sparing of the vocal cords and voice preservation. A number of randomized studies have confirmed that chemoradiation regimens are able to yield comparable survival with laryngeal preservation versus radical laryngectomy.

Cancers arising in the different subsites of the larynx have patterns of spread that reflect the anatomy of a larynx in its development and function. The malignant gradient is in reference to the horizontal midplane through the true glottis. Cancers above have

a favorable outcome and cancers below have a better prognosis for readily apparent reasons relating to the ease of detection of supraglottic compared to subglottic cancers that are obscured by the vocal cords. Cancers of the true vocal cord are detected early because they alter voice quality and lead to hoarseness. They tend to arise from the free margin, but frequently cross to the opposite cord via the anterior commissure. The vocal cords are relatively avascular and are poor in lymphatics. Consequently, lymph node involvement and distant metastases are rare.

Subglottic cancers are very uncommon because inhaling carcinogens (i.e., smoking tobacco) results in exposure of supraglottis and glottis to a larger degree. The subglottis is a relatively protected site.

A true subglottic cancer needs to arise a centimeter below the vocal cords or glottis and invade the cricoid cartilage predominantly because there is not a muscle layer and the mucosa is juxtaposed to the cartilage. Subglottic origin is clinically obscured by the vocal cords and would become symptomatic by invading the glottis. Clinically, a transglottic cancer would be interpreted to be a vocal cord cancer unless the tumor bulk was mainly in the region below the glottis. Most subglottic cancers, when discovered, tend to be bilateral and circumferential. Patterns of Spread are presented as a cancer crab that can invade in six basic directions Superior-Inferior, Medial-Lateral, Anterior-Posterior (SIMLAP) of adjacent anatomic sites (Fig. 10.2; Table 10.2).

TABLE 10.1	Histopathologic Type: Common Cancers of the Glottic Larynx

Squamous Cell Carcinoma Microscopic Variants

Keratinizing; well differentiated; moderately well differentiated; poorly differentiated

Nonkeratinizing; anaplastic squamous carcinoma

Transitional cell carcinoma

Spindle cell squamous carcinoma

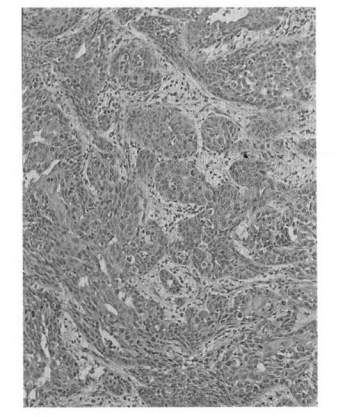

Figure 10.1 | Squamous cell carcinoma. An infiltrative neoplasm is composed of cohesive nests of tumor.

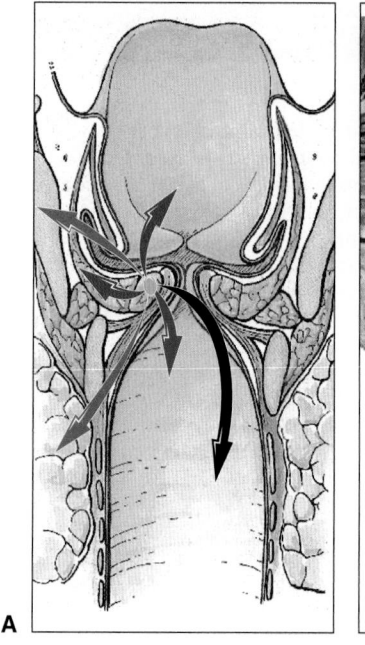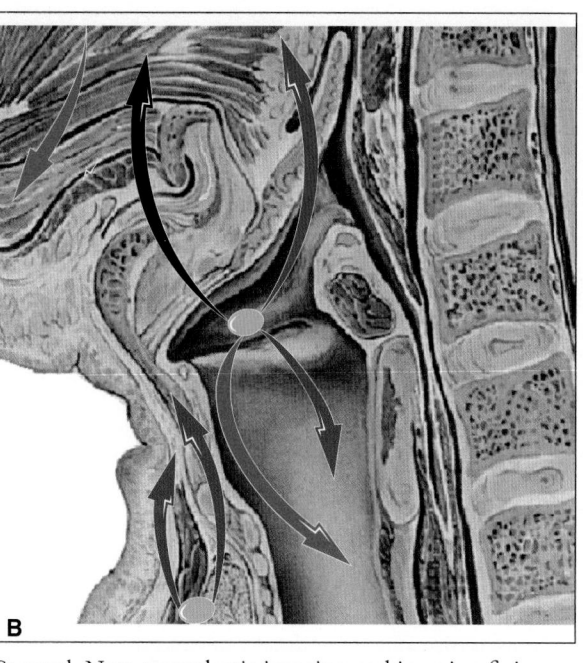

A

B

Figure 10.2 | Patterns of spread. A. Coronal. Note transglottic invasion and invasion fixing cord **B.** Sagittal. Note invasion of pre-epiglottic fat pocket invasion and subglottic extension. The primary cancer (glottic larynx) invades in various directions, which are color-coded vectors (*arrows*) representing stage of progression: Tis, yellow; T1, green; T2, blue; T3, purple; T4a, red; and T4b, black. The concept of visualizing patterns of spread to appreciate the surrounding anatomy is well demonstrated by the six directional pattern i.e. SIMLAP Table 10.2.

PATHOLOGY

The larynx is lined by pseudostratified ciliated columnar epithelium except on the superior surface of the epiglottis and vocal cords, which are covered by stratified squamous, nonker-atinized epithelium (Fig. 10.1). Most cancers are squamous cell cancers but a variety of malignancies can occur (Table 10.1). Vocal cord cancers tend to be well differentiated and supraglottic; subglottic cancers tend to be more undifferentiated.

TABLE 10.2	SIMLAP*	
Glottis (True Cord)		
S	Supraglottis, cord mobility impaired	• T2
	Deep extrinsic muscle tongue	• T4a
I	Subglottis, cord mobility impaired	• T2
	Esophagus	• T4a
M	Other true cord	• T1b
L	Paraglottic space	• T3
	Cord fixed	• T3
	Thyroid lobe	• T4a
	Carotid artery	• T4b
A	Thyroid cartilage erosion	• T3
	Through thyroid cartilage	• T4a
	Soft tissues, strap muscles neck	• T4a
P	Prevertebral space	• T4b
	Mediastinum	• T4b

*There are six basic directions or vectors (arrows): The six vectors of invasion are Superior, Inferior, Medial, Lateral, Anterior, and Posterior. The color-coded dots correlate the T stage with specific anatomic structure involved.

TNM STAGING CRITERIA

TNM STAGING CRITERIA

Glottic cancers are the most common laryngeal cancers and are three times more common than others. Glottic cancers are most often confined to the true cords along its anterior free border. However, the cancerous nodule usually is part of a field cancerization and is an alert signal to stop smoking. To halt future cancers from developing elsewhere in the respiratory and upper digestive passage, it is essential to abstain from smoking. Cancers of the true cord tend to be confined to one cord, but one third of the cases involve both cords, most often spreading across the anterior commissure where it may extend along anterior attachment (Broyles ligament) to the thyroid cartilage. Invasion of thyroid cartilage can follow with destruction of its calcified body. Posterior involvement of arytenoid cartilage is uncommon and obscures their normal double-beaded appearance.

Supraglottic cancers can arise from a variety of different locations and tend to cause few symptoms until advanced. The free surface of the epiglottis, the false cords, and the ventricles can all be involved. Transglottic cancers are usually advanced and extend from the supraglottic area, invade the vocal cords, and impair their function. These tumors spread rapidly because of the rich lymphatic network in this region. Bilateral neck nodes are often encountered. Another favored area of spread is the pre-epiglottic fat space.

Subglottic cancers, in terms of prognosis, are worse than other types. This is probably due to their tendency to invade the trachea and to reach a more advanced state before detection.

Subglottic cancers are often vocal cord lesions beginning on the inferior surface of the true cords but growing unrec-ognized. True subglottic cancers are really tracheal cancers and begin 1 cm below the vocal cords. Such cancers are rare and tend to involve the cricoid cartilage early because there is no muscle layer beneath the mucous membrane. Difficulty in breathing rather than hoarseness may be the critical complaint.

The larynx was initially staged with the development of the TNM system and appeared in the joint first edition of American Joint Committee on Cancer/International Union Against Cancer (AJCC/UICC) (1978). The basis of progression of laryngeal cancers is related to their spread patterns to subsites (T2) as well as advancement from any one major site: glottic, supraglottic, subglottic to another, and (T2) if cord mobility is preserved. Loss of cord mobility indicates T3.

SUMMARY OF CHANGES SEVENTH EDITION AJCC

The TNM stages according to the 7th Edition of AJCC are illustrated in color code of advancement (Fig. 10.3). T4 lesions have been divided into T4a (moderately advanced local disease) and T4b (very advanced local disease), leading to the stratification of Stage IV into Stage IVA (moderately advanced local/regional disease), Stage IVB (very advanced local/regional disease), and Stage IVC (distant metastatic disease).

The TNM Staging Matrix is color coded for identification of Stage Group once T and N stages are determined (Table 10.3).

TABLE 10.3	Stage Summary Matrix

	Stage T1	Stage T2	Stage T3	Stage T4a	Stage T4b
N0	I	II	III	IVA	IVB
N1	III	III	III	IVA	IVB
N2	IVA	IVA	IVA	IVA	IVB
N3	IVB	IVB	IVB	IVB	IVB
M1	IVC	IVC	IVC	IVC	IVC

- *T stage* determines stage group
  - T1 = I, T2 + II, T3 = III, T4 = IV
- *N stage* N1 = T3 and then progresses as T stage progresses
  - N1 = T3, N2 = T4a, N3 = T4b
- *M stage* is a separate stage
  - M1 = Stage IVC

GLOTTIC LARYNX

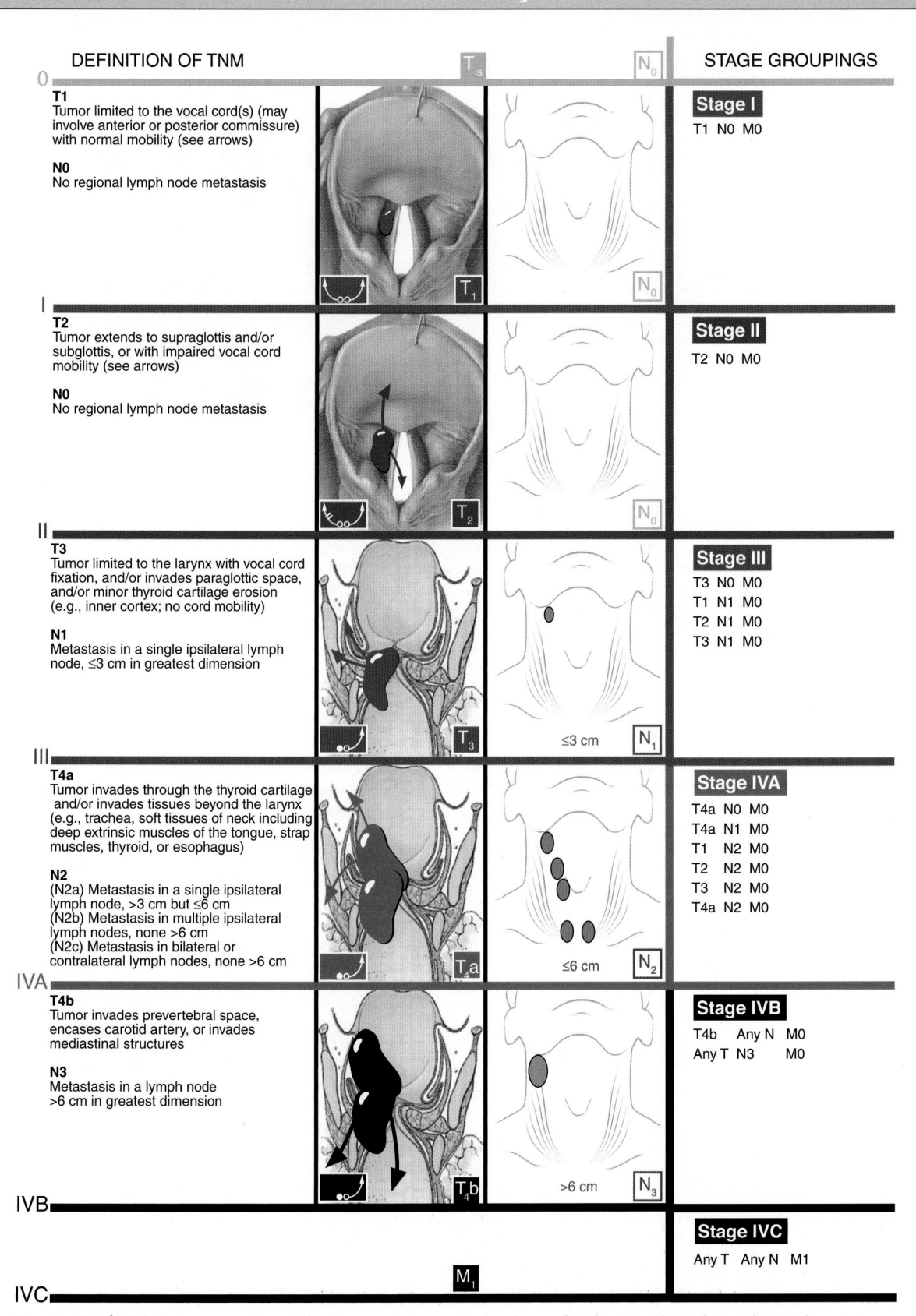

DEFINITION OF TNM	STAGE GROUPINGS

T1
Tumor limited to the vocal cord(s) (may involve anterior or posterior commissure) with normal mobility (see arrows)

N0
No regional lymph node metastasis

Stage I
T1 N0 M0

T2
Tumor extends to supraglottis and/or subglottis, or with impaired vocal cord mobility (see arrows)

N0
No regional lymph node metastasis

Stage II
T2 N0 M0

T3
Tumor limited to the larynx with vocal cord fixation, and/or invades paraglottic space, and/or minor thyroid cartilage erosion (e.g., inner cortex; no cord mobility)

N1
Metastasis in a single ipsilateral lymph node, ≤3 cm in greatest dimension

Stage III
T3 N0 M0
T1 N1 M0
T2 N1 M0
T3 N1 M0

T4a
Tumor invades through the thyroid cartilage and/or invades tissues beyond the larynx (e.g., trachea, soft tissues of neck including deep extrinsic muscles of the tongue, strap muscles, thyroid, or esophagus)

N2
(N2a) Metastasis in a single ipsilateral lymph node, >3 cm but ≤6 cm
(N2b) Metastasis in multiple ipsilateral lymph nodes, none >6 cm
(N2c) Metastasis in bilateral or contralateral lymph nodes, none >6 cm

Stage IVA
T4a N0 M0
T4a N1 M0
T1 N2 M0
T2 N2 M0
T3 N2 M0
T4a N2 M0

T4b
Tumor invades prevertebral space, encases carotid artery, or invades mediastinal structures

N3
Metastasis in a lymph node >6 cm in greatest dimension

Stage IVB
T4b Any N M0
Any T N3 M0

Stage IVC
Any T Any N M1

Figure 10.3 | TNM stage grouping. Glottic cancers are commonly confined to vocal cords producing hoarseness early, which leads to their detection. Vertical presentations of stage groupings, which follow the same color code for cancer stage advancement, are organized in horizontal lanes: Stage 0, yellow; I, green; II, blue; III, purple; IVA, red; and IVB, black. Definitions of TN on left and stage grouping on right. Note inferior box on T-oncoanatomy provides a key to vocal cord mobility.

SUBGLOTTIC CANCER LARYNX

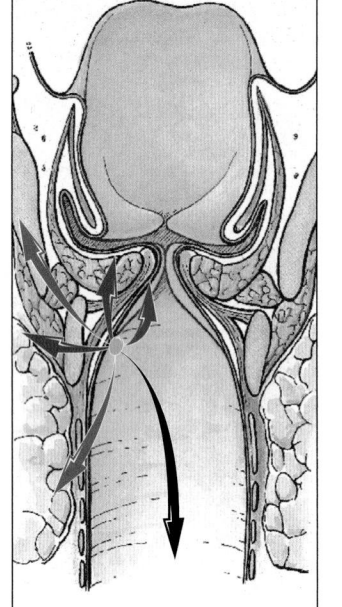

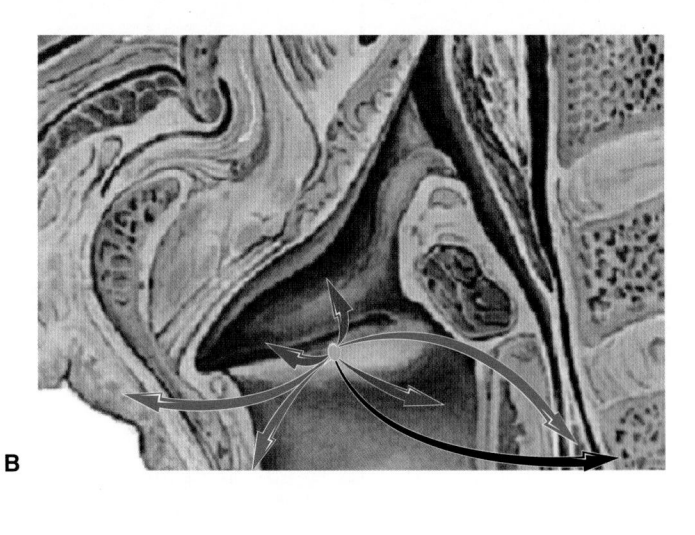

Figure 10.2A | Patterns of spread. A. Coronal: Note paralaryngeal invasion and cricoid cartilage.
B. Sagittal: Note posterior invasion into pharynx and esophagus. The primary cancer (glottic larynx) invades in various directions, which are color-coded vectors (*arrows*) representing stage of progression: Tis, yellow; T1, green; T2, blue; T3, purple; T4a, red; and T4b, black. The concept of visualizing patterns of spread to appreciate the surrounding anatomy is well demonstrated by the six directional pattern i.e. SIMLAP Table 10.2A.

TABLE 10.2A	SIMLAP	
Subglottis		
S	Glottis, impaired	• T2
	Fixed	• T3
I	Mediastinum	• T4b
M		
L	Thyroid Gland	• T4a
	Carotid Artery	• T4b
A	Through Thyroid Cartilage	• T4a
	Soft Tissue Strap Muscle Neck	• T4a
P	Through Cricord Cartilage	• T4a
	Esophagus	• T4a
	Prevertebral Space	• T4b

Histopathology: is usually squamous cell carcinoma similar to vocal cord; as are the variants (see Fig. 10.1 and Table 10.1). There are six basic directions or vectors (arrows): The 6 vectors of invasion are <u>S</u>uperior, <u>I</u>nferior, <u>M</u>edial, <u>L</u>ateral, <u>A</u>nterior, and <u>P</u>osterior. The color code dots correlate the T stage with specific anatomic structure involved.

TNM Staging Criteria: Similar to the glottis as to TNM definitions as is. The stage summary matrix:

TABLE 10.3A	Stage Summary Matrix				
	Stage T1	**Stage T2**	**Stage T3**	**Stage T4a**	**Stage T4b**
N0	I	II	III	IVA	IVB
N1	III	III	III	IVA	IVB
N2	IVA	IVA	IVA	IVA	IVB
N3	IVB	IVB	IVB	IVB	IVB
M1	IVC	IVC	IVC	IVC	IVC

- *T stage* determines stage group
  - T_1 = I, T_2 = II, T_3 = III, T_4 = IV
- *N stage* N_1 = T_3 and then progresses as T stage progresses
  - N_1 = T_3, N_2 = T_{4a}, N_3 = T_{4b}
- *M stage* is a separate stage
  - M_1 = Stage IVC

SUBGLOTTIC LARYNX

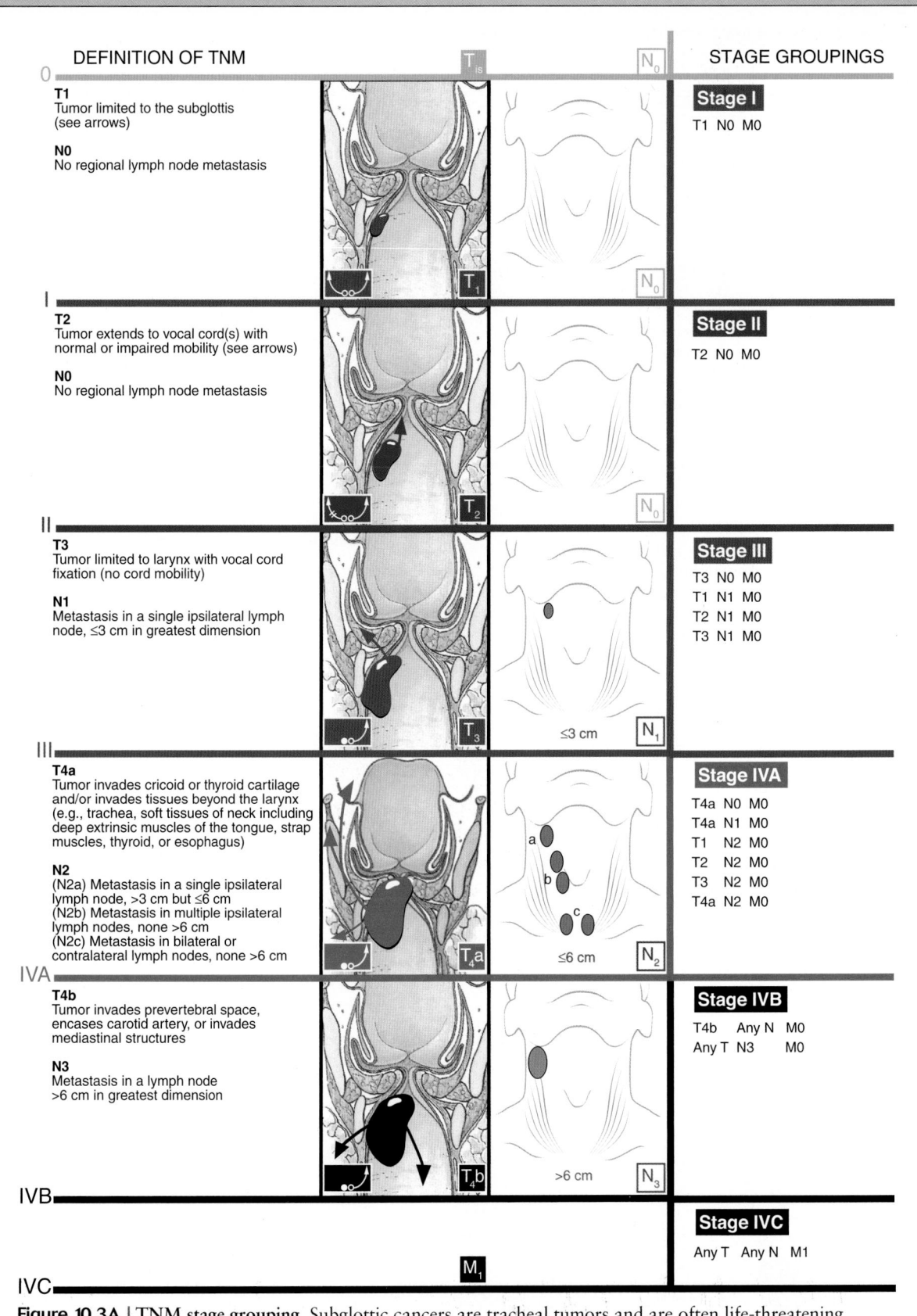

DEFINITION OF TNM

T1
Tumor limited to the subglottis
(see arrows)

N0
No regional lymph node metastasis

T2
Tumor extends to vocal cord(s) with
normal or impaired mobility (see arrows)

N0
No regional lymph node metastasis

T3
Tumor limited to larynx with vocal cord
fixation (no cord mobility)

N1
Metastasis in a single ipsilateral lymph
node, ≤3 cm in greatest dimension

T4a
Tumor invades cricoid or thyroid cartilage
and/or invades tissues beyond the larynx
(e.g., trachea, soft tissues of neck including
deep extrinsic muscles of the tongue, strap
muscles, thyroid, or esophagus)

N2
(N2a) Metastasis in a single ipsilateral
lymph node, >3 cm but ≤6 cm
(N2b) Metastasis in multiple ipsilateral
lymph nodes, none >6 cm
(N2c) Metastasis in bilateral or
contralateral lymph nodes, none >6 cm

T4b
Tumor invades prevertebral space,
encases carotid artery, or invades
mediastinal structures

N3
Metastasis in a lymph node
>6 cm in greatest dimension

STAGE GROUPINGS

Stage I
T1 N0 M0

Stage II
T2 N0 M0

Stage III
T3 N0 M0
T1 N1 M0
T2 N1 M0
T3 N1 M0

Stage IVA
T4a N0 M0
T4a N1 M0
T1 N2 M0
T2 N2 M0
T3 N2 M0
T4a N2 M0

Stage IVB
T4b Any N M0
Any T N3 M0

Stage IVC
Any T Any N M1

Figure 10.3A | TNM stage grouping. Subglottic cancers are tracheal tumors and are often life-threatening because of their vital location and present as advanced cancers. Vertical presentations of stage groupings, which follow the same color code for cancer stage advancement are organized in horizontal lanes: Stage 0, yellow; I, green; II, blue; III, purple; IVA, red; and IVB, black. Definitions of TN on left and stage grouping on right. Note inferior box on T-oncoanatomy provides a key to vocal cord mobility.

T-ONCOANATOMY

ORIENTATION OF THREE-PLANAR ONCOANATOMY

The anatomic isocenter of the true glottis is at the C5 level. The anterior surface bullet enters midway below the anterior notch of the thyroid cartilage and its inferior border (Fig. 10.4A) and the lateral bullet enters through the body of the thyroid cartilage (Fig. 10.4B).

T-oncoanatomy

The introduction to three-dimensional planar view of the larynx is best appreciated from the posterior coronal view with the constrictor musculature split.

- *Coronal plane* (Fig. 10.5A): The larynx is divided into three parts: (i) the supraglottis, (ii) the glottis, and (iii) the subglottis; these three parts are known as the vestibule, ventricle (glottis), and infraglottic cavity, respectively. The epiglottis is readily visualized at its vestibule. The opening of the larynx, referred to as the aditus larynges or the superior laryngeal aperture, can be traced from the epiglottis to the arytenoids. The aryepiglottic folds start at the free edge of the epiglottis and terminate at the corniculate and arytenoids cartilages. The false cords and true cords are sepa-

rated by the ventricle. Each acts as a sphincter that closes off the airway.

- *Sagittal plane* (Fig. 10.5B): The cartilaginous skeleton of the larynx consists of the epiglottis, thyroid, cricoid, arytenoids, corniculate cartilages, and hyoid bone. A set of fine membranes and muscles hold this cartilage together, forming a rigid structure, which is not easily destroyed by cancer invasion. The cricothyroid muscle tenses the vocal cords. The intrinsic muscles include the posterior cricoarytenoid, thyroarytenoids, vocalis, thyroepiglottis, and aryepiglottis. The essential function of these muscles is to open and close the glottis during breathing and to regulate cord tension during speaking. The true cords and false cords are separated by a ventricle. The pre-epiglottic fat-filled space can be readily infiltrated from a cancer in the supraglottic region at its base because the epiglottic cartilage sits as an upside-down paddle. These features are best appreciated in the sagittal view.

- *Transverse view* (Fig. 10.5C): The axial view illustrates the paralaryngeal space between the thyroid and epiglottal cartilage and the position of the larynx to the pharynx. The prevertebral space is separated from the larynx by the hypopharynx, and the prevertebral fascia is rarely invaded by true laryngeal malignancies.

Refer to Figure 10.5 for T-oncoanatomy for three planar sections.

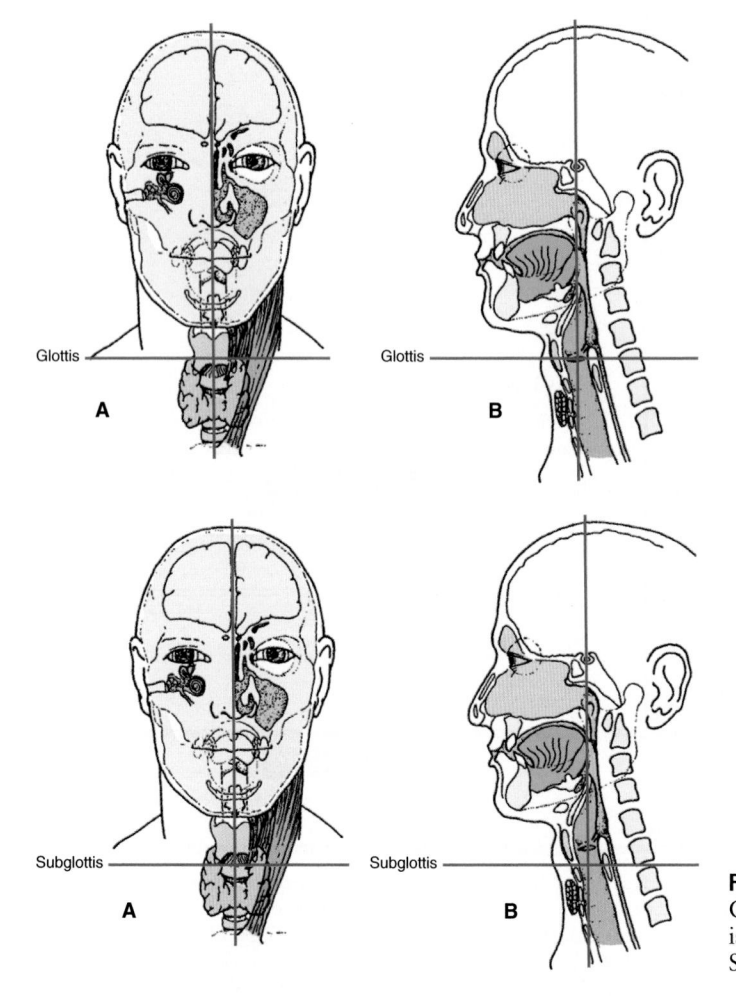

Glottis

A

Glottis

B

Subglottis

A

Subglottis

B

Figure 10.4 | Orientation of three-planar T-oncoanatomy. Glottic (**Top**). Subglottic (**Bottom**). The anatomic isocenter is at the axial level at C5/6 for Glottis, and C6/7 for Subglottis. **A.** Coronal. **B.** Sagittal.

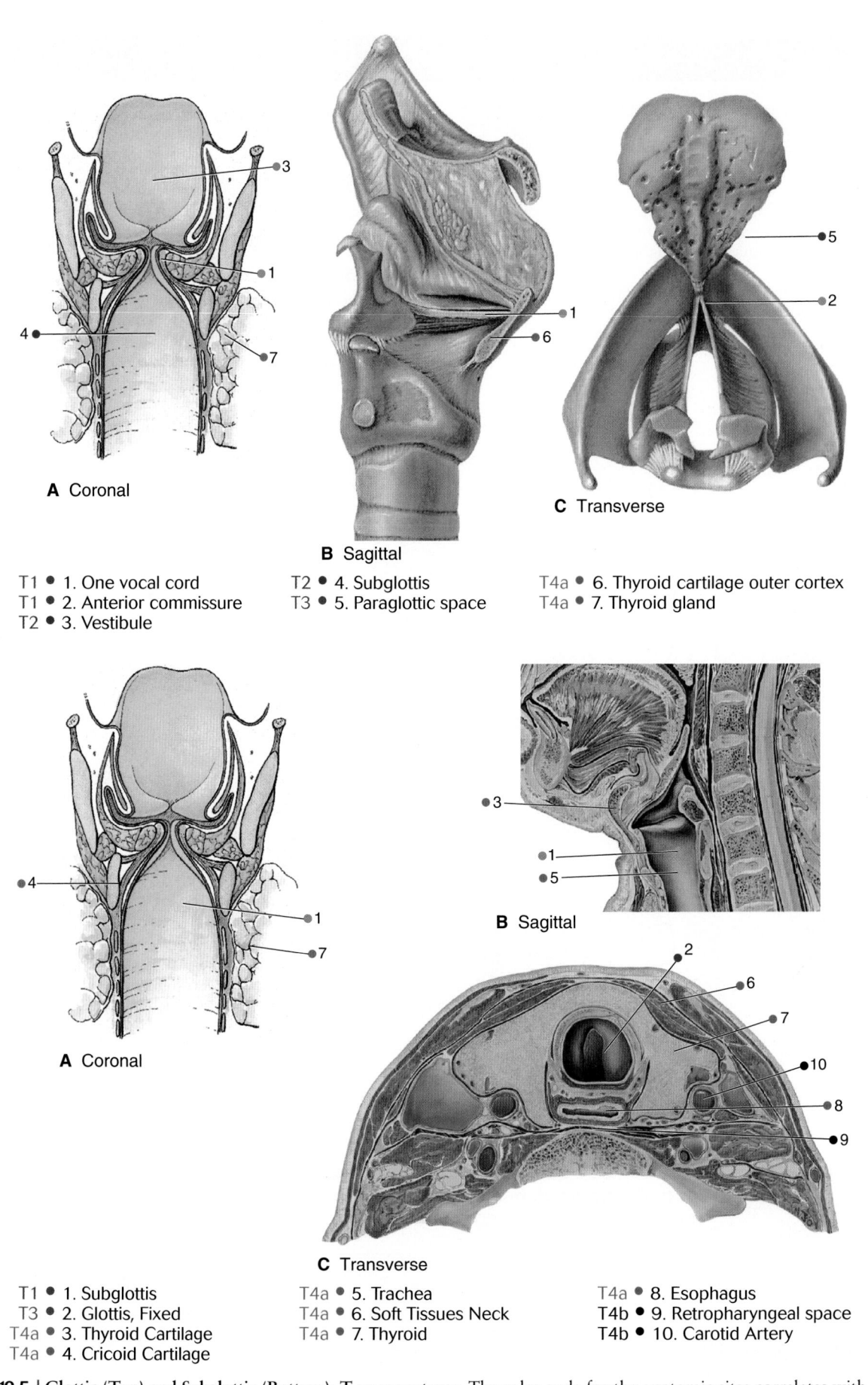

A Coronal

B Sagittal

C Transverse

T1 ● 1. One vocal cord
T1 ● 2. Anterior commissure
T2 ● 3. Vestibule

T2 ● 4. Subglottis
T3 ● 5. Paraglottic space

T4a ● 6. Thyroid cartilage outer cortex
T4a ● 7. Thyroid gland

A Coronal

B Sagittal

C Transverse

T1 ● 1. Subglottis
T3 ● 2. Glottis, Fixed
T4a ● 3. Thyroid Cartilage
T4a ● 4. Cricoid Cartilage

T4a ● 5. Trachea
T4a ● 6. Soft Tissues Neck
T4a ● 7. Thyroid

T4a ● 8. Esophagus
T4b ● 9. Retropharyngeal space
T4b ● 10. Carotid Artery

Figure 10.5 | Glottic (Top) and Subglottic (Bottom): T-oncoanatomy. The color code for the anatomic sites correlates with the color code for the stage group (Fig. 10.3 and 10.3A) and patterns of spread (Fig. 10.2 and 10.2A) and SIMLAP table (Table 10.2 and 10.2A). Connecting the dots in similar colors will provide an appreciation for the three-dimensional oncoanatomy.

N-ONCOANATOMY AND M-ONCOANATOMY

N-ONCOANATOMY

Each segment of the larynx drains to a different sentinel node (Fig. 10.6; Table 10.4). The glottis or true vocal cords are not rich in lymphatics and drain to pretracheal or paralaryngeal lymph nodes. The supraglottis is richer in lymphatics and vascularization, with drainage favoring midjugular and jugulodigastric nodes.

Subglottic cancers drain to deeper cervical nodes, the jugulo-omohyoid, and even the scalene nodes. The incidence and distribution of clinically negative neck node (N0) Figure 10.7A and Table 10.5A, and clinically positive (N+) Fig. 10.7B and Table 10.5B.

Orientation of N Oncoanatomy for Subglottic: The sentinel node is different than the glottis and is the jugulo-omohyoid. However, as the cancer advances, transglottic, the mid deep cervical nodes become involved.

M-ONCOANATOMY

The venous drainage of the larynx is by way of laryngeal veins into the internal jugular vein, brachiocephalic vein, and then into the superior vena cava. Metastases are most likely to target the lung (Figs. 10.6 and Fig. 7.7B as in Oropharynx).

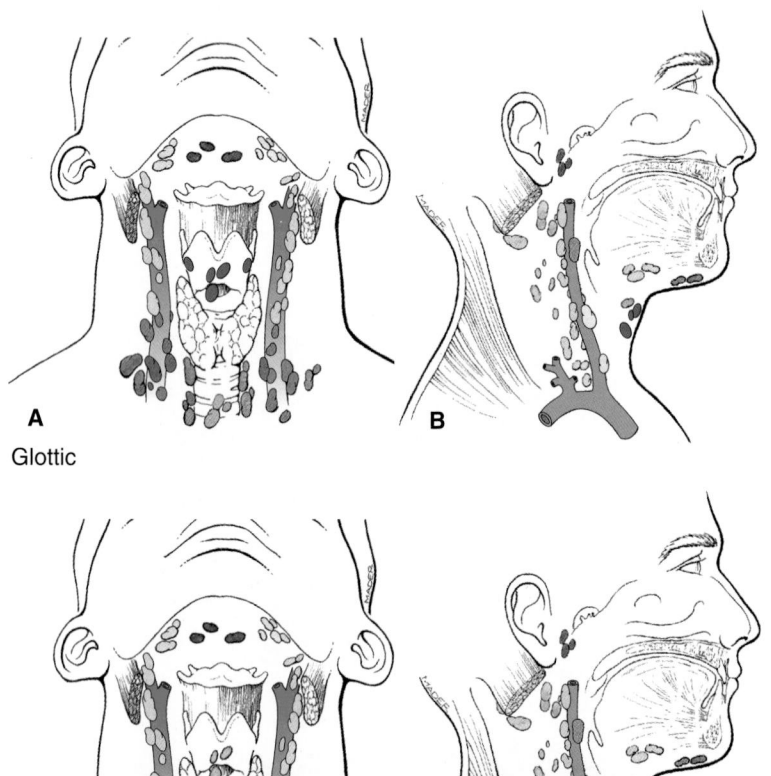

A Glottic

B

C Subglottic

D

Figure 10.6 | N-oncoanatomy. Glottic (A,B). The red node highlights the sentinel node, which is the paralaryngeal node. **Subglottic (C,D).** The red node highlights the sentinel node, which is the jugulo-omohyoid node. **A,C.** Anterior view. **B,D.** Lateral view. **M-oncoanatomy** is determined by the jugular vein, which joins with the subclavian vein to form the superior vena cava on the right, and the innominate vein, which drains into the right side of the heart and then into lung.

TABLE 10.4	Sentinel and Regional Nodes: Glottic and Subglottic Larynx (Ipsilateral)		
		Level/Location of Node(s)	
S Sentinel Node		Axial Level	AJCC Level
S1 Prelaryngeal		C5	VI
R Regional Nodes			
R1 Jugulodigastric, superior/mid deep cervical		C4–5	II
R2 Jugulo-omohyoid, inferior deep cervical		C7	IV

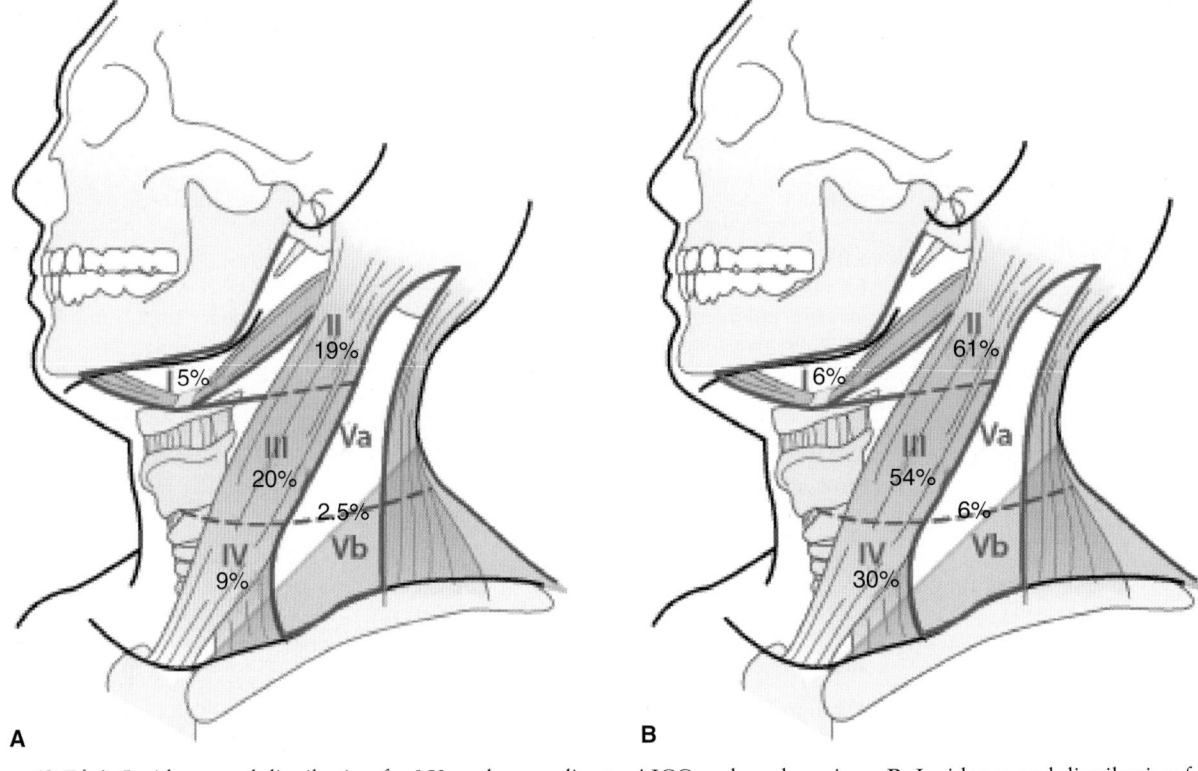

Figure 10.7 | **A.** Incidence and distribution for N0 neck according to AJCC neck node regions. **B.** Incidence and distribution for N⁺ neck according to AJCC neck regions.

TABLE 10.5A	Incidence and Distribution for N0 Neck According to AJCC Neck Node Regions

- Level I = 5%
- Level II = 19%
- Level III = 20%
- Level IV = 9%
- Level V = 2.5%

TABLE 10.5B	Incidence and Distribution for N+ Neck According to AJCC Neck Regions

Once the sentinel node is involved, the patterns of spread to the rest of the neck nodes at difference levels is due to collateralization of drainage both prograde and retrograde as well as to contralateral spread. The neck node levels (%) involved:

Level I   = 6%

Level II   = 61%

Level III = 54%

Level IV   = 30%

Level V   = 6%

Incidence and Distribution of Distant Metastases

Distant Metastases for subglottic are similar to advanced glottic cancers. Lung is the target metastatic organ.

STAGING WORKUP

TABLE 10.6	Imaging Modalities and Strategies for Diagnosis and Staging for Head and Neck: Glottic and Subglottic Larynx	
Modality	**Strategy**	**Recommended**
Primary Tumor and Nodes		
Computed tomography	Excellent for defining extent of primary depth of invasion enlargement of involved nodes. Preferred for bone invasion.	Yes—3–5 mm cuts, 3 mm for primary sites, 5 mm for neck.
Magnetic resonance imaging	Offers best 3D and 3-planar views of primary and nodes, especially soft tissue extensions. Gadolinium contrast for extensions and perineuronal spread.	Yes—$\leq$4 cm slices Gd for intracranial and perineuronal spread.
Magnetic resonance spectroscopy	Provides metabolic and biochemical analysis of tumor, choline/creatinine ratio elevated in tumor vs. normal tissues.	No.
Positron emission tomography	Functional and metabolic imaging of ^{18}FDG is based on 2-deoxy modification, which inhibits the molecule from subsequent enzymatic conversion and is "metabolically trapped" in tumor cells.	No—potential exists for distinguishing recurrence from tissue necrosis.
Single photon emission computed tomography	Thallium-201 is used to detect tumor recurrence vs. normal tissue imaging, especially central nervous system.	No—high uptake normally in salivary and thyroid glands.
Metastases		
Chest film	Search for metastases.	Yes.
Radionuclide scan	^{99m}Tc for bone metastases.	Yes—if symptomatic.

3D, three-dimensional; FDG, fluorodeoxyglucose.

RULES OF CLASSIFICATION AND STAGING

Clinical Staging and Imaging

Assessment of the larynx in its three compartments—supraglottis, glottis, and subglottis—is optimally performed with a fiberoptic laryngoscope and often requires general anesthesia, which is advised often after completion of diagnostic imaging studies. Determining vocal cord motion, namely, partial or complete paralysis, is difficult because the normal cord can cross over to meet the involved cord. Imaging studies do not supplant endoscopy and are viewed as complementary. Distinction between the three compartments is essential to staging. Computed tomography (CT) (Fig. 10.8) and magnetic resonance imaging (MRI) are often complementary (see Table 10.6).

Pathologic Staging

The gross specimen should be evaluated for margins. Unresected gross residual tumor must be included and marked with clips. All resected lymph node specimens should describe size, number, and level of involved nodes and whether there is extracapsular spread. Specimens taken after radiation, chemotherapy, or both need to be noted; specimen shrinkages may occur up to 30% after resection itself. Designations pT and pN should be used after histopathologic evaluation. Perineural invasion deserves special notation.

Oncoimaging Annotations

- After contrast administration, cross-sectional CT studies of the larynx should be performed, extending from C1 to the thoracic inlet.

- MRI should be performed before and after gadolinium enhancement.

- Extralaryngeal tumor spread, sclerosis, erosion, and lysis suggest cartilaginous cancer invasion. The negative predictive value of this combination of findings is high, but the specificity is low.

- A positive diagnosis of cartilage invasion on MRI should be made with caution because the positive predictive value of the altered signal behavior as a sign of invasion is low.

- Pretreatment CT imaging is predictive of local tumor control in patients treated with definitive radiation therapy. Tumor diameters less than 2 cm have a high likelihood of local control, whereas tumors with diameters greater than 2 cm have only a 50% chance of control.

- Both positron emission tomography with fluorine-18-labeled-deoxyglucose (FDG) and thallium-201 single photon emission computed tomography have useful potential in differentiating posttreatment radiation changes from recurrent tumor.

PROGNOSIS AND SURVIVAL

PROGNOSTIC FACTORS

- Size of lymph nodes
- Extracapsular extension from lymph nodes for head and neck
- Head and neck lymph nodes levels I-III
- Head and neck lymph nodes levels IV-V
- Head and neck lymph nodes levels VI-VII
- Other lymph node group
- Clinical location of cervical nodes
- Extracapsular spread (ECS) clinical
- Extracapsular spread (ECS) pathologic
- Human papillomavirus (HPV) status*

CANCER STATISTICS AND SURVIVAL

The survival rates for subglottic cancers are poorer than similar stage glottic and subglottic cancers. Prognostic factors are similar to glottic. Glottic cancers are found in early stage I. Therefore, survival is at 90% level. Subglottic cancers are found late stage III/IV with survival rates under 50% (Fig. 10.9).

*The foregoing passage is from Edge SB, Byrd DR, and Compton CC, et al, *AJCC Cancer Staging Manual, 7th edition.* New York, Springer, 2010, p. 65.

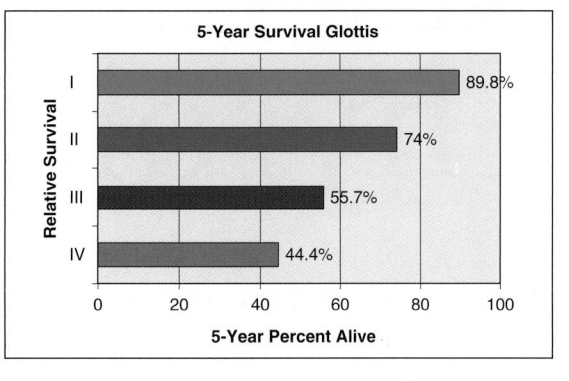

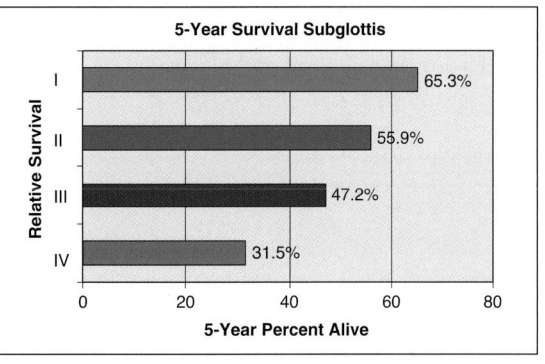

Figure 10.9 | Five-year survival rates by stage diagnosis of subglottis. (Data from Edge SB, Byrd DR, and Compton CC, et al, *AJCC Cancer Staging Manual, 7th edition.* New York, Springer, 2010.)

1. thyroid cartilage
2. cricoid cartilage
3. arytenoid cartilage
4. true vocal cord
5. ant commisure
6. laryngeal airway
7. internal jugular vein
8. common carotid art
9. sternocleidomastoid muscle
10. vertebral art
11. lymph node

1. inferior cornu thyroid cartilage
2. cricoid cartilage
3. tracheal lumen
4. thyroid gland
5. internal jugular vein
6. common carotid art
7. sternocleidomastoid muscle
8. vertebral art

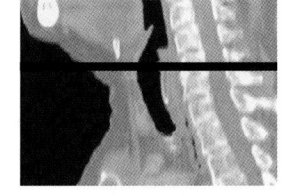
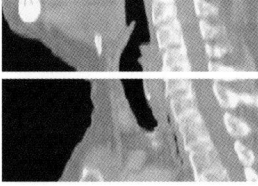
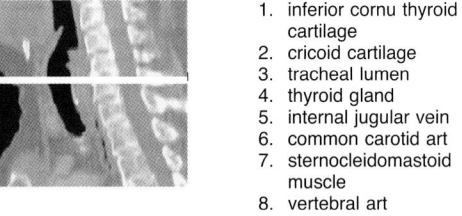
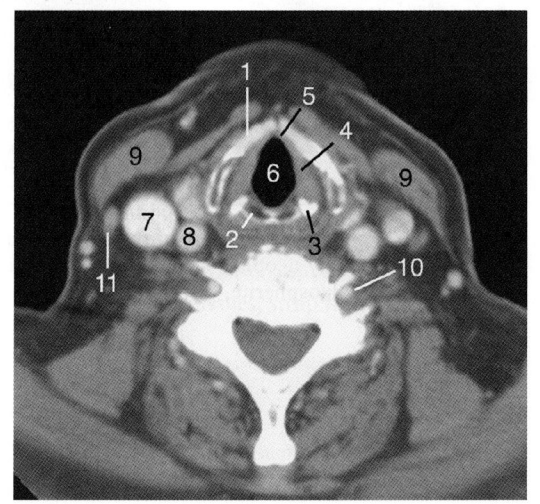

Figure 10.8 | **Glottic (left) and Subglottic (right).** Neck and Larynx—Axial CT scan. **A.** Note Thyroid cartilage encompasses true glottis and anterior commisure invasion (Broyle's ligament) erodes the calcified thyroid cartilage. **B.** Note cricoid cartilage encompasses subglottic region. The CT/MRI transverse section can be correlated with anatomy in Figure 10.5C as an assist to staging.

TNM STAGING CRITERIA

TNM STAGING CRITERIA

Histogenesis is the major factor in thyroid cancer staging because it determines behavior clinically and pathologically (Fig. 11.3). Thyroid adenomas are by far the most common tumors of this endocrine gland. They are, for the most part, low-grade carcinomas, which invade into the gland substance and are considered multicentric in origin, although intraglandular spread may seem to be similar. Nodules of the thyroid are much more common than parathyroid adenomas, and malignant degeneration similarly is a much more likely event in the thyroid. Depending on the type of thyroid malignancy, different spread patterns occur. Common types can be divided into the follicular adenocarcinoma, papillary adenocarcinoma, medullary, and anaplastic tumors, which are either small or large cell carcinomas.

Follicular carcinoma tends to be nodular and encapsulated and is more likely to displace than invade into the gland substance and its surrounding structures. Its major spread pattern is via the venous system into the systemic circulation, leading to lung and bone metastases.

Papillary adenocarcinomas are the most common tumor of the thyroid and tend to be more invasive locally, breaking through and invading the thyroid capsule into surrounding tissues. They rarely tend to be locally recurrent after their resection, indicating only low-grade local aggressiveness. Distant hematogenous spread is uncommon; these cancers tend to invade into regional lymph nodes, which can be involved bilaterally. Occasionally, the oncologic presentations can be as metastatic cervical lymph nodes of unknown origin. Neck node dissections can be more effective treatments rather than radical neck node resections.

Medullary thyroid cancers account for 10% of all thyroid cancers, can be familial, and are transmitted as an autosomal-dominant trait with high penetrance. Multiple endocrine tumors can be present as pheochromocytomas, parathyroid adenomas, or ganglioneuromatosis. These medullary thyroid cancers tend to localize between the upper third and lower two thirds of the lobe and appear on cut section as a red hard lesion consisting of C-cells, physiologically producing calcitonin. They can be locally invasive, spreading into regional nodes, or form distant metastases in liver, lung, and bones. Fortunately, these lesions tend to be slow growing.

Anaplastic small and large cell carcinomas can be very rapidly growing tumors, very invasive, and aggressive locally, leading to tracheal and/or esophageal invasion and compression. If they extend into the superior mediastinum, they can lead to compression of the superior vena cava. The recurrent laryngeal nerves are very intimately involved posterior to the thyroid gland and can be invaded; these tumors aggressively infiltrate through the capsule of the thyroid gland.

All anaplastic cancers are considered as T4. Their staging has been modified into T4a and T4b as to resectability. The size of the tumor, as in other head and neck sites, does not apply; and T3. T4a is a cancer nodule with anterior extrathyroid extension involving the sternohyoid muscle surrounding soft tissues larynx, trachea, esophagus, and recurrent laryngeal nerve. T4b is for posterior extension and invasion into the prevertebral space.

In summary, the major spread patterns are intraglandular spread; T4a, extraglandular spread into the sternocleidomastoid muscle and skin; into surrounding structures such as the trachea and esophagus; and into the recurrent laryngeal nerves, particularly on the right side. T4b is spread posteriorly into the prevertebral muscle and/or inferiorly deep into the mediastinum, carotid artery.

SUMMARY OF CHANGES SEVENTH EDITION AMERICAN JOINT COMMITTEE ON CANCER (AJCC)

The TNM stages according to the 7th Edition of AJCC are illustrated in color code of advancement (Fig. 11.3).

- Tumor staging (T1) has been subdivided into T1a (≤1 cm) and T1b (>1–2 cm) limited to thyroid.

- The descriptors to subdivide T categories have been changed to solitary tumor (s) and multifocal tumor (m).

- The terms "resectable" and "unresectable" are placed with "moderately advanced" and "very advanced."

- The TNM Staging Matrix is color coded for identification of Stage Group once T and N stages are determined (Table 11.3).

TABLE 11.3 **Stage Summary Matrix**

	N0	N1a	N1b	MI
T1	I	III	IVA	IVC
T2	II	III	IVA	IVC
T3	III	III	IVA	IVC
T4a	IVA	IVA	IVA	IVC
T4b	IVB	IVB	IVB	IVC

- *T stage* determines stage group
  - T1 = I, T2 + II, T3 = III, T4 = IV
- *N stage* N1 = T3 and then progresses as T stage progresses
  - N1 = T3, N2 = T4a, N3 = T4b
- *M stage* is a separate stage
  - M1 = Stage IVC

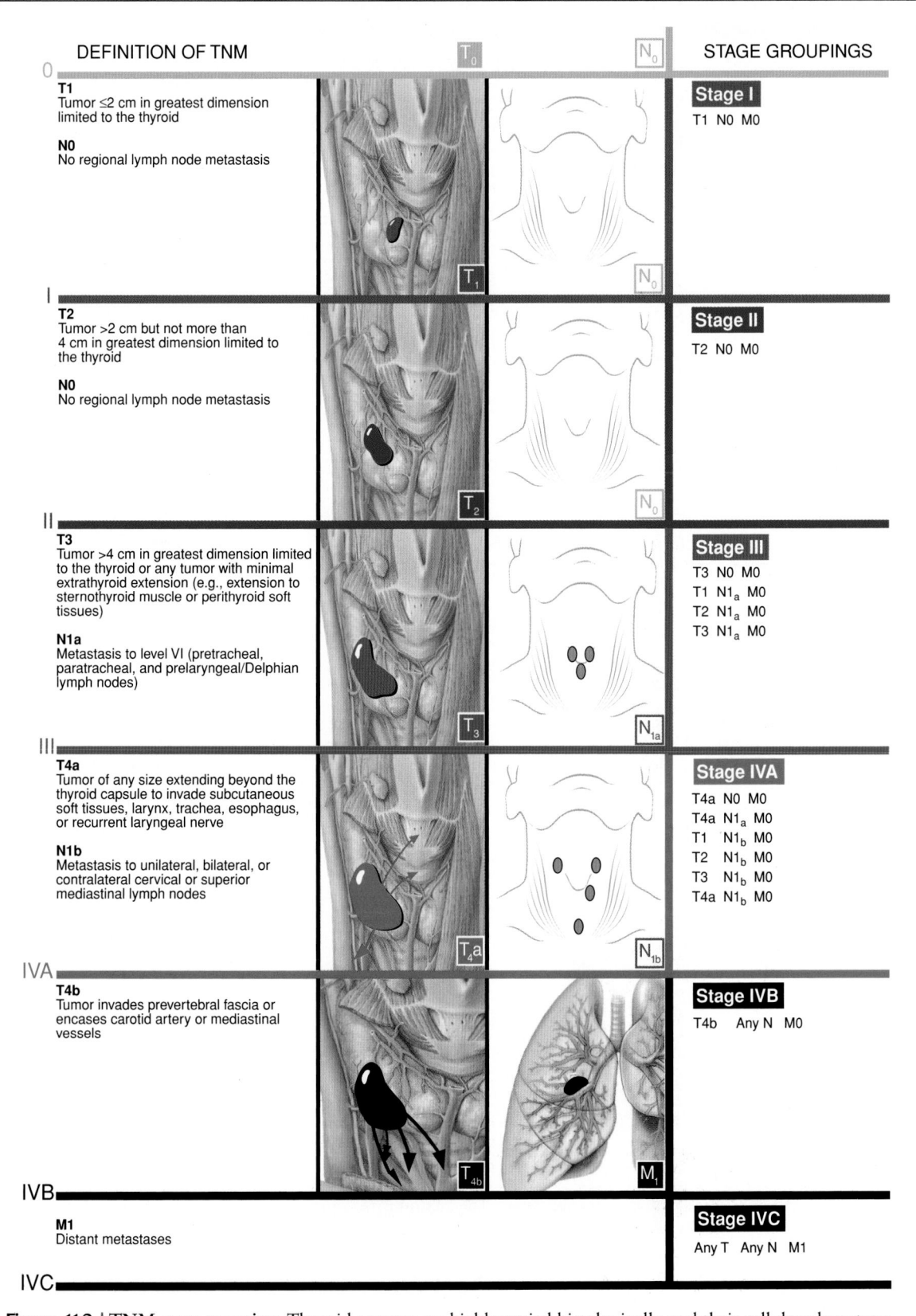

THYROID

DEFINITION OF TNM

STAGE GROUPINGS

0

T1
Tumor ≤2 cm in greatest dimension
limited to the thyroid

N0
No regional lymph node metastasis

Stage I
T1 N0 M0

I

T2
Tumor >2 cm but not more than
4 cm in greatest dimension limited to
the thyroid

N0
No regional lymph node metastasis

Stage II
T2 N0 M0

II

T3
Tumor >4 cm in greatest dimension limited
to the thyroid or any tumor with minimal
extrathyroid extension (e.g., extension to
sternothyroid muscle or perithyroid soft
tissues)

N1a
Metastasis to level VI (pretracheal,
paratracheal, and prelaryngeal/Delphian
lymph nodes)

Stage III
T3 N0 M0
T1 N1$_a$ M0
T2 N1$_a$ M0
T3 N1$_a$ M0

III

T4a
Tumor of any size extending beyond the
thyroid capsule to invade subcutaneous
soft tissues, larynx, trachea, esophagus,
or recurrent laryngeal nerve

N1b
Metastasis to unilateral, bilateral, or
contralateral cervical or superior
mediastinal lymph nodes

Stage IVA
T4a N0 M0
T4a N1$_a$ M0
T1 N1$_b$ M0
T2 N1$_b$ M0
T3 N1$_b$ M0
T4a N1$_b$ M0

IVA

T4b
Tumor invades prevertebral fascia or
encases carotid artery or mediastinal
vessels

Stage IVB
T4b Any N M0

IVB

M1
Distant metastases

Stage IVC
Any T Any N M1

IVC

Figure 11.3 | TNM stage grouping. Thyroid cancers are highly varied histologically and their cellular phenotype determines their biologic behavior, which ranges from a benign course to highly malignant. Vertical presentations of stage groupings, which follow the same color code for cancer stage advancement, are organized in horizontal lanes: Stage 0, yellow; I, green; II, blue; III, purple; IVA, red; and IVB, and IVC, black. Definitions of TN on left and stage grouping on right.

T-ONCOANATOMY

ORIENTATION OF THREE-PLANAR ONCOANATOMY

The anatomic isocenter for thyroid gland is at C7 level and inferior to the cricoid cartilage, readily palpable on swallowing when the gland moves vertically. The anterior bullet enters below the cricoid cartilage (Fig. 11.4A) and the lateral bullet through the anterior surface of the trachea (Fig. 11.4B).

T-oncoanatomy

The thyroid gland is a bilobed structure, symmetrical in size, and connected by an isthmus. It is approximately 2 to 3 cm long and wide and is shaped like a horseshoe.

- *Coronal plane* (Fig. 11.5A): From the anterior view, the gland is in close proximity to the cervical portion of the trachea, below the thyroid cartilage. It is located deep to the strap muscles of the neck, which include the sternocleidomastoid, sternohyoid, and sternothyroid muscles.

- *Sagittal plane* (Fig. 11.5B): Deep to the thyroid gland are the internal jugular vein and the common carotid artery. The recurrent laryngeal nerve lies posterior to the thyroid gland, particularly on the left side where it courses along the gland's entire length into the thorax; the right recurrent laryngeal is more lateral in its location as it hooks around the subclavian artery.

- *Transverse plane* (Fig. 11.5C): Deep to the left lobe of the thyroid is the thoracic duct, which rises into the neck and extends anteriorly, inserting into the junction of the left internal jugular and subclavian veins.

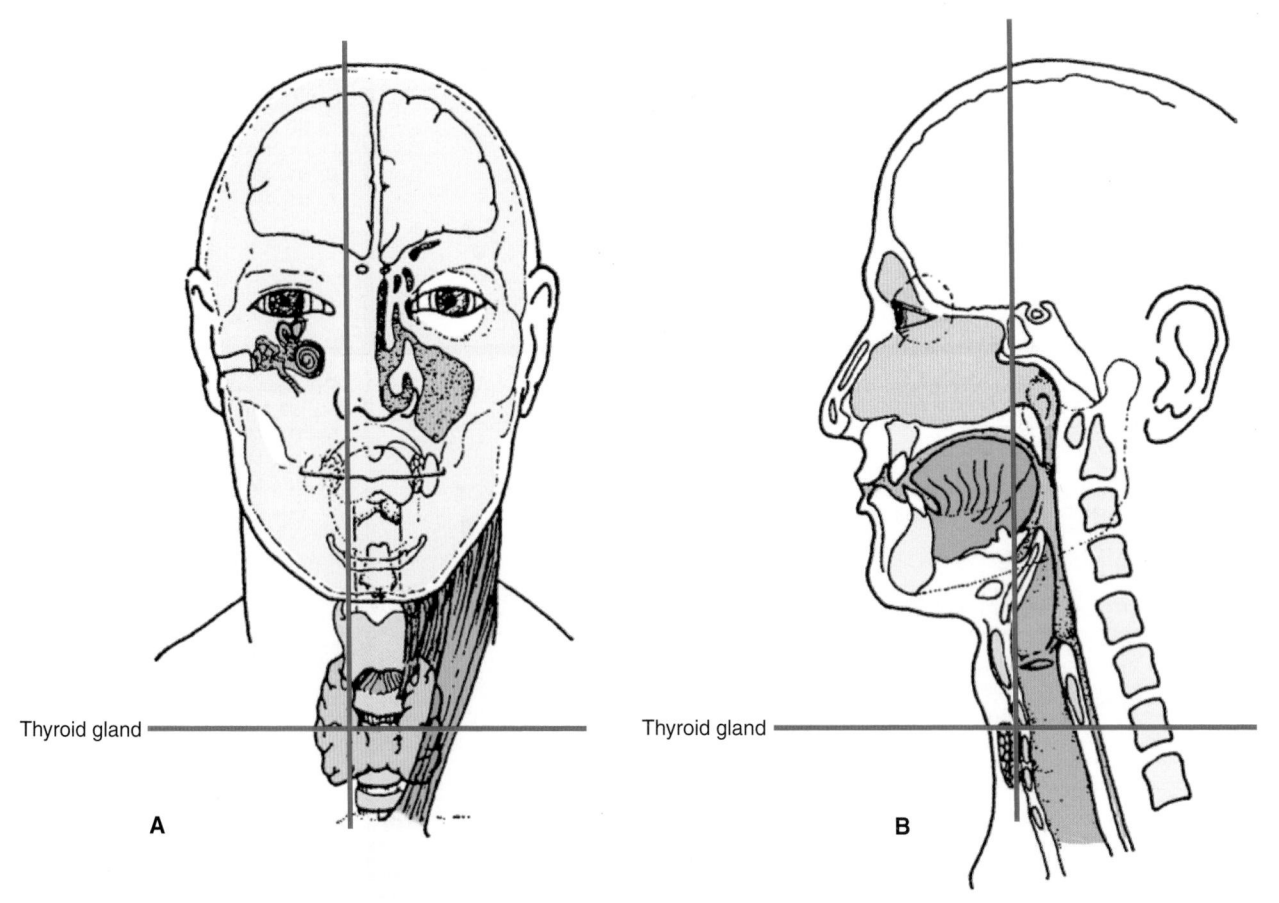

Thyroid gland

A

Thyroid gland

B

Figure 11.4 | Orientation of three-planar T-oncoanatomy. The anatomic isocenter is at the axial level at C7. **A.** Coronal. **B.** Sagittal.

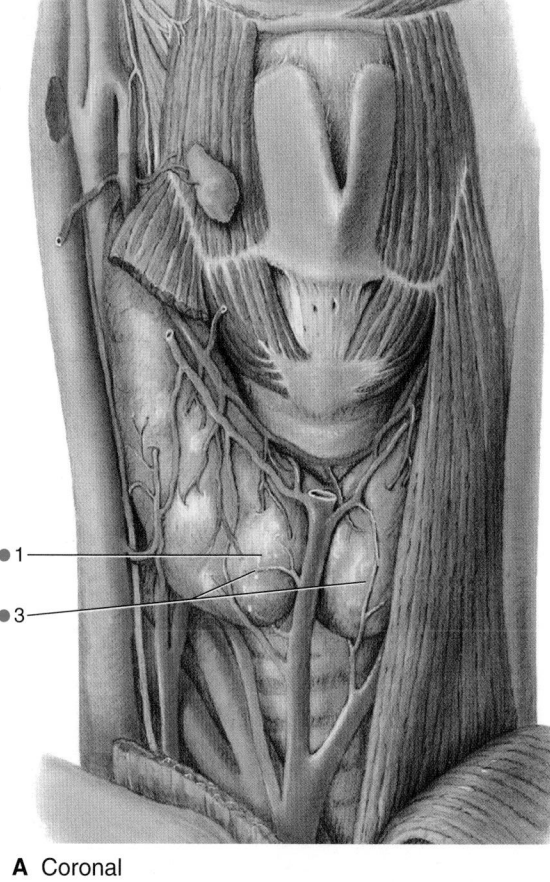

A Coronal

B Sagittal

C Transverse

T1 ●	1. Thyroid gland (lobe)	T3 ●	5. Sternothyroid muscle	T4a ●	10. Recurrent laryngeal nerve
T2 ●	2. Thyroid gland (isthmus)	T4a ●	6. Subcutaneous tissue	T4b ●	11. Retropharyngeal space
T2 ●	3. Thyroid gland (both lobes)	T4a ●	7. Larynx	T4b ●	12. Common carotid artery
T3 ●	4. Soft tissue neck (extracapsular minimal)	T4a ●	8. Trachea		
		T4a ●	9. Esophagus		

Figure 11.5 | T-oncoanatomy. The Color Code for the anatomic sites correlates with the color code for the stage group (Fig. 11.3) and patterns of spread (Fig. 11.2) and SIMLAP tables (Table 11.2). Connecting the dots in similar colors will provide an appreciation for the 3D Oncoanatomy.

N-ONCOANATOMY AND M-ONCOANATOMY

N-ONCOANATOMY

The nodal drainage of the thyroid is into the anterior and deep cervical lymph nodes. There is a small Delphic node, which sits in the midline at the superior margin of the isthmus.

In a reported series of papillary thyroid cancers, the frequency and levels of lymph node metastases are noted in Figure 11.6 and Table 11.4. The incidence for clinically negative (N0) neck, prophylactic dissection found 61% with node involvement which increased to 95.8%. (Tables 11.5A and 11.5B; Fig. 11.7A,B).

M-ONCOANATOMY

The thyroid gland is supplied by branches from the external carotid artery, superior thyroid, and subclavian artery with the inferior thyroid artery, which arises directly from the carotid artery. The venous pattern follows the arterial blood supply and drains into the internal jugular vein via superior, middle, and inferior veins (see Figs. 1.6 and 11.7B).

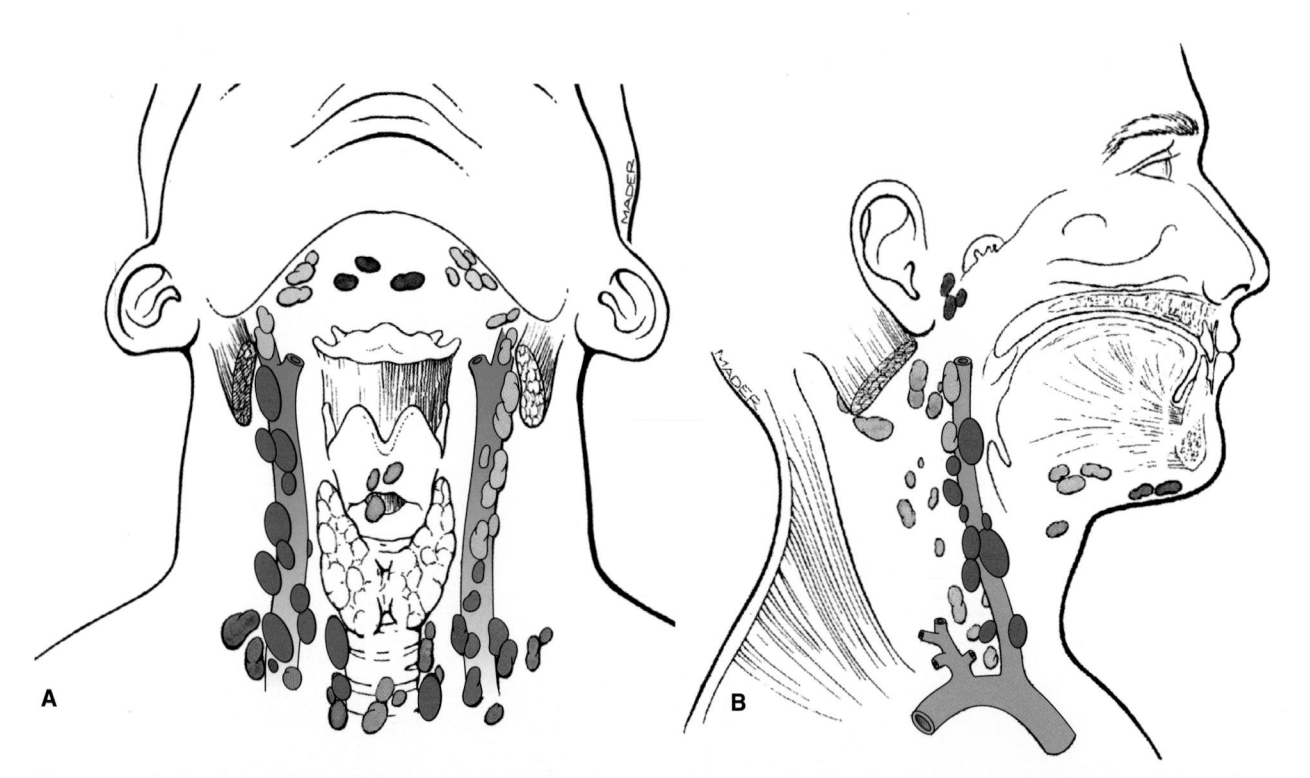

Figure 11.6 | N-oncoanatomy. The red node highlights the sentinel node, which is after the jugulo-omohyoid node but all deep cervical jugular nodes are at risk on the ipsilateral side. **A.** Anterior view. **B.** Lateral view. **M-oncoanatomy** is determined by the jugular vein, which joins with the subclavian vein to form the superior vena cava on the right, and the Innominate vein, which drains into the right side of the heart and then into lung.

TABLE 11.4	Sentinel and Regional Nodes: Thyroid (Bilateral)	
	Level/Location of Node(s)	
S Sentinel Nodes	**Axial Level**	**AJCC Level**
S1 Jugulo-omohyoid, inferior deep cervical	C7	IV
S2 Prelaryngeal Delphic	C5	VI
R Regional Nodes		
R1 Mid deep cervical	C4	III
R2 Jugulodigastric, superior deep cervical	C3	II

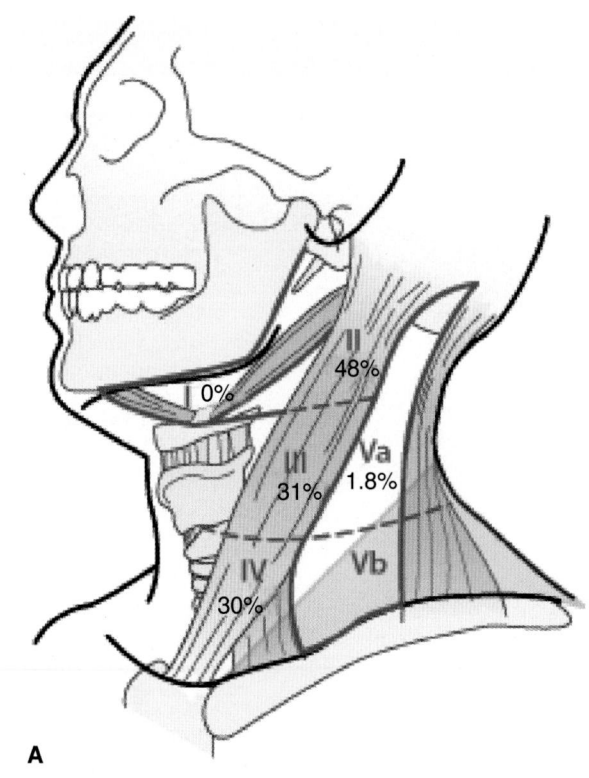
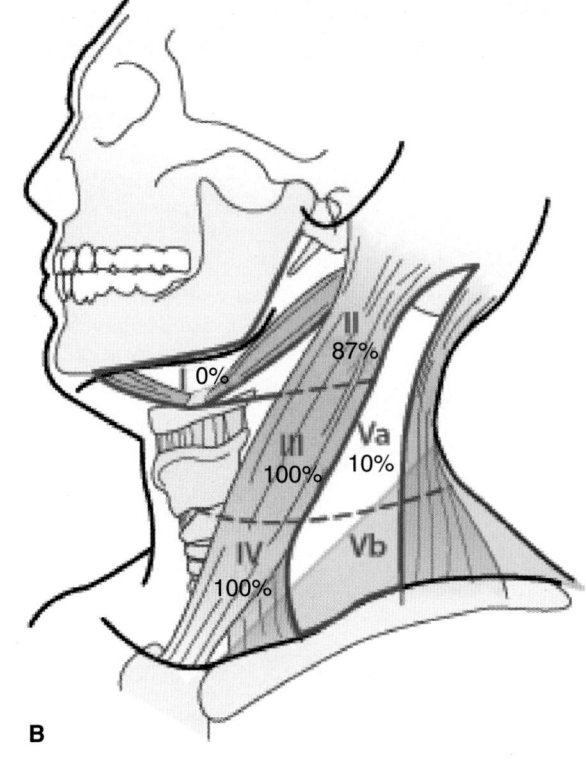

Figure 11.7 | A. Incidence and distribution of N0 neck node regional metastases. **B.** Incidence and distribution N⁺ according to AJCC neck regions.

TABLE 11.5A	Incidence and Distribution of N0 Neck Node Regional Metastases

- Level I = 0%
- Level II = 48%
- Level III = 31%
- Level IV = 30%
- Level V = 1.8%

TABLE 11.5B	Incidence and Distribution of N⁺ According to AJCC Neck Regions

Once the sentinel node is involved N+, the patterns of spread to the rest of the neck nodes at difference levels is due to collateralization of drainage both prograde and retrograde as well as contralateral spread. The neck node levels (%) involved:

Level I = 0%

Level II = 87%

Level III = 100%

Level IV = 100%

Level V = 10%

Incidence and Distribution of Distant Metastases

STAGING WORKUP

TABLE 11.6	Imaging Modalities and Strategies for Diagnosis and Staging for Head and Neck: Thyroid	
Modality	**Strategy**	**Recommended**
Primary Tumor and Nodes		
Computed tomography	Excellent for defining extent of primary depth of invasion enlargement of involved nodes. (Preferred for bone invasion.)	Yes—3–5 mm cuts, 3 mm for primary sites, 5 mm for neck. Calcifications.
Magnetic resonance imaging	Offers best 3D and 3-planar views of primary and nodes, especially soft tissue extensions. Gadolinium contrast for extensions and perineuronal spread.	Yes— ≤4 cm slices Gd for intracranial and perineuronal spread.
Magnetic ultrasound spectroscopy	Provides metabolic and biochemical analysis of tumor, choline/creatine ratio elevated in tumor vs. normal tissue.	No.
Positron emission tomography	Functional and metabolic imaging of ^{18}FDG is based on 2-deoxy modification, which inhibits the molecule from subsequent enzymatic conversion and is "metabolically trapped" in tumor cells.	No—potential exists for distinguishing recurrence from tissue necrosis.
Single photon emission computed tomography	Thallium-210 is used to detect tumor recurrence vs. normal tissue imaging, especially central nervous system.	No—high uptake normally in salivary and thyroid glands.
Metastases		
Chest film	Search for metastases/ pulmonary.	Yes.
Radionuclide scan	^{99m}Tc for bone metastases	Yes—if symptomatic.

3D, three-dimensional; FDG, fluorodeoxyglucose.

RULES OF CLASSIFICATION AND STAGING

Clinical Staging and Imaging

Assessment of thyroid tumor depends on inspection and palpation of the thyroid gland and regional neck nodes. Indirect laryngoscopy is essential to determine if vocal cord paresis or paralysis is present because of the proximity of recurrent laryngeal nerves. A large variety of imaging procedures are available, particularly the I^{131} scintiscan and uptake, which requires no iodine contrast be used before this test is done. Technetium 99M pertechnetate is currently the most widely used thyroid imaging agent. Ultrasound is the most sensitive technique for detecting focal pathology and is used for screening persons at risk. Radionuclide single photon emission computed tomography utilizing a variety of agents is recommended in Table 11.6 and Figure 11.8.

Pathologic Staging

The gross specimen should be evaluated for margins. Unresected gross residual tumor must be included and marked with clips. All resected lymph node specimens should describe size, number, and level of involved nodes and whether there is extracapsular spread. Specimens taken after radiation and/or chemotherapy need to be so noted; specimen shrinkages may occur up to 30% after resection itself. Designations pT and pN should be used after histopathologic evaluation. Perineural invasion deserves special notation.

Oncoimaging Annotations

- Microcalcifications are almost exclusively found in malignancies, mainly papillary and medullary carcinomas.

- Ultrasound is the most sensitive technique for detecting focal pathology and plays an important role in screening those at risk of developing thyroid malignancy.

- Ultrasound-guided fine-needle aspiration remains the most accurate means of distinguishing between benign and malignant lesions.

- Cystic papillary carcinomas are anechoic, with solid nodules protruding into the cyst and calcification in intracystic nodules.

- Tc^{99m} pertechnetate is the most widely used thyroid imaging agent; a solitary cold nodule is associated with malignancy in 10% to 20% of cases.

- Tc^{99m} DMSA and In-111 pentreotide are the imaging agents of choice for medullary carcinoma.

- Computed tomography or magnetic resonance imaging of the thyroid demonstrating surrounding structures (strap

PROGNOSIS AND SURVIVAL

muscles) and encasement of the great vessels and recurrent laryngeal nerve is pathognomonic for cancer.

- Enlarged cervical nodes, especially ipsilaterally, are common findings. Size per se is nonspecific, but the presence of microcalcifications or complete cystic degeneration is characteristic of cancer.

- Total body I^{131} scan is utilized in searching for functioning follicular and/or papillary metastatic pulmonary and osseous foci post total thyroidectomy.

PROGNOSTIC FACTORS

The seventh edition of the AJCC Cancer Staging Manual lists the following prognostic factors for nasal ethmoid sinus cancers:

- Size of lymph nodes
- Extracapsular extension from lymph nodes for head and neck
- Head and neck lymph nodes levels I-III
- Head and neck lymph nodes levels IV-V
- Head and neck lymph nodes levels VI-VII
- Other lymph node group
- Clinical location of cervical nodes
- Extracapsular spread (ECS) clinical
- Extracapsular spread (ECS) pathologic
- Human papillomavirus (HPV) status
- Tumor thickness
- Extra thyroid extension
- Histopathology*

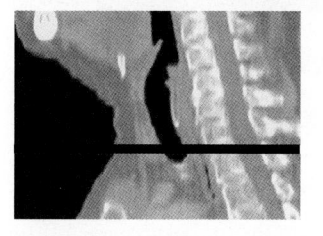

1. tracheal lumen
2. thyroid gland
3. thyroid isthmus
4. esophagus
5. internal jugular vein
6. common carotid art
7. vertebral art
8. ant scalene muscle
9. middle and post scalene muscles

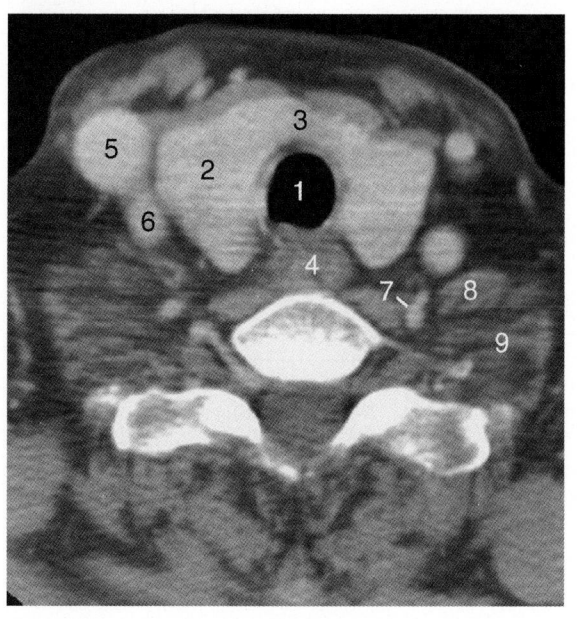

Figure 11.8 | Neck and Larynx—Axial CT scan. The CT/MRI transverse section can be correlated with the anatomy in Figure 11.5C as an assist to staging.

CANCER STATISTICS AND SURVIVAL

Specifically, the success in treating thyroid cancer is reflected in the large population of patients who are long-term survivors. The dominant papillary and follicular carcinomas yield 80% to 95% 10-year survival. Anaplastic cancers, both small and large cell varieties, are highly lethal (Figure 11.9).

*The foregoing passage is from Edge SB, Byrd DR, and Compton CC, et al, *AJCC Cancer Staging Manual, 7th edition.* New York, Springer, 2010, p. 38.

There are an estimated 45,000 new cases on Thyroid cancer in 2011 in the United States with 75% in women. The incidence rate continues to increase annually since mid 1990s and is the fastest increasing cancer in both males and females. Fortunately, Thyroid cancers are highly curable with 1,690 deaths in 2010 with death rate increasing by 1% since 1983 in men and stable in women. Risk factors are family history and radiation exposure particularly with radioactive I^{131} fallout due to nuclear power plant accidents. The 5 year survival rate for all thyroid cancer patients is 97%, 100% for localized stages, 97% regional stage and even 59% for distant metastases. As noted in Figure 11.9 for most histopathologic types, except for anaplastic cancers which are fatal.

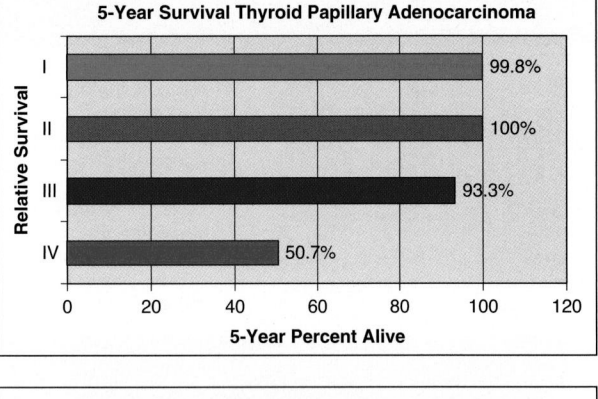

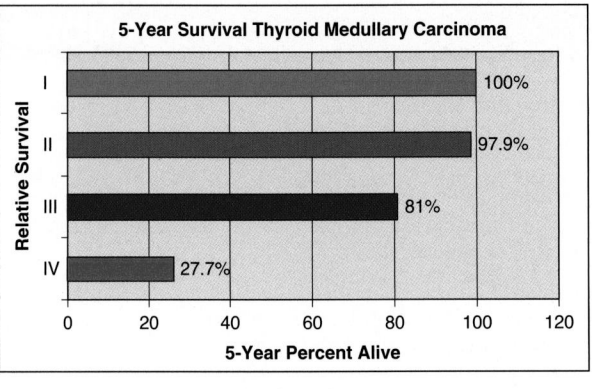

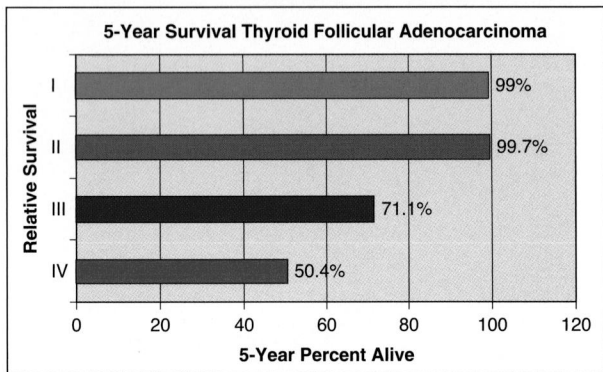

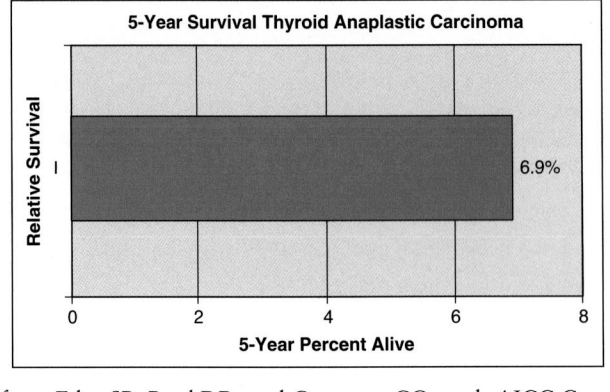

Figure 11.9 | Five-year survival rates by stage at diagnosis. (Data from Edge SB, Byrd DR, and Compton CC, et al, *AJCC Cancer Staging Manual, 7th edition.* New York, Springer, 2010.)

SECTION 2
Thorax Primary Sites

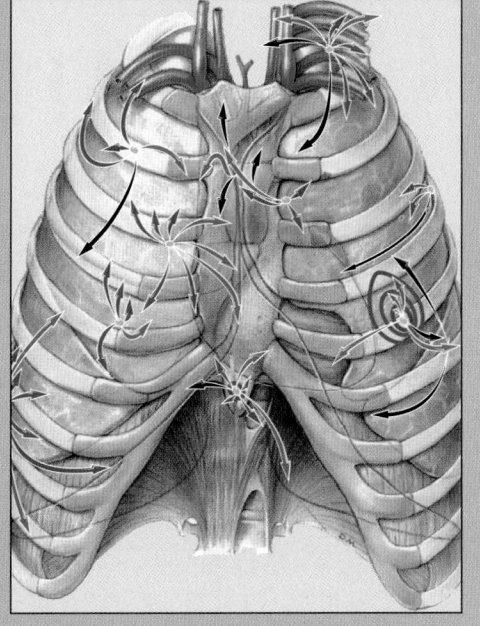

Introduction and Orientation

PERSPECTIVE AND PATTERNS OF SPREAD

The TNM lung cancer staging system reflects the oncoanatomy of the bronchial tree and its numerous divisions into pulmonary segments and functioning respiratory units, with variations in lining epithelial cell phenotypes.

PERSPECTIVE AND PATTERNS OF SPREAD

The thorax is associated with two major malignancies: pulmonary and breast cancers. To paraphrase Dickens as to the survival outcomes of these two highly prevalent cancers, one is the worst of our times and the other among the best of our times. Both organs consist of an elaborate branching ductile systems ending in a vast fine network of functioning acini. In the lung, its extensive bronchial labyrinth terminates in a huge alveolar micromesh for aeration. In the breast, its more pliable, but fine ductwork terminates in myriad compound tubuloalveolar acini that, under the stimulus of pregnancy and elevated levels of estrogens and progesterones, can expand rapidly for lactation.

Lung cancer, one of the most malignant cancers, generally strikes active men and women in the prime of their lives and is associated consistently with a 20- to 30-year history of smoking. Even the earliest signs, unfortunately, are indicative of advanced spread. A patient who presents with unresolved and recurrent pneumonia or persistent cough that leads to mild or severe chest pain often has unresectable disease. Cancers of the lung are highly invasive, rapidly metastasizing tumors. The term *lung cancer* is used in reference to many different histopathologic types, which can masquerade in the form of a large number of benign pulmonary conditions. A collage of patterns of cancer spread presents the basis for the large diversification on clinical presentations (Fig. 12.1 and Table 12.1).

Cancers of the bronchi and lung are highly lethal tumors. More than 90% of lung cancer patients do not survive this disease, and more than 50% have distant metastases at the time of diagnosis. In women, the death rate associated with lung cancer began to exceed that of breast cancer by 1987. Two million people in the United States died from lung cancer by 2000 before better diagnostic and therapeutic methods were developed. Breast cancer strikes one of every seven women in the United States, and accounts for more than 25% of all cancers in women.

With advances in diagnosis and treatment, survival rates have improved by 25% over the past five decades, ranging as high as a 97% 5-year survival for early stage node-negative disease.

If one views normal lung and lung cancers as derived from a pluripotential stem cell, then it is possible to understand its capability of expressing different features of the complex pulmonary anatomy as well as a variety of malignant phenotypes. The highly varied characteristics of each lung cancer's biologic behavior reflect their normal cell histogenic counterpart. These cells include pseudostratified epithelial reserve cells, type II pneumocytes, ciliated columnar cells, goblet cells, and neuroendocrine cells, each giving rise to a specific type of cancer. Utilizing this construct, the microscopic and macroscopic behavior of the various lung cancers and their spread patterns provides a logical basis for understanding the various staging notations and clarifications that have gradually evolved over time, while maintaining a consistently defined set of criteria for its staging. The current classification and staging was agreed to by the American Joint Committee on Cancer (AJCC)/International Union Against Cancer (UICC) in the third edition (1978); however, in subsequent editions annotations have been added to provide detailed explanations of modifications to the basic staging system, again recognizing that lung cancer is more than one disease.

Lung cancer spreads in different patterns depending on its inherent biopathology and anatomic location in the bronchial tree. Briefly, centrally located bronchial tumors tend to be **squamous cell cancers (SQCC)**, whereas tumors arising in peripheral bronchi more often are adenocarcinomas. **Bronchioloalveolar cancers** arise in alveoli and appear in a peripheral scar or as a patchy, diffuse pneumonitis and can be bilateral in distribution. **Adenocarcinomas** tend to arise in the segmental bronchi and are associated with lobar pneumonitis and atelectasis. SQCCs are true bronchogenic cancers arising in the major bronchi. **Small cell anaplastic cancers** tend to be central masses, whereas **large cell anaplastic carcinomas** are more peripheral and extensively infiltrating. No structure in the thorax or mediastinum is spared. Compression of mediastinal structures is associated invariably with advanced lymph node involvement, which can lead either to esophageal compression and difficulty in swallowing, venous compression and congestion associated with collateral circulation, or tracheal compression. Signs of metastatic disease involving such remote sites as the liver, brain, or bone are seen before any knowledge of a primary lung lesion.

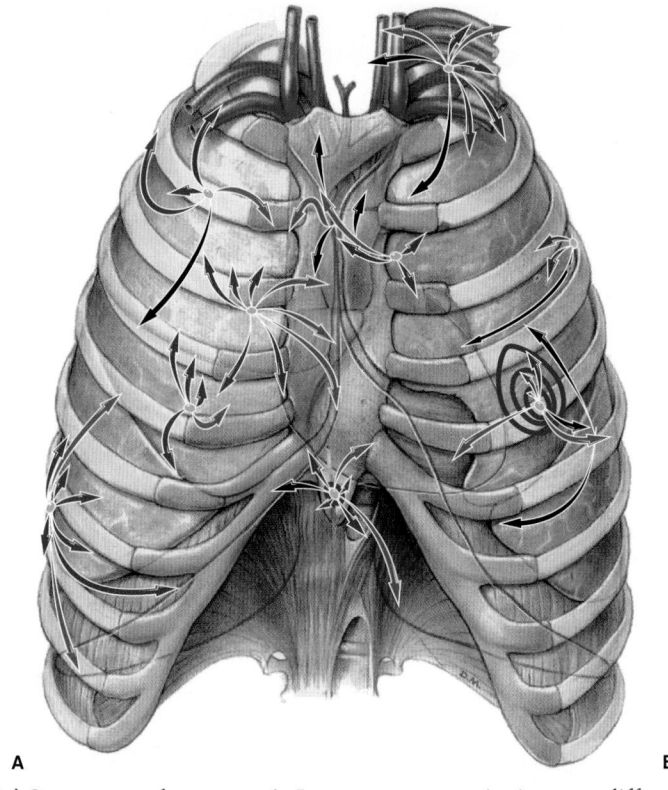
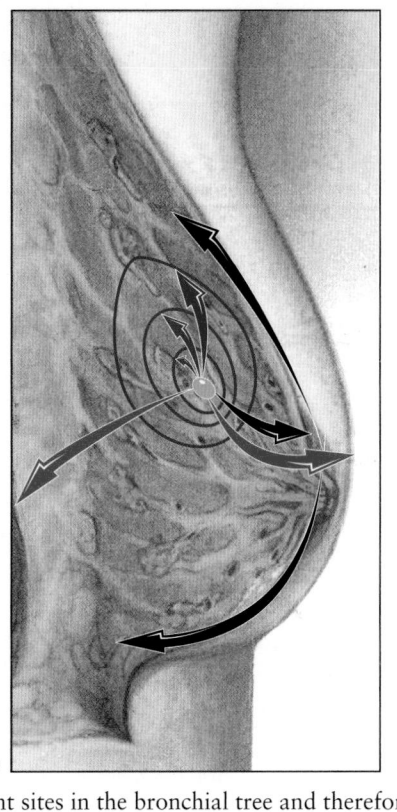

A

B

Figure 12.1 | Cancer spread patterns. A. Lung cancer can arise in many different sites in the bronchial tree and therefore presenting symptoms and signs are highly variable depending on its anatomic location. The cancer crabs are color-coded for T stage: Tis, yellow; T1, green; T2, blue; T3, purple; T4, red; and metastatic, black. **B.** Breast cancer spreads into the ductal system, stroma and ultimately invades lymphatics, skin and chest wall. The concept of visualizing patterns of spread to appreciate the surrounding anatomy is well demonstrated by the six-directional pattern i.e. SIMLAP Table 12.1.

TABLE 12.1A	SIMLAP*	
Lung Pancoast: Terminal Bronchus		
S	Superior sulcus segment	• T1
	Brachial plexus—T1, C8	• T3
	Subclavian artery	• T4
	Brachial plexus—C7+ above	• T4
I	Superior sulcus	
	Upper lobes	• T1
	Segmental atelectasis	• T2
M	Mediastinum	• T4
	Intervertebral foramen	• T4
	Spinal cord	• T4
L	1st rib	• T3
	Pleura	• T3
	Chest wall	• T3
A	1st rib	• T3
	Manubrium	• T3
	Pleura	• T3
	Chest wall	• T3
	1st rib	• T3
P	Stellate ganglion	• T3

*The six vectors of invasion are Superior, Inferior, Medial, Lateral, Anterior, and Posterior. The color-coded dots correlate the T stage with specific anatomic structure involved.

TABLE 12.1B	SIMLAP*	
Breast (Upper Outer) Quadrant		
S	UOQ	• T1
I	LOQ	• T1
M	IQ areola, nipples,	• T2
	Lactiferus Lacumae	• T3
L	UOQ	• T2
A	Skin	• T4b
	Inflammatory	• T4d
P	Pectoral fascia	• T4a
	Pectoralis major	• T4a
	Chest wall	• T4a

*The six vectors of invasion are Superior, Inferior, Medial, Lateral, Anterior, and Posterior. The color-coded dots correlate the T stage with specific anatomic structure involved.

TNM STAGING CRITERIA

TNM STAGING CRITERIA: LUNG

Lung cancer classification and staging has been stable since the first AJCC edition 1977. A major change in T categories occurred in the third edition (1988), when T3 resectable advanced disease was distinguished from T4 unresectable advanced disease. Also, N2 mediastinal nodes were divided into N2 ipsilateral and N3 contralateral nodes. Specific clarifications as to special presentations and histopathologic types were added in subsequent editions. In the third edition (1988), the AJCC introduced an elaborate numbering system for intrapulmonary and mediastinal nodes. The nodal status determines the stage grouping rather than the primary cancer status. Stage I is N0; stage II is N1; and stages IIIA and IIIB are determined by anatomic node location in the mediastinum, namely, ipsilateral or contralateral. In the fifth edition (1997), T3N0 was downstaged to stage IIB due to better survival for node-negative advanced disease patients. Then, nodal status is unresectable and assignment to stage IV would have been just as logical. Prognostic factors, including molecular, biologic, and genetic markers, are noted but are considered investigational and have not been incorporated into the staging system.

The origin of breast cancer is mainly within its glandular or ductal structure that infiltrates the lobule of its origin, then its quadrant that invades in one of two directions, toward skin or chest wall. The chest wall, for both breast and lung cancer, when involved is a sign of advancement. It is essential to understand the oncologic anatomy of the mammary gland to appreciate breast cancer's clinical manifestations and patterns of spread. Detection requires knowledge of the cancer's pathologic behavior, the surrounding structures that are commonly invaded, the location of the regional lymph nodes, and how the cancer can spread to remote sites through the breast's rich vascular network. Knowing this anatomy is a fundamental step toward the diagnosis and staging of this cancer.

With the seventh edition of the AJCC manual, dramatic changes in lung cancer staging and classification occurred. The database for the fifth and sixth editions were based on M. D. Anderson Cancer Center experience totaling 5,319 cases. The revisions currently are based on the International Association for Study of Lung Cancer (IASLC), which has amassed more than 100,000 patients of which 80,000 were used for analysis based on data from 46 centers in 19 countries, diagnosed and followed between 1990 and 2000. Summary of TNM stages are recommended for both non–small cell and small cell cancers plus carcinoid tumors.

SUMMARY OF CHANGES SEVENTH EDITION AJCC

The current staging system is now recommended for the classification of both non–small cell and small cell lung carcinomas and for carcinoid tumors of the lung (Fig. 12.2).

- The T classifications have been redefined:
  - T1 has been subclassified into T1a (≤2 cm in size) and T1b (>2–3 cm in size)
  - T2 has been subclassified into T2a (>3–5 cm in size) and T2b (>5–7 cm in size)
  - T2 (>7 cm in size) has been reclassified as T3
  - Multiple tumor nodules in the same lobe have been reclassified from T4 to T3
  - Multiple tumor nodules in the same lung but a different lobe have been reclassified from M1 to T4
- No changes have been made to the N classification. However, a new international lymph node map defining the anatomical boundaries for lymph node stations has been developed.
- The M classifications have been redefined:
  - The M1 has been subdivided into M1a and M1b
  - Malignant pleural and pericardial effusions have been reclassified from T4 to M1a
  - Separate tumor nodules in the contralateral lung are considered M1a
  - M1b designates distant metastases

Because of the magnitude of the T-category changes with shifts in both directions, that is both downstaging and upstaging, it is important to review the stage groupings of the sixth and seventh editions. The TNM Staging Matrix is color coded for identification of Stage Group once T and N stages are determined (Table 12.2).

TABLE 12.2	**Stage Summary Matrix**				
	N0	**N1**	**N2**	**N3**	**M1**
T1	IA	IIA	IIIA	IIIB	IV
T2	IB	IIB	IIIA	IIIB	IV
T3	IIB	IIIA	IIIA	IIIB	IV
T4	IIIB	IIIB	IIIB	IIIB	IV

Thorax: Lung Cancers
- N stage determines stage group
  - N0, N1, N2, N3a, N3b are stage group I, II, IIIA, IIIB
- N1 can be associated with T1 or T2
- T stage modifies substages
  - T1, T2 N0 = IA, IIB and T1, T2 N2 =IIA, IIB
- M stage is a separate stage
  - M1 = IV
- Exceptions are:
  - BAC only has T progression by definition
  - SCA is either *limited* or *extensive* (i.e., M0 or M1 independent of T or N stages)

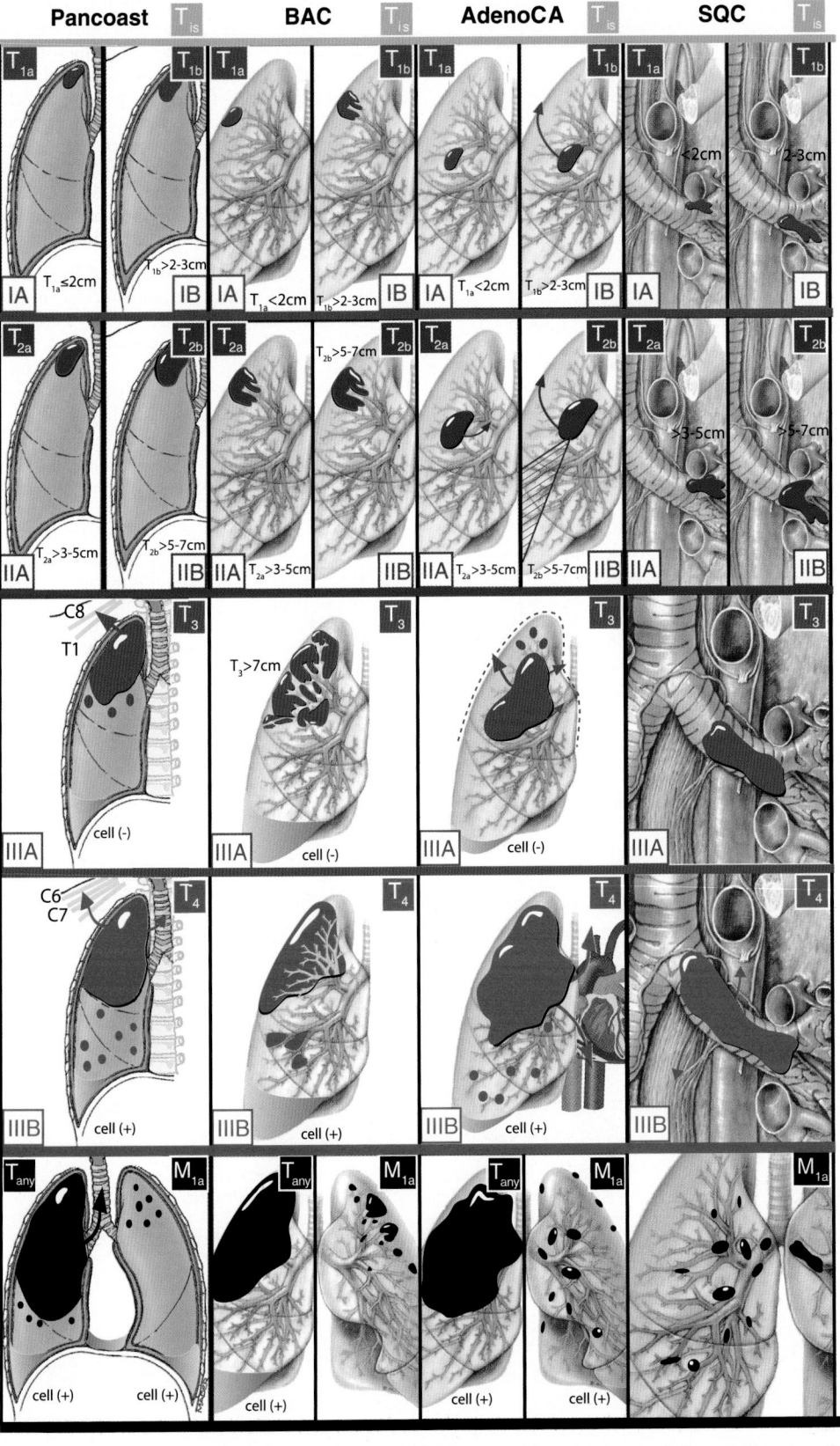

Figure 12.2 | **The T criteria are varied for each histopathologic type of lung cancer in their manifestation due to their anatomic location and origin, the bronchial tree.** Pancoast cancer arises in superior sulcus and advances by local invasion into juxta-opposed structures. Bronchioloalveolar cancer (BAC) arises in the acini peripherally and advances by lepidic spread via alveolar pores of Kohn. Adenocarcinomas (AdenoCA) arise in lobar bronchi and advance by producing lobar atelectasis and pneumonitis. Squamous cell cancers (SQC) tend to arise in main bronchi and advance to the carina. All lung cancer types can become multifocal in the lobe, they arise in T3, or spread into lung of origin T4, or spread to contralateral lung M1.

OVERVIEW OF HISTOGENESIS

In the thorax, there are three major sectors and four major cancer sites that are staged (Fig. 12.3A–D). The first sector is the lung, major bronchi, and its visceral pleura. The second sector is the chest wall, which includes the parietal pleura and breast. The third sector is anatomically the most diverse, namely, the mediastinum and its contents: the heart and great vessels, thymus gland, major intrathoracic lymph node chains, thoracic duct, and esophagus. A cancer arising in one of the sectors tends to remain localized within that sector until it spreads into regional nodes or invades hematogenously. The bony thorax and intercostal musculature are anatomic structures that surround the lung and mediastinum (Table 12.3).

- The bronchial tree (Fig. 12.3A) originates at the tracheal carina starting with the *main bronchi*; then it divides within the visceral pleura into the pulmonary parenchyma as *lobar bronchi* (secondary bronchi). The left lung is divided into two lobes and further divides into 10 bronchopulmonary segments. The right lung divides into three lobes and also into 10 bronchopulmonary segments. The segmental bronchus and its associated lung parenchyma constitute a bronchopulmonary segment. Each segment of each lobe has its own blood supply (bronchial, pulmonary arteries, and veins) and can be resected along their connective tissue septa. The bronchi undergo another five to six orders of divisions, downsizing into *terminal bronchioles* that finally end in *respiratory bronchioles*. The smallest functional unit of pulmonary structure consists of a single respiratory bronchiole, which allows for gas exchange via its acini and their multiple alveolar sacs.

- The subdivisions of the bronchial tree and summary of its histologic features are shown in Figure 12.3B. An anatomic relationship is postulated between lining epithelial cells and specific pulmonary cancers. Relating these different anatomic divisions of the bronchi to the origin of each histopathologic cancer type provides a rationale for many of the notations and clarifications for specific lung cancers and their staging features. The mesothelial pleural surfaces are barriers to cancer penetration. The lungs are encased in membranes called *visceral pleura*; the chest cavity is lined with a similar, although more fibrous, membrane called the *parietal pleura*. The potential space between these two membranes is the pleural cavity that allows for the smooth movement of lungs with respiration. Pleural mesotheliomas represent a new category that has been staged and classified for the first time in the sixth edition of the AJCC/UICC.

- The mammary gland consists of 15 to 20 lobes of glandular tissue with varying amounts of fat, in a dense fibroareolar stroma, and is attached to the anterior chest wall (Fig. 12.3C). In cross-sections starting from the nipple, there are openings of the lactiferous ducts and their lactiferous sinuses, which are the conduits for the secretions of the hormonally stimulated breast glands. These ducts are distinct and individual for each lobule; they first run dorsally from the nipple and then spread radially into the glandular tissue. The breast can be viewed three-dimensionally in terms of its anatomic relationship to other structures. As a superficial gland, it is covered by skin. Posteriorly, it is bounded by the underlying muscles of the chest. Deep to the glandular tissue there is usually a small amount of fat, which, along with the breast proper, is bounded by a deeper layer of superficial fascia. This layer can usually be dissected free from the deep fascia, investing the pectoralis major muscle. Connective tissue septa called the *suspensory ligaments* (of Cooper) form subdivisions of the breast, dividing the breast into lobes. The pectoralis major, the muscle underlying the breast, consists of two heads that arise from the clavicle, sternum, cartilages of the true ribs, and the sixth rib. The schematic of the breast dramatizes the largely ductal branched tubuloalveolar glands contained within a dense connective tissue stroma and variable amounts of adipose tissue. Each of the 15 to

---

TABLE 12.3	Orientation of Histogenesis of Primary Cancer Sites		
Primary Site Normal Anatomic Structures	**Derivative Normal Cell**	**Cancer Histopathologic Type Primary Site**	**Thorax Axial Level Assigned***
Terminal bronchiole	Simple cuboidal	Pancoast cancer (adenocarcinoma)	T1-2
Respiratory bronchiole, acini, alveoli	Type II pneumocyte	Bronchioloalveolar cancer	T2-3
Segmental bronchi	Goblet cell ciliated columnar	Adenocarcinoma with mixed subtypes	T3-4
Bronchial neuroendocrine cells	Transdifferentiated neuroendocrine	Large cell anaplastic cancer	T4-5
Main bronchi	Metaplasia of pseudostratified columnar cells	SQCC	T5-6
Lobar bronchi	Dedifferentiated stem cell ~Lung bud	Small cell cancer	T6-7
Visceral parietal pleura and space	Mesothelial cell	Mesothelioma	T7-8
Breast (chest wall)	Breast duct and lobule cells	Adenocarcinoma	T8-9
Esophagus (mediastinum and diaphragm)	Stratified squamous cell	SQCC	T9-10

SQCC, squamous cell cancer.
*Assigned thoracic axial level is designed to encompass and illustrate the different thoracic anatomic sectors and planes.

20 lobes of the breast radiates from the mammary papilla (nipple), and each is connected by a specific lactiferous duct with its own lacuna or dilated sinus (Fig. 12.3F,G).

• The esophagus consists of three principal regions (cervical, thoracic, cardiac) and it bridges the head and neck, thoracic, and abdominal oncoanatomies. Its mediastinal course allows for a rapid overview of the various organs and structures in the mediastinum, especially those contained in the posterior compartment, which include the sympathetic and parasympathetic nerves and ganglia, the spinal cord and thoracic vertebrae, the thoracic duct and the aorta, which has the longest contact with the esophagus as both of these structures descend in the chest and exit via their own diaphragmatic stoma into the abdomen. In summary, the thorax oncoanatomy is presented to encompass all the potential primary sites and their malignant gradient.

• The lung oncoanatomy rests on its bronchial tree and its order of 10 subdivisions, lung lobes, and segments and the variation in cell lining phenotypes. The malignant gradient tends to worsen as cancers in the periphery arise in more central locations (Fig. 12.3D).

• The breast oncoanatomy rests on its more pliable 15 to 20 lobules, their extensive ductal arrays with the malignant gradient tends to worsen as cancers arise in the periphery and invade into the chest wall and more rapidly into lymphatics (Fig. 12.3D).

• The esophagus is a thin-walled structure that courses through the mediastinum with a high malignant gradient throughout; cancers penetrate vital structures and viscera in the different mediastinal compartments.

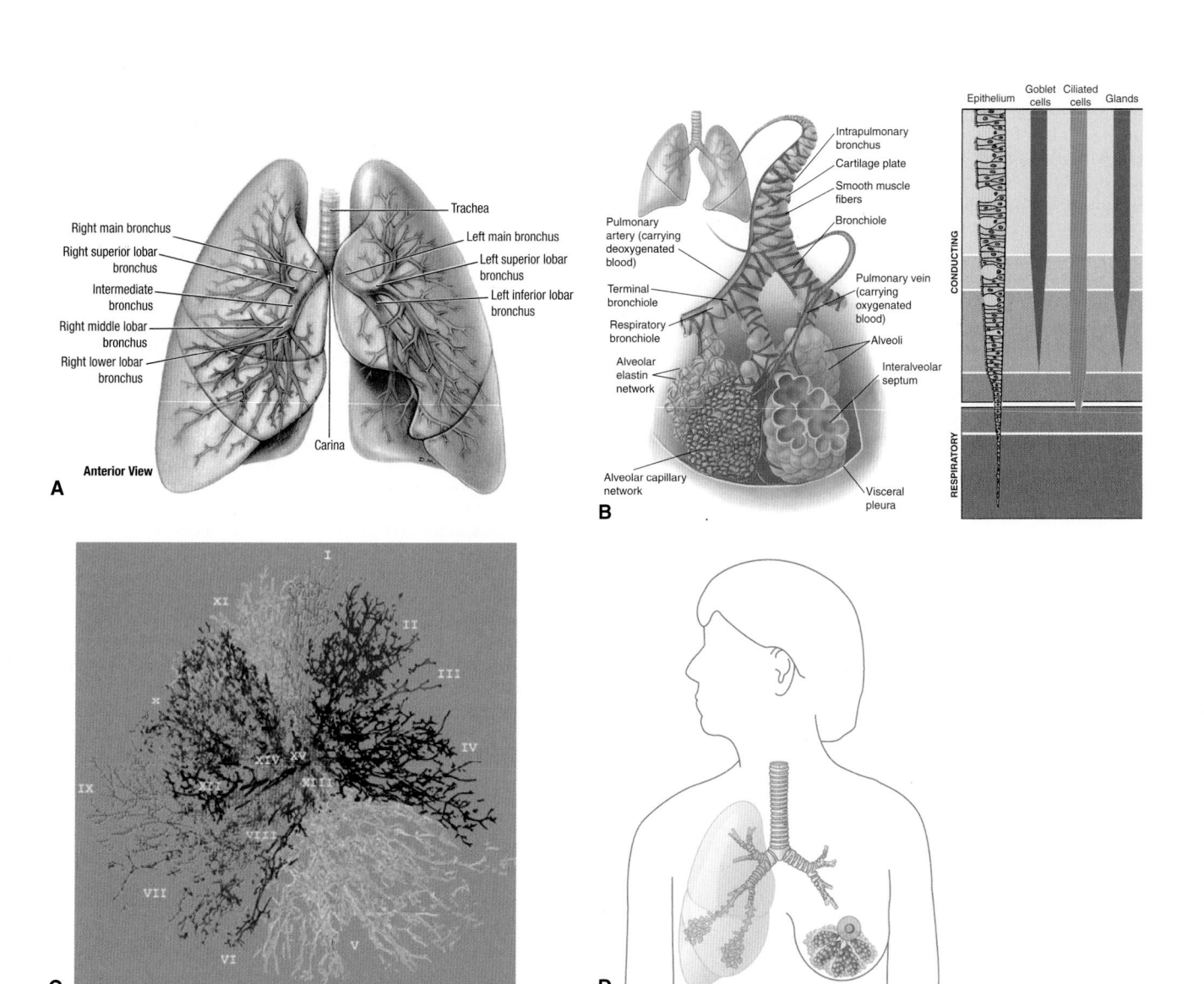

Figure 12.3 | Overview of histogenesis. A. Lung: Divisions of the Bronchial Tree. **B.** The lobar bronchi on the right and left divide into ten segmental bronchi. **C.** All ducts and their branches in an autopsy breast, viewed "en face". Each roman numerical refers to different independent duct systems for the fifteen lobules that constitute the duct system. **D.** Comparison of breast ductile system and lung bronchial tree.

T-ONCOANATOMY

ORIENTATION OF THREE-PLANAR T-ONCOANATOMY OF PRIMARY SITES

The three-planar anatomy to overcome the physiologic changes with respiratory and cardiac motion are correlated with anatomic views in dissection atlases, highlighting selected coronal and sagittal planes. The transverse planes are assigned to different lung cancers to provide a basis to encompass the complexities of thoracic anatomy. The assigned axial level is provided at 10 different levels to act as a scaffold for correlative computed tomography (CT) and cross-sectional magnetic resonance imaging (MRI).

The multiplanar diagrams in anterior (Fig. 12.4A) and lateral (Fig. 12.4B) views present the different thoracic malignancies, as variations of lung cancer histopathology and its intrinsic anatomy. Again, the biologic behavior and invasions of pulmonary cancer are determined in large part by the anatomy. To encompass the thoracic and pulmonary anatomy, the presentation of the 10 different primary site isocenters is utilized. Therefore, in Table 12.4 a specific anatomic aspect of the normal lung will be correlated with each cancer type, reinforcing concepts as to classification, staging, primary anatomy, lymph node drainage, and vascular drainage. A cephalad to caudad odyssey follows.

1. Pancoast cancers arise in the neck rather than the chest, emphasizing the apex of the lung which extends above and behind the clavicle. The symptom complex or syndrome caused by the apical cancer is readily apparent clinically since the superior sulcus of the lung is in direct contact with the inferior portion of the brachial plexus (C8 and T1). Also the stellate ganglion of the sympathetic chain is often compressed against the T1 transverse process as the cancer invades perineurally.

2. Bronchioloalveolar cancers (BACs) arise from the peripheral and most terminal part of the bronchoalveolar segment, at which point respiratory bronchioles (without cartilage) branch into an acinus consisting of alveolar sacs. BACs typically consist of large, mucus-containing cells, reminiscent of the type II pneumocytes and appear as parenchymal nodules. With their lepidic, scale-like growth pattern, they often appear in association with peripheral scars. BACs account for 5% to 9% of all lung cancers but in recent studies have increased to 20% to 24% of all lung cancers.

3. Adenocarcinomas (ADC) are the most common histopathology type of lung cancer and arise from the intrapulmonary bronchi that branch like limbs of a tree in each lung then divide into segmental and subsegmental bronchi, characterized by cartilage in their walls. They tend to be intrapulmonary in location, arising from glandular forming epithelial lining cells of bronchi. Four subtypes or variants exist and range from abundant mucus production in well-differentiated cancers and to a cancer that becomes more undifferentiated, losing the glandular arrangement. The lobar anatomy is stressed because atelectasis and obstructive pneumonitis are common and extend to the hilar area.

4. Small cell carcinoma (SCC) are the most dedifferentiated cancers and tend to be more central in location close to the mediastinum. Such cancers arise from or revert to anlage pluripotential epithelial stem cells, and one may draw an appropriate analogy to the endoderm forming cells at the time in embryogenesis when the epithelia of the future lung airways appear as right and left lung buds, giving rise to lobar and segmental airways. SCCs are extremely aggressive cancers and in the majority of presentations (80%) are central mediastinal tumors, disseminating rapidly into submucosal lymphatic vessels and regional lymph nodes, and almost always present without bronchial invasion. This pattern of spread is to hilar and mediastinal nodes with no evident primary bronchial lesion.

5. Squamous cell cancers (SQC) are true bronchogenic cancers arising in major bronchi, which are often extrapleural in location with a different blood supply, namely, bronchial arteries instead of pulmonary arteries. SQCs are common cancers, although they comprise less than 50% incidence, more in the 30% to 35% range. Smoking is invariably part of the history and, when hemoptysis is associated with a coarse hilar rhonchial wheeze, this triad is diagnostic of bronchogenic carcinoma.

6. Large cell anaplastic cancers (LCAC) are a histologic diagnosis of exclusion and behave similarly to small cell anaplastic cancers. The large cell anaplastic cancers are more proximal in location and locally tend to invade the mediastinum and its structures early. Pericardial effusion is currently categorized as T4 if malignant cells are present. The most common cardiac involvement is a pericardial malignancy secondary to pulmonary cancer, or to a lesser degree, breast cancer. If pericardial cytology is negative, an incidental viral pericarditis needs to be ruled out. Although metastatic hematogenous spread places malignant cells in direct contact with the endocardial surface of the heart, metastatic myocardial nodules are a terminal event and are most often found postmortem. Large cell anaplastic cancers behave similar to small cell cancers and are known for their rapid fatal spread.

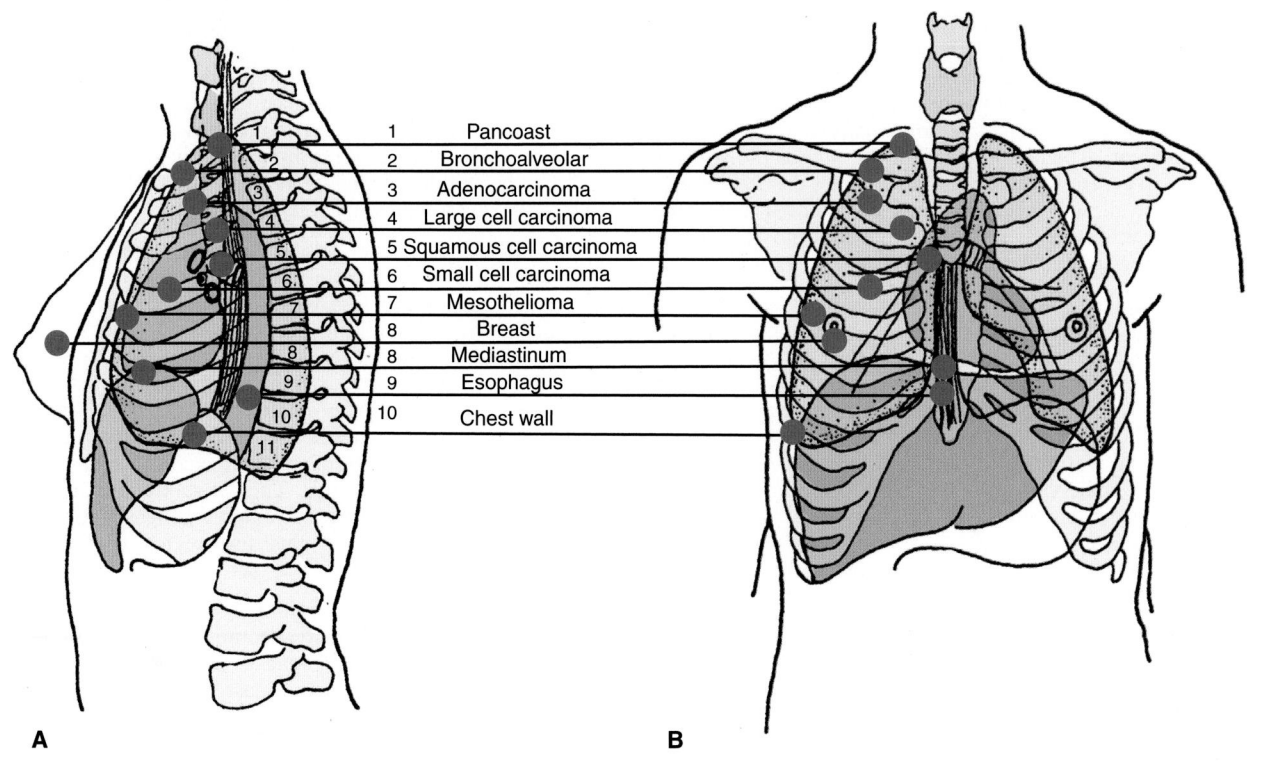

Figure 12.4 | Orientation of three-planar T-oncoanatomy of nine primary sites in the thorax. A. Anterior coronal. **B.** Lateral sagittal. Because of the angulation of the vertebrae to the convex curvature of the thoracic spine, the reference levels are between the vertebrae. *(continued)*

TABLE 12.4	Anatomic Isocenters of Primary Cancer Sites			
Normal Structure (Cancer Type)	**Relevant Anatomy**		**Thorax Axial Level Assigned***	
Terminal bronchi (superior sulcus cancer)	Supraclavicular, brachial plexus, stellate ganglion	T1-2	L/R subclavian, carotid artery	
Respiratory bronchi (bronchioloalveolar)	Surface anatomy of lung periphery, segmental/lobar arrangements	T3-4	L/R subclavian, carotid brachiocephalic trunk	
Segmental bronchi (adenocarcinoma)	Bronchial tree in situ emphasis on lobar divisions	T3-4	Arch of aorta Azygos vein	
Lobar bronchi (large cell anaplastic)	Large arteries, aorta, and innervations	T4-5	Ascending and descending aorta	
Main bronchi (SQC)	Trachea, carina, bifurcation of bronchi	T5-6	Pulmonary arteries	
Lung bud, roots (small cell anaplastic)	Large veins, SVC, and azygos and collateral hemiazygos	T6-7	Pulmonary veins	
Pleural space (mesothelioma)	Pleural space extends from neck into abdomen	T7-8	R/L auricle heart	
Mammary glands (breast cancer)	Chest wall construct: intercostal muscle, nerves, vessels	T8-9	R/L ventricle Apex of heart	
Mediastinum (esophagus)	Paraesophageal, neck through posterior mediastinum to abdomen	T9-10	Base of heart	

SQC, squamous cell cancer; SVC, superior vena cava; R, right; L, left.
*Assigned thoracic axial level is designed to encompass and illustrate the different thoracic anatomic sectors and planes.

7. Mesotheliomas are pleural-based malignancies derived from the cell lining of the pleuroperitoneal membranes of the diaphragm that separate the pleural and peritoneal cavities from each other during their embryonal development. The mesenchyme lining of these cavities differentiates into a simple single layer of squamous epithelium or mesothelium. The mesothelium of the lung is the visceral pleura. In contrast, the parietal pleura lines the diaphragm, thoracic wall, and mediastinum. Pleural-based malignancies are designated as mesotheliomas and most often are due to asbestos exposure years earlier (Fig. 12.4C).

8. Breast cancers arise in the mammary glands, an appendage on the chest wall. Cancers of the mammary gland predominate among tumors of the chest wall, which are both benign and malignant. Breast cancers can invade their rich lymphatic plexus and drain into the axillary and internal thoracic nodes (mammary or parasternal), which are essential features of its anatomic spread. As the most common female cancer, it has been thoroughly studied and analyzed. The anatomic origin is most often either intraductal or the terminal lobule. It gradually invades the lobar segments and their suspensory ligaments with dimpling of the skin due to the loss of elasticity. Extensive invasion of dermal lymphatics leads to a *peau d'orange* pitting, which is caused by the pull of multiple Cooper ligament insertions in the edematous dermal layer. Invasion into the pectoral muscle and chest wall leads to fixation of the cancer (Fig. 12.4D).

9. Mediastinal tumors can arise from any structure, encompassed between the anterior manubrial sternal boney plate and the posterior spine, which are invested in the mediastinal pleura. A multitude of malignancies arise in the different compartments of the mediastinum, which is divided into superior, anterior, middle, and posterior segments. The superior mediastinum is defined by a plane intersecting T4 with the manubriosternal junction, and the other compartments are located below with the heart in the middle mediastinum separating the anterior and posterior compartments (Fig. 12.4E).

10. Esophageal cancers arise in different anatomic regions ranging from its cervical origin to the longer longitudinal intrathoracic portion terminating at the cardia of the stomach. Although the esophagus is thought of as a thoracic organ, esophageal cancers can present in the neck and abdomen as well as in the chest. The TNM staging for esophageal cancer is presented as an introduction to gastrointestinal malignancies. Its thin muscular walls, once invaded, rapidly disseminate epithelial cancers, mistaking them for a bolus of food. The peristaltic milking activity allows for its rapid dissemination through its submucosal lymphatics and its drainage into regional lymph nodes (Fig. 12.4F).

11. The heart occupies the middle mediastinum and primary neoplasms are extremely uncommon. The most common pattern of metastatic spread is direct extension into the pericardial sac from lung, breast, and esophagus cancers, resulting in pericardial effusions and tamponage. Multiple military metastases to heart as part of diffuse metastatic spread is more often discovered at autopsy rather than clinically (Fig. 12.4F).

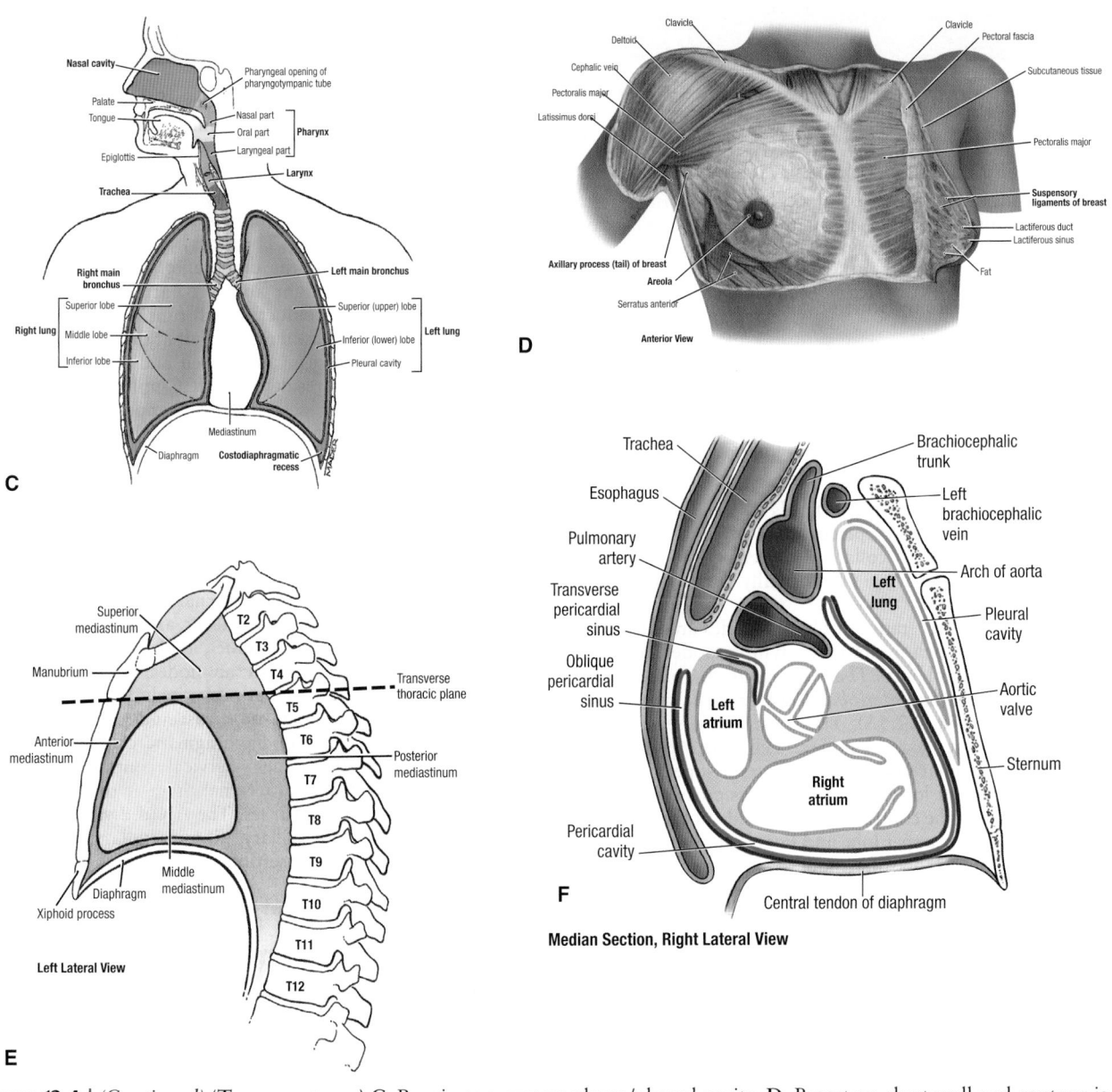

Figure 12.4 | *(Continued)* (**T-oncoanatomy**) **C.** Respiratory system pleura/pleural cavity. **D.** Breast on chest wall and contour is shaped by ligaments of Cooper. **E.** Mediastinum is divided into four compartments. **F.** Esophagus can invade different mediastinal structures depending on location.

M-ONCOANATOMY

M-ONCOANATOMY OF REGIONAL VEINS AND NEUROVASCULAR BUNDLE

The major vessels of the thorax are great vessels of the mediastinum, the aorta, and its divisions into brachiocephalic and subclavian arteries (Figs. 12.6A and 12.6B). The great veins consist of the anterior located, superior vena cava and brachiocephalic vein, the midthoracic pulmonary veins, and the azygos and hemiazygos venous complex posteriorly. The major neurovascular bundle is the vagal esophageal plexus and sympathetic gangli and nerves located in posterior mediastinum. Metastatic spread to distant organs according to the histopathologic type of lung cancer is listed in Table 12.6. The anatomic distribution of distant metastases is presented as a function of histopathologic type of lung cancer.

The lung is the most common site of metastatic cancer from other cancers due to the drainage of most sites into the superior and inferior vena cava into the right side of the heart and the flow via pulmonary artery into the lung, which acts as a filter for circulating cancer cells. For this reason, pulmonary metastases are more common than primary lung cancers. Pulmonary metastases can be the size of cannon balls on imaging and often nodules are round and well defined (see Table 31.1 *Clinical Oncology* 8th ed., p. 845).

Lung metastases can also be solitary and when detected as single or limited, the number of oligometastases can be successfully cured by surgical resection or stereotactic radiation surgery or therapy. The incidence of lung cancer metastases far exceeds diagnosis by imaging (see Table 32.1 Rubin P, Williams JP. Clinical Oncology: *A multi-Disciplinary Approach for Physicians & Students 8th edition*. Philadelphia, W.B. Saunders, 2001. p. 856).

Lymphangitic spread is less common and presents as "B lines," producing a diffuse reticular pattern from hilus to pleura, leading to shortness of breath and asphyxia.

TABLE 12.6	Anatomic Distribution of Distant Metastases of Lung			
Site of Metastasis	Squamous (%)	Small Cell Anaplastic (%)	Large Cell Anaplastic (%)	Adenocarcinoma (%)
Lymph nodes	137 (54)	163 (85)	135 (76)	42 (75)
Liver	58 (23)	122 (54)	67 (38)	26 (47)
Adrenals	54 (21)	84 (44)	69 (39)	17 (30)
Bones	59 (21)	75 (39)	53 (30)	23 (41)
Brain	26 (17)	45 (42)	30 (24)	13 (39)
Kidney	39 (15)	28 (14.5)	24 (13.5)	11 (20)
Pancreas	9 (3.5)	46 (24)	25 (14)	3 (5)
Lung	31 (12)	13 (7)	15 (8)	8 (14)
Pleura	18 (7)	21 (11)	9 (5)	3 (5)
Total	255	191	179	56

From Line DH, Deeley TJ. The necropsy findings in carcinoma of the bronchus. *Br J Dis Chest* 1971;65:238–242, with permission.

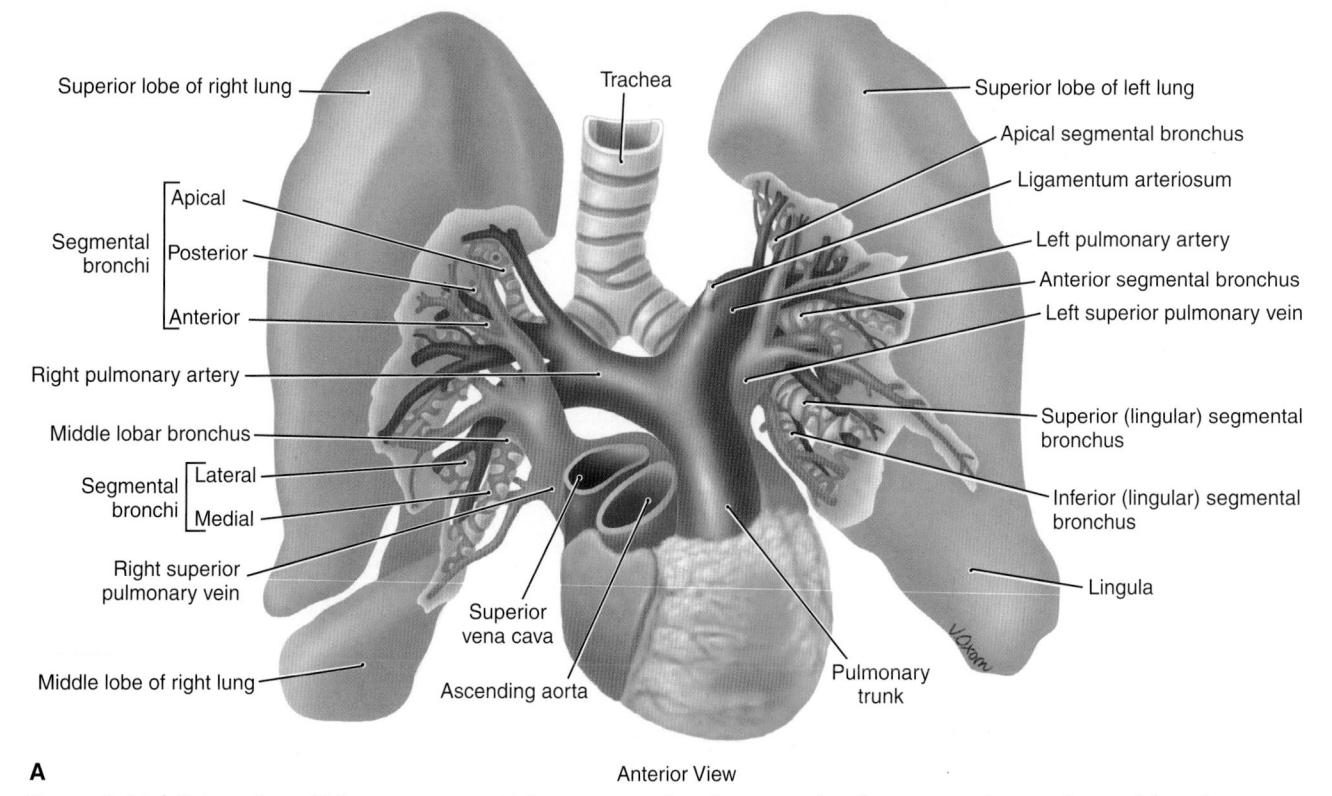

A

Anterior View

Figure 12.6A | Orientation of M-oncoanatomy. Pulmonary anterior views are related to metastatic spread to and from lung, pulmonary artery, and pulmonary vein respectively.

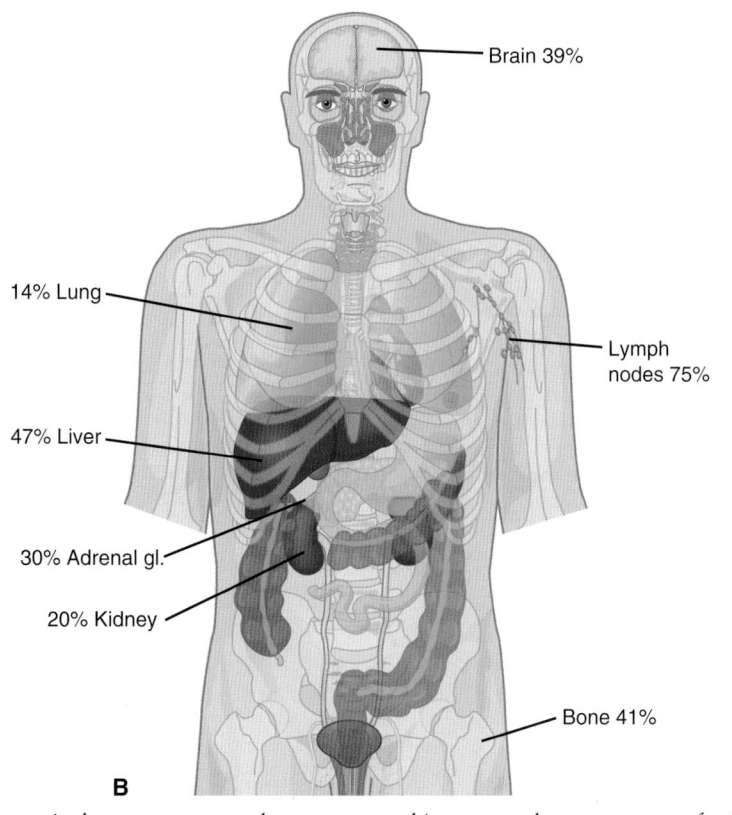

B

Figure 12.6B | Adenocarcinoma is the most common lung cancer and is presented as a prototype for lung cancers. The incidence and distribution of distant metastases are noted as percentages and correlate with Table 12.6.

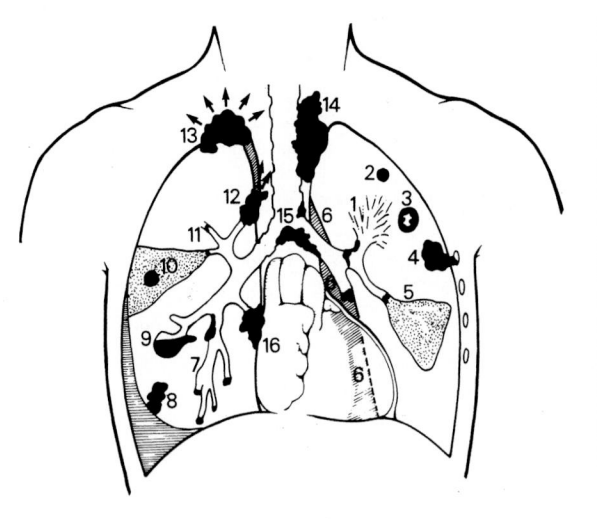

Figure 12.7 | Lung cancer imaging. The most frequent manifestation or masquerades of bronchial cancers (1) to (16). (1) Hilar lung cancer with endobronchial growth (relatively early elicitation of the cough reflex). (2) Typical round focus. (3) Tumor cavern (note the thick irregular walls). (4) Subpleural focus infiltrating the chest wall. (5) Obstructive segmental discontinuation with retention in pneumonia. (6) Atelectasis, which is hidden behind the cardiac shadow (lateral radiograph). (7) Secondary bronchiectasis due to partial stenosis. (8) Focus near to the pleura, with effusion. (9) Necrotizing tumor with draining bronchus (abscess symptom). (10) Segmental atelectasis. (11) Obstruction emphysema due to valve occlusion. (12) and (13) Outbreak of carcinoma into the mediastinum, for example, in the direction of the vena cava (upper inflow congestion) or as Pancoast tumor. (14) Lymph node involvement in the upper mediastinum and paratracheally, extending to the upper clavicular fossa. Detection by lymph node biopsy according to Daniels or by mediastinoscopy: (15) and (16) carcinoma spreading to the trachea and pericardium, respectively. Note: A bronchial carcinoma can be masked even in a normal radiograph.

Oncoimaging Annotations

- Chest radiographs seldom detect primary lung cancers in their early stages.

- Spiral CT is useful in high-risk patients to detect nodules and infiltrates.

- Positron emission tomography (PET) imaging with ^{18}FDG (fluorodeoxyglucose) appears to be of value in discriminating malignant versus benign nodules.

- CT can detect mediastinal adenopathy, but histologic verification is essential to ascertain if it is malignant.

- Determining N2 versus N3 mediastinal nodes is important; it establishes resectability.

- MRI can be of value in assessing mediastinal invasion, chest wall and rib erosion, and compromised large vein involvement.

RULES OF CLASSIFICATION AND STAGING

Clinical Staging and Imaging

Lung cancer masquerades as many different pulmonary diseases and their clinical presentations are radiologically. The most commonly used procedure for staging lung, mediastinal, and breast cancers is the spiral CT. This is utilized to define the extent of both lung and breast cancer when they are invasive and advanced MRI is useful for assessing the mediastinal malignancies or adenopathy related to pulmonary and breast lymphatic invasion. Metastatic spread workup, which is common to lung and breast cancer, includes bone scans when osseous metastases are suspected. MRI is often utilized for brain and CT liver metastases. The workup for metastatic disease is based on symptoms being present rather than electively (Table 12.7; Figure 12.7).

TABLE 12.7	Imaging Modalities for Diagnosis and Staging	
Method	Capability	Recommended
Primary tumor and regional nodes workup		
Chest films	Baseline image	Yes
CT/spiral CT	Most useful of all modalities for determining characteristics of T and N in the thorax and M in the brain and liver	Yes
MRI	Not as good as CT	No
Percutaneous needle biopsy	Guided by fluoroscopy or CT, accurate in establishing cytologic diagnosis from T (particularly peripheral lung lesions); M (especially liver or bone); less experience with N	Yes
Mediastinoscopy/ thoracoscopy	Confirmation of nodal involvement	Yes
Metastatic work-up for clinically suspected metastases		
CT/echography	For liver, adrenals	Yes
CT/MRI	For brain	Yes
Bone scan	For the bone	Yes
PET scan	Diagnosis of peripheral lesions can differentiate between cancer and benign lesions. Staging of true extent of primary and lymph node involvement.	Yes, if clinically indicated

CT, computed tomography; M, metastasis; MRI, magnetic resonance imaging; N, node; PET, positron emission tomography; T, tumor.

STAGING WORKUP, PROGNOSIS, AND CANCER SURVIVAL

PROGNOSIS AND CANCER STATISTICS AND SURVIVAL

Also of interest are biological and genetic markers that are of prognostic value based on meta-analysis data of the IASLC (Table 12.7).

The 5-year survival rates for thoracic cancer over five decades presents the best and worst achievements in controlling cancer deaths. Because breast cancer is slowly increasing in incidence and prevalence, it is anticipated that there will be more than 200,000 new diagnoses of invasive breast cancers annually in this country alone. In addition, there are 60,000 cases of highly curable preinvasive cancers. Breast cancer is currently found with mammography, mainly in noninvasive or early stage I cancers where survival rates are at the 95% mark. The improvement in breast cancer survival over the past five decades has been dramatic, with a doubling in the survival rate from 45% to 90%, also reflecting the advances in multimodal management. Breast cancer is the most common cancer in women (215,990), which translates to one third of all neoplasms diagnosed in the United States. Fortunately, most patients with breast cancer survive and only 40,110 deaths (15%) can be attributed to the malignancy.

Lung and bronchus cancers are the second most common cancers at almost 116,000 new male patients and a comparable 105,000 female patients, accounting for 15% and 14%, respectively, of cancer patients. However, lung and bronchus cancer is public enemy number one and is the leading cause of death for men 86,000 (29%) and 71,000 (26%) women. An estimated 222,500 new cases of lung cancer annually will be diagnosed by 2010, with a predicted 160,000 deaths in the same year (Tables 12.8 and 12.10). This is one of the most dismal cancer survival rates for NSCLC at 17% vs 6% for SCLC. Despite the progress of research, the causes of this disease and mortality rates have not been reduced.

Curability concepts can only be applied to breast cancer with 86% of all stages surviving 5 years, and with excellent results for all stages: 88% 5-year and an impressive 97% 5-year for localized disease and even 78% for regional nodes. For lung and esophageal cancers, most patients are in advanced stages with only 2% to 3% surviving 5 years. Although there have been improvements in multimodal approaches, only about 10% of such patients survive.

Whereas the 10% gain in lung cancer survival over five decades also represents a doubling in survival rates, it remains one of the most lethal of all cancers despite gains in knowledge. To end on a positive note, early stage I lung cancer can result in a better than 90% survival (Fig. 12.8). Although routine spiral CT scans of the thorax in high-risk patients have yielded a high number of early stage lung cancers, this procedure is too costly to apply routinely. However, it is recommended for the habitual heavy smoker on an annual basis. Large cohorts of patients have been screened, and early detection of small lung cancers have been found with an increase in their survival rate.

TABLE 12.8	Meta-analyses Published on the Prognostic Value of Biological or Genetic Markers for Survival in Lung Cancer
Biological Variable	**Prognostic Factor**
Bcl-2	Favorable
TTF1	Adverse
Cox 2	Adverse
EGFR overexpression	Adverse
EGFR mutation	Favorable
Ras	Adverse
Ki67	Adverse
HER2	Adverse
VEGF	Adverse
Microvascular density	Adverse
p53	Adverse
Aneuploidy	Adverse

EGFR, epidermal growth factor receptor; VEGF, vascular endothelial growth factor.
Adapted from Sculier JP et al. The IASLC Lung Cancer Staging Project: The impact of additional prognostic factors on survival and their relationship with the anatomical extent of disease expressed by the 6th edition of the TNM classification of malignant tumours and the proposals for the 7th edition, *J Thorac Oncol* 2008;3(4):457–466, with permission.

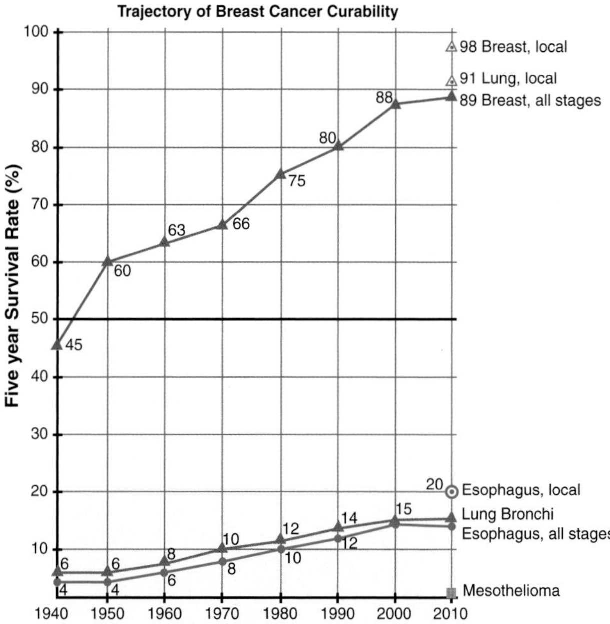

Figure 12.8 | Trajectory of Lung, Mesothelioma, Esophagus Incurability over seven decades in contrast to the high curability of breast cancer.

CHAPTER 13

Pancoast Cancer

PERSPECTIVE, PATTERNS OF SPREAD, AND PATHOLOGY

The designation of Pancoast refers to a tumor arising in the apex of lung in the neck that involves the brachial plexus and the stellate ganglion.

PERSPECTIVE AND PATTERNS OF SPREAD

The apex of the lung is in the base of the neck. The anatomy between the neck and thorax is a transitional zone because the thoracic vertebrae T1 and T2 are in the neck above the suprasternal notch. The "Pancoast" tumor refers to a symptom complex or syndrome caused by a tumor arising in the superior sulcus of the lung, which is juxtaposed with and therefore involves the inferior branches of the brachial plexus (C8 and T1) and traps the stellate ganglion of the cervical sympathetic chain which resides on the transverse process of T1 resulting in Horner's syndrome (shoulder and arm pain with ptosis, miosis, unilateral flushing, and anhidrosis).

The apical location and superior sulcus cancers in the lung apex do not present in a typical fashion with a productive cough, hemoptysis, or blood-streaked sputum, but as a progressive neuralgia with referred shoulder pain to the ulnar side of the arm. Horner's syndrome is usually subtle in onset and misleading; symptoms are related to a neurologic syndrome rather than a neoplastic process in lung. The intimate anatomic relationship of lung apex to brachial plexus and the stellate ganglion explains the onset of symptoms once the cancer spread is into the soft tissues of the neck (Fig. 13.2 and Table 13.2).

An unusual syndrome can occur with lateral invasion into the subclavian artery. Entrapment of the right recurrent laryn-

geal nerve could result in right vocal cord paresis and a thoracic inlet syndrome (TIS). TIS can be elicited by holding the patient's wrist with a finger on the radial artery pulse. As the arm is elevated, the pulse disappears due to tumor compression of the subclavian artery.

PATHOLOGY

A variety of histopathologic tumor types are possible (Table 13.1). The cells of tumor origin are in the terminal bronchioles, ranging from ciliated simple columnar to simple cuboidal cells. Cancers vary from 25% to 40% squamous cell, 25% to 60% adenocarcinoma (Fig. 13.1A and 13.1B), 5% to 15% large cell, and 2% to 5% small cell.

TABLE 13.1	Histopathologic Type
Main Pathologic Cell Type	**Variant**
Adenocarcinoma with mixed subtypes	Well-differentiated fetal adenocarcinoma
	Mucinous ("colloid" adenocarcinoma)
	Mucinous cystadenocarcinoma
	Signet ring adenocarcinoma
	Clear cell adenocarcinoma

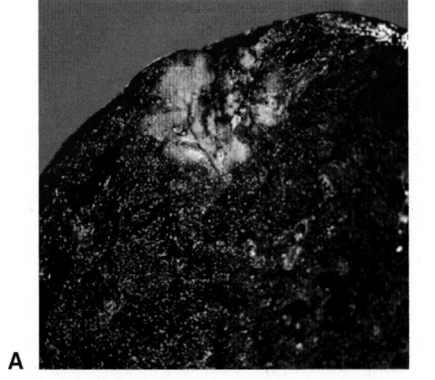

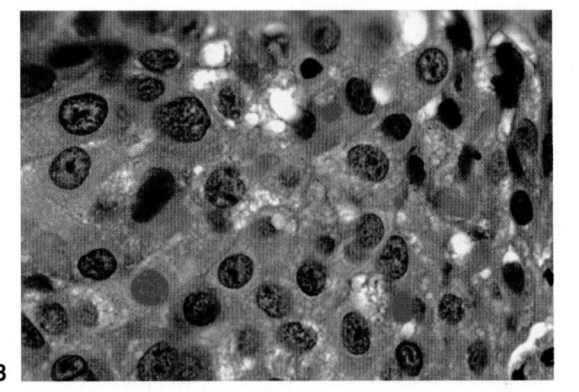

Figure 13.1 | Adenocarcinoma of the lung. A: A peripheral tumor of the right upper lobe has an irregular border and a tan or gray cut surface and causes puckering of the overlying pleura. **B.** A tumor grows in the pattern of solid adenocarcinoma with mucin formation. Several intracytoplasmic mucin droplets stain positively with the mucicarmine stain.

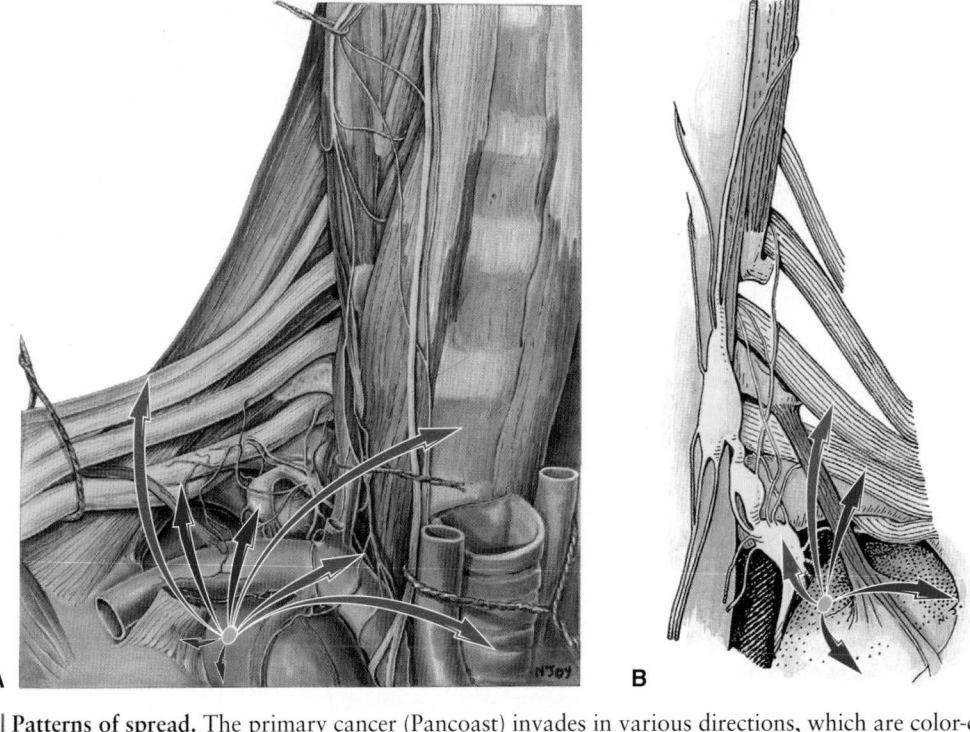

Figure 13.2 | Patterns of spread. The primary cancer (Pancoast) invades in various directions, which are color-coded vectors (arrows) representing stage of progression: Tis, yellow; T1, green; T2, blue; T3, purple; T4, red. The concept of visualizing patterns of spread to appreciate the surrounding anatomy is well demonstrated by the six-directional pattern i.e. SIMLAP Table 13.2.

TABLE 13.2	SIMLAP	
Pancoast: Terminal Bronchus		
S	Superior sulcus segment	• T1
	Brachial plexus—T1, C8	• T3
	Subclavian artery	• T4
	Brachial plexus—C7+ above	• T4
I	Superior sulcus	• T1
	Upper lobes	• T1
	Segmental atelectasis	• T2
M	Mediastinum	• T4
	Intervertebral foramen	• T4
	Spinal cord	• T4
	Esophagus	• T4
L	1st rib	• T3
	Pleura	• T3
	Chest wall	• T3
A	1st rib	• T3
	Manubrium	• T3
	Pleura	• T3
	Chest wall	• T3
P	Stellate ganglion	• T3
	1st rib	• T3

The six vectors of invasion are Superior, Inferior, Medial, Lateral, Anterior, and Posterior. The color-coded dots correlate the T stage with specific anatomic structure involved.

TNM STAGING CRITERIA

TNM STAGING CRITERIA

The designation of Pancoast tumors refers to the symptom complex or syndrome caused by a tumor arising in the superior sulcus of the lung that involves the inferior branches of the brachial plexus (C8 or T1) and the sympathetic nerve trunks, including the stellate ganglion. Some superior sulcus tumors are more anteriorly located and may cause fewer neurologic symptoms even when they are very locally advanced and encase the subclavian vessels. If there is evidence of invasion of the vertebral body or spinal canal, encasement of the subclavian vessels or unequivocal involvement of the superior branches of the brachial plexus (C8 or above), then the tumor is classified as T4. If no criteria for T4 disease pertain, the tumor is classified as T3.

Although the usual TNM criteria apply, because of the anatomic location, some exceptional findings need to be appreciated. T1 and T2 lesions less than 3 cm or greater than 3 cm are difficult to detect on routine chest films due to overlay of ribs and clavicle, which obscures small opacities in the lung. Diagnosis is most often made when the cancer reaches stage T3 because of persistent shoulder pain, which leads to discovery of chest wall invasion and posterior rib erosion on film before extensive perineural invasion, while resection is possible. Patterns of neurologic involvement vary according to which surface the cancer invades first. Thus, with superior invasion of the brachial plexus trunks of TI, C8, and C7, ribs are eroded laterally, vertebrae are invaded posteriorly, and major vessels (subclavian artery and vein) are involved anteriorly at the thoracic inlet. The difference between stages T3 and T4 is that the latter can be due to invasion of the vertebral body and unequivocal involvement of spinal cord at C8 with disastrous paraplegia or complete cord transection and quadriplegia before death. Invasion of the chest wall, pleura, and ribs imply resection is possible and therefore is considered to be T3.

SUMMARY OF CHANGES SEVENTH EDITION AJCC

- This staging system is now recommended for the classification of both non–small cell and small cell lung carcinomas and for carcinoid tumors of the lung (Fig. 13.3).
- The T classifications have been redefined:
  - T1 has been subclassified into T1a (≤2 cm in size) and T1b (>2–3 cm in size)
  - T2 has been subclassified into T2a (>3–5 cm in size) and T2b (>5–7 cm in size)
  - T2(>7 cm in size) has been reclassified as T3
  - Multiple tumor nodules in the same lobe have been reclassified from T4 to T3
  - Multiple tumor nodules in the same lung but a different lobe have been reclassified from M1 to T4
- No changes have been made to the N classification. However, a new international lymph node map defining the anatomical boundaries for lymph node stations has been developed.
- The M classifications have been redefined:
  - The M1 has been subdivided into M1a and M1b
  - Malignant pleural and pericardial effusions have been reclassified from T4 to M1a
  - Separate tumor nodules in the contralateral lung are considered M1a
  - M1b designates distant metastases

Because of the magnitude of the T-category changes with shifts in both directions, that is both downstaging and upstaging, it is important to review the stage groupings of the sixth and seventh editions. The TNM Staging Matrix is color coded for identification of Stage Group once T or N stages are determined (Table 13.3).

| TABLE 13.3 | Stage Summary Matrix |

	N0	N1	N2	N3	M1a	M1b
T1a	IA	IIA	IIIA	IIIB	IV	IV
T1b	IA	IIA	IIIA	IIIB	IV	IV
T2a	IB	IIA	IIIA	IIIB	IV	IV
T2b	IIA	IIB	IIIA	IIIB	IV	IV
T3	IIB	IIB	IIIA	IIIB	IV	IV
T4	IIIA	IIIA	IIIB	IIIB	IV	IV

Thorax: Lung Cancers
- N stage determines stage group
  - N0, N1, N2, N3a, N3b are stage group I, II, IIIA, IIIB
- N₁ can be associated with T1 or T2
- T stage modifies substages
  - T1, T2, N0 = IA, IIB; T1, T2, N2 = IIA, IIB; and T2b, N0 = IIA
- M stage is a separate stage
  - M1 = IV
- Exceptions are:
  - BAC only has T progression by definition
  - SCA is either *limited* or *extensive* (i.e., M0 or M1 independent of T or N stage)

PANCOAST CANCER

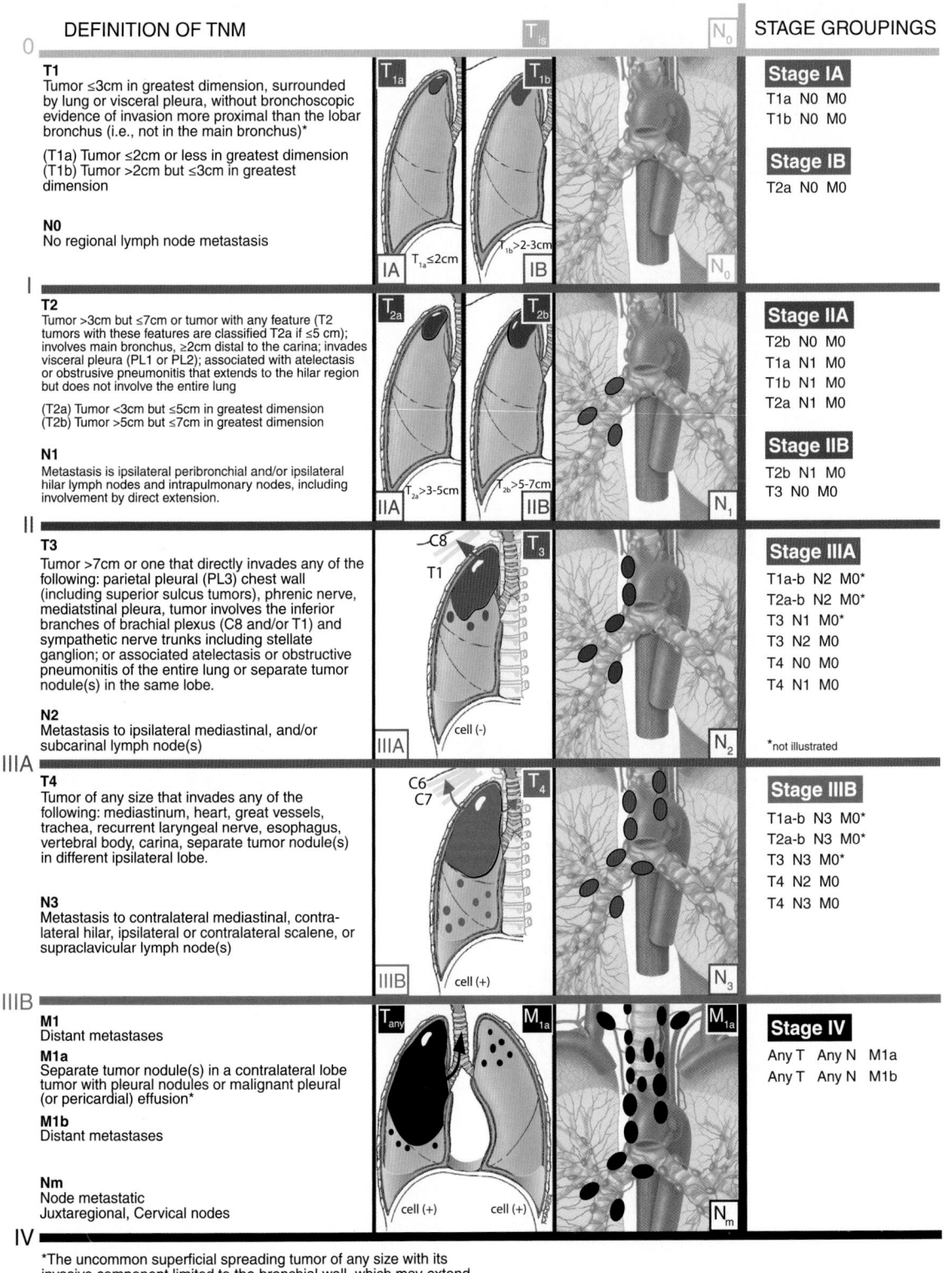

DEFINITION OF TNM	STAGE GROUPINGS

T1
Tumor ≤3cm in greatest dimension, surrounded by lung or visceral pleura, without bronchoscopic evidence of invasion more proximal than the lobar bronchus (i.e., not in the main bronchus)*

(T1a) Tumor ≤2cm or less in greatest dimension
(T1b) Tumor >2cm but ≤3cm in greatest dimension

N0
No regional lymph node metastasis

T2
Tumor >3cm but ≤7cm or tumor with any feature (T2 tumors with these features are classified T2a if ≤ 5 cm); involves main bronchus, ≥2cm distal to the carina; invades visceral pleura (PL1 or PL2); associated with atelectasis or obstructive pneumonitis that extends to the hilar region but does not involve the entire lung

(T2a) Tumor <3cm but ≤5cm in greatest dimension
(T2b) Tumor >5cm but ≤7cm in greatest dimension

N1
Metastasis is ipsilateral peribronchial and/or ipsilateral hilar lymph nodes and intrapulmonary nodes, including involvement by direct extension.

T3
Tumor >7cm or one that directly invades any of the following: parietal pleural (PL3) chest wall (including superior sulcus tumors), phrenic nerve, mediatstinal pleura, tumor involves the inferior branches of brachial plexus (C8 and/or T1) and sympathetic nerve trunks including stellate ganglion; or associated atelectasis or obstructive pneumonitis of the entire lung or separate tumor nodule(s) in the same lobe.

N2
Metastasis to ipsilateral mediastinal, and/or subcarinal lymph node(s)

T4
Tumor of any size that invades any of the following: mediastinum, heart, great vessels, trachea, recurrent laryngeal nerve, esophagus, vertebral body, carina, separate tumor nodule(s) in different ipsilateral lobe.

N3
Metastasis to contralateral mediastinal, contra-lateral hilar, ipsilateral or contralateral scalene, or supraclavicular lymph node(s)

M1
Distant metastases

M1a
Separate tumor nodule(s) in a contralateral lobe tumor with pleural nodules or malignant pleural (or pericardial) effusion*

M1b
Distant metastases

Nm
Node metastatic
Juxtaregional, Cervical nodes

*The uncommon superficial spreading tumor of any size with its invasive component limited to the bronchial wall, which may extend proximally to the main bronchus, is also classified as T1a.

Stage IA
T1a N0 M0
T1b N0 M0

Stage IB
T2a N0 M0

Stage IIA
T2b N0 M0
T1a N1 M0
T1b N1 M0
T2a N1 M0

Stage IIB
T2b N1 M0
T3 N0 M0

Stage IIIA
T1a-b N2 M0*
T2a-b N2 M0*
T3 N1 M0*
T3 N2 M0
T4 N0 M0
T4 N1 M0

*not illustrated

Stage IIIB
T1a-b N3 M0*
T2a-b N3 M0*
T3 N3 M0*
T4 N2 M0
T4 N3 M0

Stage IV
Any T Any N M1a
Any T Any N M1b

Figure 13.3 | TNM staging diagram. Pancoast cancers originate in cupula of lungs and are located in the base of the neck and spread into supraclavicular and cervical nodes. Vertical presentations of stage groupings, which follow the same color code for cancer stage advancement, are organized in horizontal lanes: Stage 0, yellow; I, green; IIIA, purple; IIIB, red; and metastatic stage IV, black. Definitions of TN are on the left and stage groupings are on the right.

T-ONCOANATOMY

ORIENTATION OF THREE-PLANAR ONCOANATOMY

The isocenter of the pulmonary apex is in the neck, around which the three-planar anatomy is presented, especially as it relates to the brachial plexus and sympathetic chain of cervical ganglion. It is important to note that T1 and T2 are above the thoracic inlet and form a transitional zone between the neck and the chest, that is, the thoracic inlet (Fig. 13.4).

T-oncoanatomy

Designated at the T1-2 level, the Pancoast tumor is fitting to introduce lung cancer as a disease with many different presentations, which masquerade the underlying cancer. The misleading signs and symptoms in the presentation of a Pancoast cancer stem from the anatomic location of the superior sulcus

of the lung in the neck and not the thorax. Grave signs are direct vertebral invasion, which can result in spinal cord encroachment and transection leading to paraplegia or entrapment of major vessels, namely, the subclavian artery and vein. The coronal and sagittal views are more revealing of the critical anatomy of the superior sulcus (Fig. 13.5).

- *Coronal:* The juxtaposition of the brachial plexus superior and posterior to the lung apex is readily seen.

- *Sagittal:* The brachial plexus and subclavian artery are appreciated as to their proximity to the lung apex posteriorly and anteriorly, respectively.

- *Transverse:* The medial location of the stellate ganglion anterior to the transverse process of T1. The spinal cord is accessible once the vertebral foramen are eroded. This is a striking view of the roof of the thoracic cavity from a diaphragmatic vantage point. The thoracic inlet is the zone that allows cancers to trap nerves, arteries, and veins and compress them against bony ribs and vertebrae; they are between the proverbial rock and a hard place.

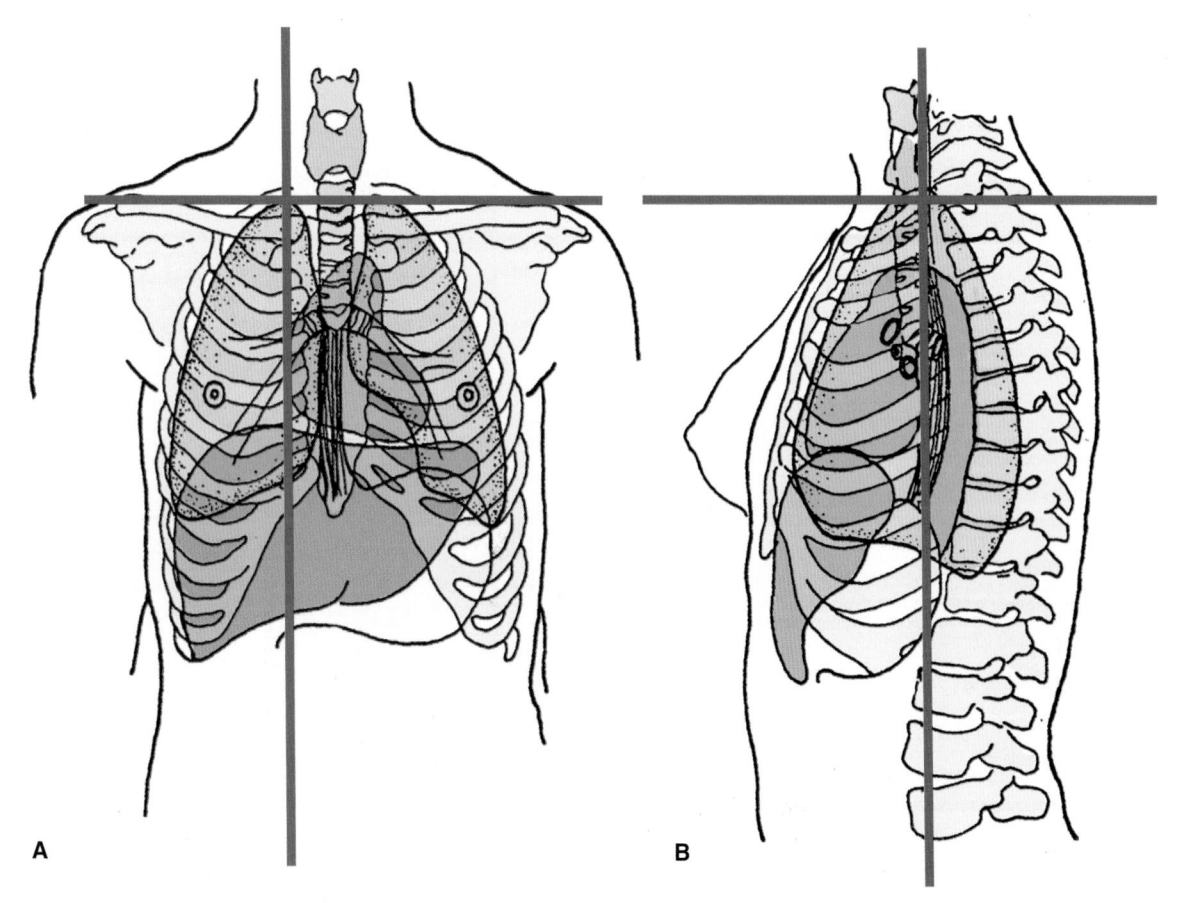

A   **B**

Figure 13.4 | Orientation of T-oncoanatomy. The anatomic isocenter is at the T1-2 level at the base of the neck in its transition to the thoracic inlet. **A.** Coronal. **B.** Sagittal.

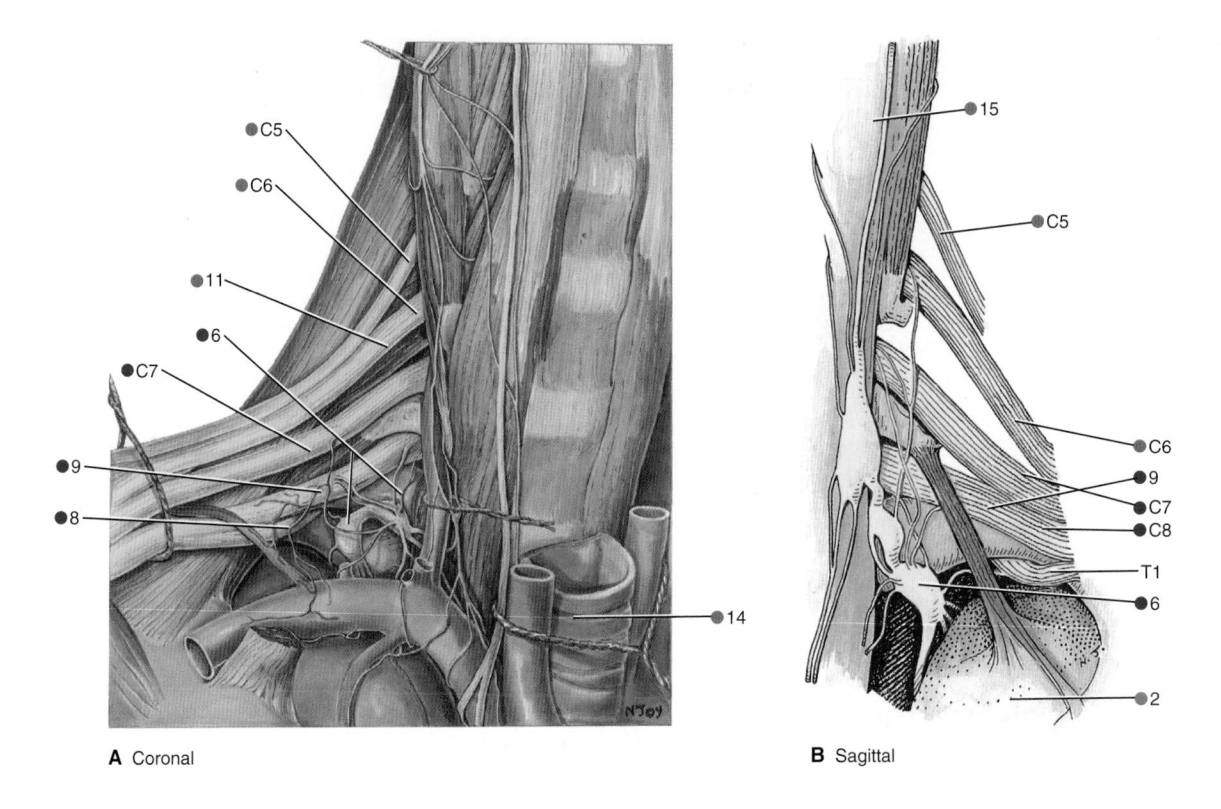

A Coronal

B Sagittal

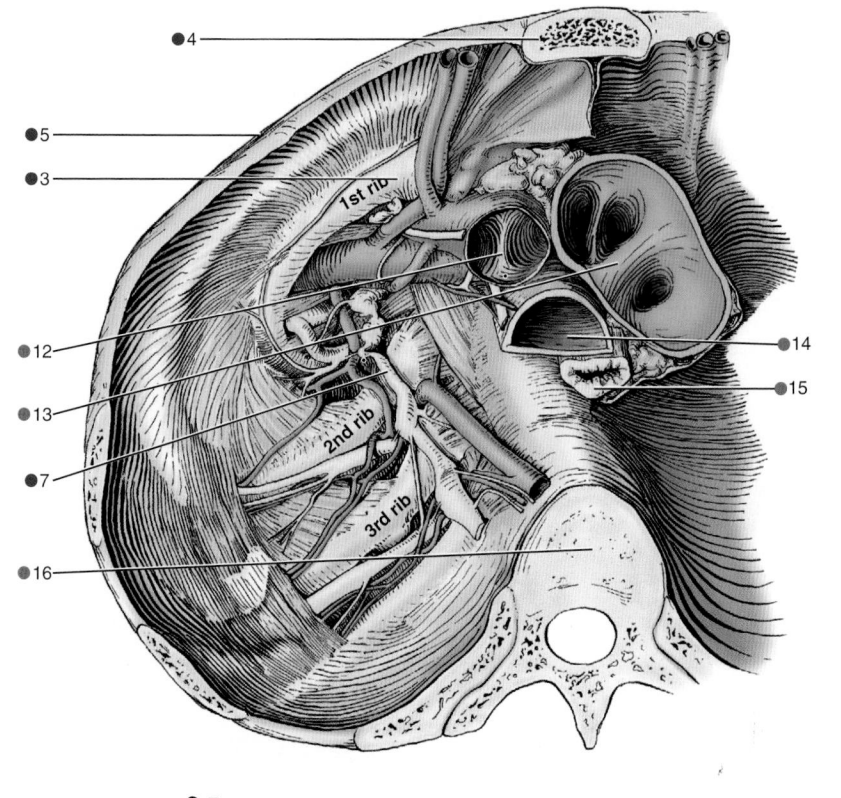

C Transverse

T₁ ● 1. Lung Superior Sulcus		T₃ ● 7. Sympathetic Trunk		T₄ ● 13. Aorta
T₂ ● 2. Pleura		T₃ ● 8. Brachial Plexus T1		T₄ ● 14. Trachea
T₃ ● 3. 1st Rib		T₃ ● 9. Brachial Plexus C8		T₄ ● 15. Esophagus
T₃ ● 4. Sternum		T₄ ● 10. Brachial Plexus C6		T₄ ● 16. Vertebrae
T₃ ● 5. Chest Wall		T₄ ● 11. Brachial Plexus C5		C = cervical nerve branch
T₃ ● 6. Stellate Ganglion		T₄ ● 12. Vena Cava		

Figure 13.5 | T-oncoanatomy. Connecting the dots: Structures are color coded for cancer stage progression. The color code for the anatomic sites correlates with the color code for the T stage group (Fig. 13.3) and patterns of spread (Fig. 13.2) and SIMLAP tables (Table 13.2). Connecting the dots in similar colors will provide an appreciation for the 3D Oncoanatomy.

N-ONCOANATOMY AND M-ONCOANATOMY

N-ONCOANATOMY

Once the pleural surface is invaded, the cancer drains into scalene or cervical nodes by way of the superior intercostal lymphatics. These lymph nodes often are the ones involved and do not deter the resectability of Pancoast cancers. Intrapulmonary nodes and hilar nodes are possibly, albeit uncommonly, involved (Figs. 13.6 and 13.7; Table 13.4). Ironically, sentinel nodes are metastatic cervical nodes.

REGIONAL LYMPH NODES

The regional lymph nodes extend from the supraclavicular region to the diaphragm. During the past three decades, three different lymph node maps have been used to describe the regional lymph node potentially involved by lung cancers. The first map was endorsed by the Japan Lung Cancer Society. The second map, the Mountain Dresler modification of the American Thoracic Society (MDATS) lymph node map, is used in North America and Europe. The nomenclature for the anatomical locations of lymph nodes differs between these two maps. Recently the International Association for the Study of Lung Cancer (IASLC) proposed a lymph node map (Figure 13.6B) that reconciles the discrepancies between these two previous maps. The IASLC lymph node map is now the recommended means of describing regional lymph node involvement for lung cancers.

There are no evidence-based guidelines regarding the *number* of lymph nodes to be removed at surgery for adequate staging. However, adequate N staging is generally considered to include sampling or dissection of lymph nodes from stations 2R, 4R, 7, 10R, and 11R for right-sided tumors, and stations 5, 6, 7, 10, L, and 11L for left-sided tumors. Station 9 lymph nodes should also be evaluated for lower lobe tumors. The more peripheral lymph nodes at stations 12-14 are usually evaluated by the pathologist in lobectomy or pneumonectomy specimens but may be separately removed when sublobar resections (e.g., segmentectomy) are performed. There is evidence to support the recommendation that histological examination of hilar and mediastinal lymphenectomy specimen(s) will ordinarily include 6 or more lymph nodes/stations. Three of these nodes/stations should be mediastinal, including the subcarinal nodes and three from N1 nodes/stations.*

M-ONCOANATOMY

Drainage into the subclavian vein, if invaded, then via the superior vena cava and pulmonary artery drain into the lung. Cancer invasion of chest wall drains into intercostal veins, then the azygos vein, and then the superior vena cava, which leads to lung dissemination. Adenocarcinoma dissemination of metastases is the most common lung cancer and is presented as the prototype for metastases into other organs (Fig. 13.7).

*Preceding passage from Edge SB, Byrd DR, and Compton CC, et al. *AJCC Cancer Staging Manual, 7th edition.* New York, Springer, 2010, pp. 254–255.

TABLE 13.4 Lymph Nodes of the Lung

Sentinel nodes are scalene and supraclavicular nodes and lower deep cervical nodes.
N1 nodes: All N1 nodes lie distal to the mediastinal pleural reflection and *within the visceral pleura.*
Hilar nodes 10
Interlobar nodes 11
Lobar nodes bronchi 12
Segmental nodes 13
Subsegmental nodes 14
N2 nodes: All N2 nodes lie within the mediastinal pleural envelope on the ipsilateral side.
Highest mediastinal nodes 1, 2R, 2L
Upper paratracheal nodes 2R, 2L
Prevascular and retrotracheal nodes 3a, 3p*
Lower paratracheal nodes 4R, 4L
Subaortic nodes (aortopulmonary window) 5
Para-aortic nodes (ascending aorta or phrenic) 6
Subcarinal nodes 7
Paraesophageal nodes (below carina) 8
Pulmonary ligament nodes 9

*3a, 3p not shown in Fig. 13.6.

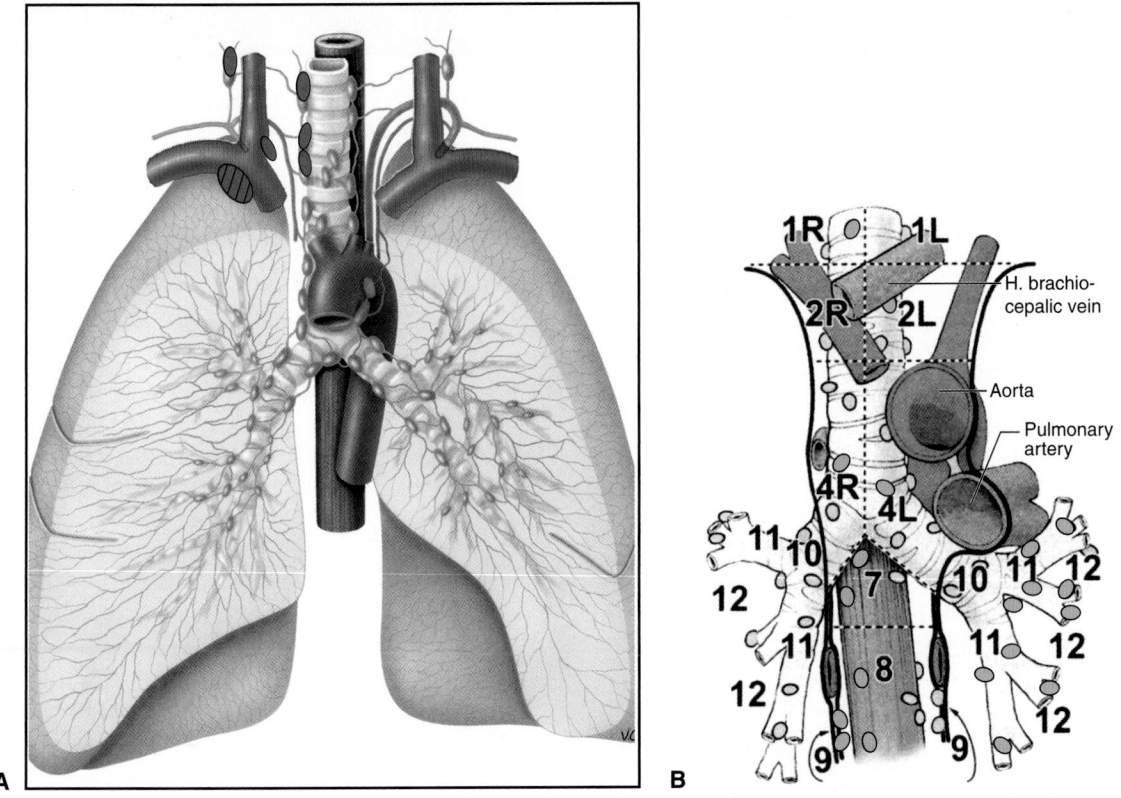

Figure 13.6 | **A. N-oncoanatomy.** Sentinel nodes are scalene and supraclavicular. **B. M-oncoanatomy:** International Association for Study of Lung Cancer (IASLC). Labels correlate with Table 13.4.

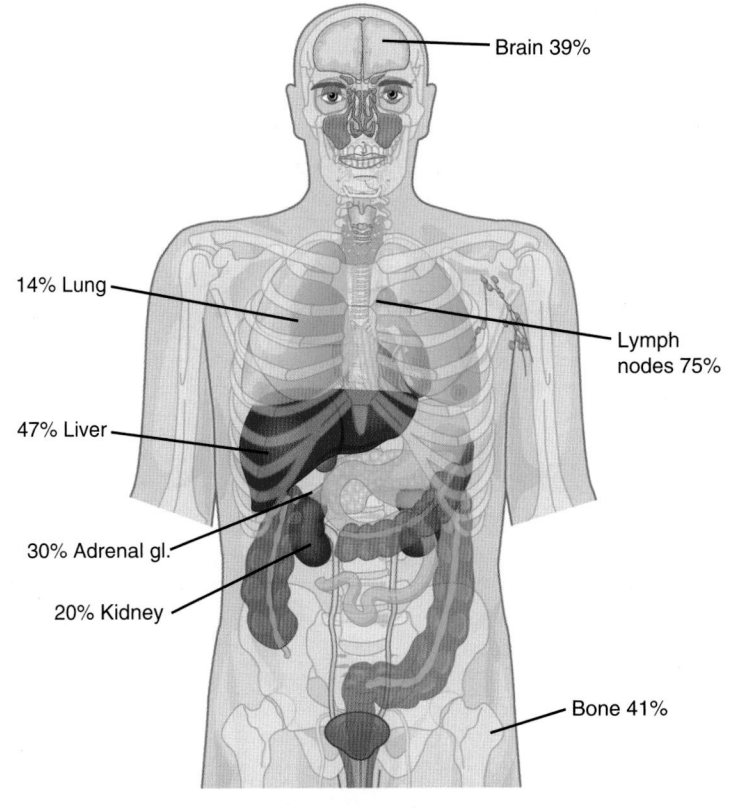

Figure 13.7 | Incidence and distribution of metastases. Adenocarcinoma is the most common lung cancer and is presented as a prototype for lung cancers.

STAGING WORKUP

RULES FOR CLASSIFICATION AND STAGING

Clinical Staging and Imaging

The TNM classification system is primarily for staging non–small cell lung cancers. The most important change dates back to the fourth edition of the American Joint Committee on Cancer (AJCC), where T3 resectable disease was distinguished from T4 unresectable disease. Simultaneously, a greater reliance on more sophisticated imaging has occurred. It is with the sixth edition that computed tomography (CT) and positron emission tomography (PET) are allowed. The imaging modalities for detection and diagnosis apply to staging (Table 13.5). Chest films and CT (preferably spiral) are essential steps in both diagnosis and staging. PET combined with CT helps to overcome motion artifacts. Magnetic resonance imaging (MRI) is useful for mediastinal evaluation. Another advantage of CT over MRI for staging is that it allows for metastatic workup of lung, liver, adrenal and for ribs, and vertebrae, especially for Pancoast cancers (Fig. 13.8).

Pathologic Staging

All pathologic specimens from clinical invasive procedures—bronchoscopy, mediastinoscopy, mediastinotomy, thoracentesis, and thoracoscopy—are applicable to pathologic stage. Thoracotomy and resection of primary and lymph nodes are the mainstay of pathologic staging. Margin status and any residual cancer need to be noted. Preferably, six nodes should be examined.

Surgical resection of primary and regional nodes needs to be carefully evaluated at bronchial stump for adequate margins. All resected nodes should be numbered according to AJCC system and assessed for tumor.

Oncoimaging Annotations

- Chest radiographs seldom detect primary lung cancers in their early stages.
- Spiral CT is useful in high-risk patients to detect nodule and infiltrates.
- PET imaging with ^{18}FDG (fluorodeoxyglucose) appears to be of value in discriminating malignant versus benign nodules.
- CT can detect mediastinal adenopathy, but histologic verification is essential to ascertain if it is malignant.
- Determining N2 versus N3 mediastinal nodes is important; it establishes resectability.
- MRI can be of value in assessing mediastinal invasion, chest wall and rib erosion, and compromised large vein involvement.
- Pancoast cancers are difficult to diagnose on routine chest films.
- CT scan using bone windows detects invasion of ribs and vertebrae.
- MRI is useful for detecting invasion of vertebrae and tumor compressing spinal cord.

TABLE 13.5	Imaging Modalities for Diagnosis and Staging	
Method	**Capability**	**Recommended**
Primary Tumor and Regional Nodes Workup		
Chest films	Baseline image	Yes
CT/spiral CT	Most useful of all modalities for determining characteristics of T and N in the thorax and M in the adrenal and liver	Yes
MRI	Superior to CT in superior sulcus tumors to determine involvement of lower branches of brachial plexus and subclavian vessels in coronal and sagittal planes.	Yes
Percutaneous needle biopsy	Guided by fluoroscopy or CT, accurate in establishing cytologic diagnosis from T (particularly peripheral lung lesions); M (especially liver or bone)	Yes
Mediastinoscopy/thoracoscopy	Confirmation of nodal involvement	Yes
Metastatic Workup for Clinically Suspected Metastases		
CT/echography	For liver, adrenals	Yes
CT/MRI	For brain	Yes
Bone scan	For the bone	Yes
PET scan	Diagnosis of peripheral lesions can differentiate between cancer and benign lesions. Staging of true extent of primary and lymph node involvement.	Yes, if clinically indicated

CT, computed tomography; M, metastasis; MRI, magnetic resonance imaging; N, node; PET, positron emission tomography; T, tumor.

PROGNOSIS AND CANCER SURVIVAL

CANCER STATISTICS AND SURVIVAL

Generally, according to Surveillance Epidemiology and End Results data based on 16,000 patients, the relative 5-year survival is 8% to 10% and 10-year survival 5% to 7%. Surprisingly, there is a small attrition for 5-year survivors with the majority (70%) remaining alive at 10 years. Female gender, good Karnofsky performance status, and cessation of smoking contribute to longer survival.

Specifically, Pancoast cancers were thought to be incurable until a fortuitous long-term survivor (27 years) was reported following preoperative radiation and resection. Nodal status is important because scalene and supraclavicular nodes may be the first involved but are not considered contraindications to surgical resection.

The ability to resect superior sulcus cancers following preoperative radiation was pioneered by Paulson, who posted a 30% 5-year survival rate with a low 3% mortality rate (Fig. 13.9). This has been reproduced by other surgical teams.

PROGNOSIS

The limited number of prognostic factors are listed in Table 13.6.

TABLE 13.6 | Prognostic Factors

Required for Staging	None
Clinically significant	Pleural/elastic layer invasion (based on H&E and elastic stains)
	Separate tumor nodules
	Vascular invasion—V classification (venous or arteriolar)

H&E, hematoxylin and eosinophilic.
From Edge SB, Byrd DR, Compton CC, et al. *AJCC cancer staging manual.* 7th ed. New York: Springer, 2010, p. 264 with permission.

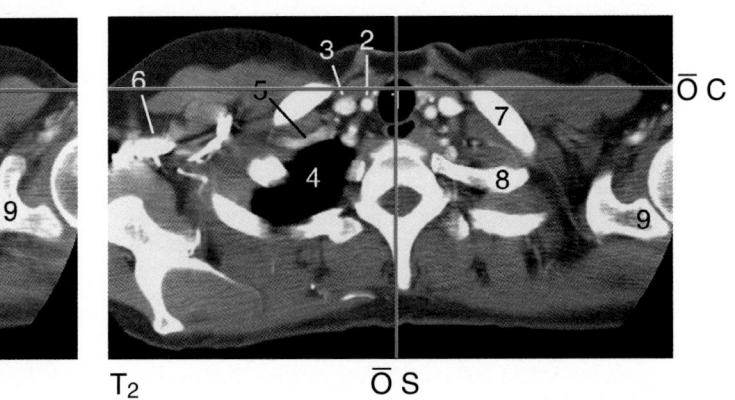

Figure 13.8 | Axial CTs of T1 and T2 level correlate with the T-oncoanatomy transverse section (Figure 13.5C). Oncoimaging with CT is commonly applied to staging lung cancers, often combined with PET to determine true extent of primary cancer and involved lymph nodes. **Left.** 1, thyroid gland; 2, trachea; 3, internal jugular vein; 4, common carotid artery; 5, esophagus; 6, vertebral artery; 7, clavicle; 8, first rib; 9, scapula. **Right.** 1, trachea; 2, common carotid artery; 3, internal jugular vein; 4, lung apex; 5, subclavian artery; 6, subclavian vein; 7, clavicle; 8, first rib; 9, scapula (glenoid).

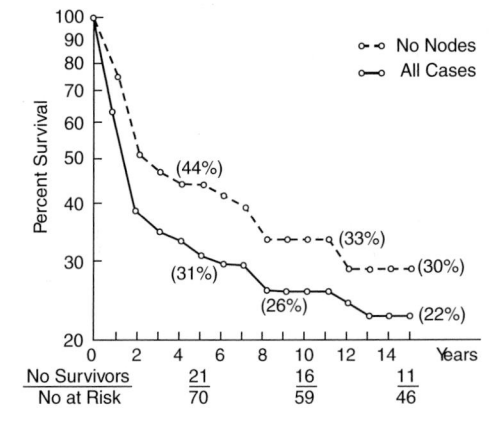

Figure 13.9 | Five-, 10-, and 15-year actuarial survival curves after combined preoperative radiation, followed by en bloc surgical resection (1956–1983) in patients with no lymph nodes involved and including those with nodal involvement. (From Movsas B, Langer CJ, Goldberg M, eds. *Controversies in lung cancer. A multidisciplinary approach.* New York: Marcel Dekker, 2001).

Bronchioloalveolar Cancer

PERSPECTIVE, PATTERNS OF SPREAD, AND PATHOLOGY

The bronchioloalveolar cancers (BACs) arise from the most peripheral respiratory bronchi branching into an acinus and alveolar sacs allowing for its lepidic spread.

PERSPECTIVE AND PATTERNS OF SPREAD

The essential cell in the evolutionary process that enabled aquatic animals to leave the sea to become air breathers is the type II pneumocyte. The cry of the newborn recapitulates that stage in our ontogeny; it ensures that air has replaced the amniotic fluid in the alveolar acini. The malignant transformation of the type II pneumocyte provides the histogenesis into a bronchioloalveolar carcinoma (BAC). BACs have three distinct patterns of presentation that have been described as clinical pathologic entities: (i) cancers in peripheral pulmonary scars; (ii) multiple primary nodules; and (iii) diffuse and extensive pneumonitis. BACs account for 5% to 10% of all lung cancers, but its incidence has doubled in more recent series as its cellular characteristics are increasingly appreciated.

BACs are true cancers of the lung since they arise from the type II pneumocytes and grow alveolar walls. They only account for 1% to 5% of all cancers (Fig. 14.2 and Table 14.2). Because they arise in segmental bronchi, they can present as a segmental pneumonitis or atelectasis in contradistinction to adenocarcinomas that tend to arise in lobar bronchi, therefore producing lobar pneumonitis or atelectasis. Alternately, BACs can appear as peripheral nodules with a characteristic "pleural tuck sign." Copious mucous sputum (bronchorrhea) is an unusual symptom and is a distinctive sign of BACs but only occurs in 5% to 10% of all presentations.

PATHOLOGY

The crucial point in understanding the concept of "lepidic" (scale-like) spread is the preexistence of a fine microcirculatory web in the alveoli walls of the terminal intrapulmonary airways or the alveolar acini and sacs (Fig. 14.1). The alveolar wall is lined by type I pneumocytes, which are singular, flat surface cells generated by the type II pneumocyte, which stores, manufactures, and secretes surfactant molecules. BACs arising in the terminal respiratory bronchiole may present as a peripheral pulmonary scar that extends to the pleural surface because a small subsegment of air sacs or alveoli collapses or becomes infiltrated by lepidic spread. Their histogenic features suggest they arise from the type II pneumocyte. (Table 14.1).

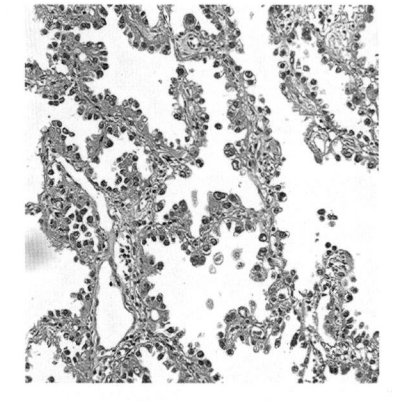

Figure 14.1 | Bronchioloalveolar carcinoma. Nonmucinous bronchioloalveolar carcinomas consist of atypical cuboidal to low columnar cells proliferating along the existing alveolar walls.

TABLE 14.1	Histopathologic Type
Main Pathologic Cell Type	**Variant**
Bronchioloalveolar carcinoma	Nonmucinous
	Mucinous
	Mixed mucinous and nonmucinous or indeterminate
	Solid adenocarcinoma with mucin formation

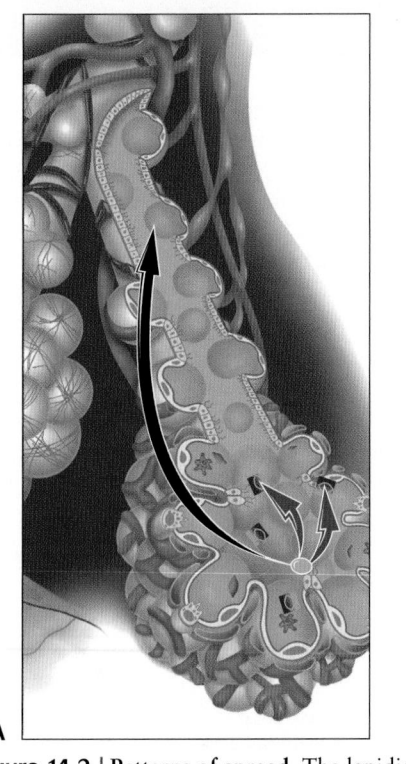
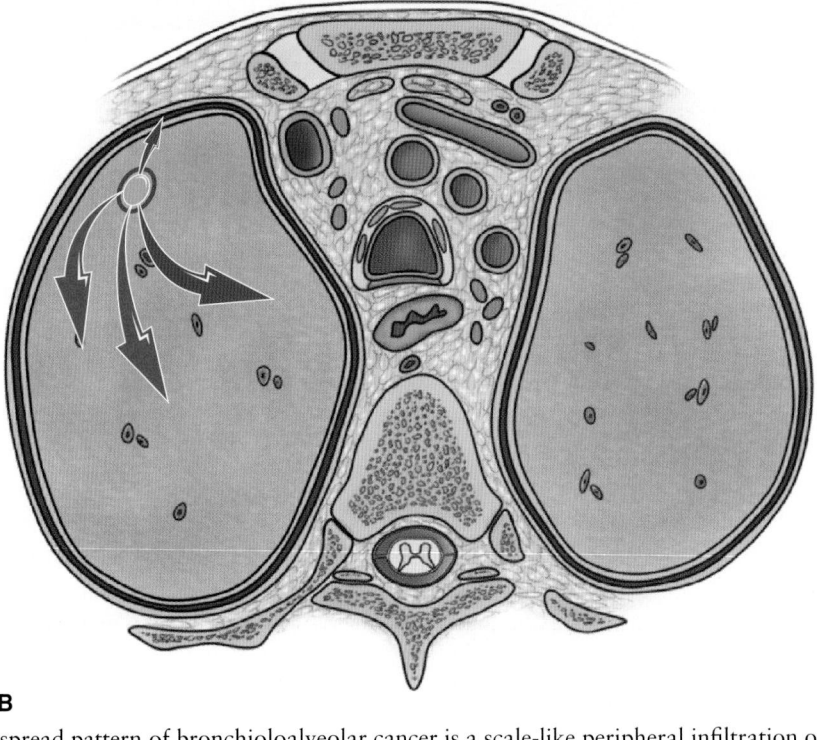

A **B**

Figure 14.2 | Patterns of spread. The lepidic spread pattern of bronchioloalveolar cancer is a scale-like peripheral infiltration of acini and alveoli through alveolar wall pores without invasion of lymphatics or microcirculation. Color code simplified: T1, peripheral nodule (*green*); cancer in a peripheral scar (*green*); and T3, dissemination. The concept of visualizing patterns of spread to appreciate the surrounding anatomy is well demonstrated by the six-directional pattern i.e. SIMLAP Table 14.2.

The International Association for Study of Lung Cancer (IASLC) has meticulously defined pleural invasion:

- P0: Tumor falls short of invading elastic layer of pleura
- P1: Tumor extends through elastic layer
- P2: Tumor extends to surface of visceral pleura
- P3: Tumor extends to parietal pleura >T3
- Direct invasion across a fissure is classified as T2a

TABLE 14.2	SIMLAP: Lung Segmental Lobe (T1), Respiration Bronchus	
Bronchioloalveolar Cancer		
S	Segmental atelectasis	• T2
	Pleura	• T2
I	Segmental atelectasis	• T2
	Pleura	• T2
M	Lobar atelectasis	• T2
	Multicentric—same lobe	• T4
L	Pleura	• T2
A	Pleura	• T2
P	Pleura	• T2

The six vectors of invasion are **S**uperior, **I**nferior, **M**edial, **L**ateral, **A**nterior, and **P**osterior. The color-coded dots correlate the T stage with specific anatomic structure involved.

TNM STAGING CRITERIA

TNM STAGING CRITERIA

Lepidic spread refers to the noninvasive nature of BACs, which is an oxymoron. This is possible because of a special feature of terminal acini. Their clusters of alveolar sacs enable surface infiltration of the preexisting pulmonary capillary bed, namely the acini that communicate through the "pores of Kohn" between their alveolar walls. This allows BACs to spread without the need for generating their own tumor neovascular bed and blood supply. If these lepidic features are not evident—that is, stromal, vascular, or pleural invasion is seen—then the cancer needs to be reclassified as adenocarcinoma. Mixed subtypes require that each subtype present be specified.

True solitary BACs carry an excellent prognosis, with a 70% 5-year survival. Another feature is its presentation as multiple primaries that are metachronous or synchronous. According to the American Joint Committee on Cancer (AJCC)/International Union Against Cancer criteria as originally proposed by Martini and Melamed: The two tumors need to be the same histologic type but in separate lobes without evidence of nodal metastasis within a common nodal drainage, that is, interlobar nodes common to upper and lower lobes. The third scenario is the pneumonitic presentation, which can be multifocal and rapidly fills intrapulmonary acinar airways, resulting in an "air bronchogram." Multiple nodules in the same lobe as the primary are considered to be metastatic and staged as T4. Survival for this multifocal disseminated form of cancer is nil.

SUMMARY OF CHANGES SEVENTH EDITION AJCC

- This staging system is now recommended for the classification of both non–small cell and small cell lung carcinomas and for carcinoid tumors of the lung. (Fig. 14.3).

- The T classifications have been redefined:
  - T1 has been subclassified into T1a (≤2 cm in size) and T1b (>2–3 cm in size)
  - T2 has been subclassified into T2a (>3–5 cm in size) and T2b (>5–7 cm in size)
  - T2 (>7 cm in size) has been reclassified as T3
  - Multiple tumor nodules in the same lobe have been reclassified from T4 to T3
  - Multiple tumor nodules in the same lung but a different lobe have been reclassified from M1 to T4
- No changes have been made to the N classification. However, a new international lymph node map defining the anatomical boundaries for lymph node stations has been developed.
- The M classifications have been redefined:
  - The M1 has been subdivided into M1a and M1b
  - Malignant pleural and pericardial effusions have been reclassified from T4 to M1a
  - Separate tumor nodules in the contralateral lung are considered M1a
  - M1b designates distant metastases

Because of the magnitude of the T-category changes with shifts in both directions, that is both downstaging and upstaging, it is important to review the stage groupings of the sixth and seventh editions. The TMN Staging Matrix is color coded for identification of Stage Group once T and N stages are determined (Table 14.3).

TABLE 14.3 Stage Summary Matrix

	N0	N1	N2	N3	M1a	M1b
T1a	IA	IIA	IIIA	IIIB	IV	IV
T1b	IA	IIA	IIIA	IIIB	IV	IV
T2a	IB	IIA	IIIA	IIIB	IV	IV
T2b	IIA	IIB	IIIA	IIIB	IV	IV
T3	IIB	IIB	IIIA	IIIB	IV	IV
T4	IIIA	IIIA	IIIB	IIIB	IV	IV

Thorax: Lung Cancers
- N stage determines stage group
  - N0, N1, N2, N3a, N3b are stage group I, II, IIIA, IIIB
- N1 can be associated with T1 or T2
- T stage modifies substages
  - T1, T2, N0 = IA, IIB; T1, T2, N2 = IIA, IIB; and T2b, N0 = IIA
- M stage is a separate stage
  - M1 = IV
- Exceptions are:
  - BAC only has T progression by definition

BRONCHIOLOALVEOLAR CANCER

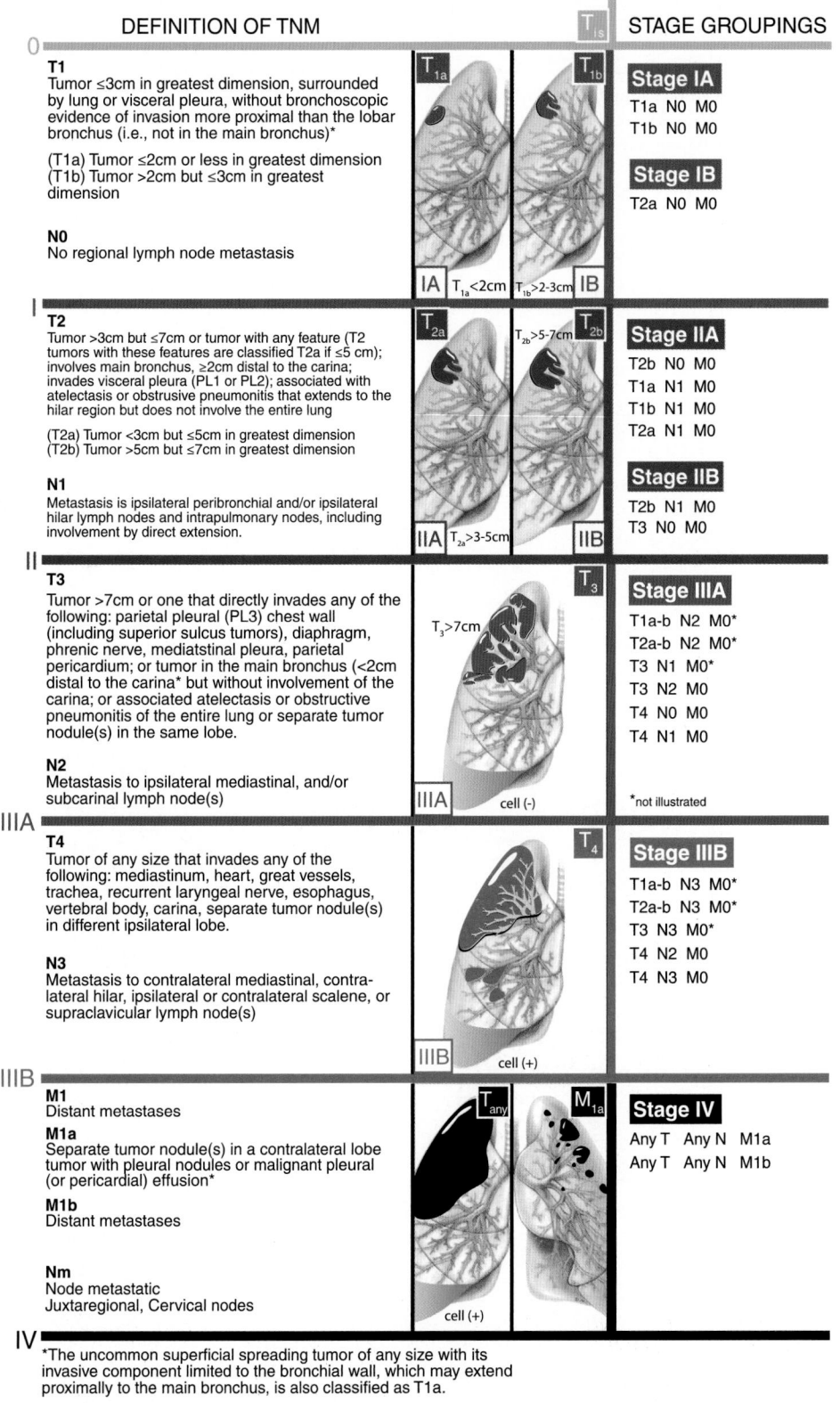

DEFINITION OF TNM

T1
Tumor ≤3cm in greatest dimension, surrounded by lung or visceral pleura, without bronchoscopic evidence of invasion more proximal than the lobar bronchus (i.e., not in the main bronchus)*

(T1a) Tumor ≤2cm or less in greatest dimension
(T1b) Tumor >2cm but ≤3cm in greatest dimension

N0
No regional lymph node metastasis

T2
Tumor >3cm but ≤7cm or tumor with any feature (T2 tumors with these features are classified T2a if ≤5 cm); involves main bronchus, ≥2cm distal to the carina; invades visceral pleura (PL1 or PL2); associated with atelectasis or obstrusive pneumonitis that extends to the hilar region but does not involve the entire lung

(T2a) Tumor <3cm but ≤5cm in greatest dimension
(T2b) Tumor >5cm but ≤7cm in greatest dimension

N1
Metastasis is ipsilateral peribronchial and/or ipsilateral hilar lymph nodes and intrapulmonary nodes, including involvement by direct extension.

T3
Tumor >7cm or one that directly invades any of the following: parietal pleural (PL3) chest wall (including superior sulcus tumors), diaphragm, phrenic nerve, mediatstinal pleura, parietal pericardium; or tumor in the main bronchus (<2cm distal to the carina* but without involvement of the carina; or associated atelectasis or obstructive pneumonitis of the entire lung or separate tumor nodule(s) in the same lobe.

N2
Metastasis to ipsilateral mediastinal, and/or subcarinal lymph node(s)

T4
Tumor of any size that invades any of the following: mediastinum, heart, great vessels, trachea, recurrent laryngeal nerve, esophagus, vertebral body, carina, separate tumor nodule(s) in different ipsilateral lobe.

N3
Metastasis to contralateral mediastinal, contra-lateral hilar, ipsilateral or contralateral scalene, or supraclavicular lymph node(s)

M1
Distant metastases
M1a
Separate tumor nodule(s) in a contralateral lobe tumor with pleural nodules or malignant pleural (or pericardial) effusion*
M1b
Distant metastases

Nm
Node metastatic
Juxtaregional, Cervical nodes

*The uncommon superficial spreading tumor of any size with its invasive component limited to the bronchial wall, which may extend proximally to the main bronchus, is also classified as T1a.

STAGE GROUPINGS

Stage IA
T1a N0 M0
T1b N0 M0

Stage IB
T2a N0 M0

Stage IIA
T2b N0 M0
T1a N1 M0
T1b N1 M0
T2a N1 M0

Stage IIB
T2b N1 M0
T3 N0 M0

Stage IIIA
T1a-b N2 M0*
T2a-b N2 M0*
T3 N1 M0*
T3 N2 M0
T4 N0 M0
T4 N1 M0

*not illustrated

Stage IIIB
T1a-b N3 M0*
T2a-b N3 M0*
T3 N3 M0*
T4 N2 M0
T4 N3 M0

Stage IV
Any T Any N M1a
Any T Any N M1b

Figure 14.3 | TNM stage grouping. Bronchioloalveolar cancers are usually detected as peripheral cancers with scarring and subsegmental collapse. They are considered non-invasive but multicentric as in T3 and Tany. When invasion occurs as in T4, it is considered to be an adenocarcinoma or mixed type. Color coding: Stage 0, yellow; I, green; II, blue; IIIA, purple; IIIB, red; IV, black (metastatic). Definitions of TN on left and stage groupings on right. Although shown, stromal, vascular and pleural invasion require reclassification as adenocarcinoma.

T-ONCOANATOMY

ORIENTATION OF THREE-PLANAR ONCOANATOMY

The respiratory bronchioles and their acini and alveoli constitute the breeding ground for BACs. Although the axial orientation is at the T2-3 level, a microscopic or macroscopic view of the intrapulmonary airways is required to appreciate the very fine bronchiole divisions as they become subsegmental, intrasegmental, lose the cartilage in their walls, and terminate as respiratory bronchioles. These respiratory bronchioles end in acini with alveolar sacs and alveoli. The intrapulmonary fine capillary meshwork is optimally designed for a lepidic cancer spread pattern due to the preconfigured microvasculature of the alveoli that BACs adopt as they extend through the pores of Kohn (Fig. 14.4).

T-oncoanatomy

The T-oncoanatomy is displayed in 3 planar views. A. Coronal, B. Sagittal, C. Transverse Axial (Fig. 14.5). The peripheral pleural anatomy of the lung is the geographic zone for the BACs. The presentation of the bronchopulmonary segmental anatomy follows:

- *Coronal:* Anterior and posterior views demonstrate the lobar and segmental anatomy of the lungs. Note the asymmetry of right and left lungs with the middle lobe on the right being equivalent to the lingula except the middle lobe bronchus arises from the lower lobe bronchus and the lingual from the upper lobe.

- *Sagittal:* Note superior segment of lower lobes appears in the upper part of the lung fields. Both the middle lobe and lingual are anterior and medial and can be obscured by the cardiac silhouette if partially collapsed.

- *Axial transverse:* At the T2-3 level and sternoclavicular joints, this shows the great vessels, trachea, esophagus, and upper lobe segments. Midline structures are bronchiocephalic arterial trunk, trachea, and esophagus with thoracic duct and nodes to left.

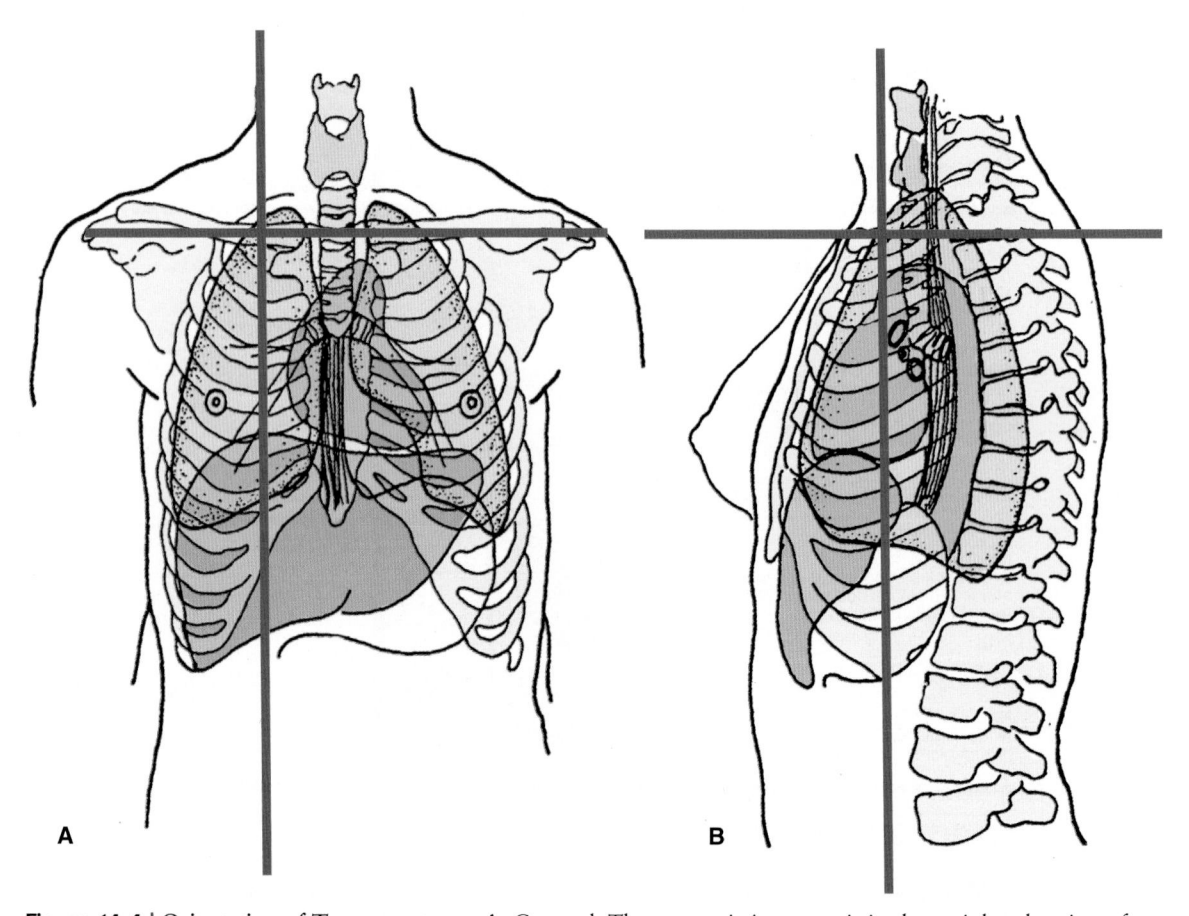

Figure 14.4 | Orientation of T-oncoanatomy. A. Coronal. The anatomic isocenter is in the peripheral region of the lung. **B.** Sagittal. The anatomic isocenter is at transverse thoracic vertebral level T2-3 at thoracic inlet.

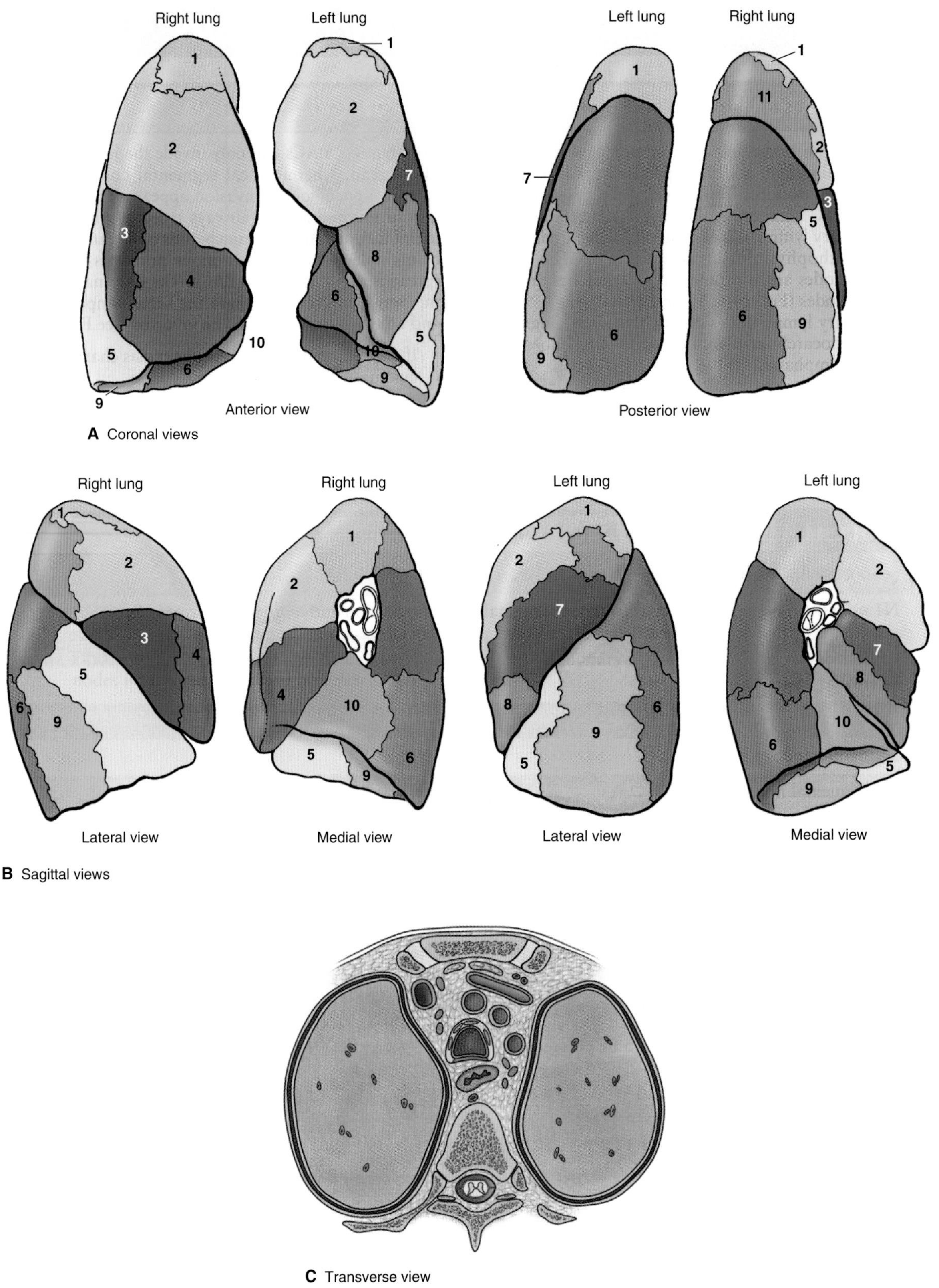

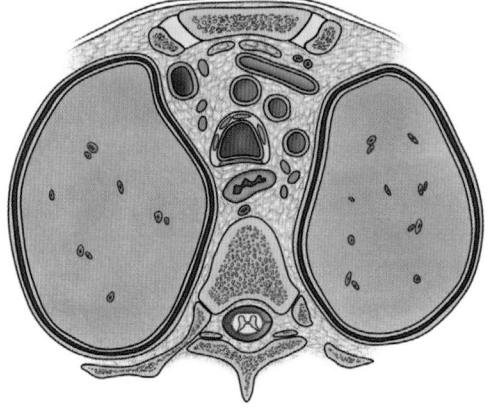

Right lung Left lung   Left lung Right lung

A Coronal views

Anterior view   Posterior view

Right lung   Right lung   Left lung   Left lung

Lateral view   Medial view   Lateral view   Medial view

B Sagittal views

C Transverse view

T₁ • 1-12. Lung Subsegment (Peripheral)   T₂ • 2-12. Pleura of Lung Segment   T₄ • Multiple Lobes

Figure 14.5 | T-oncoanatomy. The Color Code for the anatomic sites correlates with the color code for the stage group (Fig. 14.3) and patterns of spread (Fig. 14.2) and SIMLAP tables (Table 14.2). Connecting the dots in similar colors will provide an appreciation for the 3D Oncoanatomy.

STAGING WORKUP

RULES FOR CLASSIFICATION AND STAGING

Clinical Staging and Imaging

The TNM classification system is primarily for staging non–small cell lung cancers. The most important change dates back to the fourth edition of the AJCC where T3, resectable disease, was distinguished from T4, unresectable disease. Simultaneously, a greater reliance on more sophisticated imaging has occurred. It is with the sixth edition that computed tomography (CT) and positron emission tomography (PET) are allowed. The imaging modalities for detection and diagnosis apply to staging (see Table 14.5). Chest films and CT (preferably spiral) are essential steps in both the diagnosis and staging (Fig. 14.8). PET combined with CT is utilized to overcome motion artifacts. Magnetic resonance imaging (MRI) is useful for mediastinal evaluation. Another advantage of CT over MRI for staging is that it allows for metastatic workup of lung, liver, adrenal, ribs, and vertebrae, especially for Pancoast cancers.

Pathologic Staging

All pathologic specimens from clinical invasive procedures—bronchoscopy, mediastinoscopy, mediastinotomy, thoracentesis, and thorascopy—are applicable.

The thoracotomy and resection of primary and lymph nodes are the mainstay of pathologic staging. Preferably, six nodes should be examined. Surgical resection of primary and regional nodes needs to be carefully evaluated at bronchial stump for adequate margins. All resected nodes should be numbered according to AJCC system and assessed for tumor.

Oncoimaging Annotations

- Most BAC begin in peripheral nodules arising in respiratory bronchi with infiltration of the acini complex, resulting in a collapse of peripheral lung and producing a pleural tethering or tuck sign.
- Multifocal lepidic spread leads to sparing of segmental bronchi, producing an air bronchogram.
- Multiple primaries can occur in synchronous or metachronous fashion.
- Bronchi seen on an end of CT appear as small bubbles or popcorn sign.
- Presence of hilar or mediastinal nodes excludes BAC diagnosis.

TABLE 14.5	Imaging Modalities for Diagnosis and Staging	
Method	Capability	Recommended
Primary Tumor and Regional Nodes Workup		
Chest films	Baseline image	Yes
CT/spiral CT	Most useful of all modalities for determining characteristics of T and N in the thorax and M in the adrenal and liver	Yes
MRI	Not as good as CT	No
Percutaneous needle biopsy	Guided by fluoroscopy or CT, accurate in establishing cytologic diagnosis from T (particularly peripheral lung lesions); M (especially liver or bone); less experience with N	Yes
Mediastinoscopy/thoracoscopy	Confirmation of nodal involvement	Yes
Metastatic Workup for Clinically Suspected Metastases		
MRI	Not recommended unless symptomatic	No
CT/echography	Not recommended unless symptomatic	No
CT/MRI	Not recommended unless symptomatic	No
Bone scan	Not recommended unless symptomatic	No
CT/PET scan	Diagnosis of peripheral lesions can differentiate between cancer and benign lesions. Staging of true extent of primary and lymph node involvement	

CT, computed tomography; M, metastasis; MRI, magnetic resonance imaging; N, node; PET, positron emission tomography; T, tumor.

PROGNOSIS AND CANCER SURVIVAL

CANCER STATISTICS AND SURVIVAL

According to Surveillance Epidemiology and End Results data based on 16,000 patients, the relative 5-year survival is 8% to 10% and 10-year survival 5% to 7%. Surprisingly, there is a small attrition for 5-year survivors; 70% are alive at 10 years. Female gender, good Karnofsky performance status, and cessation of smoking contribute to longer survival.

Staging is a major factor in survival, and these data are presented in Tables 14.6 and 14.7. For stage IA cancers, the 90% T1N0M0 patient decreases to 61% at 5 years and stage IB 70% at 1 year is almost halved at 5 years at 38%. The 50% 5-year survival for stage I decreases to 30%, indicating metastatic disease is highly likely. Stage IIIA represents the most favorable advanced disease patients, with 50% 1-year survival and, despite vigorous chemoradiation, only decreases to 10%. Surgically staged IIIA patients do better, as expected, with 25% alive at 5 years. BACs have the best 5-year survival rates (65%) as compared to other histologies (Table 14.7).

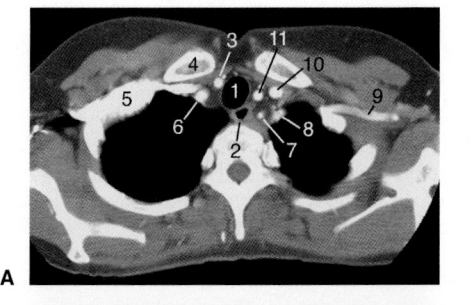

A

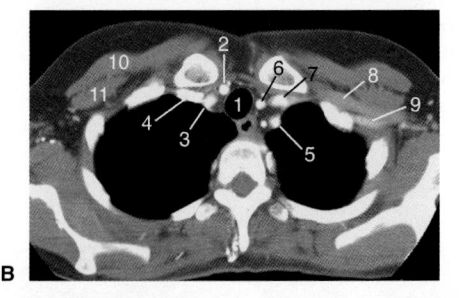

B

BAC is characterized by the nuclear anaplasia and pleomorphism of type II pneumocytes or clara cells. The spread pattern is in a monolayer over acinar alveoli and can, when extensive (T3, T4), interfere with gas exchange and result in a right to left intrapulmonary shunt. Five subtypes have been described. Types A and B have a 100% survival and are noninvasive. Type C is transitional into an adenocarcinoma and has an 80% survival rate. Types D and E have angiolymphatic invasion to lymph nodes and beyond with higher mortality rates similar to adenocarcinomas with regional nodal invasion survival of 25% to 30% and with distant metastases of 5%.

PROGNOSIS

The limited number of prognostic factors are listed in Table 14.6.

TABLE 14.6	Prognostic Factors	
Required for Staging	None
Clinically significant	Pleural/elastic layer invasion (based on H&E and elastic stains)
	Separate tumor nodules
	Vascular invasion—V classification (venous or arteriolar)

H&E, hematoxylin and eosinophilic.
From Edge SB, Byrd DR, Compton CC, et al. *AJCC cancer staging manual.* 7th ed. New York: Springer, 2010:264, with permission.

Figure 14.8 | Axial CTs of T2 and T3 level correlate with the T-oncoanatomy transverse section (Figure 14.5C). Oncoimaging with CT is commonly applied to staging lung cancers, often combined with PET to determine true extent of primary cancer and involved lymph nodes **A.** 1, trachea; 2, esophagus; 3, right common carotid artery; 4, head of clavicle; 5, subclavian vein; 6, right subclavian artery; 7, left vertebral artery; 8, left subclavian artery; 9, left subclavian (axillary) artery; 10, internal jugular vein; 11, left common carotid artery. **B.** 1, trachea; 2, right common carotid artery; 3, right subclavian artery; 4, right brachiocephalic vein; 5, left subclavian artery; 6, left common carotid artery; 7, left brachiocephalic vein; 8, subclavian vein (unopacified); 9, subclavian artery; 10, pectoralis major muscle; 11, pectoralis minor muscle.

TABLE 14.7	Five-Year Relative Survival Rates for Non–Small Cell Lung Cancer by Histology				
		5-Year Survival (%)			
Histologic Type	**No. of Cases**	**All Stages**	**Local**	**Regional**	**Distant**
All carcinomas	87,128	13.9	39.6	14.4	1.5
Squamous cell carcinoma	26,407	16.5	34.3	14.9	1.5
Adenocarcinoma, NOS	20,991	46.6	49.9	16.1	1.5
Bronchioloalveolar carcinoma	**2,382**	**42.1**	**65.1**	**31.8**	**4.2**
Papillary adenocarcinoma	568	23.7	57.4*	25.8	5.4
Adenosquamous carcinoma	1,056	21.6	49.6	19.1	2.2
Small cell carcinoma	10,656	4.6	12.3	7.5	1.4
Large cell carcinoma	7,592	11.4	34.8	13.2	1.6

NOS, not otherwise specified.
*Standard error >5% and ≤10%.

Adenocarcinoma

PERSPECTIVE, PATTERNS OF SPREAD, AND PATHOLOGY

The adenocarcinomas (ADCs) arise from the intrapulmonary bronchi that branch like limbs of a tree in each lung, dividing into segmental and subsegmental bronchi.

PERSPECTIVE AND PATTERNS OF SPREAD

Adenocarcinomas (ADC) are the most common histopathologic type of lung cancer (Fig. 15.1), and they have gradually exceeded squamous cell cancers in incidence in the past two decades. The mucosal lining of the respiratory epithelium of the major bronchi is a pseudostratified ciliated columnar epithelium with goblet cells, which constitute 30% of the total cell population. They produce the mucinogen secretions and provide the mucin lubrication when released in an aqueous environment. These gland-forming ADC cells tend to give rise to four subtypes or variants ranging from well-differentiated ADCs with abundant mucous production to undifferentiated varieties that tend to lose their glandular arrangement (Table 15.1).

These cancers tend to be pulmonary in the more peripheral regions, arising in the lobar bronchi (Fig. 15.2; Table 15.2), which is also a major factor in determining their clinical presentation. They are the predominant female lung cancers (69%) and constitute 45% of male lung cancers. ADCs arise in lobar bronchi, which is the key determinant in their clinical presentation and pattern of spread. Because the lobar and segmental bronchi are the scaffolding for the lung, such cancers trigger segmental or lobar collapse or obstructive pneumonitis, which are more peripheral in location and do not extend beyond the lung hilus.

Cavitation produces a thickened wall with an air fluid level. The wall is irregular and its thickness is the key to whether it is benign or malignant. A wall thickness of 4 mm or less is 92% benign, between 5 to 10 mm it is 51%, and greater than 15 mm it drops to 5%. Cavitation is more common in squamous cell cancer and large cell anaplastic cancers; small cell anaplastic cancers do not cavitate.

PATHOLOGY

The precursor lesion for pulmonary adenocarcinoma is believed to be atypical alveolar hyperplasia (AAH), typically a coincidental finding in resected lung lobes. AAH is composed of proliferating type II pneumocytes and associated with bronchioloalveolar cancer. Genetic and cytologic features often overlap, making histologic distinction between bronchioloalveolar cancer and adenocarcinoma difficult. Only 1% to 5% of AAH cases progress to adenocarcinoma over a period of years.

The findings of a lung nodule that is more peripheral than central in location is a common presentation. The increased incidence in women of adenocarcinoma is 70% as opposed to men, where it is only 57%, and in both, it is more than 50%. Because of its peripheral location, extension to pleura is more common than squamous cell cancer.

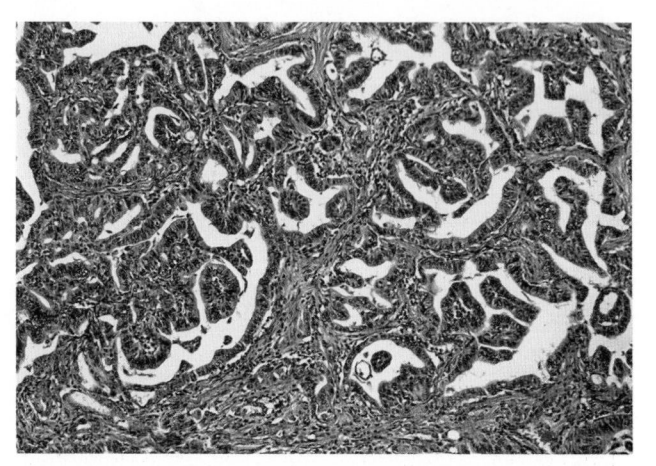

Figure 15.1 | Adenocarcinoma of the lung. A papillary adenocarcinoma consists of malignant epithelial cells growing along thin fibrovascular cores.

TABLE 15.1	Histopathologic Type
Main Pathologic Cell Type	**Variant**
ADC	Acinar
ADC with mixed subtypes	Papillary
	Well-differentiated fetal ADC
	Mucinous ("colloid") ADC
	Mucinous cystadenocarcinoma
	Signet ring ADC
	Clear cell ADC

ADC, adenocarcinoma.

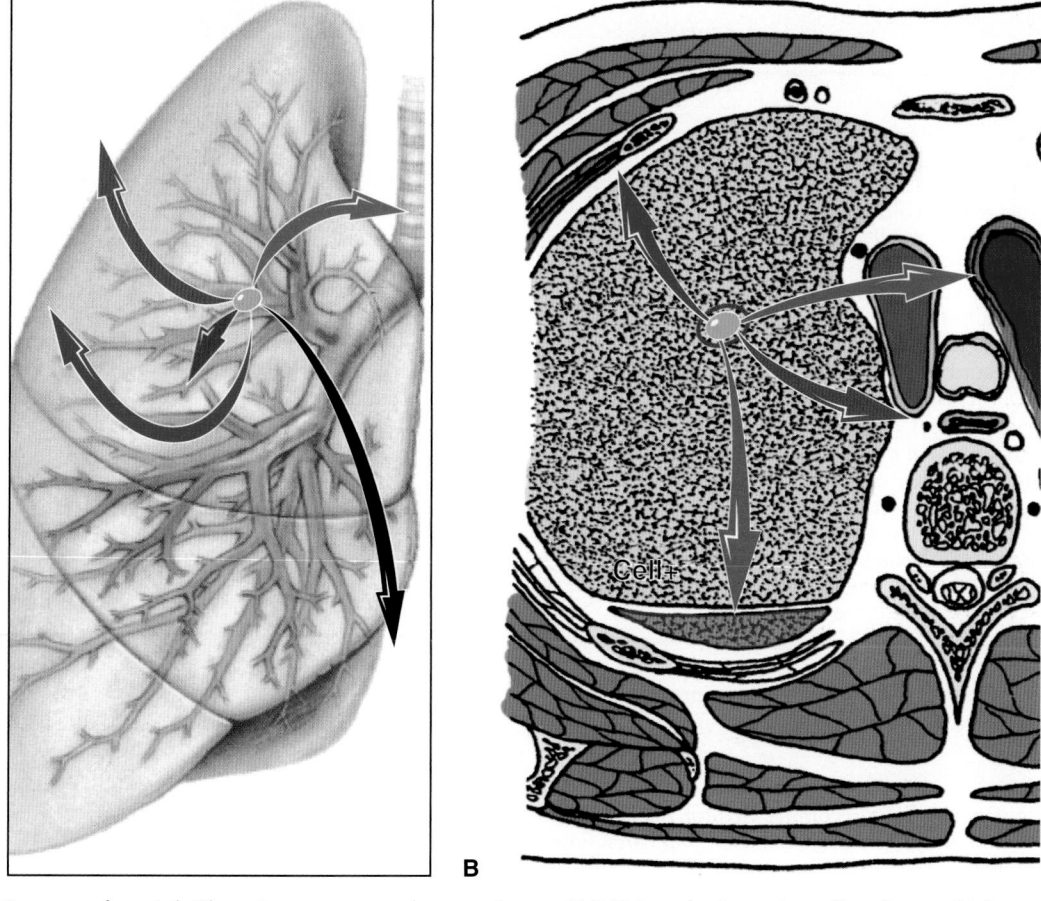

Figure 15.2 | Patterns of spread. The primary cancer adenocarcinoma (ADC) invades in various directions, which are color coded for T stage: Tis, yellow; T1, green; T2, blue; T3, purple; T4, red; and metastatic, black. The concept of visualizing patterns of spread to appreciate the surrounding anatomy is well demonstrated by the six-directional pattern i.e. SIMLAP Table 15.2.

TABLE 15.2	SIMLAP	
Adenocarcinoma (T1), Lobar Bronchi		
S	Segmental/lobar atelectasis	• T2
	Pleura	• T2
I	Segmental/lobar atelectasis	• T2
	Pleura	• T2
M	Lobar atelectasis	
	Involves main bronchus <2 cm	• T3
	Mediastinum	• T4
L	Pleura	• T2
	Pleural effusion—cell (−)	• T3
	cell (+)	• T4
A	Pleura	• T2
	Pleural effusion—cell (−)	• T3
	cell (+)	• T4
P	Pleura	• T2
	Pleural effusion—cell (−)	• T3
	cell (+)	• T4

The six vectors of invasion are Superior, Inferior, Medial, Lateral, Anterior, and Posterior. The color-coded dots correlate the T stage with specific anatomic structure involved.

TNM STAGING CRITERIA

TNM STAGING CRITERIA

In their earliest stages, ADCs can be detected as pulmonary lesions T1 (<3 cm) or T2 (>3 cm) that are intrapulmonary. The lung segments that collapse or consolidate do not extend beyond the hilar region medially. Such cancers lead to persistence or recurrence of symptoms and signs, namely, obstructive pneumonitis. The pathology does not extend beyond the visceral pleura laterally. Their stage categories have been consistent over the past decade and their associated findings are highlighted in Figure 15.3. The color code corresponds to a basic key, but T4 lesions are noted in red and black, with the malignant gradient being highest with mediastinal visceral invasions. The distinction between T3 and T4 occurred in the American Joint Committee on Cancer's (AJCC) fourth edition (1992). T3 cancers do not extend to the chest wall parietal pleura and are limited in extent to the visceral pleura. The stigmata of T4, unresectable cancer, are due to invasion of mediastinal viscera as heart, esophagus, and vital structures such as the great vessels, aorta, and vena cava.

SUMMARY OF CHANGES SEVENTH EDITION AJCC

- This staging system is now recommended for the classification of both non–small cell and small cell lung carcinomas and for carcinoid tumors of the lung.

- The T classifications have been redefined (Fig. 15.3):
  - T1 has been subclassified into T1a ($\leq$2 cm in size) and T1b (>2–3 cm in size)
  - T2 has been subclassified into T2a (>3–5 cm in size) and T2b (>5–7 cm in size)
  - T2 (>7 cm in size) has been reclassified as T3
  - Multiple tumor nodules in the same lobe have been reclassified from T4 to T3
  - Multiple tumor nodules in the same lung but a different lobe have been reclassified from M1 to T4

- No changes have been made to the N classification. However, a new international lymph node map defining the anatomical boundaries for lymph node stations has been developed.

- The M classifications have been redefined:
  - The M1 has been subdivided into M1a and M1b
  - Malignant pleural and pericardial effusions have been reclassified from T4 to M1a
  - Separate tumor nodules in the contralateral lung are considered M1a
  - M1b designates distant metastases

The TNM Staging Matrix is color coded for identification of Stage Group once T and N stages are determined (Table 15.3).

TABLE 15.3 | **Stage Summary Matrix**

	N0	N1	N2	N3	M1a	M1b
T1a	IA	IIA	IIIA	IIIB	IV	IV
T1b	IA	IIA	IIIA	IIIB	IV	IV
T2a	IB	IIA	IIIA	IIIB	IV	IV
T2b	IIA	IIB	IIIA	IIIB	IV	IV
T3	IIB	IIB	IIIA	IIIB	IV	IV
T4	IIIA	IIIA	IIIB	IIIB	IV	IV

Thorax: Lung Cancers
- N stage determines stage group
  - N0, N1, N2, N3a, N3b are stage group I, II, IIIA, IIIB
- N1 can be associated with T1 or T2
- T stage modifies substages
  - T1, T2, N0 = IA, IIB; T1, T2, N2 = IIA, IIB; and T2b, N0 = IIA
- M stage is a separate stage
  - M1 = IV

ADENOCARCINOMA

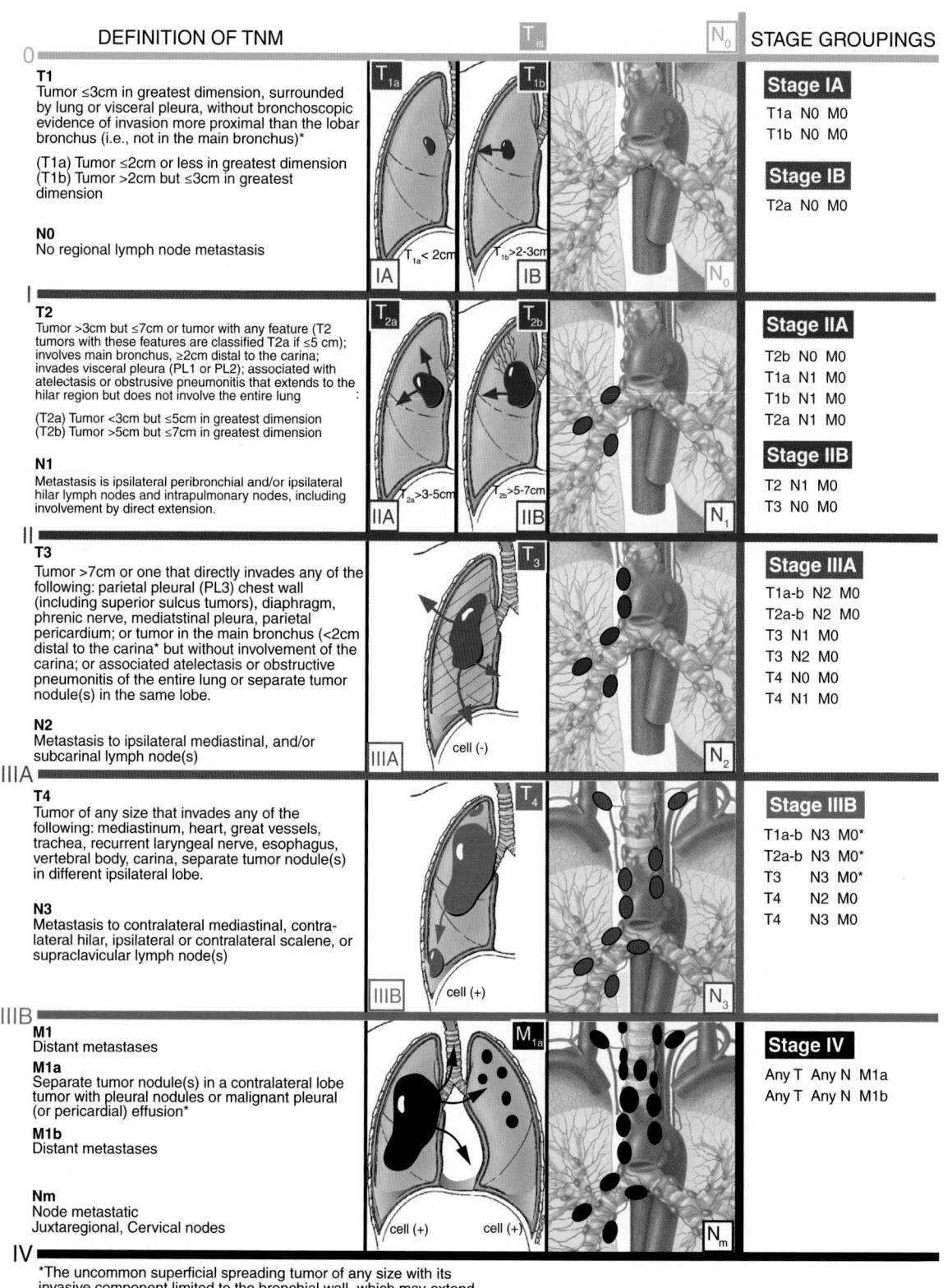

DEFINITION OF TNM

T1
Tumor ≤3cm in greatest dimension, surrounded by lung or visceral pleura, without bronchoscopic evidence of invasion more proximal than the lobar bronchus (i.e., not in the main bronchus)*

(T1a) Tumor ≤2cm or less in greatest dimension
(T1b) Tumor >2cm but ≤3cm in greatest dimension

N0
No regional lymph node metastasis

T2
Tumor >3cm but ≤7cm or tumor with any feature (T2 tumors with these features are classified T2a if ≤ 5 cm); involves main bronchus, ≥2cm distal to the carina; invades visceral pleura (PL1 or PL2); associated with atelectasis or obstrusive pneumonitis that extends to the hilar region but does not involve the entire lung :

(T2a) Tumor <3cm but ≤5cm in greatest dimension
(T2b) Tumor >5cm but ≤7cm in greatest dimension

N1
Metastasis is ipsilateral peribronchial and/or ipsilateral hilar lymph nodes and intrapulmonary nodes, including involvement by direct extension.

T3
Tumor >7cm or one that directly invades any of the following: parietal pleural (PL3) chest wall (including superior sulcus tumors), diaphragm, phrenic nerve, mediatstinal pleura, parietal pericardium; or tumor in the main bronchus (<2cm distal to the carina* but without involvement of the carina; or associated atelectasis or obstructive pneumonitis of the entire lung or separate tumor nodule(s) in the same lobe.

N2
Metastasis to ipsilateral mediastinal, and/or subcarinal lymph node(s)

T4
Tumor of any size that invades any of the following: mediastinum, heart, great vessels, trachea, recurrent laryngeal nerve, esophagus, vertebral body, carina, separate tumor nodule(s) in different ipsilateral lobe.

N3
Metastasis to contralateral mediastinal, contra-lateral hilar, ipsilateral or contralateral scalene, or supraclavicular lymph node(s)

M1
Distant metastases
M1a
Separate tumor nodule(s) in a contralateral lobe tumor with pleural nodules or malignant pleural (or pericardial) effusion*
M1b
Distant metastases

Nm
Node metastatic
Juxtaregional, Cervical nodes

*The uncommon superficial spreading tumor of any size with its invasive component limited to the bronchial wall, which may extend proximally to the main bronchus, is also classified as T1a.

STAGE GROUPINGS

Stage IA
T1a N0 M0
T1b N0 M0

Stage IB
T2a N0 M0

Stage IIA
T2b N0 M0
T1a N1 M0
T1b N1 M0
T2a N1 M0

Stage IIB
T2 N1 M0
T3 N0 M0

Stage IIIA
T1a-b N2 M0
T2a-b N2 M0
T3 N1 M0
T3 N2 M0
T4 N0 M0
T4 N1 M0

Stage IIIB
T1a-b N3 M0*
T2a-b N3 M0*
T3 N3 M0*
T4 N2 M0
T4 N3 M0

Stage IV
Any T Any N M1a
Any T Any N M1b

Figure 15.3 | TNM staging diagram. Adenocarcinomas are peripheral arising in segmental bronchi and tend to be associated with atelectasis or obstructive pneumonitis. Vertical presentation of stage groupings, which follow the same color code for cancer advancement, are organized in horizontal lanes: Stage 0, yellow; I, green; II, blue; IIIA, purple; IIIB, red; and metastatic stage IV, black. Definitions of TN are on the left and stage groupings is on the right. Major stage group progression is dominated by the N stage progression.

T-ONCOANATOMY

ORIENTATION OF THREE-PLANAR ONCOANATOMY

The isocenter chosen relates to the branching lobar and segmental bronchi. The three-planar levels are chosen at thorax T3-4 level. The plane at this level divides the superior and inferior mediastinum. It is central to understanding the thoracic anatomy (Fig. 15.4).

T-oncoanatomy

The bronchial tree in which ADCs arise branches throughout the pulmonary parenchyma undergoing 10 orders of division. The trachea, which lies in the superior mediastinum, divides into right and left main stem bronchi that extend into the right and left lungs. At that point, they divide into lobar bronchi for the upper, middle, and lower lobes on the right, and the upper and lower lobes on the left. Each lobar bronchus divides into segmental bronchi (Fig. 15.5).

The lobes of the lung are divided into bronchopulmonary segments (10 per lung) and are defined by the branching of the segmental bronchi. The mucosa lining the bronchus is the usual site of origin for cancer of the lung, although cancer also may arise in the more peripheral areas of the bronchiolar tree.

Of particular interest are both the symmetry and asymmetry that exist between various portions of the left and right lungs and the bronchial trees. The projection of the lower lobe lesions in the upper half of the lung emphasizes the need to understand this complex anatomy. It is important to be familiar with the lung lobes in different projections when viewed anteriorly and posteriorly as well as their lateral and medial faces to recognize obstructive pneumonitis on chest films.

The right lung has three lobes and the left lung has two lobes. The middle lobe in the right side arises from the lower lobe bronchus, whereas the lingula, or the left side, which corresponds to the middle lobe, arises from the upper lobe bronchus. Major and segmental bronchi are presented in Figure 15.5A.

- *Coronal:* Anterior view demonstrates the lobar and segmental anatomy of the bronchial tree. Note the asymmetry of right and left lungs with the middle lobe on the right being equivalent to the lingula except the middle lobe bronchus arises from the lower lobe bronchus and the lingual from the upper lobe.

- *Transverse (Fig. 15.5):* This T3-4 level is at the plane dividing the mediastinum. Note broadening of the trachea at the carina, the azygos vein arching into the superior vena cava on the left and the arch of the aorta, and the entry of its three major arteries—the brachiocephalic, common carotid, and subclavian. The thoracic duct is in the left.

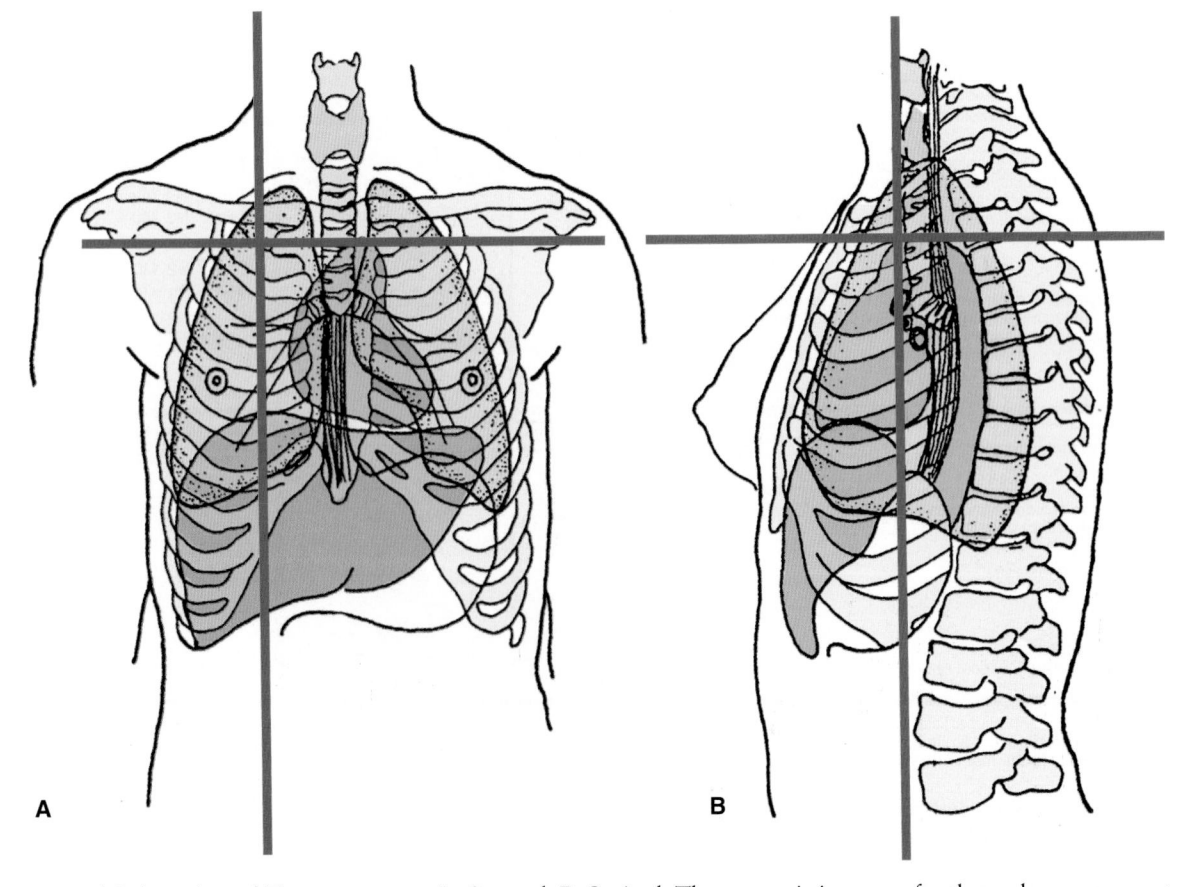

Figure 15.4 | Orientation of T-oncoanatomy. A. Coronal. **B.** Sagittal. The anatomic isocenter for three-planar oncoanatomy is placed at the thoracic vertebral level T3-4.

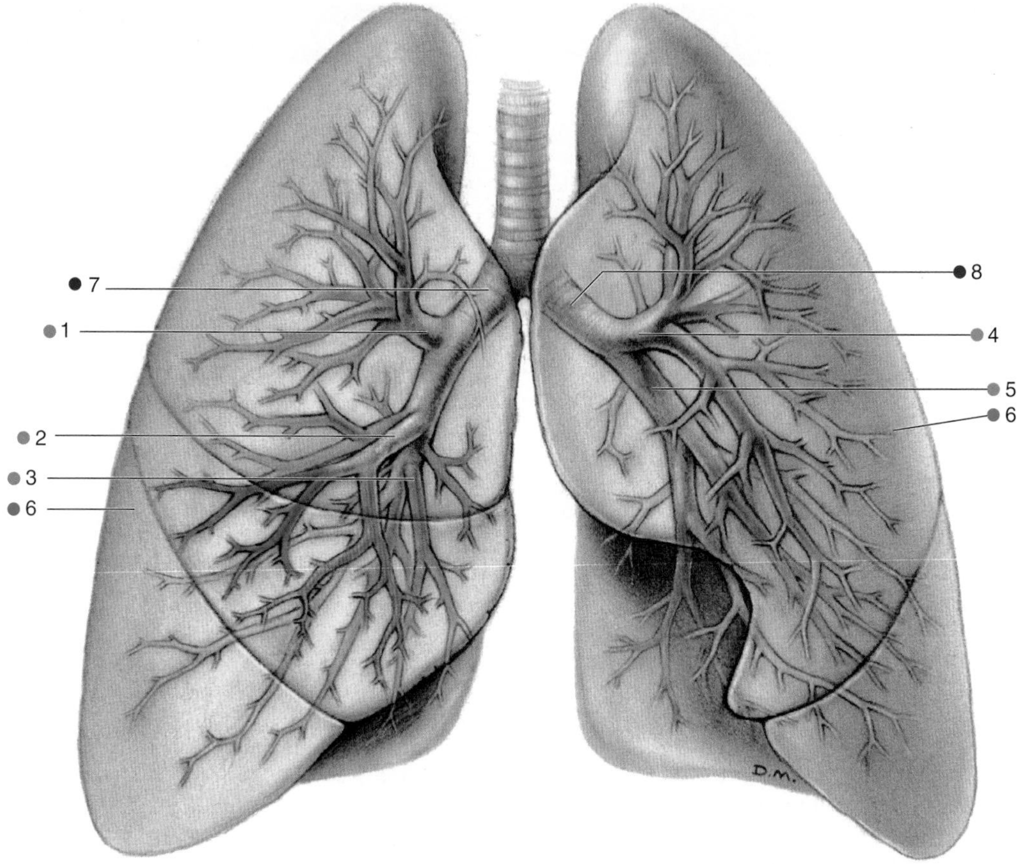

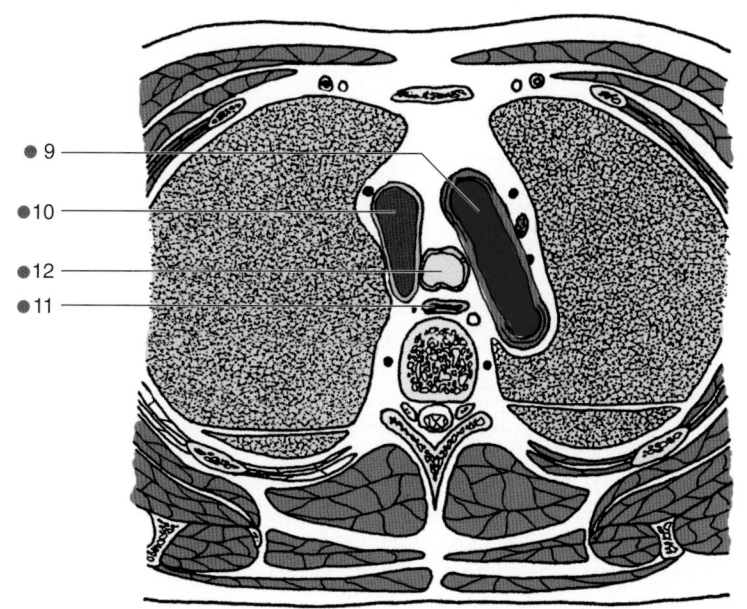

A Coronal

B Transverse

T₁	● 1. Right Superior Lobar Bronchus	T₁	● 5. Left Inferior Lobar Bronchus	T₄	● 9. Aortic Arch
T₁	● 2. Right Middle Lobar Bronchus	T₂	● 6. Pleura	T₄	● 10. Superior Vena Cava
T₁	● 3. Right Lower Lobar Bronchus	T₃	● 7. Right Main Bronchus	T₄	● 11. Esophagus
T₁	● 4. Left Superior Lobar Bronchus	T₃	● 8. Left Main Bronchus	T₄	● 12. Trachea

Figure 15.5 | T-oncoanatomy. The Color Code for the anatomic sites correlates with the color code for the stage group (Fig. 15.3) and patterns of spread (Fig. 15.2) and SIMLAP tables (Table 15.2). Connecting the dots in similar colors will provide an appreciation for the 3D Oncoanatomy.

N-ONCOANATOMY AND M-ONCOANATOMY

N-ONCOANATOMY

The intrapulmonary lymph nodes are designated by their relationship to the bronchial tree and are referred to as lobar nodes bronchi on interlobar lymph nodes, which then drain to hilar nodes (Fig. 15.6). The tabulation of regional nodes is noted in Table 15.4.

REGIONAL LYMPH NODES

The regional lymph nodes extend from the supraclavicular region to the diaphragm. During the past three decades, three different lymph node maps have been used to describe the

TABLE 15.4 Lymph Nodes of Lung

Interlobar bronchial nodes and hilar nodes are sentinel nodes within visceral pleura.

N1 nodes: All N1 nodes lie distal to the mediastinal pleural reflection and *within the visceral pleura.*

Hilar nodes 10

Interlobar nodes 11

Lobar nodes bronchi 12

Segmental nodes 13

Subsegmental nodes 14

N2 nodes: All N2 nodes lie within the mediastinal pleural envelope on the ipsilateral side.

Highest mediastinal nodes 1, 2R, 2L

Upper paratracheal nodes 2R, 2L

Prevascular and retrotracheal nodes 3a, 3p*

Lower paratracheal nodes 4R, 4L

Subaortic nodes (aortopulmonary window) 5

Para-aortic nodes (ascending aorta or phrenic) 6

Subcarinal nodes 7

Paraesophageal nodes (below carina) 8

Pulmonary ligament nodes 9

*3a, 3p not shown in Fig. 15.6.

regional lymph node potentially involved by lung cancers. The first map was endorsed by the Japan Lung Cancer Society. The second map, the Mountain Dresler modification of the American Thoracic Society (MDATS) lymph node map, is used in North America and Europe. The nomenclature for the anatomical locations of lymph nodes differs between these two maps. Recently the International Association for the Study of Lung Cancer (IASLC) proposed a lymph node map (Figure 15.6B) that reconciles the discrepancies between these two previous maps. The IASLC lymph node map is now the recommended means of describing regional lymph node involvement for lung cancers.

There are no evidence-based guidelines regarding the *number* of lymph nodes to be removed at surgery for adequate staging. However, adequate N staging is generally considered to include sampling or dissection of lymph nodes from stations 2R, 4R, 7, 10R, and 11R for right-sided tumors, and stations 5, 6, 7, 10L, and 11L for left-sided tumors. Station 9 lymph nodes should also be evaluated for lower lobe tumors. The more peripheral lymph nodes at stations 12–14 are usually evaluated by the pathologist in lobectomy or pneumonectomy specimens but may be separately removed when sublobar resections (e.g., segmentectomy) are performed. There is evidence to support the recommendation that histological examination of hilar and mediastinal lymphenectomy specimen(s) will ordinarily include 6 or more lymph nodes/stations. Three of these nodes/stations should be mediastinal, including the subcarinal nodes and three from N1 nodes/stations.*

M-ONCOANATOMY

Drainage into the subclavian vein, if invaded, then via the superior vena cava and pulmonary artery drain into the lung. Cancer invasion of chest wall drains into intercostal veins, then the azygos vein, and then the superior vena cava, which leads to lung dissemination. Adenocarcinoma dissemination of metastases is the most common lung cancer and is presented as the prototype for metastases into other organs (Fig. 15.7).

The M-oncoanatomy emphasizes the pulmonary venous drainage, which is oxygenated, drains the pulmonary parenchymal cancers and disseminates cells to many remote anatomic states by way of the left side of the heart. Virtually every remote organ site can be involved and include liver, adrenal, bones, and brain.

*Preceding passage from Edge SB, Byrd DR, and Compton CC, et al. *AJCC Cancer Staging Manual, 7th edition.* New York, Springer, 2010, pp. 254–255.

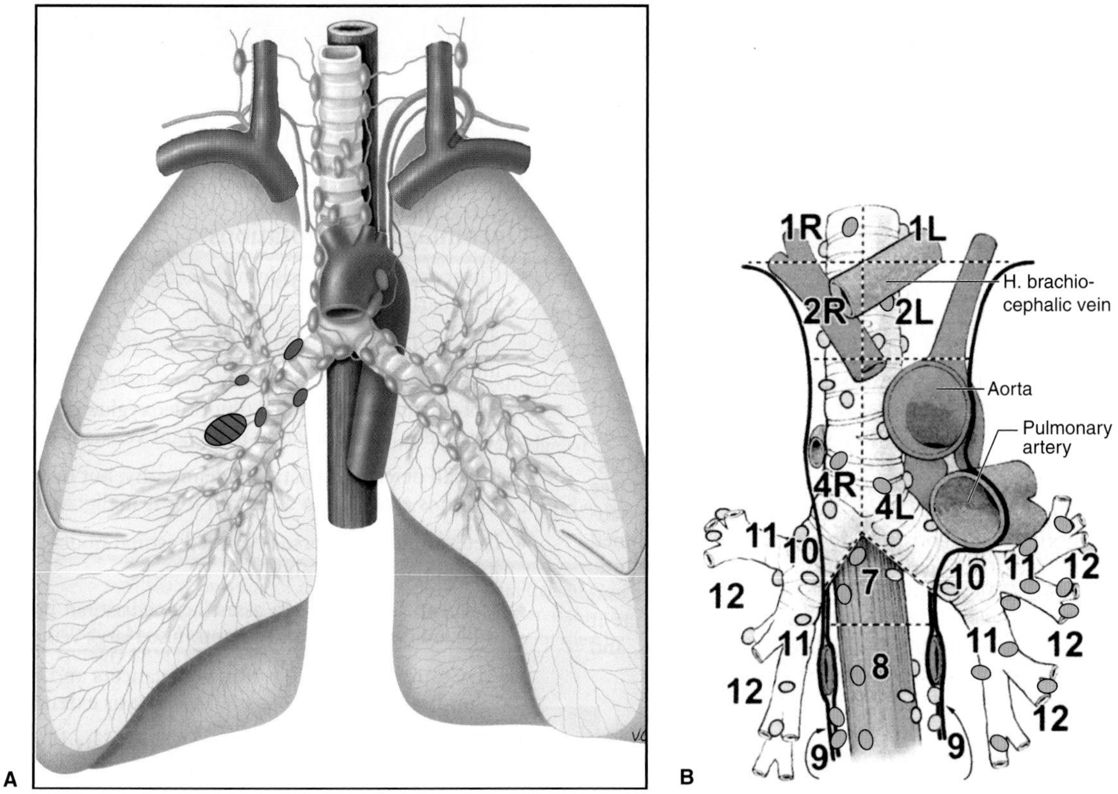

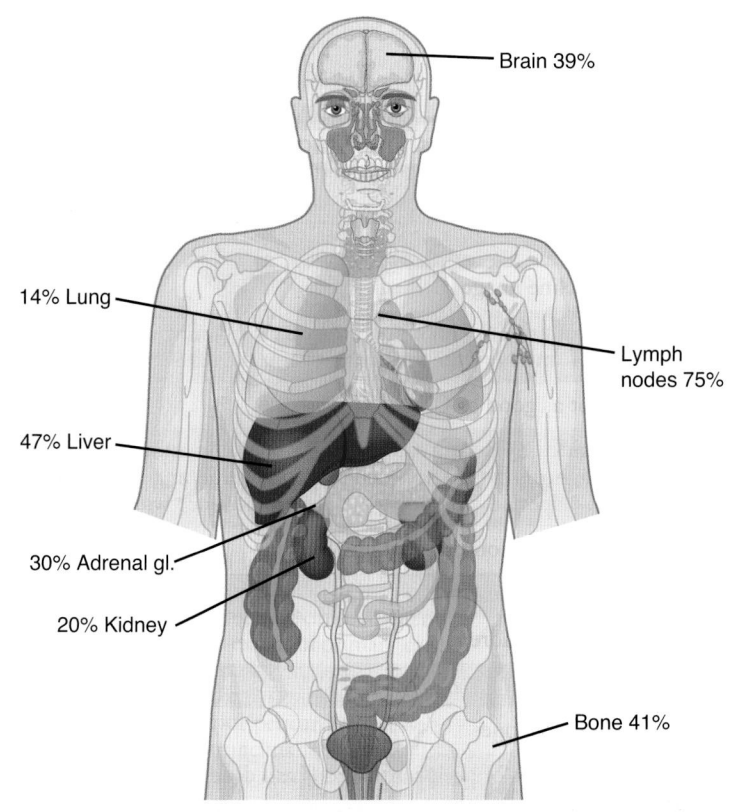

Figure 15.6 | A. N-oncoanatomy. Interlobar bronchial nodes and hilar nodes are sentinel nodes within visceral pleura. **B. M-oncoanatomy.** International Association for the Study of Lung Cancer (IASLC). Labels correlate with Table 15.4.

Figure 15.7 | Incidence and distribution of metastases. Adenocarcinoma is the most common lung cancer and is presented as a prototype for lung cancers. The incidence and distribution of distant metastases are noted as percentages and correlate with Table 12.6.

Large Cell Anaplastic Cancer

PERSPECTIVE, PATTERNS OF SPREAD, AND PATHOLOGY

Large cell anaplastic cancers arise in more proximal bronchi and have a proclivity to invade mediastinal structures early.

PERSPECTIVE AND PATTERNS OF SPREAD

Large cell anaplastic (LCA) cancers are those cancers that are distinguished from small cell anaplastic cancers by numerous morphologic variants: large cell neuroendocrine, basaloid carcinoma, lymphoepithelioma-like and clear cell, or large cell with rhabdoid phenotype (Table 16.1; Fig. 16.1). It is not a common cancer type, accounting for 5% to 10% of lung cancers, distinguished by its propensity to invade the mediastinum pleura and pericardium. A paradox to ponder is the resistance of the heart to direct invasion despite circulating cancer cells, especially from lung cancers, recognizing that the endocardium is never seeded and that myocardial nodulation is more often recognized and found only postmortem. Because most LCAs are undifferentiated, vascular infiltration occurs with rapid systemic dissemination to remote sites (Fig. 16.2; Table 16.2).

Superior vena caval obstruction (SVCO) is a dreaded syndrome that can be rapid or slow in onset. It begins with facial edema, most apparent at the eyelids, plethora, headache or confusion (brain edema), and arm edema; caput medusa dilation of veins on chest wall and abdomen can occur.

A rapid onset is an emergent situation, especially if there is difficulty breathing, suggesting tracheal compression. A slow onset and compensating altered blood flow patterns can be discerned clinically by compressing a prominent chest wall vein to determine if flow is in a caudal or cranial direction.

- SVCO above the azygos vein allows blood to flow inferiorly via hemiazygous vein into the vena cava.
- SVCO below the azygos vein allows blood to flow superiorly around the shoulder and to flow inferiorly via internal thoracic (mammary) and chest and abdominal wall veins into the inferior vena cava. Leg edema may result.
- SVCO and azygos vein obstructed shunts blood caudally from internal thoracic (mammary) veins to superior or inferior epigastric veins.

PATHOLOGY

LCA cancers with large pleomorphic nuclei spread in sheets, are often large and bulky masses, and can compress mediastinal structures as do small cell anaplastic (SCA) cancers. Variants are listed in Table 16.1.

TABLE 16.1	Histopathologic Type
Main Pathologic Cell Type	**Variant**
Large cell carcinoma	Large cell neuroendocrine carcinoma
	Combined large cell neuroendocrine carcinoma
	Basaloid carcinoma
	Lymphepithelioma-like carcinoma
	Clear cell carcinoma
	Large cell carcinoma with rhabdoid phenotype

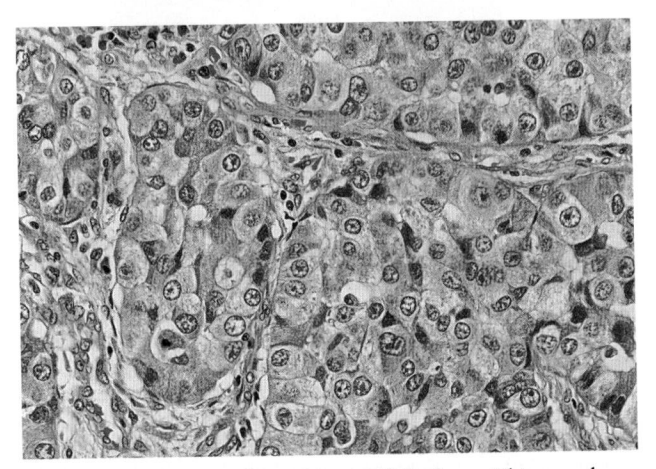

Figure 16.1 | Large cell carcinoma of the lung. This poorly differentiated tumor grows rapidly. The tumor cells are large and contain ample cytoplasm and prominent nucleoli.

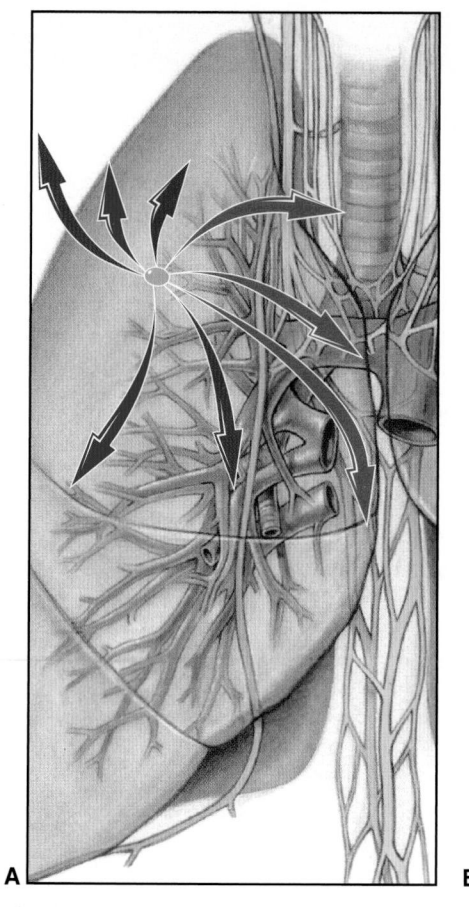
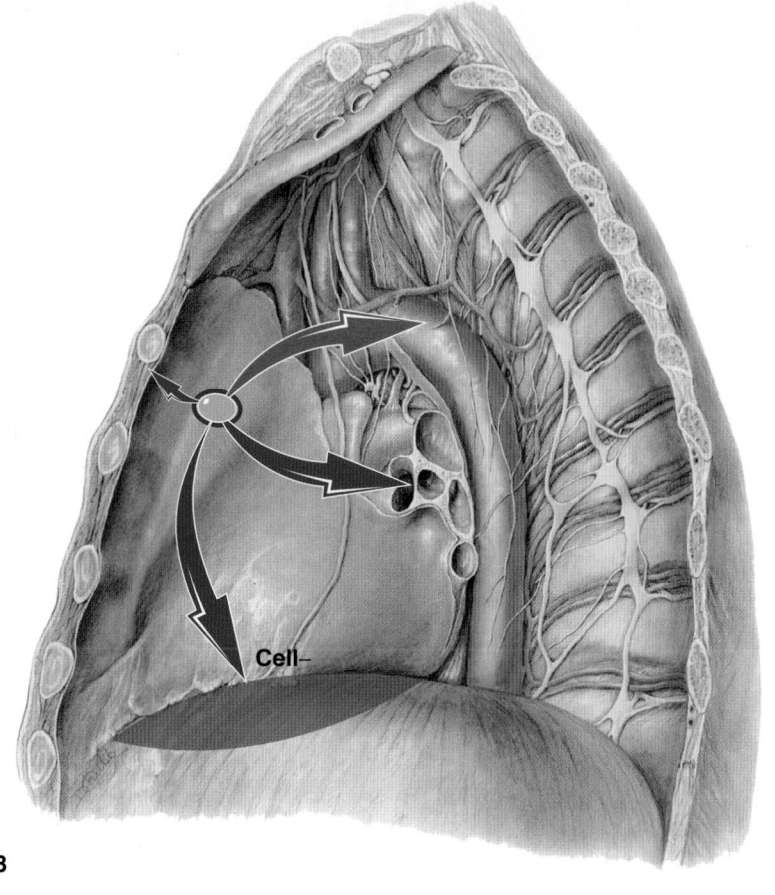

Figure 16.2 | Patterns of spread. The primary cancer invades in various directions, which are color coded for T stage: Tis, yellow; T1, green; T2, blue; T3, purple; T4, red; and when metastatic, black. The concept of visualizing patterns of spread to appreciate the surrounding anatomy is well demonstrated by the six-directional pattern i.e. SIMLAP Table 16.2.

TABLE 16.2	SIMLAP	
Large Cell Anaplastic Cancer: Lobar Bronchi		
S	Segmental/lobar atelectasis	• T2
	Pleura	• T2
I	Segmental/lobar atelectasis	• T2
	Pleura	• T2
M	Lobar atelectasis	• T2
	Involves main bronchus >2 cm	• T3
	Mediastinum	• T4
L	Pleura	• T2
	Pleural effusion—cell (−)	• T3
	cell (+)	• T4
A	Pleura	• T2
	Pleural effusion—cell (−)	• T3
	cell (+)	• T4
P	Pleura	• T2
	Pleural effusion—cell (−)	• T3
	cell (+)	• T4

The six vectors of invasion are Superior, Inferior, Medial, Lateral, Anterior, and Posterior. The color-coded dots correlate the T stage with specific anatomic structure involved.

TNM STAGING CRITERIA

TNM STAGING CRITERIA

As thoracic surgery improved, the need for defining criteria of unresectability became evident. The distinction between T3 and T4 entered the American Joint Committee on Cancer (AJCC)/International Union Against Cancer staging in its fourth edition (1982), as did more researched biologic and molecular markers to distinguish small cell anaplastic cancers from its variants. T4 stage applies to any tumor regardless of size that invaded any of the following: mediastinum, heart, great vessels, trachea, esophagus, vertebral body, or malignant effusion with positive cells identified after both pleural and pericardial taps.

SUMMARY OF CHANGES SEVENTH EDITION AJCC

- This staging system is now recommended for the classification of both non–small cell and small cell lung carcinomas and for carcinoid tumors of the lung (Fig. 16.3).
- The T classifications have been redefined:
  - T1 has been subclassified into T1a (≤2 cm in size) and T1b (>2–3 cm in size)
  - T2 has been subclassified into T2a (>3–5 cm in size) and T2b (>5–7 cm in size)
  - T2 (>7 cm in size) has been reclassified as T3
  - Multiple tumor nodules in the same lobe have been reclassified from T4 to T3
  - Multiple tumor nodules in the same lung but a different lobe have been reclassified from M1 to T4
- No changes have been made to the N classification. However, a new international lymph node map defining the anatomical boundaries for lymph node stations has been developed.
- The M classifications have been redefined:
  - The M1 has been subdivided into M1a and M1b
  - Malignant pleural and pericardial effusions have been reclassified from T4 to M1a
  - Separate tumor nodules in the contralateral lung are considered M1a
  - M1b designates distant metastases

Because of the magnitude of the T-category changes with shifts in both directions, that is both downstaging and upstaging, it is important to review the stage groupings of the sixth and seventh editions. The TNM Staging Matrix is color coded for identification of Stage Group once T and N stages are determined (Table 16.3).

TABLE 16.3 | Stage Summary Matrix

	N0	N1	N2	N3	M1a	M1b
T1a	IA	IIA	IIIA	IIIB	IV	IV
T1b	IA	IIA	IIIA	IIIB	IV	IV
T2a	IB	IIA	IIIA	IIIB	IV	IV
T2b	IIA	IIB	IIIA	IIIB	IV	IV
T3	IIB	IIB	IIIA	IIIB	IV	IV
T4	IIIA	IIIA	IIIB	IIIB	IV	IV

Thorax: Lung Cancers
- N stage determines stage group
  - N0, N1, N2, N3a, N3b are stage group I, II, IIIA, IIIB
- N1 can be associated with T1 or T2
- T stage modifies substages
  - T1, T2, N0 = IA, IIB; T1, T2, N2 = IIA, IIB; and T2b, N0 = IIA
- M stage is a separate stage
  - M1 = IV

LARGE CELL ANAPLASTIC CANCER

DEFINITION OF TNM

STAGE GROUPINGS

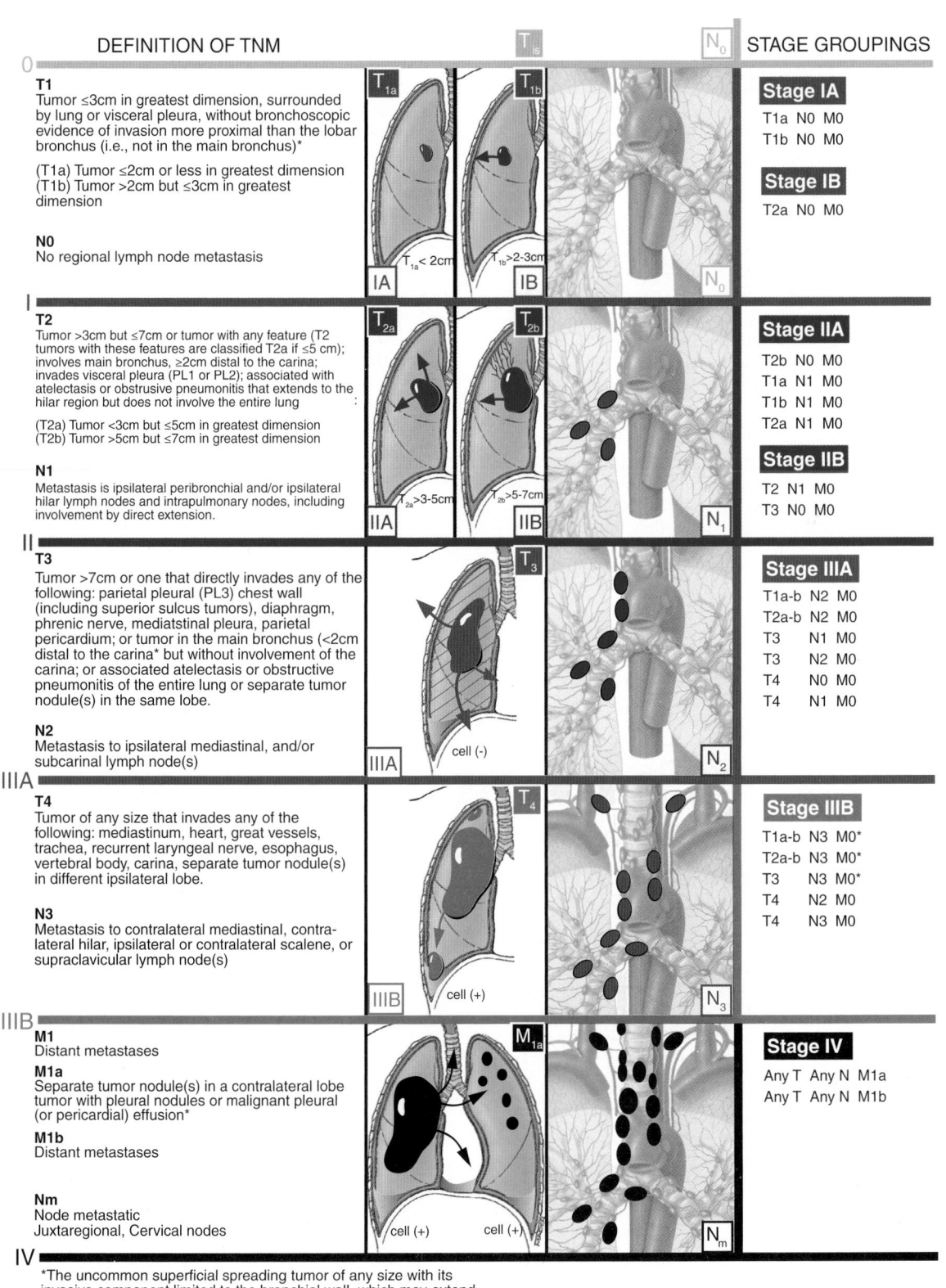

T1
Tumor ≤3cm in greatest dimension, surrounded by lung or visceral pleura, without bronchoscopic evidence of invasion more proximal than the lobar bronchus (i.e., not in the main bronchus)*

(T1a) Tumor ≤2cm or less in greatest dimension
(T1b) Tumor >2cm but ≤3cm in greatest dimension

N0
No regional lymph node metastasis

T2
Tumor >3cm but ≤7cm or tumor with any feature (T2 tumors with these features are classified T2a if ≤5 cm); involves main bronchus, ≥2cm distal to the carina; invades visceral pleura (PL1 or PL2); associated with atelectasis or obstrusive pneumonitis that extends to the hilar region but does not involve the entire lung

(T2a) Tumor <3cm but ≤5cm in greatest dimension
(T2b) Tumor >5cm but ≤7cm in greatest dimension

N1
Metastasis is ipsilateral peribronchial and/or ipsilateral hilar lymph nodes and intrapulmonary nodes, including involvement by direct extension.

T3
Tumor >7cm or one that directly invades any of the following: parietal pleural (PL3) chest wall (including superior sulcus tumors), diaphragm, phrenic nerve, mediatstinal pleura, parietal pericardium; or tumor in the main bronchus (<2cm distal to the carina* but without involvement of the carina; or associated atelectasis or obstructive pneumonitis of the entire lung or separate tumor nodule(s) in the same lobe.

N2
Metastasis to ipsilateral mediastinal, and/or subcarinal lymph node(s)

T4
Tumor of any size that invades any of the following: mediastinum, heart, great vessels, trachea, recurrent laryngeal nerve, esophagus, vertebral body, carina, separate tumor nodule(s) in different ipsilateral lobe.

N3
Metastasis to contralateral mediastinal, contra-lateral hilar, ipsilateral or contralateral scalene, or supraclavicular lymph node(s)

M1
Distant metastases

M1a
Separate tumor nodule(s) in a contralateral lobe tumor with pleural nodules or malignant pleural (or pericardial) effusion*

M1b
Distant metastases

Nm
Node metastatic
Juxtaregional, Cervical nodes

Stage IA
T1a N0 M0
T1b N0 M0

Stage IB
T2a N0 M0

Stage IIA
T2b N0 M0
T1a N1 M0
T1b N1 M0
T2a N1 M0

Stage IIB
T2 N1 M0
T3 N0 M0

Stage IIIA
T1a-b N2 M0
T2a-b N2 M0
T3   N1 M0
T3   N2 M0
T4   N0 M0
T4   N1 M0

Stage IIIB
T1a-b N3 M0*
T2a-b N3 M0*
T3   N3 M0*
T4   N2 M0
T4   N3 M0

Stage IV
Any T Any N M1a
Any T Any N M1b

*The uncommon superficial spreading tumor of any size with its invasive component limited to the bronchial wall, which may extend proximally to the main bronchus, is also classified as T1a.

Figure 16.3 | TNM staging diagram. Large cell anaplastic cancers are variants and aggressive cancers with invasive qualities often with neuroendocrine effects. Vertical presentation of stage groupings, which follow the same color code for cancer advancement, is organized in horizontal lanes: Stage 0, yellow; I, green; II, blue; IIIA, purple; IIIB, red; and metastatic stage IV, black. Definitions of TN are on the left and stage grouping is on the right. Major stage group progression is dominated by the N stage progression.

T-ONCOANATOMY

ORIENTATION OF THREE-PLANAR ONCOANATOMY

LCA cancers can arise throughout the bronchial tree, and its isocenter has been assigned to thoracic T4-5 level posteriorly and to the fourth rib articulation with the sternum at the level of the horizontal fissure on the right and the cardiac contour on the left (Fig. 16.4).

T-oncoanatomy

T-oncoanatomy focuses on the left side of the mediastinum featuring the ascending aorta and descending aorta. The major nerves coursing into the thorax are the focus of the three-planar views, indicating where they are vulnerable to compression or invasion (Fig. 16.5).

- Coronal: At the thoracic inlet the vagus nerve (cranial nerve X) enters the chest, but the recurrent laryngeal loops around the right subclavian; whereas on the left it loops around the aortic arch. Compression on the right is anticipated with metastatic right supraclavicular and scalene nodes. On the

left, the more common event is for mediastinal nodes to invade the recurrent laryngeal at the aortic pulmonary window. The anterior and posterior pulmonary plexuses receive sympathetic contributions from the right and left sympathetic trunks (second to fifth thoracic ganglia) and parasympathetic contributions from the right and left vagus nerves. The right and left vagus nerves pass inferiorly from the posterior pulmonary plexus to contribute fibers to the esophageal plexus. Branches from the pulmonary plexuses continue along the bronchi and pulmonary vasculature to the lungs. The phrenic nerve passes anterior to the root of the lung to the diaphragm.

- Sagittal: The left side of the mediastinum is the "red side," dominated by the arch and descending portion of the aorta and the left common carotid and subclavian arteries, which obscures the trachea from view. The left vagus nerve passes posterior to the root of the lung, sending its recurrent laryngeal branch around the ligamentum arteriosum inferior, then medial to the aortic arch. The phrenic nerve passes anterior to the root of the lung and penetrates the diaphragm more anteriorly than on the right side.

- Transverse: Note the juxtaposition of the ascending and descending aorta with the carina at the T4-5 level.

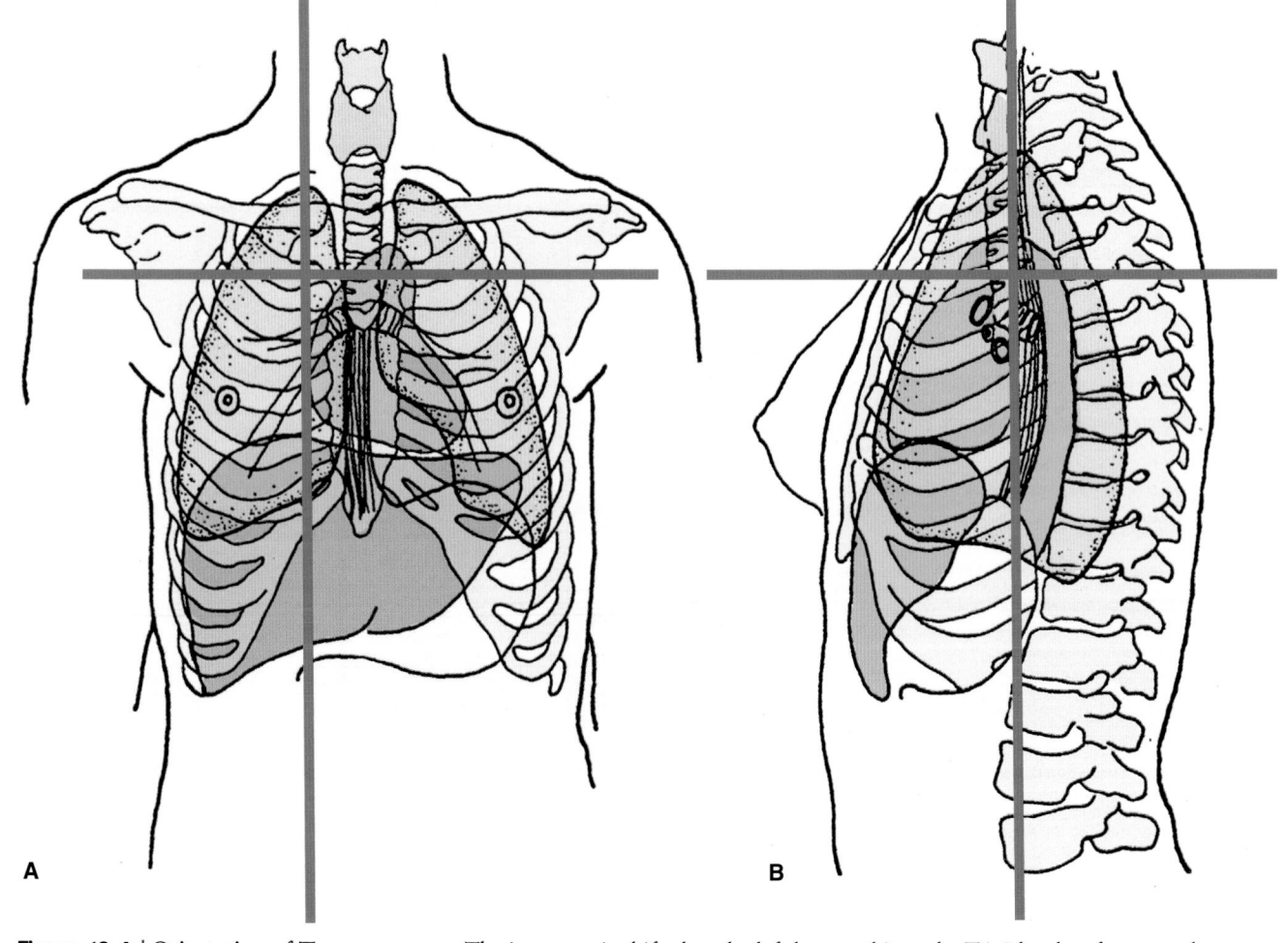

A **B**

Figure 16.4 | Orientation of T-oncoanatomy. The isocenter is shifted to the left lung and is at the T4-5 level to focus on the nerves entering the thorax and their course. **A.** Coronal. **B.** Sagittal.

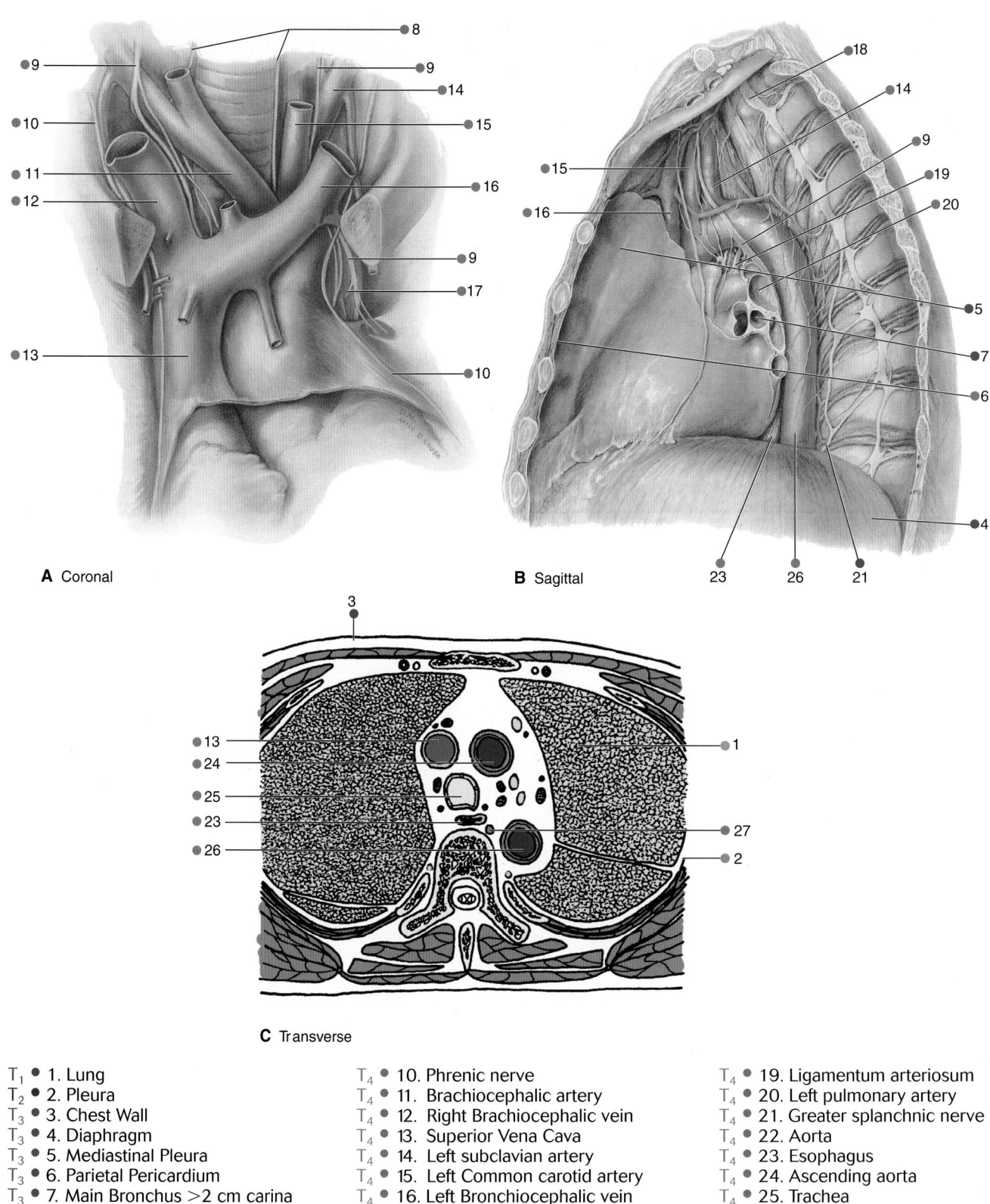

A Coronal

B Sagittal

C Transverse

T₁	1. Lung	T₄	10. Phrenic nerve	T₄	19. Ligamentum arteriosum
T₂	2. Pleura	T₄	11. Brachiocephalic artery	T₄	20. Left pulmonary artery
T₃	3. Chest Wall	T₄	12. Right Brachiocephalic vein	T₄	21. Greater splanchnic nerve
T₃	4. Diaphragm	T₄	13. Superior Vena Cava	T₄	22. Aorta
T₃	5. Mediastinal Pleura	T₄	14. Left subclavian artery	T₄	23. Esophagus
T₃	6. Parietal Pericardium	T₄	15. Left Common carotid artery	T₄	24. Ascending aorta
T₃	7. Main Bronchus >2 cm carina	T₄	16. Left Bronchiocephalic vein	T₄	25. Trachea
T₄	8. Recurrent Laryngeal nerves	T₄	17. Left Recurrent Laryngeal nerve	T₄	26. Descending aorta
T₄	9. Vagus Nerve	T₄	18. Sympathetic Trunk	T₄	27. Thoracic (lymphatic) duct

Figure 16.5 | T-oncoanatomy. The Color Code for the anatomic sites correlates with the color code for the stage group (Fig. 16.3) and patterns of spread (Fig. 16.2) and SIMLAP tables (Table 16.2). Connecting the dots in similar colors will provide an appreciation for the 3D Oncoanatomy.

N-ONCOANATOMY AND M-ONCOANATOMY

N-ONCOANATOMY

The first station lymph nodes are the intrapulmonary, pulmonary, and bronchopulmonary lymph nodes, which are contained within the visceral pleural reflection. There are three major collecting trunks: the superior, middle, and inferior trunks. These drain into 10 to 15 peribronchial nodes and then to hilar nodes. Second station lymph nodes are those in the mediastinum and may be paraesophageal, subcarinal, or paratracheal and pretracheal or retrotracheal in location. Involvement of scalene, cervical, supraclavicular, and axillary nodes is considered distant metastases (Fig. 16.6A; Table 16.4).

REGIONAL LYMPH NODES

The regional lymph nodes extend from the supraclavicular region to the diaphragm. During the past three decades, three different lymph node maps have been used to describe the regional lymph node potentially involved by lung cancers. The first map was endorsed by the Japan Lung Cancer Society. The second map, the Mountain Dresler modification of the American Thoracic Society (MDATS) lymph node map,

is used in North America and Europe. The nomenclature for the anatomical locations of lymph nodes differs between these two maps. Recently the International Association for the Study of Lung Cancer (IASLC) proposed a lymph node map (Figure 16.6B) that reconciles the discrepancies between these two previous maps. The IASLC lymph node map is now the recommended means of describing regional lymph node involvement for lung cancers.

There are no evidence-based guidelines regarding the *number* of lymph nodes to be removed at surgery for adequate staging. However, adequate N staging is generally considered to include sampling or dissection of lymph nodes from stations 2R, 4R, 7, 10R, and 11R for right-sided tumors, and stations 5, 6, 7, 10, L, and 11L for left-sided tumors. Station 9 lymph nodes should also be evaluated for lower lobe tumors. The more peripheral lymph nodes at stations 12–14 are usually evaluated by the pathologist in lobectomy or pneumonectomy specimens but may be separately removed when sublobar resections (e.g., segmentectomy) are performed. There is evidence to support the recommendation that histological examination of hilar and mediastinal lymphenectomy specimen(s) will ordinarily include 6 or more lymph nodes/stations. Three of these nodes/stations should be mediastinal, including the subcarinal nodes and three from N1 nodes/stations.*

M-ONCOANATOMY

The vasculature of the lung is rich. The microcirculation is intimately organized into the alveolar matrix and originates from two separate circulations—the bronchial arteries and the pulmonary arteries. However, all the blood is gathered and returned by the pulmonary veins (Fig. 16.6B). The anatomic distribution of distant metastases is shown in Table 16.5.

There is a major difference between the bronchial and pulmonary arteries. The pulmonary arteries are essentially venous blood carrying the right heart output into the lungs for aeration. Similarly, the pulmonary vein, unlike other veins in the body, has well-oxygenated blood carrying blood from the lungs to the left heart for injection into the general circulation. The bronchial arteries rise from the aorta and, therefore, carry oxygenated blood. An important feature of staging is the difference between T3 and T4 cancers.

Drainage into the subclavian vein, if invaded, then via the superior vena cava and pulmonary artery drain into the lung. Cancer invasion of chest wall drains into intercostal veins, then the azygos vein, and then the superior vena cava, which leads to lung dissemination.

*Preceding passage from Edge SB, Byrd DR, and Compton CC, et al. *AJCC Cancer Staging Manual, 7th edition.* New York, Springer, 2010, pp. 254–255.

TABLE 16.4 Lymph Nodes of Lung

The hilar and coronal nodes are the sentinel nodes. However, if lower lobe cancers invade the mediastinum directly, the posterior mediastinal nodes are at risk.

N1 nodes: All N1 nodes lie distal to the mediastinal pleural reflection and *within* the visceral pleura.

Hilar nodes 10

Interlobar nodes 11

Lobar nodes bronchi 12

Segmental nodes 13

Subsegmental nodes 14

N2 nodes: All N2 nodes lie within the mediastinal pleural envelope on the ipsilateral side.

Highest mediastinal nodes 1, 2R, 2L

Upper paratracheal nodes 2R, 2L

Prevascular and retrotracheal nodes 3a, 3p*

Lower paratracheal nodes 4R, 4L

Subaortic nodes (aortopulmonary window) 5

Para-aortic nodes (ascending aorta or phrenic) 6

Subcarinal nodes 7

Paraesophageal nodes (below carina) 8

Pulmonary ligament nodes 9

*3a, 3p not shown in Fig. 16.6.

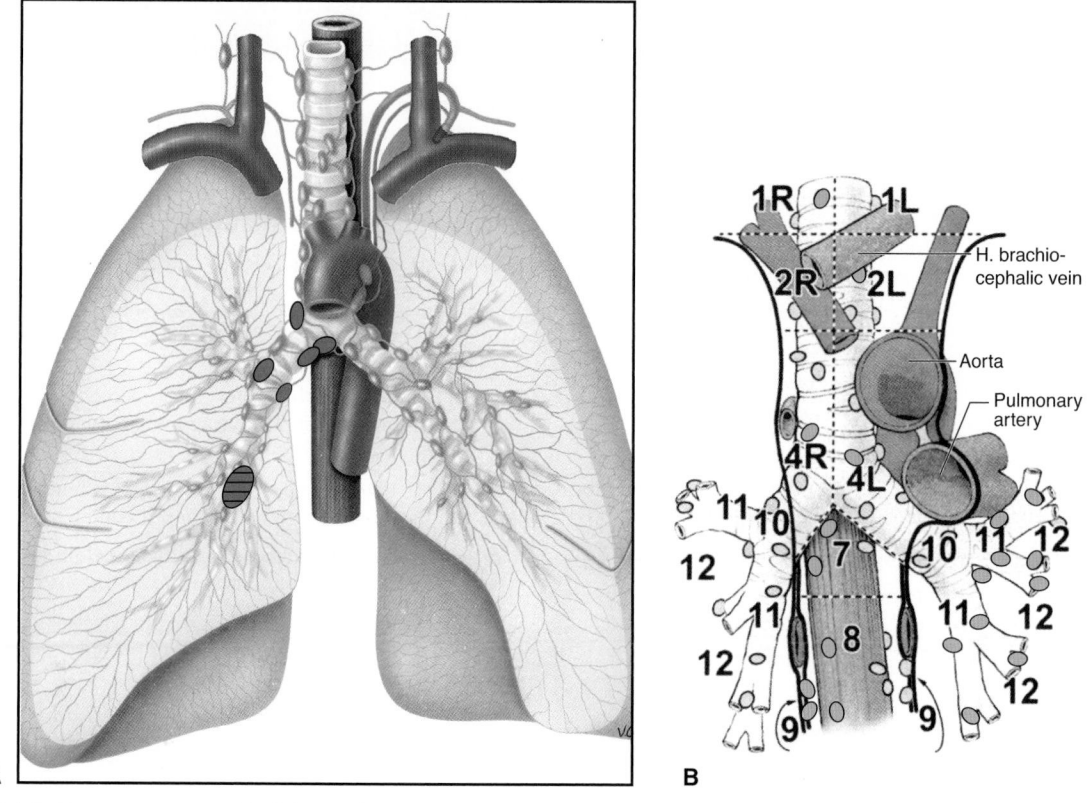

Figure 16.6 | **A. N-oncoanatomy.** The hilar and coronal nodes are the sentinel nodes. However, if lower lobe cancers invade the mediastinum directly, the posterior mediastinal nodes are at risk. If the diaphragm is invaded directly, posterior and inferior mediastinal nodes are the sentinel nodes. **B. M-oncoanatomy.** International Association for the Study of Lung Cancer (IASLC). Labels correlate with Table 16.4.

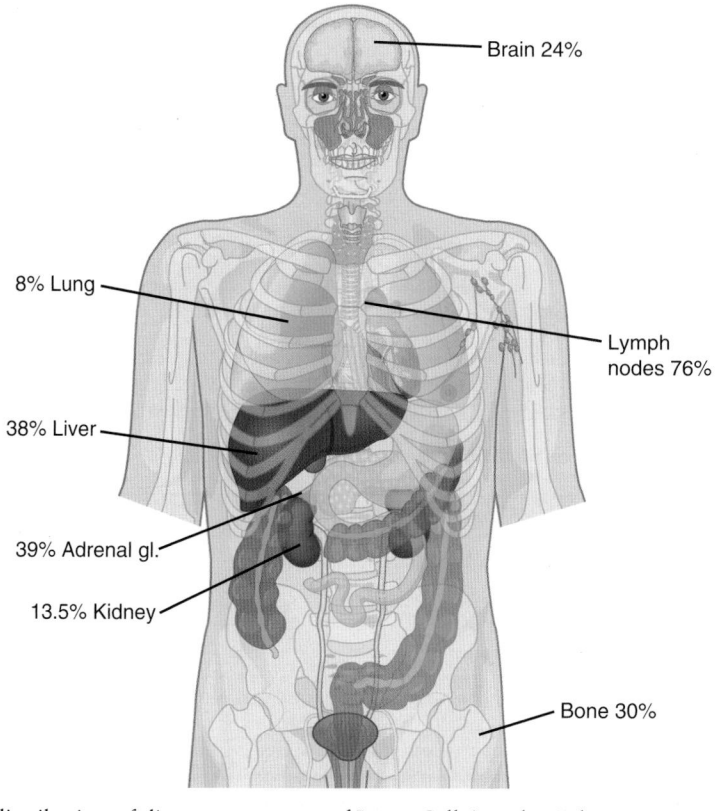

Figure 16.7 | Incidence and distribution of distant metastases of Large Cell Anaplastic lung cancer correlates with Table 16.6.

STAGING WORKUP

RULES FOR CLASSIFICATION AND STAGING

Clinical Staging and Imaging

The TNM classification system is primarily for staging non–small cell lung cancers. The most important change dates back to the fourth edition of the AJCC, where T3, resectable disease, was distinguished from T4, unresectable disease. Simultaneously, a greater reliance on more sophisticated imaging has occurred. It is with the sixth edition that computed tomography (CT) and positron emission tomography (PET) are allowed. The imaging modalities for detection and diagnosis apply to staging (Table 16.5). Chest films and CT (preferably spiral) are essential steps in both diagnosis and staging. PET combined with CT is utilized to overcome motion artifacts. Magnetic resonance imaging (MRI) is useful for mediastinal evaluation. Another advantage of CT over MRI for staging is that it allows for metastatic workup of lung, liver, adrenal, ribs, and vertebrae, (Fig. 16.8).

Pathologic Staging

All pathologic specimens from clinical invasive procedures—bronchoscopy, mediastinoscopy, mediastinotomy, thoracentesis, and thorascopy—are applicable to pathologic stage. Thoracotomy and resection of primary and lymph nodes are the mainstay of pathologic staging. Margin status and any residual cancer need to be noted. Preferably, six nodes should be examined.

Oncoimaging Annotations

- Chest radiographs seldom detect primary lung cancers in their early stages.
- Spiral CT is useful in high-risk patients to detect nodule and infiltrates.
- PET imaging with [18]FDG (fluorodeoxyglucose) appears to be of value in discriminating malignant versus benign nodules.
- CT can detect mediastinal adenopathy, but histologic verification is essential to ascertain if it is malignant.
- Determining N2 versus N3 mediastinal nodes is important; it establishes resectability.
- MRI can be of value in assessing mediastinal invasion, chest wall and rib erosion, and compromised large vein involvement.
- CT staging should include liver and adrenal glands by extending chest examinations. Most adrenal enlargements are benign and require biopsy or MRI to establish metastatic cancer.

Also of interest are biological and genetic markers that are of prognostic value based on meta-analysis data of the International Association for Study of Lung Cancer (IASLC).

TABLE 16.5	Imaging Modalities for Diagnosis and Staging	
Method	Capability	Recommended
Primary Tumor and Regional Nodes Workup		
Chest films	Baseline image	Yes
CT/spiral CT	Most useful of all modalities for determining characteristics of T and N in the thorax and M in the adrenal and liver	Yes
MRI	Not as good as CT	No
Percutaneous needle biopsy	Guided by fluoroscopy or CT, accurate in establishing cytologic diagnosis from T (particularly peripheral lung lesions); M (especially liver or bone); less experience with N	Yes
Mediastinoscopy/thoracoscopy	Confirmation of nodal involvement	Yes
Metastatic Workup for Clinically Suspected Metastases		
CT/echography	For liver, adrenals	Yes
CT/MRI	For brain	Yes
Bone scan	For the bone	Yes
PET scan	Diagnosis of peripheral lesions can differentiate between cancer and benign lesions. Staging of true extent of primary and lymph node involvement.	Yes, if clinically indicated

CT, computed tomography; M, metastasis; MRI, magnetic resonance imaging; N, node; PET, positron emission tomography; T, tumor.

PROGNOSIS AND CANCER SURVIVAL

PROGNOSIS

The limited number of prognostic factors are listed in Table 16.6.

TABLE 16.6	Prognostic Factors
Required for Staging	None
Clinically significant	Pleural/elastic layer invasion (based on H&E and elastic stains)
	Separate tumor nodules
	Vascular invasion – V classification (venous or arteriolar)

H&E, hematoxylin and eosinophilic.
From Edge SB, Byrd DR, Compton CC, et al. *AJCC Cancer Staging Manual.* 7th ed. New York: Springer, 2010, p. 264, with permission.

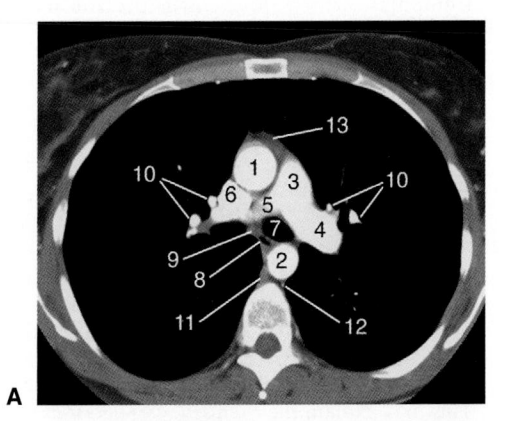

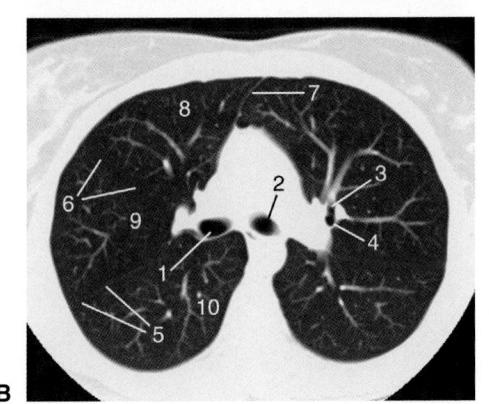

Figure 16.8 | Axial CTs of T4 and T5 level correlate with the T-oncoanatomy transverse section (Figure 16.5C). Oncoimaging with CT is commonly applied to staging lung cancers, often combined with PET to determine true extent of primary cancer and involved lymph nodes. **A.** Mediastinal window. 1, ascending aorta; 2, descending aorta; 3, main pulmonary artery; 4, left pulmonary artery; 5, right pulmonary artery; 6, superior vena cava; 7, left main bronchus; 8, esophagus; 9, normal subcarinal lymph node; 10, superior pulmonary veins; 11, azygos vein; 12, hemiazygos vein branch; 13, thymus. **B.** Lung window. 1, bronchus intermedius; 2, left main bronchus; 3, anterior segment LUL bronchus; 4, apical-posterior segment LUL bronchus; 5, major fissure; 6, minor fissure; 7, anterior junction line; 8, RUL; 9, RML; 10, RLL.

CANCER STATISTICS AND SURVIVAL

According to American Cancer Society facts and figures 2010, the age adjusted Cancer Death Rates for the more common cancers is striking in that cancer of lung and bronchus is the only cancer site that increases over the last 2 decades where as others decrease or plateau. (ACS Figure P3)

The number of new cases in the USA, exceed 220,000 new cases and result in approximately 157,000 deaths almost equally divided between genders with males exceeding females in incidence and mortality rates. Lung cancer constitutes of 15% of all cancer in males and is the second most common cancer, exceeded only by prostate cancer. Similarly in females, it constitutes 14% of all cancer cases and second only to breast cancer.

- Lung cancer remains the most lethal of all cancers accounting for 29% of male cancer deaths vs. 26% for female deaths.
- Smoking cigarettes remains the major risk factor and increases with quantity and duration. Other risk factors are second hand smoke, occupational or environmental exposure to radon, asbestos, and certain metals (chromium, cadmium, and arsenic).
- The value of CT screening in detecting early stage cancer in high risk patients is encouraging and is still undergoing clinical trial investigation.
- The 1 year survival for lung cancer increased from 35% in the seventies to 42% in 2000–2005.
- Generally the 5 year survival for NSCLC is 13% vs. 6% SCLC.
- Survival, according to stage: localized is 53%, regional nodes is 24% and for metastatic distant disease is 4%.
- According to the IASLC lung database, a series of survival curves, plotted by stage group demonstrates the median survival for combination of clinical and pathologic staging, and illustrates the decrement of survival with stage (F25.5). Histopathology is a major factor and (F25.4) NSCLC vs. SCLC demonstrates the increasing mortality as anticipated.

The impact of both stage and histopathology is well demonstrated in T14.7 illustrating the 5 year relative survival rates for different lung cancers. Although 5 year survival rates have improved with early detection and surgery in localized stages and current radiation chemotherapy regimens, the outcome for each subset is presented in the graph.

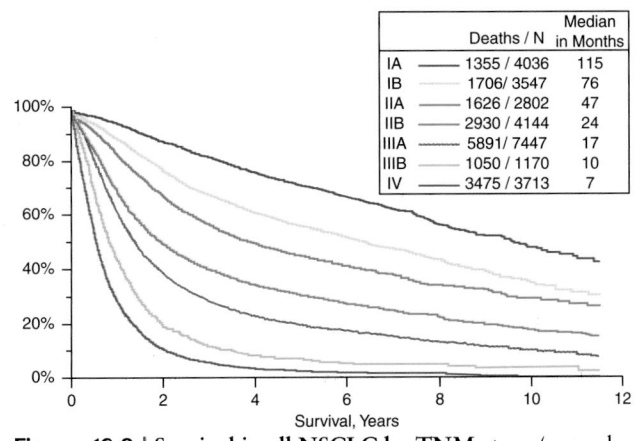

Figure 16.9 | Survival in all NSCLC by TNM stage (according to "best" based on a combination of clinical and pathologic staging). (From Edge SB, Byrd DR, Compton CC, et al. *AJCC Cancer Staging Manual.* 7th ed. New York: Springer, 2010, p. 261, with permission.)

17

Squamous Cell Cancer

PERSPECTIVE, PATTERNS OF SPREAD, AND PATHOLOGY

Squamous cell cancers are true bronchogenic carcinomas arising in major bronchi, which are extrapleural in location with an oxygenated arterial blood supply.

PERSPECTIVE AND PATTERNS OF SPREAD

Squamous cell lung cancers (SQC) are often extrapulmonary cancers arising in the major bronchi—located in the mediastinum rather than lung parenchyma. The normal pseudo-stratified ciliated columnar epithelium with its different cell types undergoes metaplastic changes, losing its ciliation, secretory goblets, brush cells, and serous cells due to smoking and its pollutants, leading to a dry hacking "smoker's cough." As the patient's mucous thickens, his or her lungs and cough produce plugs of phlegm. The metaplastic changes in the columnar and cuboidal basal cells lead to stratified squamous dysplasia and, over time, to squamous cell neoplasia with malignant transformation. The epithelial surface breaks down with fine ulcerations and then rust-streaked sputum appears. The triad of coarse rhonchial breathing over a major bronchus, hemoptysis, and a long history of smoking virtually ensures a diagnosis of SQC, which can be readily confirmed with a chest film. Although SQCs at one time were the most common lung cancers (50%), they have been surpassed by adenocarcinomas, which now constitute the majority of histopathologic types. The patterns of cancer invasion in major bronchi can result in dramatic obstruction, that is, complete atelectasis and collapse of one lung (Fig. 17.2; Table 17.2).

PATHOLOGY

Squamous cell cancers tend to arise in the main bronchi, and the distance from the carina determines whether it is T2 greater than 2 cm or T3 less than 2 cm. Unlike other more peripheral locations, they are supplied by the bronchial artery (oxygenated blood) versus pulmonary artery (unoxygenated blood). This may explain their tendency to necroses once their blood supply is invaded. An irregular, shaggy walled abscess, with wall thickness exceeding 15 mm strongly suggests a diagnosis of squamous cell cancer (Table 17.1; Fig. 17.1).

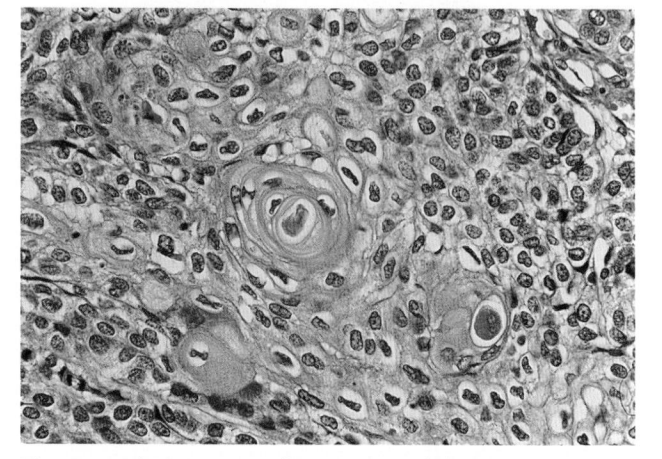

Figure 17.1 | Squamous cell carcinoma of the lung. A photomicrograph shows well-differentiated squamous cell carcinoma with a keratin pearl composed of cells with brightly eosinophilic cytoplasm.

TABLE 17.1	Histopathologic Type
Main Pathologic Cell Type	**Variant**
Squamous cell carcinoma	Papillary
	Clear cell
	Small cell
	Basaloid

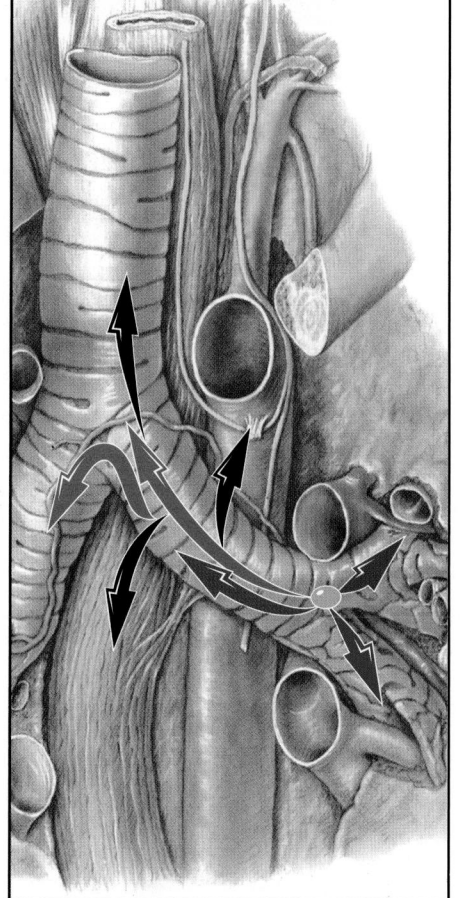
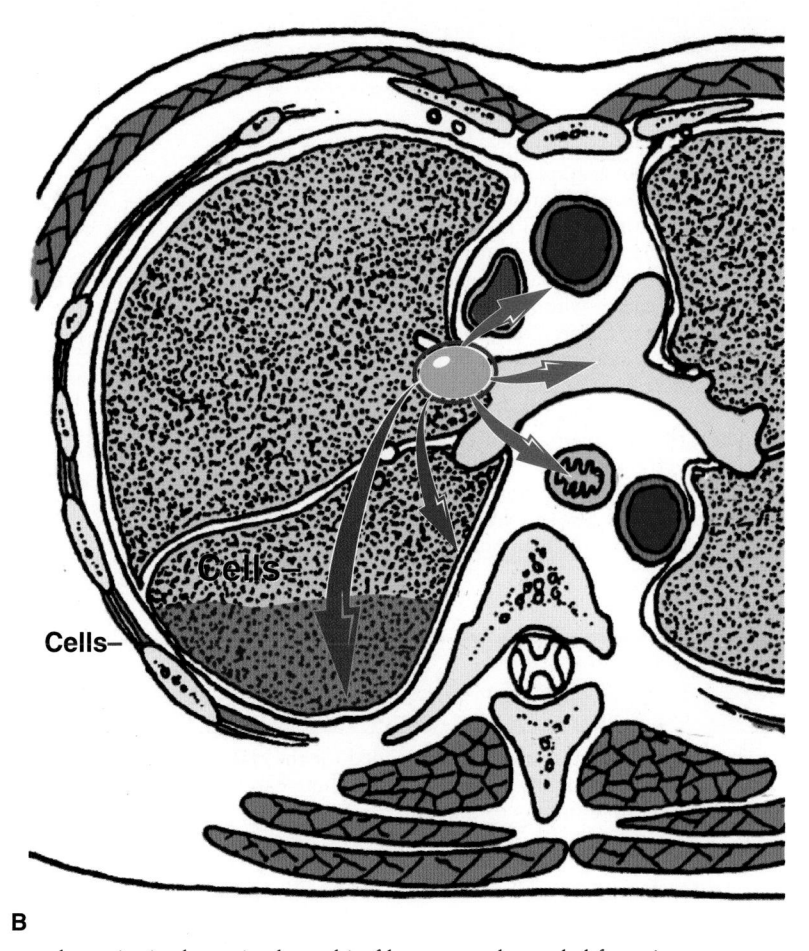

Figure 17.2 | Patterns of spread. Squamous cell cancers that arise in the major bronchi of lung are color coded for primary tumor spread to carina: Tis, yellow; T1, green (>2 cm); T2, blue (>2 cm) without obstruction of bronchus; T3, purple (<2 cm of carina with obstruction leading to complete lung collapse); T4, red (invading carina); M1, black (invading mediastinal structures). The concept of visualizing patterns of spread to appreciate the surrounding anatomy is well demonstrated by the six directional pattern i.e. SIMLAP Table 17.2.

TABLE 17.2	SIMLAP	
Squamous Cell: Main Bronchi		
S	Trachea, mediastinum	• T4
I	Pericardium	• T4
	Pleura effusion (−)	• T3
M	>2 cm carina	• T3
	<2 cm carina	• T4
	Cavitation	• **T2**
L	Into lobar bronchi/atelectasis	• T3
	Lung collapse	• T3
A	Vena cava, pulmonary artery	• T4
	Vein, aorta	• T4
P	Esophagus	• T4
	Thoracic duct	• T3
	Chylous effusion	• T3

The 6 vectors of invasion are Superior, Inferior, Medial, Lateral, Anterior, and Posterior. The color code dots correlate the T stage with specific anatomic structure involved.

TNM STAGING CRITERIA

TNM STAGING CRITERIA

SQCs arise from metaplastic bronchial epithelium in major bronchi, which is specifically addressed in the staging system in relationship to the carina. T1 is an early intraluminal lesion less than 3 cm in diameter and greater than 2 cm from the carina. T2 is of larger size (greater than 3 cm in diameter) and is less than 2 cm from the carina without bronchial obstruction. Cavitation may occur due to the necrosis and most often occurs in SQC. T3 tumors may occlude major stem bronchi, which may cause unilateral atelectasis or pneumonitis with complete collapse of an entire lung. When the cancer involves the carina or trachea, it becomes T4 and invariably invades paracarinal mediastinal nodes directly or subcarinal or contralateral nodes. The resectability of an entire lung depends on producing a well-healed stump and also providing a reasonable margin when SQC of the major bronchi approach the carina.

SUMMARY OF CHANGES SEVENTH EDITION AJCC

- This staging system is now recommended for the classification of both non–small cell and small cell lung carcinomas and for carcinoid tumors of the lung.
- The T classifications have been redefined:
  - T1 has been subclassified into T1a (≤2 cm in size) and T1b (>2–3 cm in size)
  - T2 has been subclassified into T2a (>3–5 cm in size) and T2b (>5–7 cm in size)
  - T2 (>7 cm in size) has been reclassified as T3
  - Multiple tumor nodules in the same lobe have been reclassified from T4 to T3
  - Multiple tumor nodules in the same lung but a different lobe have been reclassified from M1 to T4
- No changes have been made to the N classification. However, a new international lymph node map defining the anatomical boundaries for lymph node stations has been developed.
- The M classifications have been redefined:
  - The M1 has been subdivided into M1a and M1b
  - Malignant pleural and pericardial effusions have been reclassified from T4 to M1a
  - Separate tumor nodules in the contralateral lung are considered M1a
  - M1b designates distant metastases

Because of the magnitude of the T category changes with shifts in both directions, that is both downstaging and upstaging, it is important to review the stage groupings of the sixth and seventh editions. The TNM Staging Matrix is color coded for identification of Stage Group once T and N stages are determined (Table 17.3).

TABLE 17.3 | Stage Summary Matrix

	N0	N1	N2	N3	M1a	M1b
T1a	IA	IIA	IIIA	IIIB	IV	IV
T1b	IA	IIA	IIIA	IIIB	IV	IV
T2a	IB	IIA	IIIA	IIIB	IV	IV
T2b	IIA	IIB	IIIA	IIIB	IV	IV
T3	IIB	IIB	IIIA	IIIB	IV	IV
T4	IIIA	IIIA	IIIB	IIIB	IV	IV

Thorax: Lung Cancers
- N stage determines stage group
  - N0, N1, N2, N3a, N3b are stage group I, II, IIIA, IIIB
- N1 can be associated with T1 or T2
- T stage modifies substages
  - T1, T2, N0 = IA, IIB; T1, T2, N2 = IIA, IIB; and T2b, N0 = IIA
- M stage is a separate stage
  - M1 = IV

SQUAMOUS CELL CANCER

DEFINITION OF TNM

STAGE GROUPINGS

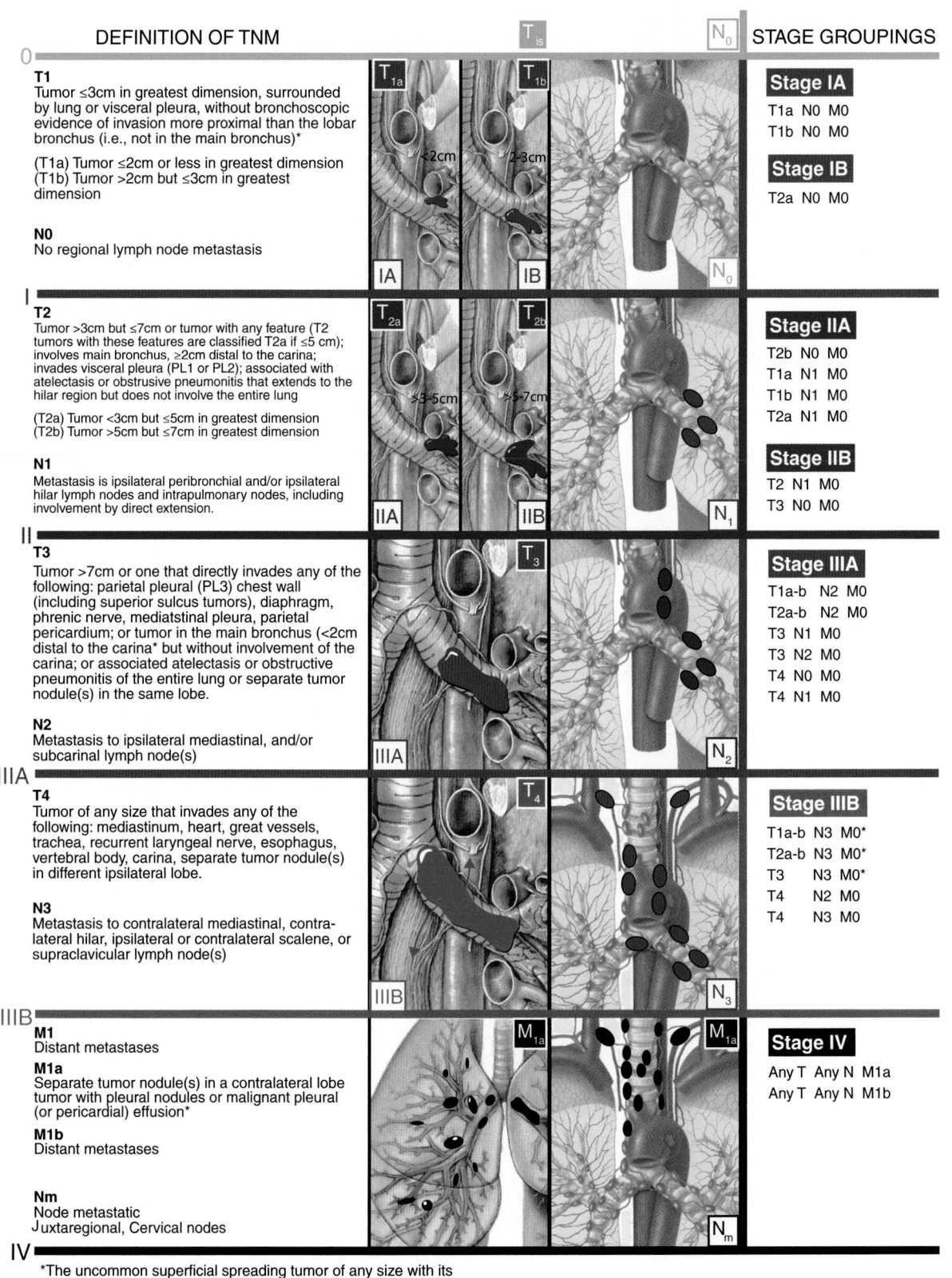

T1
Tumor ≤3cm in greatest dimension, surrounded by lung or visceral pleura, without bronchoscopic evidence of invasion more proximal than the lobar bronchus (i.e., not in the main bronchus)*

(T1a) Tumor ≤2cm or less in greatest dimension
(T1b) Tumor >2cm but ≤3cm in greatest dimension

N0
No regional lymph node metastasis

Stage IA
T1a N0 M0
T1b N0 M0

Stage IB
T2a N0 M0

T2
Tumor >3cm but ≤7cm or tumor with any feature (T2 tumors with these features are classified T2a if ≤5 cm); involves main bronchus, ≥2cm distal to the carina; invades visceral pleura (PL1 or PL2); associated with atelectasis or obstrusive pneumonitis that extends to the hilar region but does not involve the entire lung

(T2a) Tumor <3cm but ≤5cm in greatest dimension
(T2b) Tumor >5cm but ≤7cm in greatest dimension

N1
Metastasis is ipsilateral peribronchial and/or ipsilateral hilar lymph nodes and intrapulmonary nodes, including involvement by direct extension.

Stage IIA
T2b N0 M0
T1a N1 M0
T1b N1 M0
T2a N1 M0

Stage IIB
T2 N1 M0
T3 N0 M0

T3
Tumor >7cm or one that directly invades any of the following: parietal pleural (PL3) chest wall (including superior sulcus tumors), diaphragm, phrenic nerve, mediatstinal pleura, parietal pericardium; or tumor in the main bronchus (<2cm distal to the carina* but without involvement of the carina; or associated atelectasis or obstructive pneumonitis of the entire lung or separate tumor nodule(s) in the same lobe.

N2
Metastasis to ipsilateral mediastinal, and/or subcarinal lymph node(s)

Stage IIIA
T1a-b N2 M0
T2a-b N2 M0
T3 N1 M0
T3 N2 M0
T4 N0 M0
T4 N1 M0

T4
Tumor of any size that invades any of the following: mediastinum, heart, great vessels, trachea, recurrent laryngeal nerve, esophagus, vertebral body, carina, separate tumor nodule(s) in different ipsilateral lobe.

N3
Metastasis to contralateral mediastinal, contra-lateral hilar, ipsilateral or contralateral scalene, or supraclavicular lymph node(s)

Stage IIIB
T1a-b N3 M0*
T2a-b N3 M0*
T3 N3 M0*
T4 N2 M0
T4 N3 M0

M1
Distant metastases
M1a
Separate tumor nodule(s) in a contralateral lobe tumor with pleural nodules or malignant pleural (or pericardial) effusion*

M1b
Distant metastases

Nm
Node metastatic
Juxtaregional, Cervical nodes

Stage IV
Any T Any N M1a
Any T Any N M1b

*The uncommon superficial spreading tumor of any size with its invasive component limited to the bronchial wall, which may extend proximally to the main bronchus, is also classified as T1a.

Figure 17.3 | TNM staging diagram. Squamous cell cancers arise in main and lobar bronchi in dysplastic epithelia that becomes neoplastic. Vertical presentation of stage groupings, which follow the same color code for cancer advancement, are organized in horizontal lanes: Stage 0, yellow; I, green; II, blue; IIIA, purple; IIIB, red; metastatic stage IV, black. Definitions of TN are on the left and stage grouping is on the right. Major stage group progression is dominated by the N stage progression.

T-ONCOANATOMY

ORIENTATION OF THREE-PLANAR ONCOANATOMY

The isocenter of the respiratory system is at the carina of the trachea and the origin of the main stem bronchi. The isocenter of the main stem bronchi is inferior to the manubriosternal angle anteriorly, and posteriorly the plane is at the thoracic vertebral level T5-6. The carina and 2 cm of the major bronchi are within the mediastinal pleural. The relationships of the bifurcation of the trachea to other mediastinal structures, which are from the midline to superficial, are super imposed (Fig. 17.4).

T-oncoanatomy

The T-oncoanatomy is displayed in three planar views. A. Coronal, B. Sagittal, C. Traverse Axial (Fig. 17.5). SQC are often bronchogenic cancers involving the major bronchi, which are at the T5 level positioned inferior to the manubriosternal angle. A unique feature of this location is

that the SQC are unlike other lung cancers, because they are supplied by oxygenated blood. The blood supply for SQCs is derived from the bronchial artery directly arising from the thoracic aorta. Cavitation may be more common in SQCs because its vascular attenuation may lead to severe hypoxia and necrosis. Other lung cancers, such as adenocarcinoma, are supplied with unoxygenated pulmonary arterial blood and may be more accustomed to hypoxic conditions.

- *Coronal view:* The extrapulmonary portion of the bronchial tree is seen arising from the trachea at the carina. The left major bronchi is longer than the right, which immediately divides into right middle lobe, the bronchus intermedius, and right lower lobe with its own bronchi.

- *Sagittal view:* The hilus is highly trafficked with pulmonary vessels anterior to the bronchi.

- *Axial view:* Pulmonary arteries dominate the middle mediastinum at the T5-6 level along with the ascending aorta in the midline and the thoracic duct in the midline. The azygos vein enters the superior vena cava posteriorly. The descending aorta is the most posterior structure and on the left side in mediastinum.

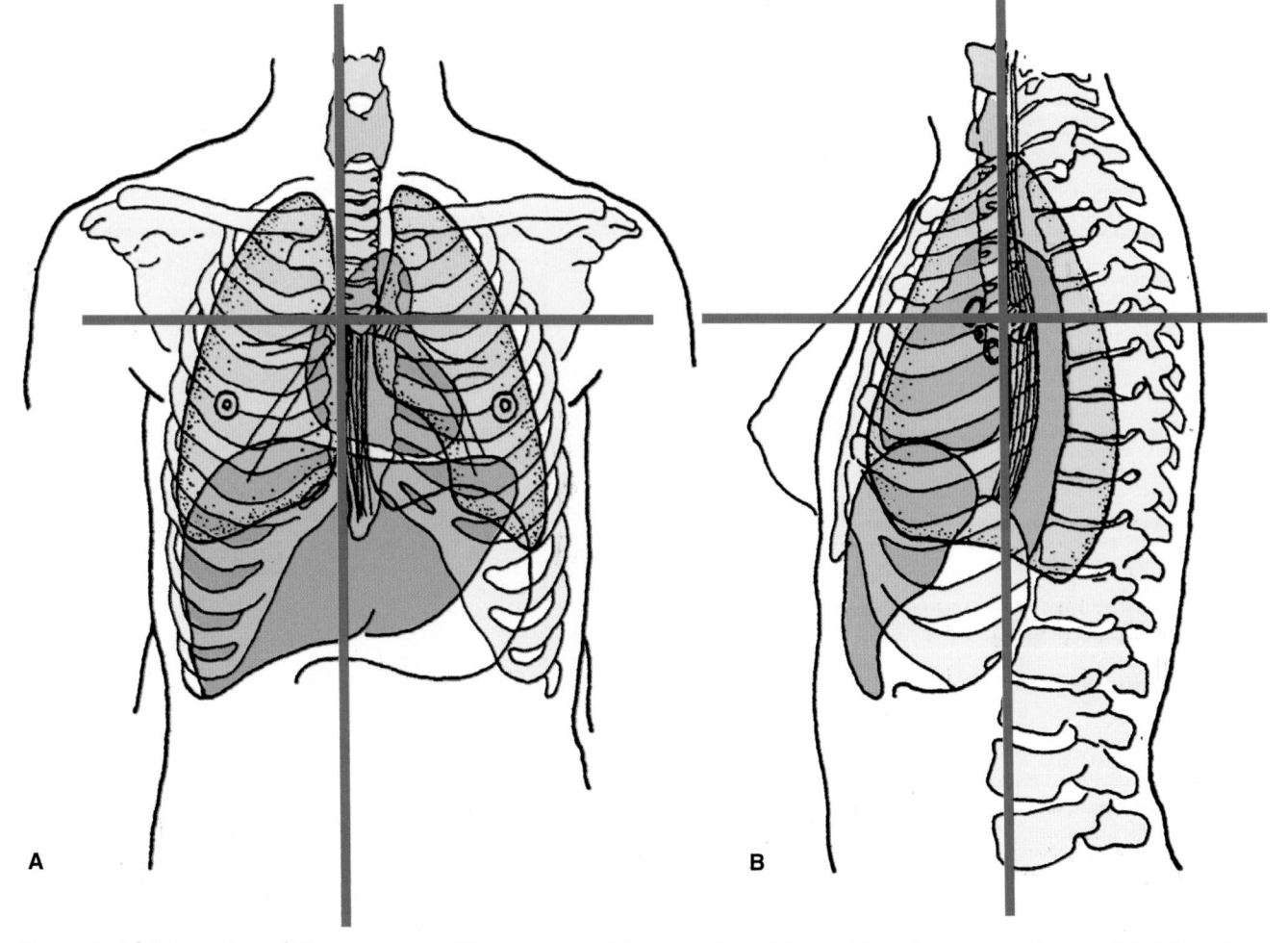

A

B

Figure 17.4 | Orientation of T-oncoanatomy. The isocenter of the major bronchi are mid-mediastinum and at the T5-6 thoracic level. **A.** Coronal. **B.** Sagittal.

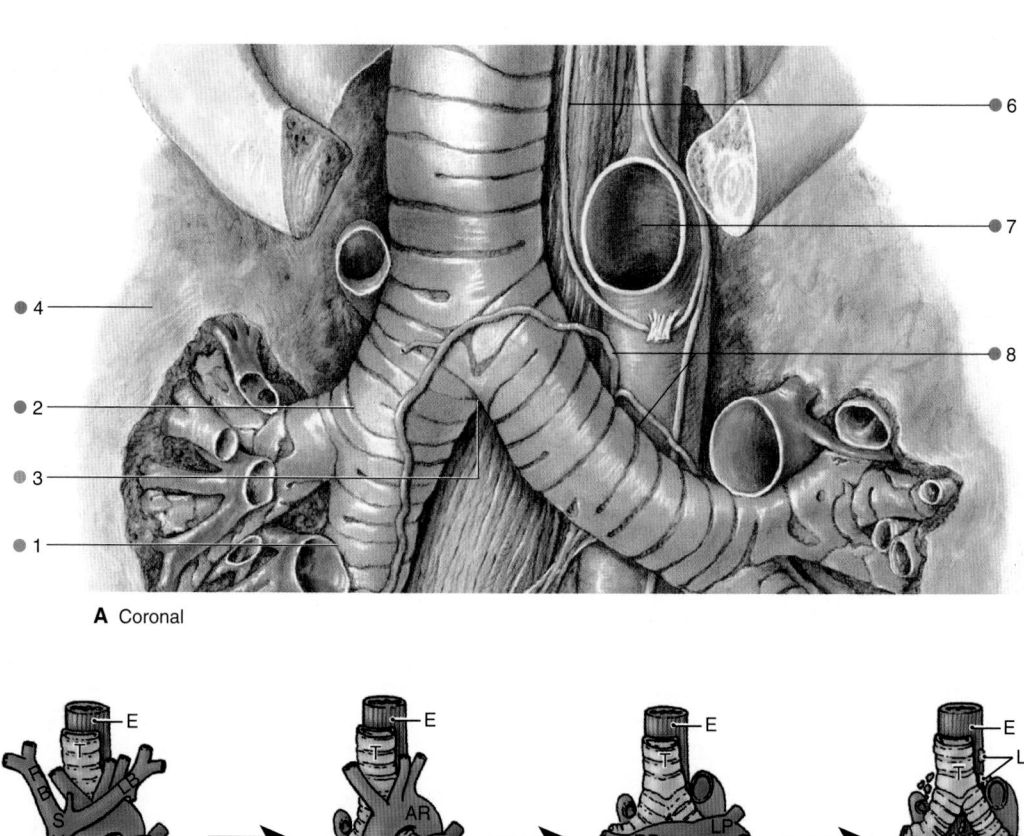

A Coronal

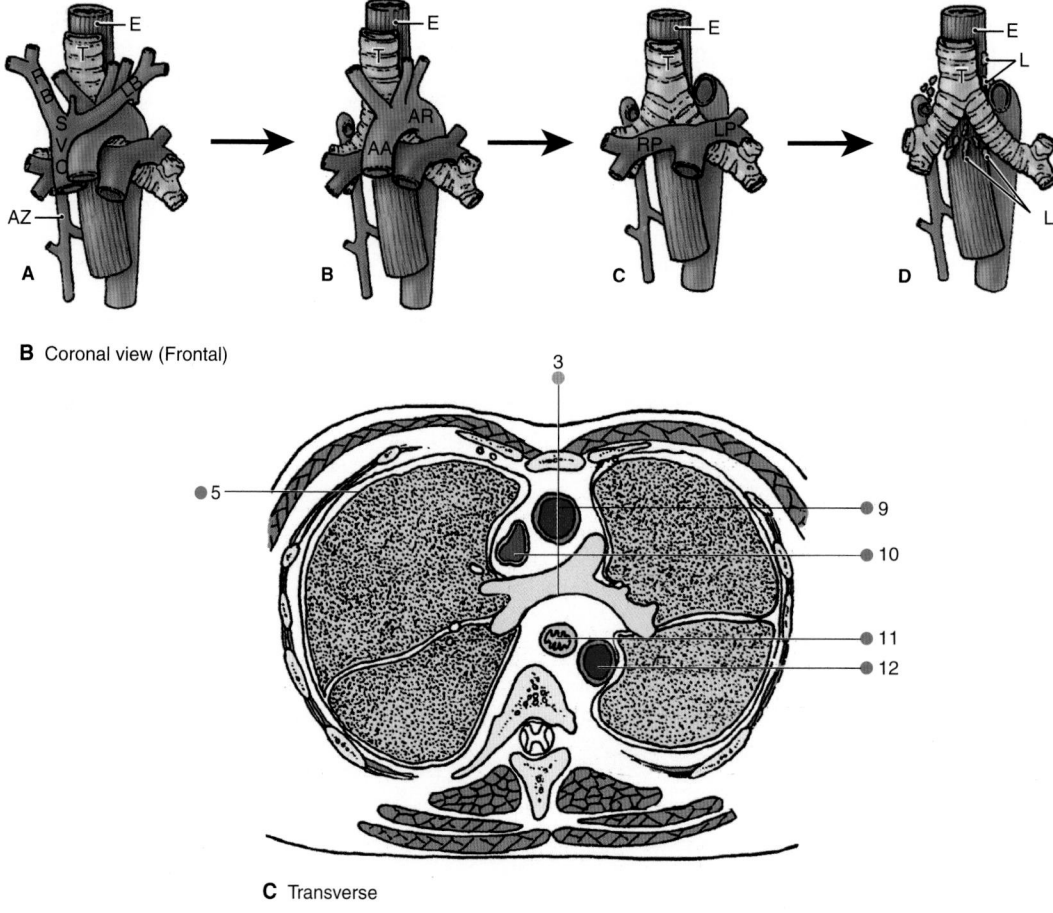

B Coronal view (Frontal)

C Transverse

T₁	● 1. Intermediate Bronchus	T₄	● 5. Visceral pleura	T₄	● 9. Ascending aorta
T₂	● 2. Rt. Main Bronchus	T₄	● 6. Left recurrent laryngeal nerve	T₄	● 10. Superior vena cava
T₃	● 3. Tracheal Bifurcation	T₄	● 7. Arch of aorta	T₄	● 11. Esophagus
T₄	● 4. Lung	T₄	● 8. Bronchial artery	T₄	● 12. Descending aorta

Figure 17.5 | **T-oncoanatomy.** The Color Code for the anatomic sites correlates with the color code for the stage group (Fig. 17.3) and patterns of spread (Fig. 17.2) and SIMLAP tables (Table 17.2). Connecting the dots in similar colors will provide an appreciation for the 3D Oncoanatomy.

N-ONCOANATOMY AND M-ONCOANATOMY

N-ONCOANATOMY

Mediastinal supracarinal and subcarinal nodes rather than hilar nodes may be the first sentinel nodes because these cancers tend to be extrapulmonary and mediastinal in location. The three-planar views depict the mediastinal lymph nodes in the region of the major bronchi and carina are depicted in Figure 17.6 and Table 17.4).

REGIONAL LYMPH NODES

The regional lymph nodes extend from the supraclavicular region to the diaphragm. During the past three decades, three different lymph node maps have been used to describe the regional lymph node potentially involved by lung cancers. The first map was endorsed by the Japan Lung Cancer Society. The second map, the Mountain Dresler modification of the American Thoracic Society (MDATS) lymph node map, is used in North America and Europe. The nomenclature for the anatomical locations of lymph nodes differs between these two maps. Recently the International Association for the Study of Lung Cancer (IASLC) proposed a lymph node map (Figure 17.6B) that reconciles the discrepancies between these two previous maps. The IASLC lymph node map is now the recommended means of describing regional lymph node involvement for lung cancers.

There are no evidence-based guidelines regarding the *number* of lymph nodes to be removed at surgery for adequate staging. However, adequate N staging is generally considered to include sampling or dissection of lymph nodes from stations 2R, 4R, 7, 10R, and 11R for right-sided tumors, and stations 5, 6, 7, 10, L, and 11L for left-sided tumors. Station 9 lymph nodes should also be evaluated for lower lobe tumors. The more peripheral lymph nodes at stations 12–14 are usually evaluated by the pathologist in lobectomy or pneumonectomy specimens but may be separately removed when sublobar resections (e.g., segmentectomy) are performed. There is evidence to support the recommendation that histological examination of hilar and mediastinal lymphenectomy specimen(s) will ordinarily include 6 or more lymph nodes/stations. Three of these nodes/stations should be mediastinal, including the subcarinal nodes and three from N1 nodes/stations.*

M-ONCOANATOMY

The venous drainage is into the azygos system by bronchial veins with entry of circulating metastatic cells to the lung. The anatomic distribution of distant metastases is shown in Figure 17.7.

Drainage into the subclavian vein, if invaded, then via the superior vena cava and pulmonary artery drain into the lung. Cancer invasion of chest wall drains into intercostal veins, then the azygos vein, and then the superior vena cava, which leads to lung dissemination. Adenocarcinoma dissemination of metastases is the most common lung cancer and is presented as the prototype for metastases into other organs.

*Preceding passage from Edge SB, Byrd DR, and Compton CC, et al. *AJCC Cancer Staging Manual, 7th edition.* New York, Springer, 2010, pp. 254–255.

TABLE 17.4	Lymph Nodes of Lung
Paracarinal and subcarinal nodes as well as hilar nodes are sentinel nodes.	
N1 nodes: All N1 nodes lie distal to the mediastinal pleural reflection and *within the visceral pleura.*	
Hilar nodes 10	
Interlobar nodes 11	
Lobar nodes bronchi 12	
Segmental nodes 13	
Subsegmental nodes 14	
N2 nodes: All N2 nodes lie within the mediastinal pleural envelope on the ipsilateral side.	
Highest mediastinal nodes 1, 2R, 2L	
Upper paratracheal nodes 2R, 2L	
Prevascular and retrotracheal nodes 3a, 3p*	
Lower paratracheal nodes 4R, 4L	
Subaortic nodes (aortopulmonary window) 5	
Para-aortic nodes (ascending aorta or phrenic) 6	
Subcarinal nodes 7	
Paraesophageal nodes (below carina) 8	
Pulmonary ligament nodes 9	

*3a, 3p not shown in Fig. 17.6.

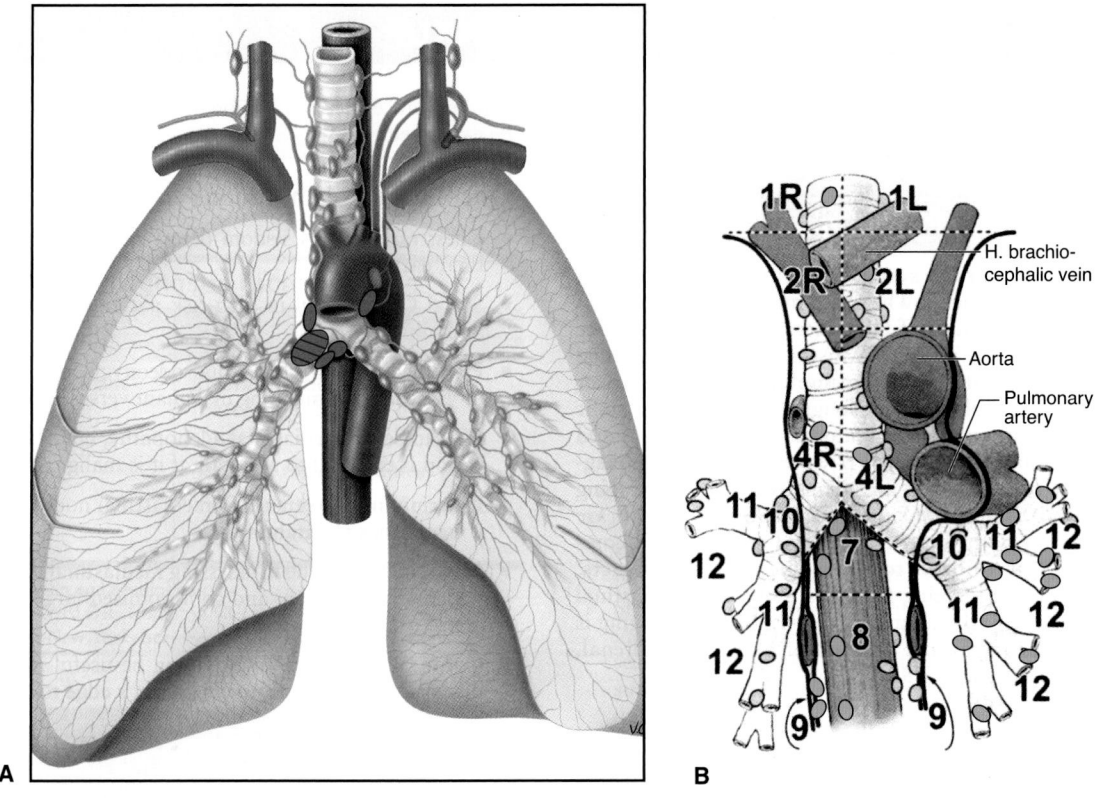

Figure 17.6 | **A: N-oncoanatomy.** Paracarinal and subcarinal nodes as well as hilar nodes are sentinel nodes. **B: M-oncoanatomy.** International Association for the Study of Lung Cancer (IASLC). Labels correlate with Table 17.4.

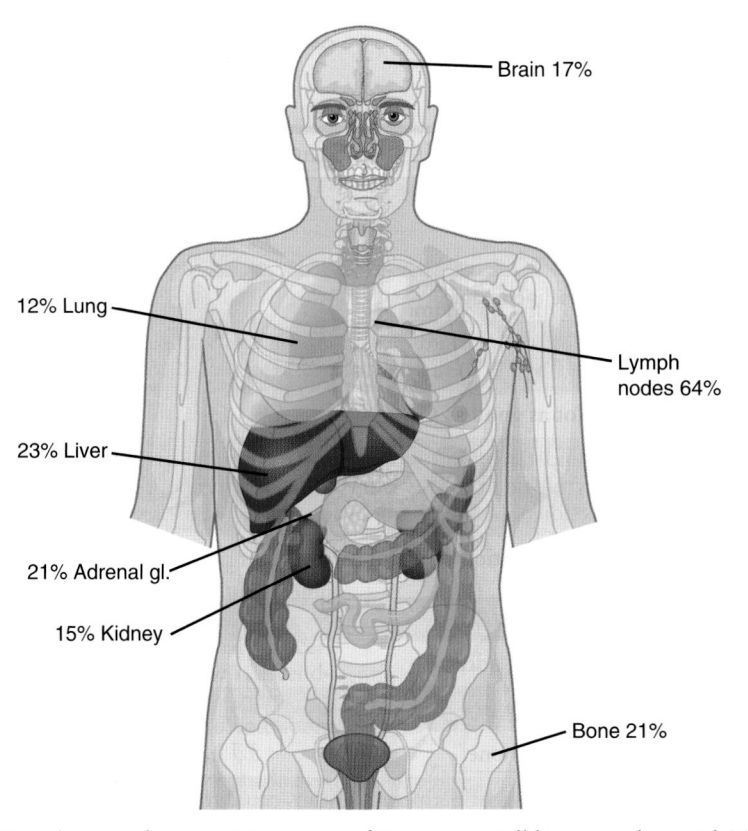

Figure 17.7 | Incidence and Distribution of Distant Metastases of Squamous Cell lung correlate with Table 12.6.

Small Cell Anaplastic Cancer

PERSPECTIVE, PATTERNS OF SPREAD, AND PATHOLOGY

Small cell anaplastic cancer's favored site is mostly central or proximal lung root, reminiscent of the embryonic origin of the multipotential cells of lung buds, which form the anlage of lung endoderm.

PERSPECTIVE AND PATTERNS OF SPREAD

Small cell anaplastic (SCA) cancers are the most undifferentiated cancers. Their origin is mostly in central airways juxtaposed to the mediastinum. It is the most dedifferentiated and highly invasive lung cancer, entering into lymphatics and commonly presents as a large mediastinal nodal mass. Superior vena caval obstruction as a low-pressure thin wall is more vulnerable to compression than other mediastinal structures, such as the aorta, esophagus, and trachea. These cancers are notorious for being metastatic on presentation. The derepression of chromosomes leads to a variety of neuroendocrine and paraneoplastic syndromes including Cushing disease, severe lymphedema due to antidiuretic hormone excess, and neuromyopathic conditions. Their favored site is mostly central or proximal lung root, reminiscent of the embryonal origin of the multipotential cells of lung buds, which form the anlage of lung endoderm. Unlike most lung cancers, SCA cancer tends to infiltrate submucosally and distort the bronchus by extrinsic and submucosal compression. Their pattern of spread tends to create mediastinal masses (Fig. 18.2; Table 18.2).

Research advances in genetic and molecular biology have uncovered new markers that were recognized in the American Joint Committee on Cancer's (AJCC) fifth and sixth edition with their tabulation. However, the results were insufficient to recommend their incorporation into their staging system. In fact, in the seventh edition (2010) there is emphasis of molecular markers except to note "the marker needs to bear a strong relationship to patient prognosis" but not included in staging.

The dedifferentiation of SCA derepresses the cell, resulting in paraneoplastic syndromes that are expressed in 10% to 20% of cases.

PARANEOPLASTIC SYNDROMES

Extrapulmonary manifestations of lung cancer may be recognized before the lung cancer itself produces any symptoms. Approximately 2% of patients present with a paraneoplastic syndrome. These may be categorized as follows:

- Metabolic: Cushing's syndrome, hypercalcemia, excessive antidiuretic hormone, and carcinoid syndrome
- Neuromuscular: peripheral neuritis, cortical or cerebellar degenerations, and myopathy
- Dermatologic: acanthosis nigricans and dermatomyositis
- Skeletal: pulmonary hypertrophic osteoarthropathy, including clubbing of fingers
- Vacular: migratory thrombophlebitis and nonbacterial verrucous endocarditis
- Hematologic: anemia and disseminated intravascular coagulopathy*

PATHOLOGY

Of the many solid cancers, SCAs have been genetically classified as classic versus variants depending on their biologic characteristics. Frequently expressed mutations in tumor suppressor genes include 3P, RB, and TP_{53} (Fig. 18.1; Table 18.1).

*Preceding passage from Rubin P, Williams JP. *Clinical Oncology: A Multi-Disciplinary Approach for Physicians & Students*, 8th edition. Philadelphia, W.B. Saunders. 2001, p. 825.

TABLE 18.1	Histopathologic Type
Main Pathologic Cell Type	**Small Cell Variant**
Small cell carcinoma	Oat cell carcinoma
	Intermediate cell type
	Fusiform cell type
	Combined cell types

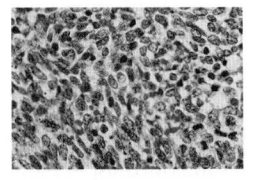

Figure 18.1 | Small cell carcinoma of the lung. This tumor consists of small oval to spindle-shaped cells with scant cytoplasm, finely granular nuclear chromatin, and conspicuous mitoses.

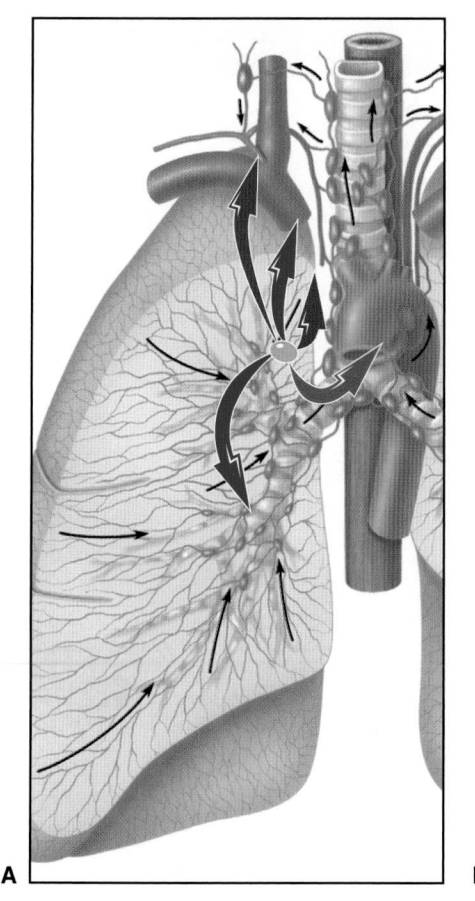
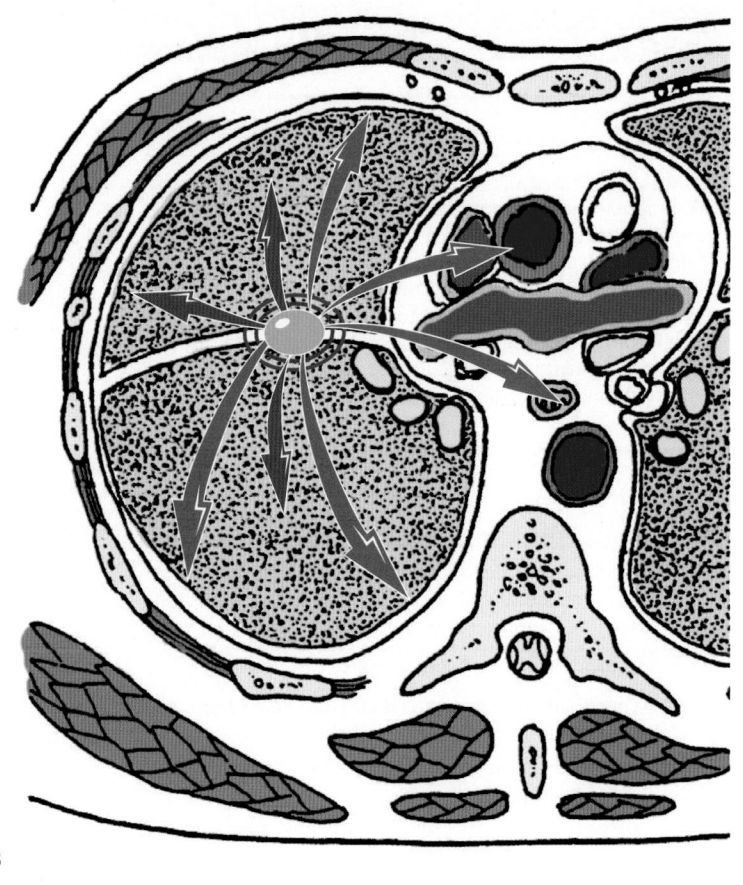

Figure 18.2 | Patterns of spread. The proximal location of the small cell cancer and its rapid dissemination via lymphatics is stressed. Although color coded, all T and N stages are referred to as "limited" if they are confined to the thorax. The concept of visualizing patterns of spread to appreciate the surrounding anatomy is well demonstrated by the six-directional pattern i.e. SIMLAP Table 18.2.

TABLE 18.2	SIMLAP	
Small Cell Anaplastic Cancer: Hilar Bronchi Anlage		
Central Mass		
S	Superior vena cava	• T4
I	Pericardial, diaphragms	• T4
M	Mediastinal	• T4
	Rec. laryngeal node	• T4
	Trachea	• T4
	Esophagus	• T4
L	Lobar/lung collapse	• T3
A	Pleural effusion Cell (+)	• T4
	Chest Wall	• T3
P	Pleural effusion Cell (+)	• T4
	Chest wall	• T3

The six vectors of invasion are **S**uperior, **I**nferior, **M**edial, **L**ateral, **A**nterior, and **P**osterior. The color-coded dots correlate the T stage with specific anatomic structure involved.
*T3, T4 Considered Limited.

TNM STAGING CRITERIA

TNM STAGING CRITERIA

The common criteria of size in staging lung cancer do not apply to SCA. Pragmatically, all intrathoracic T stages and N categories are lumped together into "limited" stage intrathoracic disease. The "extensive" stage is applied to metastatic dissemination, which is all too common and, until shown otherwise, bone marrow invasion, liver, bone, and brain foci need to be excluded. For practical purposes, the staging is based on M0 versus M1 and the mainstay of treatment is systemic first because of the high likelihood of occult micrometastases.

SUMMARY OF CHANGES SEVENTH EDITION AJCC

- This staging system is now recommended for the classification of both non–small cell and small cell lung carcinomas and for carcinoid tumors of the lung (Fig. 18.3).
- The T classifications have been redefined:
  - T1 has been subclassified into T1a ($\leq$2 cm in size) and T1b (>2–3 cm in size)
  - T2 has been subclassified into T2a (>3–5 cm in size) and T2b (>5–7 cm in size)
  - T2 (>7 cm in size) has been reclassified as T3
  - Multiple tumor nodules in the same lobe have been reclassified from T4 to T3
  - Multiple tumor nodules in the same lung but a different lobe have been reclassified from M1 to T4
- No changes have been made to the N classification. However, a new international lymph node map defining the anatomical boundaries for lymph node stations has been developed.
- The M classifications have been redefined:
  - The M1 has been subdivided into M1a and M1b
  - Malignant pleural and pericardial effusions have been reclassified from T4 to M1a
  - Separate tumor nodules in the contralateral lung are considered M1a
  - M1b designates distant metastases

Because of the magnitude of the T-category changes with shifts in both directions, that is both downstaging and upstaging, it is important to review the stage groupings of the sixth and seventh editions. The TNM Staging Matrix is color coded for identification of Stage Group once T and N stages are determined (Table 18.3).

TABLE 18.3 Stage Summary Matrix

	N0	N1	N2	N3	M1a	M1b
T1a	IA	IIA	IIIA	IIIB	IV	IV
T1b	IA	IIA	IIIA	IIIB	IV	IV
T2a	IB	IIA	IIIA	IIIB	IV	IV
T2b	IIA	IIB	IIIA	IIIB	IV	IV
T3	IIB	IIB	IIIA	IIIB	IV	IV
T4	IIIA	IIIA	IIIB	IIIB	IV	IV

Thorax: Lung Cancers
- N stage determines stage group
  - N0, N1, N2, N3a, N3b are stage group I, II, IIIA, IIIB
- N$_1$ can be associated with T1 or T2
- T stage modifies substages
  - T1, T2, N0 = IA, IIB; T1, T2, N2 = IIA, IIB; and T2b, N0 = IIA
- M stage is a separate stage
  - M1 = IV
  - SCA is either *limited* or *extensive* (i.e., M0 or M1 independent of T or N stage)

SMALL CELL ANAPLASTIC CANCER

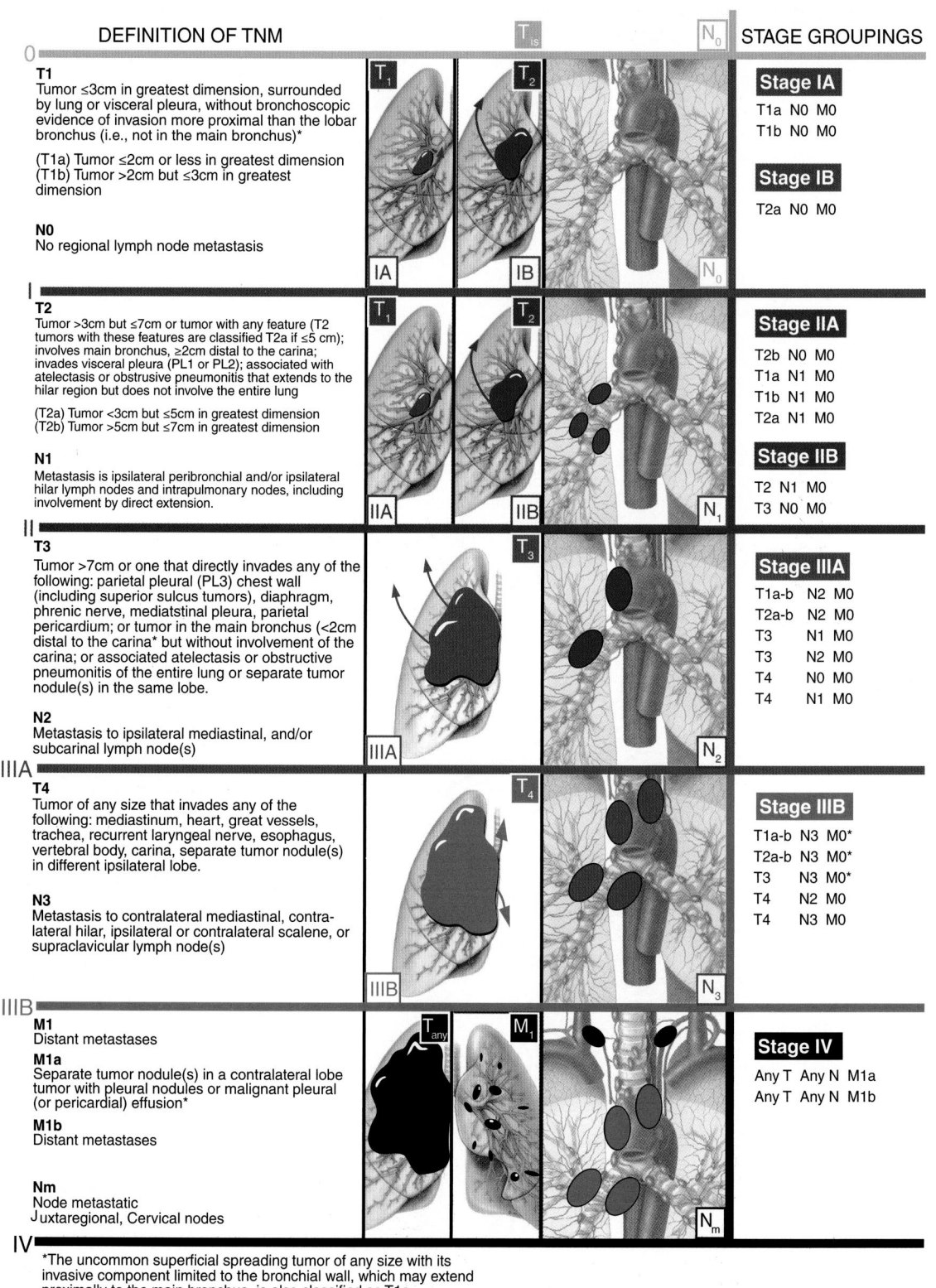

DEFINITION OF TNM

T1
Tumor ≤3cm in greatest dimension, surrounded by lung or visceral pleura, without bronchoscopic evidence of invasion more proximal than the lobar bronchus (i.e., not in the main bronchus)*

(T1a) Tumor ≤2cm or less in greatest dimension
(T1b) Tumor >2cm but ≤3cm in greatest dimension

N0
No regional lymph node metastasis

T2
Tumor >3cm but ≤7cm or tumor with any feature (T2 tumors with these features are classified T2a if ≤5 cm); involves main bronchus, ≥2cm distal to the carina; invades visceral pleura (PL1 or PL2); associated with atelectasis or obstrusive pneumonitis that extends to the hilar region but does not involve the entire lung

(T2a) Tumor <3cm but ≤5cm in greatest dimension
(T2b) Tumor >5cm but ≤7cm in greatest dimension

N1
Metastasis is ipsilateral peribronchial and/or ipsilateral hilar lymph nodes and intrapulmonary nodes, including involvement by direct extension.

T3
Tumor >7cm or one that directly invades any of the following: parietal pleural (PL3) chest wall (including superior sulcus tumors), diaphragm, phrenic nerve, mediastinal pleura, parietal pericardium; or tumor in the main bronchus (<2cm distal to the carina* but without involvement of the carina; or associated atelectasis or obstructive pneumonitis of the entire lung or separate tumor nodule(s) in the same lobe.

N2
Metastasis to ipsilateral mediastinal, and/or subcarinal lymph node(s)

T4
Tumor of any size that invades any of the following: mediastinum, heart, great vessels, trachea, recurrent laryngeal nerve, esophagus, vertebral body, carina, separate tumor nodule(s) in different ipsilateral lobe.

N3
Metastasis to contralateral mediastinal, contra-lateral hilar, ipsilateral or contralateral scalene, or supraclavicular lymph node(s)

M1
Distant metastases

M1a
Separate tumor nodule(s) in a contralateral lobe tumor with pleural nodules or malignant pleural (or pericardial) effusion*

M1b
Distant metastases

Nm
Node metastatic
Juxtaregional, Cervical nodes

*The uncommon superficial spreading tumor of any size with its invasive component limited to the bronchial wall, which may extend proximally to the main bronchus, is also classified as T1a.

STAGE GROUPINGS

Stage IA
T1a N0 M0
T1b N0 M0

Stage IB
T2a N0 M0

Stage IIA
T2b N0 M0
T1a N1 M0
T1b N1 M0
T2a N1 M0

Stage IIB
T2 N1 M0
T3 N0 M0

Stage IIIA
T1a-b N2 M0
T2a-b N2 M0
T3 N1 M0
T3 N2 M0
T4 N0 M0
T4 N1 M0

Stage IIIB
T1a-b N3 M0*
T2a-b N3 M0*
T3 N3 M0*
T4 N2 M0
T4 N3 M0

Stage IV
Any T Any N M1a
Any T Any N M1b

Figure 18.3 | TNM staging diagram. Small cell cancers have a tendency to metastasize early. They arise in central hilar locations with mediastinal invasion and they often present as large masses causing superior vena cava obstruction. Although shown in stages similar to other lung cancers, the typical stages are clustered as *limited* (M0), which includes all stages from IA, IB, to IIIA,B. *Extensive* applies to overt metastases M1 stage IV. Small cell cancer stage I/II/IIIA/B are color coded green/blue/red but are lumped together as M0 *limited* to thorax. Stage IV is metastatic black and referred to as *extensive*. Major stage group progression is dominated by the N stage progression.

T-ONCOANATOMY

ORIENTATION OF THREE-PLANAR ONCOANATOMY

The orientation diagrams are at the T6-7 level and the key anatomic feature is their central locations as their point of origin akin to lung bud anlage. The isocenter for SCA is at the hilar area, which is at the thoracic T6-7 level (Fig. 18.4). The three main branches of each major bronchus are within the visceral pleura.

T-oncoanatomy

The rich lymphatic submucosal network ensures the cancer's rapid spread to the visceral pleura and crosses the mediastinal pleura. The three-planar views (Fig. 18.5) emphasize the right pulmonary mediastinal surfaces and the juxtaposed right mediastinum because mediastinal mass formation and invasion are common presentations.

- *Sagittal plane:* The lung bud anlage is superior imposed on the bronchial tree. The mediastinal structures that are com-

monly compressed include the low-pressure, thin-walled superior vena cava or brachiocephalic vein and their entrapment between metastatic matted mediastinal masses of nodes and arteries. Plugs of tumor, when entering the thoracic duct or metastatic lymph nodes, can also compress and block the lymphatic flow, which can lead to chylous or pseudochylous effusions. Similarly, pulmonary venous compression results in serous pleural effusions. It is critical in staging to send cytospins of pleural effusions for evaluation to determine if they are positive for cancer cells or whether they are cytologically negative.

- *Coronal view:* The medial aspects of the lung reflect the structures into the superior and inferior mediastinum by virtue of anatomic position. A rapidly growing neoplasm penetrates the mediastinal pleura and invades mediastinal lymphatics and nodes directly.

- *Transverse view:* The T6-7 level is a critical level to appreciate. The arch of the aorta is defined, the trachea is bifurcating, and the branches of the sympathetics and parasympathetics, particularly the cardiac branches, are streaming alongside the trachea to form the cardiac plexuses, which, when invaded, can lead to cardiac arrhythmias.

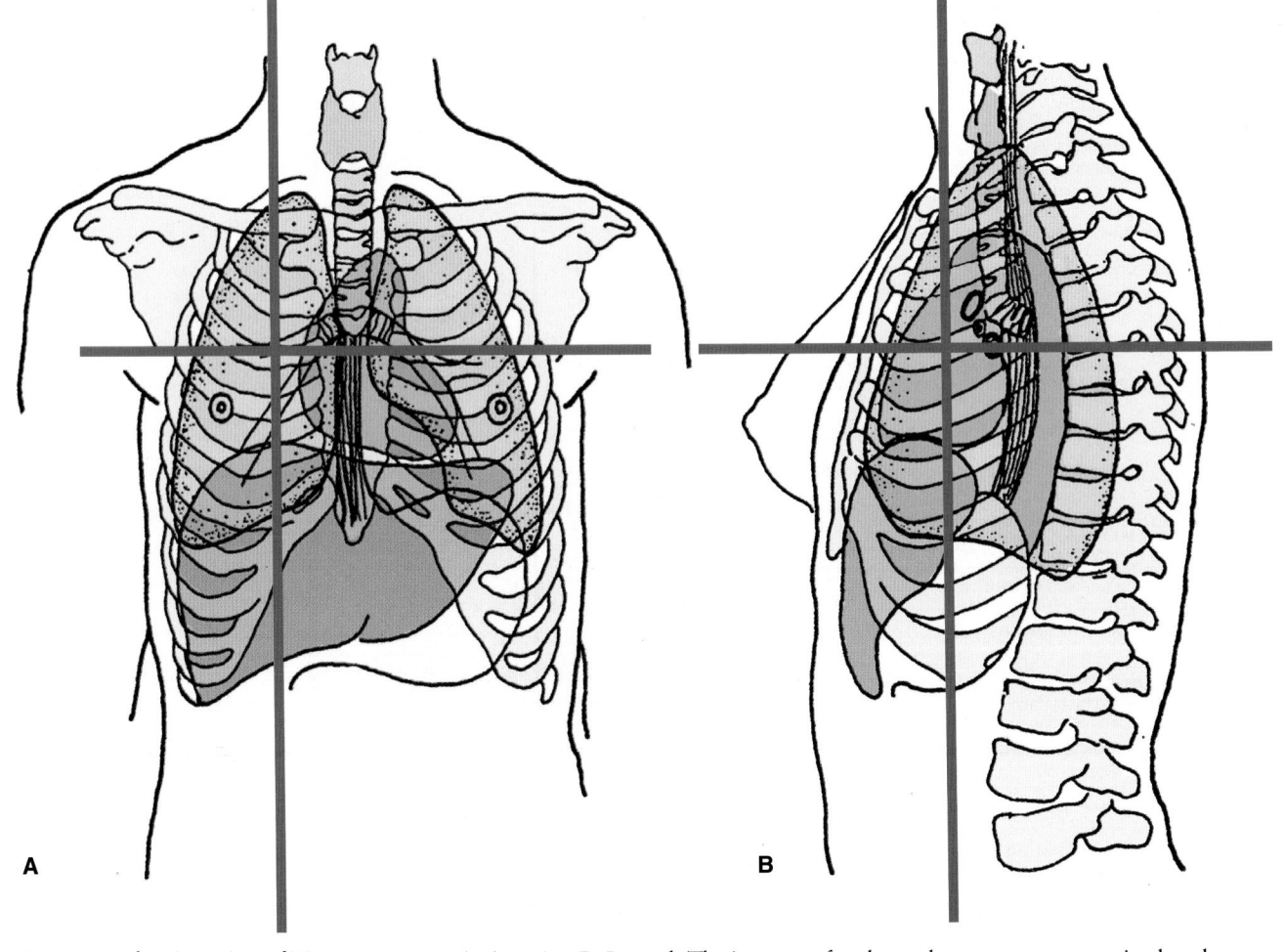

A

B

Figure 18.4 | Orientation of T-oncoanatomy. A. Anterior. **B.** Lateral. The isocenter for three-planar oncoanatomy is placed centrally at the lung root and transversely at the thoracic vertebral level T6-7.

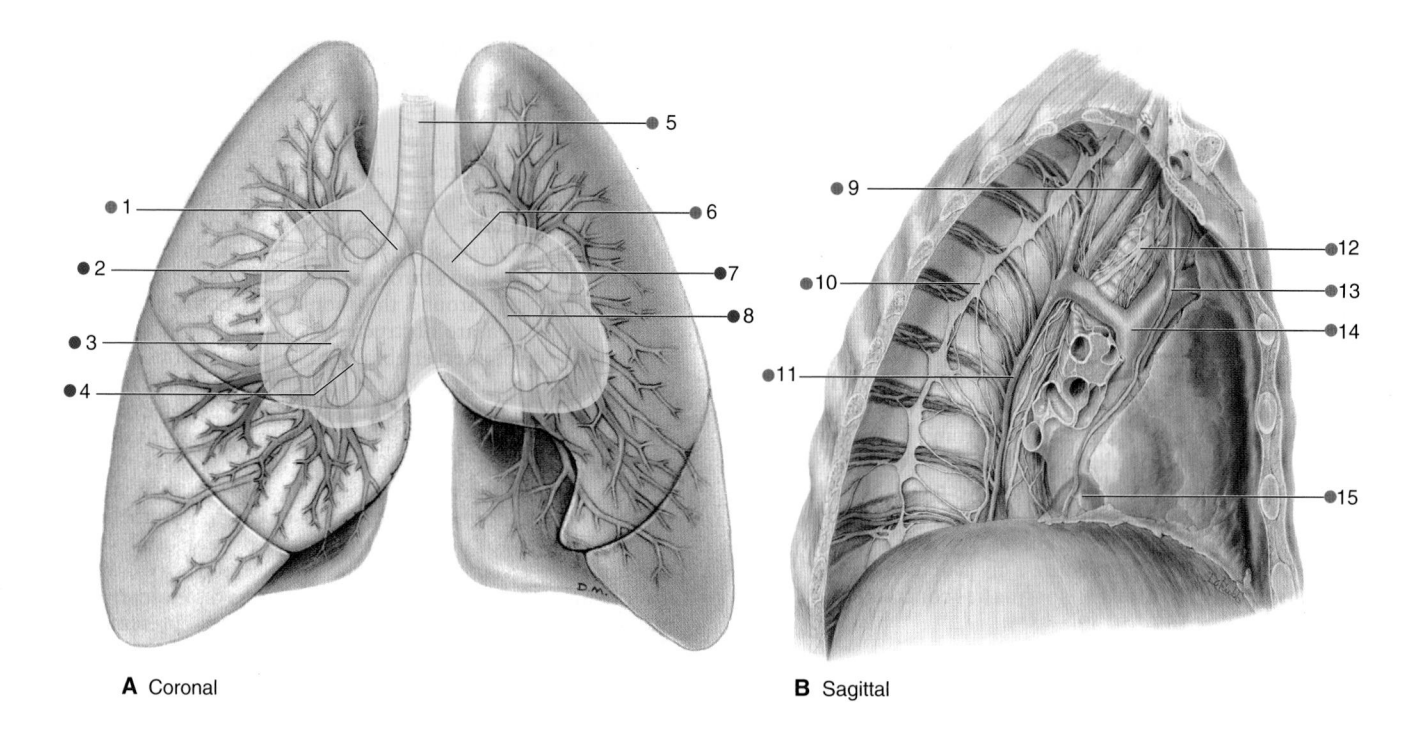

A Coronal

B Sagittal

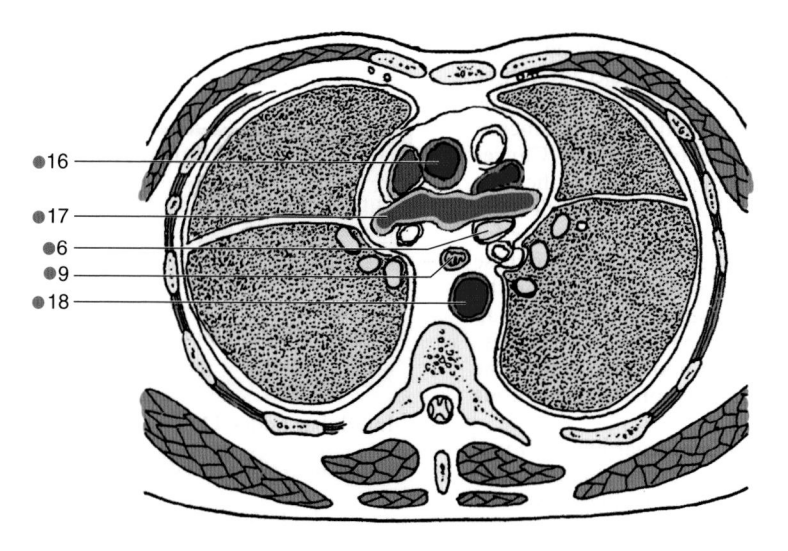

C Transverse

T_3 • 2. Right superior lobar bronchus	T_4 • 5. Trachea	T_4 • 13. Phrenic nerve
T_3 • 3. Right middle lobar bronchus	T_4 • 6. Left main bronchus	T_4 • 14. Superior vena cava
T_3 • 4. Right lower lobar bronchus	T_4 • 9. Esophagus	T_4 • 15. Inferior vena cava
T_3 • 7. Left superior lobar bronchus	T_4 • 10. Sympathetic trunk	T_4 • 16. Ascending aorta
T_3 • 8. Left inferior lobar bronchus	T_4 • 11. Azygos vein	T_4 • 17. Pulmonary trunk
T_4 • 1. Right main bronchus	T_4 • 12. Vagus nerve	T_4 • 18. Descending aorta

Figure 18.5 | **T-oncoanatomy.** The Color Code for the anatomic sites correlates with the color code for the stage group (Fig. 18.3) and patterns of spread (Fig. 18.2) and SIMLAP tables (Table 18.2). Connecting the dots in similar colors will provide an appreciation for the 3D Oncoanatomy.

TNM STAGING CRITERIA

TNM STAGING CRITERIA

The AJCC has adopted the staging system of the International Mesothelioma Interest Group (IMIG) and is based on patterns of spread of this aggressive thoracic malignancy. The pleura is like the peritoneum; although it consists of only a single layer of cells, it acts as a barrier to cancer spread. Thus, T1 tumors are focal nodular lesions of parietal pleura; T2 indicates spread to visceral pleura and lung; and T3 is deeper invasion of the chest wall and mediastinum, but potentially resectable. The major feature of unresectability are T4 criteria and include destruction of the chest wall ribs or vertebra or mediastinal, visceral infiltration, and extension through the diaphragm into the peritoneal cavity, the contralateral pleural space, or the brachial plexus in the neck.

SUMMARY OF CHANGES SEVENTH EDITION AJCC

- Peridiaphragmatic lymph nodes have been added to the N2 category (Fig. 19.3).

The TNM staging matrix is color coded for identification of stage group once T and N stages are determined (Table 19.3).

TABLE 19.3 Stage Summary Matrix

	N0	N1	N2	N3	M1
T1a	IA	III	III	IV	IV
T1b	IB	III	III	IV	IV
T2	II	III	III	IV	IV
T3	III	III	III	IV	IV
T4	IV	IV	IV	IV	IV

Thorax: Mesothelioma
- T stage determines stage group
  - T1a/b = IA,B, T2 = II, T3 = III, T4 = IV
- N stage modifies stage group progression
  - N1,2 = T3 = III, N3 = IV
- M stage is equivalent to advance T+N, not separate
  - M1 = T4, N3 = IV

MESOTHELIOMA

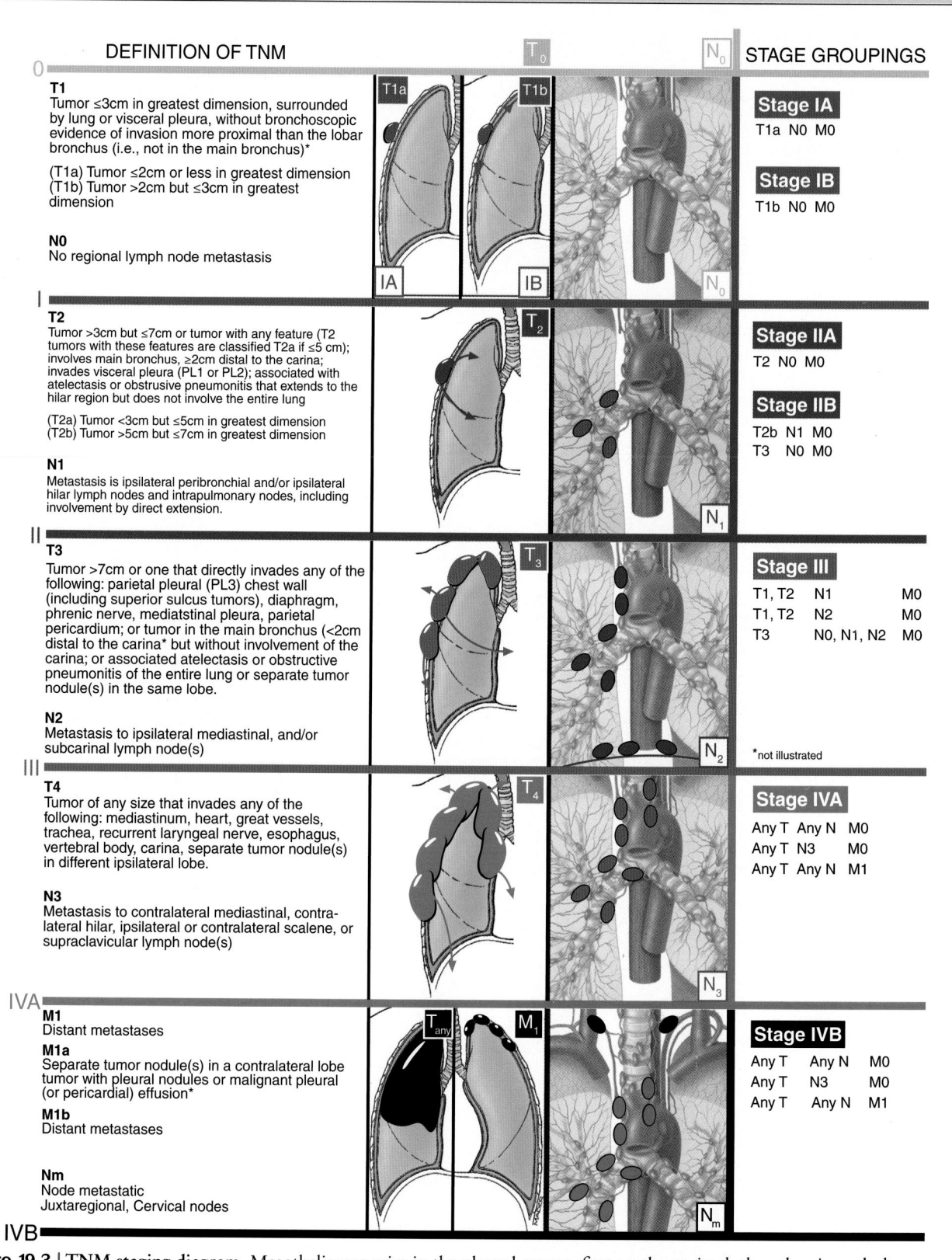

DEFINITION OF TNM

T1
Tumor ≤3cm in greatest dimension, surrounded by lung or visceral pleura, without bronchoscopic evidence of invasion more proximal than the lobar bronchus (i.e., not in the main bronchus)*

(T1a) Tumor ≤2cm or less in greatest dimension
(T1b) Tumor >2cm but ≤3cm in greatest dimension

N0
No regional lymph node metastasis

T2
Tumor >3cm but ≤7cm or tumor with any feature (T2 tumors with these features are classified T2a if ≤5 cm); involves main bronchus, ≥2cm distal to the carina; invades visceral pleura (PL1 or PL2); associated with atelectasis or obstrusive pneumonitis that extends to the hilar region but does not involve the entire lung

(T2a) Tumor <3cm but ≤5cm in greatest dimension
(T2b) Tumor >5cm but ≤7cm in greatest dimension

N1
Metastasis is ipsilateral peribronchial and/or ipsilateral hilar lymph nodes and intrapulmonary nodes, including involvement by direct extension.

T3
Tumor >7cm or one that directly invades any of the following: parietal pleural (PL3) chest wall (including superior sulcus tumors), diaphragm, phrenic nerve, mediastinal pleura, parietal pericardium; or tumor in the main bronchus (<2cm distal to the carina* but without involvement of the carina; or associated atelectasis or obstructive pneumonitis of the entire lung or separate tumor nodule(s) in the same lobe.

N2
Metastasis to ipsilateral mediastinal, and/or subcarinal lymph node(s)

T4
Tumor of any size that invades any of the following: mediastinum, heart, great vessels, trachea, recurrent laryngeal nerve, esophagus, vertebral body, carina, separate tumor nodule(s) in different ipsilateral lobe.

N3
Metastasis to contralateral mediastinal, contra-lateral hilar, ipsilateral or contralateral scalene, or supraclavicular lymph node(s)

M1
Distant metastases

M1a
Separate tumor nodule(s) in a contralateral lobe tumor with pleural nodules or malignant pleural (or pericardial) effusion*

M1b
Distant metastases

Nm
Node metastatic
Juxtaregional, Cervical nodes

STAGE GROUPINGS

Stage IA
T1a N0 M0

Stage IB
T1b N0 M0

Stage IIA
T2 N0 M0

Stage IIB
T2b N1 M0
T3   N0 M0

Stage III
T1, T2   N1   M0
T1, T2   N2   M0
T3   N0, N1, N2 M0

*not illustrated

Stage IVA
Any T Any N M0
Any T N3   M0
Any T Any N M1

Stage IVB
Any T Any N M0
Any T N3   M0
Any T Any N M1

Figure 19.3 | TNM staging diagram. Mesotheliomas arise in the pleural spaces, first on the parietal, then the visceral pleura, and continue invading into fissures. Then the aggressive malignancy spreads into the parietal pleura, chest wall and mediastinal pleura, and mediastinal structures. Unlike lung cancers, stage IVA is T4N3M0 and stage IVB M1 is metastatic. Vertical presentations of stage groupings, which follow the same color code for cancer stage advancement, are organized in horizontal lanes: Stage 0, yellow; I, green; II, blue; III, purple; IVA, red; and metastatic stage IVB, black. Definitions of TN are on the left and stage groupings are on the right.

T-ONCOANATOMY

ORIENTATION OF THREE-PLANAR ONCOANATOMY

The pleural space is coated by the visceral and parietal pleura of the chest wall and mediastinal pleura. This is presented at the thoracic T7-8 level (Fig. 19.4).

T-Oncoanatomy

The T-oncoanatomy is displayed in 3 planar views. A. Coronal, B. Sagittal, C. Transverse Axial. (Figure 19.5).

The pleural space is readily recognized during pathologic states as a pleural effusion or pneumothorax; in its normal state, it is invisible but shown in reference to the lung in expiration (Fig. 19.4).

- *Coronal:* Anterior and posterior views, the pleura extends into the neck and enters the costadiaphragmatic recess. The visceral pulmonary pleura faces the parietal pleural on the chest wall and medially the mediastinal pleura. The horizontal and oblique fissures are due to visceral pleural invagination on the right side and, similarly, the oblique fissure of the left lung as constituted by visceral pleura.

- *Sagittal:* The pleura invaginates its layers to form fissures. In the lateral view, pleural recesses are more shallow.

- *Transverse:* The diaphragmatic surface can be viewed as separating the pleural and peritoneal cavities.

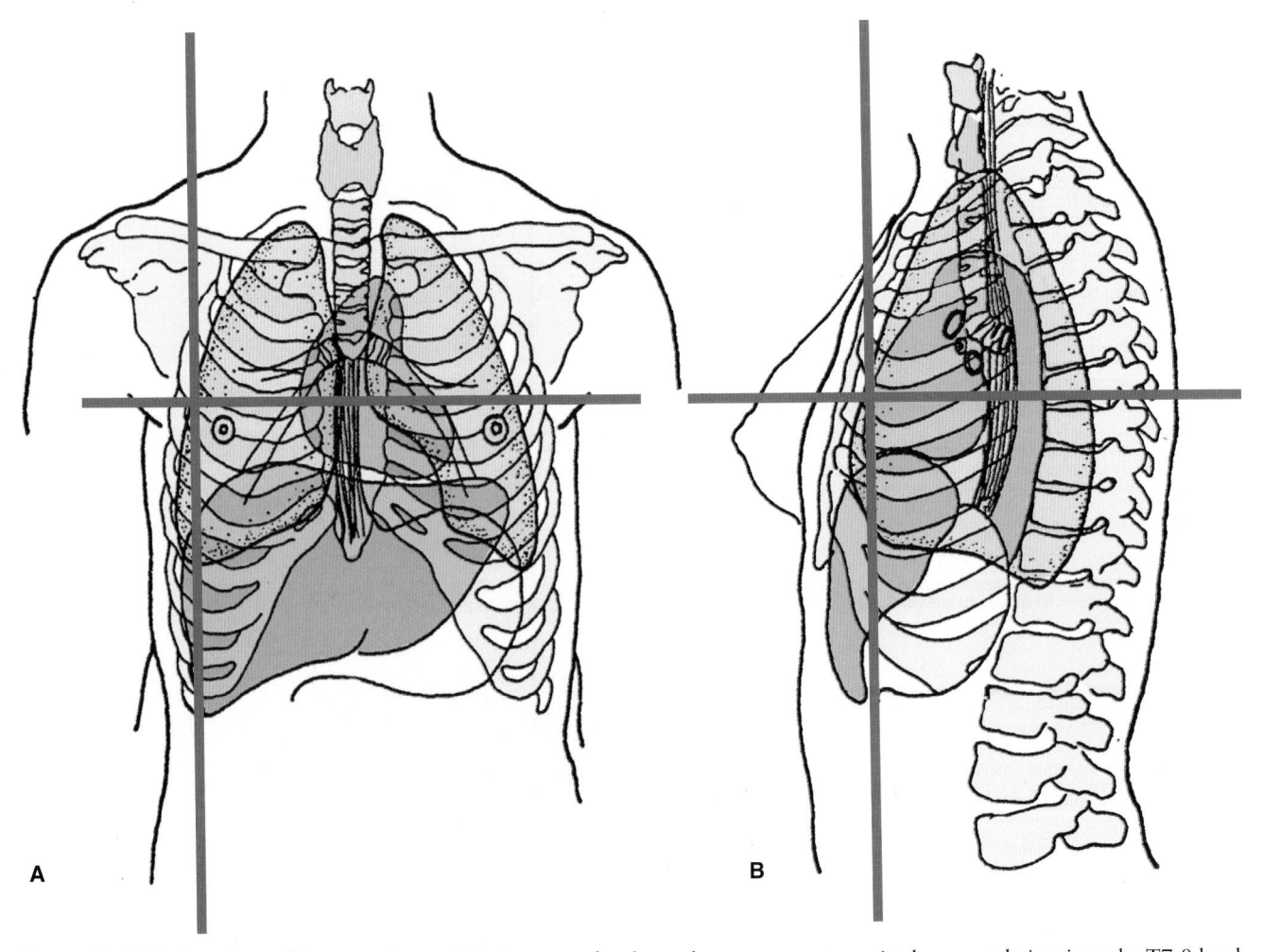

A

B

Figure 19.4 | Orientation of T-oncoanatomy. The isocenter for three-planar oncoanatomy in the coronal view is at the T7-8 level. A. Coronal. B. Sagittal.

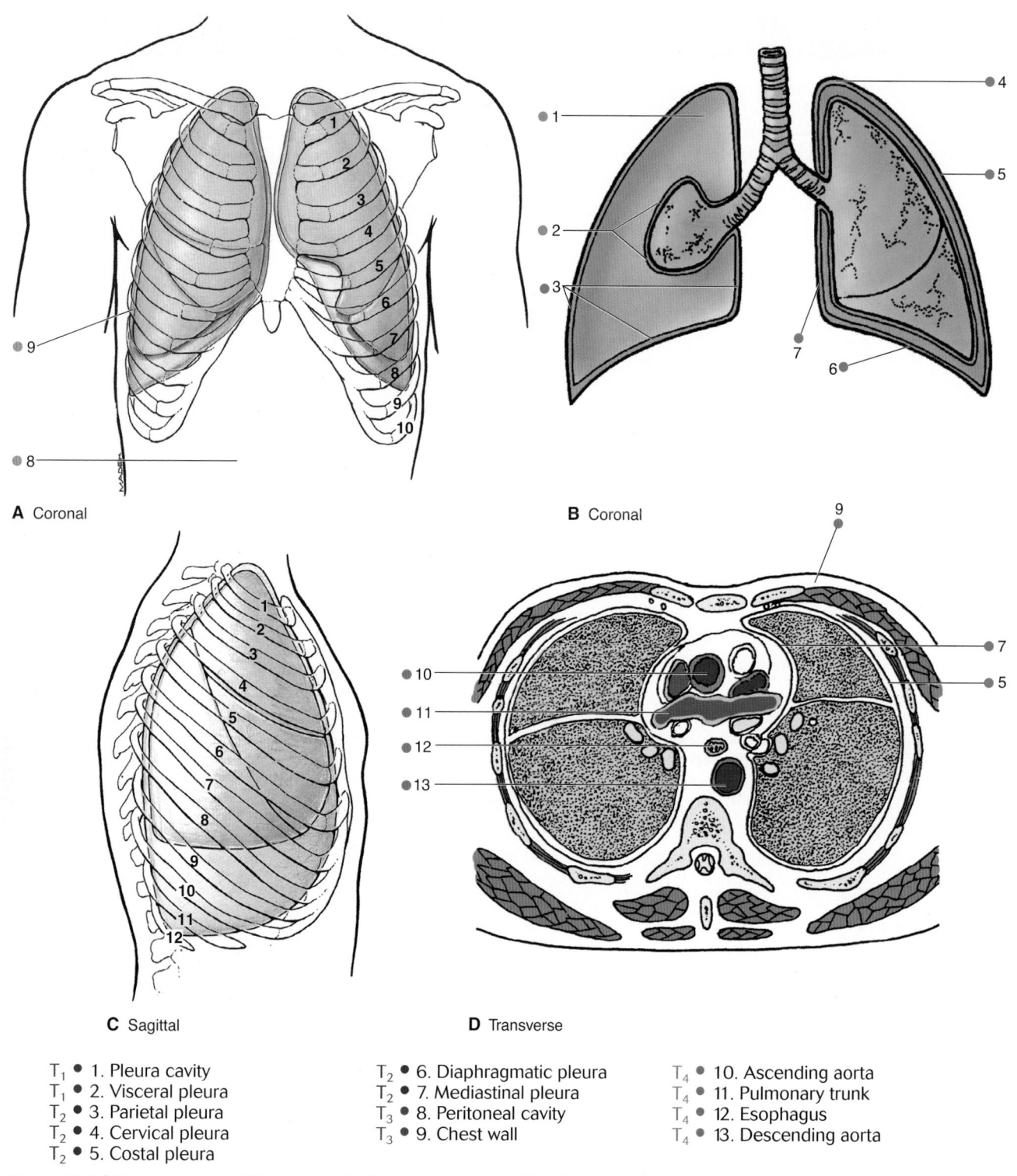

A Coronal

B Coronal

C Sagittal

D Transverse

T_1 • 1. Pleura cavity	T_2 • 6. Diaphragmatic pleura	T_4 • 10. Ascending aorta
T_1 • 2. Visceral pleura	T_2 • 7. Mediastinal pleura	T_4 • 11. Pulmonary trunk
T_2 • 3. Parietal pleura	T_3 • 8. Peritoneal cavity	T_4 • 12. Esophagus
T_2 • 4. Cervical pleura	T_3 • 9. Chest wall	T_4 • 13. Descending aorta
T_2 • 5. Costal pleura		

Figure 19.5 | T-oncoanatomy. The color code for the stage group (Fig. 19.3) and the patterns of spread (Fig. 19.2) and SIMLAP table (Table 19.2). Connecting the dots in similar colors will provide an appreciation for the 3D oncoanatomy.

N-ONCOANATOMY AND M-ONCOANATOMY

N-ONCOANATOMY

The regional lymph nodes are dependent on invasion patterns. Generally, they are mediastinal nodes, but with lung invasion, pulmonary and hilar nodes are at risk, and with chest wall invasion, costal nodes and internal thoracic nodes are at risk. The AJCC notes regional nodes are similar to lymph node map, nomenclature, and numbering for lung cancers (Fig. 19.6A; Table 19.4).

REGIONAL LYMPH NODES

The regional lymph nodes include:

- Intrathoracic
- Scalene
- Supraclavicular
- Internal mammary
- Peridiaphragmatic

The regional lymph node map and nomenclature adopted for the mesothelioma staging system is identical to that used for lung cancer. A detailed list of intrathoracic lymph nodes can be found in *AJCC Cancer Staging Manual*, 7th edition (Chapter 25). For pN, histologic examination of a mediastinal lymphadenectomy or lymph node sampling specimen will ordinarily include regional nodes taken from the ipsilateral N1 and N2 nodal stations. In addition, mesotheliomas often metastasize to lymph nodes not involved by lung cancers, most commonly the internal mammary and peridiaphragmetic nodes. These latter two regions also are classified as N2 nodal stations. Contralateral mediastinal and supraclavicular nodes may be available if a mediastinoscopy or node biopsy is also performed. If involved by metastatic disease these would be staged as N3 (Fig. 19.6B).*

M-ONCOANATOMY

The chest wall has a rich venous network of intercostals veins, azygos and hemiazygos veins interdigitating with intervertebral veins. Metastases to spinal cord and brain, contralateral spread to opposite chest, and lung can occur. Most common metastatic sites are on the mesothelial surfaces as opposed to pleura, pericardial, and peritoneal cavity. With dissemination, uncommon sites such as thyroid and prostate have been noted (Fig. 19.7).

*Preceding passage from Edge SB, Byrd DR, and Compton CC, et al. *AJCC Cancer Staging Manual, 7th edition*. New York, Springer, 2010, pp. 271.

TABLE 19.4	Lymph Nodes of Lung

With pulmonary invasion, intrapulmonary and interbronchial nodes are involved. With extension to mediastinal pleura, the mediastinal nodes are at risk.

N1 nodes: All N1 nodes lie distal to the mediastinal pleural reflection and *within the visceral pleura.*

Hilar nodes 10

Interlobar nodes 11

Lobar nodes bronchi 12

Segmental nodes 13

Subsegmental nodes 14

N2 nodes: All N2 nodes lie within the mediastinal pleural envelope on the ipsilateral side.

Highest mediastinal nodes 1, 2R, 2L

Upper paratracheal nodes 2R, 2L

Prevascular and retrotracheal nodes 3a, 3p*

Lower paratracheal nodes 4R, 4L

Subaortic nodes (aortopulmonary window) 5

Para-aortic nodes (ascending aorta or phrenic) 6

Subcarinal nodes 7

Paraesophageal nodes (below carina) 8

Pulmonary ligament nodes 9

*3a, 3p not shown in Fig 19.6.

A
B
1R
1L
H. brachio-
cephalic vein
2R
2L
Aorta
Pulmonary
artery
4R
4L
11
10
12
7
10
11
12
11
8
11
12
12
12
9
9

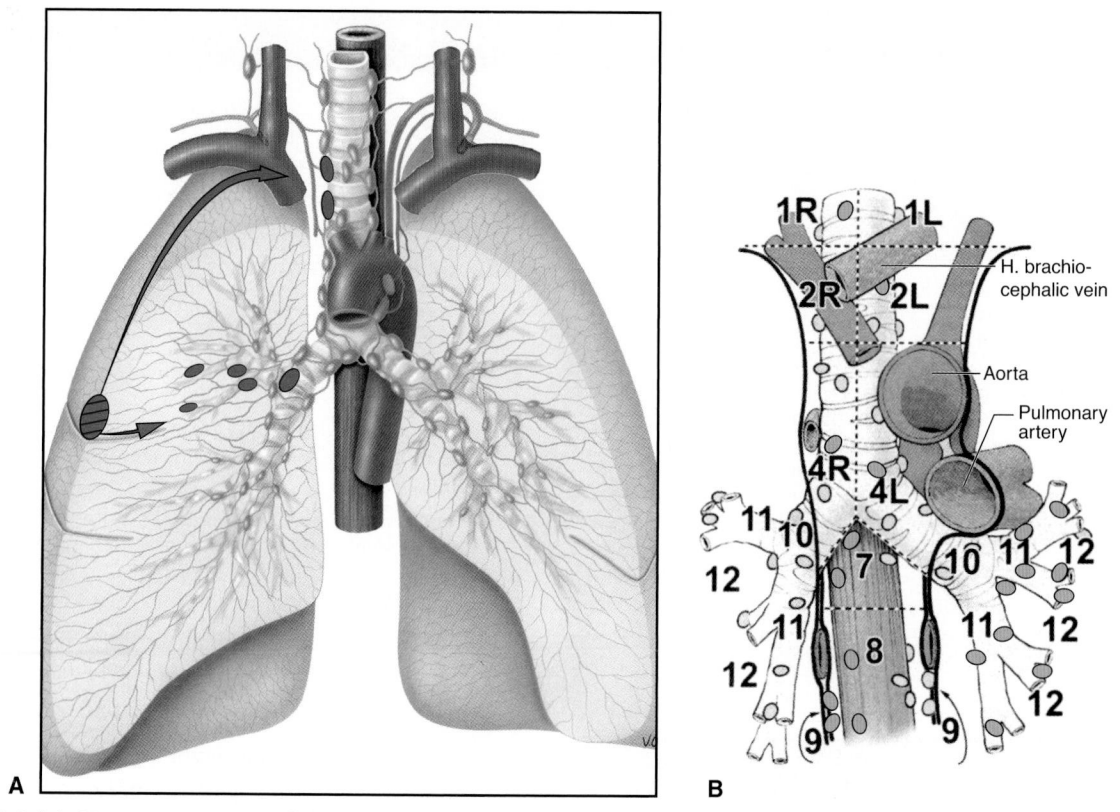

Figure 19.6 | **A. N-oncoanatomy.** With pulmonary invasion, intrapulmonary and interbronchial nodes are involved. With extension to mediastinal pleura, the mediastinal nodes are at risk. **B. M-oncoanatomy.** International Association for the Study of Lung Cancer (IASLC). Labels correlate with Table 19.4.

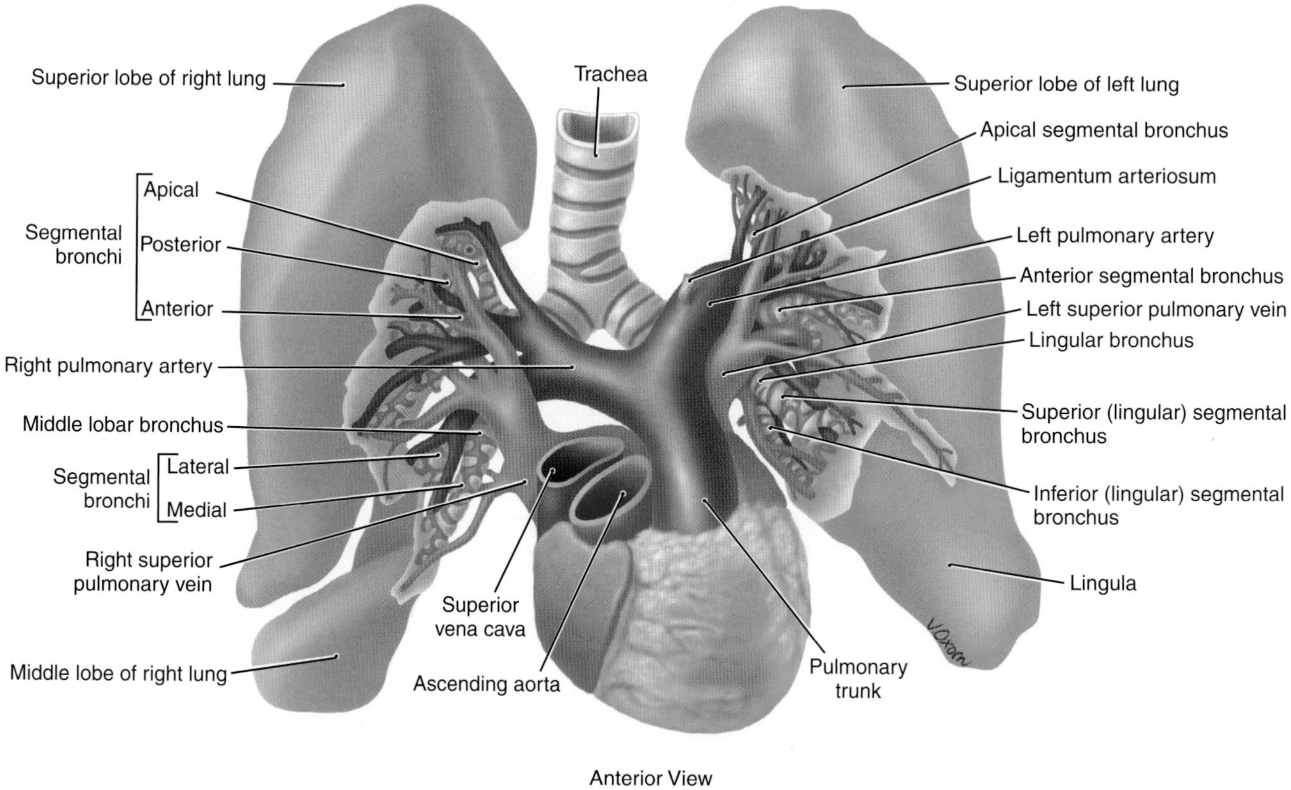

Superior lobe of right lung
Trachea
Superior lobe of left lung
Apical segmental bronchus
Ligamentum arteriosum
Segmental
bronchi
Apical
Posterior
Anterior
Left pulmonary artery
Anterior segmental bronchus
Left superior pulmonary vein
Lingular bronchus
Right pulmonary artery
Middle lobar bronchus
Superior (lingular) segmental
bronchus
Segmental
bronchi
Lateral
Medial
Inferior (lingular) segmental
bronchus
Right superior
pulmonary vein
Lingula
Superior
vena cava
Middle lobe of right lung
Ascending aorta
Pulmonary
trunk
Anterior View

Figure 19.7 | **Orientation of M-oncoanatomy.** Pulmonary anterior views are related to metastatic spread to and from lung, respectively.

STAGING WORKUP

RULES FOR CLASSIFICATION AND STAGING

Clinical Staging and Imaging

The TNM classification system is primarily for staging non–small cell lung cancers. The most important change dates back to the fourth edition of the AJCC where T3, resectable disease, was distinguished from T4, unresectable disease. Simultaneously, a greater reliance on more sophisticated imaging has occurred. It is with the sixth edition that computed tomography (CT) and positron emission tomography (PET) are allowed. The imaging modalities for detection and diagnosis apply to staging (see Table 19.5). Chest films and CT (preferably spiral) are essential steps in both diagnosis and staging. PET combined with CT is utilized to overcome motion artifacts. Magnetic resonance imaging (MRI) is useful for mediastinal evaluation. Another advantage of CT over MRI for staging is that it allows for metastatic workup of lung, liver, adrenal, ribs, and vertebrae (Fig. 19.8).

Pathologic Staging

All pathologic specimens from clinical invasive procedures—bronchoscopy, mediastinoscopy, mediastinotomy, thoracentesis, and thorascopy—are applicable to pathologic stage.

Thoracotomy and resection of primary and lymph nodes are the mainstay of pathologic staging. Margin status and any residual cancer need to be noted. Preferably, six nodes are examined.

Oncoimaging Annotations

- Chest radiographs seldom detect primary mesotheliomas in their early stages.
- Spiral CT is useful in high-risk patients to detect nodule and infiltrates.
- PET imaging with ^{18}FDG (fluorodeoxyglucose) appears to be of value in discriminating malignant versus benign nodules.
- CT can detect mediastinal adenopathy, but histologic verification is essential to ascertain if it is malignant.
- Determining N2 versus N3 mediastinal nodes is important; it establishes resectability.
- MRI can be of value in assessing mediastinal invasion, chest wall and rib erosion, and compromised large vein involvement.
- Small pleural plaques and subpleural spread can be compatible with asbestosis inhalation.
- Extension along diaphragmatic curare can lead to peritoneal invasion across the diaphragm.

TABLE 19.5	Imaging Modalities for Diagnosis and Staging	
Method	Capability	Recommended
Primary Tumor and Regional Nodes Workup		
Chest films	Baseline image	Yes
CT/spiral CT	Most useful of all modalities for determining characteristics of T and N in the thorax and M in the adrenal and liver	Yes
MRI	Is superior to CT in detecting mediastinal invasion	No
Percutaneous needle biopsy	Guided by fluoroscopy or CT, accurate in establishing cytologic diagnosis from T (particularly peripheral lung lesions); M (especially liver or bone); less experience with N	Yes
Mediastinoscopy/thoracoscopy	Confirmation of nodal involvement	Yes
Metastatic Workup for Clinically Suspected Metastases		
CT/echography	For liver, adrenals	Yes
CT/MRI	For brain	Yes
Bone scan	For the bone	Yes
PET scan	Diagnosis of peripheral lesions can differentiate between cancer and benign lesions. Staging of true extent of primary and lymph node involvement.	Yes, if clinically indicated

CT, computed tomography; M, metastasis; MRI, magnetic resonance imaging; N, node; PET, positron emission tomography; T, tumor.

PROGNOSIS AND CANCER SURVIVAL

CANCER STATISTICS AND SURVIVAL

It is difficult to find a malignancy more lethal than lung cancer, especially small cell cancers, which comprise overall about 5% of cases. However, mesotheliomas have virtually no 5-year survivors. Most reports with radical extrapleural pneumonectomy with chemoradiation are yielding median survival of less than 1 year (9 months) with high complication rates with mortality rates down to 10% or less. Elegant radiation using three-dimensional conformal techniques with intensity modulation has not been able to alter the dismal course of this disease.

PROGNOSIS

Prognostic factors are mainly related to histopathology subtypes (Table 19.6).

TABLE 19.6	Prognostic Factors
Required for Staging	None
Clinically significant	Histological subtype (epithelioid, mixed or biphasic, sarcomatoid, desmoplastic)
	History of asbestos exposure
	Presence or absence of chest pain
	FDG-PET SUV

FDG-PET, fluorodeoxyglucose positron emission tomography; SUV, standardized uptake value.
From Edge SB, Byrd DR, Compton CC, et al. *AJCC Cancer Staging Manual*. 7th ed. New York: Springer, 2010, p. 276, with permission.

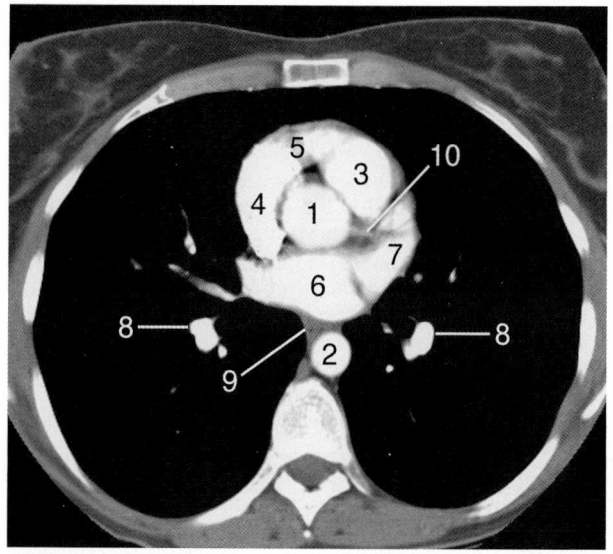
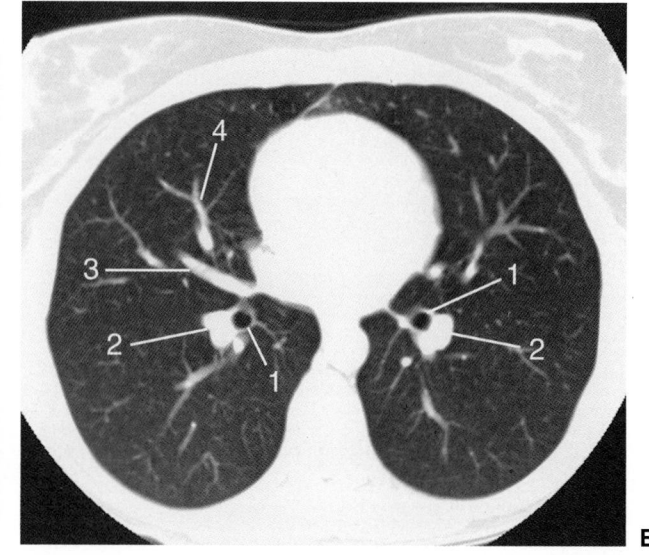

Figure 19.8 | Axial CTs of T7 and T8 level correlate with the T-oncoanatomy transverse section (Fig. 19.5C). Oncoimaging with CT is commonly applied to staging cancers, often combined with PET to determine true extent of primary cancer and involved lymph nodes. **A.** Mediastinal window. 1, ascending aorta; 2, descending aorta; 3, right ventricular outflow tract; 4, right atrium; 5, right atrial appendage; 6, left atrium; 7, left atrial appendage; 8, basal lower lobe artery; 9, esophagus; 10, left coronary artery. **B.** Lung window. 1, basal trunk lower lobe bronchus; 2, basal lower lobe artery; 3, RML vein; 4, medial segment RML artery.

Breast Cancer

PERSPECTIVE, PATTERNS OF SPREAD, AND PATHOLOGY

Cancers of the mammary gland predominate among tumors of the chest wall, and their oncoanatomy emphasizes their rich lymphatics and microvasculature.

PERSPECTIVE AND PATTERNS OF SPREAD

Breast cancer is the most prevalent female malignancy and exceeds the incidence of the next two common cancers of lung and colorectal areas combined. At an annual rate of 215,000 new patients and a death rate of 40,000, virtually everyone has a family member or friend who has encountered or experienced breast cancer. With the widespread use of mammography, most cancers are detected in early stages that often are not palpable. Especially important is the ability to identify preinvasive carcinomas in situ.

The patterns of spread account for the physical signs associated with breast cancer (Fig. 20.2; Table 20.2). Most commonly, a small palpable nodule, often without tenderness, appears to be a thickening or swelling, which is freely movable. If the lesion causes skin wrinkling with positional changes, Cooper's suspensory ligaments are involved. Lactiferous ductal invasion can result in expression of a bloody secretion from the nipple or even nipple inversion. Loss of mobility strongly suggests invasion of the pectoralis major or chest wall. When loss of mobility occurs with muscle flexion, it is due to muscle invasion; chest wall infiltration leads to a permanent loss of mobility (Fig. 20.2; Table 20.2).

PATHOLOGY

The majority (85%) are ductal carcinomas in situ and the rest are lobular cancer in situ, which run a more benign course. The histopathologic varieties of breast cancer are tabulated in Table 20.1; Figure 20.1. It is recommended that all invasive breast cancers be graded utilizing the Nottingham system, in which point scores based on specific features are equated with grades 1 to 3. A comprehensive review of the literature of histologic grade and outcome in early stage breast cancer in the current American Joint Committee on Cancer (AJCC) sixth edition indicates its robustness as a prognostic factor. It seems certain that emerging data will support its incorporation into staging in the future editions, similar to the Gleason grade for prostate cancer staging.

TABLE 20.1	Histopathologic Type: Common Cancers of the Breast

Type
In situ carcinomas
NOS
Intraductal
Paget disease and intraductal
Invasive carcinomas
NOS
Ductal
Inflammatory
Medullary, NOS
Medullary with lymphoid stroma
Mucinous
Papillary (predominantly micropapillary pattern)
Tubular
Lobular
Paget disease and infiltrating
Undifferentiated
Squamous cell
Adenoid cyst
Secretory
Cribriform

NOS, not otherwise specified.
From Edge SB, Byrd DR, Compton CC, et al. *AJCC Cancer Staging Manual.* 7th ed. New York, Springer, 2010, p. 362, with permission.

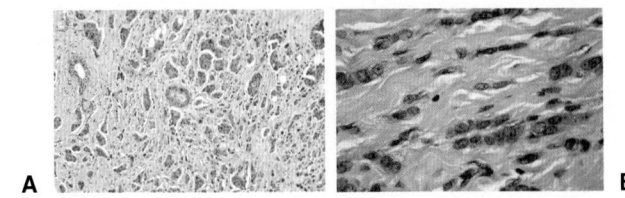

Figure 20.1 | A: Carcinoma of the breast. Ductal carcinoma cells invading stroma showing irregular cords and nests of invasive. B: Lobular carcinoma. Invasive lobular carcinoma. In contrast to invasive ductal carcinoma, the cells of lobular carcinoma tend to form single strands that invade between collagen fibers in a single pattern. The tumor cells are similar to those seen in lobular carcinoma in situ.

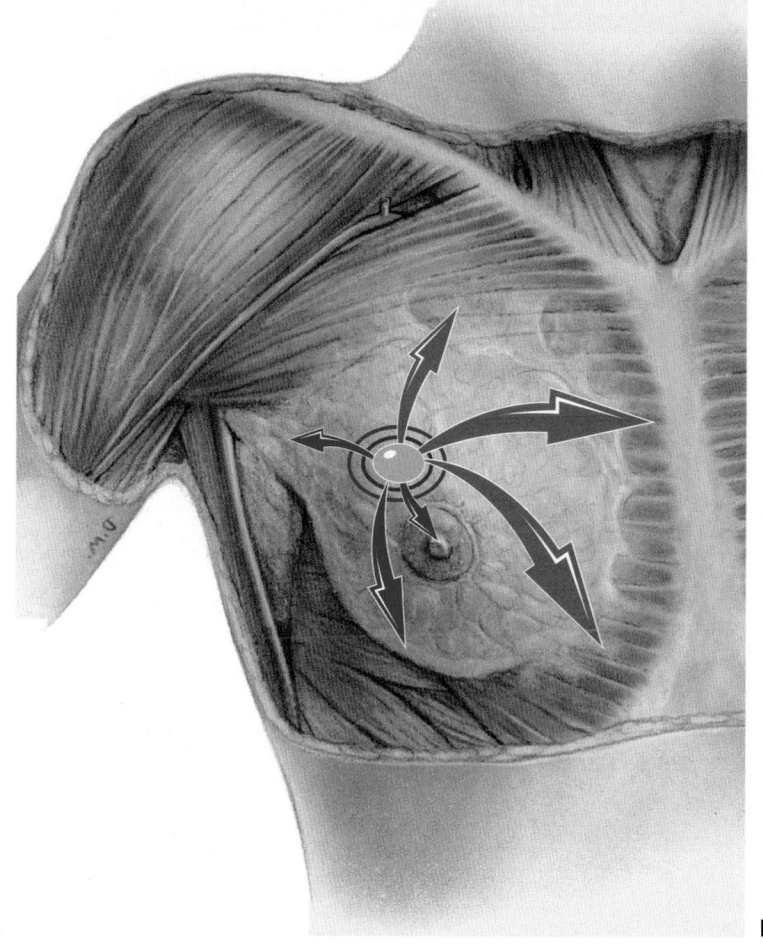

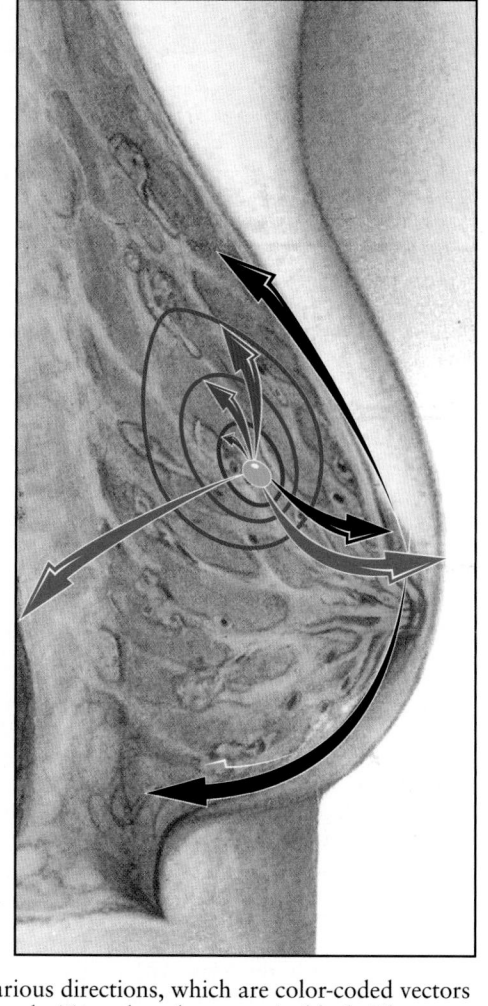

A

B

Figure 20.2 | Patterns of spread. The primary cancer (breast cancer) invades in various directions, which are color-coded vectors (*arrows*) representing stage of progression: Tis, yellow; T1, green; T2, blue; T3, purple; T4, red; and metastatic, black. The concept of visualizing patterns of spread to appreciate the surrounding anatomy is well demonstrated by the six-directional pattern i.e. SIMLAP Table 20.2.

TABLE 20.2	SIMLAP	
Breast (Upper Outer) Uquadrant		
S	UOQ	• T1
I	LOQ	• T1
M	IQ areola, nipples, lactiferus lacumae	• T2 • T3
L	UOQ	• T2
A	Skin Inflammatory	• T4b • T4d
P	Pectoral fascia Pectoralis major Chest wall	• T4a • T4a • T4a

The six vectors of invasion are <u>S</u>uperior, <u>I</u>nferior, <u>M</u>edial, <u>L</u>ateral, <u>A</u>nterior, and <u>P</u>osterior. The color-coded dots correlate the T stage with specific anatomic structure involved.

TNM STAGING CRITERIA

TNM STAGING CRITERIA

Breast cancer has been among the earliest cancers staged utilizing the TNM system and was proposed in 1954 by the International Union Against Cancer (UICC). Agreement by both UICC/AJCC (the first joint publication in 1968) has enabled the staging criteria to remain constant over the past three decades. The modifications relate to the frequent use of surgical findings and their histopathologic examination. The clinical basis for primary breast cancer staging is size: T1, less than 2 cm; T2, 2 to 5 cm; and T3, greater than 5 cm in any dimension. Evidence of fixation to the chest wall appeared as a modifier in each stage, that is, A or B. The lymph node staging applied to axillary nodes mainly.

In the fourth edition (1992), the impact of mammography was acknowledged and tumor size was so noted and used to create subcategories for stage I: T1A, 0.5 cm; T1B, 0.5 to 1 cm; T1C, 1 to 2 cm; and extension to skin or chest wall is applied to T4 cancers only.

In the fifth edition (1997), clinical measurement of size applied to both physical examination and mammography, and pathologic tumor size for T applied "only to the invasive component." Cellular and molecular markers were tabulated, acknowledging that 80 putative variables were reported in the literature. Although three prognostic groupings were noted, no specific incorporation of biomarkers was made by the American College of Pathologists. In the sixth edition (2003), microinvasion is defined at the primary site and regional nodes. The use of scintigraphy for determining the sentinel node(s) has been allowed. More subcategories exist for the primary and regional nodes, but the general parameters of size have remained stable. There have been considerable new data presented for the interested investigator in the latest AJCC 7th edition for evidence-based changes. These are covered in the rules for classification section. Histopathologic evaluation of surgical specimens can yield a long list of histopathologic types.

The importance of specific imaging modalities to estimate tumor size includes mammograms, sonograms, and magnetic resonance imaging (MRI), as noted at the beginning of the seventh edition summary of changes. Most of the changes relate to microinvasive disease and identifying the invasive components, mostly for accurate pathologic stages. An increasing array of categories and definitions include (Fig. 20.3B):

- DIN: ductal intraepithelial neoplasia
- DCIS: ductal cancer in situ
- LIN: lobular neoplasia
- LCIS: lobular cancer in situ
- Paget's disease

The TNM staging matrix is color coded for identification of stage group once T and N stages are determined (Table 20.3)

SUMMARY OF CHANGES SEVENTH EDITION AJCC

Tumor (T)

- Identified specific imaging modalities that can be used to estimate clinical tumor size, including mammography, ultrasound, and MRI (Fig. 20.3A).

- Made specific recommendations that (i) microscopic measurement is the most accurate and preferred method to determine pathologic staging (pT) with a small invasive cancer that can be entirely submitted in one paraffin block, and (ii) the gross measurement is the most accurate and preferred method to determine pT with larger invasive cancers that must be submitted in multiple paraffin blocks.

- Made the specific recommendation to use the clinical measurement thought to be most accurate to determine the clinical T of breast cancers treated with neoadjuvant therapy. Pathologic (posttreatment) size should be estimated based on the best combination of gross and microscopic histological findings.

- Made the specific recommendation to estimate the size of invasive cancers that are unapparent to any clinical modalities or gross pathologic examination by carefully measuring and recording the relative positions of tissue samples submitted for microscopic evaluation and determining which of these contain tumor.

| TABLE 20.3 | Stage Summary Matrix |

	N0	N1	N2	N3	M1
T1	I	IIA	IIIA	IIIC	IV
T2	IIA	IIB	IIIA	IIIC	IV
T3	IIB	IIIA	IIIA	IIIC	IV
T4	IIIB	IIIB	IIIB	IIIC	IV

Thorax: Breast Cancer
Both T and N progress and determine stage progression. T stage and N stage combined determine substage progression. Subscript T and N additionally provide guide to substage progression.

- I = T1N0 = 1
- IIA = T1N1 = 2
- IIB = T2N1 = 3, T2N2 = 4
- IIIA = T3N2 = 5
- IIIB = T4N2 = 6
- IIIC = T4N3 = 7
- M Stage is a separate stage, IV

BREAST CANCER

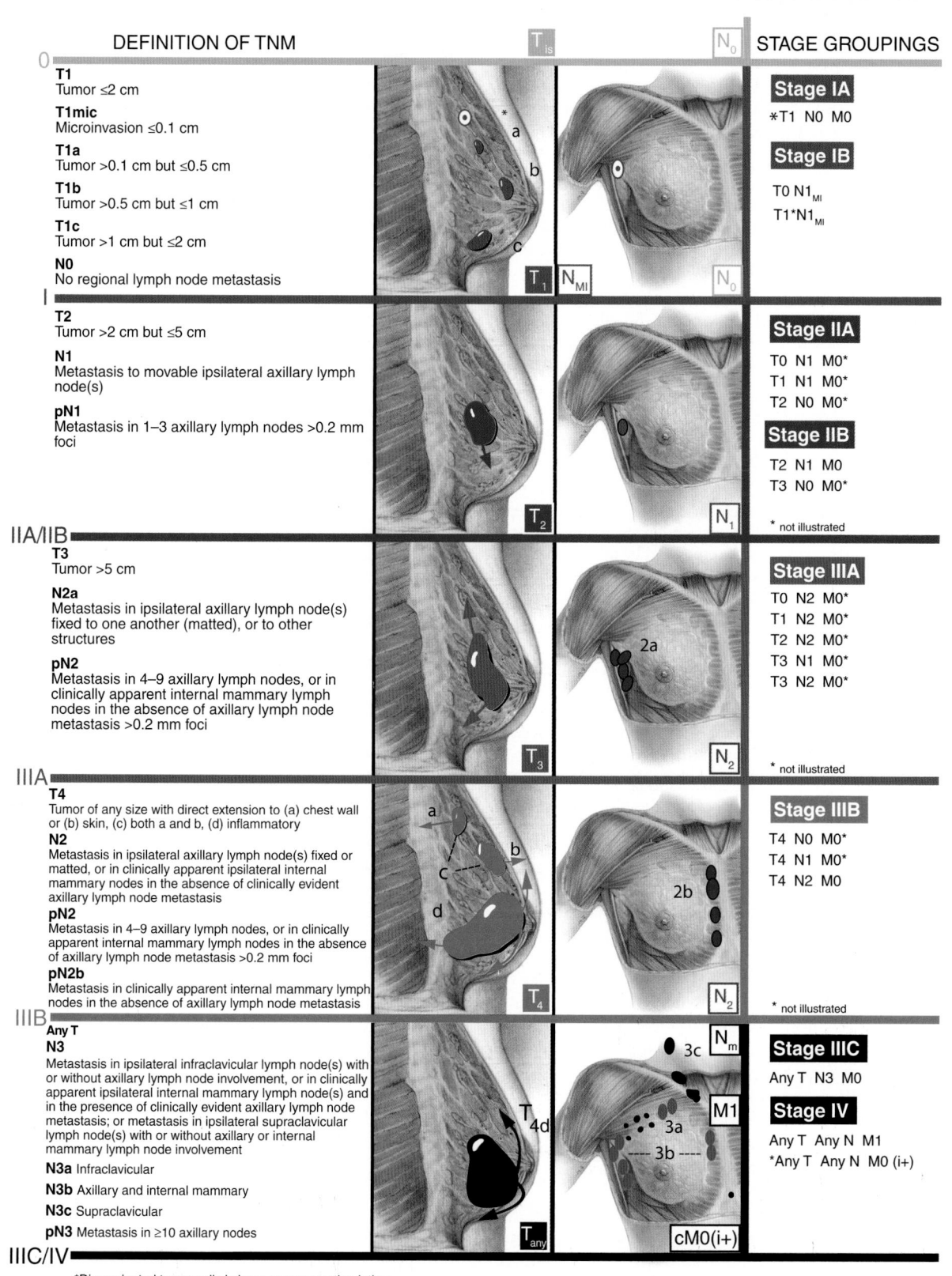

DEFINITION OF TNM

0

T1
Tumor ≤2 cm

T1mic
Microinvasion ≤0.1 cm

T1a
Tumor >0.1 cm but ≤0.5 cm

T1b
Tumor >0.5 cm but ≤1 cm

T1c
Tumor >1 cm but ≤2 cm

N0
No regional lymph node metastasis

I

T2
Tumor >2 cm but ≤5 cm

N1
Metastasis to movable ipsilateral axillary lymph node(s)

pN1
Metastasis in 1–3 axillary lymph nodes >0.2 mm foci

IIA/IIB

T3
Tumor >5 cm

N2a
Metastasis in ipsilateral axillary lymph node(s) fixed to one another (matted), or to other structures

pN2
Metastasis in 4–9 axillary lymph nodes, or in clinically apparent internal mammary lymph nodes in the absence of axillary lymph node metastasis >0.2 mm foci

IIIA

T4
Tumor of any size with direct extension to (a) chest wall or (b) skin, (c) both a and b, (d) inflammatory

N2
Metastasis in ipsilateral axillary lymph node(s) fixed or matted, or in clinically apparent ipsilateral internal mammary nodes in the absence of clinically evident axillary lymph node metastasis

pN2
Metastasis in 4–9 axillary lymph nodes, or in clinically apparent internal mammary lymph nodes in the absence of axillary lymph node metastasis >0.2 mm foci

pN2b
Metastasis in clinically apparent internal mammary lymph nodes in the absence of axillary lymph node metastasis

IIIB

Any T

N3
Metastasis in ipsilateral infraclavicular lymph node(s) with or without axillary lymph node involvement, or in clinically apparent ipsilateral internal mammary lymph node(s) and in the presence of clinically evident axillary lymph node metastasis; or metastasis in ipsilateral supraclavicular lymph node(s) with or without axillary or internal mammary lymph node involvement

N3a Infraclavicular

N3b Axillary and internal mammary

N3c Supraclavicular

pN3 Metastasis in ≥10 axillary nodes

IIIC/IV

*Disseminated tumor cells in bone marrow or circulating cells in blood or excised tissue as ovary <0.2mm.

STAGE GROUPINGS

Stage IA
*T1 N0 M0

Stage IB
T0 N1_MI
T1*N1_MI

Stage IIA
T0 N1 M0*
T1 N1 M0*
T2 N0 M0*

Stage IIB
T2 N1 M0
T3 N0 M0*

* not illustrated

Stage IIIA
T0 N2 M0*
T1 N2 M0*
T2 N2 M0*
T3 N1 M0*
T3 N2 M0*

* not illustrated

Stage IIIB
T4 N0 M0*
T4 N1 M0*
T4 N2 M0

* not illustrated

Stage IIIC
Any T N3 M0

Stage IV
Any T Any N M1
*Any T Any N M0 (i+)

Figure 20.3A | TNM staging diagram. Breast cancers are mammary gland cancers, and because of the effectiveness of mammography screening the classification has become more of a pathologic staging system for both primary and lymph nodes. Note stage III is divided into A/B/C as distinct from stage IV. Vertical presentation of stage groupings, which follows the same color code for cancer advancement, are organized in horizontal lanes: Stage 0, yellow; I, green; II, blue; IIIA, purple; IIIB, red; and metastatic stage IIIC and IV, black. Definitions of TN are on the left and stage groupings are on the right.

- Acknowledged DIN as uncommon, and still not widely accepted, terminology encompassing both DCIS and atypical ductal hyperplasia (ADH), and clarification that only cases referred to as DIN containing DCIS (+/– ALH) are classified as Tis (DCIS) (Fig. 20.3B).

- Acknowledged LIN as uncommon, and still not widely accepted, terminology encompassing both LCIS and atypical lobular hyperplasia (ALH), and clarification that only cases referred to as LIN containing LCIS (+/– ALH) are classified as Tis (LCIS).

- Clarification that only Paget's disease *not* associated with an underlying noninvasive (i.e., DCIS or LCIS) or invasive breast cancer should be classified as Tis (Paget's) and that Paget's disease associated with an underlying cancer be classified according to the underlying cancer (Tis, T1, etc.).

- Made the recommendation to estimate the size of noninvasive carcinomas (DCIS and LCIS), even though it does not currently change their T classification, because noninvasive cancer size may influence therapeutic decisions, acknowledging that providing a precise size for LCIS may be difficult.

- Acknowledged that the prognosis of microinvasive carcinoma is generally thought to be quite favorable, although the clinical impact of multifocal microinvasive disease is not well understood at this time.

- Acknowledged that it is not necessary for tumors to be in separate quadrants to be classified as multiple simultaneous ipsilateral carcinomas, providing that they can be unambiguously demonstrated to be macroscopically distinct and measurable using available clinical and pathologic techniques.

- Maintained that the term "inflammatory carcinoma" be restricted to cases with typical skin changes involving a third or more of the skin of the breast. While the histologic presence of invasive carcinoma invading dermal lymphatic is supportive of the diagnosis, it is not required, nor is dermal lymphatic invasion without typical clinical findings sufficient for a diagnosis of inflammatory breast cancer.

- Recommended that all invasive cancer should be graded using the Nottingham combined histologic grade (Elston-Ellis modification of Scarff-Bloom-Richardson grading system).

Nodes (N)

- Classification of isolated tumor cell clusters and single cells is more stringent. Small clusters of cells not greater than 0.2 mm, or nonconfluent or nearly confluent clusters of cells not exceeding 200 cells in a single histologic lymph node cross-section are classified as isolated tumor cells.

- Use of the (sn) modifier has been clarified and restricted. When six or more sentinel nodes are identified on gross examination of pathology specimens the (sn) modifier should be omitted.

- Stage I breast tumors have been subdivided into stage IA and stage IB; stage ID includes small tumors (T1) with exclusively micrometastases in lymph nodes (N1mi).

Metastases (M)

- Created new M0 (i+) category, defined by presence of either disseminated tumor cells detectable in bone marrow or circulating tumor cells or found incidentally in other tissues (such as ovaries removed prophylactically) if not exceeding 0.2 mm. However, this category does not change

the stage grouping. Assuming that they do not have clinically or radiographically detectable metastases, patients with M0 (i+) are staged according to T and N.

Postneoadjuvant Therapy (yc or ypTNM)

- In the setting of patients who received neoadjuvant therapy, pretreatment clinical T (cT) should be based on clinical or imaging findings.

- Postneoadjuvant therapy T should be based on clinical or imaging (ycT) or pathologic findings (ypT).

- A subscript will be added to the clinical N for both node negative and node positive patients to indicate whether the N was derived from clinical examination, fine-needle aspiration, core needle biopsy, or sentinel lymph node biopsy.

- The posttreatment ypT will be defined as the largest contiguous focus of invasive cancer as defined histopathologically with a subscript to indicate the presence of multiple tumor foci. Note: Definition of posttreatment ypT remains controversial and an area in transition.

- Posttreatment nodal metastases no greater than 0.2 mm are classified as ypN0 (i+) as in patients who have not received neoadjuvant systemic therapy. However, patients with this finding are not considered to have achieved a pathologic complete response (pCR).

- A description of the degree of response to neoadjuvant therapy (complete, partial, no response) will be collected by the registrar with the posttreatment ypTNM. The registrars are requested to describe how they defined response (by physical examination, imaging techniques—mammograms, ultrasound, MRI—or pathologically).

- Patients will be considered to have M1 (and therefore stage IV) breast cancer if they have had clinically or radiographically detectable metastases, with or without biopsy, prior to neoadjuvant systemic therapy, regardless of their status after neoadjuvant systemic therapy.

Breast cancer staging is equally weighted more to lymph node progression and the primary tumor (Fig. 20.2). This is evident in stage I N0, stage II N1, stage IIIA N2, and stage IIIC N3. The pathologic staging is more detailed with each N category being further subdivided into N1a/b/c based mainly on the number of nodes microscopically involved and the number of locations (i.e., axillary and internal mammary).

There are a number of important and interesting definitions for a lymph node to be considered positive. Definitions of microdeposits began in breast cancer staging:

- ITC: isolated tumor cell clusters in lymph nodes less than 0.2 mm (approximately 1,000 cells).

- Micromets: greater than 0.2 mm to less than or equal to 2.0 mm deposits in nodes

- NB: size of largest deposit, not sum of deposits

- pN0 (mol+): refers to use of molecular markers (reverse transcription-polymerase chain reaction [RT-PCR])

- SN: refers to sentinel nodes

- yP: prefix refers to posttreatment assessment of disease

- c M0(i+): refers to molecular or microdeposits of circulating tumor cells (CTC) or in bone marrow.

Although histopathologic grading systems are discussed, they are to be noted but not included in staging as in prostate cancer. The Nottingham combined histologic grade is recommended (Table 20.4).

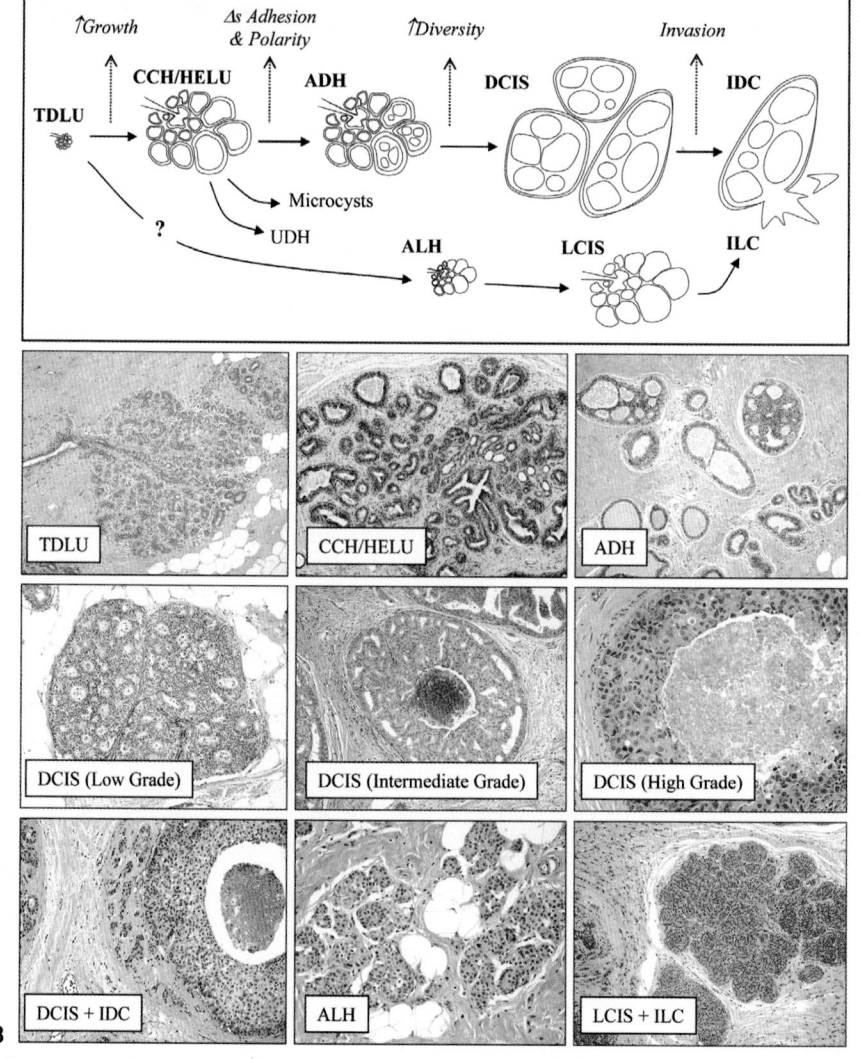

Figure 20.3B | The Wellings-Jensen model of breast cancer evolution proposes that the cellular origin of breast cancers occurs in the normal terminal duct lobular unit (TDLU) and that the putative precursors represent a nonobligatory series of increasingly abnormal stages that progress to cancer over long periods of time, probably decades in most cases. Briefly, the key stages in the so-called ductal lineage (representing about 80% of all breast cancers) are referred to as columnar cell hyperplasia (CCH) or hyperplastic enlarged lobular units (HELUs), atypical ductal hyperplasia (ADH), ductal carcinoma *in situ* (DCIS), and invasive ductal carcinoma (IDC). The stages in the so-called lobular lineage (representing the remaining 20% of carcinomas) are referred to as atypical lobular hyperplasia (ALH), lobular carcinoma *in situ* (LCIS), and invasive lobular carcinoma (ILC).

T-ONCOANATOMY

ORIENTATION OF THREE-PLANAR ONCOANATOMY

The isocenter for the breast three-planar anatomy is customarily at the thoracic T8-9 level. The planes for regional lymph nodes are midaxillary, midclavicular, and parasternal (Fig. 20.4).

T-Oncoanatomy

The mammary gland consists of 15 to 20 lobes of glandular tissue with varying amounts of fat in a dense fibroareolar stroma and is attached to the anterior chest wall by pectoral fascia. In cross-sections starting from the nipple, there are openings of the lactiferous ducts and their lactiferous sinuses, which are the conduits for the secretions of the hormonally stimulated breast glands. These ducts are distinct and individual for each lobule; they first run dorsally from the nipple and then spread radially into the glandular tissue.

The *three-planar views* illustrate the breast three-dimensionally in terms of its anatomic relationships to other structures (Fig. 20.5). As a superficial structure, the mammary gland is covered by skin. Posteriorly, the underlying pectoral muscles bind the breast to the chest wall. Deep to the glandular tissue, there is usually a small amount of fat, which, along with the breast proper, is bounded by a deeper layer of superficial fascia. This layer can usually be dissected free from the deep fascia invaginating the pectoralis major muscle. Connective tissue septa called the suspensory ligaments

(of Cooper) form subdivisions of the breast, dividing the breast into lobes.

The pectoralis major, the muscle underlying the breast, consists of two heads that arise from the clavicle, sternum, and cartilages of the first six ribs, and it inserts as a bilaminar structure on the anterolateral aspect of the humeral shaft.

The entire chest and breast must be considered as an anatomic unit. This requires knowledge of the underlying bony architecture, the muscles, as well as the nerves and vessels of the region.

- *Coronal:* As a superficial appendage of the chest wall, the mammary gland is covered by skin, and its glandular structures are compartmentalized between connective tissue septa—15 to 20 lobes that have their own lacunae and duct opening on the alveolar area of the nipple. Note the axillary tail (of Spence) of the breast.

- *Sagittal:* Most of the breast consists of fat; a region of loose connective tissue between the pectoral fascia muscle and breast—the retromammary space—permits mobility because the suspensory ligaments of Cooper allow alteration of shape with movement.

- *Axial:* The T8-9 level demonstrates the relationship of the breast to chest wall. The diagram is simplified by showing nerves on the right and arteries on the left. The three musculomembranous layers are the external intercostals muscle and membrane, internal intercostals muscle and membrane, and the innermost intercostals, transverse thoracic muscle, and the membrane connecting them. The intercostal nerves are the anterior rami of spinal nerves T1 to T11; the anterior ramus of T12 is the subcostal nerve.

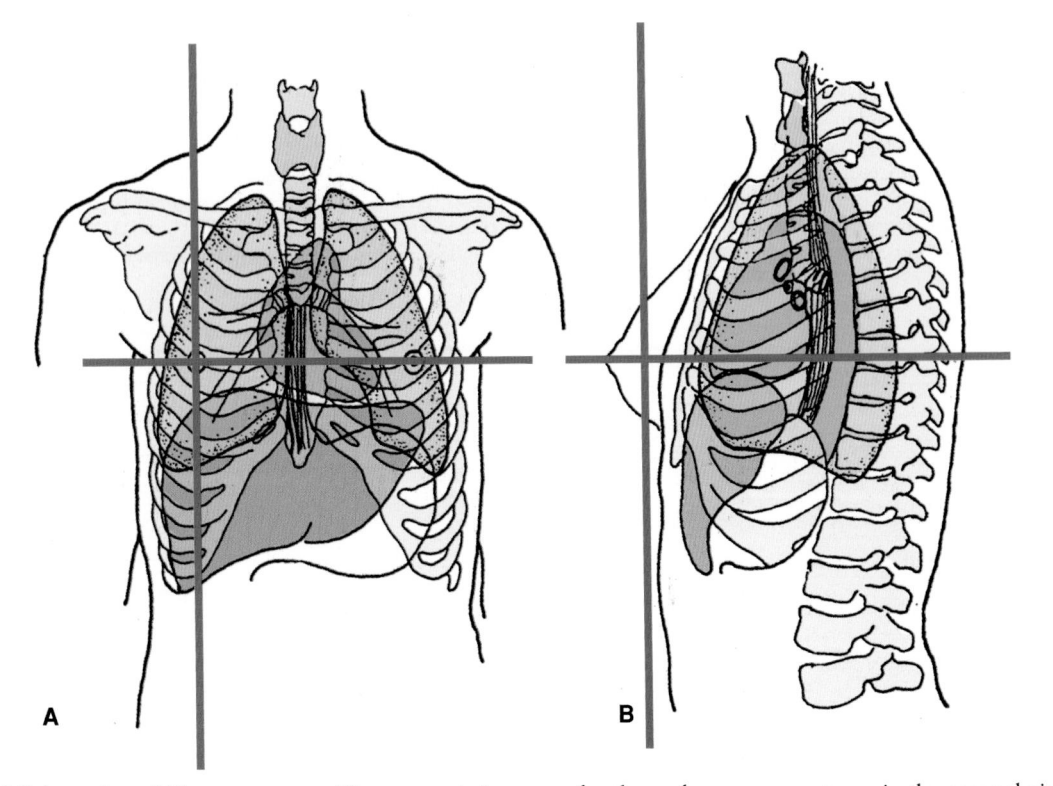

A　　　　**B**

Figure 20.4 | Orientation of T-oncoanatomy. The anatomic isocenter for three-planar oncoanatomy in the coronal view is placed lateral to midline over the breast and in the sagittal view anterior to the chest wall with the transverse view at the T8-9 level.

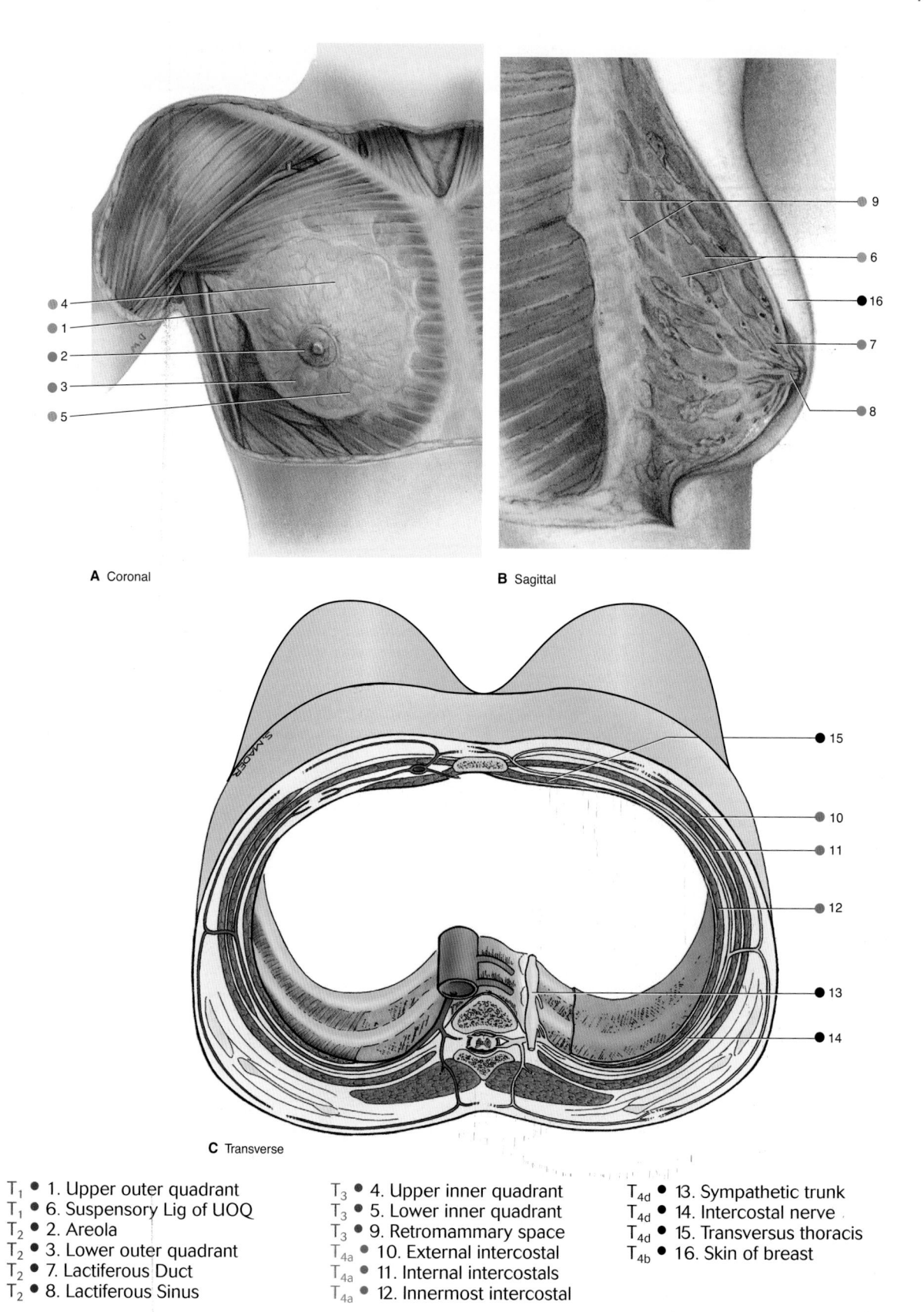

A Coronal

B Sagittal

C Transverse

T_1	● 1. Upper outer quadrant	T_3	● 4. Upper inner quadrant	T_{4d}	● 13. Sympathetic trunk
T_1	● 6. Suspensory Lig of UOQ	T_3	● 5. Lower inner quadrant	T_{4d}	● 14. Intercostal nerve
T_2	● 2. Areola	T_3	● 9. Retromammary space	T_{4d}	● 15. Transversus thoracis
T_2	● 3. Lower outer quadrant	T_{4a}	● 10. External intercostal	T_{4b}	● 16. Skin of breast
T_2	● 7. Lactiferous Duct	T_{4a}	● 11. Internal intercostals		
T_2	● 8. Lactiferous Sinus	T_{4a}	● 12. Innermost intercostal		

Figure 20.5 | T-oncoanatomy. Connecting the dots: Structures are color coded for cancer stage progression. The color code for the anatomic sites correlates with the color code for the stage group (Fig. 20.3) and patterns of spread (Fig. 20.2) and SIMLAP table (Table 20.2). Connecting the dots in similar colors will provide an appreciation for the 3D Oncoanatomy.

N-ONCOANATOMY AND M-ONCOANATOMY

N-ONCOANATOMY

The breast lymphatics drain via four major routes—axillary, transpectoral, internal thoracic parasternal (mammary) trunks, and intercostal into numerous surrounding regional nodes, such as axillary (low, middle), axillary apex, supraclavicular, internal thoracic parasternal, interpectoral, and subclavicular nodes. Other pathways include crossover lymphatic channels to the opposite breast and inferior drainage into diaphragmatic and subdiaphragmatic channels. (Note: Subclavicular nodes are considered juxtaregional on the ipsilateral side.) Disease involvement in all other nodes—cervical, contralateral, supraclavicular, and contralateral internal thoracic, and mammary nodes—is equivalent to distant metastases (Fig. 20.6; Table 20.4).

The axilla is a crucial area to multidisciplinary oncologic decision making. Thorough knowledge of the axillary nodal status requires surgical sampling or dissection by the surgical oncologist. The presence of positive axillary nodes often determines the use of adjuvant chemotherapy. And, if the axilla is to be treated by radiation therapy, it needs to be encompassed in its entirety.

The axillary contents consist of a variety of important structures. Damage to vessels can occur if they are injured during dissection. The major vessels include axillary veins, the cephalic vein and its branches, and the axillary artery and its branches. There is a close association between the brachial plexus and these vessels. Although perineural invasion by tumor is uncommon, it can occur.

Although anatomic knowledge of the region of the mammary nodes is quite important in oncologic decision making, internal thoracic (mammary or parasternal) nodes are most commonly identified in the first three intercostal spaces or the xiphisternal angle. These nodes lie laterally to the sternum in an approximately 1- to 2-cm-wide strip and are 3 cm deep to the chest wall. The deeper lymphatics within the thoracic cavity and mediastinum are important pathways for dissemination. They include the pleural, vertebral, and mediastinal nodes and the thoracic duct. Of equal importance clinically are the major lymphatic routes. The lymphatic circulation empties into the general circulation at the junction of the internal jugular and subclavian veins. Therefore, lymphatic metastases often become blood borne metastases, as if direct vascular invasion occurred.

REGIONAL LYMPH NODES

The breast lymphatics drain by way of three major routes: axillary, transpectoral, and internal mammary (Fig. 20.6). Intramammary lymph nodes reside within breast tissue and are coded as axillary lymph nodes for staging purposes. Supraclavicular lymph nodes are classified as regional lymph nodes for staging purposes. Metastases to any other lymph node, including cervical or contralateral internal mammary or axillary lymph nodes, are classified as distant (M1). The regional lymph nodes are as follows:

1. Axillary (ipsilateral): interpectoral (Rotter's) nodes and lymph nodes along the axillary vein and its tributaries that may be (but are not required to be) divided into the following levels:

   a. Level I (low-axilla): lymph nodes lateral to the lateral border of pectoralis minor muscle.

   b. Level II (mid-axilla): lymph nodes between the medial and lateral borders of the pectoralis minor muscle and the interpectoral (Rotter's) lymph nodes.

   c. Level III (apical axilla): lymph nodes medial to the medial margin of the pectoralis minor muscle and inferior to the clavicle. These are also known as apical or infraclavicular nodes. Metastases to these nodes portend a worse prognosis. Therefore, the infraclavicular designations will be used hereafter to differentiate these nodes from the remaining (level I, II) axillary nodes.

2. Internal thoracic (mammary) (ipsilateral): lymph nodes in the intercostal spaces along the edge of the sternum in the endothoracic fascia.

3. Supraclavicular: lymph nodes in the supraclavicular fossa, a triangle defined by the omohyoid muscle and tendon (lateral and superior border), the internal jugular vein (lower border). Adjacent lymph nodes outside of this triangle are considered to be lower cervical nodes (M1).

4. Intramammary: lymph nodes within the breast; these are considered axillary lymph nodes for purposes of N classification and staging.*

M-ONCOANATOMY

The rich plexus of veins parallel the lymphatics, with the outer quadrants draining into the axillary veins and the inner quadrants draining into the internal thoracic (mammary) veins. The axillary veins enter the subclavian, and the internal thoracic veins enter the brachiocephalic veins, which form the superior vena cava (Fig. 20.7). Metastatic breast cancer will result in an estimated death toll of almost 40,000 patients. The identification of circulating cancer cells for disseminated cancer cells in the blood or bone marrow has been designated M0(i+) in the 7th edition as a precursor state for metastases, but does not change the stage group. Monoclonal antibodies to epithelial cytokeratine or membrane glycoproteins can be used to detect bone marrow spread. Micro metastases are detected in 30% of patients, most often with negative prognostic factors as ERC-S, PRC-S, HER-2(+). If micro metastases are detected survival is poorer in multivariate outcome.

*Preceding passage from Edge SB, Byrd DR, and Compton CC, et al. *AJCC Cancer Staging Manual, 7th edition*. New York: Springer, 2010, pp. 352.

TABLE 20.4	Lymph Nodes of Breast	
Sentinel Nodes		**Juxtaregional Nodes**
Axillary		Supraclavicular
Internal mammary		Lateral axilla
		Parasternal contralateral
Regional Nodes		
Axillary, low		
Axillary, lateral		
Axillary, mid		
Axillary, apex		
Internal mammary (parasternal)		
Interpectoral		
Infraclavicular		

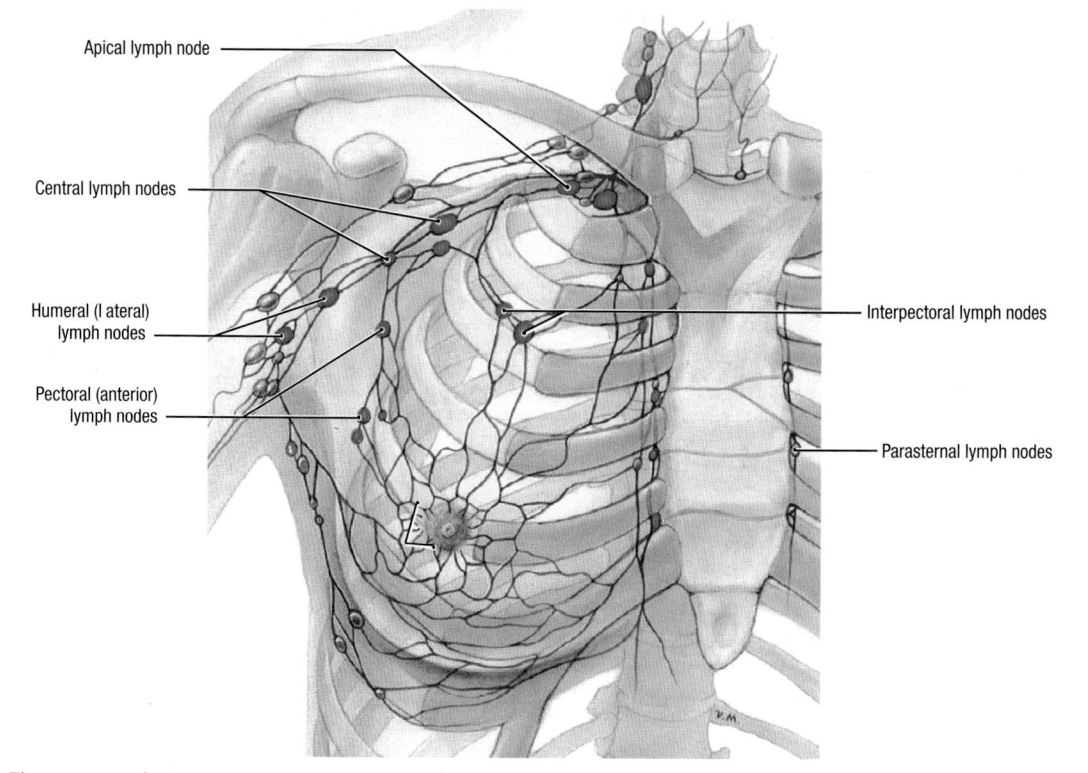

Figure 20.6 | N-oncoanatomy. Lymph drained from the upper limb and breast passes through nodes arranged irregularly in groups. Pectoral, along the inferior border of the pectoralis muscle. Subscapular, along the subscapular artery and veins. Brachial, along the distal part of the axillary vein. Central, at the base of the axilla embedded in axillary fat. Apical, along the axillary vein between the clavicle and the pectoralis minor muscle.

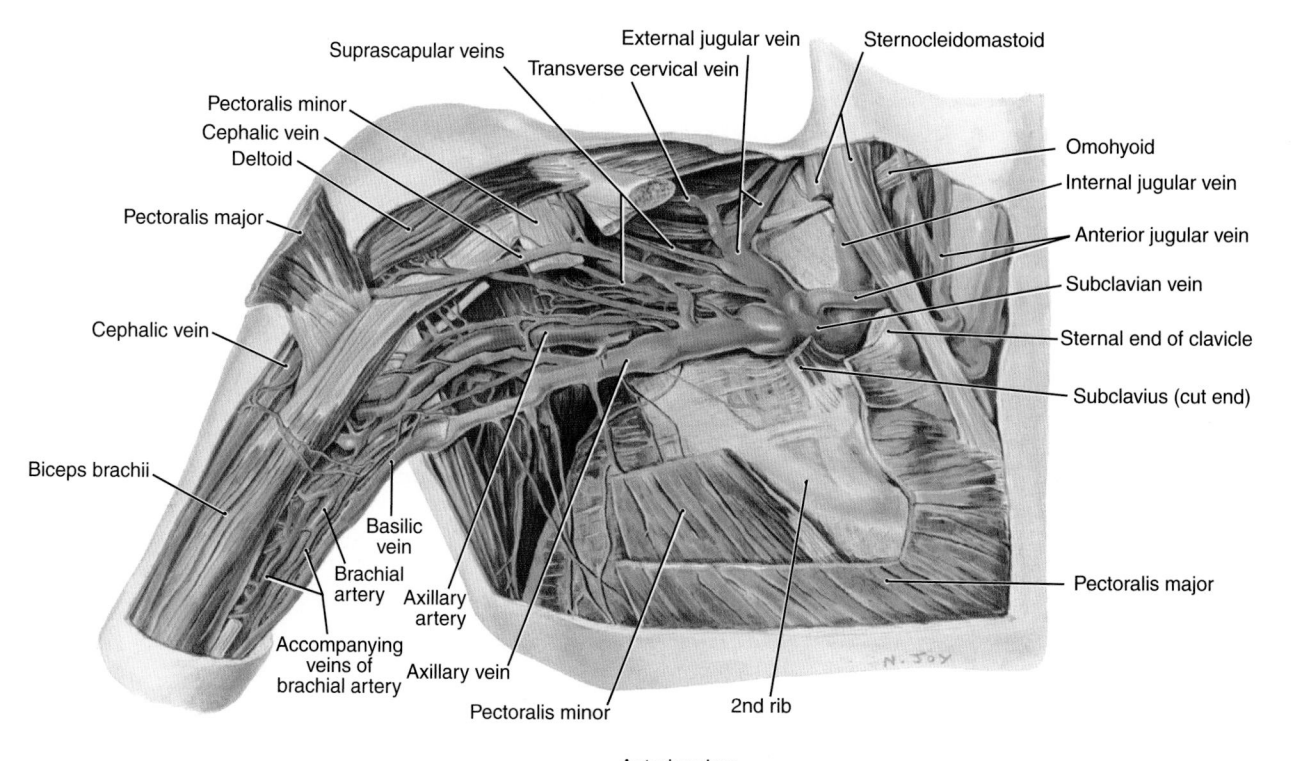

Anterior view

Figure 20.7 | M-oncoanatomy. The basilic vein joins the accompanying veins of the brachial artery to become the axillary vein at the inferior border of teres major, the axillary vein becomes the subclavian vein at the lateral border of the first rib, and the subclavian joins the internal jugular to become the brachiocephalic vein posterior to the sternal end of the clavicle. Observe the three suprascapular veins: One entering the axillary vein and two entering the external jugular vein.

RULES FOR CLASSIFICATION AND STAGING

Clinical Staging

With early and subclinical detection of breast cancer by screening mammography and further evaluation by MRI, the clinical staging that relied on physical examination, consisting of careful palpation and inspection of the mammary glands and draining lymph nodes, has been supplemented by image-guided biopsy of the breast and suspicious nodes. The key feature in staging is in determining the size of the invasive component within 4 months of diagnosis and in the absence of disease progression (Table 20.5; Fig. 20.8).

Pathologic Staging

The importance of pathologic staging (pT) is in its ability to truly assess the invasive component of a nodule and evaluate lymph node involvement, often as sentinel nodes determined by scintigraphy. The nodule needs to be completely excised for pT, only microscopic positive margins are allowed, not macroscopic. The intraductal component is not added to the invasive component. Microinvasion is defined as extension beyond the basement membrane, with no focus more than 0.1 cm in diameter. When multiple foci exist, the size of the largest is used to classify microinvasion. Similarly, for multiple primaries only the largest is given a T stage, no stage is assigned to smaller cancers.

- T1a is greater than 1 mm and less than or equal to 5 mm in greatest dimension;

- T1b is greater than 5 mm and less than or equal to 10 mm in greatest dimension; and

- T1c is greater than 10 mm and less than or equal to 20 mm in greatest dimension.

Curiously, microinvasion first defined in cervical uterine cancers is noted differently: $T1a_1$ is stromal invasion 3 mm in depth <7 mm horizontally and $T1a_2$ is greater than 3 mm × less than or equal to 7 mm, respectively.

The pN categories are the most detailed in the AJCC manual, noting both the size of micrometastases in nodes, as pN1Mi is greater than 0.2 mm to less than 2 mm, and the number of nodes involved as well as their geographic location. Each pN stage is modified into three subcategories, creating 9 to 12 possibilities. At issue awaiting more data and analysis are:

- Isolated tumor cells (ITCs) detected by immunohistochemical techniques may be as small as 1 mm or 500,000 cells; however, confirmatory hematoxylin and eosin stains are advised.

- ITC is defined as less than or 0.2 mm and micrometastases as greater than 0.2 mm but less than or 2 mm.

- RT-PCR can identify isolated cancer cells, but pN0 is advised with an appended designation of (mol+) or (mol−) as appropriate.

- The number of positive nodes is well supported by large series: 1 to 3 positive, 4 to 10 positive, and 10 positive show a progressive decline in survival as a function of the number of positive nodes.

- Supraclavicular lymph nodes (SCLN) are considered N3 and not M1 because survival is better with isolated SCLN without disseminated metastatic foci.

- Maturation of 80 potential prognostic variables remains under study, namely, p53, HER2/neu, and Ki-67.

Oncoimaging Annotations

- There are no pathognomonic mammographic signs that a lesion is either benign or malignant. The more irregular a mass is, the greater the likelihood of malignancy. Spiculated masses, however, can be caused by radial scars, postoperative scars, fat necrosis, desmoid tumors, hemorrhage, or abscesses.

- Approximately 10% of breast cancers are not mammographically visible. Only about two thirds of recurrent cancers in the treated breast are visible mammographically.

- On ultrasound, malignancies are typically ill defined, irregular, hypoechoic, taller than wide, and have posterior acoustic shadowing.

- MRI is the most reliable imaging study for assessing the presence of cancer. Contrast enhancement is not needed for this study. Dynamic contrast enhancement is, however, critical in the MRI evaluation of breast masses.

- Calcification per se is not a sign of malignancy and may be associated with firm adenomas, fibrocystic processes, and sclerosing adenosis.

- Highly suspicious calcifications are divided into two groups: pleomorphic or heterogeneous (granular) similar to a crushed stone pattern.

- Fine linear or branching in a discontinuous dot dash pattern are suspicious.

- Branching points in a duct produce Y-shaped patterns that can appear bizarre and are the most suspicious types seen on mammography.

TABLE 20.5	Diagnostic Capabilities of Current Imaging Modalities in Breast Cancer	
Method	Diagnosis and Staging Capability	Recommended for Use
Primary Tumor and Regional Nodes		
Mammography	Visualizes approximately 90% of breast cancers	Film/screen and xeromammography have similar diagnostic accuracies.
Ultrasound (dedicated)	Limited to identification of cystic lesions and evaluation of dense breast	Dedicated units are expensive and not suitable for stand-alone screening.
CT	Limited to evaluation of chest wall and internal mammary node involvement	Use of dedicated CT breast imaging systems had been abandoned.
MRI	Good for discrete lesions; calcifications are difficult to distinguish	Dedicated units are expensive. Useful for follow-up and for women with implants.
Metastatic Breast Cancer (as required)		
Chest x-ray film	Adequate for diagnosis; CT usually not needed	Essential for all tumor types.
Radionuclide bone scans	Essential for baseline verification and evaluation of symptomatic patients	Abnormal bone scans require film.
Liver and adrenal imaging	Indicated with abnormal chemistries or symptoms	Initial imaging study: radionuclide scan (requires validation of abnormal scan by ultrasound or CT).

CT, computed tomography; MRI, magnetic resonance imaging.
Modified from Bragg DG, Youker JE, eds. *Oncologic imaging.* Elmsford, NY: Pergamon, 1985.

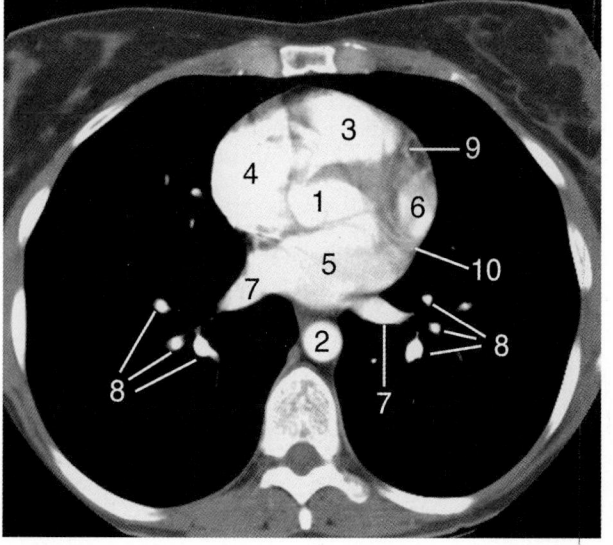
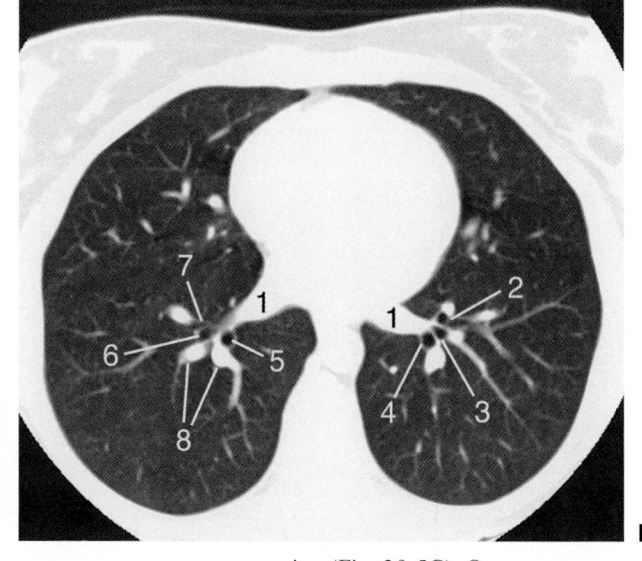

A   B

Figure 20.8 | Axial CTs of T8 and T9 level correlate with the T-oncoanatomy transverse section (Fig. 20.5C). Oncoanatomy with CT is commonly applied to staging cancers, often combined with PET to determine true extent of primary cancer and involved lymph nodes. **A.** Mediastinal window. 1, ascending aorta; 2, descending aorta; 3, right ventricle; 4, right atrium; 5, left atrium; 6, left atrial appendage; 7, inferior pulmonary vein; 8, segmental lower lobe artery; 9, left anterior descending coronary artery; 10, circumflex coronary artery. **B.** Lung window. 1, inferior pulmonary vein; 2, anteromedial segment LLL bronchus; 3, lateral segment LLL bronchus; 4, post segment LLL bronchus; 5, post segment RLL bronchus; 6, lateral segment RLL bronchus; 7, antior segment RLL bronchus; 8, segmental pulmonary artery.

PROGNOSIS

The limited number of prognostic factors are listed in Table 20.6.

TABLE 20.6	Prognostic Factors
Required for Staging	None
Clinically significant	Paget's disease
	Tumor grade (Scarff-Bloom-Richardson system)
	Estrogen receptor and test method (IHC, RT-PCR, other)
	Progesterone receptor and test method (IHC, RT-PCR, other)
	HER2 status and test method (IHC, FISH, CISH, RT-PCR, other)
	Method of lymph node assessment (e.g., clinical, fine needle aspiration; core biopsy; sentinel lymph node biopsy)
	IHC of regional lymph nodes
	Molecular studies regional lymph nodes
	Distant metastases method of detection (clinical, radiographic, biopsy)
	Circulating tumor cells (CTC) and method of detection (RT-PCR, immunomagnetic separation, other)
	Disseminated tumor cells (DTC; bone marrow micrometastases) and method of detection (RT-PCR, immunohistochemical, other)
	Multigene signature score
Response to neoadjuvant therapy	Will be collected in the registry but does not affect the postneoadjuvant stage
Complete response (CR)	Pathologic complete response can only be determined by histopathologic evaluation and is defined by the absence of invasive carcinoma in the breast and lymph nodes.
	Residual in situ cancer, in the absence of invasive disease, constitutes a pCR.
	Patients with isolated tumor foci in lymph nodes are not classified as having a CR. The presence of axillary nodal tumor deposits of any size, including cell clusters less than or equal to 0.2 mm, excludes a complete response. These patients will be categorized as ypN0(i+).
Partial response (PR)	A decrease in either or both the T or N category compared to the pretreatment T or N, and no increase in either T or N. After chemotherapy, one should use the method that most clearly defines tumor dimensions at baseline for this comparison, although prechemotherapy pT cannot be measured.
	Clinical (pretreatment) T will be defined by clinical and radiographic findings. y pathologic (posttreatment) T will be determined by pathologic size and extension.
	Nodal response should be determined by physical examination or radiologic evaluation, if the nodes are palpable or visible before chemotherapy. If prechemotherapy pathologic lymph node involvement is demonstrated by fine-needle aspiration, core biopsy, or sentinel node biopsy, it should be recorded as such. Absence of posttreatment pathologic nodal involvement should be used to document pathologic complete response, and should be recorded, but does not necessarily represent a true "response" since one does not know whether lymph nodes removed surgically postchemotherapy were involved prior to chemotherapy.
No response (NR)	No apparent change in either the T or N categories compared to the clinical (pretreatment) assignment or an increase in the T or N category at the time of y pathologic evaluation.
	Clinical (pretreatment) T will be defined by clinical and radiographic findings.
	yp (posttreatment) T will be determined by pathologic size.
	The response category will be appended to the y stage description. For example: ypTisypN0cM0CR; ypT1ypN0cM0PR; ypT-2ypN1cM0NR

IHC, immunohistochemistry; RT-PCR, reverse transcription-polymerase chain reaction; FISH, fluorescence in situ hybridization; CISH, chromogenic in situ hybridization.
From Edge SB, Byrd DR, Compton CC, et al. *AJCC Cancer Staging Manual.* 7th ed. New York: Springer, 2010, p. 361, with permission.

PROGNOSIS AND CANCER SURVIVAL

CANCER STATISTICS AND SURVIVAL

Breast cancer death rates have been decreasing since 1990, after 5 decades with minimal change. The dramatic improvement in breast cancer survival is due to multiple factors including early detection and improved multimodal treatments, often with breast conservation. There are more than 200,000 new cases of breast cancer diagnosed in the USA, which constitutes 28% of all female cancers and is the most common female cancer. Nevertheless, breast cancer accounts for approximately 40,000 deaths, 15% of all cancer deaths in females, and are the second most common female death exceeded only by lung cancer.

Early detection, by mammography on average will detect 80 to 90% of breast cancers in women without symptoms. MRI is recommended for women at high risk, i.e., family history of breast cancer, have BRAC1 and BRAC2 gene expression, use of combined estrogen and progesterone, and high radiation dose in young women survivors with Hodgkin's disease.

The five year survival rates have improved from 60% in the 1950's to 90% currently. Also, five year survival for Stage I cancer is 98%, decreases with regional node involvement to 84%, and decrements with metastases to 23%. All stages combined are 82% at ten years, and 75% at 15 years. The observed survival rates of breast cancer based on the National Cancer Database (271,645 cases) as shown in Figure 20.10, which is presented at 5 year rates.

The impact of two important prognostic factors are:

- Diameter of primary tumor (cm) <2 cm − >5 cm.
- Nodal involvement 1–3+ nodes, and 4+ nodes (Fig. 20.11).

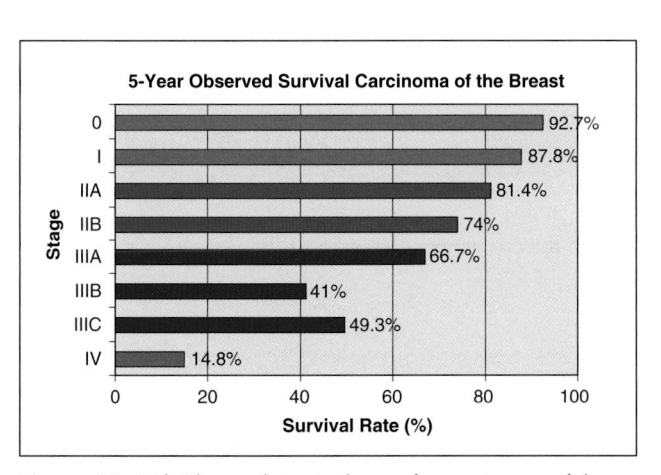

Figure 20.10 | Observed survival rates for carcinoma of the breast. Data from the National Cancer Data Base (Commission on Cancer of the American College of Surgeons and the American Cancer Society). Diagnosed in years 2001–2002.

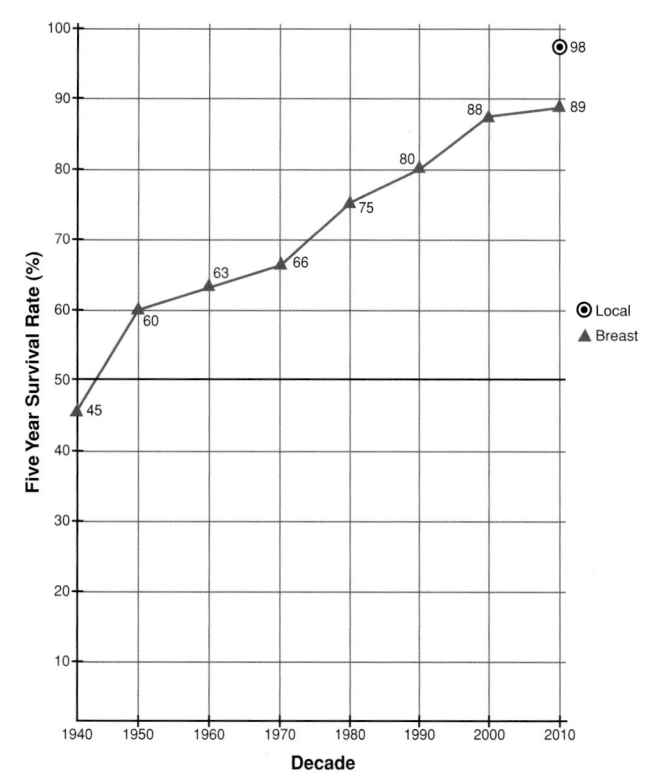

Figure 20.9 | Trajectory for breast cancer curability.

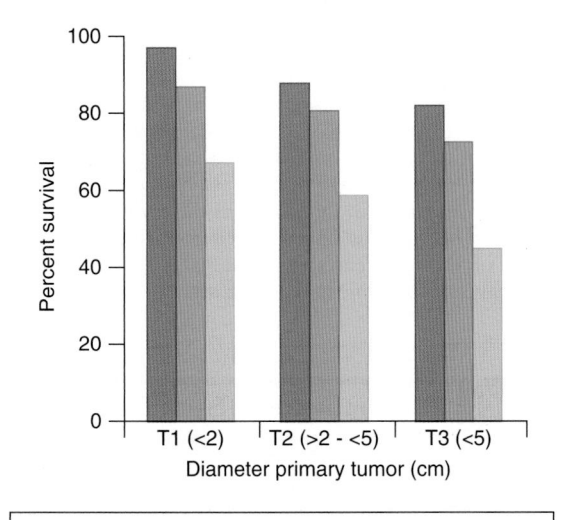

Figure 20.11 | Impact of tumor diameter and nodal involvement on breast cancer survival.

21
Thoracic Esophagus

PERSPECTIVE, PATTERNS OF SPREAD, AND PATHOLOGY

Although the esophagus is thought of as a thoracic organ, cancers of the esophagus can arise in the neck and abdomen as well as the chest.

PERSPECTIVE AND PATTERNS OF SPREAD

Esophageal cancers vary in their presentation, depending on the anatomic site of origin: cervical, thoracic, or abdominal. This long, tubular structure is subject to a variety of stresses beginning with smoking and alcohol abuse and terminating with acid reflux and hiatal hernia. The histopathologic types reflect their histogenic origin (Table 21.2).

The incidence of esophageal cancers is approximately 16,640 new cases with an appalling 80% mortality rate unless the cancer is detected in its early stages. In some regions of the world, there is a very high prevalence, namely, northern provinces of China (20% of all cancer deaths), the Transkei province in South America (50% of all cancers), and the Gonbad region of northern Iran (200 times that of the United States). Numerous risk factors exist as aforementioned. Of interest is the early esophageal staging system. The Japanese have evolved an early staging system because of their increased and intensive screening and because this cancer is endemic in the Far East.

The concern for esophageal cancer is ulceration and perforation, which can lead to numerous disastrous complications, depending on the surrounding anatomy: in the upper third, tracheoesophageal fistulas, in the middle third, aortoesophageal perforation can lead to a fatal and rapid exsanguination, and in the lower third, pericardial tamponade can result in pulsus paradoxus and heart failure (Fig. 21.2; Table 21.2).

The malignant gradient is high throughout, with more survivors in the cervical segment decreasing intrathoracically and least at the gastroesophageal junction because of the ease of cancer spread to infradiaphragmatic sites.

There are a wide variety of mediastinal tumors due to different origins of many tissues. The mediastinum is divided into four distinct compartments and each are prone to specific neoplasms. The anterior superior compartment contains the thymus and lymph nodes. Thus thymomas, thymic carcinomas, Hodgkin's lymphoma (HL), and non-Hodgkin's lymphomas are more common. The middle compartment contains the heart, which uncommonly is involved in neoplastic transformation into sarcomas. The anterior inferior compartment may give rise to germ cell tumors or germinomas that differentiate into different cell lives. The posterior compartment is prone to neurogenic tumors, from pediatric neuroblastomas to neurofibromas.

The esophagus transverses the posterior mediastinum and is the major site prone to develop squamous cell cancers, and at the cardia junction, to develop stomach adenocarcinomas.

TABLE 21.1	Histopathologic Type: Common Cancers of the Esophagus
Type	
Squamous cell carcinoma	
Adenocarcinoma	

Note: The classification applies to all carcinomas. Sarcomas are not included. Worldwide, squamous cell carcinomas are the most common, but the incidence of adenocarcinoma is increasing. In North America and Europe, adenocarcinomas are more common than squamous cell carcinomas. Adenocarcinomas arising from Barrett esophagus are included in the classification. From Edge SB, Byrd DR, and Compton CC, et al. (eds). *AJCC Cancer Staging Manual, 7th edition.* New York: Springer, 2010, p. 111.

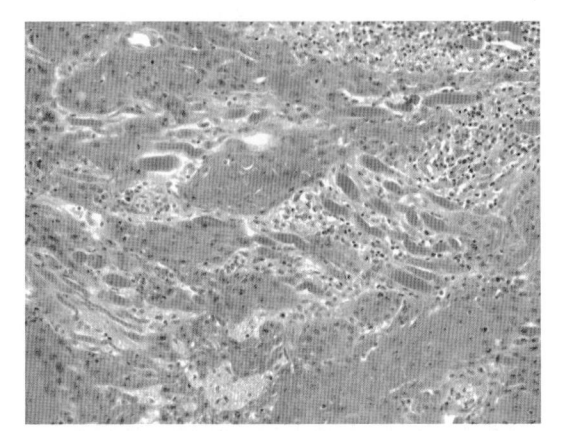

Figure 21.1 | A squamous cell carcinoma with a typical pattern of infiltration.

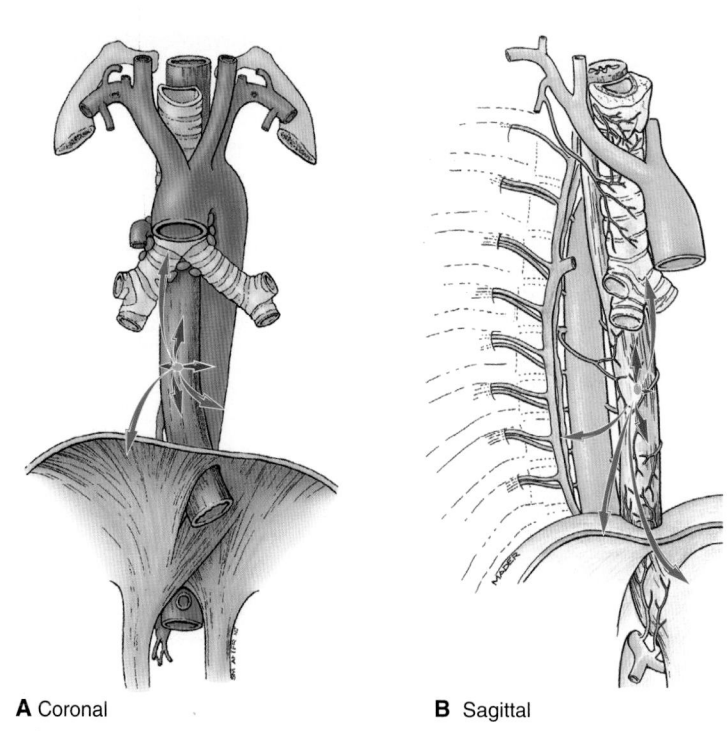

A Coronal   **B** Sagittal

Figure 21.2 | Patterns of spread. T categories. The patterns of spread and the primary tumor classification are similarly color coded: Tis, yellow, cancer in situ of mucosa; T1, green (infiltrates the submucosa); T2, blue (penetrates to the muscularis propria); T3, purple (reaches the subserosa); and T4, red (invades through the serosa into a neighboring viscera). **A.** Coronal: Invasion into trachea and bronchi. **B.** Sagittal: Invasion into aorta. The concept of visualizing patterns of spread to appreciate the surrounding anatomy is well demonstrated by the six-directional pattern i.e. SIMLAP Table 21.2.

PATHOLOGY

The thoracic esophagus is largely a stratified squamous epithelium that gives rise to squamous cell carcinomas and is similar to the mucous membrane of the upper digestive passage, which has a rich network of submucosal lymphatics and capillary loops. The lower esophagus is prone to develop adenocarcinoma owing to Barrett epithelial islands of gastric mucosa (Fig. 21.1; Table 21.1). This variety of cancer is presented separately, with digestive system cancers of the abdomen.

TABLE 21.2	SIMLAP	
Thoracic Esophagus		
S	Submucosal lymphatics (longitudinal layer of muscularis propria)	• T2
	Aortic arch	• T4
	Azygos vein	• T4
I	Submucosal lymphatics (longitudinal layer of muscularis propria)	• T2
	Mediastinal lymph nodes	• **N1**
M	Mediastinal lymph nodes	• **N1**
	Submucosa	• T1
	(circular layer of muscularis propria)	• T2
L	Mediastinal lymph nodes	• **N1**
	(circular layer of muscularis propria)	• T2
	Right or left main bronchus	• T4
A	Adventitia of esophagus (Tracheoesophageal fistula)	• T3
	Pericardium	• T4
	Inferior vena cava	• T4
P	Descending aorta	• T4
	Thoracic duct	• T4
	Vertebral body	• T4
	Spinal cord	• T4

The six vectors of invasion are <u>S</u>uperior, <u>I</u>nferior, <u>M</u>edial, <u>L</u>ateral, <u>A</u>nterior, and <u>P</u>osterior. The color-coded dots correlate the T stage with specific anatomic structure involved.

TNM STAGING CRITERIA

TNM STAGING CRITERIA

Esophageal staging has remained consistent with some changes in T and N categories. The only histologic difference from other hollow digestive system sites is the presence of an adventitia instead of a serosa. This allows for distensibility of the esophagus to accommodate a food bolus because, in its normal collapsed state, it appears on computed tomography (CT) to have a straw-like lumen of a few millimeters. T1 is mucosal, T2 muscular, T3 adventitial, and T4 is into the surrounding structures (Fig. 21.2).

SUMMARY OF CHANGES SEVENTH EDITION AJCC

- Tumor location is simplified, and esophagogastric junction and proximal 5 cm of stomach are included.
- Tis is redefined and T4 is subclassified into T4a resectable, T4b unresectable.
- Regional lymph nodes are redefined. N is subclassified according to the number of regional lymph nodes containing metastasis.
- M is redefined.
- There are separate stage groupings for squamous cell carcinoma and adenocarcinoma.
- Stage groupings are reassigned using T, N, M, and G classifications.
- Thoracic esophagus addressed the T-oncoanatomy of the mediastinum, and in turn emphasizes the importance of mediastinal lymph nodes (Fig. 21.3A). The more common neoplasms of the mediastinum include Hodgkin's (H) lymphoma, NH lymphomas. The esophageal tube is a hollow serial organ that encompasses the entire thorax, entering at the thoracic inlet and exits at the diaphragm. The T stage refers to depth of penetration of its wall:

- T1 submucosa
- T2 muscularis propria (externa)
- T3 adventitia
- T4 adjacent structures

- N stage criteria have changed and depend on node number.
- Stage groups are different with the four stage groups mushrooming into eight stage groups.
- Histopathology: Squamous cell cancer and adenocarcinoma each have their separate staging systems.
- Tumor grade and tumor location have been added, introducing more parameters into the staging system.

The TNM Staging Matrix is color coded for identification of Stage Group once T and N stages are determined (Table 21.3).

TABLE 21.3 | **Stage Summary Matrix**

	N0	N1	N2	N3	M1
T1	I*	IIB	IIIA	IIIC	IV
T2	II**	IIB	IIIA	IIIC	IV
T3	II**	III	IIIB	IIIC	IV
T4	III	III	IIIC	IIIC	IV

Location	X	1	2	3
X	IB	IB	IIA	IIA
Lower	IB	IB	IIA	IIA
Middle	IIA	IIA	IIB	IIB
Upper	IIA	IIA	IIB	IIB

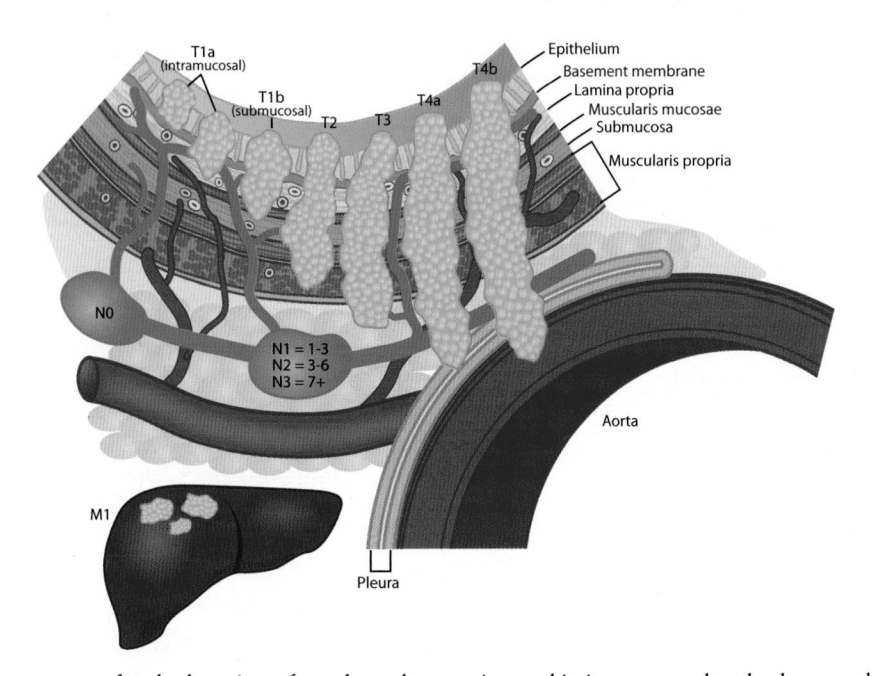

Figure 21.3A | The importance of early detection of esophageal cancer is noted in intramucosal and submucosal phases.

THORACIC ESOPHAGUS SQUAMOUS CELL

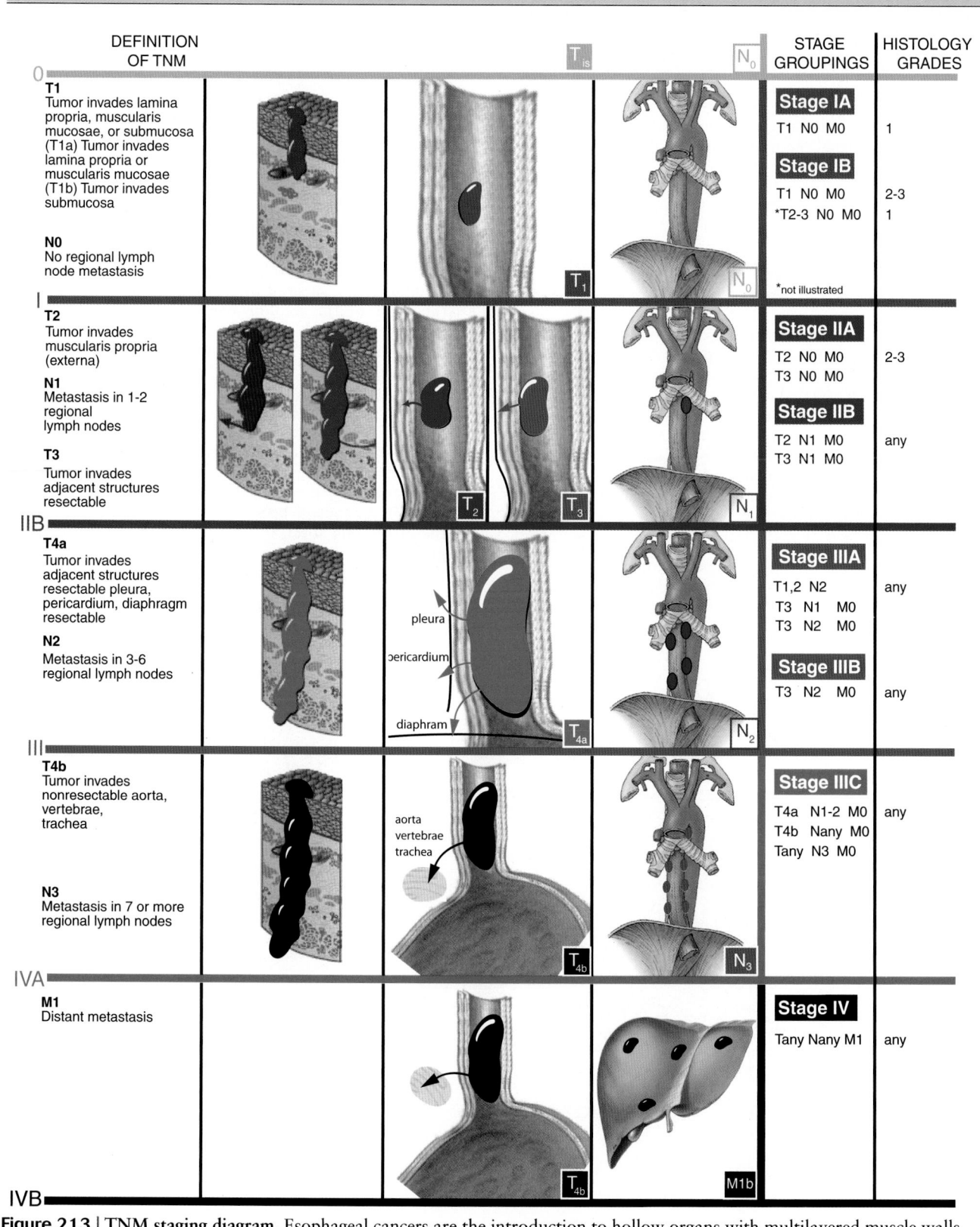

Figure 21.3 | TNM staging diagram. Esophageal cancers are the introduction to hollow organs with multilayered muscle walls lined by an epithelial mucosa on the inside and adventitia or serosa outside. Vertical presentation of stage groupings, which follow the same color code for cancer advancement, are organized in horizontal lanes: Stage 0, yellow; I, green; II, blue; III, purple; IVA, red; and metastatic stage IVB, black. Definitions of TN are on left and stage grouping is on the right. The histologic section of the esophageal wall illustrates the cancer invasion into and through the wall layers (Fig. 21.1). Note the nodal distribution is from the neck to the abdomen although the esophagus is a thoracic organ.

T-ONCOANATOMY

ORIENTATION OF THREE-PLANAR ONCOANATOMY

The isocenter chosen for the esophagus is at the thoracic T9/T10 level to signal the termination of primary sites in the thorax and simultaneously introduce the beginning of the digestive system. T9/T10 is the level of the esophageal opening in the diaphragm; T8 is for the level of the opening for the vena cava; and T12 is the stomal opening for the aorta (Fig. 21.4).

T-oncoanatomy

- *Coronal:* The T-oncoanatomy of the esophagus consists of three principal regions: cervical, thoracic, and cardiac portions (Fig. 21.5). The cervical esophagus extends from the pharyngeal–esophageal junction (the cricopharyngeal sphincter) inferiorly to the level of the thoracic inlet, about 18 cm from the upper incisor teeth. The upper and midthoracic esophagus extends from the thoracic inlet to a point 10 cm above the esophagogastric junction, which is usually at the level of the lower border of the esophagus to the cardiac orifice of the stomach, which is about 40 cm from the upper incisor teeth (Fig. 21.5A).
- *Sagittal:* The esophagus is a muscular tube consisting of two layers of smooth muscle, one longitudinal and the other horizontal, and this is carried through into the rest of the gastrointestinal system. Peristalsis is initiated with swallowing and the major function is to propel food into the stomach. There are two sphincters in the esophagus: the cricopharyngeal muscle and the cardiac sphincter at the cardia of the stomach. These sphincters have been extensively studied from the physiologic point of view and are common sites of both benign and neoplastic disease (Fig. 21.5B).
- *Transverse:* The esophageal opening of the diaphragm is anterior and to the left (T10) of the aorta (T12); note the esophagus in between the right and left layer of the mediastinum. The course of the esophagus is from slightly to the right of the midline to the left as it pierces the diaphragm through its own opening. It is in continual contact with the right lung; on the left side, the aorta is in continual contact with the left lung. The azygos vein provides a partial shield on the right side and posteriorly. Pulmonary veins are expected to be in more intimate contact because they drain to the left atrium, which is posterior to the ventricle. The thoracic duct is posterior to the esophagus along its course, which is the reverse of the esophagus coursing from the right side of midline to the left as it ascends. When the esophagus comes in front of the descending aorta, it is suspended by the mesoesophagus, which allows it to curve forward before its passes through the diaphragm (Fig. 21.5C).

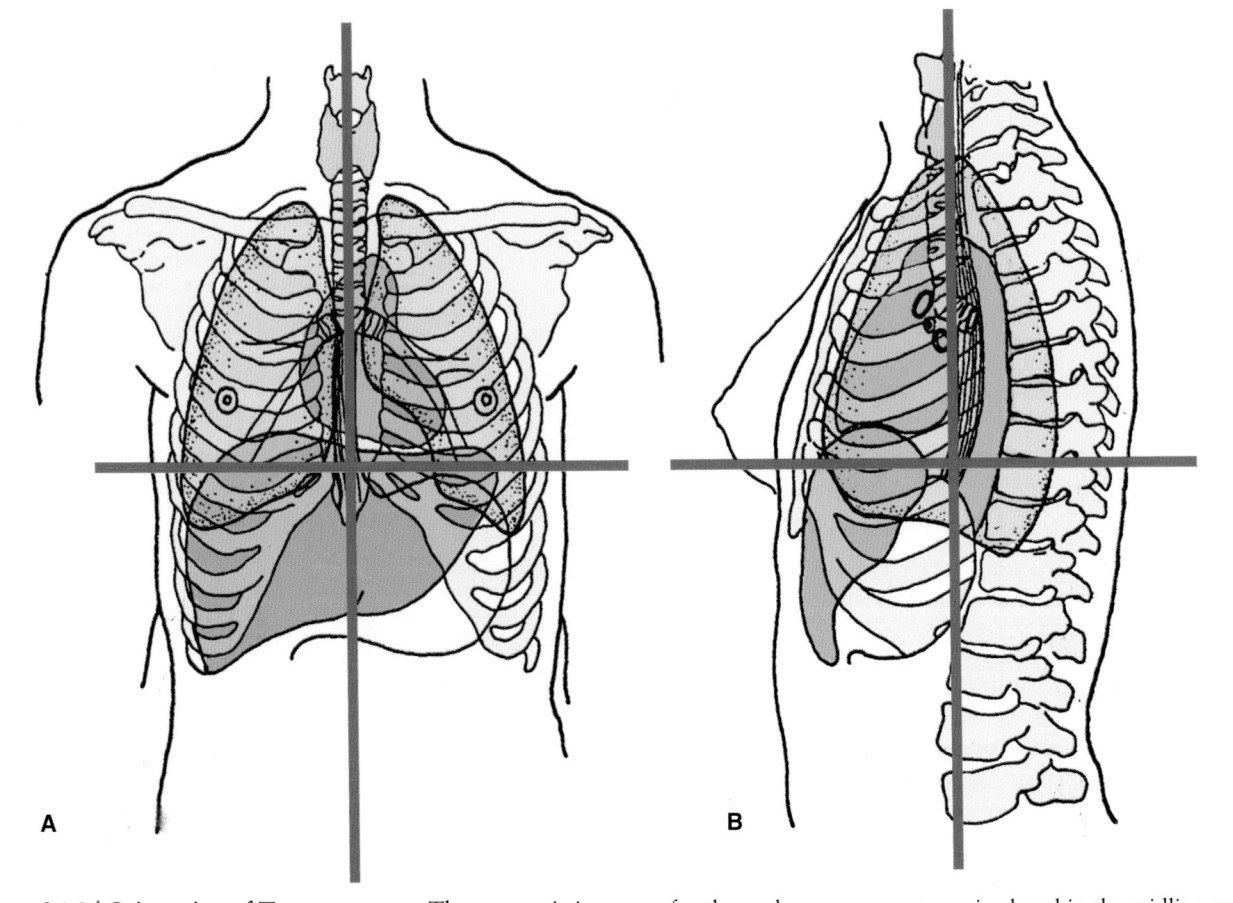

Figure 21.4 | Orientation of T-oncoanatomy. The anatomic isocenter for three-planar oncoanatomy is placed in the midline and at the T9/T10 level at the dome of the diaphragm. **A.** Coronal. **B.** Sagittal.

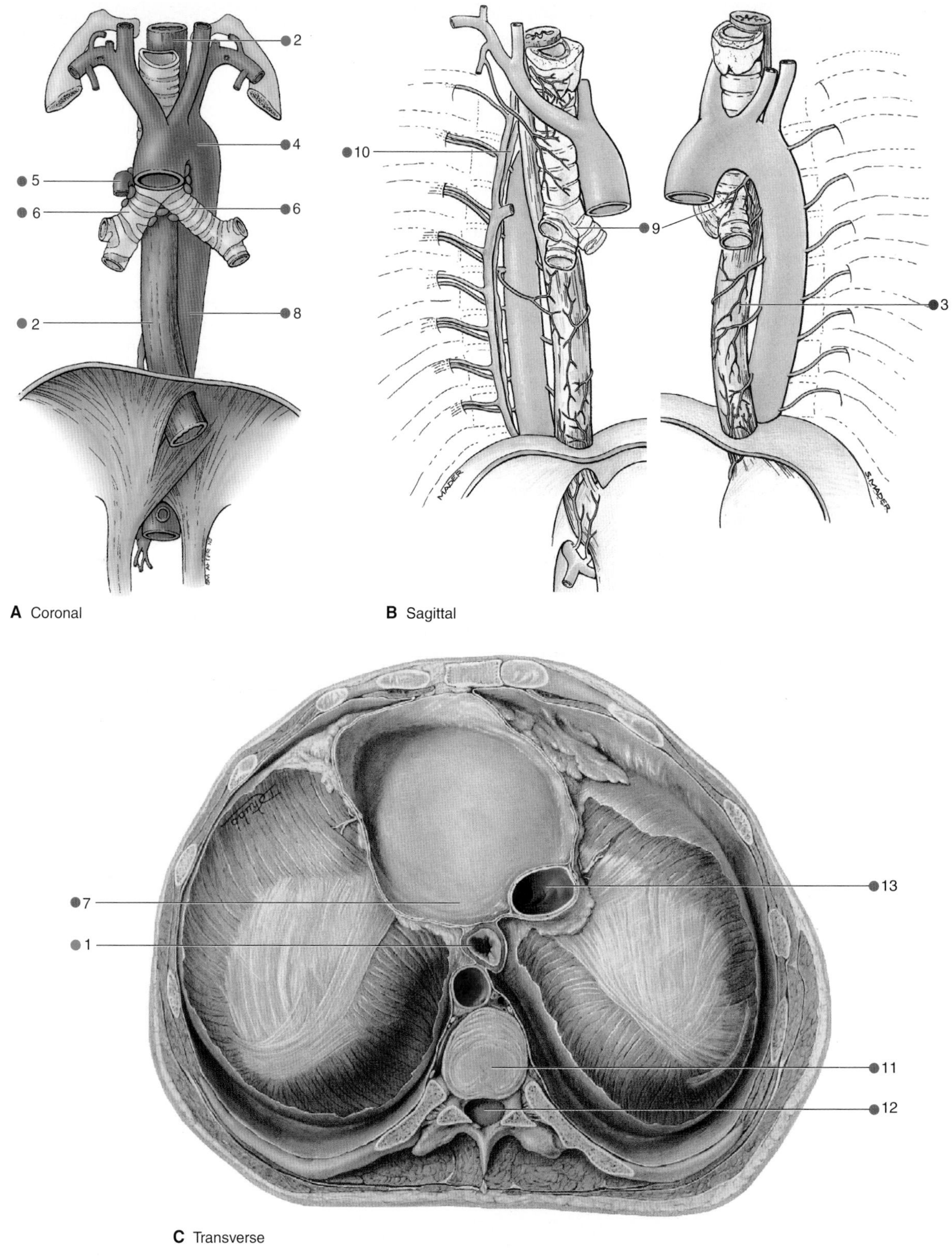

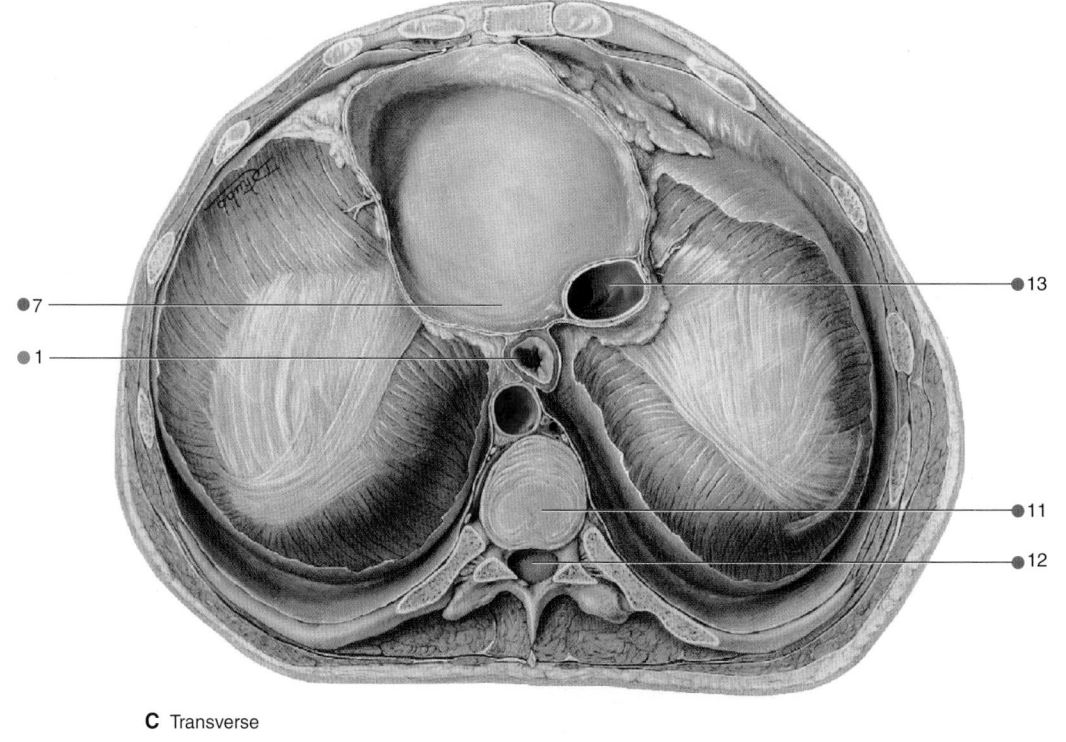

A Coronal   **B** Sagittal

C Transverse

T_1 ● 1. Submucosa	T_4 ● 6. Right and Left Main Bronchus T_4 ● 11. Vertebral Body
T_2 ● 2. Esophagus	T_4 ● 7. Percardium T_4 ● 12. Spinal Cord
T_3 ● 3. Adventitia of Esophagus	T_4 ● 8. Descending Aorta T_4 ● 13. Inferior Vena Cava
T_4 ● 4. Aortic Arch	T_4 ● 9. Trachea Burification
T_4 ● 5. Azygos Vein Arch	T_4 ● 10. Thoracic Duct

Figure 21.5 | T-oncoanatomy. Connecting the dots: Structures are color coded for cancer stage progression. The Color Code for the anatomic sites correlates with the color code for the stage group (Figure 21.3B) and patterns of spread (Figure 21.2) and SIMLAP table (Table 21.2). Connecting the dots in similar colors will provide an appreciation for the 3D Oncoanatomy.

N-ONCOANATOMY AND M-ONCOANATOMY

N-ONCOANATOMY

The American Joint Committee on Cancer (AJCC)/International Union Against Cancer numbering of cervical mediastinal lymph nodes is consistent with IASLC lymph node map for lung cancers. Abdominal lymph nodes are numbered separately, and it differs from the International Anatomic Terminology.

The regional lymph nodes for the cervical esophagus are the cervical and supraclavicular nodes. For the thoracic esophagus, the regional nodes are the adjacent mediastinal lymph nodes. Non regional nodal involvement is considered distant metastasis. Retrograde and prograde lymphatic spread usually places all of the lymph node stations in the neck, mediastinum, and abdomen at risk. One of the major problems with control of this cancer is the frequency with which lymph node invasion occurs and the rapidity of its dissemination to the other distant anatomic areas. Esophageal cancer is therefore not only a disease of the chest, but also of the neck and abdomen. Because of its lymphatic drainage, esophageal cancer is a formidable tumor to encompass by locoregional modalities of therapy (Fig. 21.6; Table 21.4).

Since the esophagus extends the entire vertical length of the thorax, the patterns of spread vary with the segment in which the cancer arises. Customarily the thoracic esophagus is divided into three segments: The upper third extends from the thoracic inlet to the level of the tracheal bifurcation; the middle third lies between the carina and 5 cm above the diaphragm; and the lower third includes the esophagogastric junction.

M-ONCOANATOMY

A rich plexus of venous anastomoses exists with stomach, liver, pancreas, and adrenals. Therefore, the liver, lung, and adrenals are the most common sites of distant metastases. Remote metastasis from the carcinoma of the esophagus, although ultimately fatal, often carries a better prognosis than when the primary lesion has extended locally outside the esophagus into mediastinal structures, a condition that is rapidly fatal.

TABLE 21.4	Sentinel and Regional Lymph Nodes (LN)
Thoracic Esophagus	
Upper Thoracic (Cervical) Esophagus	
Sentinel LN:	Scalene, supraclavicular (1)
	LT and RT paratracheal (2R/2L)
Regional LN:	Mid and upper Cervical
	Upper mediastinal periesophageal (3P)
	Carinal (7)
	Paratracheal (10R+10L)
	Aortopulmonary (5)
	Anterior mediastinal (6)
Mid Thoracic Esophagus	
Sentinel LN:	Mid periesophageal posterior mediastinal (3P)
	RT + LT lower tracheobronchial nodes (4R/4L)
	Carinal, subcarinal (7)
Lower Thoracic Esophagus	
Sentinel LN:	Mid paraesophageal (8M)
	Lower paraesophageal (8L)
Regional LN:	Pulmonary ligament (9)
	Diaphragmatic (15)
	Paracardial (16)
	Left gastric (17)
	Common hepatic (18)
	Splenic nodes (19)
	Coeliac nodes (20)

Nomenclature and numbers are from Edge SB, Byrd DR, and Compton CC, et al. *AJCC Cancer Staging Manual, 7th edition*. New York, Springer, 2010, pp.106–107, 10.3C.

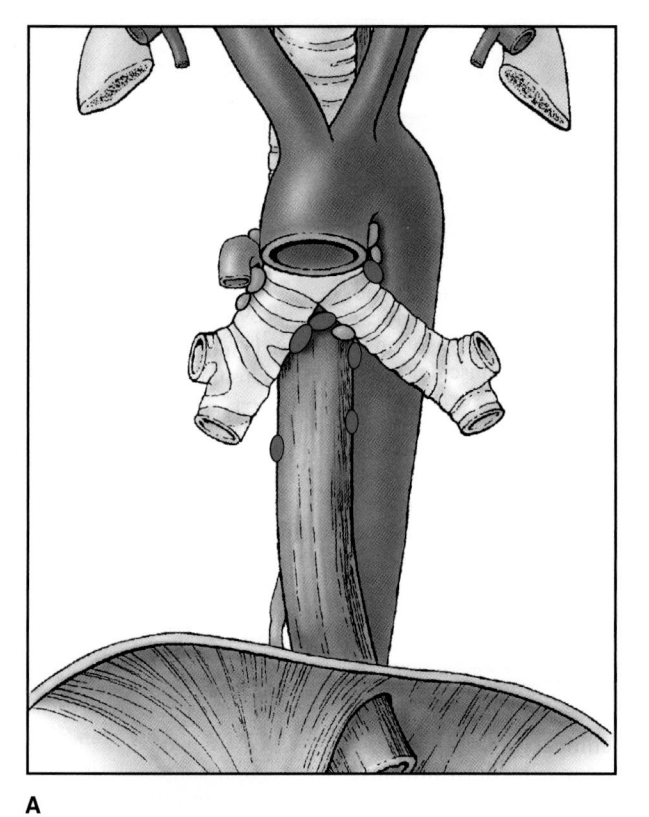

A

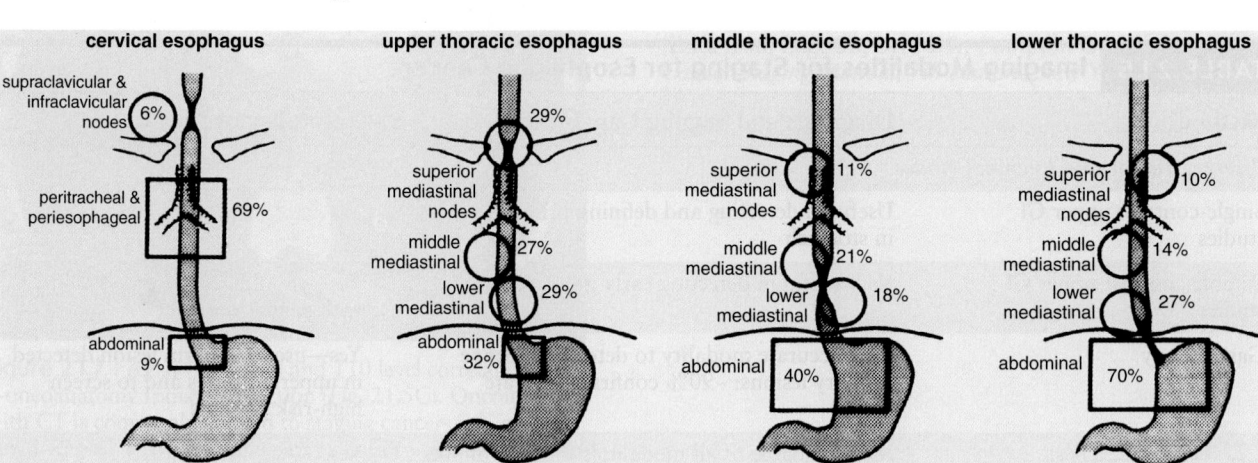

B

Figure 21.6 | Orientation of N-oncoanatomy. A. Mediastinal sentinel nodes vary depending on location of cancer. Paracarinal and subcarinal nodes are frequently involved. **B.** The percentage of positive lymph nodes found at surgery for esophageal carcinoma in the upper, middle, and lower esophagus. (B: From Akiyama H, Tsurumaru M, Kawamura T. Principles of surgical treatment of carcinoma of the esophagus: Analysis of lymph node involvement. *Ann Surg* 1981;194(4):438–446, with permission.)

TNM STAGING CRITERIA

CLASSIFICATION AND STAGING

TNM Staging Criteria

Gastrointestinal Tract

The pattern of hollow viscous invasion varies with the anatomic location or site of origin of the cancer in the GIT. The size of the lumen and the proximity of the tumor to sphincters determine whether obstruction is an early expression of malignant activity or a sign of an extensive tumor. Adjacent structures are invaded first, particularly those in direct proximity. The bowel loops with mesenteries are more mobile than those that are fixed and can spread their cancer cells intraperitoneally more readily. Tumor behavior is a function of the anatomy and physiology at each of the major sites in the alimentary tract. The GIT is a hollow tubular organ. The cancer's depth of penetration of the wall of bowel is the commonality for staging at all sites, T1, T2, T3, and T4—mucosal, muscularis, serosa, and adjacent viscera, respectively (Fig. 22.3). This is also the rule for most other hollow organs in other systems—for example, gallbladder and bile ducts (Table 22.2). Staging in solid organs (pancreas and liver) is based on tumor size T1, T2 and capsular invasion T3 and major vessels invasion is T4.

The lymphoid drainage of the digestive system and that of major digestive glands (MDGs) overlap and reflect both the arterial blood supply and venous drainage, which are not always parallel. The small intestine is a major extranodal site with its Peyer patches, and the appendix is an analog for the bursa of Fabricius, the origin for B cells in lower vertebrates. The mesenteric nodes are not acknowledged in the lymphoma staging as a node-bearing region. The para-aortic and paracaval locations for lymph nodes relate to the roots of origin of visceral arteries as the celiac, superior, and inferior mesenteric arteries. Smooth metastatic nodules in the pericolic and perirectal fat are considered lymph node metastases and counted in N staging. Irregular nodules are considered as vascular invasion and are either V1 (microscopic) or V2 (macroscopic) when viewed histopathologically.

The sentinel lymph nodes for each primary site are also noted.

When the visceral vessels drain into the inferior vena cava, the retroperitoneal lymph nodes cluster along the abdominal aorta and inferior vena cava vessels. When these nodes are involved, they are juxtaregional and can be considered metastatic nodes. The staging of nodes in the gastrointestinal region is extremely varied, and one can only speculate as to the lack of more uniform criteria in the sixth edition AJCC. At most major primary sites, there is only an N1 designation independent of size and number of nodes involved. Thus, N1 is simply a positive node and applies to esophagus, small intestine, liver, pancreas, gallbladder, extrahepatic ducts, and ampulla of Vater.

The colon and rectum are similar to the breast in that N1 is one to three nodes and N2 is more than four nodes. The stomach was the most distinct site, with an elaborate nodal classification: N1, 1 to 6 nodes; N2, 7 to 15 nodes; and N3, ≥15 nodes. This has been revised in the seventh edition.

Major Digestive Glands and Ducts

The major feature in staging cancer of the liver and pancreas is size of the cancer(s) and venous invasion or entrapment of major arteries and veins that render such malignancies unresectable with conventional radical surgery. However, the increasing use of liver transplantation and/or liver–pancreas transplants with their connecting extrahepatic ducts may require the criteria of unresectability to be revamped. For the liver a size of 5 cm and for the pancreas a size of 2 cm divides lesions between early (T1) and advanced (T2, T3; Fig. 22.3). The gallbladder and extrahepatic duct cholangiocarcinomas, and the rare cancer of the hepatopancreatic ampulla (of Vater) masquerade as gallstones, presenting with obstructive jaundice. If detected when those duct cancers are contained within their walls, it is T1 or T2, and the possibility of resection and cure is real. However, once their walls are penetrated by cancer (T3) or enter and invade adjacent and surrounding organs (T4), their resectability decreases and their patient's survival is compromised.

SUMMARY OF CHANGES

Generally, there is no overarching principle or context design for the digestive system (GIT) or MDG as to stage groupings. For gastrointestinal system and major digestive glands there are no overarching rules as to stage groups and definitions of nodal categories. The T categories are consistent for hollow tubular multilayered digestive system sites, i.e., T1 mucosa, T2 submucosa, T3 muscularis, T4 serosa. N1 is the only nodal category in 7 of 10 sites but is variously assigned from stage I to stage III. Stage subgroups A/B are variously assigned in stage I, II, III, IV with an occasional C. The major basis for stage subgroups are supportive survival data, justifying the amalgams of T and N. The color code for progression of stage groups generally defines resectable (purple) versus unresectable (red) cancers and black is reserved for metastatic. Stages are frequently expanded to six by subdividing a stage into A and B. The T and N categories are assigned to a stage grouping, specifically for division of a stage into a (A) more favorable versus a (B) less favorable grouping. This occurs at different stages for different sites. N1 is the only nodal category in 7 of 10 sites but is variously assigned from I, II, III, and IV. There is an anatomic basis for T-stage assignment to N, as a function of primary tumor extent, that is, the T stage progression and depth of invasion is equal to where nodes are located.

Colon	Small Intestine	Liver	Pancreas

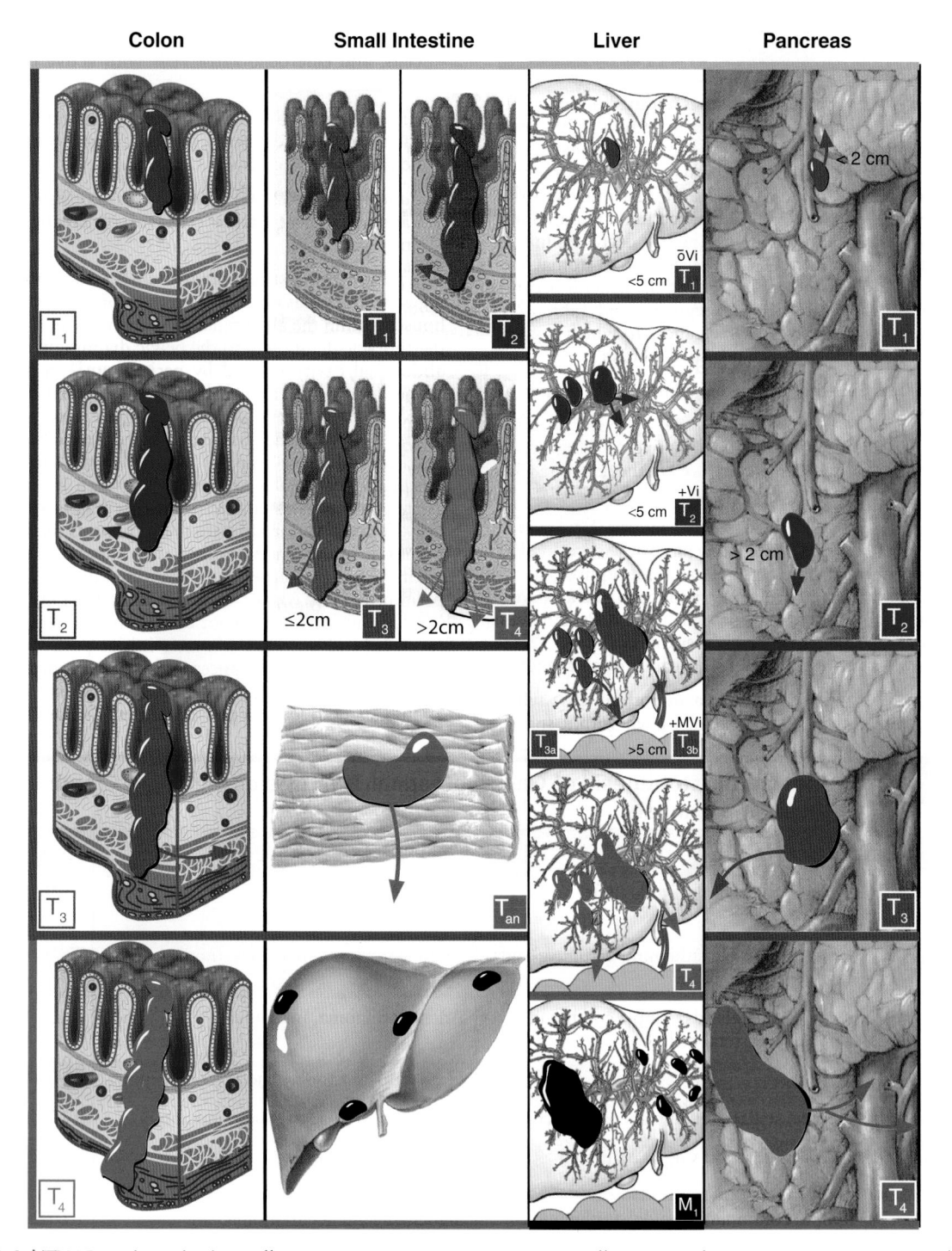

Figure 22.3 | TNM staging criteria. Hollow organ prototype. Tis (mucosa), yellow; T1 (submucosa), green; T2 (muscularis externa), blue; T3 (serosa), purple; and T4 (perforates into another organ), red. Solid organ (pancreas). T1, green; T2, blue; T3, purple; and T4, red.

T-ONCOANATOMY

THREE-PLANAR ONCOANATOMY

Orientation of T-oncoanatomy

There are 11 primary cancer sites, including the 7 GIT hollow structures: esophagus, stomach, small intestine, appendix (new), colon, rectum, and anus. In addition, there are 7 primary sites arising in the MDG: liver, intrahepatic bile ducts (new), gallbladder, extrahepatic bile ducts (hilar and distal), the ampulla of Vater, and pancreas. There are 2 major anatomic sectors and 11 major primary cancer sites. The abdomen is divided into two sectors based on the peritoneum, that is, the structures are intraperitoneal or extraperitoneal. With the exception of the pancreas, lower rectum, and anus, all major primary sites are intraperitoneal except for that portion of the bowel that is directly attached to the posterior wall of the abdomen and has no mesentery.

The abdomen superiorly extends under the diaphragm into the lower third of the thorax and inferiorly extends into the pelvis. The GIT and the MDG are the frequent sites of adenocarcinomas. To interweave these 11 primary sites, which are largely intraperitoneal, a multiplanar orientation follows (Fig. 22.5A, B). The presentation of primary site isocenters starts at T11 and T12 near the diaphragmatic insertion and progresses to L1 to L5 and then onto the pelvis S1, S2, and S3.

- *Esophagus*: The gastroesophageal junction is at the diaphragmatic level, and islands of Barrett mucosa can occur. The ectopic location of gastric mucosa in the distal esophagus is vulnerable for forming adenocarcinomas. The cardioesophageal junction has become increasingly notorious for adenocarcinomas that spread into the thorax as well as the epigastrium.

- *Stomach*: The stomach is divided into three regions: upper, middle, and lower third. To delineate these regions, the lesser and greater curves of the stomach are divided; the upper third is the cardiac area and fundus, the middle third is the body, and the lower third is the antrum. Gastric cancers can become large before they produce obstructive symptoms. Avid and aggressive screening in at-risk populations (Japan) has led to detection of early gastric cancers.

- *Small intestine*: The small intestine extends from the pylorus of the stomach to the ileocecal valve. It is approximately 25 feet long and is divided into three sections: the duodenum, jejunum, and ileum. The duodenum is essentially a midline structure approximately 1 foot long. It provides some of the most complex anatomy in the upper abdomen as it conforms to and surrounds the head of the pancreas. The small intestine, despite its length, gives rise to few cancers. Instead, a large variety of neoplastic syndromes occur, and unusual tumors is its hallmark.

- *Colon*: The large intestine is the most prevalent site for cancer, particularly with its numerous (eight) subsites at high risk. The large intestine or colon picture frames the abdominal content and is 60 cm long and is divided into an ascending, transverse, descending, and sigmoid colon with a hepatic flexure on the right and splenic flexure on the left. Favored subsites for malignancy include the cecum, sigmoid, and rectum. The colon is vulnerable to polyposis and chronic inflammatory disease, which can lead to carcinomas.

- *Rectum*: The rectum is the most common site in GIT for malignancies. It is about 12 cm long and extends from a point opposite the third sacral vertebra down to the apex of the prostate in the male and to the apex of the perineal body in the female, that is, to a point 4 cm anterior to the tip of the coccyx. It may be arbitrarily defined as the distal 10 cm of the large intestine, as measured by preoperative sigmoidoscopy from the anal verge. The rectum has no epiploic appendages, no haustrations, and no taeniae. It is covered by peritoneum in front and on both sides in its upper third and on the anterior wall only in its middle third; there is no peritoneal covering in the lower third.

- *Anus*: About 4 cm long, the anal canal courses downward and backward from the apex of the prostate or the perineal body. The anocutaneous line, or white line of Hilton, at the base of the rectal columns marks the site of the original anal membrane that separated the endodermal gut from the ectodermal proctoderm. With the high incidence of anal viral infection—both human papilloma virus and human immunodeficiency virus—the risk of anal cancers is increasing in the homosexual population.

The MDG constitute seven more primary sites, a number of which are quite uncommon cancers (Table 22.2):

- *Liver*: By virtue of its weight, the liver is the largest organ in the body. When filled with cancerous nodules, it is often the greatest repository of neoplastic disease, exceeding the primary tumors in the quantity of malignant cells. To understand the anatomy of the liver, it is important to be aware of its internal structure as a gland of compound tubular design. Each lobule is shaped like a cylinder or tubule, with a central vein that drains a rich anatomic sinusoidal network derived from the fine hepatic arterioles and portal vessels. The hepatocyte elaborates both an external/exocrine secretion and an internal/endocrine secretion of enzymes into the blood. The former is referred to as bile and is collected by biliary canaliculi.

- *Intrahepatic bile ducts*: cholangiocarcinomas is new.

- *Gallbladder*: The gallbladder is a small, saccular organ located inferior to the liver in its own fossa. It is a harbinger for gallstones and it can undergo dysplastic and then neoplastic changes. As a hollow, pear-shaped organ it simulates bowel, with an epithelial mucosa, smooth muscle layer, and serosa. In contrast to the intestine, there is no submucosa, and there is only one muscle layer, muscularis externa.

- *Extrahepatic bile ducts*: The extrahepatic bile ducts are a continuation of the intrahepatic ducts. The confluence of right and left hepatic ducts is the site of most cholangiocarcinomas and has been added as a new site. Symptoms of obstructive jaundice are invariably present.

- *Ampulla of Vater*: The ampulla of Vater is another confluence junction of both the pancreatic duct and extrahepatic bile ducts as it enters the second part of the duodenum. This is perhaps the least common malignancy of the MDG.

- *Pancreas*: The pancreas is a long, lobulated structure that lies transversely in the posterior abdomen located retroperitoneally in the concavity of the duodenum on its right end and touching the spleen on its left end. The shape of the pancreas may be compared with the letter J placed sideways. It is divisible into a head with an uncinate process, neck, body, and tail. Each of these sites, when afflicted with cancer, produces a specific set of characteristic signs and symptoms.

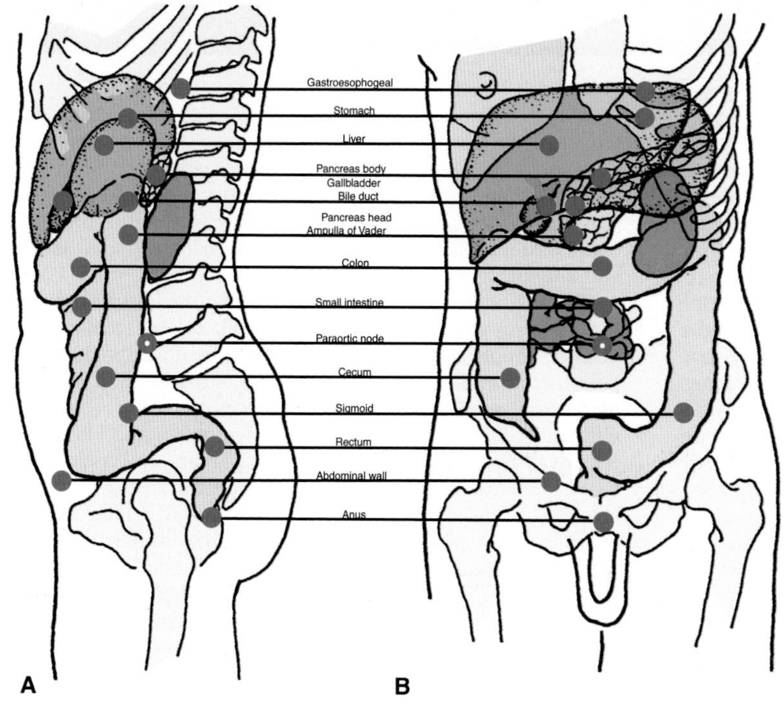
Gastroesophogeal
Stomach
Liver
Pancreas body
Gallbladder
Bile duct
Pancreas head
Ampulla of Vader
Colon
Small intestine
Paraortic node
Cecum
Sigmoid
Rectum
Abdominal wall
Anus
A
B

Figure 22.5 | Orientation of three-planar T-oncoanatomy. Anatomic isocenter of multiple GIT primary sites. **A.** Sagittal lateral. **B.** Coronal anterior. A cephalad-to-caudad GIT and MDG tabulation of the cancers, the vertebral levels, and the adjacent anatomic structures to be aware of at the transverse axial level assists in presenting the classification and staging process of the digestive tract cancers. Most GIT and MDG organs occupy many vertebral levels; the three planar views and the axial vertebral assignment is designed to be at the anatomic isocenter of the structure. The anatomic isocenters (Fig. 22.5) for the gastrointestinal tract are displayed in sections transversely at a specific vertebral levels, recognizing there is a variability.

TABLE 22.2 Overview of T-oncoanatomy of Gastrointestinal Tract/Major Digestive Glands

Primary Site	Three-planar Coronal	Sagittal	Transverse	Axial Level
Esophagus (see thorax)	Posterior mediastinum, descending aorta	Sympathetics, parasympathetics	Diaphragmatic stoma	T9/T10
Esophagogastric junction	Zigzag line	Lesser omental bursa, liver	Lesser omental bursa, spleen	T9/T10
Stomach	Fundus, body, pylorus	Lesser and greater omentum	Liver, spleen, kidneys	T10/T11/T12
Liver	Right and left lobes of liver	Eight sectors of liver divided by scissures	H-shaped fissures and fossae, caudate and quadratic lobes	T10/T11/ T12, L1
Gallbladder	Gallbladder, cystic duct, bile ducts	Junction of cystic and hepatic ducts	Inferior to liver	T12, L1
Extrahepatic ducts	Extrahepatic bile ducts and pancreatic ducts	Portal triad of bile duct, hepatic artery and portal vein	Relationship to first and second parts of duodenum	L1/L2
Pancreas	Head, body, and tail of pancreas	Retroperitoneal	Head and uncinate process wrap around superior mesenteric artery	L1/L2
Ampulla	Relationship of pancreatic duct and bile duct in development	Variation in fusion of bile and pancreatic ducts	Relationship of ventral and dorsal pancreatic bud	L2
Colon	Picture frames abdomen and its intestinal contents	Greater omentum relationship to colon, stomach, and pancreas	Anterior and lateral locations, mesentery	L2/L3/L4/L5
Small intestine	Circular folds variation, duodenum, jejunum, and ileum	Intraperitoneal and mesenteric roots	Fill most of abdomen at this level	L3/L4/L5
Sigmoid colon and rectum	Transition to pelvis exit into sacral hollow	Dorsal vein of male and female pelvis organ	Prostate and bladder anterior Denonvilliers fascia	S1–S5
Anus	Anorectal line, column of Morgagni, pectinate line	Perineal, postanal, presacral, deep, and superficial spaces	Bladder neck, urethra	Pubic bone, femoral head

N-ONCOANATOMY AND M-ONCOANATOMY

Orientation of N-oncoanatomy

The coronal planar oncoanatomy of lymph nodes will present the arrays of regional lymph nodes (Fig. 22.6). The lymphoid drainage of the digestive system and major digestive glands (MDG) overlap and reflect both the arterial blood supply and venous drainage, which are not always parallel. The small intestine is a major extranodal site with its Peyer patches and the appendix is an analog for the bursa of Fabricius, the origin for B cells in lower vertebrates. The mesenteric nodes are not acknowledged in the lymphoma staging as a node-bearing region. The para-aortic and paracaval location for lymph nodes relate to the roots of origin of visceral arteries as the celiac, superior, and inferior mesenteric arteries. Smooth metastatic nodules in the pericolic and perirectal fat are considered lymph node metastases and counted in N staging. Irregular nodules are considered as vascular invasion and are either V1 (microscopic) or V2 (macroscopic) when viewed histopathologically.

The lymphatics and major lymph node stations of the digestive tract are rich and directly related to the vascular arcades that characterize the extensive arterial and venous network. In the upper abdomen, the celiac axis of arteries supplies the stomach along its lesser and greater curvatures and the hepatic and pancreaticosplenic arteries, liver, and pancreas along with its ductal systems. The major lymphatic collecting trunks are parallel with the left gastric artery, splenic artery, and hepatic artery.

The major first station nodes are along the lesser gastropyloric, suprapyloric, pancreatoduodenal, celiac, splenic, and hepatic lymph nodes. The second station nodes include the para-aortic nodes. However, it is the superior and inferior mesenteric arterial and venous arcades that one associates with the GIT's rich lymphatics and lymph nodes. The intestinal wall is impregnated with Peyer patches and a rich network of lacteals in villi that provide robust drainage of chyme into the cisterna chili and then onto the thoracic duct. Each of these regional lymph nodes is discussed separately with the GIT/MDG organ of interest. The sentinel nodes for each site are listed in Table 22.3. The spleen can function as a major systemic lymph node and plays an important immunologic role.

TABLE 22.3	N-oncoanatomy: Primary Cancer Sites and Sentinel Nodes		
Cancer Type	**Axial Level**	**Adjacent Anatomic Structure/Site**	**Sentinel Nodes**
Esophagogastric junction	T9/T10	Diaphragm, pericardium, thoracic duct	Lesser curvature and celiac nodes
Stomach	T10/T11/T12	Crura, liver, spleen, pancreas, greater omentum	Lesser and greater curvature nodes
Liver	T10/T11/T12, L1	Diaphragm, spleen, stomach, lesser omentum sac	Paracaval nodes, porta hepatis nodes
Gallbladder	T12, L1	Liver and intrahepatic and extrahepatic bile ducts, portal vein	Porta hepatis nodes
Extrahepatic bile ducts	L1/L2	Porta hepatic, extrahepatic bile ducts, pancreas, and ampulla of Vater	Porta hepatis nodes
Pancreas	L1/L2	Duodenum, bile ducts, ampulla of Vater, and spleen	Pancreaticoduodenal, pancreaticosplenic nodes
Ampulla of Vater	L2	Duodenum, bile ducts, ampulla of Vater, and spleen	Pancreaticoduodenal nodes
Colon, transverse	L2/L3	Greater omentum, hepatic and splenic flexures, and mesentery	Pericolic, superior and inferior mesenteric nodes
Small intestine	L3/L4/L5	Mesentery, superior mesentery arteries	Superior mesenteric nodes
Cecum	L5	Appendix, sigmoid, small intestine, and ileocecal valve	Iliocecal and pericolic nodes
Sigmoid	S1	Mesentery, small intestine, and gynecologic organs	Pericolic and inferior mesenteric nodes
Rectum	S1–S5	Bladder, male genitourinary, prostate, and vas deferens vs. female uterus	Perirectal and sacral nodes
Anus	Pubic bone and femoral head	Perineum/vagina or vulva urethra	Inguinal nodes

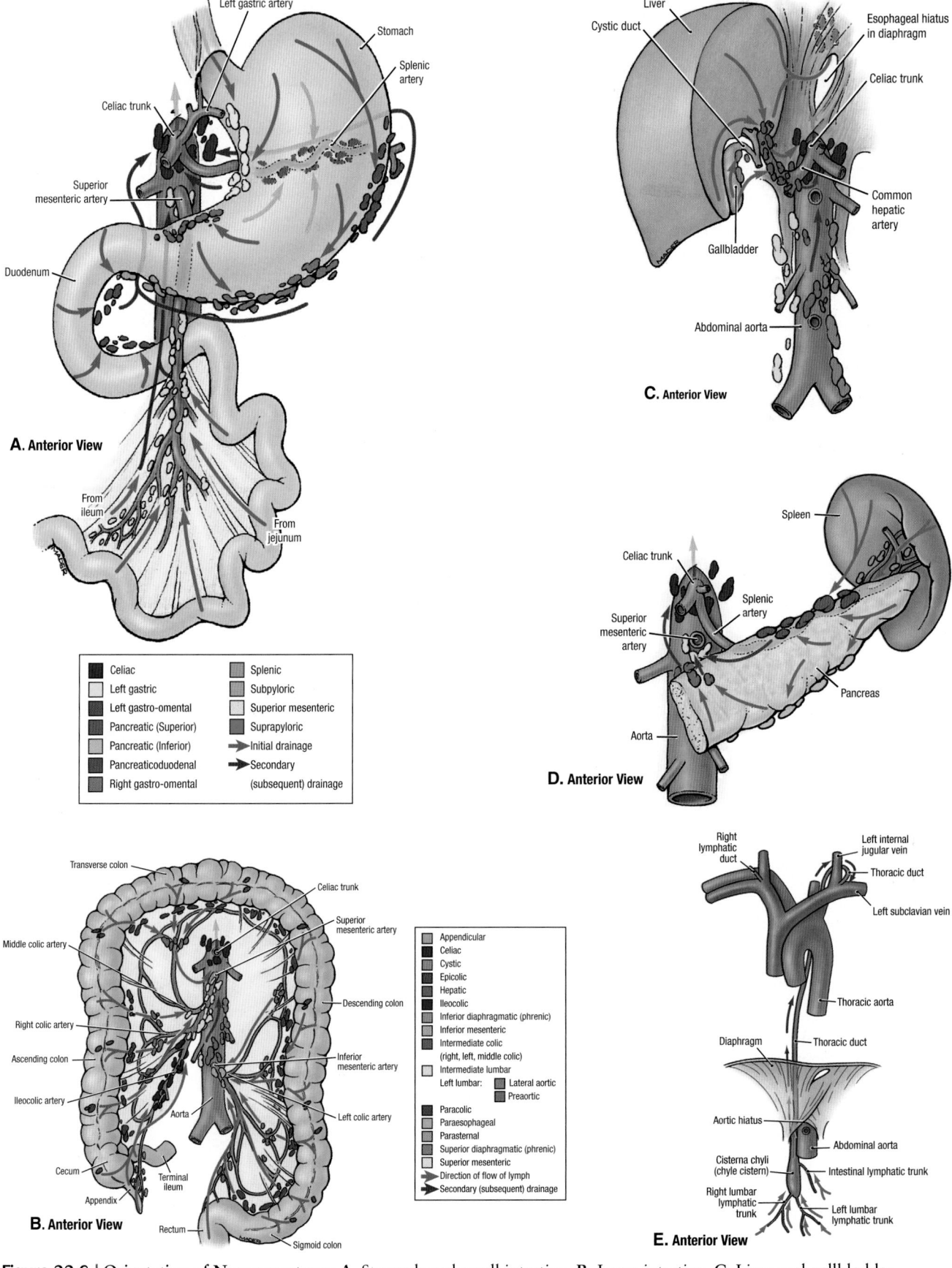

Figure 22.6 | Orientation of N-oncoanatomy. A. Stomach and small intestine. **B.** Large intestine. **C.** Liver and gallbladder. **D.** Spleen and pancreas. **E.** Drainage from lumbar and intestinal lymphatic trunks. Lymph from the abdominal nodes drains into the cistern chyli, origin of the inferior end of the thoracic duct. The thoracic duct receives all lymph that forms inferior to the diaphragm and left upper quadrant (thorax and left upper limb) and empties into the junction of the left subclavian and left internal jugular veins.

Orientation of M-oncoanatomy

The entire portal circulation should be considered as a unit in regard to the venous anatomy of the GIT below the diaphragm (Fig. 22.7A.) The two major trunks are the inferior mesenteric and superior mesenteric veins. The inferior mesenteric vein drains the left colon and sigmoid colon tributaries, which covers the vascular drainage to the left of the midline originating from the superior rectal veins. On the right side, the superior mesenteric vein originates from the tributaries draining the ileum, jejunum, and ileocolic and right colic veins. The inferior mesenteric vein usually joins the splenic vein, which coalesces with the superior mesenteric vein and forms the portal vein. The splenic vein, which is a major tributary of the portal system in addition, drains much of the stomach along its greater curvature and includes the short gastric veins and left gastroepiploic and right gastric epiploic veins. The right gastroepiploic also flows into the superior mesenteric vein. The entire drainage of the lesser curvature of the stomach, including the left and right gastric veins, drains directly into the portal vein. Because the portal vein then drains directly into the liver, it is the target metastatic organ and the most commonly involved organ in hematogenous spread pattern from the venous system of the GIT as compared with other parts of the body, where the drainage is directly into the lung by way of the caval system (Fig. 22.7; Table 22.4).

THE ABDOMINAL PERITONEAL CAVITY

The abdominal cavity is lined by peritoneum, an areolar membrane covered with a single layer of mesothelial cells. The peritoneal cavity is a physiologically complex structure containing fluid secretions, which bathe and lubricate the bowel surfaces, and anatomically consists of numerous sacs and folds. Normally, the fluid is absorbed, but when it accumulates as ascites, malignancy with peritoneal seeding is a concern clinically. A double layer of peritoneum connects the stomach with the lesser omentum (from the lesser curvature) and with the greater omentum (from the greater curvature). The numerous peritoneal folds consist of mesenteries for gut, arteries, and veins, although some do not contain tubes. Peritoneal fossae, recesses, and gutters determine initial pathways of tumor spread both for bowel cancer and ovarian cancer. In addition to the omental bursae, there is a duodenal fossa, a cecal fossa, an intersigmoid fossa, a pelvic fossa, and a paracolic fossa (Figure 22.7B,C).

The origin of the abdominal cavity and the gastrointestinal contents is essential to understand metastatic seeding in the abdomen. Embryologically, the gastrula folds into a tube with a foregut, midgut, and hindgut, suspended by a dorsal mesentery into the abdominal cavity lined by a simple squamous parietal peritoneal lining over the abdominal wall and a visceral peritoneum over the gut. As the gut rotates clockwise, the viscera are suspended by "ligaments" that create separate pockets, that is, lesser and greater peritoneal sacs, as well as the omentum.

The diaphragm develops from the septum transversum that partitions the thoracic and abdominal cavities; its muscle, derived from cervical somite myotones, carries with it the phrenic nerve, that is, referring abdominal inflammation to the shoulder and neck. The infradiaphragmatic lymphatics drain the peritoneal fluid, which is secreted with flow patterns determined by visceral movement and ligamentous attachments.

Once gastrointestinal cancer penetrates the gut wall serosa, it can do the following:

- Seed out into the abdominal cavity and lead to the omental or visceral deposits of cancer.

- Form masses; a dramatic illustration is stomach-seeding ovarian masses—Krukenberg tumors.

- Lead to peritoneal fluid formation, resulting in ascites, that is, mucinous peritoneal due to goblet cell proliferations.

- Cause diaphragmatic lymphatic obstruction, resulting in serous exudates or, if the cisternachyli is invaded, a chylous ascites.

- Lead to omental cakes, which can lead to mass formation that in turn invades the abdominal wall.

- Directly invade another segment of the small intestine and colon, resulting in stricture and bowel obstruction.

- Lead to perforation of visceral peritoneum, which can lead to fistula and to abscess formation localized to the cancer site or migrate leading to subdiaphragmatic abscess.

- Lead to acute peritonitis with an acute abdomen: air accumulating under the diaphragm due to ulceration and perforation.

TABLE 22.4	Incidence of Liver Metastases from Various Primary Tumors at Autopsy
Primary Site	**Percentage with Liver Metastases**
Esophagus	30–100
Stomach	38–100
Colorectal	40–100
Pancreas	50–73
Bile ducts and gallbladder	15–80
Small cell lung cancer	38–67
Breast	19–73
Melanoma	69
Ovary	48–68
Uterus	21–75
Renal cell cancer	40
Urothelial cancer	37–38
Thyroid	20
Prostate	9–71

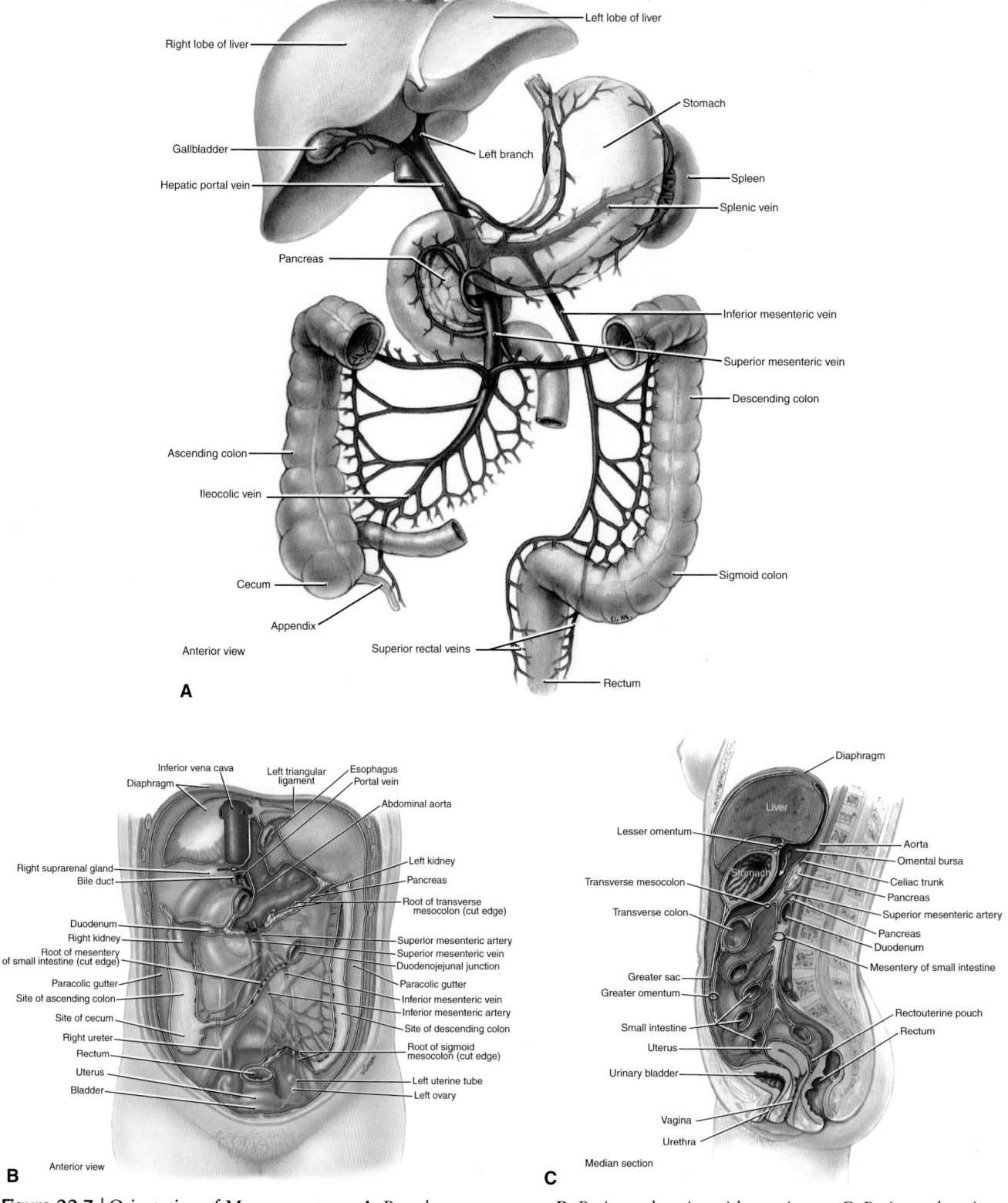

Figure 22.7 | Orientation of M-oncoanatomy. A. Portal venous system. B. Peritoneal cavity without viscera. C. Peritoneal cavity with viscera.

STAGING WORKUP

RULES FOR CLASSIFICATION AND STAGING

Clinical Staging and Imaging

Most of the digestive system and MDG are inaccessible to physical examination to detect and diagnose cancer formation and invasion. Endoscopic viewing provides the diagnosis, but to probe and biopsy the wall carries the hazard of perforation. The role and importance of sophisticated imaging are essential to staging. Endoscopic ultrasound can visualize the multilayered wall as rings of hyperechoic and hypoechoic bands and their signal distortion by tumor invasion. Virtual endoscopy, like colonoscopy, is an improving modality with more accurate computer displays and reconstructions. Computed tomography (CT) and magnetic resonance imaging (MRI) are valuable for assessing solid organs such as liver and pancreas, as well as adenopathy. Three-planar viewing is widely adopted and available for staging the primary tumor and regional nodes. Hepatic metastases are the greatest concern for all GIT and MDG sites, and CT and MRI are excellent modes for searching and identifying lesions. Positron emission tomographic scanning is a sensitive means to total body scan for occult dissemination (Table 22.5). Endorectal ultrasounds is useful in defining depth of wall invasion (Fig. 22.8). The arterial phase can be useful to determine tumor blood supply in various abdominal organs (Fig. 22.9A, B).

Pathologic Staging

The surgically resected portion of the GIT and associated lymph nodes removed are noted, numbered, and assessed for tumor. Tumor extension and location of both primary and nodes should be documented. Residual cancer can be R1, microscopic, or R2, macroscopic.

TABLE 22.5	Imaging Modalities for Staging for Abdominal Organs	
Method	Diagnosis and Staging Capability	Recommended for Use
Primary Tumor ± Regional Nodes		
Barium enema	Very useful in detecting and defining primary lesions in the colon	Yes
Endoscopy	Single-contrast study may be less sensitive than double-contrast in detecting polyps	Yes, if used to confirm lesion detected on barium enema or to screen high-risk patients
Endorectal ultrasound or coil	Very accurate modality for detecting and defining primary lesions in rectum, sigmoid (flex sigmoidoscopy), or remaining colon (colonoscopy)	
Magnetic resonance imaging	Useful in defining depth of penetration of the primary lesion	Yes, if preoperative chemoradiation is considered
Computed tomography (CT)	Most valuable of all modalities for determining extrarectal or extracolonic local invasion and nodal metastases	Yes
Positron emission tomography	Not useful for staging primary cancer	No
Metastases		
Chest film ± CT	Chest film—best for metastasis screening; CT chest—rules out multiple metastases	Yes
CT abdomen	Most useful study to define para-aortic node enlargement or liver metastases	Yes
Liver ultrasound	Can differentiate between cystic and solid lesions	Yes

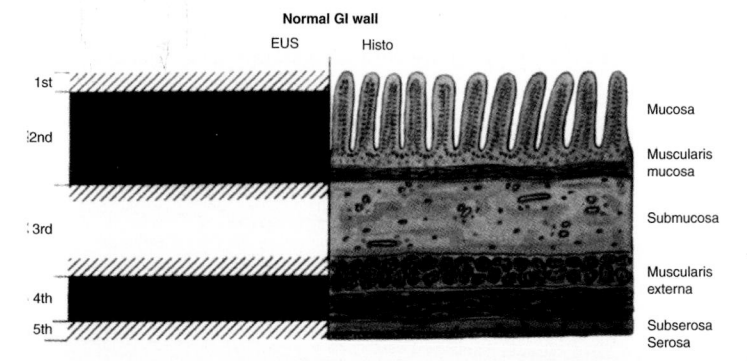

Figure 22.8 | Schematic representation of endoscopic ultrasound appearance of the typical five-layered wall pattern and the histologic correlation.

PROGNOSIS AND CANCER SURVIVAL

CANCER STATISTICS AND SURVIVAL

The majority of digestive systems neoplasms are successfully treated with multimodal treatment. The number of new patients with cancers are 275,000 of which 50% (140,000) survive. The incidence is slightly greater in males than females 54% vs. 46% i.e., 150,000 vs. 1260,000. The death rates over the past five decades have most dramatically decreased in stomach and colon rectum cancers and are unchanged for pancreas and liver. The deaths are also greater in males than females: 56% vs. 44% i.e. 80,000 vs. 60,000.

An overview of digestive system cancers and their incidence of new patients and their death rates are tabulated according to ACS Cancer Facts and Figures 2010 (Tables 22.6 and 22.7).

The largest gains in survival are in colon and rectum, followed by stomach. The poorest results are those in pancreas and liver. The gains other sites vary depending on early detection of cancer in a localized stage in esophago-gastric junction or where chemoradiation is very effective i.e. anal cancers.

TABLE 22.6 5-Year Survival

	All Stages	Localized	Regional	Distant
Colon Rectum	65%	91%	70%	11%
Esophagus	17%	37%	19%	3%
Liver	13%	26%	9%	2%
Pancreas	6%	22%	9%	2%
Stomach	26%	63%	27%	3%

American Cancer Society, Inc., "Cancer Facts and Figures 2010." http://www.cancer.org/Research/CancerFactsFigures/CancerFactsFigures/cancer-facts-and-figures-2010.

TABLE 22.7

Digestive System	New Cases	Deaths
Esophagus	16,640 (6%)	14,500 (10%)
Stomach	21,000 (7%)	10,570 (7.5%)
Small Intestine	6,960 (2%)	1,100 (<1%)
Colon	102,900 (38%)	51,370 (37%)
Rectum	39,670 (15%)	—
Anus	5,260 (2%)	720 (<1%)
Liver/Intrahepatic Bile Duct	24,120 (8%)	18,910 (14%)
Gall Bladder/Bile Duct	9,760 (4%)	36,800 (26%)
Pancreas	43,140 (15%)	3,320 (3%)
Other	4,880 (3%)	2,290 (1%)

American Cancer Society, Inc., "Cancer Facts and Figures 2010." http://www.cancer.org/Research/CancerFactsFigures/CancerFactsFigures/cancer-facts-and-figures-2010.

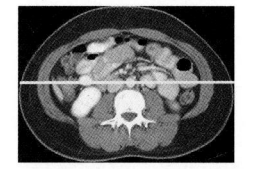
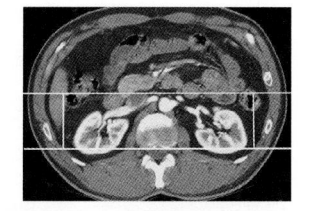
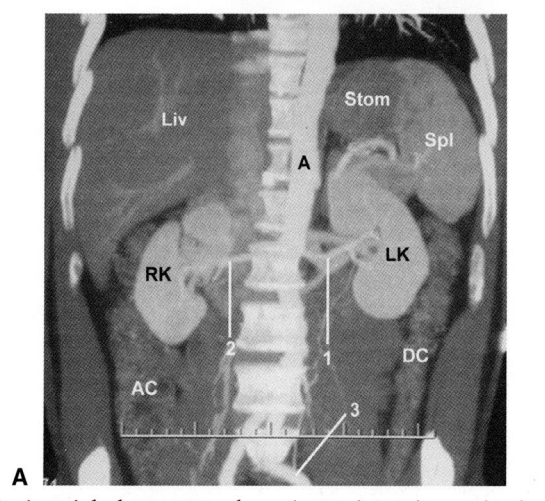
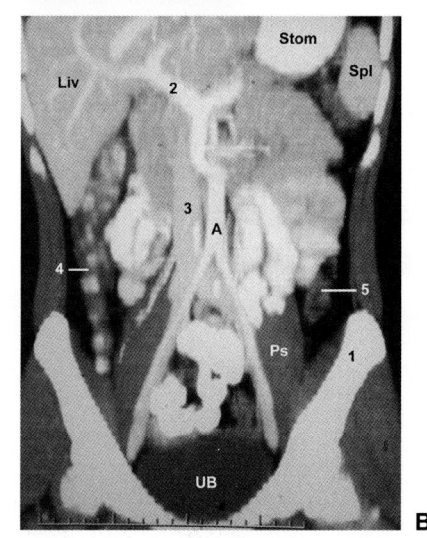

Figure 22.9 | A. Arterial phase coronal maximum intensity projection image. 1. left renal art 2. right renal art 3. left common iliac art. A, abdominal aorta; AC, ascending colon; DC, descending colon; Liv, liver; LK, left kidney; RK, right kidney; Spl, spleen; Stom, stomach. **B. Coronal abdomen.** 1. left iliac bone 2. main portal vein 3. inferior vena cava 4. ascending colon 5. descending colon. A, abdominal aorta; Liv, liver; Ps, psoas muscle; Spl, spleen; Stom, stomach; UB, urinary bladder.

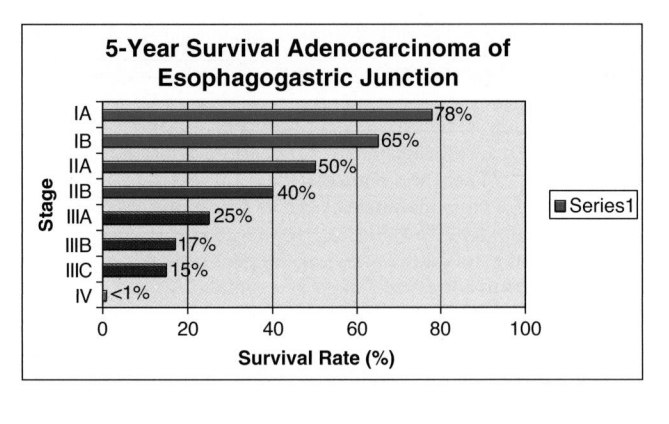

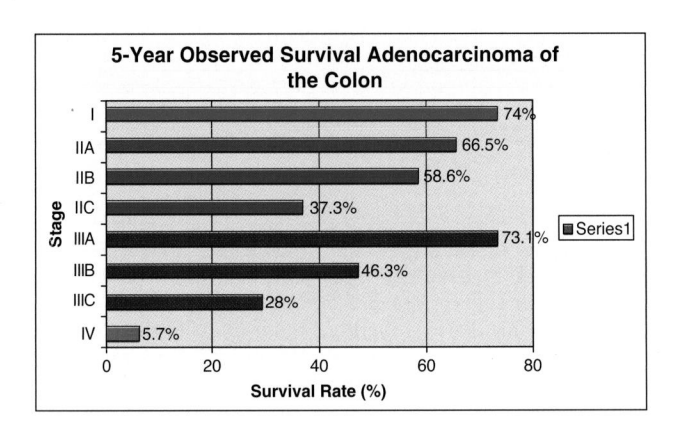

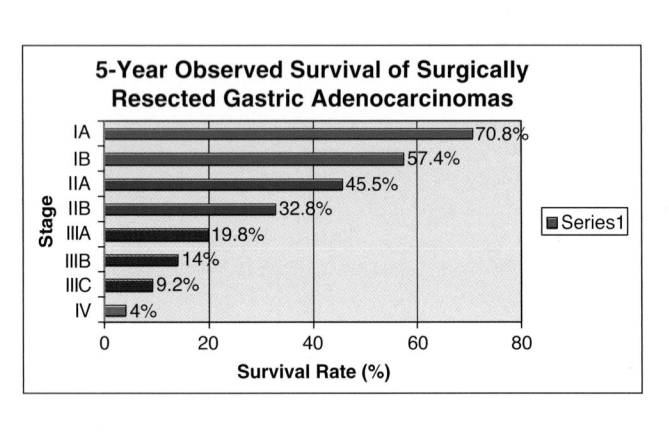

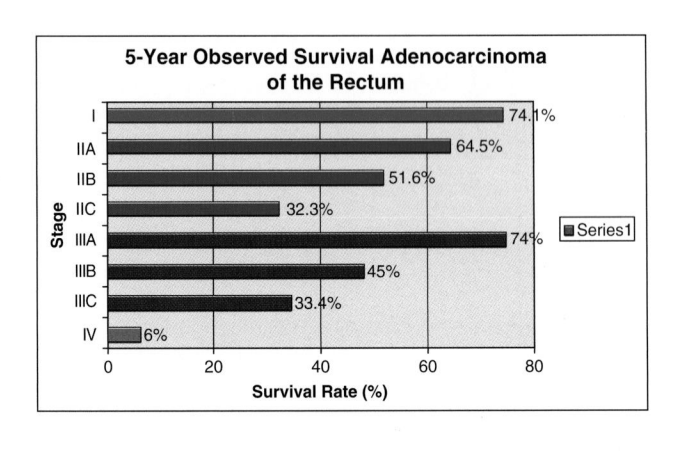

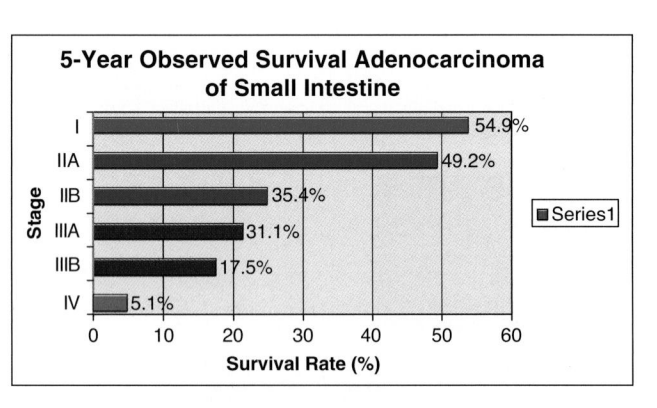

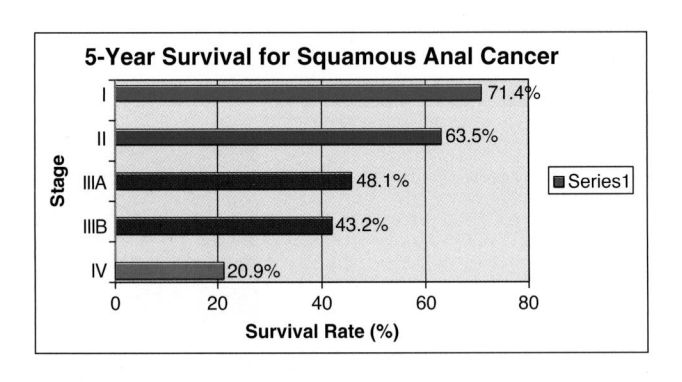

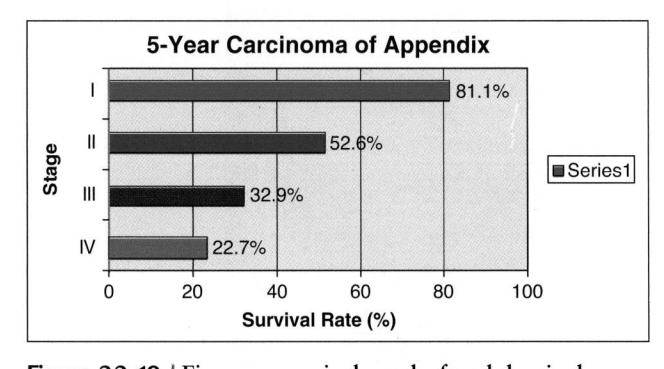

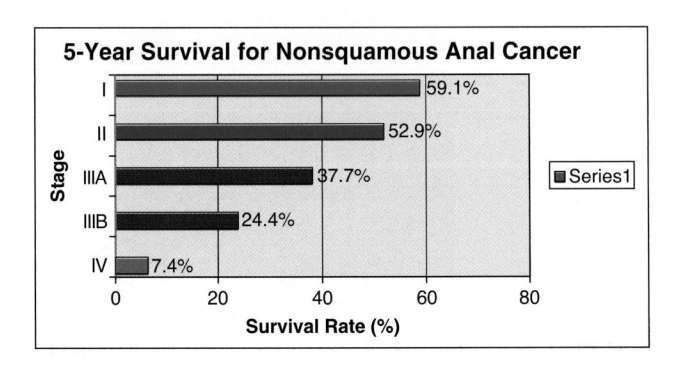

Figure 22.10 | Five-year survival graphs for abdominal cancers. (Data from Edge SB, Byrd DR, and Compton CC, et al, *AJCC Cancer Staging Manual, 7th edition.* New York: Springer, 2010.) *(continued)*

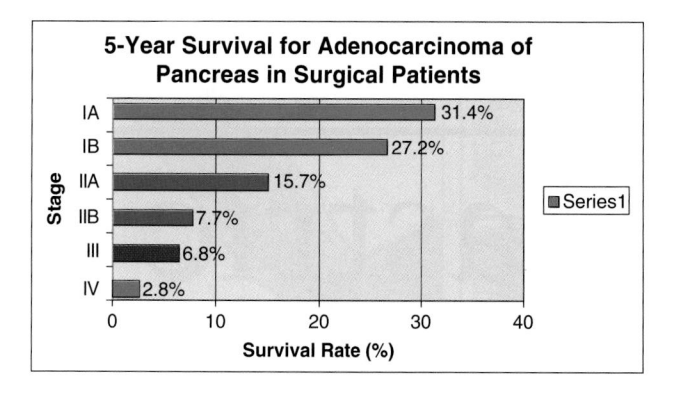

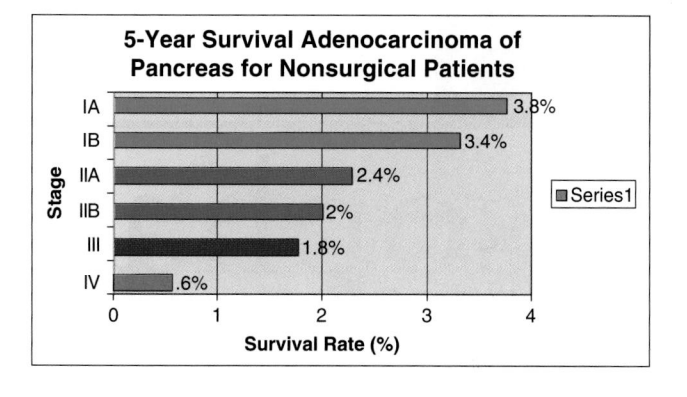

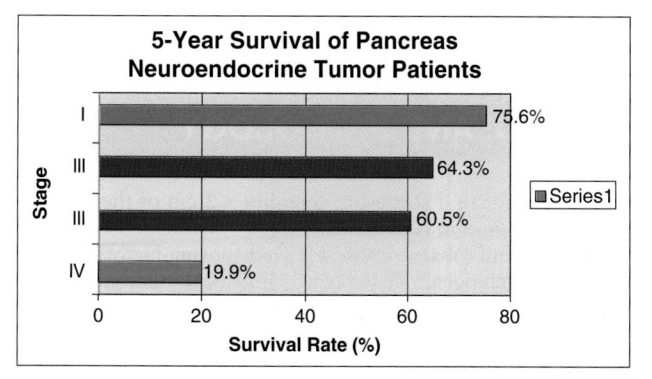

Figure 22.10 | Five-year survival graphs for abdominal cancers. (Data from Edge SB, Byrd DR, and Compton CC, et al, *AJCC Cancer Staging Manual,* *7th edition.* New York: Springer, 2010.)

TNM STAGING CRITERIA

TNM STAGING CRITERIA

The normal EGJ is a zigzag line, which divides the whitish stratified esophageal squamous mucous membranes from the pinkish glandular gastric mucosa. The longitudinal esophageal folds fade into the gastric rugal folds. Spasm, obstruction, and regurgitation occur with cardia dysfunction. Eventually, persistent inflammation results with the mucosal transformation to malignancy. Perforation is rare because thickening of the dual muscular layers of the distal esophagus is reinforced as in muscle layers of the stomach. The staging of esophageal cancers has not changed and relates to the standard hollow organ model in which depth of penetration of the wall rather than size determines stage—that is, T1, mucosa; T2, muscular; T3, serosa; and T4, extraesophageal (Fig. 23.3). Dysplastic Barrett mucosa is substaged in terms of length: short versus long segment based on whether the lesion is <3 cm or >3 cm long, respectively, from the zigzag line of the EGJ.

Generally, there is no overarching principle or context design for the digestive system (gastrointestinal tract) or major digestive glands. Stages are frequently expanded to six by subdividing a stage into A and B. The T and N categories are assigned to a stage grouping, specifically for division of a stage into more (a) versus less (b) favorable groupings. This occurs at different stages for different sites.

The esophagogastric junction has 6 to 8 stages; Stages I and II have A and B categories. Stage III has three substages, A, B and C. The initial-stage progression (I/II/III) is due to advancement of the primary, and the late-stage progression (III/IV) is by nodal involvement: IIB is N1. Regional nodes are either stage II or III, and nonregional nodes are stage IV. There are 3 nodal categories, N1, N2, N3.

The staging system for esophagogastric adenocarcinoma is entirely new in the seventh edition AJCC and differs not only in the specific T and N definitions but in stage grouping them from esophageal squamous cell cancer. Thus, the main features relate to the clustering of T and N categories and to the additional cancer grade (Table 23.3).

SUMMARY OF CHANGES SEVENTH EDITION AJCC

- Tumor location is simplified, and esophagogastric junction and proximal 5 cm of stomach are included.
- Tis is redefined and T4 is subclassified.
- Regional lymph nodes are redefined. N is subclassified according to the number of regional lymph nodes containing metastasis.
- M is redefined.
- Separate stage groupings for squamous cell carcinoma and adenocarcinoma.
- Stage groupings are reassigned using T, N, M, and G classifications.

The TNM Staging Matrix is color coded for identification of Stage Group once T and N stages are determined (Table 23.3).

TABLE 23.3	Stage Summary Matrix				
	N0	N1	N2	N3	M1
T1	IA	IIB	IIIA	IIIC	IV
T2	IB	IIB	IIIA	IIIC	IV
T3	IIA	IIIA	IIIB	IIIC	IV
T4a/b	IIIA	IIIC	IIIC	IIIC	IV

Both T and N progress and determine stage progression. T stage and N stage combined determine substage progression. However, survival data has lead to further modifications.

ESOPHAGOGASTRIC JUNCTION ADENOCARCINOMA

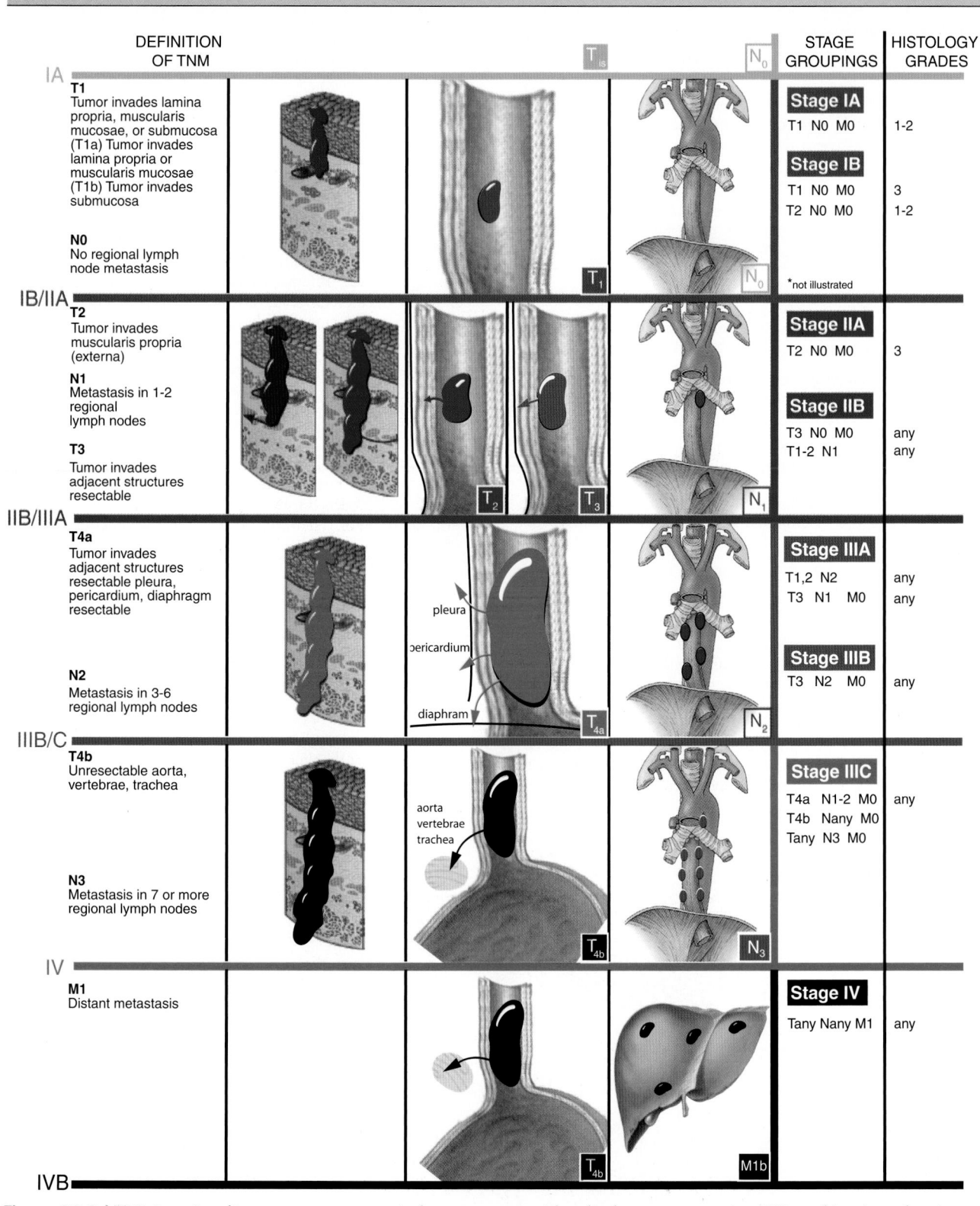

Figure 23.3 | TNM staging diagram presents a vertical arrangement with color bars encompassing TN combinations showing progression. Esophagogastric junction cancers are adenocarcinomas. Note juxtaregional nodes as M_{1a}; celiac nodes, although considered metastatic when resected, offer a better chance for 5-year survival (10%) than visceral metastases (black). Stage 0, yellow; stage I, green; stage II, blue; stage III, purple; stage IV, red; and stage IV (metastatic), black. Definitions of TN on left and stage grouping on right.

T-ONCOANATOMY

ORIENTATION OF THREE-PLANAR ONCOANATOMY

The anatomic isocenter for the EGJ cancers is at T9/T10. These EGJs are posterior in location for both the mediastinum and the abdominal cavity (Fig. 23.4).

T-oncoanatomy

The T-oncoanatomy is displayed in three planar views. A. Coronal, B. Sagittal, C. Transverse axial (Fig. 23.5).

The esophagus consists of three principal regions: the cervical, thoracic, and cardiac portions.

- Cervical esophagus extends from the pharyngeal–esophageal sphincter to the level of the thoracic inlet, about 18 cm from upper incisor teeth (UIT).

- Upper thoracic esophagus extends from the thoracic inlet to the level of the tracheal bifurcation, about 24 cm from UIT.

- Midthoracic esophagus extends from the tracheal bifurcation toward the esophagogastric junction, about 32 cm from UIT.

- Lower thoracic esophagus is ductal, 3 to 8 cm in length, includes the esophageal gastric junction, and is about 40 cm from UIT.

The esophagus is a muscular tube that consists of two layers of smooth muscle—one longitudinal and the other circular—and this is carried through into the rest of the gastrointestinal system. Peristalsis is initiated with swallowing, and the major function is to propel food into the stomach. There are two sphincters in the esophagus, and these are at the cricopharyngeous muscle at its inlet and the cardiac sphincter at the cardia of the stomach. These sphincters have been extensively studied from the physiologic point of view and are common sites of both benign and neoplastic disease.

The course of the esophagus is from slightly to the right of the midline to the left as it pierces the diaphragm through its own opening. It is in continual contact with the right lung; on the left side, the descending aorta is in continual contact. The azygos vein provides a partial shield on the right and posteriorly. Pulmonary veins would be expected to be in more intimate contact because they drain to the left auricle, which is posterior to the ventricle. The thoracic duct is posterior to the esophagus along its course, which is the reverse of the esophagus coursing from the right side of midline to the left as it ascends. When the esophagus comes anterior to the descending aorta, it is suspended by the mesoesophagus, which allows it to curve forward before it passes through the diaphragm (Fig. 23.4).

- *Coronal*: The EGJ is usually located to the left of the midline, at the 11th thoracic vertebra, and the pylorus is usually located at the L1 vertebral level to the right of the midline at the transpyloric plane; the angular incisura separates the body from the pyloric region of the stomach.

- *Sagittal*: The peritoneal cavity consists of the greater sac and omental bursa. The superior recess of the omental bursa is between the liver and the posterior attachment of the diaphragm. The inferior recess of the omental bursa is between the two double layers of the greater omentum. In the adult, the inferior recess usually only extends inferiorly as far as the transverse colon because of fusion of the two double peritoneal layers at birth.

- *Transverse*: The gastrosplenic and splenorenal ligaments tether the spleen in place between the stomach and the kidney; the ligaments from a pedicle (stalk) through which blood vessels run to and from the hilum of the spleen. These ligaments are double layers of peritoneum that form the left boundary of the omental bursa (lesser sac); the inner layer consists of peritoneum lining the omental bursa, and the outer layer consists of peritoneum lining the peritoneal cavity (greater sac).

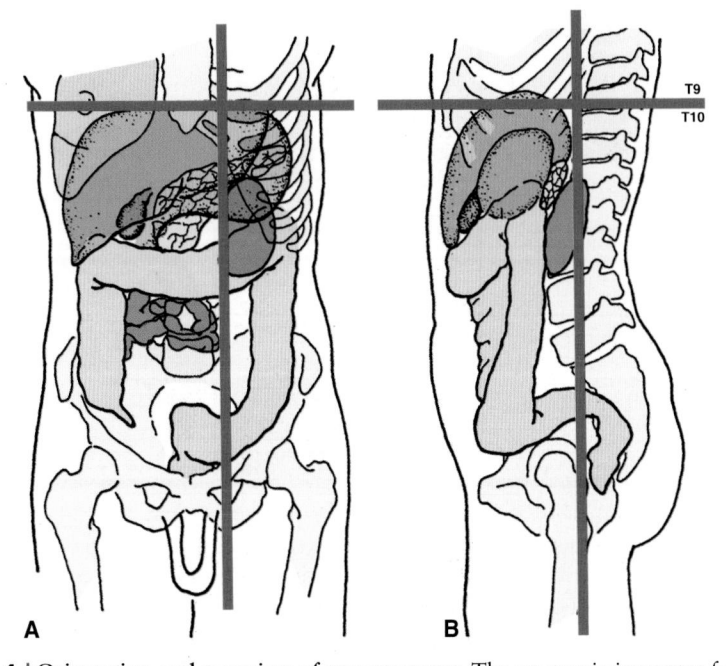

Figure 23.4 | Orientation and overview of oncoanatomy. The anatomic isocenter for the esophagogastric junction (EGJ) cancers is at T9/T10. **A.** Coronal. **B.** Sagittal.

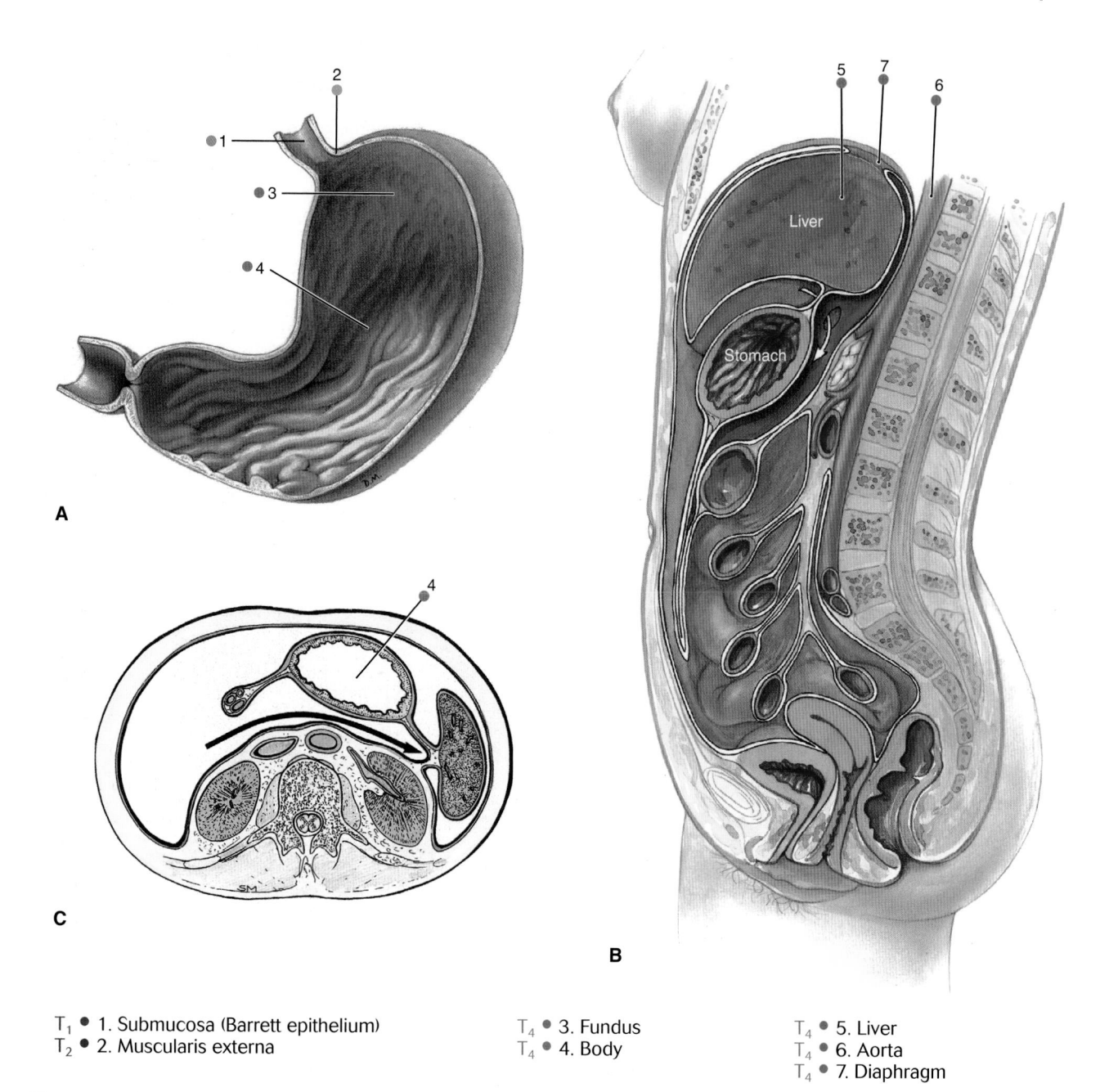

T_1 • 1. Submucosa (Barrett epithelium)	T_4 • 3. Fundus	T_4 • 5. Liver
T_2 • 2. Muscularis externa	T_4 • 4. Body	T_4 • 6. Aorta
		T_4 • 7. Diaphragm

Figure 23.5 | T-oncoanatomy. Connecting the dots: Structures are color coded for cancer stage progression. The color code for the anatomic sites correlates with the color code for the stage group (Fig. 23.3) and patterns of spread (Fig. 23.2) and SIMLAP table (Table 23.2). Connecting the dots in similar colors will provide an appreciation for the 3D oncoanatomy.

N-ONCOANATOMY AND M-ONCOANATOMY

N-ONCOANATOMY

Esophagogastric cancers frequently lead to lymphatic involvement not only of mediastinal nodes, but also of celiac and para-aortic nodes (Table 23.4). The AJCC/International Union

TABLE 23.4	Lymph Nodes of Esophagogastric Junction
Sentinel Nodes include Lesser Curvature and Celiac Nodes	
Regional Nodes	**Juxtaregional Nodes**
Lower esophageal	Internal jugular
Left gastric	Cervical
Posterior mediastinal	Para-aortic
Pericardial	
Diaphragmatic	

Against Cancer numbering of mediastinal and abdominal nodes is unique and is different from the International Anatomy Terminology. The percentage of positive lymph nodes in the celiac area increases as the cancer location migrates from the upper esophagus to the EGJ (Fig. 23.6A), namely, from 32% to 70%.

The regional lymph nodes for the cervical esophagus are the cervical and supraclavicular nodes. For the thoracic esophagus, the regional nodes are the adjacent mediastinal lymph nodes. Involvement of more distant nodes is considered distant metastasis. Retrograde and prograde lymphatic spread usually places all of the lymph node stations in the neck, mediastinum, and abdomen at risk.

One of the major problems with control of this cancer is the frequency with which lymph node invasion occurs and the rapidity of its dissemination to other, distant anatomic areas. Esophageal cancer is therefore a disease not only of the chest, but also of the neck and abdomen. Because of its lymphatic drainage, esophageal cancer is a formidable tumor to encompass by locoregional modalities of therapy. The percentage of positive nodes found at surgery staging—both mediastinal and abdominal—indicates that at all levels of the primary, infradiaphragmatic nodes are frequently involved (Fig. 23.6B).

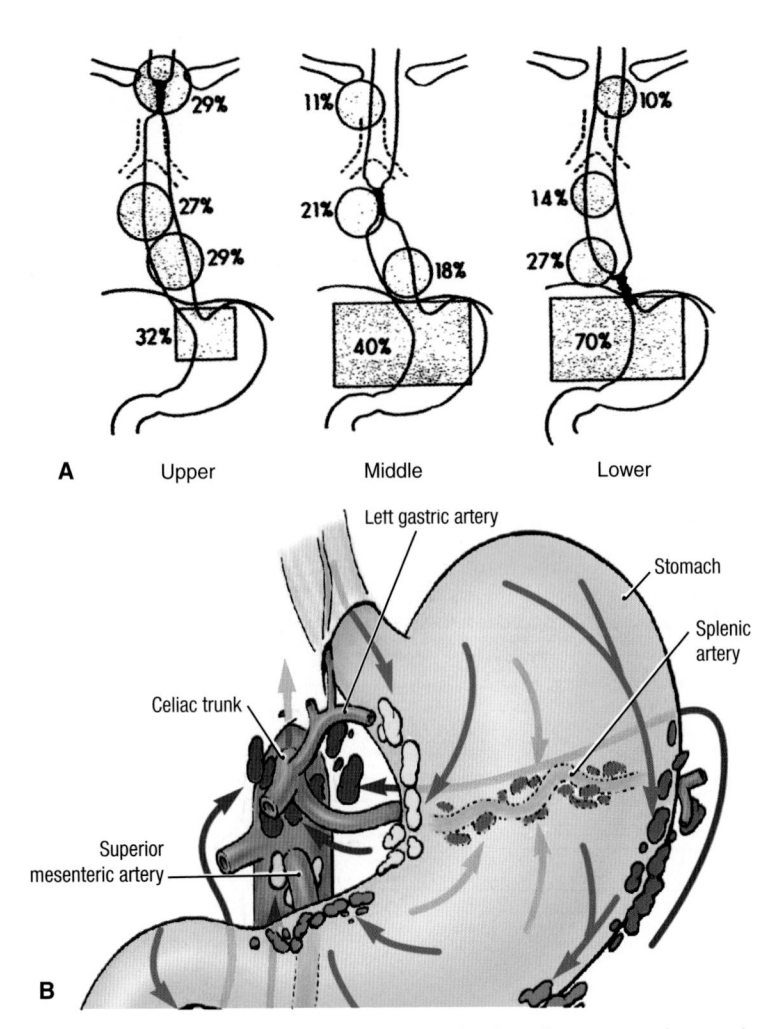

Figure 23.6 | N-oncoanatomy. **A.** The percentage of positive lymph nodes found at surgery for esophageal carcinoma in the upper, middle, and lower esophagus. **B.** Sentinel nodes of esophagogastric junction include thoracic and abdominal nodes. *(continued)*

A rich plexus of venous anastomoses exists with stomach, liver, pancreas, and adrenals (Fig. 23.6C). Therefore, the liver, lung, and adrenals are the most common sites of distant metastases. Remote metastasis from the carcinoma of the esophagus, although ultimately fatal, often carries a better prognosis than when the primary lesion has extended locally outside the esophagus into mediastinal structures, a condition that is rapidly fatal. The incidence of liver metastases exceeds that of other sites. According to a variety of reports in the literature, the range is 30% to 100% at autopsy. Other sites are mainly bone metastases (20% to 35%) and lung metastases (40% to 60%), with only occasional metastases to brain.

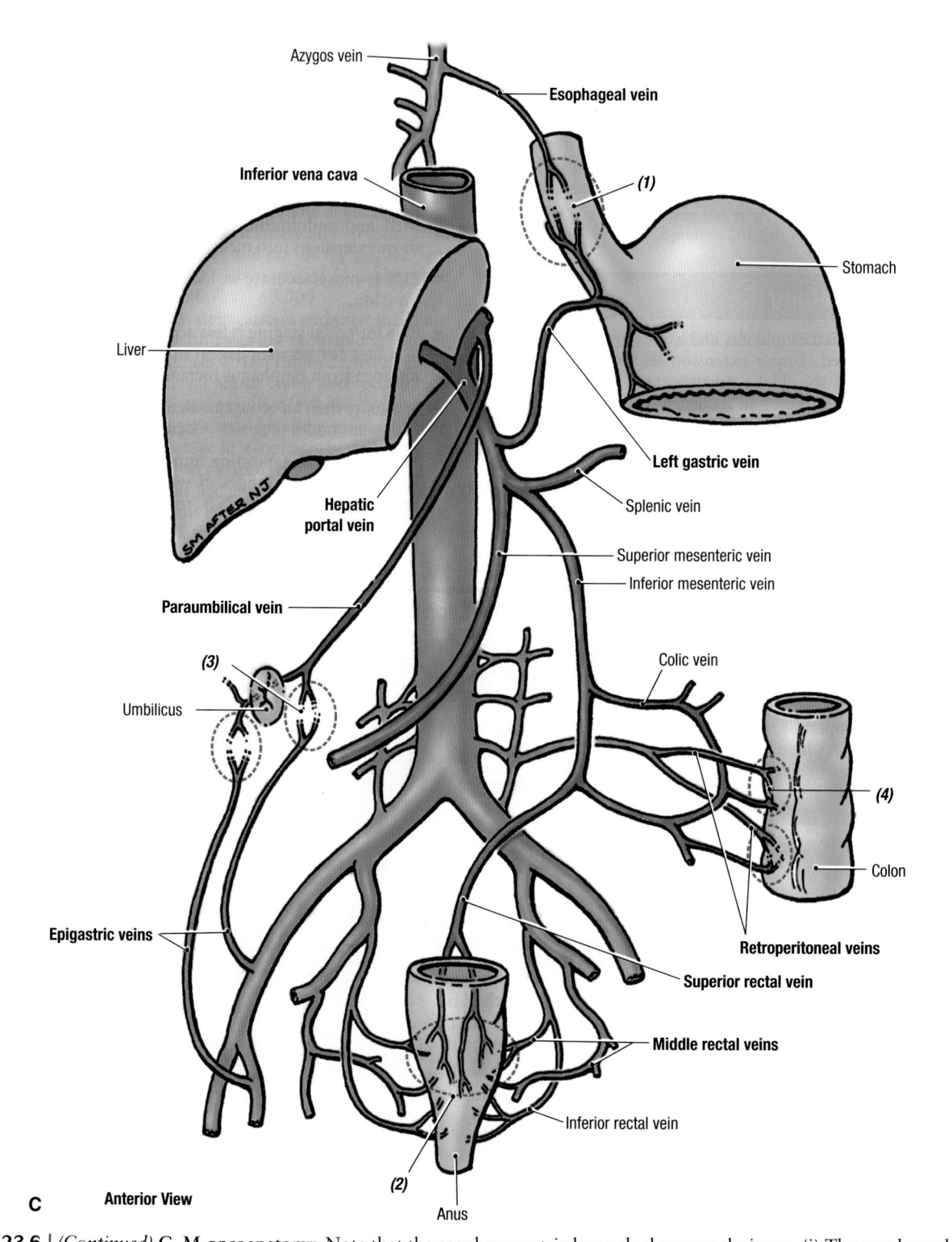

Figure 23.6 | *(Continued)* **C. M-oncoanatomy.** Note that the esophagogastric has a duel venous drainage. (i) The esophageal vein connects with the azygos vein and drains into the right heart, resulting in lung metastases. (ii) The left gastric vein drains the junction of esophagus and stomach, which in turn drains into the portal vein, resulting in liver metastases.

Stomach Cancer and Stromal Tumors

PERSPECTIVE, PATTERNS OF SPREAD, AND PATHOLOGY

The predisposing carcinogenic factors are atrophic gastric mucosa and intestinal metaplasia that transit into neoplasia from Ménétrier disease or hypertrophic gastritis. The predominant cancer is adenocarcinoma. Gastrointestinal stromal tumors (GISTs) are presented for staging in the seventh edition of the *AJCC Cancer Staging Manual* and is being presented here with stomach cancers, although they can occur elsewhere in the gastrointestinal tract (GIT). GISTs are the most common mesenchymal tumors in the GIT.

PERSPECTIVE AND PATTERNS OF SPREAD

Gastric cancers have undergone a decline in deaths and incidence since the 1950s; however, their status as aggressive and highly malignant neoplasms has not changed. In the United States and the Western world, although they have steadily declined in incidence. There is a tremendous variation worldwide; Japan has the highest incidence, accounting for 20% to 30% of all stomach cancers. The predisposing factors remain atrophic gastric mucosa and intestinal metaplasia that transit into neoplasia from Ménétrier disease or hypertrophic gastritis. Fundic and adenomatous polyps as in Gardner and Peutz–Jeghers syndromes tend to undergo carcinogenic

TABLE 24.1	Histopathologic Type: Common Cancers of the Esophagogastric and Junction and Stomach

Type
Adenocarcinoma
Papillary adenocarcinoma
Mucinous adenocarcinoma
Tubular adenocarcinoma
Signet ring cell carcinoma
Adenosquamous carcinoma
Squamous cell carcinoma
Small cell carcinoma
Undifferentiated carcinomas

Data from Edge SB, Byrd DR, Compton CC, et al. *AJCC Cancer Staging Manual, 7th ed.* New York, Springer, 2010, p. 111.

change. Because of the large, saclike nature of the stomach, this part of the digestive system can accommodate large neoplasms before onset of symptoms. Presentations range from fungating and ulcerative process to a widely infiltrative process resulting in a linitis plastica, stomach almost devoid of peristalsis. The patterns of invasion into and through the stomach wall are shown in Fig. 24.2 and Table 24.2.

Early diagnosis is essential to cure, and when camera imaging and frequent endoscopic screens are employed, as in Japan, precancerous and small lesions are found. An Early Gastric Cancer (ECG) classification of minimal microscopic lesions has been introduced. ECG in Japan constitutes 25% to 50% of all gastric adenocarcinomas as compared to 5% to 15% in Western countries. ECG is noted to have three types of presentation: Type I (elevated) protrudes in lumen >5 cm; type II are superficial lesions with elevations or depressions; and type III resembles ulcers or craters and amputate gastric folds. The staging recommendations apply to carcinomas, not lymphomas or sarcomas. A tabulation of cell types reflects the varied surface epithelia and secretory glandular cells. Once the mucosa is breeched, invasion of the muscle cell wall occurs with dissemination along these muscle layers (see Table 24.1).

A unique feature of the stomach is the attachment of suspensory ligaments consisting of two layers of peritoneum, that is, gastrohepatic ligament along the lesser curvature and the gastrocolic ligament along the greater curvature. Thus cancer penetrates the muscular propria and invades the ligaments (subserosally) without breeching the serosa. Gastric cancer invasion of the lesser and greater omentum is T3, not T4. Perforation of the visceral peritoneum is required to be T4.

Likewise, the uniquely high number of nodes invaded also are due to lymph nodes along the lesser and greater curvature and located inside the aforementioned ligaments (subserosal) and not external to the serosa cover as in the small intestine and colon.

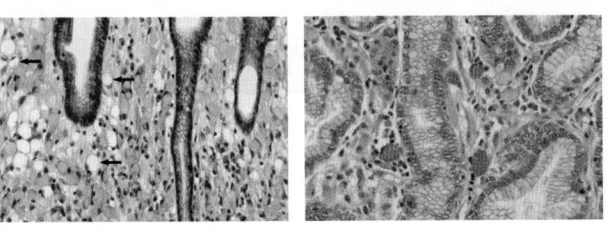

A   B

Figure 24.1 A,B | Infiltrating gastric carcinoma. A. Numerous signet ring cells (*arrows*) infiltrate the lamina propria between intact crypts. **B.** Mucin stains highlight the presence of mucin within the neoplastic cells.

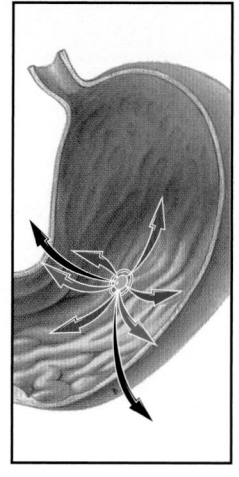

Figure 24.2 | Patterns of spread. The patterns of spread and the primary tumor classification are similarly color coded: Tis (cancer in situ of mucosa), yellow; T1 (infiltrates the submucosa), green; T2 (penetrates the muscularis externa), blue; T3 (reaches the subserosa), purple; and T4 (invades through the serosa into a neighboring viscera), red. The concept of visualizing patterns of spread to appreciate the surrounding anatomy is well demonstrated by the six-directional pattern, i.e., SIMLAP, Table 24.2.

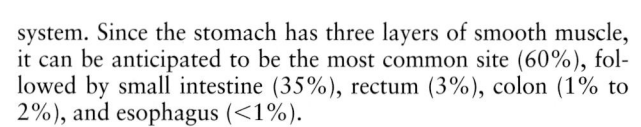

TABLE 24.2	SIMLAP		
Stomach (body)			
S	Fundus of stomach	• T1	• T2a
I	Antrum	• T1	• T2a
M	Lesser omentum	• T2b	
	Hepatoduodenal ligament	• T2b	
L	Greater omentum, spleen	• T2b	
A	Liver, left lobe	• T4	
P	Lesser omental bursa	• T3	
	Body and tail pancreas	• T4	

The six vectors of invasion are <u>S</u>uperior, <u>I</u>nferior, <u>M</u>edial, <u>L</u>ateral, <u>A</u>nterior, and <u>P</u>osterior. The color-coded dots correlate the T stage with specific anatomic structure involved.

PATHOLOGY

Patients with familial adenomatus polyposis have gastric adenomas that transform into cancers at a tenfold higher risk than the general population. Patients with hereditary nonpolyposis colorectal cancer have a 10% risk; juvenile polyposis has 15% to 20% risk of cancer. Numerous genetic abnormalities are associated with gastric adenocarcinoma. P53 is the most common association in 60% to 70% of gastric adenocarcinomas.

Cancer syndromes vary with size, location, and cancer progression. Submucosal T1 cancers are usually asymptomatic; T2 patients, muscularis propria, often have dyspepsia and weight loss; T3 patients often ulcerate and bleed and have melena; T4 patients can have feculent emesis or undigested food due to a gastrocolic fistula. More unusual symptoms and syndromes include the following:

- Pyloric outlet obstruction: early satiety and vomiting versus cardiac lesions where dysphagia predominates

- Paraneoplastic syndromes, such as thrombophlebitis (Trousseau's sign), neuropathies, nephritic syndromes, and less often dermatologic changes as hyperpigmented patches in axilla.

Unusual metastatic manifestations include the following:

- Krukenberg tumors of ovary

- Rectal shelf of Blumer due to pouch of Douglas invasion

- St. Joseph nodule at umbilicus

GIST refers to a wide spectrum of mesenchymal tumors, from leiomyomas to leiomyosarcomas, with varying combinations and permutations that include tumor size, mitotic activity, mitotic rate (mitosis/high-power field [HPF]) and are clustered into a range of prognostic groups. GIST can arise from smooth muscle walls of muscularis propria, which is ubiquitous in the GIT, it is not surprising that they can occur throughout this system. Since the stomach has three layers of smooth muscle, it can be anticipated to be the most common site (60%), followed by small intestine (35%), rectum (3%), colon (1% to 2%), and esophagus (<1%).

Lymph nodes and lymphatic spread do not occur as a rule. Metastases tend to be intra-abdominal (omental deposits) and to the liver, but other nonabdominal sites include bone, lung, and skin. Solitary omental and mesenteric tumors can be primaries. Multiple GIST can occur in neurofibromatosis type I (familiar GIST). Symptoms include GIT bleeding, dyspepsia, or obstructions. As a group they represent 1% of gastric tumors.

Gastric cancer can be subdivided into two forms:

- The *intestinal form* is characterized by tubular gland-like structures mimicking intestinal villi and is declining worldwide.

- The *diffuse form* is poorly differentiated, infiltrative, and lacks any semblance of glands.

There is evidence that gastric cancers are a multistep process similar to colon cancer. The initiation and progression are attributed to *Helicobacter pylori* that causes a chronic gastritis and gastric ulcers.

Intestinal metaplasias consist of three types: Type I is similar to normal morphology, Type II lacks enterocytes secretes siglomucins and Type III secretes sulfamucins. Progression to severe cysplasia and cancer is 10-20%, 20–40%, and 75–100% respectively for Types I, II, II. Gastric polyps tend to be hyperplastic and malignancy unlike colon is low: <1% in contrast to gastric adenomas transform in 11%.

GISTs arise from "pacemaker cells" and are so classified based on molecular and immunohistology, specifically express KIT protein, tyrosine kinase receptor, or its gene (PDG FRA). Histologically, the cells are composed of plump spindle cells with permanent cytoplasmic vacuoles enmeshed within a myoid stroma.

TNM STAGING CRITERIA

TNM STAGING CRITERIA

T size is the key factor, not depth of invasion as in epithelial adenocarcinomas, that is, <5, 5 to 10, >10 cm, and is modified by mitotic rate/HPF that assigns a prognostic group (score), which in turn provides a rate of tumor progression. Gastric cancers are confined and accommodated in the stomach and can reach large size as compared with other, narrower parts of the intestine. Bormans originally described the various appearances of advanced cancer, including the criteria to distinguish a malignant versus a benign gastric ulcer: I, polypoid; II, ulcerative; III, infiltrative ulcerated; and IV, linitis plastica.

The major American Joint Committee on Cancer (AJCC) staging criteria are based on depth of invasion of a hollow viscus: T1 (mucosal) invades lamina propria; T2 has been modified as T2a (invades muscularis propria) and T2b (subserosa). Subserosal stage applies to tumors extending into gastrocolic or gastrohepatic ligament or lesser or greater omentum. The omentum consists of two layers of peritoneum. An infiltrating cancer sandwiched between the two layers of omental peritoneum is considered subserosal despite being extragastric because the serosa is not penetrated. T3 means penetration of serosa or visceral peritoneum, and T4 implies invasion of surrounding viscera such as spleen, transverse colon, liver, diaphragm, pancreas, or other structure (Fig. 24.3A).

Intramural extension to esophagus or duodenum follows the depth-of-invasion rules for staging rather than advancing in stage.

Generally, there is no overarching principle or context design for stage groupings in the digestive system (gastrointestinal tract) or major digestive glands. Stages are frequently expanded to six by subdividing stages into A and B. The T and N categories are assigned to a stage grouping, specifically for division of a stage into more (a) versus less (b) favorable groupings. This occurs at different stages for different sites.

Specifically, this site has the most unorthodox staging with its eight stages. Stage III is divided into A, B, and C. It is the only anatomic site in which positive nodes (T1 N1) are still stage I, assigned to IB. The T and N progression together advances stages II, III, and IV. Adding subscript numbers to T and N categories together correlates with stage; that is, stage IA = 1, stage IB = 2, stage II = 3, stage IIIA = 4, stage IIIB = 5, and stage IV > 5. The nodal categories are unique: N1, 1 to 2 nodes; N2, 3 to 6 nodes; and N3a 7–15 nodes, N3b has ≥ 16 nodes, >15 nodes. In comparison to many digestive system sites where N1 encompasses all nodal categories, the stomach is the most elaborate. Nevertheless, there are survival curve data supporting subdividing I and III into A and B (see last section).

Gastric cancer can be subdivided into two forms:

- The *intestinal form* is characterized by tubular gland-like structures mimicking intestinal villi and is declining worldwide.

- The *diffuse form* is poorly differentiated and infiltrative and lacks any semblance of glands.

There is evidence that gastric cancers are a multistep process similar to colon cancers. The initiation and progression are attributed to *Helicobacter pylori* that causes a chronic gastritis and gastric ulcers.

Intestinal metaplasias consist of three types: Type I is similar to normal morphology, type II lacks enterocytes secreting siglomucins, and type III secretes sulfamucins. Rates of progression to severe cysplasia and cancer are 10% to 20%, 20% to 40%, and 75% to 100%, respectively, for types I, II, and III. Gastric polyps tend to be hyperplastic, and malignancy, unlike those of the colon, is low: <1%, in contrast to gastric adenomas, which transform in 11% of cases.

SUMMARY OF CHANGES SEVENTH EDITION AJCC

Major changes include subdividing T1 into T1a muscularis mucosa T1b submucosa invasion; T2, T3, T4 are the same N categories are major new definitions for N1, N2, N3 (6th edition). N1 1–2 (1–6), N3 3–6 (7–15), N3 ≥ 7 (>15 nodes).

M1 includes positive peritoneal cytology, which differs from staging.

- Tumors arising at the esophagogastric junction, or arising in the stomach ≤5cm from the esophagogastric junction and crossing the esophagogastric junction are staged using the TNM system for esophageal adenocarcinoma.

- T categories have been modified to harmonize with T categories of the esophagus and small and large intestine.

  - T1 lesions have been subdivided into T1a and T1b

  - T2 is defined as a tumor that invades the muscularis propria

  - T3 is defined as a tumor that invades the subserosal connective tissue

  - T4 is defined as a tumor that invades the serosa (visceral peritoneum) or adjacent structures

- N categories have been modified, with N1 = 1–2 positive lymph nodes, N2 = 3–6 positive lymph nodes, N3 = 7 or more positive lymph nodes

- Positive peritoneal cytology is classified as M1

- Stage groupings have been changed

The TNM Staging Matrix is color coded for identification of stage group once T and N stages are determined (Table 24.3).

| TABLE 24.3 | **Stage Summary Matrix** | | | |

	N0	N1	N2	N3	M1
T1	IA	IB	IIA	IIB	IV
T2	IB	IIA	IIB	IIIA	IV
T3	IIA	IIB	IIIA	IIIB	IV
T4a	IIB	IIIA	IIIB	IIIC	IV
T4b	IIIB	IIIB	IIIC	IIIC	IV

Both T and N progression determine Stage Group and substage
T stage progression $T_1, T_2, T_3, T_4 = $ IA, IB, II, IIIA
N stage progression $N_0, N_1, N_2, N_3 = $ IA, IB, IIA, B, IIIA, B, and IV

- $N_0 = $ IA, $N_1 = $ IB, $N_2 = $ II, IIIA, B, $N_3 = $ IV

Subscript Addition of T + N determines stage and substage progression generally:

- *Stage IA = 1 = T_1N_0*
- *IB = 2 = T_2N_0 or T_1N_1*
- *II = 3 = T_3N_0, T_2N_1, T_1N_2*
- *IIIA = 4 = T_2N_2, T_0N_1*
- *IIIB = 5 = T_3N_2*
- *IIIC = 6 = T_4N_2 or 7 = T_4N_3*

STOMACH ADENOCARCINOMA

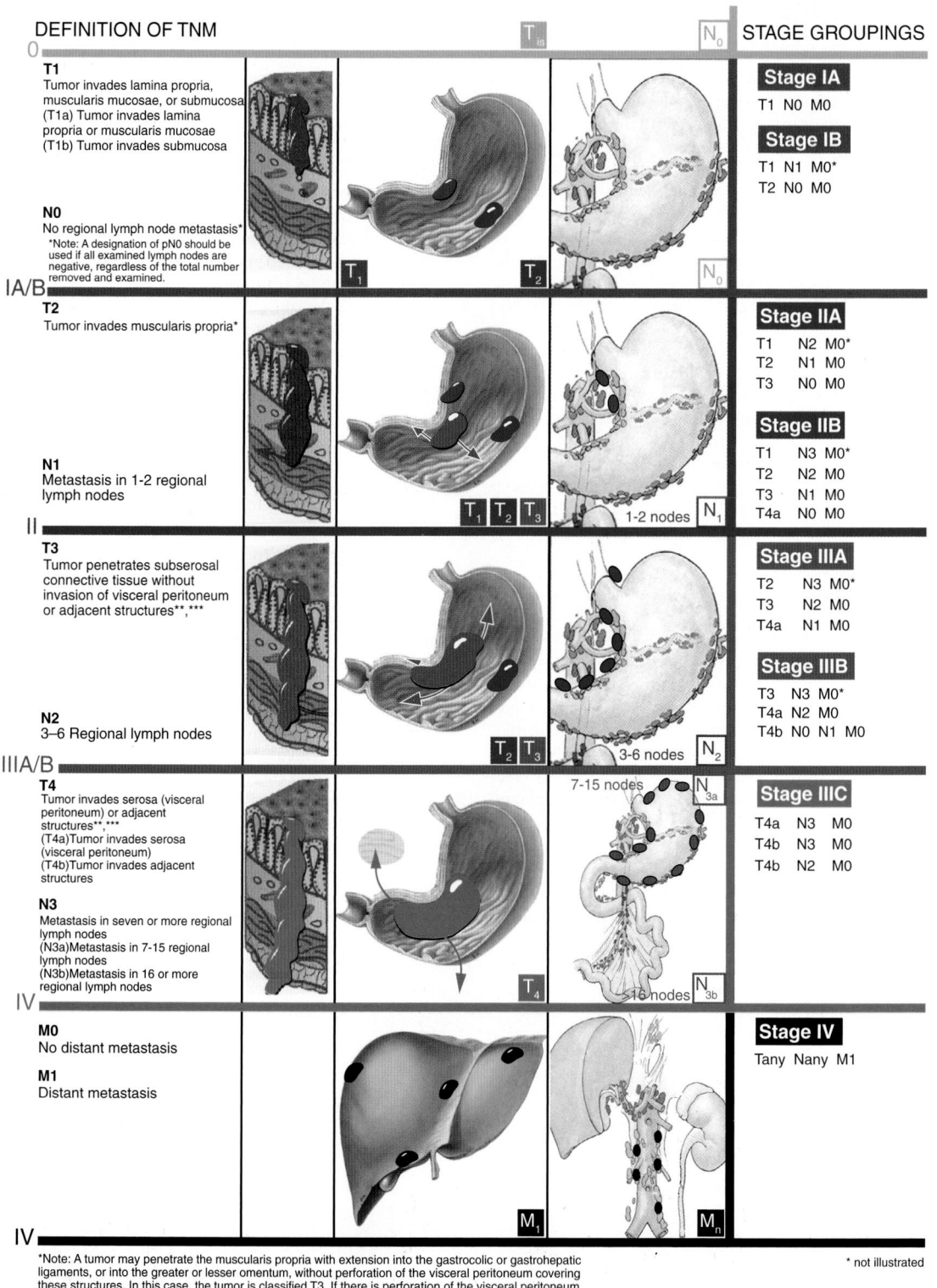

DEFINITION OF TNM

T1
Tumor invades lamina propria, muscularis mucosae, or submucosa
(T1a) Tumor invades lamina propria or muscularis mucosae
(T1b) Tumor invades submucosa

N0
No regional lymph node metastasis*
*Note: A designation of pN0 should be used if all examined lymph nodes are negative, regardless of the total number removed and examined.

T2
Tumor invades muscularis propria*

N1
Metastasis in 1-2 regional lymph nodes

T3
Tumor penetrates subserosal connective tissue without invasion of visceral peritoneum or adjacent structures**,***

N2
3–6 Regional lymph nodes

T4
Tumor invades serosa (visceral peritoneum) or adjacent structures**,***
(T4a) Tumor invades serosa (visceral peritoneum)
(T4b) Tumor invades adjacent structures

N3
Metastasis in seven or more regional lymph nodes
(N3a) Metastasis in 7-15 regional lymph nodes
(N3b) Metastasis in 16 or more regional lymph nodes

M0
No distant metastasis

M1
Distant metastasis

STAGE GROUPINGS

Stage IA
T1 N0 M0

Stage IB
T1 N1 M0*
T2 N0 M0

Stage IIA
T1 N2 M0*
T2 N1 M0
T3 N0 M0

Stage IIB
T1 N3 M0*
T2 N2 M0
T3 N1 M0
T4a N0 M0

Stage IIIA
T2 N3 M0*
T3 N2 M0
T4a N1 M0

Stage IIIB
T3 N3 M0*
T4a N2 M0
T4b N0 N1 M0

Stage IIIC
T4a N3 M0
T4b N3 M0
T4b N2 M0

Stage IV
Tany Nany M1

* not illustrated

*Note: A tumor may penetrate the muscularis propria with extension into the gastrocolic or gastrohepatic ligaments, or into the greater or lesser omentum, without perforation of the visceral peritoneum covering these structures. In this case, the tumor is classified T3. If there is perforation of the visceral peritoneum covering the gastric ligaments or the omentum, the tumor should be classified T4.
**The adjacent structures of the stomach include the spleen, transverse colon, liver, diaphragm, pancreas, abdominal wall, adrenal gland, kidney, small intestine, and retroperitoneum.
***Intramural extension to the duodenum or esophagus is classified by the depth of the greatest invasion in any of these sites, including the stomach.

Figure 24.3A | TNM staging diagram presents a vertical arrangement with color bars encompassing TN combinations showing progression. The stomach has the most elaborate nodal staging categories, and despite <15 or >15 regional nodes (N2/N3), resections allow for 20% versus 8% 5-year survival, that is, IIIA ≠ B versus IV or purple versus red lane, respectively. Stage 0, yellow; I, green; II, blue; III, purple; IV, red; and IV (metastatic), black. Definitions of TN on left, and stage grouping on right.

GASTROINTESTINAL STROMAL TUMORS

Perspective and Patterns of Spread

Gastrointestinal stromal tumors (GIST) had been regarded as an obscure entity, but with uncovering of its molecular mechanism and improved diagnosis and reporting, a dramatic increase in incidence after 2000 has been found. In the United States, the annual reported incidence of 15 cases increased after 2000 to approximately 5000 cases per year. The majority of GISTs arise in the stomach (60% to 70%), and so it is presented and discussed at this anatomic site. The other site of some incidence is the small intestine (20% to 30%); for the rest of the digestive system, it is only 10%. Even more uncommon are extraintestinal sites, that is, omentum, mesentery, and retroperitoneum.

Clinical presentations vary with site of occurrence and tumor size, that is, >5 cm, with palpable mass, abdominal pain, and altered digestive peristalsis manifesting as nausea, anorexia, or vomiting. Most frightening is acute hemorrhage, which can occur in 40% of patients. Rupture can lead to peritoneal irritation and acute abdominal pain with splinting.

Several clinical syndromes have been described in association with GIST, characterized by multifocal tumors in other organs, for example, lung or adrenal gland, and linkages to neurofibromatosis.

Histopathology

Typically, GISTs were lumped with leiomyomas and, if mitotic activity was high, leiomyosarcomas, before availability of molecular markers. It was recognized that these tumors had similarities to "pacemaker cells" of the digestive system, that is, interstitial cells of Cajal, which coordinates peristalsis. This led to the observation of the role played by KIT receptor tyrosine kinase (RTK). GISTs express CD117, and immunochemical staining distinguishes them from leiomyosarcomas and desmoid tumors.

TNM Staging Criteria

According to consensus by pathologists, two important criteria are the hallmark for staging: size and number of mitosis. Less important are cell phenotype and cell pleomorphism. The AJCC TN categories are illustrated in Table 24.4.

Detection and Diagnosis

Most symptomatic lesions are identified endoscopically as a smooth protrusion of the mucosa. To establish a diagnosis, deep biopsy often is required but may be deferred to avoid tumor rupture. Endoscopic ultrasonograms are useful, revealing a hypoechoic mass contiguous with either muscularis mucosa or, more often, the muscularis propria. If margins are irregular or cystic degeneration is present, these signs suggest malignancy; lesions >4 cm also are most often malignant. Computed tomography (CT) imaging is superior to magnetic resonance imaging (MRI) and more accurately provides tumor extent. Positron emission tomography (PET) scans with 18-fluorodeoxyglucose can provide functional imaging to supplement CT and is believed due to overactive KIT/RTK. PET is also effective in finding metastasis foci in the liver and peritoneal cavity.

Management

Surgical resection is advised for accessible GIST tumors. Radiation therapy is not advised because of the dose-limiting tolerance of stomach, intestine, and liver. Cytotoxic chemotherapy is universally futile. Most intriguing and exciting are the use and effectiveness of molecular targeted therapy with imatinib mesylate for unresectable and metastatic foci. Numerous clinical trials have shown clinical benefit and response in 45% to 89% of cases. PET scanning can demonstrate decrease in tumor avidity in 24 hours, predicting CT responses months later. The optimal dose of imatinib remains to be determined in future clinical trials.

TABLE 24.4	Disease Progression in GISTs			
Stage	Tumor Size (cm)	Mitotic Rate	Prognostic Group[a]	Observed Rate of Progressive Disease[a]
Stage IA	≤5	Low	1, 2	0%–2%
Stage IB	>5–10	Low	3a	3%–4%
Stage II	>5–10	High	4	Insufficient data
	>5–10	High	5	15%
	>10	Low	3b	12%
Stage IIIA	>5–10	High	6a	49%
IIIB	>10	High	6b	86%

[a]From Miettinen M, Sobin LH, Lasota J. Gastrointestinal stromal tumors of the stomach: a clinicopathologic, immunohistochemical, and molecular genetic studies of 1765 cases with long-term follow-up. *Am J Surg Pathol* 2005;29:52–68. With permission from Lippincott Williams & Wilkins.

GASTRIC STROMAL SARCOMA

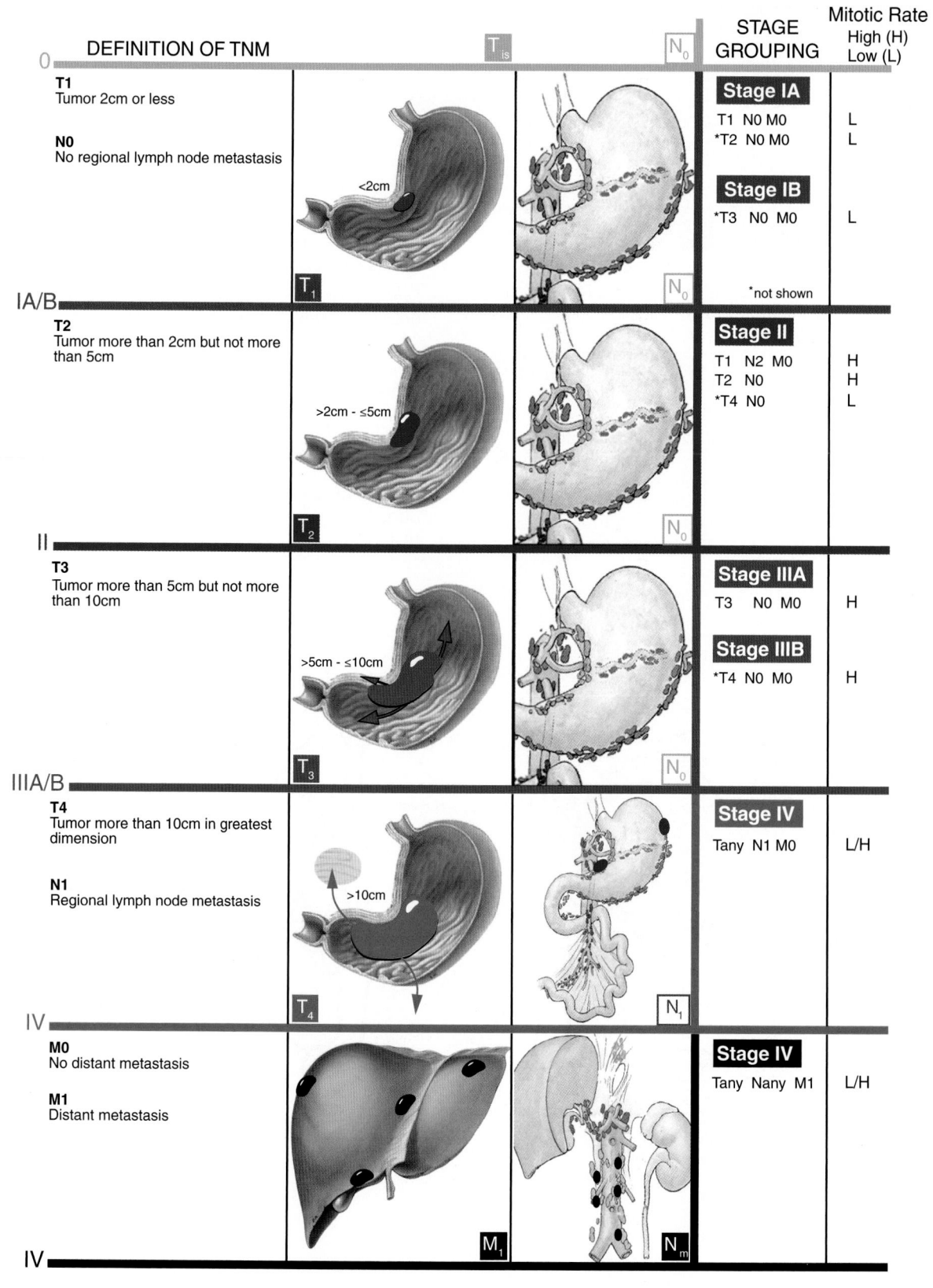

DEFINITION OF TNM

T1
Tumor 2cm or less

N0
No regional lymph node metastasis

T2
Tumor more than 2cm but not more than 5cm

T3
Tumor more than 5cm but not more than 10cm

T4
Tumor more than 10cm in greatest dimension

N1
Regional lymph node metastasis

M0
No distant metastasis

M1
Distant metastasis

STAGE GROUPING

Mitotic Rate
High (H)
Low (L)

Stage IA
T1 N0 M0   L
*T2 N0 M0   L

Stage IB
*T3 N0 M0   L

*not shown

Stage II
T1 N2 M0   H
T2 N0   H
*T4 N0   L

Stage IIIA
T3 N0 M0   H

Stage IIIB
*T4 N0 M0   H

Stage IV
Tany N1 M0   L/H

Stage IV
Tany Nany M1 L/H

Figure 24.3B | TNM staging criteria are color-coded bars for T advancement: Tis, yellow; T1, green; T2, blue; T3, purple; T4, red.

T-ONCOANATOMY

ORIENTATION OF THREE-PLANAR ONCOANATOMY

The isocenter for the three-planar anatomy is to the left of the midline anteriorly and at the T10/T11 level posteriorly (Fig. 24.4).

T-oncoanatomy

The T-oncoanatomy is displayed in three planar views. A. Coronal, B. Sagittal, C. Transverse axial (Figure 24.5).

The stomach is divided into three regions: upper, middle, and lower third. To delineate these regions, the lesser and greater curves of the stomach are divided; the upper third is the cardia and the fundus, the middle third is the body, and the lower third is the antrum.

The stomach is an organ with numerous metamorphic shapes: Hypertonic contracted stomach is often high in the upper quadrant; hypotonic to atonic viscus drops into the pelvis; and normal orthotonic viscus reaches to the umbilicus. The stomach mucosa begins at the zigzag line of the cardia defined by the pinkish glandular mucosa with its chief and parietal cells (Fig. 24.6).

- *Coronal*: The body of the stomach has a lesser and a greater curvature, a fundus superior to the body, and a pyloric region divided into an antrum and a pyloric canal. Extensions into adjacent or contiguous structures such as esophagus or duodenum are staged according to the depth of invasion in their wall. Gastric rugae or Magenstrasse are the villous mucosal folds with their secretory epithelia with parietal (HCl), chief (pepsinogen), and mucous (mucin) cells, which constitute them and their varied secretions. In addition to an inner circular layer and an outer longitudinal layer, there is a middle zone of both circular and oblique muscle layers. The cardia and pylorus have sphincteric activity and control the entry and departure of swallowed food.

- *Sagittal*: The arrow passes from the greater sac into the omental foramen into the lesser sac or omental bursa (Fig. 24.5C).

- *Transverse*: The gastrosplenic and splenorenal ligaments tether the spleen in place between the stomach and the kidney; the ligaments form a pedicle (stalk), through which blood vessels run to and from the hilum of the spleen. These ligaments are double layers of peritoneum that form the left boundary of the omental bursa (lesser sac); the inner layer consists of peritoneum lining the omental bursa, and the outer layer consists of peritoneum lining the peritoneal cavity (greater sac).

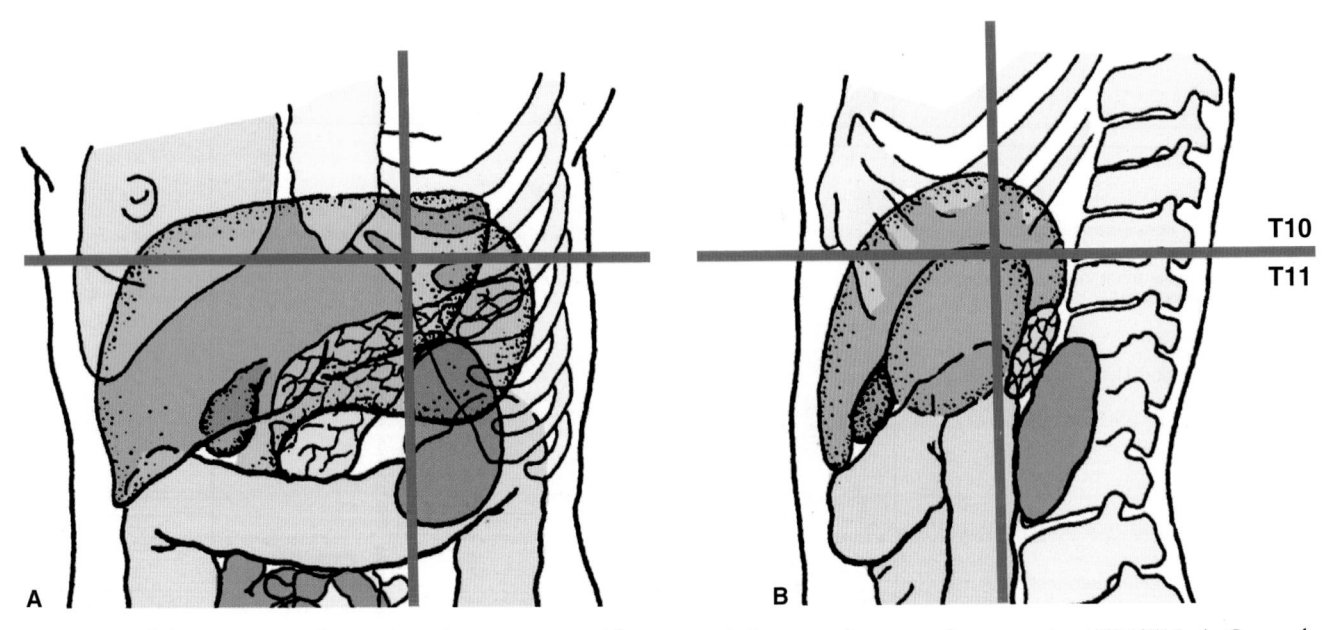

Figure 24.4 | **Orientation and overview of oncoanatomy.** The anatomic isocenter for stomach cancers is at T10/T11. **A.** Coronal. **B.** Sagittal.

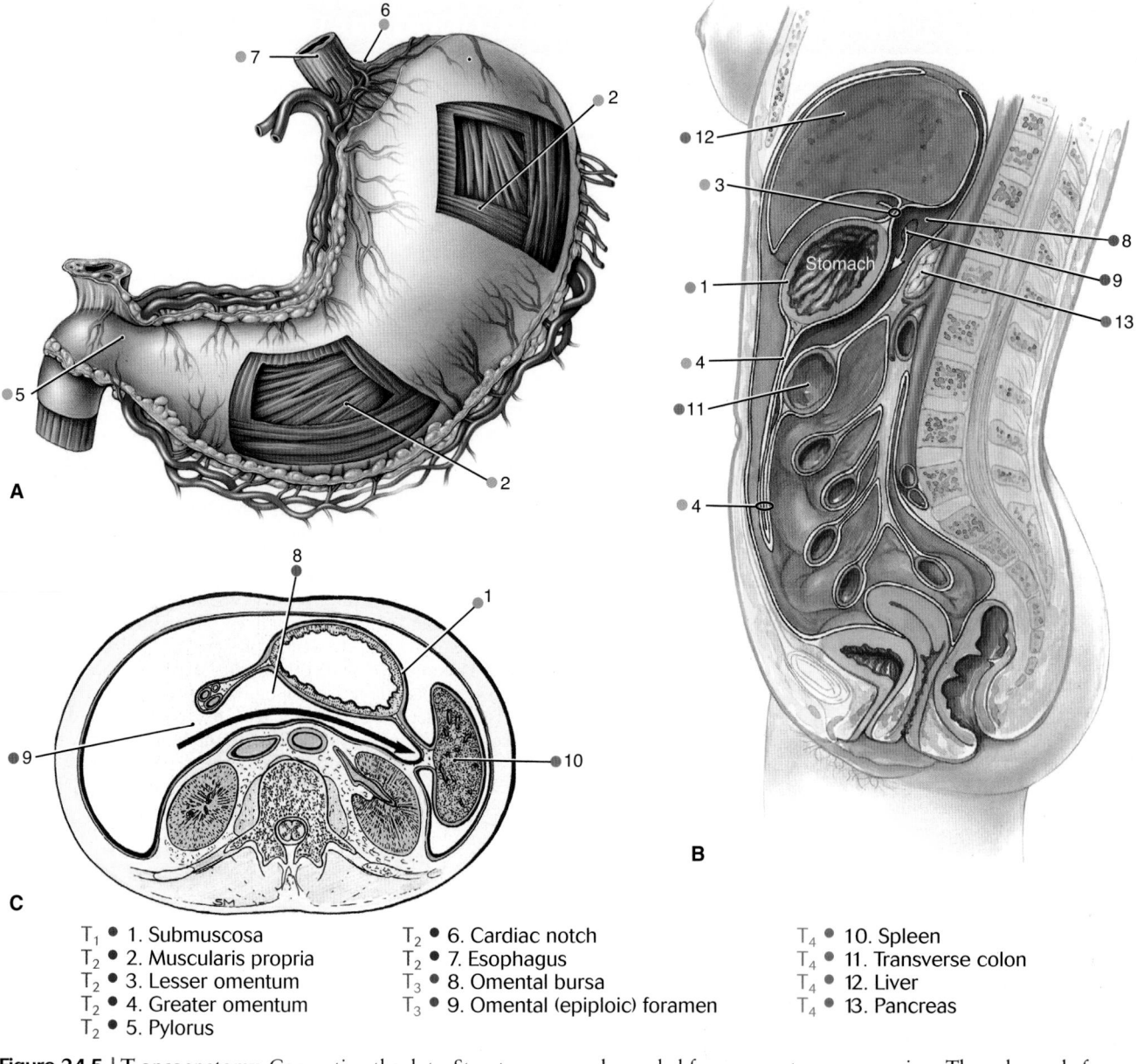

T1	●	1. Submuscosa	T2	●	6. Cardiac notch	T4	●	10. Spleen
T2	●	2. Muscularis propria	T2	●	7. Esophagus	T4	●	11. Transverse colon
T2	●	3. Lesser omentum	T3	●	8. Omental bursa	T4	●	12. Liver
T2	●	4. Greater omentum	T3	●	9. Omental (epiploic) foramen	T4	●	13. Pancreas
T2	●	5. Pylorus						

Figure 24.5 | T-oncoanatomy. Connecting the dots. Structures are color coded for cancer stage progression. The color code for the anatomic sites correlates with the color code for the stage group (Fig. 24.3) and patterns of spread (Fig. 24.2) and SIMLAP tables (Table 24.2). Connecting the dots in similar colors will provide an appreciation for the 3D oncoanatomy.

N-ONCOANATOMY AND M-ONCOANATOMY

N-ONCOANATOMY

Regional Lymph Nodes

Several groups of regional lymph nodes drain the wall of the stomach. These perigastric nodes are found along the lesser and greater curvatures. Other major nodal groups follow the main arterial and venous vessels from the aorta and the portal circulation. Adequate nodal dissection of these regional nodal areas is important to ensure appropriate designation of the pN determination. Although it is suggested that at least 16 regional nodes be assessed pathologically, a pN0 determination may be assigned on the basis of the actual number of nodes evaluated microscopically (Table 24.5, Fig. 24.6).

Involvement of other intra-abdominal lymph nodes, such as the hepatoduodenal, retropancreatic, mesenteric, and para-aortic, is classified as distant metastasis. The specific nodal areas are as follows:

- *Greater curvature of stomach*: Greater curvature, greater omental, gastroduodenal, gastroepiploic, pyloric, and pancreaticoduodenal

- *Pancreatic and splenic area*: Pancreaticolienal, peripancreatic, splenic

- *Lesser curvature of stomach*: Lesser curvature, lesser omental, left gastric, cardioesophageal, common hepatic, celiac, and hepatoduodenal

- *Distant nodal groups*: Retropancreatic, para-aortic, portal, retroperitoneal, mesenteric.*

*Preceding passage from Edge SB, Byrd DR, and Compton CC, et al, *AJCC Cancer Staging Manual, 7th edition*. New York, Springer, 2010, p. 119.

M-ONCOANATOMY

The entire portal circulation should be considered as a unit in regard to the venous anatomy of the gastrointestinal tract below the diaphragm (Fig. 24.6B). The two major trunks are the inferior mesenteric and superior mesenteric veins. The inferior mesenteric vein drains the left colon and sigmoid colon tributaries, which covers the vascular drainage to the left of the midline originating from the superior rectal veins. On the right side, the superior mesenteric vein originates from the tributaries draining the ileum, jejunum, and the ileocolic and right middle colic veins. The inferior mesenteric vein usually joins the splenic vein, which coalesces with the superior mesenteric vein and forms the portal vein. The splenic vein, which is a major tributary of the portal system, also drains much of the stomach along its greater curvature and includes the short gastric veins and left and right gastric epiploic veins. The right gastric epiploic also flows into the superior mesenteric vein. The entire drainage of the lesser curvature of the stomach including the left and right gastric veins drains directly into the portal vein. Because the portal vein then drains directly into the liver, it is the target metastatic organ and the most commonly involved organ in hematogenous spread pattern from the venous system of the gastrointestinal tract, as compared with other parts of the body, where the drainage is directly into the lung by way of the caval system.

The incidence of liver metastases exceeds that of other sites. According to a variety of reports in the literature, the range is 38% to 100% at autopsy. Other sites are mainly bone metastases, 20% to 35%, and lung metastases, 40% to 60%, with only occasional metastases to brain.

TABLE 24.5	**Lymph Nodes of Stomach**
Sentinel Nodes include Lesser and Greater Curvature Nodes	
Regional Nodes	**Juxtaregional Nodes**
Celiac	Para-aortic
Left gastropancreatic	Mediastinal
Lesser curvature	Retrocaval
Juxtacardiac	
Splenic	
Hepatic	
Gastroduodenal	
Right gastropyloric	
Suprapyloric	
Pancreatic–duodenal	

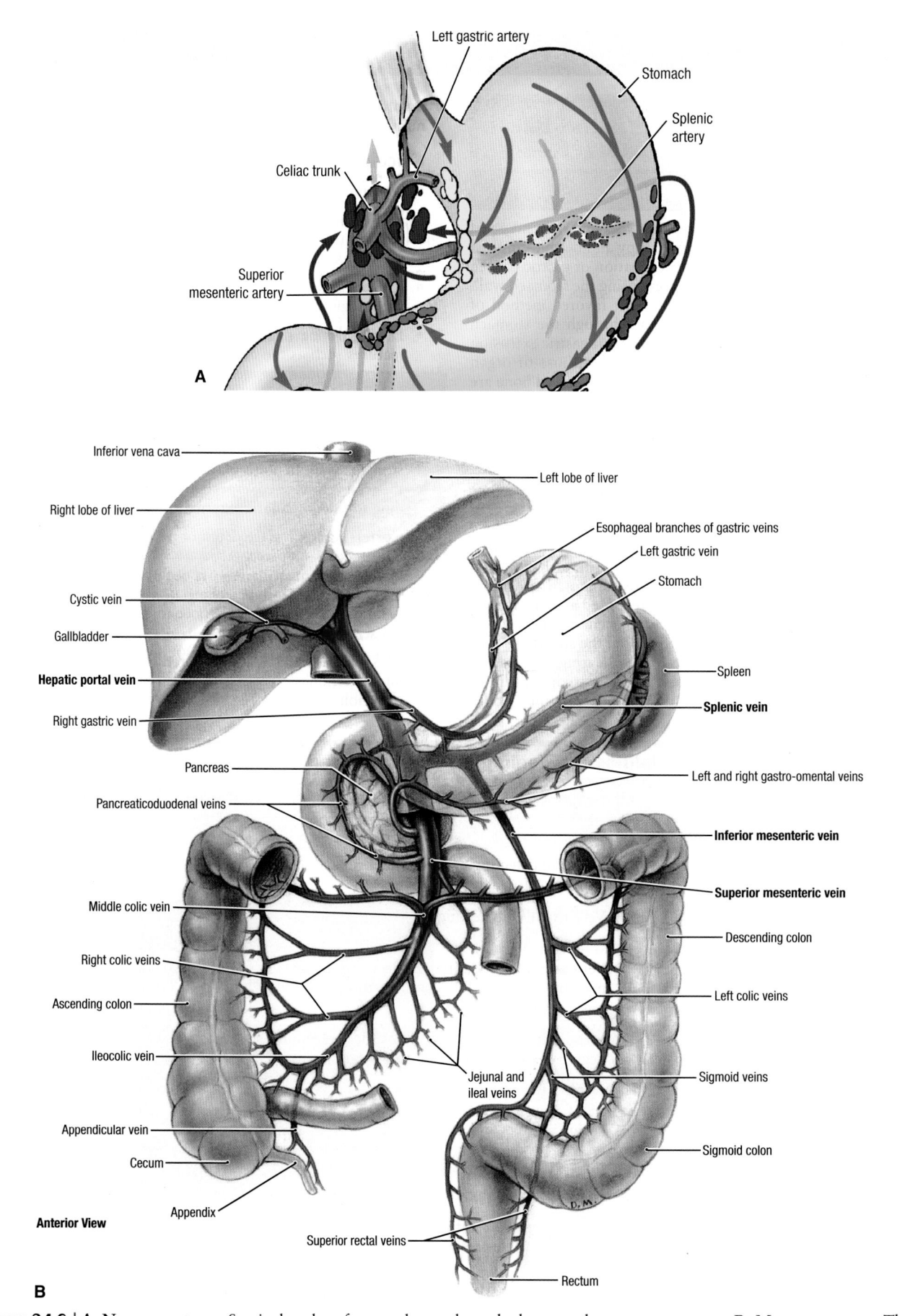

Figure 24.6 | A. N-oncoanatomy. Sentinel nodes of stomach are along the lesser and greater curvatures. **B. M-oncoanatomy.** The left and right gastric veins drain into the portal venous system, leading to liver metastases predominantly.

Liver and Intrahepatic Bile Ducts

PERSPECTIVE, PATTERNS OF SPREAD, AND PATHOLOGY

Because of the higher incidence of hepatitis B viral infections, wider ingestion of aflatoxins from moldy peanuts, and intestinal parasites such as schistosomiasis, hepatocellular cancers are extremely common among Asians and the Bantu of Africa.

PERSPECTIVE AND PATTERNS OF SPREAD

Cancers of the major digestive glands (MDGs) remain a challenge to diagnose and treat. The 5-year survival rates have remained at 1% to 2% for decades, reflecting the advanced stages at which this disease is detected. Masquerading as nonspecific complaints such as epigastric fullness or mild distress, vague abdominal or back pain, or unexplained weight loss, it is no surprise that these neoplasms are not recognized until they have become extensive, replacing much of their organ of origin. Both cancer of the pancreas and cancer of the liver are increasing in incidence. Incidence of pancreatic cancers has tripled over the last 40 years, and they are the second-most-common tumor in the alimentary tract. By contrast, liver neoplasms are relatively uncommon in North America; however, in Southeast Asia and Africa, because of the higher incidence of hepatitis B viral infections, wider ingestion of aflatoxins from moldy peanuts, and intestinal parasites such as schistosomiasis, hepatocellular cancers are extremely common among Asians and the Bantu. In fact, the high incidence of hepatomas in China and Asia makes this tumor, by sheer size of the population involved, a common cancer globally.

Clinical features and presentations include abdominal pain (59% to 95%), abdominal swelling (28% to 43%), and eventually severe weight loss and weakness. Hepatomegaly (54% to 98%), splenomegaly (27% to 42%), and ascites (35% to 61%) are common. With hepatic vein and inferior vena cava tumor invasion or compression, severe pitting edema accompanies ascites. Paraneoplastic syndromes are uncommon but rare enough to suggest hepatocellular carcinoma (HCC).

- Severe hypoglycemia (type B) can occur due to defective processing of precursor to insulin growth factor II (pro-IGFII).

- Polycythemia occurs in 10% of cases, and, if associated cirrhosis exists, hepatocellular cancer is a highly probable cause and is known to produce erythropoietin-like substances.

- Hypercalcemia in the absence of osteolytic metastases can be due to parathyroid hormone–related protein due to HCC.

- Sudden elevated cholesterol levels can be manifested in one third of wasted patients.

TABLE 25.1 Histopathologic Type: Common Cancers of the Liver

Type	Incidence (%)
Hepatocellular carcinoma (liver cell carcinoma)[a]	85–95
Fibrolamellar variant of hepatocellular carcinoma	
Cholangiocarcinoma (intrahepatic bile duct carcinoma)	5–15
Mixed hepatocellular cholangiocarcinoma	<1
Undifferentiated	<1

[a]Hepatocellular carcinoma is by far the more common of the two types of primary carcinoma of the liver. The staging classification does not apply to primary sarcomas or metastatic tumors and no longer applies to tumors of the bile ducts (cholangiocarcinomas including mixed hepatocholangiocarcinoma), which are now considered in a separate, new staging system (see AJCC Cancer Staging Manual, 7th ed., Chapter 19). The histologic type and subtype should be recorded since they may provide prognostic information. Edge SB, Byrd DR, Compton CC, et al., AJCC Cancer Staging Manual, 7th edition. New York. Springer, p. 194 and p. 204.

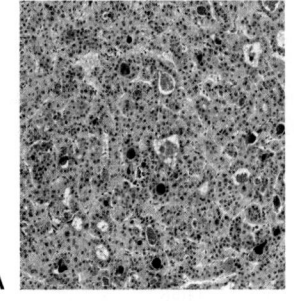

A

Figure 25.1A | A photomicrograph of the tumor shows a trabecular pattern of malignant hepatocytes. Many cells are arranged in an acinar pattern and surround concretions of inspissated bile.

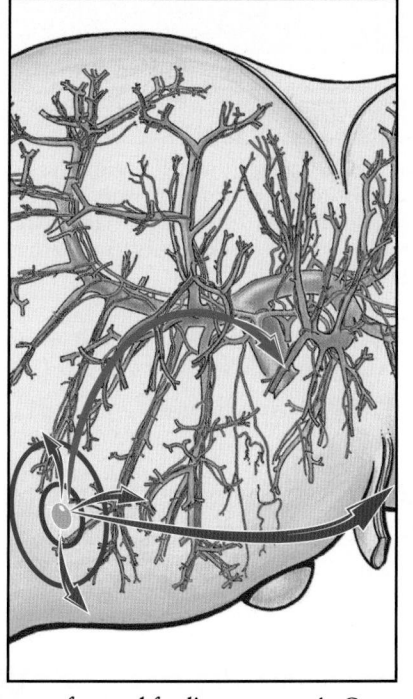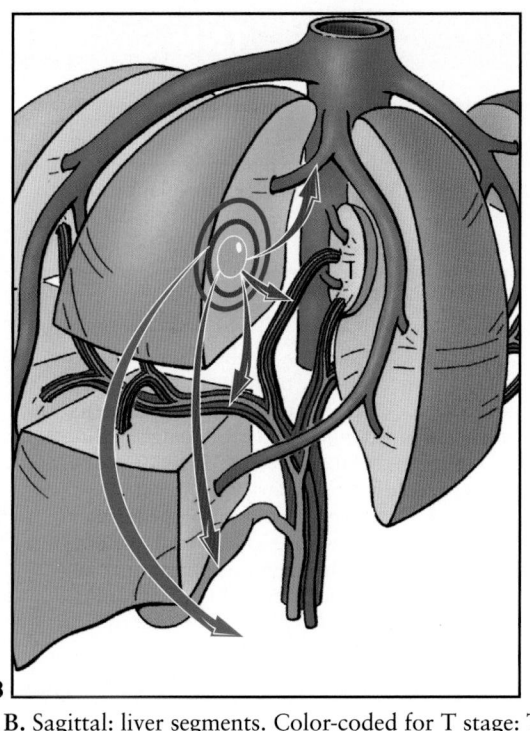

Figure 25.2 | **Patterns of spread for liver cancer. A.** Coronal. **B.** Sagittal: liver segments. Color-coded for T stage: Tis, yellow; T1, green; T2, blue; T3, purple; and T4, red. The concept of visualizing patterns of spread to appreciate the surrounding anatomy is well demonstrated by the six-directional pattern, i.e., SIMLAP Table 25.2.

- Elevation of alpha fetoprotein suggests HCC in Chinese and African populations.

- Dermatopathic lesions such as pityriasis rotunda manifest as rashes with single or multiple oval or round scaly and hyperpigmental lesions on trunk or thigh; this is an especially useful indication in black Africans as to HCC.

- If a person is infected with both hepatitis B virus (HBV) and hepatitis C virus (HCV), then HCC is three times higher than for each alone.

- Hemachromatosis and Wilson disease with alpha-1-antitrypsin deficiency increase risk of HCC.

With an annual rate over 20,000 new patients, liver cancers are becoming a major problem in the United States. Most patients succumb to either the hepatoma or the cirrhotic liver induced by hepatitis virus B and C. Liver failure is inevitable. Patterns of spread are mainly into adjacent liver lobules and then into its vasculature and major vessels, i.e., portal vein, hepatic artery, and then the surrounding viscera (Fig. 25.2; Table 25.2).

PATHOLOGY

The genome of HBV is integrated into the DNA of HCC and probably transforms liver cells into malignancy. HCC can be solitary or clusters of multiple nodules either as a function of multicentricity or metastatic spread. Vascular invasion is common in both the portal vein and hepatic vein since the majority of the circulation is venous (70% to 80%). The histologic types range widely from well, to mixed, to poorly differentiated.

- In the differentiated trabecular variety, hepatocytes grow in sheets separated by inconspicuous sinusoids.

- In the undifferentiated variety, the cells are pleomorphic and vary in size and shape; bizarre giant cells are present.

- Moderate differentiation can appear as a mixture and appear solid, scirrhous, or clear celled.

- Fibrolamellar HCC is a unique variant that occurs in adolescents and young adults and has eosinophilic tumor cells in a lamellar pattern.

The histopathology of hepatic malignancy originates from either hepatocytes or intrahepatic duct lining cells, that is, HCC or cholangiocarcinoma, respectively (Fig. 25.1; Table 25.1). Propagation and proliferation of cancers spread within the liver, pursuing paths infiltrating low-pressure zones such as central veins or into bile ducts.

TABLE 25.2	SIMLAP	
Liver (right lobe)		• T1
S	Diaphragm	• T4
I	Gall bladder, transverse colon	• T3
	Hepatic flexure	• T3
M	Laudate/quadrate lobes	• T3
	Stomach	• T4
	Porta hepatis	• T3
L	Abdominal wall	• T4
A	Diaphragm	• T4
P	Hepatic vein, inferior vena cava	• T3

The six vectors of invasion are Superior, Inferior, Medial, Lateral, Anterior, and Posterior. The color-coded dots correlate the T stage with specific anatomic structure involved.

TNM STAGING CRITERIA

CLASSIFICATION AND STAGING

The only viable alternative most often is liver transplantation.

TNM STAGING CRITERIA

Hepatomas or hepatocellular cancers of the liver tend to remain localized in the liver for long periods of time. They often tend to invade various lobes of the liver, deep into its substance, entering sinusoidal channels and producing satellite lesions. Although some encapsulation occurs, it tends to be diffuse and does not respect lobar boundaries.

As the liver substance is replaced, the cancer penetrates through Glisson's capsule. It can invade other vital viscera, such as the stomach and intestine, although this is very uncommon. The size of the liver nodules and their volume have influenced the establishment of a staging system. The size of T1 cancer is solitary, <5 cm, and lacks vascular invasion. T2 are multiple nodules in aggregates <5 cm in size but with vascular invasion. T3 are multiple tumors >5 cm, or evidence of invasion of a major branch of the portal or hepatic system must be present. T4 is penetration of the visceral peritoneum or direct invasion of surrounding abdominal viscera excluding the gallbladder (Fig. 25.3A).

Specifically, there is a direct relationship of T category advancement and stage. Stage III is divided into A/B/C: IIIA = T3, IIIB = T4, and IIIC = N1.

SUMMARY OF CHANGES SEVENTH EDITION AJCC

There are major changes. The seventh edition AJCC includes only hepatocellular carcinomas (Fig 25.3A), and cholangiocarcinomas (Fig. 25.3B) have their own TNM criteria.

Intrahepatic bile ducts are no longer included in this staging chapter. The staging of liver cancer now includes only hepatocellular carcinoma.

T Category Changes

- In the T3 category, patients with invasion of major vessels are distinguished from patients with multiple tumors, of which any are >5 cm, but lack major vessel invasion because of the markedly different prognosis of these subgroups.
  - T3a includes multiple tumors, any >5 cm.
  - T3b includes tumors of any size involving a major portal vein or hepatic vein.
- T4 category is unchanged.

N Category Changes

- Inferior phrenic lymph nodes were reclassified to regional lymph nodes from distant lymph nodes

Stage Grouping Changes

- Changes in T3 classification led to changes in Stage III groupings.
  - Stage IIIA now includes only T3a; patients with major vessel invasion are removed from the IIIA stage grouping.
  - Stage IIIB now includes only T3b (major vessel invasion).
  - T4 is shifted to Stage IIIC.
- Stage IV includes all patients with metastasis, whether nodal or distant, separated into IVA and B to permit identification of each subgroup.
  - Stage IVA now includes node-positive disease (N1).
  - Stage IVB now includes distant metastasis (M1).

The TNM Staging Matrix is color coded for identification of Stage Group once T and N stages are determined (Table 25.3).

TABLE 25.3	Stage Summary Matrix		
	N0	**N1**	**M1**
T1	I	IIIC	IV
T2	II	IIIC	IV
T3a/b	IIIA/B	IIIC	IV
T4	IIIC	IIIC	IV

Sequential Progression of T stage and then N stage determines stage group progression:
- *T stage T_1 = I, T_2 = II, T_3 = IIIA/B, T_4 = IIIC*
- *N stage N_1 = T_4 and advances to IIIC*
- *M stage is separate*

LIVER HEPATOMA

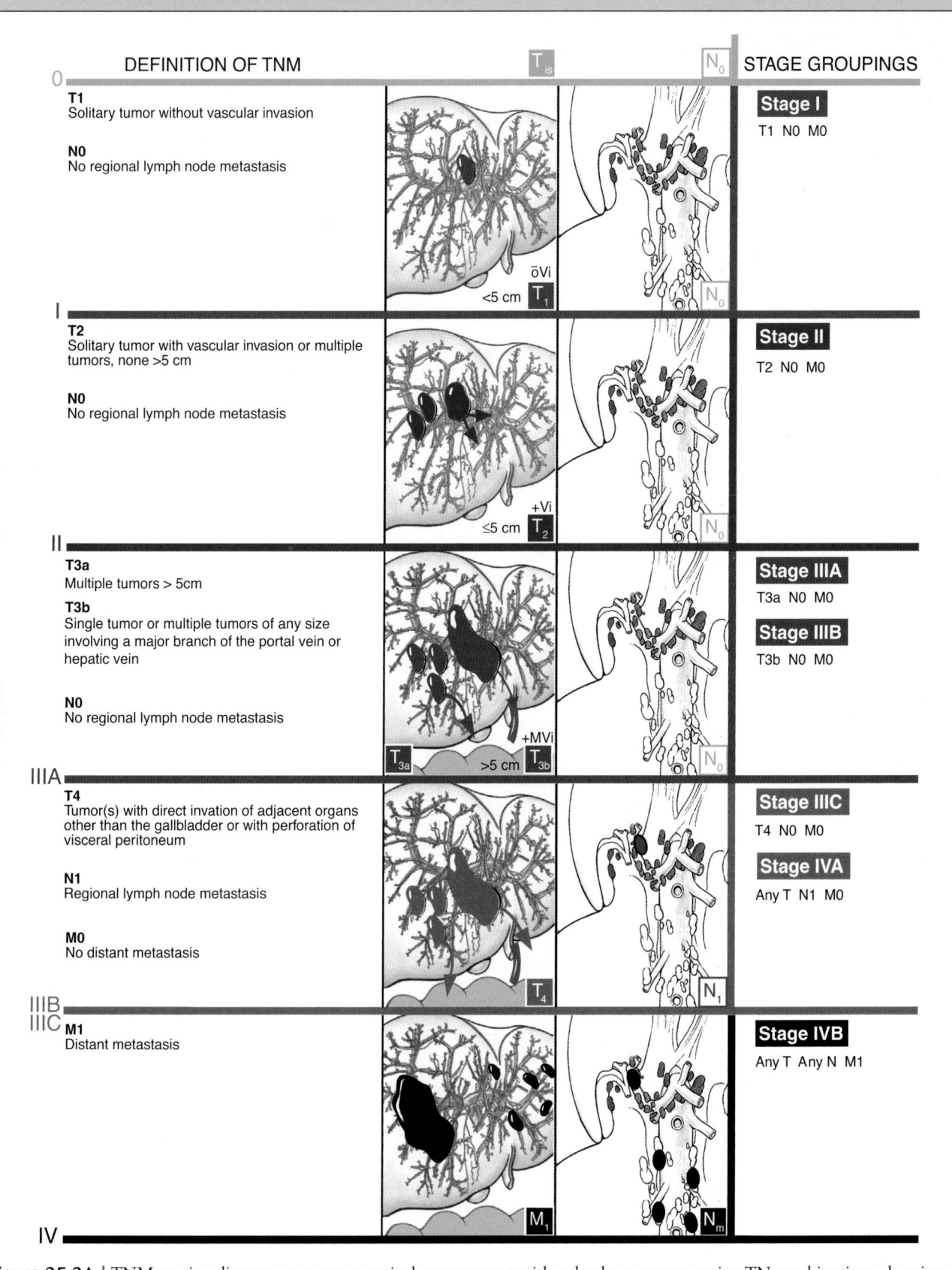

DEFINITION OF TNM

T1
Solitary tumor without vascular invasion

N0
No regional lymph node metastasis

T2
Solitary tumor with vascular invasion or multiple tumors, none >5 cm

N0
No regional lymph node metastasis

T3a
Multiple tumors > 5cm

T3b
Single tumor or multiple tumors of any size involving a major branch of the portal vein or hepatic vein

N0
No regional lymph node metastasis

T4
Tumor(s) with direct invation of adjacent organs other than the gallbladder or with perforation of visceral peritoneum

N1
Regional lymph node metastasis

M0
No distant metastasis

M1
Distant metastasis

STAGE GROUPINGS

Stage I
T1 N0 M0

Stage II
T2 N0 M0

Stage IIIA
T3a N0 M0

Stage IIIB
T3b N0 M0

Stage IIIC
T4 N0 M0

Stage IVA
Any T N1 M0

Stage IVB
Any T Any N M1

Figure 25.3A | TNM staging diagram presents a vertical arrangement with color bars encompassing TN combinations showing progression. Liver cancers are generally advanced stages. Stage IIIA is borderline resectable (purple), stage IIIB (red) is unresectable, as is stage IV metastatic (black). Stage 0, yellow; I, green; II, blue; III, purple; IV, red; and IV (metastatic), black. Definitions of TN on left and stage grouping on right.

INTRAHEPATIC CHOLANGIOCARCINOMA

Perspective and Patterns of Spread

Intrahepatic cholangiocarcinomas are less common than HCC and show geographic variation. Their frequency rate varies from 15% to 20% of hepatic cancers. Higher ratios are found in the Far East—Thailand, Laos, and Cambodia. Chronic infestation of the biliary tree with liver flukes is causally related. Additional risk factors include sclerosing cholangitis, biliary atresia, von Meyenburg complexes, Caroli disease, cholidochocyst, and intrahepatic cholethiasis. HBV and HCV infections and alcoholic cirrhosis are not factors. The incidence has been rising over the last two decades in Europe and North America. They occur in older patients between 50 and 65 years old; they are equal for male and female patients and peak in the ninth decade.

- *Jaundice* is more frequent and prominent and occurs earlier than HCC; the liver is not as large, and ascites, fever, and metastatic spread are less frequent. Hepatic bruit is absent.

- *Laboratory values* are raised for CA 19-9 levels and CEA as well.

- *Molecular level* changes are most frequently mutations of the K-ras gene and p53, p16, and p73.

- *Histopathology* (Fig. 25.1B) shows that Cholangiocarcinomas are composed of cubic cells arranged in duct-like and glandular configurations.

- *Differential diagnosis* includes metastatic liver cancers since they can form masses.

CLASSIFICATION AND STAGING

Summary of Changes Seventh Edition AJCC

- This is a novel staging system that is independent of the staging system for hepatocellular carcinoma and independent of the staging system for extrahepatic bile duct malignancy, including hilar bile duct cancers. The rare combined hepatocellular and cholangiocarcinoma (mixed hepatocholangiocarcinomas) are included with the intrahepatic bile duct cancer staging classification (Fig. 25.3B).

- The tumor category (T) is based on three major prognostic factors including tumor number, vascular invasion, and direct extrahepatic tumoral extension.

- The nodal category (N) is a binary classification based on the presence or absence of regional lymph node metastasis.

- The metastasis category (M) is a binary classification based on the presence or absence of distant disease.

- Recommend collection of preoperative or pretreatment serum CA19.9

Regional Lymph Nodes

Compared with primary hepatocellular carcinoma, regional lymph node metastases are more commonly associated with intrahepatic cholangiocarcinoma. The lymph node drainage patterns from the intrahepatic bile ducts demonstrate laterality. Tumors in the left lateral bisegment (segments 2 to 3) of the liver may preferentially drain to lymph nodes along the lesser curvature of the stomach and subsequently to the celiac nodal basin. In contrast, intrahepatic cholangiocarcinomas of the right liver (segments 5 to 8) may primarily drain to hilar lymph nodes and subsequently to caval and periaortic lymph nodes.

For right liver (segments 5 to 8) intrahepatic cholangiocarcinomas, the regional lymph nodes include the hilar (common bile duct, hepatic artery, portal vein, and cystic duct), periduodenal, and peripancreatic lymph nodes. For left liver (segment 2 to 4) intrahepatic cholangiocarcinomas, regional lymph nodes include hilar and gastrohepatic lymph nodes. For intrahepatic cholangiocarcinomas, disease spread to the celiac and/or periaortic and caval lymph nodes is considered distant metastasis (M1). Inferior phrenic nodes are considered regional, not distant nodes.

Intrahepatic bile duct carcinoma tends to involve lymph nodes more than HCC and varies depending on the location of the primary.

Right lobe segments 5 to 8 drain to hilar lymph nodes and then the paracaval and periaortic nodes.

Left lobe segments 2 to 4, after hilar nodes, tend to drain along lesser curvature stomach and celiac nodes.

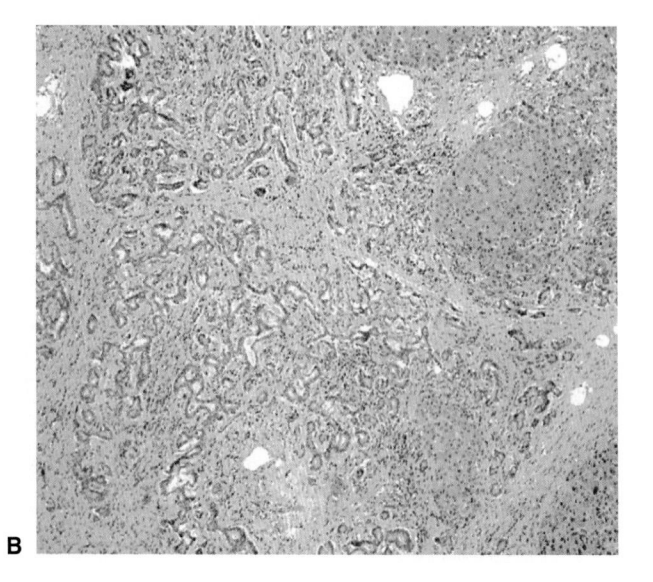

B

Figure 25.1B | Cholangiocarcinoma. Well-differentiated neoplastic glands are embedded in a dense fibrous stroma.

INTRAHEPATIC BILE DUCT

DEFINITION OF TNM

STAGE GROUPINGS

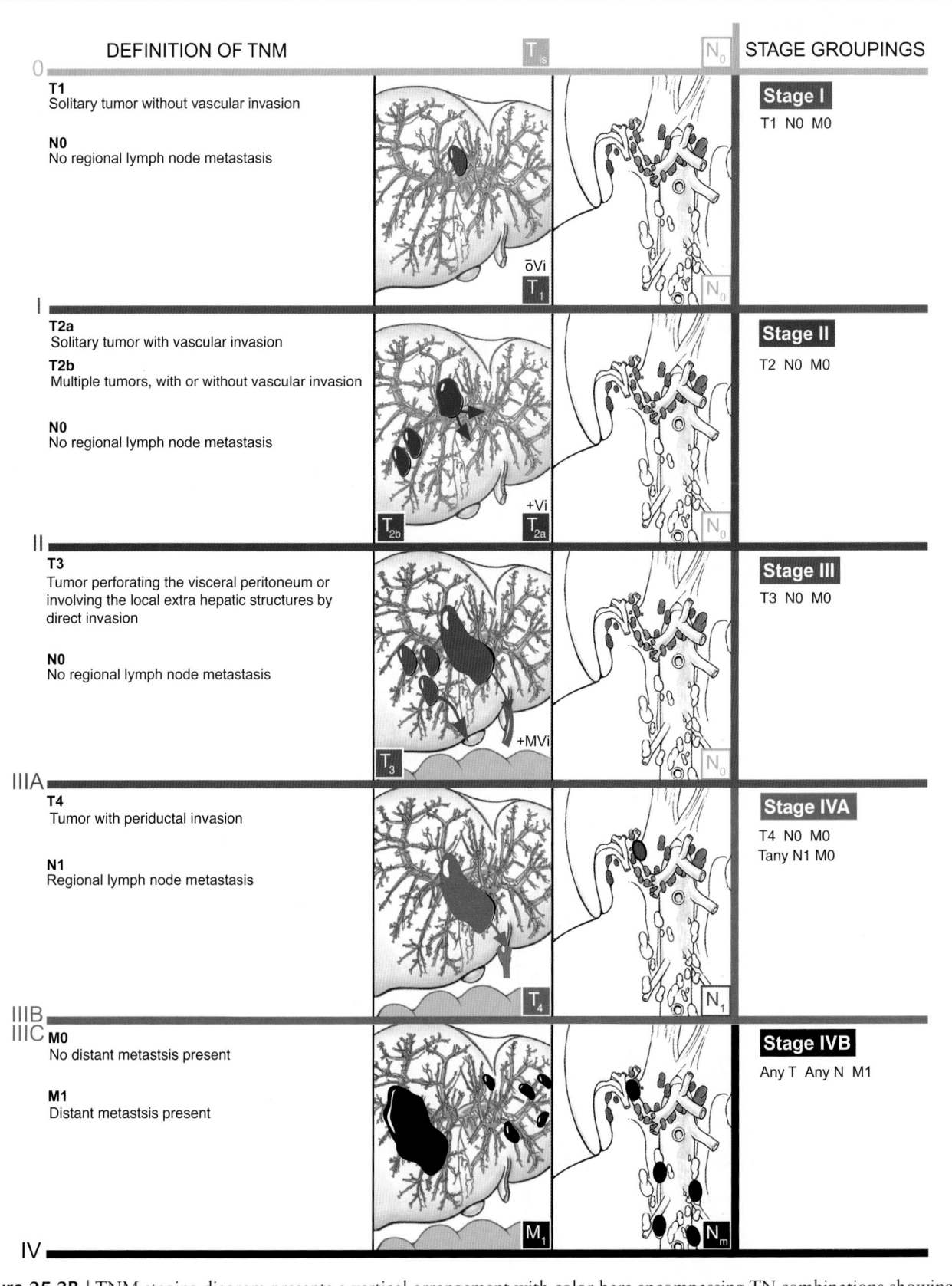

T1
Solitary tumor without vascular invasion

N0
No regional lymph node metastasis

Stage I
T1 N0 M0

T2a
Solitary tumor with vascular invasion
T2b
Multiple tumors, with or without vascular invasion

N0
No regional lymph node metastasis

Stage II
T2 N0 M0

T3
Tumor perforating the visceral peritoneum or involving the local extra hepatic structures by direct invasion

N0
No regional lymph node metastasis

Stage III
T3 N0 M0

T4
Tumor with periductal invasion

N1
Regional lymph node metastasis

Stage IVA
T4 N0 M0
Tany N1 M0

M0
No distant metastsis present

M1
Distant metastsis present

Stage IVB
Any T Any N M1

Figure 25.3B I TNM staging diagram presents a vertical arrangement with color bars encompassing TN combinations showing progression. Liver cancers are generally advanced stages. Stage IIIA is borderline resectable (purple), stage IIIB (red) is unresectable as is stage IV metastatic (black). Stage 0, yellow; I, green; II, blue; III, purple; IV, red; and IV (metastatic), black. Definitions of TN on left and stage grouping on right.

T-ONCOANATOMY

ORIENTATION OF THREE-PLANAR ONCOANATOMY

The anatomic isocenter for the liver is to right of the midline at the T10 to T12 level (Fig. 25.4).

T-oncoanatomy

The T-oncoanatomy is displayed in three planar views. A. Coronal, B. Sagittal, C. Transverse axial (Figure 25.5).

By virtue of its weight, the liver is the largest visceral organ in the body. When filled with cancerous nodules, it is often the greatest repository of neoplastic disease, exceeding primary tumors in the quantity of malignant cells. To understand the anatomy of the liver, it is important to be aware of its internal structure as a gland of compound tubular design. Each lobule is shaped like a cylinder or tubule, with a central vein that drains a rich anatomic sinusoidal network derived from the fine hepatic arterioles and portal vessels (Fig. 25.4). The hepatocyte elaborates both an external/exocrine secretion and an internal/endocrine secretion of enzymes into the blood. The former is referred to as bile and is collected by biliary canaliculi.

At the porta hepatis, the bile ducts coalesce into a right and a left main duct via the common hepatic duct to the gallbladder and the cystic ducts below, as common bile duct courses toward the second portion of the duodenum, where it fuses with the pancreatic duct at the ampulla of Vater. The gallbladder and its cystic duct are to the right and below the porta hepatis.

The liver sits under and is virtually surrounded by the diaphragm superiorly, most of which is covered by peritoneum. Inferiorly, it is partially attached to the retroperitoneum. Abdominal viscera are in contact with its undersurface.

There are two major vascular systems in the liver. The major blood supply to the organ consists of the hepatic artery and vein. The portal system results from a fusion of the splenic vein with the superior mesenteric vein to form a portal vein that also enters the liver parenchyma via the porta hepatis. This brings the products of the intestine for detoxification and metabolic activation. The lymphatics follow the hepatic and portal veins and drain into the high para-aortic nodes, particularly around the celiac axis.

The new anatomic terminology refined by Couinaud is based on dividing the liver into four sectors by virtual/oblique planes referred to as scissura. The sectors are divided by a horizontal scissura, thereby increasing the number of liver segments to eight. The eight segments are numbered clockwise in the frontal plane (Fig. 25.5).

• *Coronal:* The liver is divided into a right and a left half, if one judges by its blood supply, for both the hepatic artery and portal veins bifurcate at the porta hepatis. The left side usually includes the quadrate and caudate lobes of the liver.

• *Sagittal:* The new anatomic terminology refined by Couinaud is based on dividing the liver into four sectors by virtual/oblique planes referred to as scissura. The sectors are divided by a horizontal scissura, thereby increasing the number of liver segments to eight. The eight segments are numbered in a clockwise manner in the frontal plane and are based on hepatic vein branching, and determine portal liver resections.

• *Transverse:* There is an H-shaped group of fissures and fossae that describe these aforementioned lobes on either side of the H, with other lobes positioned on the right and left sides. The porta hepatis represents the letter's crossbar, where the hepatic artery, portal vein, and major bile ducts enter, as well as nerves and lymphatics. The falciform ligament holds the liver in its position anteriorly and is attached to the superior and anterior surfaces as well as the dome of the diaphragm. The stomach and bowel are in contact on its inferior surface.

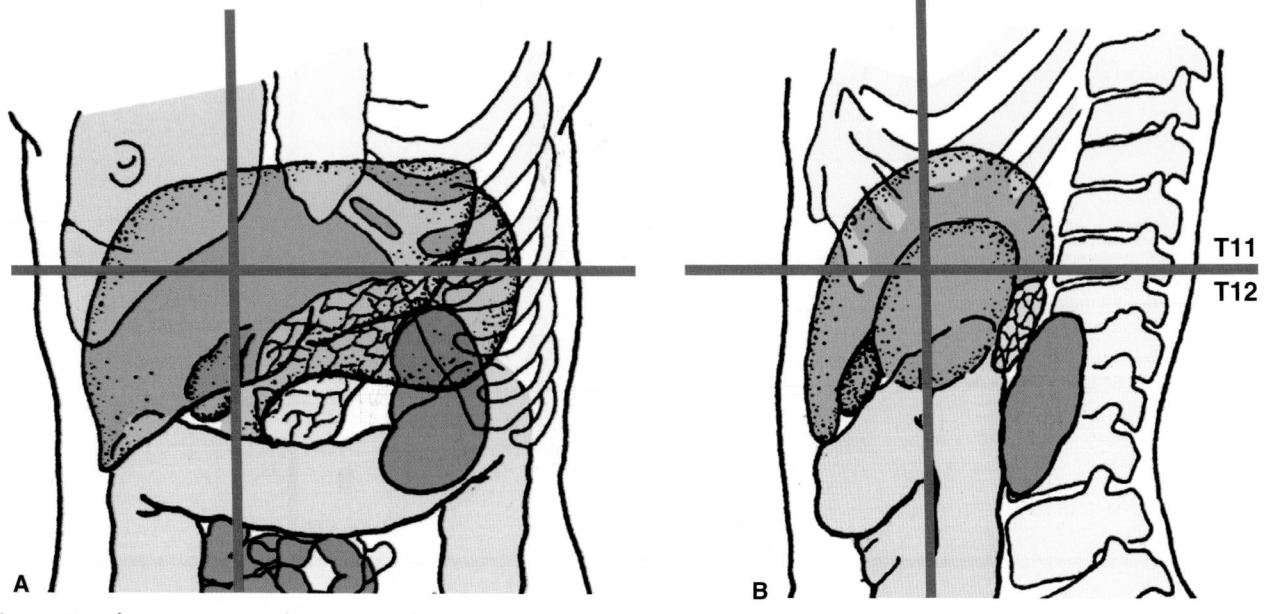

Figure 25.4 | Orientation and overview of oncoanatomy. The anatomic isocenter of the three-planar anatomy is placed to the right in the epigastrium and between T11 and T12 posteriorly. **A.** Coronal. **B.** Sagittal.

*This only applies to hepatocellular carcinomas.

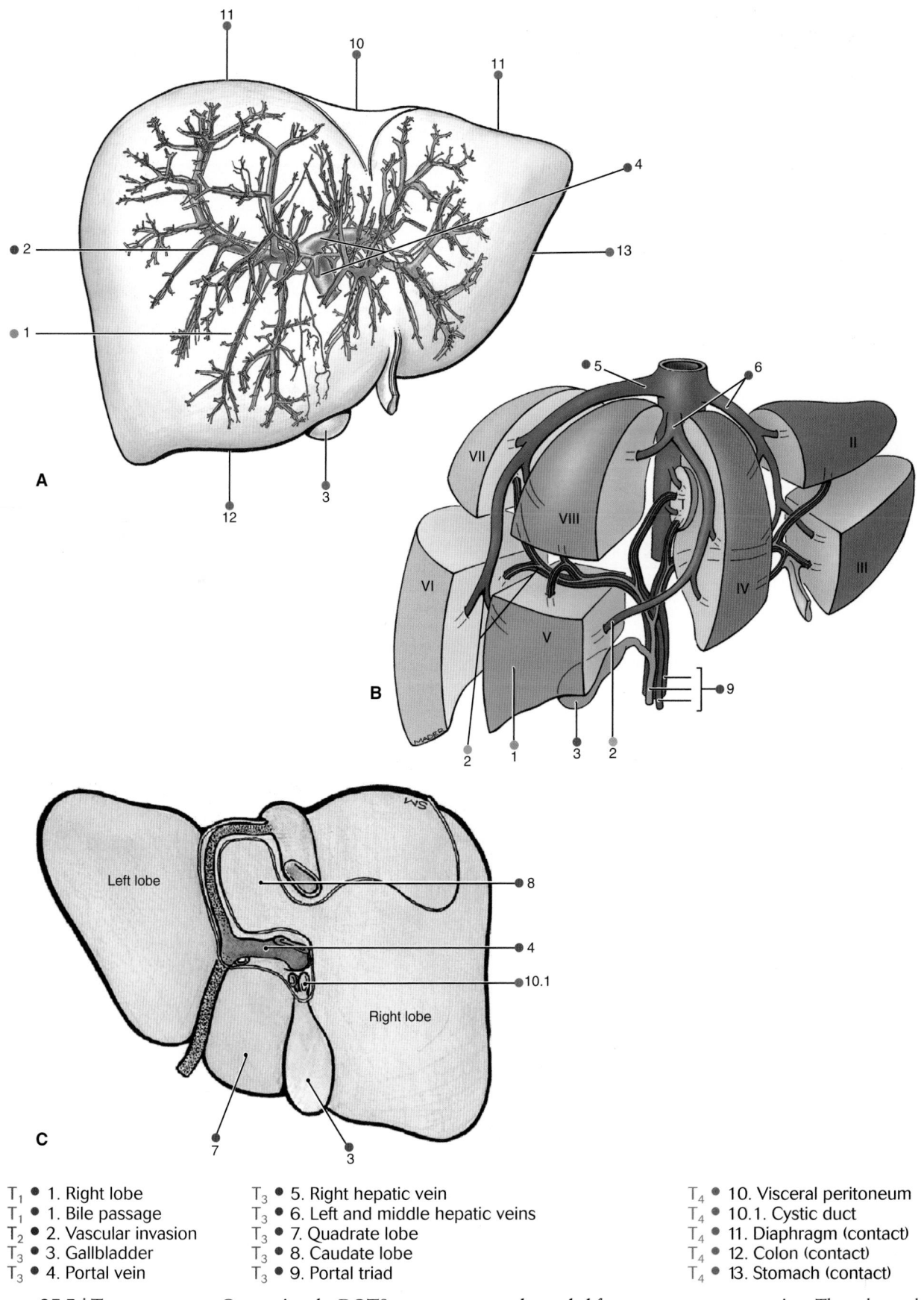

T₁	● 1. Right lobe	T₃	● 5. Right hepatic vein	T₄	● 10. Visceral peritoneum
T₁	● 1. Bile passage	T₃	● 6. Left and middle hepatic veins	T₄	● 10.1. Cystic duct
T₂	● 2. Vascular invasion	T₃	● 7. Quadrate lobe	T₄	● 11. Diaphragm (contact)
T₃	● 3. Gallbladder	T₃	● 8. Caudate lobe	T₄	● 12. Colon (contact)
T₃	● 4. Portal vein	T₃	● 9. Portal triad	T₄	● 13. Stomach (contact)

Figure 25.5 | T-oncoanatomy. **Connecting the DOTS: structures are color coded for cancer stage progression.** The color code for the anatomic sites correlates with the color code for the stage group (Fig. 25.3) and patterns of spread (Fig. 25.2) and SIMLAP tables (Table 25.2). Connecting the dots in similar colors will provide an appreciation for the 3D oncoanatomy.

N-ONCOANATOMY AND M-ONCOANATOMY

N-ONCOANATOMY

The lymphatics follow the hepatic and portal veins and drain into the para-aortic or paracaval nodes, particularly around the celiac axis (Fig. 25.6A; Table 25.4).

Regional Lymph Nodes

The regional lymph nodes are the hilar, hepatoduodenal ligament, inferior phrenic, and caval lymph nodes, among which the most prominent are the hepatic artery and portal vein lymph nodes. Nodal involvement should be coded as N1. Nodal involvement is now considered stage IV disease.

TABLE 25.4	Lymph Nodes of Liver
Sentinel Nodes Include Paracaval and Porta Hepatis Nodes	
Regional Nodes	**Juxtaregional Nodes**
Hepatic vein	Mediastinal
Paracaval	Iliac
Celiac	Superior mesentery
	Pericardial and diaphragmatic

M-ONCOANATOMY

The entire portal circulation should be considered as a unit with regard to the venous anatomy of the gastrointestinal tract below the diaphragm (see Fig. 25.6B). The two major trunks are the inferior mesenteric and superior mesenteric veins. The inferior mesenteric vein drains the left colon and sigmoid colon tributaries, which cover the vascular drainage to the left of the midline originating from the superior rectal veins. On the right side, the superior mesenteric vein originates from the tributaries draining the ileum, the jejunum, and the ileocolic and right and middle colic veins. The inferior mesenteric vein usually joins the splenic vein, which coalesces with the superior mesenteric vein and forms the portal vein. The splenic vein, which is a major tributary of the portal system, also drains much of the stomach along its greater curvature and includes the short gastric veins and left and right gastric epiploic veins. The right gastroepiploic also flows into the superior mesenteric vein. The entire drainage of the lesser curvature of the stomach, including the left and right gastric veins, drains directly into the portal vein. Because the portal vein then drains directly into the liver, it is the target metastatic organ and the most commonly involved organ in a hematogenous spread pattern from the venous system of the gastrointestinal tract, as compared with other parts of the body, where the drainage is directly into the lung by way of the caval system.

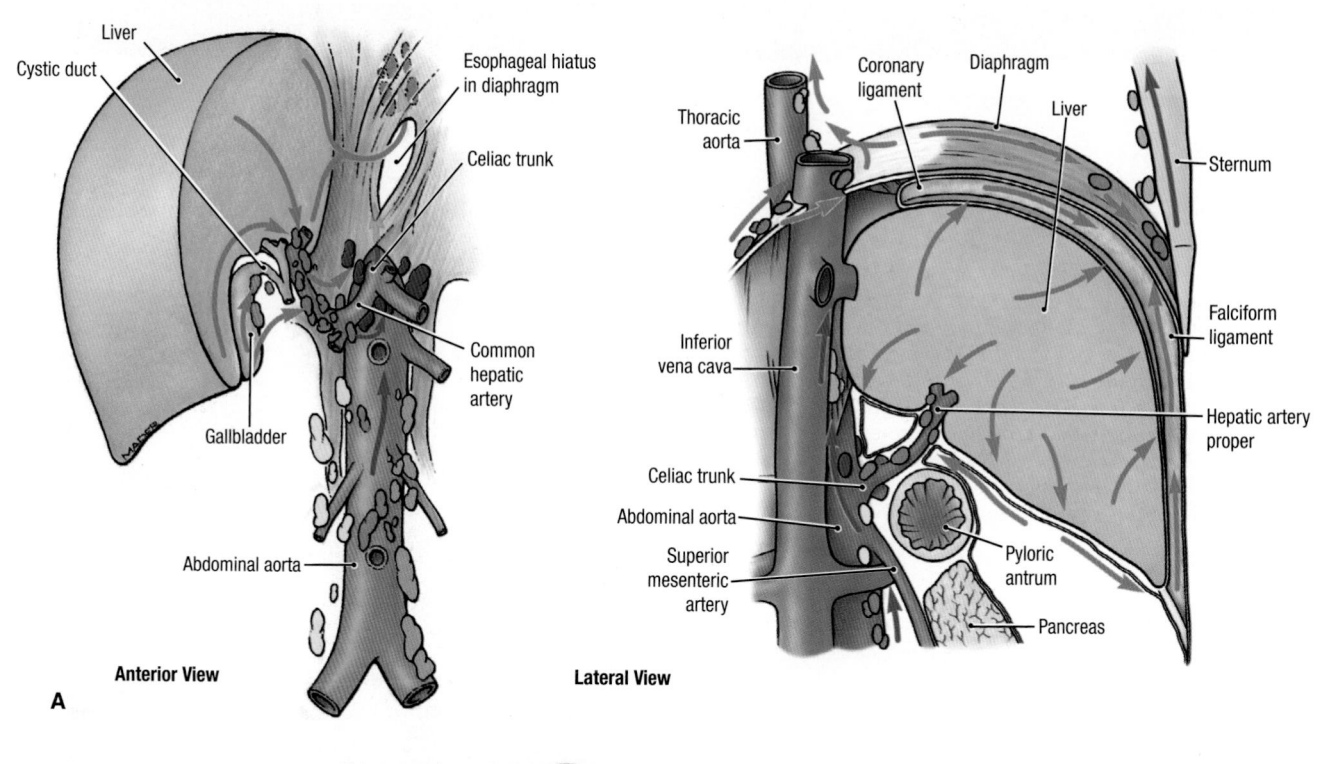

A

Anterior View

Lateral View

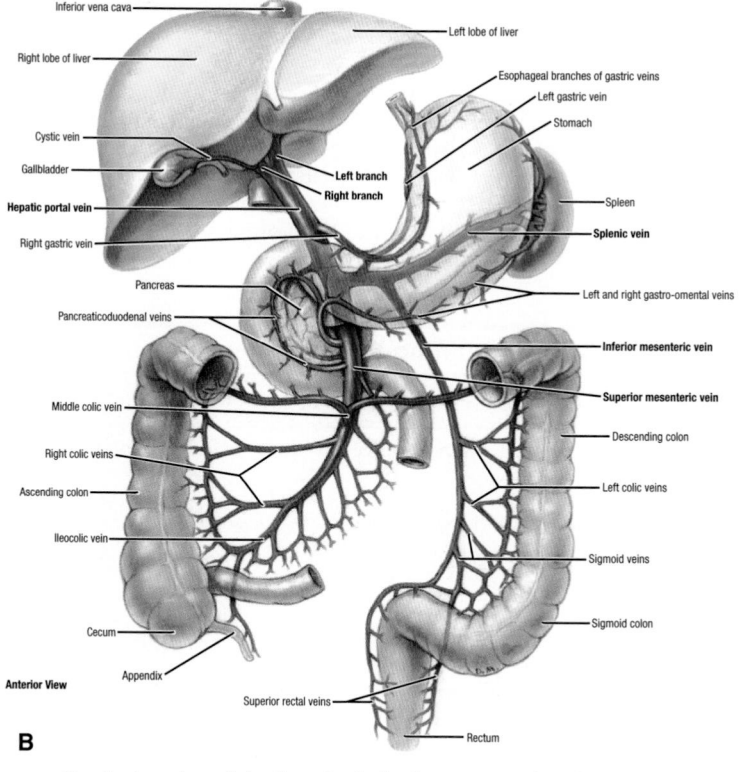

B

Anterior View

Figure 25.6 | A. N-oncoanatomy. Sentinel nodes of the liver include the paracaval and para-aortic nodes. **B. M-oncoanatomy.** Both hepatomas and cholangiocarcinomas tend to spread directly into the liver or can be multifocal, similar to metastatic spread. Since the liver drains into the central vein, which in turn drains into the inferior vena cava, spread of metastases will be into the lung as well.

STAGING WORKUP

RULES OF CLASSIFICATION AND STAGING

Clinical Staging and Imaging

Imaging is essential for clinical staging of HCC. Because the liver is diseased due to hepatitis B and C infection and its associated cirrhosis, it is a challenge to uncover dysplastic nodules believed to be precursors to HCC. Computed tomography is favored to determine tumor size and if vascular invasion is present. Only 10% to 20% of HCC patients are surgically resected, preferably with T1 nodules, preferably <2 cm and not >5 cm. Numerous additional adverse factors can be found to contraindicate surgery, namely, presence of nodules in other lobes, lymphadenopathy, or major vessel invasion (Table 25.5; Fig. 25.7).

Pathologic Staging

The surgically resected liver segments and associated lymph nodes removed are assessed. Tumor extension and location of both primary and nodes should be documented. Complete surgical staging consists of evaluation of primary tumor and underlying associated liver disease as severity of fibrosis/cirrhosis (F_0 = Ishak score 0–4; F_1 = Ishak score 5–6) for better versus worse prognosis. Histologic grade and lymph node, if any, are recorded. If surgical margins are not released, total hepatectomy and liver transplantation are required for survival.

Oncoimaging Annotations

- HCC nodules receive blood via hepatic artery versus dysplastic nodules supplied by portal veins.
- HCC is classified on imaging as nodular, massive, and diffuse.

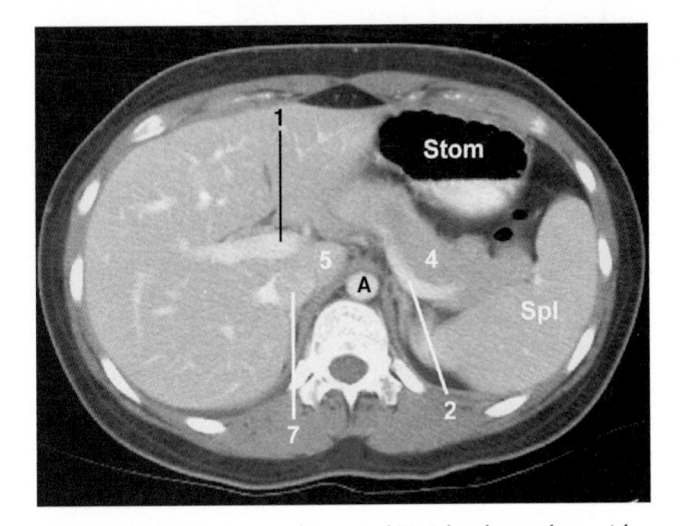

Figure 25.7 | Axial CTs of T11 and T12 level correlate with the T-oncoanatomy transverse section (Figure 25.5C). Oncoimaging with CT is commonly applied to staging cancers, often combined with PET to determine true extent of primary cancer and involved lymph nodes. **1.** Main portal vein. 2. Splenic vein. 4. Pancreas (body) 5. Caudate lobe of liver. 7. Inferior vena cava A, abdominal aorta; Spl, spleen; Stom, stomach.

TABLE 25.5	Imaging Modalities for Evaluating Carcinoma of the Liver	
Method	Capability	Recommended for Use
CT	CT with IV contrast using dynamic changes in tumor enhancement multiphase	Yes; helical CT preferred
MRI	Dynamic study increases specificity to 85%–95% using gadolinium (T1 and T2 weighted).	Yes
CT	CT arterial portography for determining major vessel invasion	No
Ultrasonography	Ultrasonography is useful for guiding needle biopsies, also Doppler and ultrasound angiography	Yes

CT, computed tomography; IV, intravenous; MRI, magnetic resonance imaging.

PROGNOSIS AND CANCER SURVIVAL

PROGNOSIS

The limited number of prognostic factors are listed in Tables 25.6A and Table 25.6B.

CANCER STATISTICS AND SURVIVAL

The digestive system or gastrointestinal tract, which includes MDGs, accounts for 255,640 new patients annually, with colon and rectum responsible for >50%, or about 147,000 new diagnoses annually. Approximately half of these patients eventually die of these cancers. MDG cancers as a group are more lethal; only a handful of patients become long-term survivors. Fortunately, colon and rectal cancers are the most common, with the majority of patients becoming 5-year survivors (63%) responding to chemoradiation programs often with the sparing of the rectal sphincter with conservative surgery. Anal cancers are the most responsive to chemoradiation (5-fluorouracil and cisplatin), eliminating the need for surgery, and 5-year survival is >90%, with anal sphincter preservation. This regimen has been proven to be very effective in clinical trials and to result in more long-term survivors, which is currently reflected in the literature. Liver, bile duct, and pancreatic cancers are among the poorest in the terms of survival, often measured in months rather than years.

Specifically, the liver accounted for 24,120 new cancer cases and 18,910 cancer deaths (88%), with a 5-year survival rate improvement over the last three decades of 10%. Currently, relative 5-year survival for all stages is 14%, but, when localized, it improves to 16.3% (see Table 24.5).

Overall survival at 5 years has steadily improved with total hepatectomy and liver transplantation, from 30% survival in 1988 to 57% today. For all liver transplantations in the United States, a 74% 5-year survival is reported (Fig. 25.8).

TABLE 25.6A	Prognostic Factors
Required for staging	None
Clinically significant	Alpha fetoprotein
	Fibrosis score
	Hepatitis serology
	Creatinine[a]
	Bilirubin[a]
	Prothrombin time, International Normalized Ratio[a]

[a]Part of the Model for End-Stage Liver Disease score.
Reprinted with permission from Edge SB, Byrd DR, Compton CC, et al. *AJCC Cancer Staging Manual, 7th edition.* New York, Springer, 2010, p. 197.

TABLE 25.6B	Prognostic Factors: Intrahepatic Cholangiocarcinoma
Required for staging	None
Clinically significant	Tumor growth pattern
	Primary sclerosing cholangitis
	CA 19-9

Reprinted with permission from Edge SB, Byrd DR, Compton CC, et al. *AJCC Cancer Staging Manual, 7th edition.* New York, Springer, 2010, p. 207.

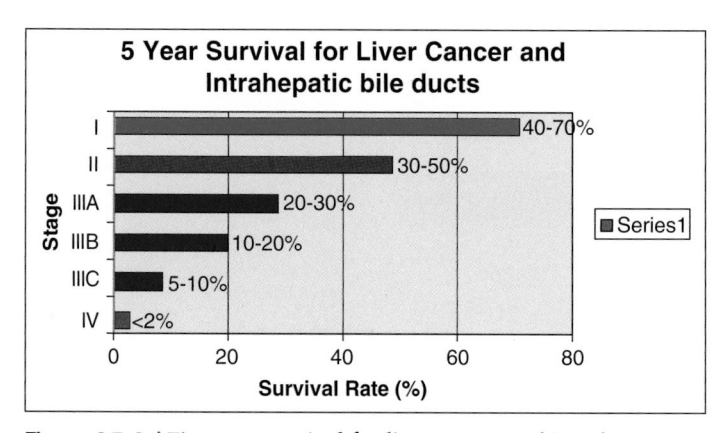

Figure 25.8 | Five-year survival for liver cancer and intrahepatic bile ducts. (Data from Edge SB, Byrd DR, Compton CC, et al., *AJCC Cancer Staging Manual, 7th edition.* New York, Springer, 2010.)

26

Extrahepatic Bile Ducts

PERSPECTIVES, PATTERNS OF SPREAD, AND PATHOLOGY

The commonest site for cancers of the extrahepatic bile ducts is at the confluence of the right and left ducts—the Klatskin tumor or hilar cholangiocarcinoma.

PERSPECTIVE AND PATTERNS OF SPREAD

The onset of jaundice is the common provocative symptom that requires attention and may lead to an early diagnosis of an extrahepatic cholangiocarcinoma. An unusually high serum bilirubin (>10 to 20 mg) should suggest malignancy because bilirubin levels of 2 to 4 mg are normal for obstructive cholelithiasis. This uncommon malignant entity is a disease of elderly populations, peaking late in 80-year-olds. As with hepatocellular carcinoma, for which hepatitis B and C virus infec-

tions are predisposing factors, the presence of infection in the form of primary sclerosing cholangitis is most often associated with cholangiocarcinoma. Primary sclerosing cholangitis is an autoimmune process and produces multifocal strictures in both extrinsic and intrinsic hepatic bile ducts. Although the incidence of cancer is only detected in 10% of infected patients, it can be as high as 30% to 40% at autopsy. Another source of chronic infection, especially in the Far East, is biliary parasites, which can increase the risk of cholangiocarcinomas via hepatolithiasis. These parasites can lead to hepatic pigment stone formation to strictures, then to recurrent cholangitis and carcinogenesis. Another well-recognized risk factor is Canoli disease or congenital choledochal cysts. Canoli disease patients have a predisposition for harboring infection, which has been shown in adults and even when excised to have incidental rates of 15% to 20% bile duct cancers.

Patterns of spread depend on the site of origin in the biliary tree (Fig. 26.2; Table 26.2). Extrahepatic cholangiocarcinoma

TABLE 26.1 | **Histopathologic Type: Common Cancers of the Gallbladder and the Bile Duct**

Type	Incidence (%)
Carcinoma	96
Adenocarcinoma	86
Adenocarcinoma, NOS	71
Papillary adenocarcinoma	6
Mucinous and mucin producing	5
Other adenocarcinoma	4
Squamous cell carcinoma	0.2
Carcinoma, NOS	7
Other specific carcinomas	0.5
Sarcoma	0.2
Other unspecified	0.8

NOS, not otherwise specified.
Modified from Carriaga MT, Henson DE: Liver, gallbladder, extrahepatic bile ducts, and pancreas. *Cancer* 1995;75(Suppl):171.

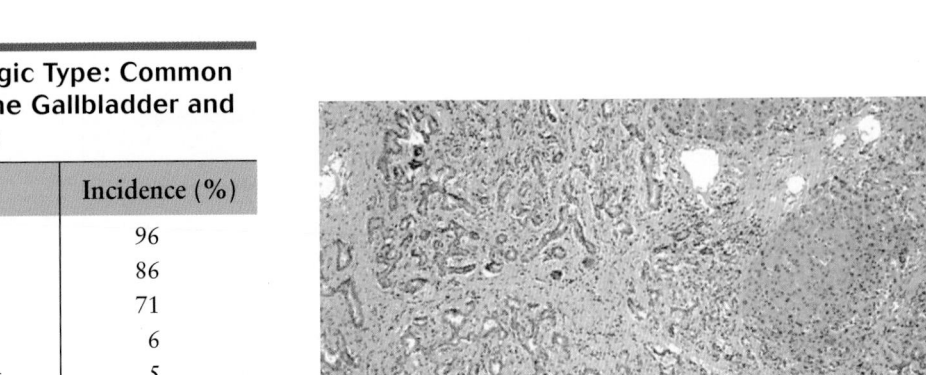

Figure 26.1 | Cholangiocarcinoma. Well-differentiated neoplastic glands are embedded in a dense fibrous stroma.

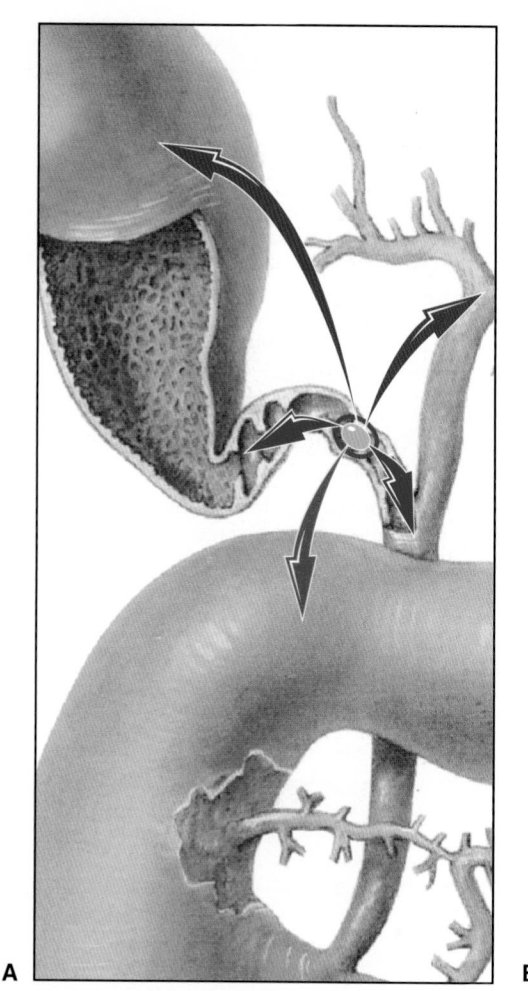 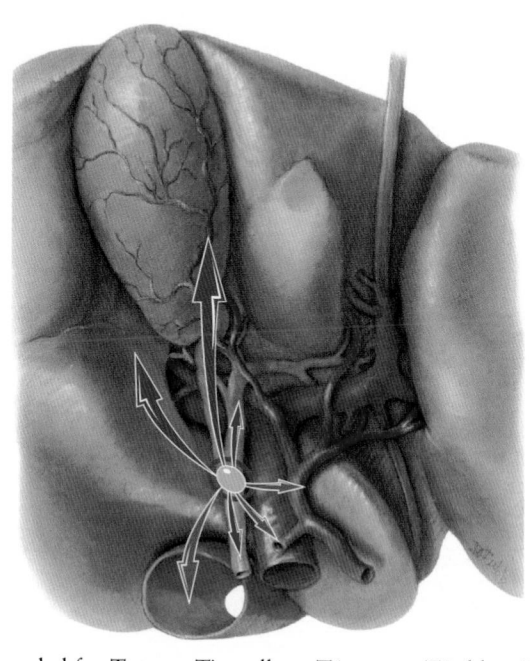

Figure 26.2 | Patterns of spread for extrahepatic bile ducts. Color coded for T stage: Tis, yellow; T1, green; T2, blue; T3, purple; and T4, red. The concept of visualizing patterns of spread to appreciate the surrounding anatomy is well demonstrated by the six-directional pattern, i.e., SIMLAP Table 26.2.

can arise anywhere along its length. By far the commonest site is at the confluence of the right and left hepatic ducts, which has an incidence of 40% to 60% and includes Klatskin tumor or hilar cholangiocarcinoma. Multifocality is rare, with ≤10% occurring throughout the biliary tree. The overwhelming majority are well-differentiated, mucin-producing adenocarcinomas (see Table 26.1).

Hilar or confluens cholangiocarcinomas can readily penetrate through the thin muscular walls of extrahepatic bile ducts and have immediate access to the major vessels of the porta hepatis, portal vein, and hepatic artery. Distal biliary duct cancers represent the other 20% to 30% of cholangiocarcinomas; midduct occurrence is rare. These cancers are discussed with periampullary cancers or cancers of the ampulla of Vater.

PATHOLOGY

There are numerous histopathologic types, but the overwhelming majority are well-differentiated, mucin-producing adenocarcinomas (Table 26.1; Figure 26.1).

TABLE 26.2	SIMLAP	
Extrahepatic Bile Ducts		
S	Intrahepatic bile duct	
	Liver	• T3
I	Ampulla of Vater	• T3
M	Sphincter of Oddi, second part of duodenum	• T3
L	Cystic duct, gallbladder	• T2
A	First part of duodenum, liver	• T4
P	Pancreas	• T3
	L1, L2	• T4

The six vectors of invasion are Superior, Inferior, Medial, Lateral, Anterior, and Posterior. The color-coded dots correlate the T stage with specific anatomic structure involved.

TNM STAGING CRITERIA

TNM STAGING CRITERIA

The TNM staging in the seventh edition of the American Joint Committee on Cancer (AJCC) *AJCC Cancer Staging Manual* has added perihilar bile ducts (PBD) (Klatskin tumor) as new and distinct from distal bile ducts (DBD). This division changes the descriptors for T but in so doing clarifies adjacent structures at risk for invasion, particularly for vascular invasion patterns. Thus DBD has been simplified but has major changes. A single classification is offered for both the clinical and pathologic staging. This site was added in the fourth edition (1992) of the *AJCC Manual*. The extrahepatic bile duct on cross section is lined by a single layer of columnar cells. In its collapsed state, the mucosa is pleated with longitudinal folds, and a thin subepithelial layer of fibrous and muscle cells is surrounded by serosal cells. For these reasons, T1 is confined to the bile duct, T2 is tumor beyond its confines, and both require histologic verification. T3 relates to the immediate surrounding anatomy in the porta hepatis being invaded as liver, gallbladder, and unilateral branches of the hepatic artery and portal vein, whereas T4 is further spread into the common portal vein or hepatic artery or into colon, stomach, or duodenum—essentially the other viscera.

For distal bile ducts, nodal involvement N1 refers to the hilar nodes near the gallbladder and around the portal vein, hepatic artery, cystic ducts.

SUMMARY OF CHANGES SEVENTH EDITION AJCC

Distal Bile Duct

- Extrahepatic bile duct was a single chapter in the sixth edition. This has been divided into two chapters for the seventh edition [Distal Bile Duct (Fig. 26.3A) and Perihilar Bile Ducts (Fig. 26.3B)].

- Two site-specific prognostic factors, preoperative or pretreatment serum carcinoembryonic antigen and CA19.9, are recommended for collection.

The TNM Staging Matrix is color coded for identification of stage group once T and N stages are determined (Tables 26.3A and 26.3B).

TABLE 26.3B Stage Summary Matrix for Perihilar Bile Ducts

	N0	N1	N2	M1
T1	*I	IIIB	IVB	IVB
T2a,b	II	IIIB	IVB	IVB
T3	IIIA	IIIB	IVB	IVB
T4	IVA	IVA	IVB	IVB

TABLE 26.3A Stage Summary Matrix for Distal Bile Ducts

	N0	N1	M1
T1	IA	IIB	IV
T2	IB	IIB	IV
T3	IIA	IIB	IV
T4	III	III	IV

Sequential Progression of T stage and then N stage determines stage group progression:
- *T stage T_1 = I, T_2 = II, T_3 = IIIA, T_4 = IIIB*
- *N stage N_1 = T_4 and advances to IIIC*
- *M stage is separate*

DISTAL BILE DUCT

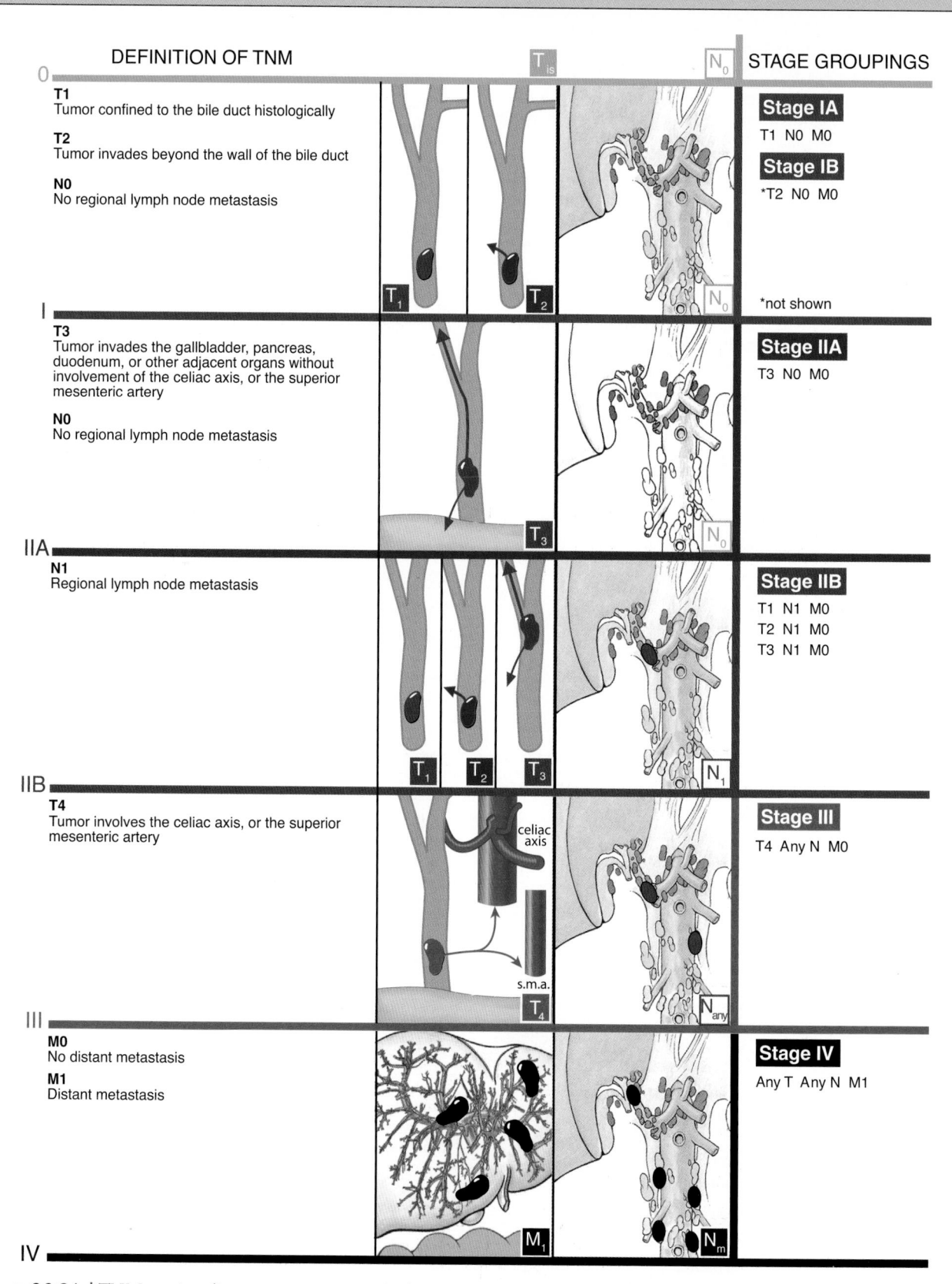

DEFINITION OF TNM

T1
Tumor confined to the bile duct histologically

T2
Tumor invades beyond the wall of the bile duct

N0
No regional lymph node metastasis

T3
Tumor invades the gallbladder, pancreas, duodenum, or other adjacent organs without involvement of the celiac axis, or the superior mesenteric artery

N0
No regional lymph node metastasis

N1
Regional lymph node metastasis

T4
Tumor involves the celiac axis, or the superior mesenteric artery

M0
No distant metastasis
M1
Distant metastasis

STAGE GROUPINGS

Stage IA
T1 N0 M0
Stage IB
*T2 N0 M0

*not shown

Stage IIA
T3 N0 M0

Stage IIB
T1 N1 M0
T2 N1 M0
T3 N1 M0

Stage III
T4 Any N M0

Stage IV
Any T Any N M1

Figure 26.3A | TNM staging diagram presents a vertical arrangement with color bars encompassing TN combinations showing progression. Note that stages I and II are divided into substages A/B. Resectability is possible with stage IA/B and stage IIA and decreases with stage IIB (purple) when nodes are involved and invasion of gallbladder occurs. Stage III is unresectable, and stage IV is metastatic and not treatable. Stage 0, yellow; I, green; II, blue; III, purple; IV, red; and stage IV (metastatic), black. Definitions of TN on left and stage grouping on right.

PERIHILAR CHOLANGIOCARCINOMA BILE DUCT

Perspective and Patterns of Spread

The Klatskin tumor is the most common cancer of the biliary tree and is at the bifurcation of the left and right hepatic ducts. The distal bile duct is the second-most-common cancer, and intrahepatic bile duct is the least common. Of all the bile duct cancers, this is regarded as the most challenging to treat because of the juxtaposition of vital vascular structures in the portahepatic. This is a rare cancer, occurring at a rate of 1 to 2 per 100,000 in the United States, but it comprises 50% to 70% of cholangiocarcinomas (Table 26.3B).

The pattern of spread predominantly is direct invasion of the liver and occurs in 85% of presentations. The next structure invaded commonly is the portal vein. Extension along the biliary tree, cystic duct, and gallbladder also can occur.

Histopathology

The staging system applies to a large variety of histopathologic types of carcinomas (98%), but sarcomas and carcinoids are excluded.

- Carcinomas in situ
- Adenocarcinoma
- Adenocarcinoma, intestinal type
- Clear cell adenocarcinoma
- Mucinous carcinoma
- Signet ring cell carcinoma
- Squamous cell carcinoma
- Adenosquamous carcinoma
- Small cell carcinoma (grade 4 by definition)
- Undifferentiated carcinoma (grade 4 by definition)
  - Spindle and giant cell types
  - Small cell types
- Papillomatosis
- Papillary carcinoma, noninvasive
- Papillary carcinoma, invasive
- Carcinoma, not otherwise specified*

Summary of Changes Seventh Edition AJCC

- Extrahepatic bile duct tumors have been separated into perihilar (proximal) and distal groups and separate staging classifications defined for each (Fig. 26.3B).
- T1 (confined to bile duct) and T2 (beyond the wall of the bile duct) have been specified histologically.
- T2 includes invasion of adjacent hepatic parenchyma.
- T3 is defined as unilateral vascular invasion.
- T4 is defined on the basis of bilateral biliary and/or vascular invasion.
- Lymph node metastasis has been reclassified as stage III (upstaged from stage II).

*Preceding passage from Edge SB, Byrd DR, Compton CC, et al., *AJCC Cancer Staging Manual, 7th edition*. New York, Springer, 2010, pp. 221–222.

The stage IV groupings define unresectability based on local invasion (IVA) or distant lymph nodes (N2) and metastatic disease (IVB).

T-oncoanatomy

The perihilar bile duct region is at the portahepatic and is surrounded by numerous vital structures. The right and left hepatic veins parallel the major right and left bile ducts, as does the right and left hepatic arteries. The juxtaposition to the quadrate lobe of the liver and gallbladder is evident. The anatomy of the portahepatic region is also highly variable.

N-oncoanatomy

The portahepatic lymph nodes are the sentinel lymph nodes; in addition, pericholodochal nodes in the hepatoduodenal ligament are involved.

Regional Lymph Nodes
In perihilar cholangiocarcinoma, the prevalence of lymphatic metastasis increases directly with T category and ranges from 30% to 53% overall. Hilar and pericholedochal nodes in the hepatoduodenal ligament are most often involved.[†]

M-oncoanatomy

The major spread pattern is to the juxtaposed liver via intrahepatic duct extension or invasion of portal vein. Extrahepatic metastases are uncommon, but lung, brain, and bone metastases have been noted.

RULES FOR STAGING

There are a variety of imaging methodologies. The most dramatic and clear visualization is by percutaneous transhepatic cholangiography outlining the biliary tree. However, computed tomography (CT) and magnetic resonance (MR) are required to determine cancer extensions. MR cholangiopancreatography is recommended. The most accurate staging is most often at surgery, and, if unresectable, biopsy of suspected extensions is advised.

PROGNOSIS AND SURVIVAL

The adverse effect of vascular invasion is shown and clearly demonstrates the superior survival of partial hepatectomy versus concomitant resection of portal vein. For localized disease, a 5-year survival rate of 20% to 40% can be achieved.

MANAGEMENT

Surgical resection is preferred for early stages; in advanced stages, neoadjuvant chemoradiation regimens and liver transplantation are the only options. There is significant perioperative morbidity (30% to 50%) and mortality (5% to 10%).

†Preceding passage from Edge SB, Byrd DR, Compton CC, et al., *AJCC Cancer Staging Manual, 7th edition*. New York, Springer, 2010, p. 228.

PERIHILAR BILE DUCT

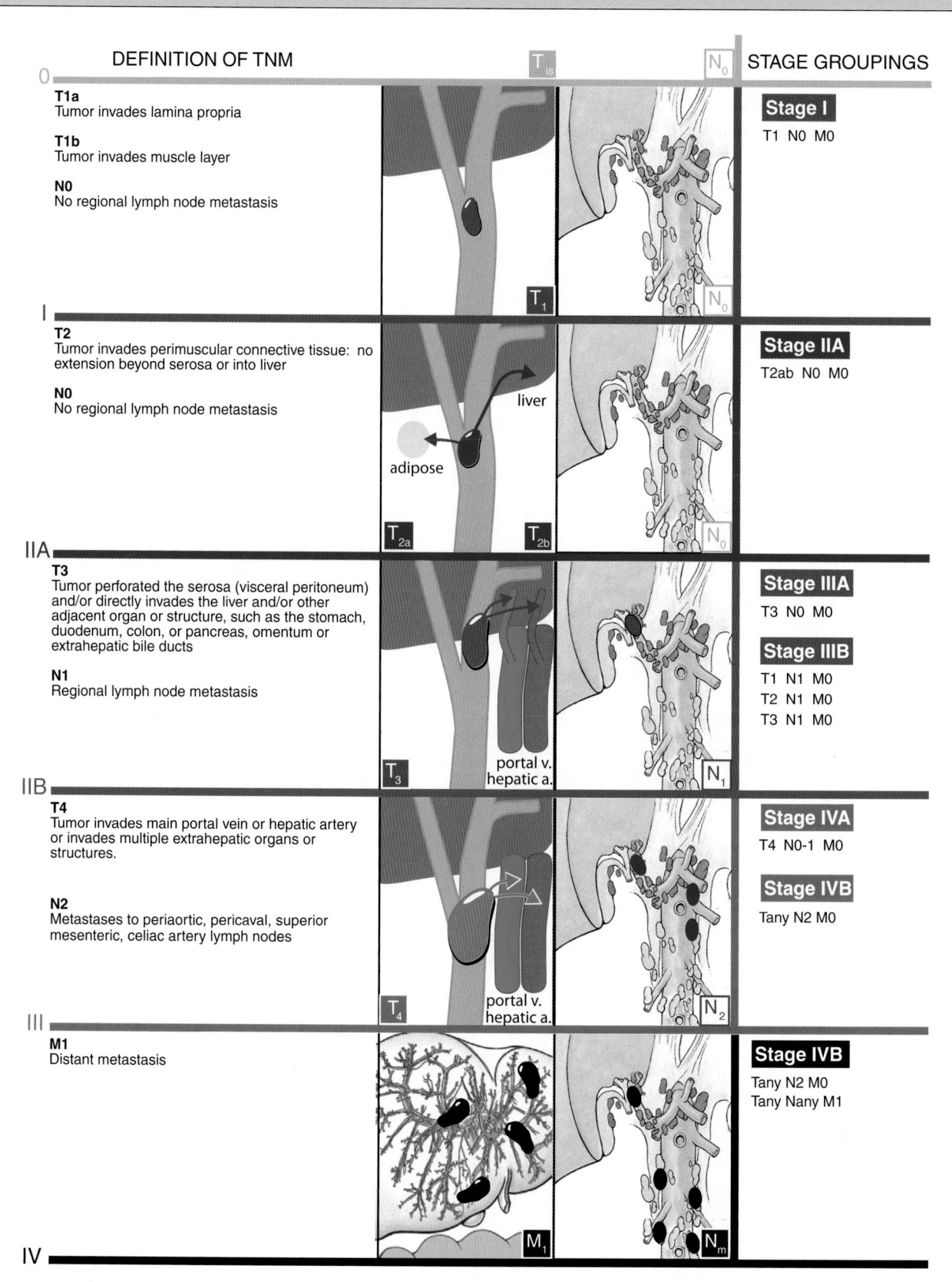

Figure 26.3B | TNM staging diagram presents a vertical arrangement with color bars encompassing TN combinations showing progression. Note that stages I and II are divided into substages A/B. Resectability is possible with stage IA/B and stage IIA and decreases with stage IIB (purple) when nodes are involved and invasion of gallbladder occurs. Stage III is unresectable, and stage IV is metastatic and not treatable. Stage 0, yellow; I, green; II, blue; III, purple; IV, red; and stage IV (metastatic), black. Definitions of TN on left and stage grouping on right.

T-ONCOANATOMY

ORIENTATION OF THREE-PLANAR ONCOANATOMY

The anatomic isocenter for the extrahepatic biliary tree is at the hilar level, and (i) the bullet is to the right of the midsagittal plane, and (ii) in the midcoronal plane, the bullet is anterior to the 12th rib (Fig. 26.4).

T-oncoanatomy

The complexity in understanding the oncoanatomy of the extrahepatic biliary tree relates to the precise details in each individual, given the potential variations in the arrangements of the gallbladder, cystic duct, and the confluens, which can be a low or high union or swerving in its course (Fig. 26.5). In addition, resectability relates to the arrangement of the hepatic artery and the portal vein, as well as to their branching. Optimally, a confluens carcinoma with a low-lying union and separation of the right and left hepatic artery would be more resectable than a high union with the main hepatic artery lying anterior to the confluens.

- *Coronal*: The extrahepatic bile ducts, pancreatic bile ducts, and pancreatic ducts are dissected free. The left and right hepatic ducts collect bile from the liver and unite with the cystic duct superior to the pancreas and the duodenum (Fig. 26.5A).

- *Sagittal*: The extrahepatic bile duct lies posterior to the gallbladder and passes posterior to the first part of the duodenum at the porta hepatis. The portal triad of the common bile duct, hepatic artery, and portal vein lies in the hepatoduodenal ligament, at the entrance to the lesser omental sac.

- *Transverse*: The inferior surface of the liver exposes the intimate relationship at the porta hepatis of the cystic duct to the common bile duct and its confluens in addition to medially placed hepatic artery and portal vein (Fig. 26.5B).

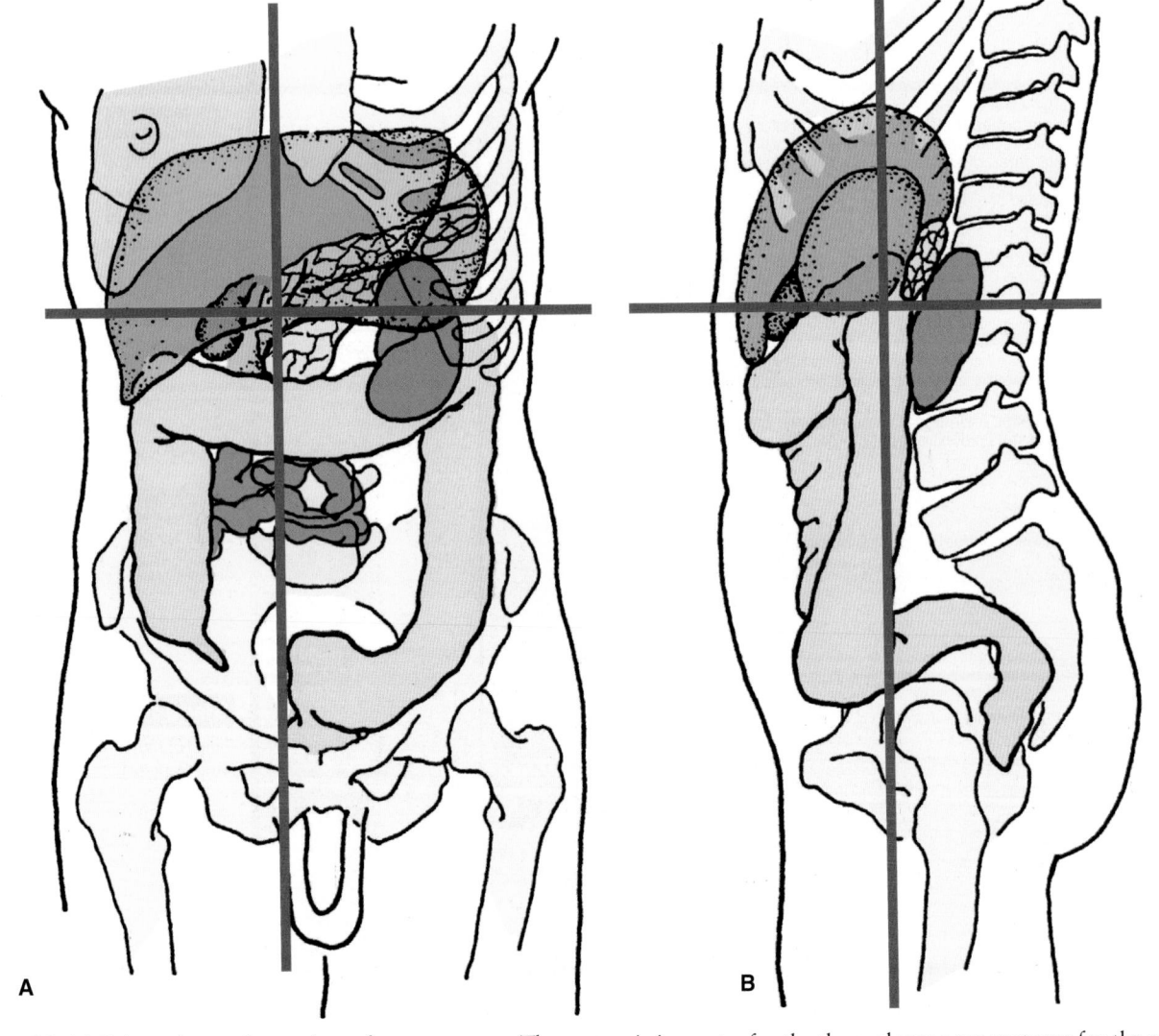

A   **B**

Figure 26.4 | **Orientation and overview of oncoanatomy.** The anatomic isocenter for the three-planar oncoanatomy for the gallbladder is the right of the midline (pararectus plane) at the subcostal region anteriorly and L1/L2 posteriorly. The bile ducts are in a similar locale but inferior at L1/L2. **A.** Coronal. **B.** Sagittal.

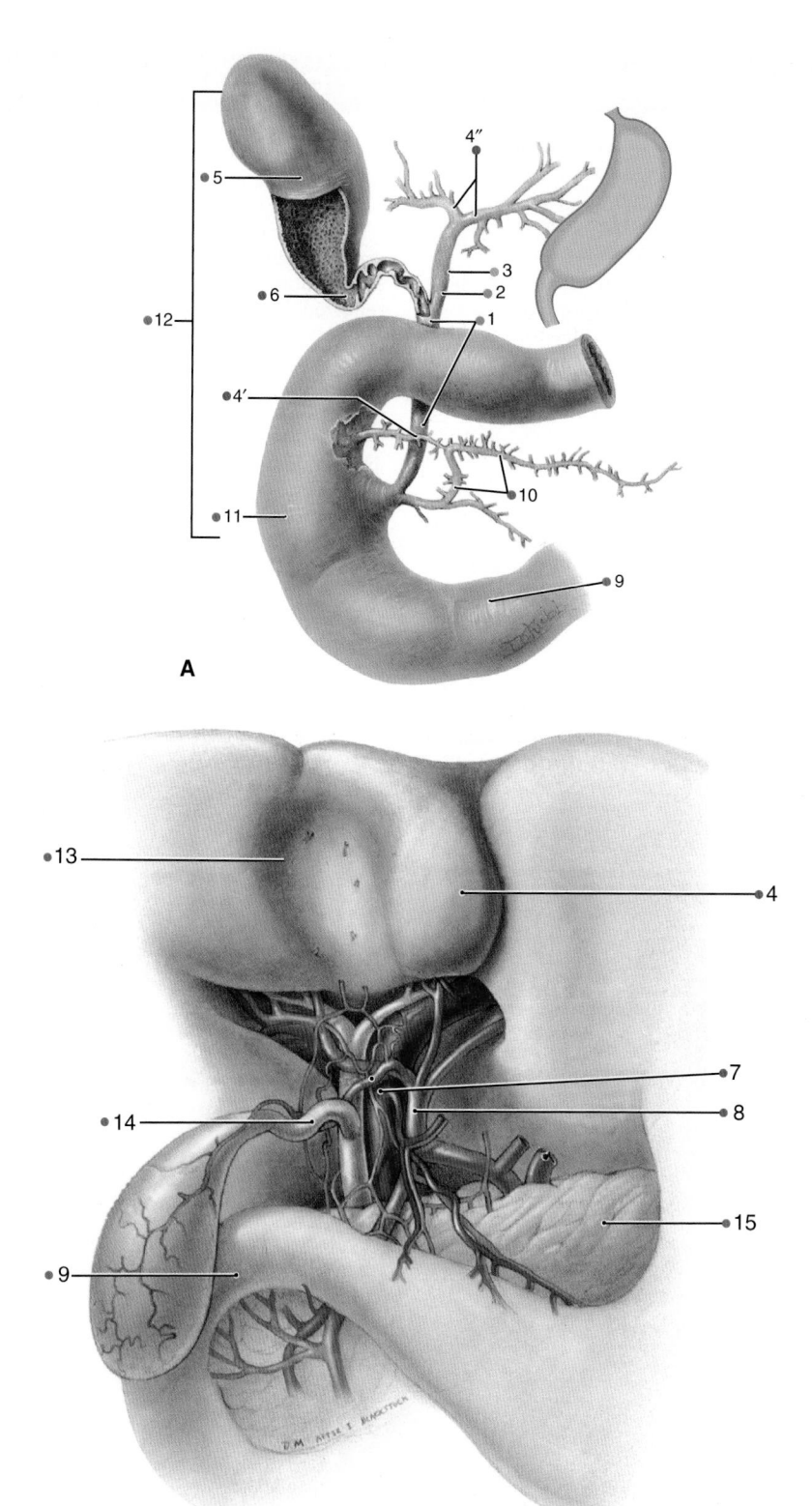

A

B Anterior View, Liver Reflected Superiorly

T_1 • 1. Common Bile Duct	T_3 • 5. Gallbladder	T_4 • 11. Second part of duodenum
T_1 • 2. Common hepatic duct	T_3 • 6. Neck of gallbladder	T_4 • 12. Abdominal wall
T_2 • 3. Beyond Wall	T_3 • 7. Portal vein	T_4 • 13. Fossa for gallbladder
T_3 • 4. Liver	T_3 • 8. Proper hepatic artery	T_4 • 14. Cystic duct
T_3 • 4′. Accessory pancreatic duct	T_4 • 9. Duodenum	T_4 • 15. Pancreas
T_3 • 4″. Right and left hepatic ducts	T_4 • 10. Pancreatic ducts	

Figure 26.5 | T-oncoanatomy. Connecting the dots. Structures are color coded for cancer stage progression. The color code for the anatomic sites correlates with the color code for the stage group (Fig. 26.3) and patterns of spread (Fig. 26.2) and SIMLAP table (Table 26.2). Connecting the dots in similar colors will provide an appreciation for the 3D oncoanatomy.

N-ONCOANATOMY AND M-ONCOANATOMY

DISTAL BILE DUCTS

N-oncoanatomy

The lymphatic drainage of the extrahepatic bile duct is via the lymph nodes at the porta hepatis and include hilar, celiac, periduodenal, and peripancreatic nodes as well as nodes around the gallbladder and the hepatic triad. The sentinel nodes are the porta hepatis nodes. Nodal metastases are common and occur in 30% of cases (Fig. 26.6A; see Table 26.4).

Regional Lymph Nodes

Accurate tumor staging requires that all removed lymph nodes be analyzed. Optimal histologic examination of a pacreaticoduodenectomy specimen should include analysis of a minimum of 12 lymph nodes. If the resected lymph node is negative but this number of examined nodes is not met, pN0 should still be assigned. The regional lymph nodes are the same as those resected for cancers of the head of the pancreas, that is,

nodes along the common bile duct, hepatic artery, and back toward the celiac trunk, the posterior and anterior pancreaticoduodenal nodes, and the nodes along the superior mesenteric vein and the right lateral wall of the superior mesenteric artery. Anatomic division of regional lymph nodes is not necessary; however, separately submitted lymph nodes should be reported as submitted.*

M-oncoanatomy

The venous drainage of the extrahepatic bile ducts joins the cystic vein and drains into the right gastric vein and posterior superior pancreaticoduodenal vein and then into the portal vein, returning to the liver. In addition to hematogenous spread, perineural and neural invasion are common (see Fig. 26.6B).

*Preceding passage from Edge SB, Byrd DR, Compton CC, et al., *AJCC Cancer Staging Manual, 7th edition.* New York, Springer, 2010.

TABLE 26.4	Lymph Nodes of Gallbladder and the Bile Duct
Sentinel Nodes Include Porta Hepatis Nodes	
Regional Nodes	**Juxtaregional Nodes**
Hepatic vein	Mediastinal
Paracaval	Iliac
Celiac	Superior mesentery
	Pericardial and diaphragmatic

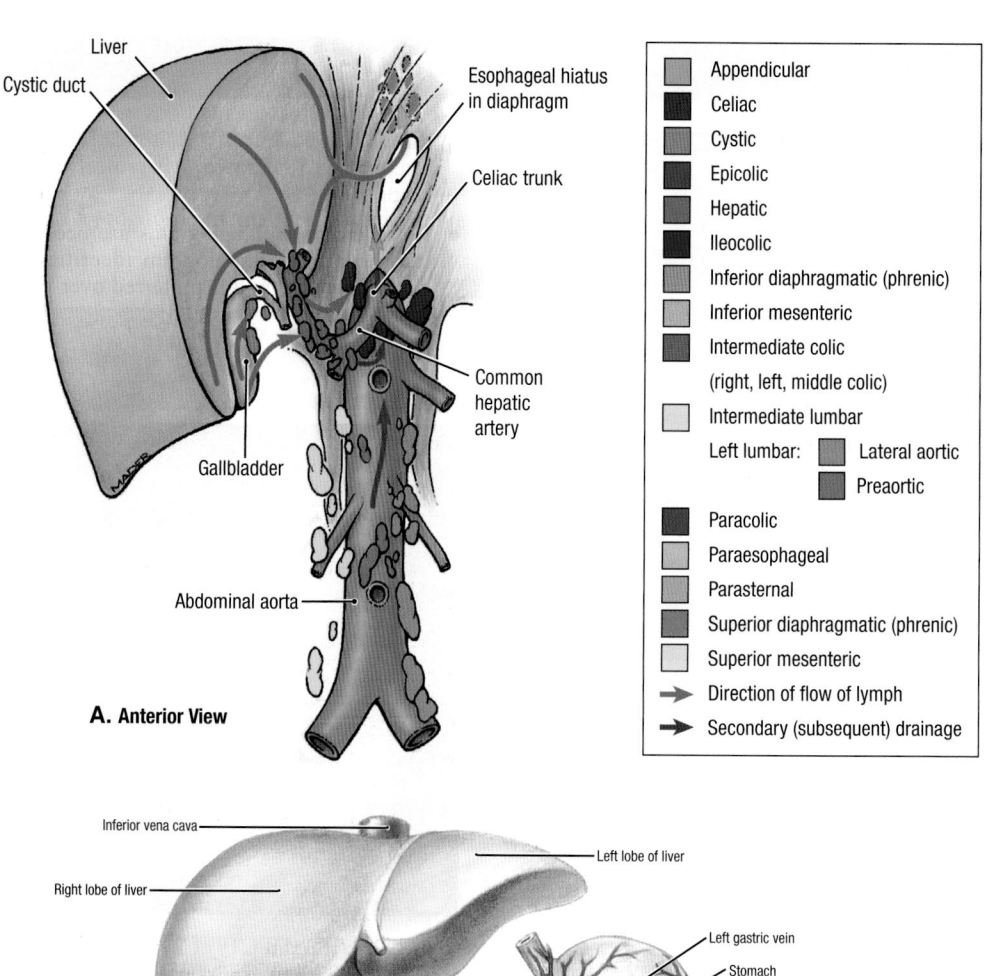

A. Anterior View

Liver
Cystic duct
Esophageal hiatus in diaphragm
Celiac trunk
Common hepatic artery
Gallbladder
Abdominal aorta

Appendicular
Celiac
Cystic
Epicolic
Hepatic
Ileocolic
Inferior diaphragmatic (phrenic)
Inferior mesenteric
Intermediate colic
(right, left, middle colic)
Intermediate lumbar
Left lumbar: Lateral aortic
Preaortic
Paracolic
Paraesophageal
Parasternal
Superior diaphragmatic (phrenic)
Superior mesenteric
→ Direction of flow of lymph
⟹ Secondary (subsequent) drainage

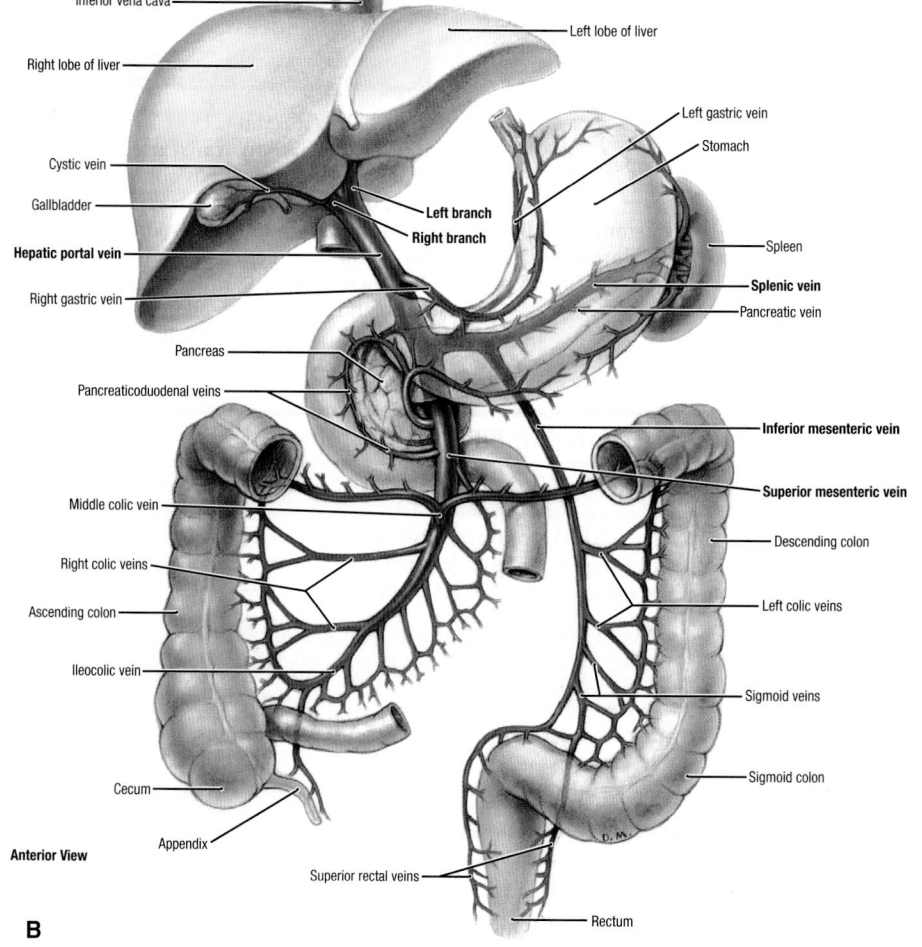

Anterior View

Inferior vena cava
Right lobe of liver
Left lobe of liver
Left gastric vein
Stomach
Cystic vein
Gallbladder
Left branch
Right branch
Hepatic portal vein
Spleen
Splenic vein
Pancreatic vein
Right gastric vein
Pancreas
Pancreaticoduodenal veins
Inferior mesenteric vein
Superior mesenteric vein
Middle colic vein
Descending colon
Right colic veins
Ascending colon
Left colic veins
Ileocolic vein
Sigmoid veins
Cecum
Sigmoid colon
Appendix
Superior rectal veins
Rectum

B

Figure 26.6 | A. N-oncoanatomy. Sentinel nodes of the bile ducts include the porta hepatis nodes. **B. M-oncoanatomy.** The venous drainage of the extrahepatic bile ducts joins the cystic vein and drains into the right gastric vein and posterior superior pancreaticoduodenal vein and then into the portal vein, returning to the liver, resulting in liver metastases.

Gallbladder

PERSPECTIVE, PATTERNS OF SPREAD, AND PATHOLOGY

Cancer of the gallbladder is insidious in onset and is associated with gallstones in 75% of presentations.

PERSPECTIVE AND PATTERNS OF SPREAD

An elaborate bile ductal system originates in the liver, which becomes extrahepatic at the porta hepatis. The gallbladder can be viewed as a bile reservoir that responds to fat in meals and is connected by a cystic duct to the common bile duct (CBD). The CBD joins the pancreatic duct and forms an ampulla within the head of the pancreas referred to as the ampulla of Vater, which terminates in a papilla that empties into the second part of the duodenum. This complex of branching bile ducts and fusion with the pancreatic duct is best appreciated diagrammatically. These sites give rise to a variety of cancers, but the most common are adenocarcinomas.

The gallbladder and the extrahepatic biliary ducts account for 960 new cancer cases annually, and approximately 50% of these patients survive. Cancer of the gallbladder is insidious in onset and is associated with gallstones in 75% of presentations. Many gallbladder cancers are unsuspected and found incidentally by the surgeon, who may be operating because of cholelithiasis. Although extrahepatic bile duct cancers can arise anywhere in its network, it is worth noting that 70% to 80% are found at the confluence of the right and the left hepatic ducts, and the other 20% to 30% arise more distally. Obstructive jaundice is a frequent consequence and can occur even with small tumors. The main reason for identifying the ampulla of Vater separately is that obstruction at the site induces severe pain and causes jaundice and a most disconcerting reflux pancreatitis. Patterns of spread are into bile ducts, liver, and adjacent viscera (Table 27.2; Fig. 27.2).

Gallbladder cancer (GBC) is the sixth-most-common cancer of the digestive system, but only accounts for 3% to 4% of all gastrointestinal (GIT) cancers. GBC occurs in the elderly and is three times more common in females. Gallstones lead to chronic inflammation; larger stones (>3 cm) are associated with 10 times higher risk of cancer. The calcified gallbladder, so-called porcelain wall, is associated with a very high risk, ranging from 20% to 50%, of leading to cancer. Thus, symptoms and signs are usually nonspecific initially; as the cancer advances, right upper quadrant pain becomes continuous and there is a palpable mass and eventually jaundice, pruritis, and weight loss. Hepatomegaly and ascites suggest liver invasion. Laboratory data include elevated alkaline phosphatase, bilirubin, and aminotransferase.

PATHOLOGY

Adenocarcinomas are the most common cancer type and can vary from differentiated to anaplastic cancer, often with a desmoplastic reaction.

The histopathology of gallbladder cancers are largely adenocarcinomas and the variety of cancers are listed in Table 27.1 and Fig. 27.1 illustrates the typical pathology with gallstones.

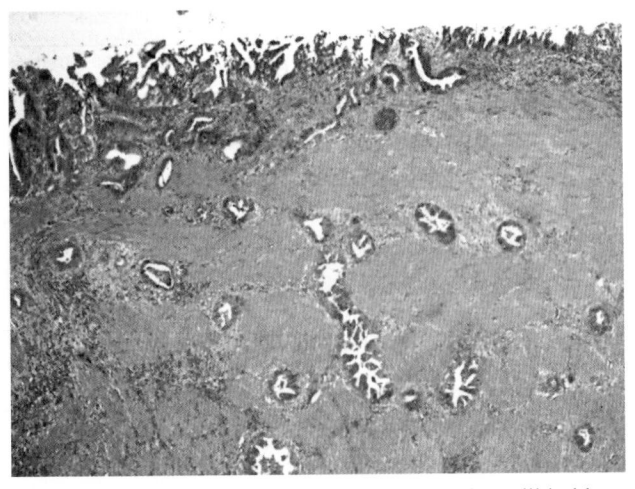

Figure 27.1 | Carcinoma of the gallbladder. The gallbladder wall is infiltrated by a moderately differentiated adenocarcinoma, which has stimulated a desmoplastic response.

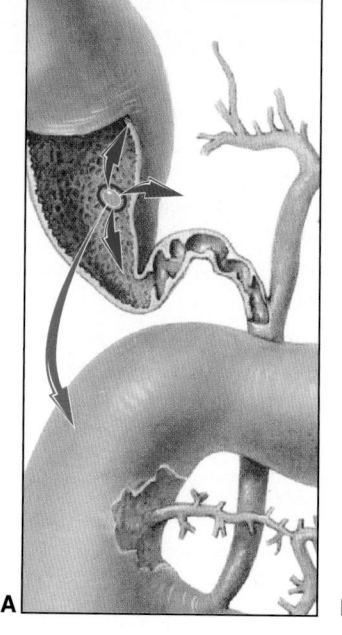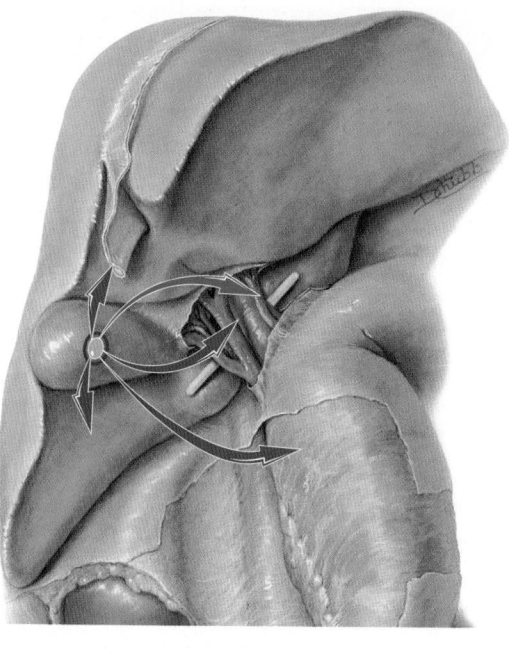

Figure 27.2 | Patterns of spread for gallbladder. Color coded for T stage: Tis, yellow; T1, green; T2, blue; T3, purple; T4, red. The concept of visualizing patterns of spread to appreciate the surrounding anatomy is well demonstrated by the six-directional pattern, i.e., SIMLAP Table 27.2.

TABLE 27.1 Histopathologic Type: Common Cancers of the Gallbladder and the Bile Duct

Type	Incidence (%)[a]	Seventh Edition AJCC
Carcinoma	96	Carcinoma in situ
Adenocarcinoma	86	Adenocarcinoma, NOS
Adenocarcinoma, NOS	71	Papillary carcinoma
Papillary adenocarcinoma	6	Adenocarcinoma, intestinal type
Mucinous and mucin producing	5	Clear cell adenocarcinoma
Other adenocarcinoma	4	Mucinous carcinoma
Squamous cell carcinoma	0.2	Signet ring cell carcinoma
Carcinoma, NOS	7	Squamous carcinoma
Other specific carcinomas	0.5	Adenosquamous carcinoma
Sarcoma	0.2	Small cell carcinoma[b]
Other unspecified	0.8	Undifferentiated carcinoma[b] Spindle and giant cell types Small cell types Carcinoma, NOS Carcinosarcoma Other (specify)

[a]Data from Carriaga MT, Henson DE. Liver, gallbladder, extrahepatic bile ducts, and pancreas. *Cancer* 1995;75(Suppl):171.
[b]Grade 4 by definition.
NOS, not otherwise specified.

TABLE 27.2 SIMLAP

	Gallbladder	• T1
S	Right lobe liver	• T3
I	Duodenum, first, second	• T3
M	Cystic	• T2
	Bile ducts	• T3
	Porta hepatis	• T4
	Portal vein	• T4
L	Right lobe liver	• T3
A	Transverse colon	• T3
	Hepatic flexure	• T3
P	Portal vein, inferior vena cava	• T4
	Hepatic artery	• T4
	Pancreas	• T3

The six vectors of invasion are Superior, Inferior, Medial, Lateral, Anterior, and Posterior. The color-coded dots correlate the T stage with specific anatomic structure involved.

TNM STAGING CRITERIA

TNM STAGING CRITERIA

The gallbladder and the extrahepatic bile ducts terminating at the ampulla of Vater share a hollow structure with thin walls. With the exception of the gallbladder, most bile duct cancers can obstruct and still be small. Whereas cancer of the ampulla of Vater can be confused with primary duodenal and/or pancreatic cancer of the head of the gland, their relative infrequency suggests that this diagnosis may be made by exclusion.

Each of these staging systems has been revised and simplified. Each primary site is of hollow structure with muscular walls, and they share common staging criteria (Fig. 27.3). T1 is a tumor that invades the lamina propria muscle layer and is contained within the wall. In stage T2, the tumor penetrates to the serosa. T3 tumor invades and penetrates the wall through the serosa to a surrounding structure as liver or pancreas. T4 is an advanced cancer with invasion of multiple adjacent sites and into blood vessels. The staging criteria attempt to stage cancers of extrahepatic ducts as T3 to indicate resectability versus T4, which are nonresectable. Two of these three cancer sites are presented together to enable comparisons.

The malignant gradient of the gallbladder is highest at the surface in contact with the liver and decreases on the free side and the cystic duct. For the extrahepatic ducts, the malignant gradient is close to liver at the confluence of the right and left hepatic ducts and decreases peripherally.

Generally, there is no overarching principle or context design for the digestive system (gastrointestinal tract) or major digestive glands (MDGs). Stages are frequently expanded to six by subdividing stages into A and B. The T and N categories are assigned to a stage grouping, specifically for division of a stage into more (a) versus less (b) favorable groupings. This occurs at different stages for different sites.

Specifically, there is a direct relationship between T categories and stage progression; that is, T1 = IA, T2 = IIA, T3 = IIB, and T4 = IV.

SUMMARY OF CHANGES SEVENTH EDITION AJCC

- The cystic duct is now included in this classification scheme.

- The N classification now distinguishes hilar nodes (N1: lymph nodes adjacent to the cystic duct, bile duct, hepatic artery, and portal vein) from other regional nodes (N2: celiac, periduodenal, and peripancreatic lymph nodes and those along the superior mesenteric artery).

- Stage groupings have been changed to better correlate with surgical resectability and patient outcome; locally unresectable T4 tumors have been reclassified as Stage IV.

- Lymph node metastasis is now classified as Stage IIIB (N1) or Stage IVB (N2).

- The T categories are the same and N categories are divided N1, N2.

- The major change is the assignment to a stage group, although the T/N clusters are the same.

6th Edition	7th Edition
IA	I T1 N0
IB	II T2 N0
IIA	IIIA T3 N0
IIB	IIIB T3 N1
IV	IVA T4 N1
	IVB T4 N2 (new)

The TNM Staging Matrix is color coded for identification of Stage Group once T and N stages are determined (Table 27.3).

TABLE 27.3 Stage Summary Matrix

	N0	N1	N2	M1
T1a,b	IA*	IIIB	IVB	IVB
T2	II	IIIB	IVB	IVB
T3	IIIA	IIIB	IVB	IVB
T4	IVA	IVA	IVB	IVB

Sequential progression of T stage and then N stage determines stage group progression:
- *T stage T$_1$ = I, T$_2$ = II, T$_3$ = IIIA, T$_4$ = IVA*
- *N stage N$_1$ = T$_3$ advances all to stage IIIB*
- *M stage is separate*

GALLBLADDER

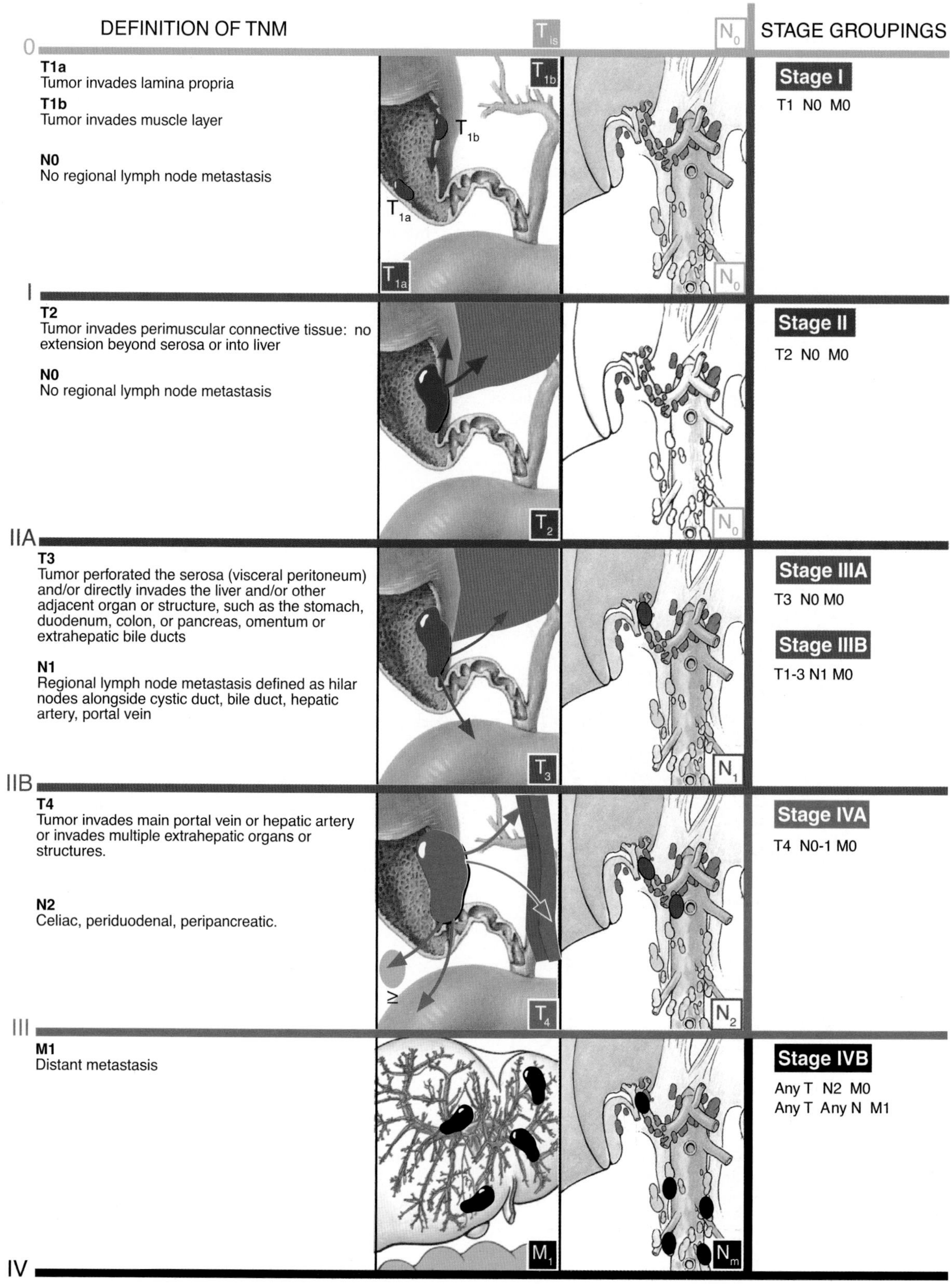

Figure 27.3 | TNM staging diagram presents a vertical arrangement with color bars encompassing TN combinations showing progression. Gallbladder cancers are discovered incidentally to gallstones, with stage IIA (blue) being most resectable; stage IIB (purple), borderline N1 nodes; and stage III (red), unresectable. Stage 0, yellow; I, green; II, blue; III, purple; IV, red; and IV (metastatic), black. Definitions of TN on left and stage grouping on right.

T-ONCOANATOMY

ORIENTATION OF THREE-PLANAR ONCOANATOMY

The anatomic isocenter for the three-planar oncoanatomy for the gallbladder is to the right of the midline (pararectus plane) at the subcostal region anteriorly and T12/L1 posteriorly (Fig. 27.4). The bile ducts are in a similar locale but inferior at L1/L2.

T-oncoanatomy

Figure 27.5 provides the orientation of three-planar views of these interrelated sites, anatomically as well as functionally; **A.** Coronal, **B.** Sagittal, **C.** Transverse axial.

- *Coronal:* The gallbladder is a pearlike organ with four layers: a lining epithelium, which is simple columnar consist-

ing of common clear cells and occasional brush cells; the lamina propria, a layer of smooth muscle with connective tissue and cone of a serosa on the free caudad tail side; and the adventitia on the cephalad head side juxtaposed to the liver. When empty, the gallbladder is folded into tall parallel ridges; when it is filled, the folds are reduced.

- *Sagittal:* The extrahepatic ducts unite with the cystic duct to become the CBD. Again, there are four layers or sphincter muscles of Oddi that control the flow of bile and move pancreatic secretions in the correct directions without reflux of bile into the pancreas. The ampulla of Vater opens at a duodenal papilla to always maintain a prograde flow into the small bowel.

- *Transverse:* The gallbladder is at the inferior margin of the right lobe of the liver to which it is juxtaposed on its superior surface and to the bowel on its inferior surface. The cystic duct drains to the left, toward the midline, where it coalesces with the extrahepatic bile ducts to form the CBD at the porta hepatis.

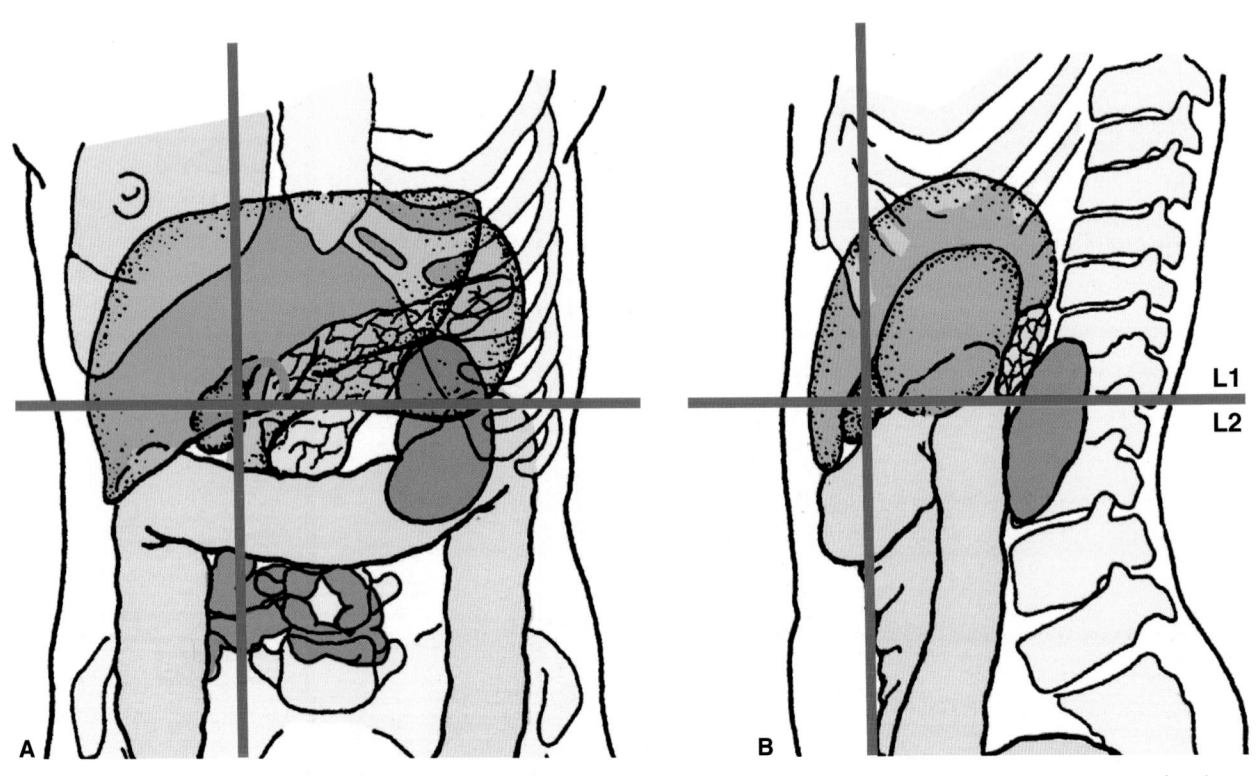

Figure 27.4 | Orientation and overview of oncoanatomy. The anatomic isocenter for the three-planar oncoanatomy for the gallbladder is the right of the midline (pararectus plane) at the subcostal region anteriorly and L1/L2 posteriorly. **A.** Coronal. **B.** Sagittal.

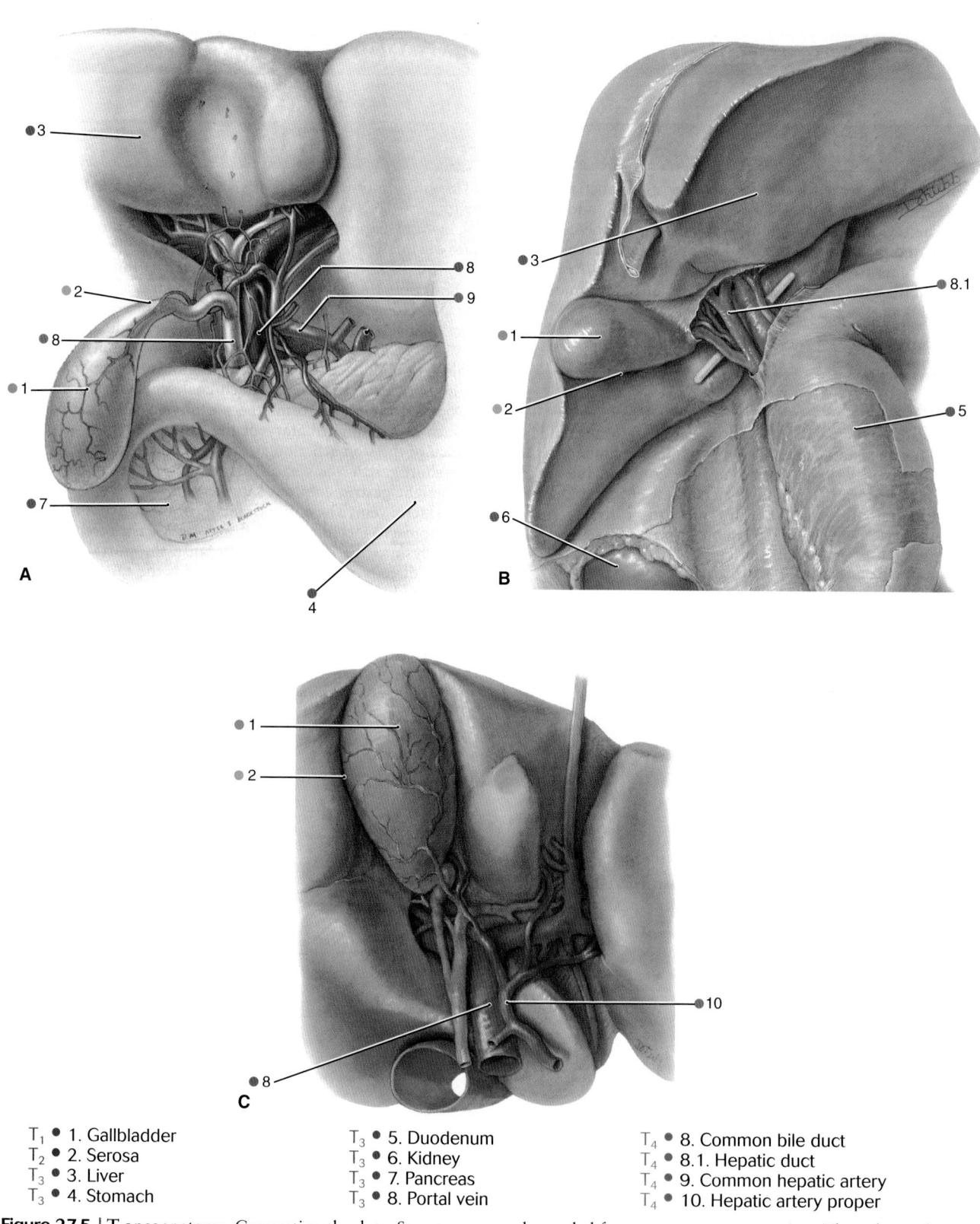

T_1	• 1. Gallbladder	T_3	• 5. Duodenum	T_4	• 8. Common bile duct
T_2	• 2. Serosa	T_3	• 6. Kidney	T_4	• 8.1. Hepatic duct
T_3	• 3. Liver	T_3	• 7. Pancreas	T_4	• 9. Common hepatic artery
T_3	• 4. Stomach	T_3	• 8. Portal vein	T_4	• 10. Hepatic artery proper

Figure 27.5 | T-oncoanatomy. Connecting the dots. Structures are color coded for cancer stage progression. The color code for the anatomic sites correlates with the color code for the stage group (Fig. 27.3) and patterns of spread (Fig. 27.2) and SIMLAP tables (Table 27.2). Connecting the dots in similar colors will provide an appreciation for the 3D oncoanatomy.

TABLE 28.2	Histopathologic Type: Common Cancers of the Pancreas
Type	
Severe ductal dysplasia/carcinoma in situ (pancreatic intraepithelial neoplasia)	Intraductal papillary mucinous carcinoma with or without invasion
Ductal adenocarcinoma	Acinar cell carcinoma
Mucinous noncystic carcinoma	Acinar cell cystadenocarcinoma
Signet ring cell carcinoma	Mixed acinar–endocrine carcinoma
Adenosquamous carcinoma	Pancreaticoblastoma
Undifferentiated carcinoma, spindle and giant cell types, small cell types	Solid pseudopapillary carcinoma
Mixed ductal–endocrine carcinoma	Borderline (uncertain malignant potential) tumors Mucinous cystic tumor with moderate dysplasia Intraductal papillary–mucinous tumor with moderate dysplasia Solid pseudopapillary tumor
Osteoclast-like giant cell tumor	Composite carcinoid (combined with adenocarcinoma)
Serous cystadenocarcinoma	Adenocarcinoid tumor
Mucinous cystadenocarcinoma	Mixed islet cell and exocrine adenocarcinoma Islet cell carcinoma Insulinoma Glucagonoma Gastrinoma Vipoma Somatostatinoma Enteroglucagonoma

Reprinted with permission from Edge SB, Byrd DR, Compton CC, et al. *AJCC Cancer Staging Manual*, 7th ed. New York: Springer, 2010, p. 245.

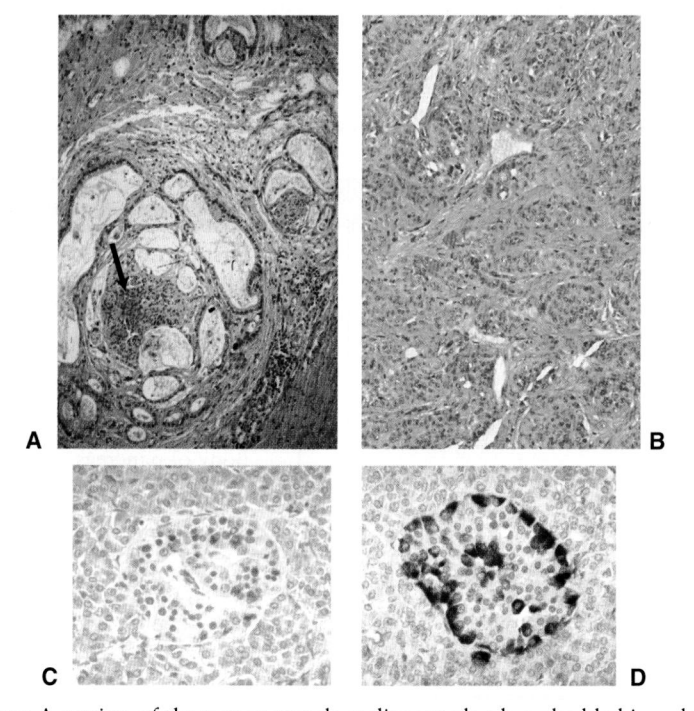

Figure 28.2A-D | **A. Carcinoma:** A section of the tumor reveals malignant glands embedded in a dense fibrous stroma. A nerve (*arrow*) shows perineural invasion. **B. Insulinoma:** Nests of tumor cells are surrounded by numerous capillaries. **C. Somatostatinoma:** somatostatin in sparsely distributed delta cells. **D. Glucagonoma:** glucagon in alpha cells at the periphery of the islet. *(continued)*

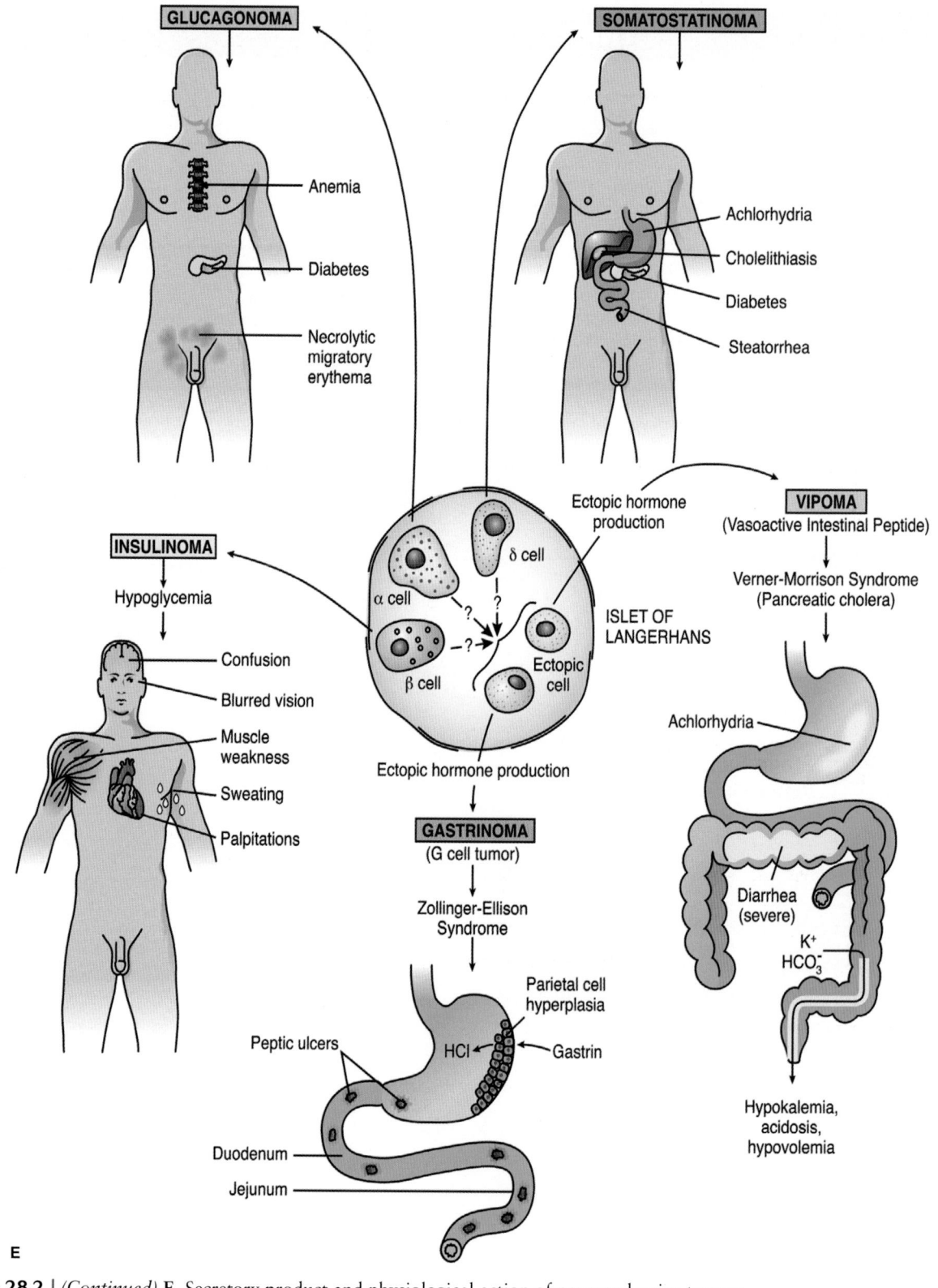

Figure 28.2 | *(Continued)* **E.** Secretory product and physiological action of neuroendocrine tumors.

Neuroendocrine tumors although uncommon are currently staged in a similar fashion as carcinomas, whether they are considered benign or malignant. Their secretary product and physiological action are noted in Fig. 28.1E. Because they are rare, factors other than T and N stage as age, degree of differentiation, impact of functional status on host are prognostic factors.

TNM STAGING CRITERIA

TNM STAGING CRITERIA

The pancreas is both intraperitoneal and retroperitoneal in location. Situated in the epigastrium, the cancer can and does invade adjacent structures. Size is the major factor in staging: T1, <2 cm and T2, >2 cm, limited to pancreas. Involvement of the celiac axis and superior mesenteric artery (SMA) renders the cancer T4 and nonresectable (Fig. 28.3A).

Each section of the pancreas has a critical adjacent structure that determines the clinical course as mentioned, but does not affect staging. Despite the intimate contact anteriorly with stomach, duodenum, colon, spleen, and kidneys, pancreatic cancers rarely invade these viscera; however, peritoneal seeding is common and can lead to massive ascites.

Generally, there is no overarching principle or context design for the digestive system (gastrointestinal tract) or major digestive glands (MDGs). Stages are frequently expanded to six by subdividing stages into A and B. The T and N categories are assigned to a stage grouping—specifically for division of a stage into more (a) versus less (b) favorable groupings. This occurs at different stages for different sites.

There is a direct relationship between N category and stage II progression with stage: IIA = N0 and IIB = N1.

The distinction between T3 and T4 reflects the border between resectable and unresectable cancers, respectively. M1 has been expanded to include positive peritoneal washings and ascites cells and for cancer seeding.

SUMMARY OF CHANGES SEVENTH EDITION AJCC

- Pancreatic neuroendocrine tumors (including carcinoid tumors) are now staged by a single pancreatic staging system.
- Survival tables and figures have been added for adenocarcinoma and neuroendocrine tumors.
- The definitions of TNM and the Anatomic Stage/Prognostic Groupings for this chapter have not changed from the sixth edition for exocrine tumors.

The TNM Staging Matrix is color coded for identification of Stage Group once T and N stages are determined (Table 28.3).

| TABLE 28.3A | Stage Summary Matrix: Pancreas |

	N0	N1	M1
T1	IA	IIB	IV
T2	IB	IIB	IV
T3	IIA	IIB	IV
T4	III	III	IV

Sequential progression of T stage and then N stage determines stage group progression:

- *T stage T_1 = I, T_2 = II, T_3 = IIIA, T_4 = IIIB*
- *N stage N_1 = T_3 advances all to Stage IIIC*
- *M stage is separate*

PANCREAS

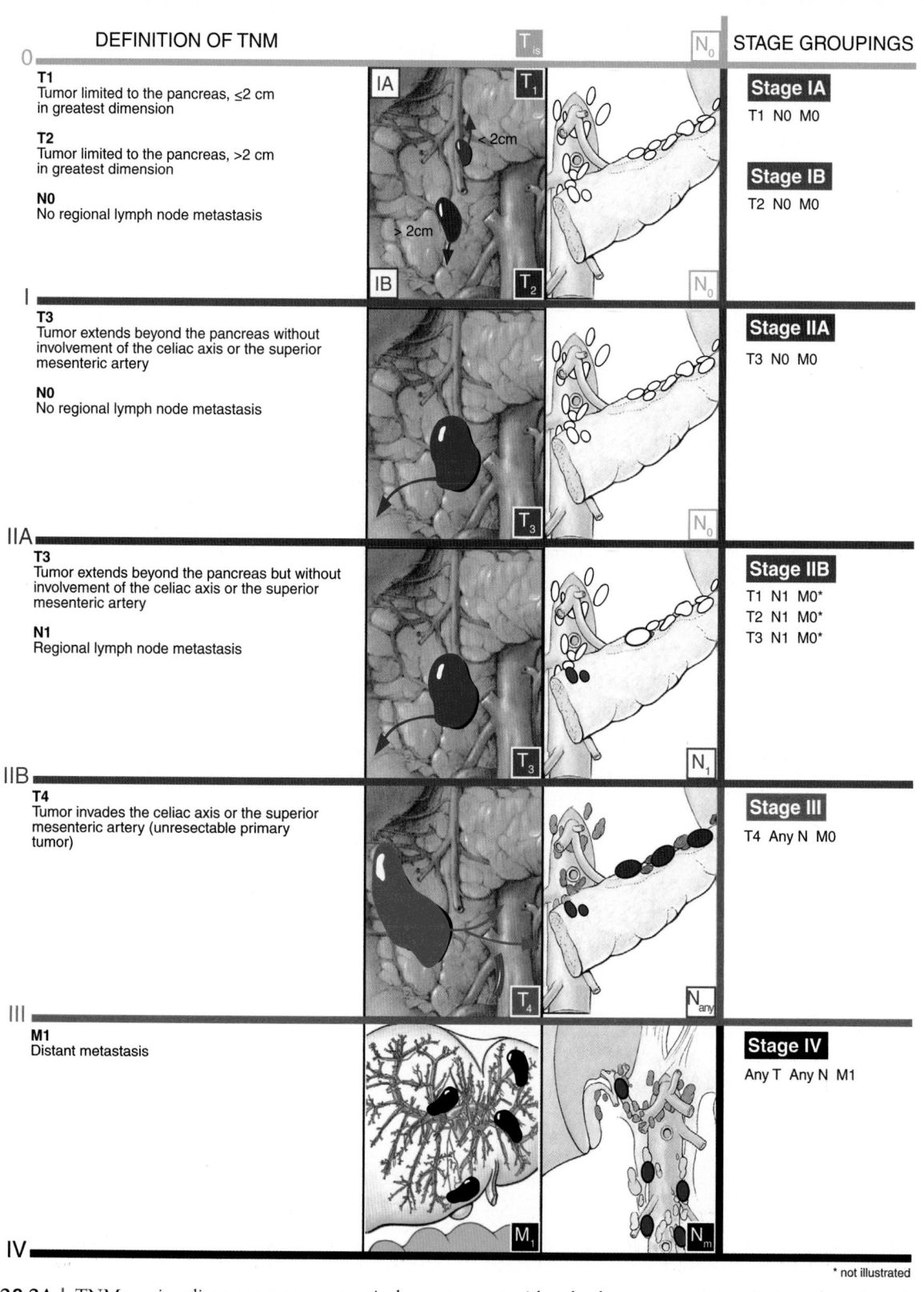

DEFINITION OF TNM

T1
Tumor limited to the pancreas, ≤2 cm in greatest dimension

T2
Tumor limited to the pancreas, >2 cm in greatest dimension

N0
No regional lymph node metastasis

T3
Tumor extends beyond the pancreas without involvement of the celiac axis or the superior mesenteric artery

N0
No regional lymph node metastasis

T3
Tumor extends beyond the pancreas but without involvement of the celiac axis or the superior mesenteric artery

N1
Regional lymph node metastasis

T4
Tumor invades the celiac axis or the superior mesenteric artery (unresectable primary tumor)

M1
Distant metastasis

STAGE GROUPINGS

Stage IA
T1 N0 M0

Stage IB
T2 N0 M0

Stage IIA
T3 N0 M0

Stage IIB
T1 N1 M0*
T2 N1 M0*
T3 N1 M0*

Stage III
T4 Any N M0

Stage IV
Any T Any N M1

* not illustrated

Figure 28.3A I TNM staging diagram presents a vertical arrangement with color bars encompassing TN combinations showing progression. Pancreatic cancers are generally advanced, stage IIB (purple), and N1 borderline resectable. Stage III (red) are unresectable, and stage IV (black) are metastatic. Stage 0, yellow; I, green; IIA, blue; IIB, purple; III, red; and stage IV (metastatic), black. Definitions of TN on left and stage grouping on right.

AMPULLA OF VATER

Perspective and Patterns of Spread

Carcinomas of the ampulla of Vater reflect its complex anatomy although it is only 1.5 cm long. Remarkably, it has the highest rate of malignant transformation in the small intestine, likely due to interactions of bile, pancreatic enzymes, and duodenal content. Neoplastic transformation is similar to that of the colon, with transition of adenomas to adenocarcinomas with evidence of biassociation of 80% to 90%, that is, the adenocarcinoma is surrounded by benign adenoma. The average for adenomas is 50 years of age and of adenocarcinomas is 60 years of age, adding credence for the evolution to cancer.

Cancers in the distal portion of the bile duct at its confluens with the pancreatic duct are uncommon. The reason to be aware of these periampullary cancers is that they may offer a better chance for survival than that of the more common cancer in their neighborhood, cancer of the pancreas. The onset is insidious and unexplained persistent itching; slight alterations in the color of stool and urine are the precursors to frank jaundice. Mirizzi syndrome, idiopathic focal stenosis, or sclerosing cholangitis, referred as the "malignant masquerade," is a hopeful entity in the differential diagnosis. Classically, Mirizzi syndrome is caused by a large gallstone impacted in the neck of the gallbladder causing biliary obstruction because of periductal inflammation.

- *Familial adenomatous polyposis* and *Peutz–Jeghers syndrome* have higher incidence of ampullary adenomas, ranging from 50% to 86%.

- *Obstructive jaundice* is seen in 80% of cases, and weight loss, abdominal pain, and occult bleeding occur.

- *Silver stools* are due to blood without bile.

Classification and Staging

Three distinct macroscopic subtypes occur: sclerosing, nodular, and papillary. With the sclerosing variety, diffuse or annular thickening or stricturing of the bile duct occurs, often associated with inflammatory disease. Nodular cancers project into the lumen, and papillary cancers are soft and friable but with a better prognosis because transmural invasion is less often seen. These tumors are more often encountered in the ductal part of the bile duct. Adenocarcinomas are most frequent at the site and have been referred to as periampullary or peripapillary, reflecting the normal anatomy (Fig. 28.2A; Table 28.2).

TABLE 28.3B	Stage Summary Matrix: Ampulla of Vater		
	N0	**N1**	**M1**
T1	IA	IIB	IV
T2	IB	IIB	IV
T3	IIA	IIB	IV
T4	III	III	IV

Sequential progression of T stage and then N stage determines stage group progression:

- *T stage $T_1 = I$, $T_2 = II$, $T_3 = IIIA$, $T_4 = IIIB$*
- *N stage $N_1 = T_4$ and advances to IIIC*
- *M stage is separate*

TNM Staging Criteria

The accuracy in staging is most often apparent after resection and dissection of the specimen. T1 is limited to the ampulla of Vater or the sphincter of Oddi, T2 invades the duodenal wall, T3 invades the pancreas, and T4 invades more extensively in peripancreatic tissues and adjacent organs and structures such as stomach, colon, and small intestines (Fig. 28.3B).

The nodal designation is simply N1, and the sentinel nodes are the pancreaticoduodenal lymph nodes. The regional nodes are in the porta hepatis region surrounding the hepatic artery and portal vein and juxtaregional paracaval and para-aortic nodes.

Summary of Changes Seventh Edition AJCC

- This staging system is the same for the seventh edition.

The TMN Staging Matrix is color coded for identification of Stage Group once T and N stages are determined (Table 28.3B).

T-ONCOANATOMY

The anatomic isocenter is at the L2 level surrounded by pancreas and duodenum. (i) The anterior bullet enters to right of the midline at the subcostal plane and (ii) the lateral bullet enters at the midcoronal plane anterior to the bodies of the upper lumbar vertebrae (Fig. 28.4).

The variation in the pancreatic duct and bile duct fusion are understandable if one reviews the developmental stages of this region (Fig. 28.4).

- *Coronal*: The gallbladder, bile duct, and ventral pancreas bud rotate when the duodenum rotates clockwise on its long axis during embryonic development. The fusion of the ventral and dorsal pancreatic buds results in numerous possible unions of the bile duct and pancreatic duct as it forms the ampulla of Vater.

- *Transverse*: The clockwise rotation is best appreciated in this view as the ventral pancreatic bud, which becomes the uncinate process, and the dorsal pancreatic bud forms the head, body, and tail of the pancreas.

- *Sagittal*: A variety of ampulla of Vater formations are shown, emphasizing the different fusions of the common bile duct and the main and accessory pancreatic ducts.

RULES FOR CLASSIFICATION AND STAGING

Clinical Staging and Imaging

The inability to evaluate the gallbladder, its ducts, and the ampulla of Vater has led the American Joint Committee on Cancer to simplify the staging so that both clinical and surgical criteria are the same. Imaging procedures include abdominal ultrasound, which is surpassed by computed tomography (CT) in defining biliary obstruction. Endoscopic retrograde cholangiopancreatography (ERCP) and percutaneous transhepatic cholangiography define biliary tree anatomy. Magnetic resonance imaging with gadolinium is also useful (see Table 28.5).

AMPULLA OF VATER

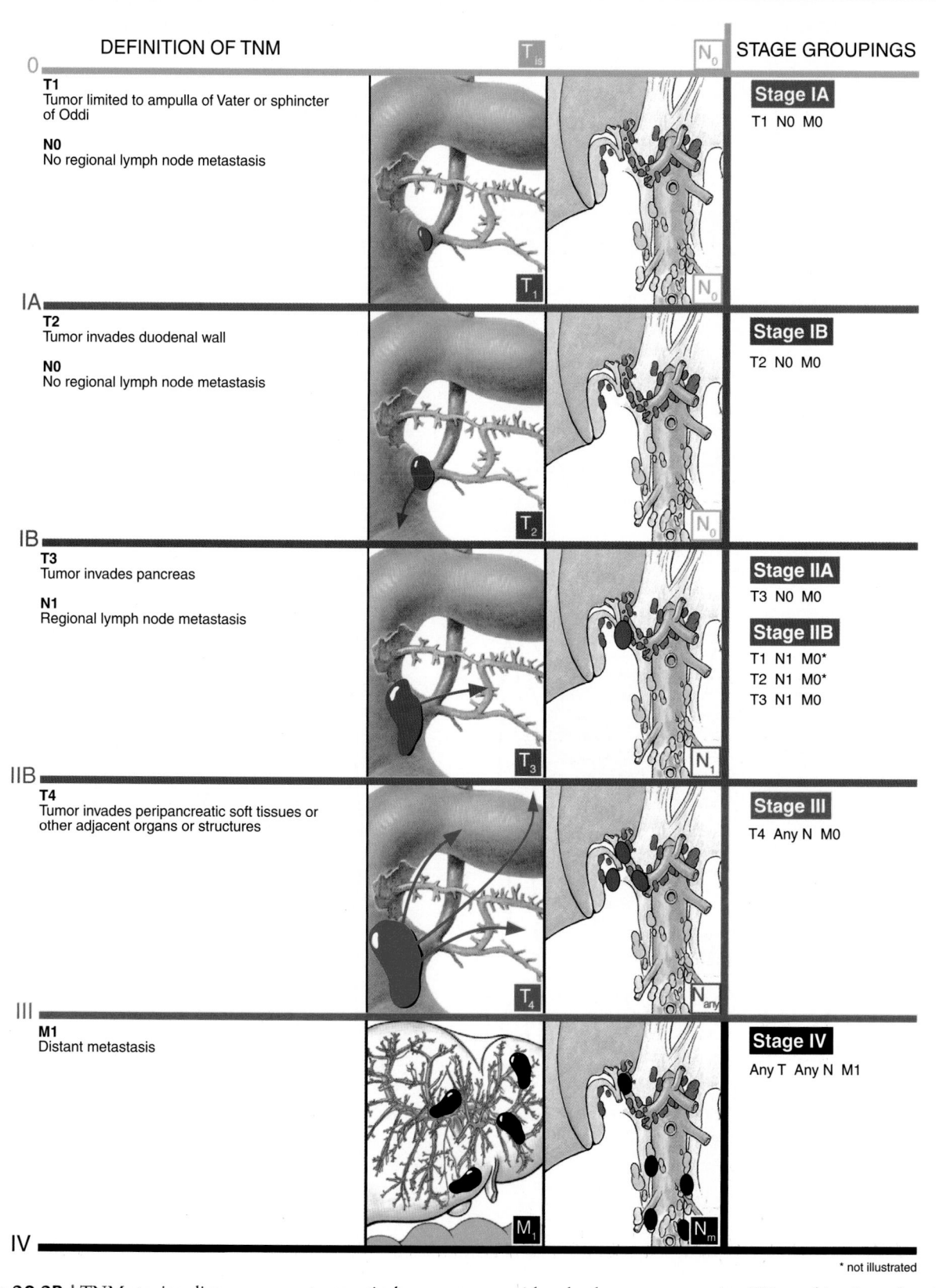

DEFINITION OF TNM

T1
Tumor limited to ampulla of Vater or sphincter of Oddi

N0
No regional lymph node metastasis

T2
Tumor invades duodenal wall

N0
No regional lymph node metastasis

T3
Tumor invades pancreas

N1
Regional lymph node metastasis

T4
Tumor invades peripancreatic soft tissues or other adjacent organs or structures

M1
Distant metastasis

STAGE GROUPINGS

Stage IA
T1 N0 M0

Stage IB
T2 N0 M0

Stage IIA
T3 N0 M0

Stage IIB
T1 N1 M0*
T2 N1 M0*
T3 N1 M0

Stage III
T4 Any N M0

Stage IV
Any T Any N M1

* not illustrated

Figure 28.3B | TNM staging diagram presents a vertical arrangement with color bars encompassing TN combinations showing progression. Ampulla of Vater cancers masquerade as pancreatic head cancers and are resectable as stage I and IIA, with stage IIB (purple) borderline resectable. Stage III (red) is often unresectable, and stage IV is metastatic (black). Stage 0, yellow; IA, green; IB, blue; IIB, purple; III, red; and IV (metastatic), black. Definitions of TN on left and stage grouping on right.

T-ONCOANATOMY

ORIENTATION OF THREE-PLANAR ONCOANATOMY

The anatomic isocenter for the three-planar oncoanatomy for the pancreas is at the L1/L2 level deep in the epigastrium (Fig. 28.4).

T-oncoanatomy

The T-oncoanatomy is displayed in three planar views. **A.** Coronal, **B.** Sagittal, **C.** Transverse axial (Fig. 28.5A).

Pancreas

- *Coronal*: The pancreas is a long, lobulated structure that lies transversely in the posterior abdomen, located retroperitoneally in the concavity of the duodenum on its right end and touching the spleen on its left end. The shape of the pancreas may be compared to the letter J placed sideways. It is divisible into a head with an uncinate process, a

neck, a body, and a tail (Fig. 28.6A). The acinous glands of the pancreas secrete into a branching ductal network, which forms the main horizontal pancreatic duct that runs the length of the pancreas and terminates in the second portion of the duodenum after it creates a common junction with the hepatic duct at the ampulla of Vater. There is often a small accessory pancreatic duct, which has a separate opening into the duodenum. The uncinate process of the head wraps around the SMA and is hugged by the duodenum (Fig. 28.5B).

- *Sagittal*: The midsagittal plane shows the intimate relationship of the head of the pancreas to the SMA inferiorly. Note the retroperitoneal location of the pancreas posterior to the lesser omental bursa. However, the transverse mesocolon arising from its anterior surface allows pancreatic cancers to spread intraperitoneally and seed the peritoneal surface, once invaded.

- *Transverse*: The pancreas lies in the midcoronal plane and is at the divide of the retroperitoneum from the peritoneal cavity. The pancreas stretches from right kidney hilum to splenic and left renal hilum.

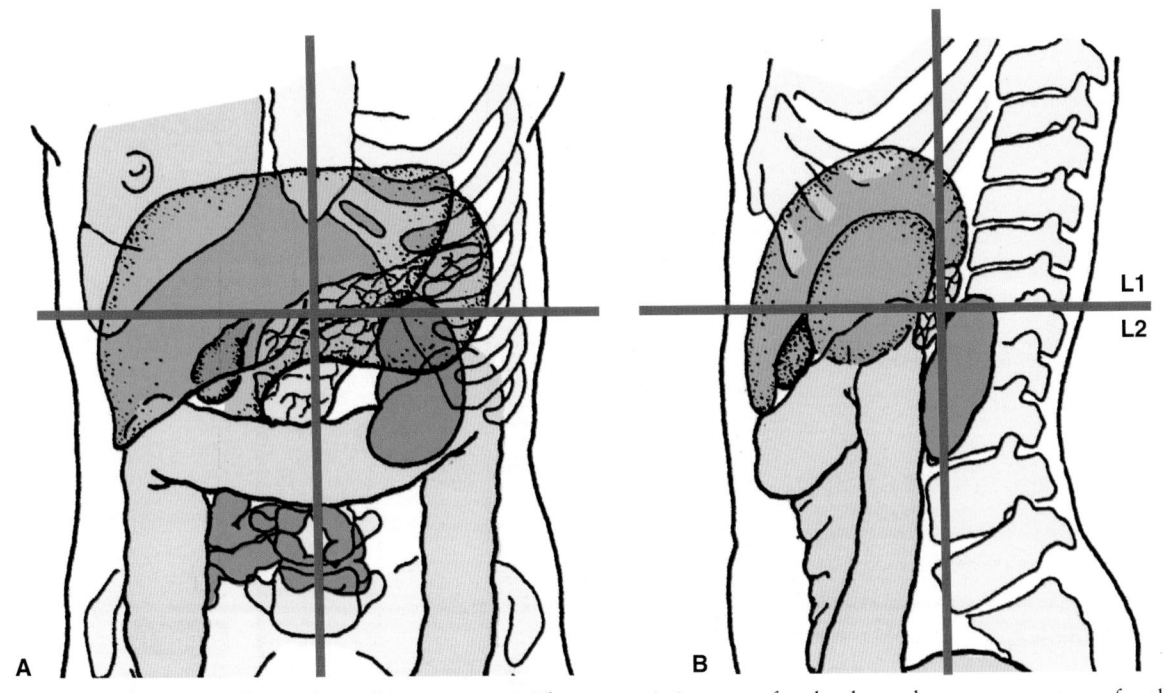

Figure 28.4 | Orientation and overview of oncoanatomy. The anatomic isocenter for the three-planar oncoanatomy for the pancreas and ampulla of Vater is at the L1/L2 level, deep in the epigastrium. **A.** Coronal. **B.** Sagittal. Same for ampulla of Vater.

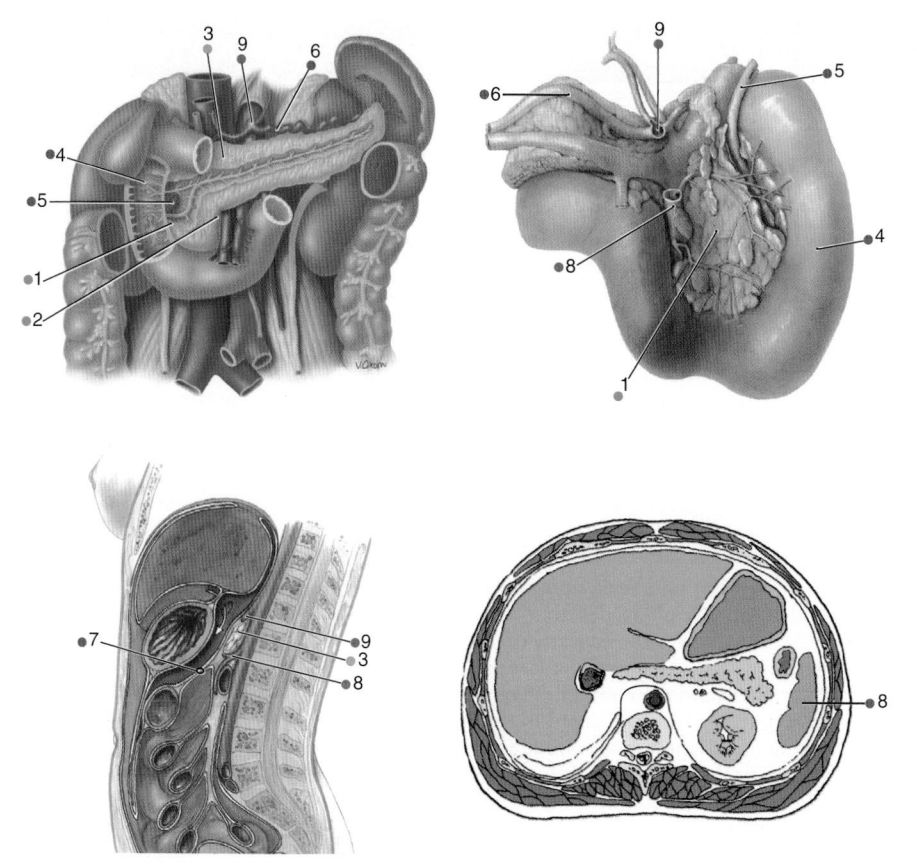

T$_1$ ● 1. Head		T$_3$ ● 5. Common bile duct		T$_4$ ● 8. Superior mesenteric artery
T$_1$ ● 2. Uncinate process		T$_3$ ● 6. Splenic artery		T$_4$ ● 9. Celiac trunk
T$_2$ ● 3. Pancreas body		T$_3$ ● 7. Transverse mesocolon		T$_4$ ● 10. Portal vein
T$_3$ ● 4. Second part of duodenum		T$_3$ ● 8. Spleen		

Figure 28.5A | Pancreas T-oncoanatomy. Connecting the dots. Structures are color coded for cancer stage progression. The color code for the anatomic sites correlates with the color code for the stage group (Fig. 28.3A) and patterns of spread (Fig. 28.2A) and SIMLAP table (Table 28.2). Connecting the dots in similar colors will provide an appreciation for the 3D oncoanatomy.

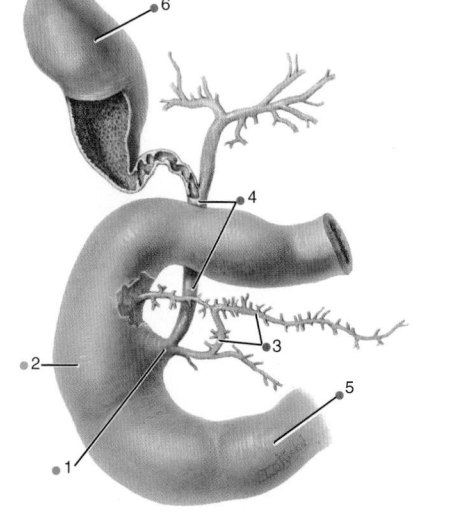

T$_1$ ● 1. Hepatopancreatic ampulla of Vater	T$_3$ ● 3. Main pancreatic duct		T$_4$ ● 4. Common bile duct
T$_2$ ● 2. Second part of duodenum			T$_4$ ● 5. Duodenum (4th part)
			T$_4$ ● 6. Gallbladder

Figure 28.5B | Ampulla of Vater T-oncoanatomy. Connecting the dots. Structures are color coded for cancer stage progression. The color code for the anatomic sites correlates with the color code for the stage group (Fig. 28.3B) and patterns of spread (Fig. 28.2B) and SIMLAP table (Table 28.2). Connecting the dots in similar colors will provide an appreciation for the 3D oncoanatomy.

N-ONCOANATOMY AND M-ONCOANATOMY

N-ONCOANATOMY

A rich lymphatic network surrounds the pancreas, with a left splenic and superior and inferior right-side truncal drainage. The first station nodes include the celiac, splenic, suprapancreatic, left gastropancreatic, and hepatic arteries, and inferior pancreatic, juxta-aortic, anterior pancreatic duodenal, and posterior pancreatic duodenal lymph nodes. Juxtaregional nodes include the inferior portion of the para-aortic nodal drainage and mediastinal and mesenteric nodes (Fig. 28.6A; Table 28.4).

Regional Lymph Nodes

A rich lymphatic network surrounds the pancreas, and accurate tumor staging requires that all lymph nodes that are removed be analyzed. Optimal histologic examination of a pancreaticoduodenectomy specimen should include analysis of a minimum of 12 lymph nodes. The standard regional lymph node basins and soft tissues resected for tumors located in the head and neck of the pancreas include lymph nodes along the common bile duct, common hepatic artery, portal vein, and posterior and anterior pancreaticoduodenal arcades and along the superior mesenteric vein and right lateral wall of the superior mesenteric artery. For cancers located in body and tail, regional lymph node basins include lymph nodes along the common hepatic artery, celiac axis, splenic artery, and splenic hilum. Anatomic division of regional lymph nodes is not necessary. However, separately submitted lymph nodes should be reported as labeled by the surgeon.*

*Preceding passage from Edge SB, Byrd DR, and Compton CC, et al., *AJCC Cancer Staging Manual*, 7th edition. New York. Springer, 2010, p. 242.

M-ONCOANATOMY

The rich venous anastomoses of pancreas and its juxtaposition to the liver make portal vein invasion and liver metastases the favored target organs. The entire portal circulation should be considered as a unit with regard to the venous anatomy of the gastrointestinal tract below the diaphragm (see Fig. 28.6B). The two major trunks are the inferior and superior mesenteric veins. The inferior mesenteric vein drains the left colon and sigmoid colon tributaries, which cover the vascular drainage to the left of the midline originating from the superior rectal veins. On the right side, the superior mesenteric vein originates from the tributaries draining the ileum, jejunum, and ileocolic and right middle colic veins. The inferior mesenteric vein usually joins the splenic vein, which coalesces with the superior mesenteric vein and forms the portal vein. The splenic vein, which is a major tributary of the portal system, also drains much of the stomach along its greater curvature and includes the short gastric veins and left and right gastroepiploic veins. The right gastroepiploic also flows into the superior mesenteric vein. The entire drainage of the lesser curvature of the stomach, including the left and right gastric veins, drains directly into the portal vein. Because the portal vein then drains directly into the liver, it is the target metastatic organ and the most commonly involved organ in the hematogenous spread pattern from the venous system of the gastrointestinal tract, as compared with other parts of the body, where the drainage is directly into the lung by way of the caval system.

The incidence of liver metastases exceeds that of other sites. According to a variety of reports in the literature, the range is 45% to 80% at autopsy. Other sites are mainly bone metastases (20% to 35%) and lung metastases (40% to 60%), with only occasional metastases to the brain.

The position of the pancreas often leads to direct invasion of the mesentery and omentum, with studding out of the peritoneal cavity with diffuse carcinomatosis and ascites.

Distant spread occurs mainly to liver and lungs, with a lesser degree of involvement of bones and brain, as well as to other anatomic sites.

TABLE 28.4	Lymph Nodes of Pancreas	
Sentinel Nodes Include Pancreatic Duodenal and Pancreatosplenic Nodes		
Regional Nodes	**Juxtaregional Nodes**	
Splenic hilum	Mediastinal	
Suprapancreatic	Mesenteric	
Left gastropancreatic fold	Iliac	
Hepatic artery		
Inferior pancreatic		
Juxta-aortic		
Anterior pancreatic–duodenal		
Posterior pancreatic–duodenal		
Celiac		

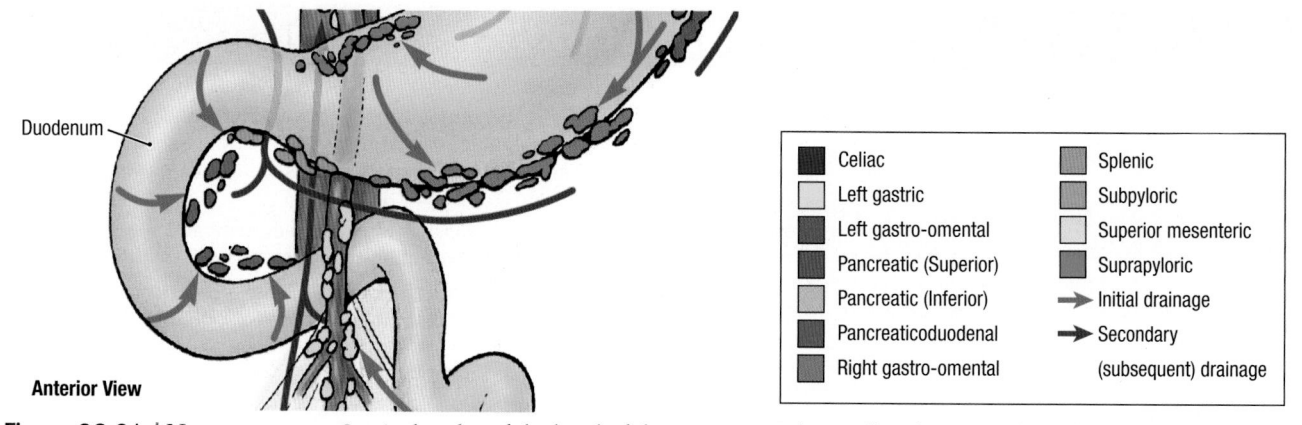

Figure 28.6A | N-oncoanatomy. Sentinel nodes of the head of the pancreas and ampulla of Vater include the pancreatic duodenal nodes, as shown in a circle on the right, and those of the body and tail of the pancreas, as shown on the left.

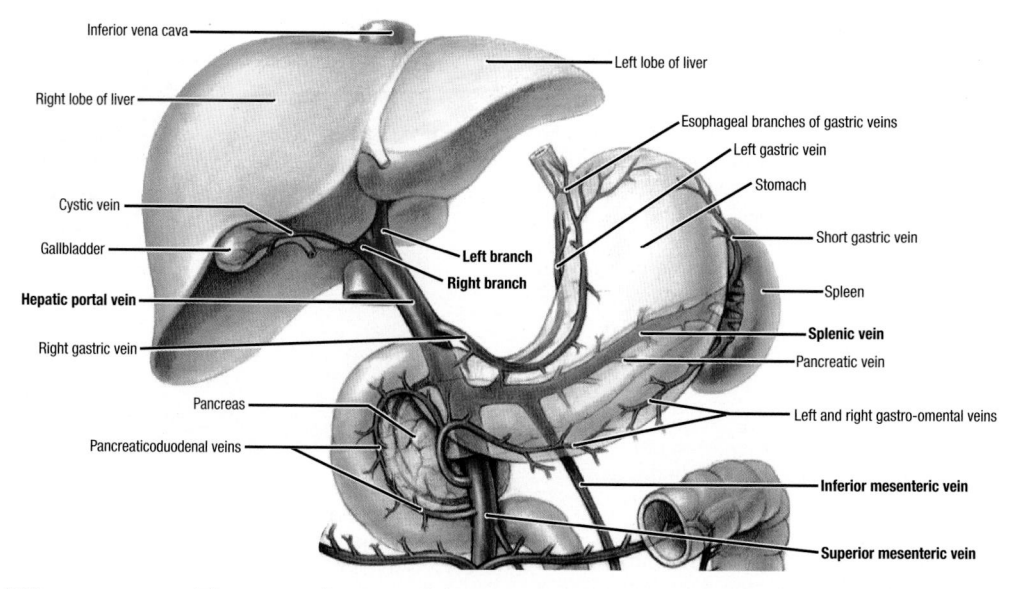

Figure 28.6B | M-oncoanatomy. The venous drainage of the pancreas is complex in view of its length. The head of the pancreas drains into pancreatic to adrenal veins and then into the left gastro-omental veins. The body and tail drain into the splenic vein along its superior border, and all of the venous drainage enters into the portal system ultimately, resulting in liver metastases.

STAGING WORKUP

RULES FOR CLASSIFICATION AND STAGING

Clinical Staging and Imaging

Clinical and pathologic classifications have been combined into a single staging system. It is important to distinguish resectable (T1, T2, and T3) from unresectable (T4). The critical feature is reliance on contrast-enhanced CT to assess whether the adjacent arterial structures—namely, the SMA or celiac axes—are involved. Portal vein involvement can also occur. Endoscopic ultrasound can be used for guiding needle biopsies. Laparoscopy is useful for detecting peritoneal seeding. ERCP is useful to place shunts when obstructions of bile ducts are present. Surgical pathologic staging requires definition of margins (Table 28.5; Fig. 28.7).

Pathologic Staging

Both partial and complete resections of pancreas and regional nodes, as well as of bile ducts and pancreatic ducts, need to be examined for margins and include the common bile duct, pancreatic neck, retroperitoneal margin, other soft tissue margins (such as posterior pancreatic), duodenum, and stomach. Special attention is required to the retroperitoneal margin adjacent to SMA. The uncinate process of head should be marked. The microscopic clearance of tumor should be recorded in millimeters. The completeness of resection depends on the clearing of the deepest point of invasion: R0, complete; R1, microscopic; and R2, macroscopic.

Oncoimaging Annotations

- When combined with needle biopsy, *EUS* is highly sensitive and specific. It yields the correct diagnosis with >95% accuracy.
- *Multiplanar CT* is highly effective in determining arterial and venous involvement and for staging. Unresectability is >76% accurate.
- *Magnetic resonance imaging with gadolinium* is excellent for defining extrapancreatic spread. Unresectability of >90% with gadolinium obviates the need for angiography.

- *ERCP* in combination with other imaging approaches is very valuable for distinguishing bile duct versus pancreatic cancer. Double duct strictures (bile duct/pancreatic duct) are associated with PCC.
- *CT-guided biopsy* is essential; sensitivity and specificity range from 57% to 96%; however, there are few to no false positives.
- *Laparoscopy* is advocated to ascertain peritoneal implants and seeding and obtain washings for cells and is essential to rule out M1.
- Staging is excellent with either *CT* or *magnetic resonance imaging*.
- Ultrasound initially reveals a dilated extrahepatic duct and intrahepatic duct system >90%.
- When direct cholangiograms are needed, a percutaneous transhepatic cholangiogram identifies the common bile duct cancer site and is preferred to ERCP.

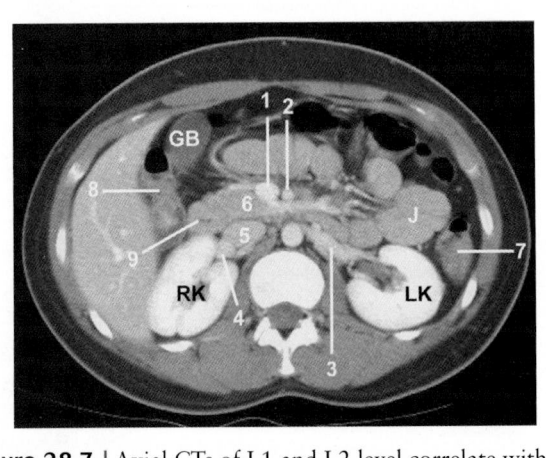

Figure 28.7 | Axial CTs of L1 and L2 level correlate with the T-oncoanatomy transverse section (Figure 28.5A). Oncoimaging with CT is commonly applied to staging cancers, often combined with PET to determine true extent of primary cancer and involved lymph nodes. 1. Superior mesenteric vein. 2. Superior mesenteric art. 3. Left renal vein. 4. Right renal vein. 5. Inferior vena cava. 6. Pancreas. 7. Descending colon. 8. Ascending colon. 9. Duodenum. GB, gallbladder; J, jejunum; LK, left kidney; RK, right kidney.

TABLE 28.5	Imaging Modalities for Evaluating Carcinoma of the Pancreas and Ampulla of Vater	
Method	**Diagnosis and Staging Capability**	**Recommended for Use**
Abdominal ultrasound	Helpful in defining primary tumor and evaluating dilated bile ducts and ascites; useful for evaluating suspected abdominal metastases, especially hepatic	Yes
CT	Most useful of all imaging modalities for determining local invasion and distant metastases	Yes
ERCP/PTC	Very accurate in defining deformity of bile and pancreatic duct and localizing site of obstruction	No
MRI	Useful in jaundiced patient; morphologic imaging of pancreas and peripancreatic duct for distant metastases	No

CT, computed tomography; ERCP/PTC, endoscopic retrograde cholangiopancreatography/percutaneous transhepatic cholangiography; MRI, magnetic resonance imaging.

PROGNOSIS AND CANCER SURVIVAL

PROGNOSIS

The limited number of prognostic factors are listed in Table 28.6. The prognostic factors for pancreas (Table 28.6A) differ from Ampulla of Vater (Table 28.6B).

CANCER STATISTICS AND SURVIVAL

The digestive system (gastrointestinal tract), which includes the MDG, accounts for 274,330 new patients annually, with colon and rectum responsible for >50%, with about 142,500 new diagnoses annually. Approximately half of these patients eventually die of these cancers. MDG cancers as a group are more lethal; only a handful of patients become long-term survivors. Fortunately, colon and rectal cancers are the most common, with the majority of patients becoming 5-year survivors (63%) responding to chemoradiation programs, often with the sparing of the rectal sphincter with conservative surgery. Anal cancers are the most responsive to chemoradiation (5-fluorouracil and cisplatin), eliminating the need for surgery. The 5-year survival rate is >90%, with anal sphincter preservation. This regimen has been proven to be very effective in clinical trials and to result in more long-term survivors, which is currently reflected in the literature. Liver, bile duct, and pancreatic cancers are among the poorest in terms of survival, which is often measured in months rather than years.

Specifically, the pancreas accounted for 43,140 new cancer cases and 36,800 cancer deaths (85%), with a survival (5-year) rate improvement over the last five decades of 3.4%. Currently, the 5 year survival for surgical resection vs.

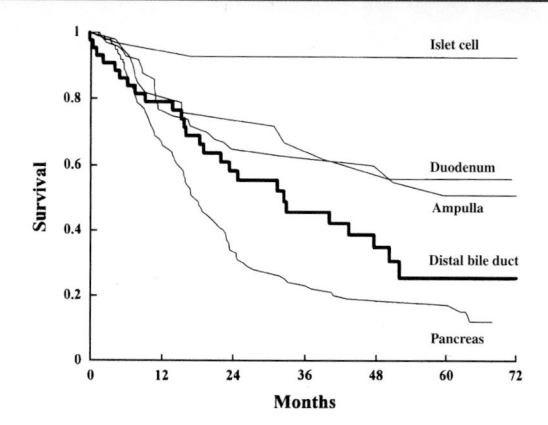

Figure 28.8 | Survival for patients with various peripancreatic tumors.

chemoradiation is: Stage IA, IB, 31-27% respectively vs. nonsurgical Stage IA/B patients is a dismal 3-4% (Fig. 28.9A/B). More hopeful survival outcomes improves for neuroendocrine tumors if found in Stage I is 75.6%, especially islet cell and for Ampulla of Vater (Fig. 28.8 and Fig. 28.9C).

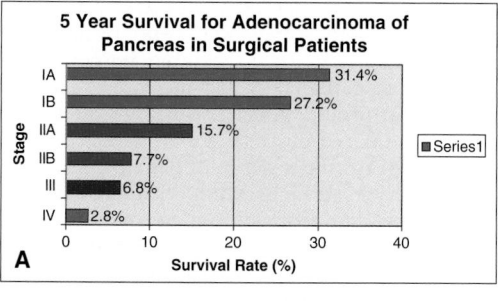

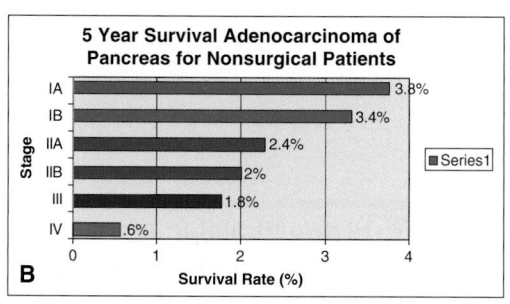

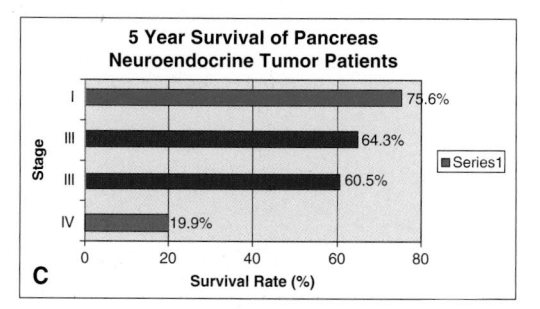

Figure 28.9 | **A.** Five-year survival for adenocarcinoma of the pancreas in surgical patients. **B.** Five-year survival for adenocarcinoma of pancreas in nonsurgical patients. **C.** Five-year survival of pancreatic neuroendocrine tumor patients. (Data from Edge SB, Byrd DR, Compton CC, et al. *AJCC Cancer Staging Manual*, 7th ed. New York: Springer, 2010, p. 244.)

TABLE 28.6A	Prognostic Factors for Pancreas
Required for staging	None
Clinically significant	Preoperative CA 19.9
	Preoperative carcinoembryonic antigen (CEA)
	Preoperative plasma chromogranin A level (CgA) (endocrine pancreas)
	Mitotic count (endocrine pancreas)

Reprinted with permission from Edge SB, Byrd DR, Compton CC, et al. *AJCC Cancer Staging Manual*, 7th ed. New York: Springer, 2010, p. 248.

TABLE 28.6B	Prognostic Factors for Ampulla of Vater
Required for staging	None
Clinically significant	Preoperative plasma chromogranin A level (CgA)
	Urinary 5-hydroxyindolacetic acid (5-HIAA) level
	Mitotic count

Reprinted with permission from Edge SB, Byrd DR, Compton CC, et al. *AJCC Cancer Staging Manual*, 7th ed. New York: Springer, 2010, p. 239.

Colon

PERSPECTIVE, PATTERNS OF SPREAD, AND PATHOLOGY

There are multiple steps in gene and mutational events: a series of deletions and mutations that result in carcinogenesis.

PERSPECTIVE AND PATTERN OF SPREAD

The colon, including the rectum, accounts for the majority of digestive system cancers. There has been intensive study of adenomas in relation to genetic defects that lead to their transformation from benign polyps to dysplasia and neoplasia. Portions of chromosomes 5, 17, and 18 are mutated or deleted. The gene deletion associated with the multistep process leading to malignancy and metastases has been documented by Fearon and Vogelstein. Large intestine has no villi, and the feathered mucosa is characterized by haustral markings. Except for the absence of Paneth cells, the cellular makeup of the crypts of Lieberkühn is similar. The number of goblet cells increases from cecum to sigmoid colon. The major colon function is to absorb water and electrolytes; it also compacts feces. The array of histopathology is largely similar to intestinal tumors, but the staging system applies only to carcinomas, not lymphomas, sarcomas, or carcinoids (Table 29.1).

The Ras oncogene, the deleted in colorectal cancer (DCC) gene, the p53 tumor suppressor gene, and DNA mismatch repair leads to carcinogenesis.

This paradigm of adenoma to adenocarcinoma has been modified and applied to other gastrointestinal sites—stomach and small intestine—in addition to colon and rectum.

Genetic conditions that increase the risk of developing colon cancer include the following:

- Genetic conditions that increase the risk of developing a large bowel cancer include familial adenomatous polyposis syndrome (FAP) and its variants and hereditary nonpolyposis colorectal cancer. FAP is a hereditary disease with an autosomal dominant transmission pattern characterized by pancolonic adenomatous polyps. It is not treated by surgical removal of the large bowel, and most patients die of colorectal cancer before age 60 years.

- The incidence and distribution of colon cancers are as follows: cecum, ascending colon (25%), transverse (15%), descending (5%), sigmoid (25%), rectosigmoid (10%), and rectum (20%). Incidence of inflammatory conditions, such as ulcerative colitis, with a disease duration of 7 years, increases 10% per decade, reaching approximately 30% at 25 years.

TABLE 29.1	Histopathologic Type: Common Cancers of the Colon
Type	
Adenocarcinoma in situ	Squamous cell (epidermoid) carcinoma
Adenocarcinoma	Adenosquamous carcinoma
Medullary carcinoma	Small cell carcinoma
Mucinous carcinoma (colloid type; >50% mucinous carcinoma)	Undifferentiated carcinoma
Signet ring cell carcinoma (>50% signet ring cell)	Carcinoma, NOS

NOS, not otherwise specified.
Reprinted with permission from Edge SB, Byrd DR, Compton CC, et al. *AJCC Cancer Staging Manual*, 7th ed. New York: Springer, 2010, p. 156.

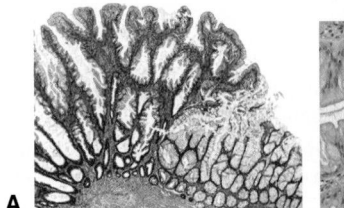
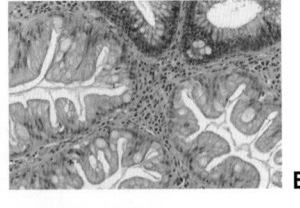
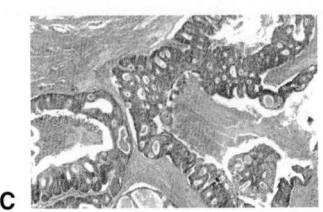

Figure 29.1 | Variants of hyperplastic polyps. A. Microscopically, sessile serrated adenoma features irregular, asymmetric crypts that are often dilated by mucin. **B.** Mixed hyperplastic adenomatous polyp. Two adenomatous crypts in the upper right contrast with the three hyperplastic crypts. **Adenocarcinoma of the colon. C.** Microscopically, this colon adenocarcinoma consists of moderately differentiated glands with a prominent cribriform pattern and frequent central necrosis.

- Gardner syndrome includes desmoid tumors, osteomas, and fibromas in addition to colorectal adenomas. The risk for developing adenocarcinoma is similar to that of patients with FAP.
- Peutz–Jeghers syndrome and juvenile polyposis are also associated with an increased risk of developing large bowel or other gastrointestinal cancers.

Inherited familial cancer syndromes also have been described in which affected members have fewer polyps than are seen with FAP. The genetic condition is inherited in an autosomal dominant pattern and includes Lynch syndromes I and II. Patients are typically young, have multiple large bowel lesions, and have a higher incidence of other intra-abdominal malignancies.

The Patterns of Spread are similar in different parts of the colon with invasion of a multilayered wall or retro colon area of posterior abdominal wall. The major difference is dependent on the anatomic segment of the colon when the wall is penetrated and cancer invades adjacent to viscera (Figure 29.2; Table 29.2).

PATHOLOGY

The array of histopathology is largely similar to intestinal tumors, but the staging system applies only to carcinomas, not lymphomas, sarcomas, or carcinoids (Table 29.1; Figure 29.1). The vast majority of colon tumors are adenocarcinomas (>90%), and neuroendocrine neoplasms occur and are staged separately. It is recommended that low-grade (G1, G2, well to moderately differentiated) and high-grade (G3, G4, poorly to undifferentiated) designations be used.

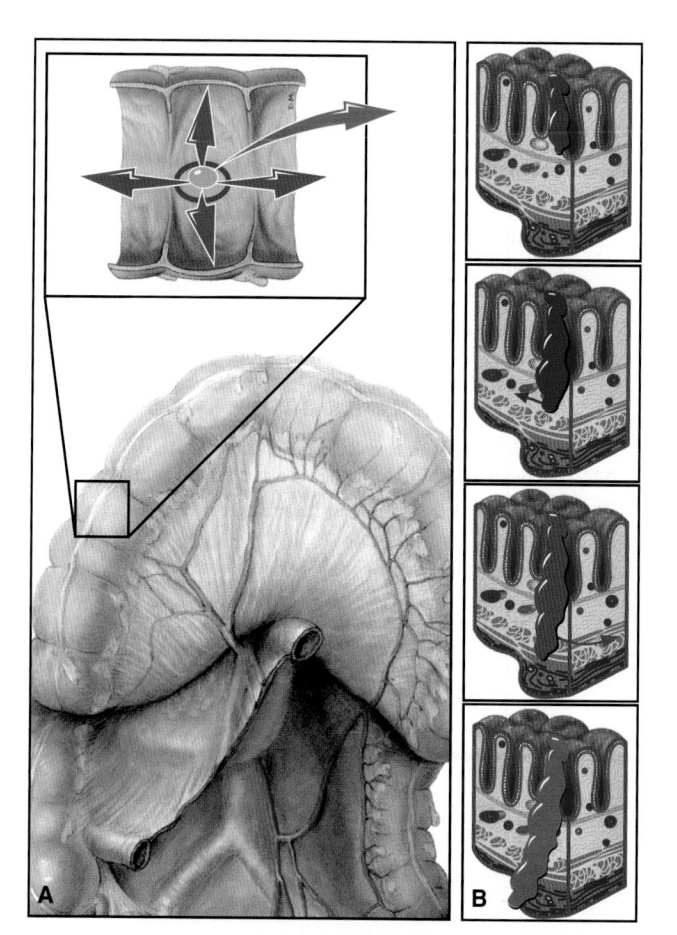

Figure 29.2 | A. Colon cancer patterns of spread. B. T categories. The patterns of spread and the primary tumor classification are similarly color coded: Tis (cancer in situ of mucosa), yellow; (infiltrates the submucosa), green; T2 (penetrates the muscularis externa), blue; T3 (reaches the subserosa), purple; and T4 (invades through the serosa into a neighboring viscera), red. The six patterns of spread–superior, inferior, medial, lateral, anterior, and posterior—are presented in SIMLAP Table 29.2 under ascending, transverse, and descending colon, respectively. The concept of visualizing patterns of spread to appreciate the surrounding anatomy is well demonstrated by the six-directional pattern, i.e., SIMLAP Table 29.2.

TABLE 29.2	SIMLAP	
Colon (Ascending)		
S	Right hepatic flexure	• T3
	Liver right lobe	• T4
I	Cecum, appendix	• T3
	Ileocecal valve	• T3
M	Supermesenteric artery, vein	• T4
	Pericolic lymph nodes	**N1**
L	Paracolic gutter	• T2
A	Small intestine	• T4
P	Retroperitoneum and abdominal wall	• T3
Colon (Transverse)		
S	Transversal mesocolon	• T3
I	Greater omentum	• T3
	Small intestine	• T4
M	Colon	• T2
L	Colon right, left (hepatic/splenic flexure)	• T2
A	Greater omentum	• T3
P	Retroperitoneum, abdominal wall	• T3
Colon (Descending)		
S	Splenic flexure	• T3
I	Sigmoid colon	• T3
M	Inferior mesenteric artery/vein	• T4
	Pericolic nodes	• T4
L	Paracolic gutter	• T3
A	Small intestine	• T4
P	Retroperitoneum, abdominal wall	• T3

The six vectors of invasion are Superior, Inferior, Medial, Lateral, Anterior, and Posterior. The color-coded dots correlate the T stage with specific anatomic structure involved.

T-ONCOANATOMY

ORIENTATION OF THREE-PLANAR ONCOANATOMY

The three-planar anatomic isocenter for the colon occupies the L2/L3 level in the abdomen (Fig. 29.4).

T-oncoanatomy

The T-oncoanatomy is displayed in three planar views. **A.** Coronal, **B.** Sagittal, **C.** Transverse axial (Figure 29.5).

- *Coronal*: The colon is a large structure that frames the entire abdominal visceral contents. It begins at the cecum and continues as the right ascending, transverse, left descending, and sigmoid segments of the colon. The colon is partially covered by a peritoneal surface. Tumors arise on the mucosal surface and penetrate into the muscularis and the serosa; therefore, their manifestations relate to their location. Depending on where the cancer arises, it can invade surrounding structures such as the liver at the

hepatic flexure, which is at the junction of the ascending and the transverse colon. The stomach and spleen are at risk when the cancer arises at the splenic flexure or the junction of the transverse and the descending colon. The large intestine, or colon, extends from the terminal ileum to the anal canal. It may be subdivided into sections, exclusive of the rectum: right, middle, and left, or ascending, transverse, descending, and sigmoid portions, respectively. The large intestine may also be divided into the intraperitoneal colon and the rectum.

- *Sagittal*: The peritoneal cavity consists of the greater sac and omental bursa. The superior recess of the omental bursa is between the liver and the posterior attachment of the diaphragm. The inferior recess of the omental bursa is between the two double layers of the greater omentum. In the adult, the inferior recess usually only extends inferiorly as far as the transverse colon because of fusion of the two double peritoneal layers at birth.

- *Transverse*: The transverse colon is located anteriorly, with the ascending colon on the right and the descending colon on the left. Note that this is at the lower pole of the kidney.

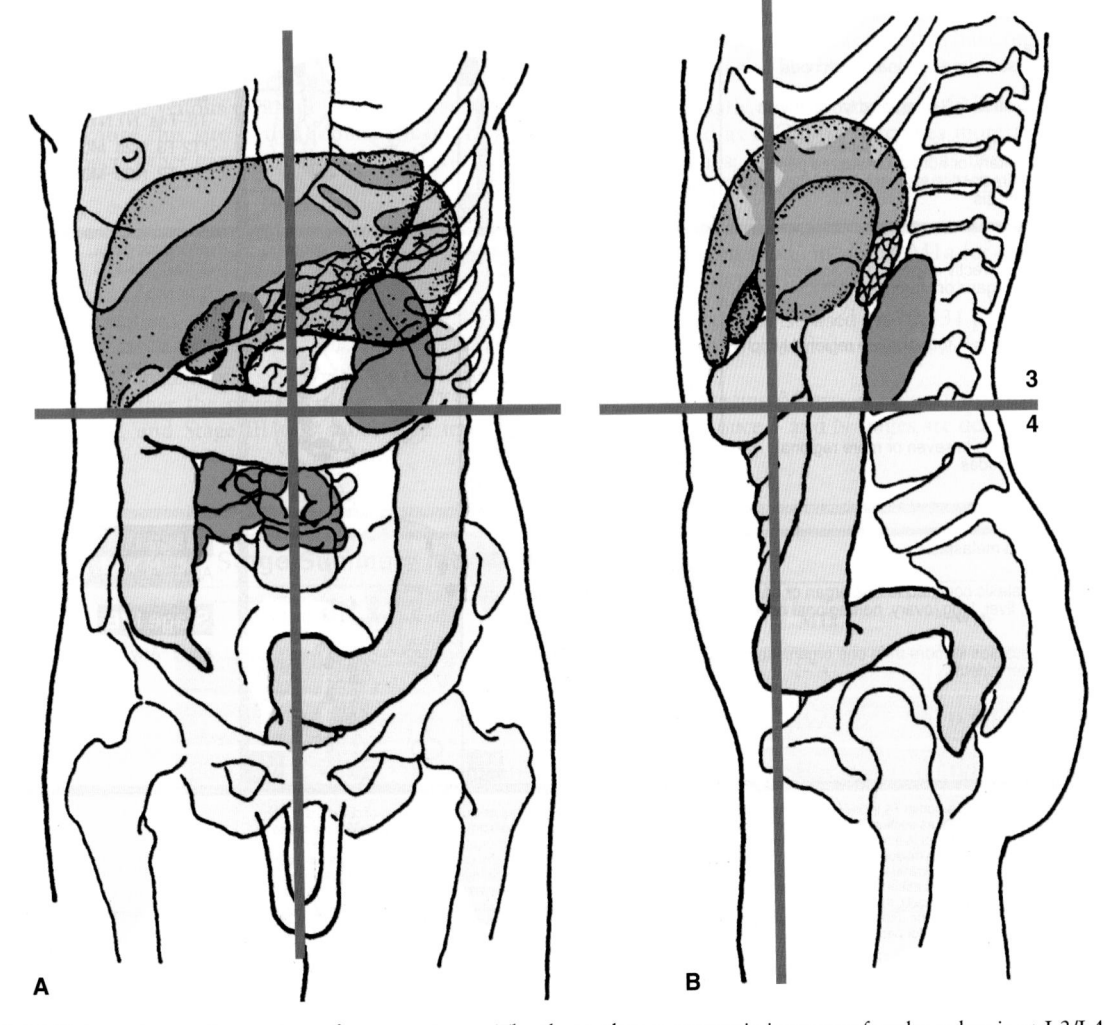

A   B

Figure 29.4 | Orientation and overview of oncoanatomy. The three-planar anatomic isocenter for the colon is at L3/L4. **A.** Coronal. **B.** Sagittal.

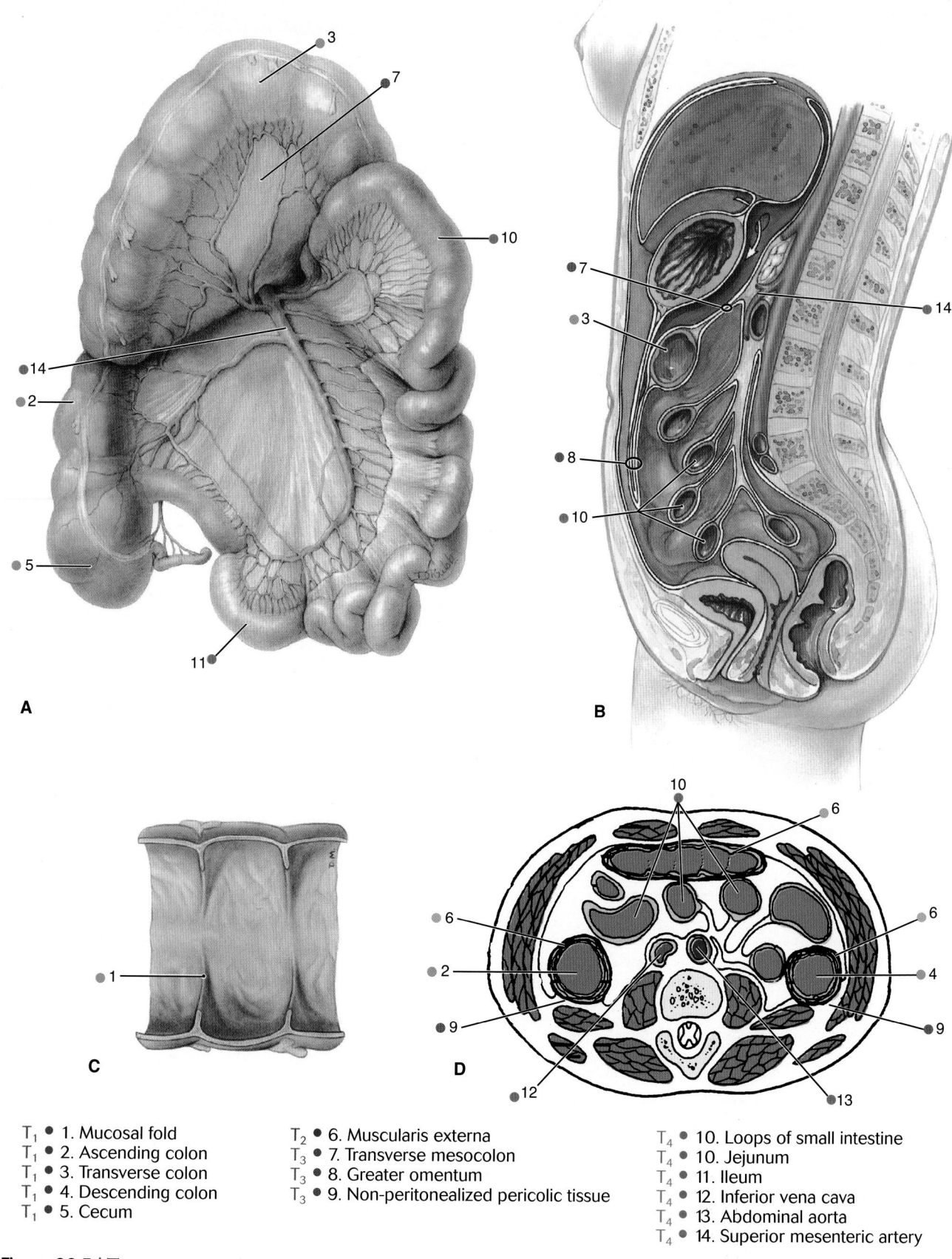

Figure 29.5 | T-oncoanatomy. Connecting the dots. Structures are color coded for cancer stage progression.

T_1 ● 1. Mucosal fold
T_1 ● 2. Ascending colon
T_1 ● 3. Transverse colon
T_1 ● 4. Descending colon
T_1 ● 5. Cecum

T_2 ● 6. Muscularis externa
T_3 ● 7. Transverse mesocolon
T_3 ● 8. Greater omentum
T_3 ● 9. Non-peritonealized pericolic tissue

T_4 ● 10. Loops of small intestine
T_4 ● 10. Jejunum
T_4 ● 11. Ileum
T_4 ● 12. Inferior vena cava
T_4 ● 13. Abdominal aorta
T_4 ● 14. Superior mesenteric artery

N-ONCOANATOMY AND M-ONCOANATOMY

N-ONCOANATOMY

Regional nodes follow the vascular arcades for each colon segment along its marginal arteries on the mesocolic border. Specifically, the regional lymph nodes for each segment are shown and listed. The recent major revisions in staging relate to nodules in the pericolic fat: If such nodules are smooth, they are considered to be nodes; if irregular, they are considered to be vascular or venous invasion (Fig. 29.6A; Table 29.4).

Regional Lymph Nodes

Regional lymph nodes are located (i) along the course of the major vessels supplying the colon and rectum, (ii) along the vascular arcades of the marginal artery, and (iii) adjacent to the colon—that is, located along the mesocolic border of the colon. Specifically, the regional lymph nodes are the pericolic and perirectal nodes and those found along the ileocolic, right colic, middle colic, left colic, inferior mesenteric, superior rectal (hemorrhoidal), and internal iliac arteries.

In the assessment of pN, the number of lymph nodes sampled should be recorded. The number of nodes examined from an operative specimen has been reported to be associated with improved survival, possibly because of increased accuracy in staging. It is important to obtain at least 10 to 14 lymph nodes in radical colon and rectum resections in patients without neoadjuvant therapy, but in cases in which tumor is resected for palliation of patients who have received preoperative radiation, fewer lymph nodes may be removed or present. In all cases, however, it is essential that the total number of regional lymph nodes recovered from the resection specimen be described since that number is prognostically important. A pN0 determination is assigned when these nodes are histologically negative, even though fewer than the recommended number of nodes has been analyzed. However, when fewer than the number of nodes recommended by the College of American Pathologists have been found, it is important that pathologists report the degree of diligence of their effort to find the lymph nodes in the specimen.*

M-ONCOANATOMY

The entire portal circulation should be considered as a unit with regard to the venous anatomy of the gastrointestinal tract below the diaphragm (see Fig. 29.6B). The two major trunks are the inferior mesenteric and superior mesenteric veins. The inferior mesenteric vein drains the left colon and sigmoid colon tributaries, which covers the vascular drainage to the left of the midline originating from the superior rectal veins. On the right side, the superior mesenteric vein originates from the tributaries draining the ileum, jejunum, and ileocolic right and middle colic veins. The inferior mesenteric vein usually joins the splenic vein, which coalesces with the superior mesenteric vein and forms the portal vein. The splenic vein, which is a major tributary of the portal system, also drains much of the stomach along its greater curvature and includes the short gastric veins and left and right gastric epiploic veins. The right gastroepiploic vein also flows into the superior mesenteric vein. The entire drainage of the lesser curvature of the stomach, including the left and right gastric veins, drains directly into the portal vein. Because the portal vein then drains directly into the liver, it is the target metastatic organ and the most commonly involved organ in hematogenous spread from the venous system of the gastrointestinal tract, as compared with other parts of the body, where the drainage is directly into the lung by way of the caval system.

The incidence of liver metastases exceeds that of other sites. According to a variety of reports in the literature, the range is 40% to 100% at autopsy. Other sites are mainly bone metastases 20% to 35% and lung metastases 40% to 60%, with only occasional metastases to brain.

*Preceding passage from Edge SB, Byrd DR, and Compton CC, et al., *AJCC Cancer Staging Manual, 7th edition.* New York, Springer, 2010, pp. 145–146.

TABLE 29.4	Sentinel and Regional Lymph Nodes
Segment	**Regional Lymph Nodes**
Cecum	Pericolic, anterior cecal, posterior cecal, ileocolic, right colic
Ascending colon	Pericolic, ileocolic, right colic, middle colic
Hepatic flexure	Pericolic, middle colic, right colic
Transverse colon	Pericolic, middle colic
Splenic flexure	Pericolic, middle colic, left colic, inferior mesenteric
Descending colon	Pericolic, left colic, inferior mesenteric, sigmoid
Sigmoid colon	Pericolic, inferior mesenteric, superior rectal (hemorrhoidal), sigmoidal, sigmoid mesenteric
Rectosigmoid	Pericolic, perirectal, left colic, sigmoid mesenteric, sigmoidal, inferior mesenteric, superior rectal (hemorrhoidal), middle rectal (hemorrhoidal)
Rectum	Perirectal, sigmoid mesenteric, inferior mesenteric, lateral sacral presacral, internal iliac, sacral promontory, internal iliac, superior rectal (hemorrhoidal), middle rectal (hemorrhoidal), inferior rectal (hemorrhoidal)

Reprinted with permission from Edge SB, Byrd DR, Compton CC, et al. *AJCC Cancer Staging Manual,* 7th ed. New York: Springer, 2010, p.145–146.

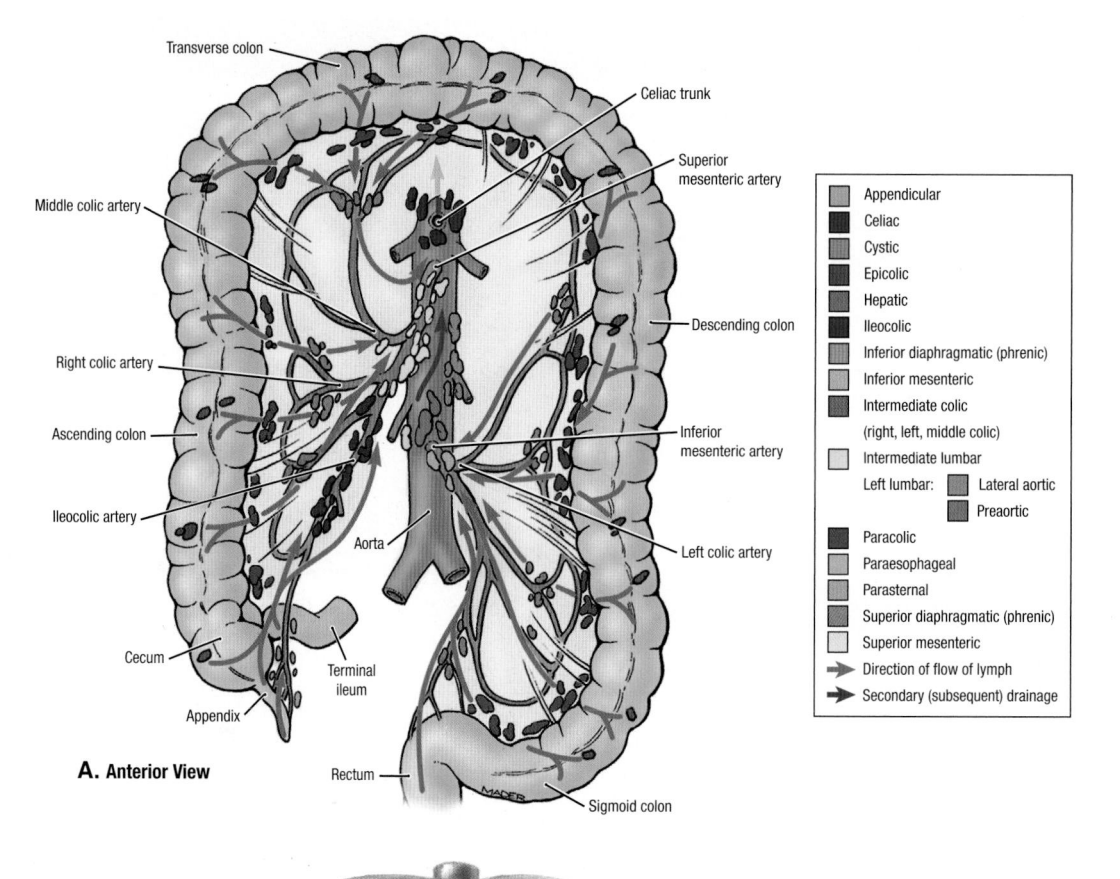

Appendicular
Celiac
Cystic
Epicolic
Hepatic
Ileocolic
Inferior diaphragmatic (phrenic)
Inferior mesenteric
Intermediate colic
(right, left, middle colic)
Intermediate lumbar
Left lumbar: Lateral aortic
               Preaortic
Paracolic
Paraesophageal
Parasternal
Superior diaphragmatic (phrenic)
Superior mesenteric
→ Direction of flow of lymph
→ Secondary (subsequent) drainage

A. Anterior View

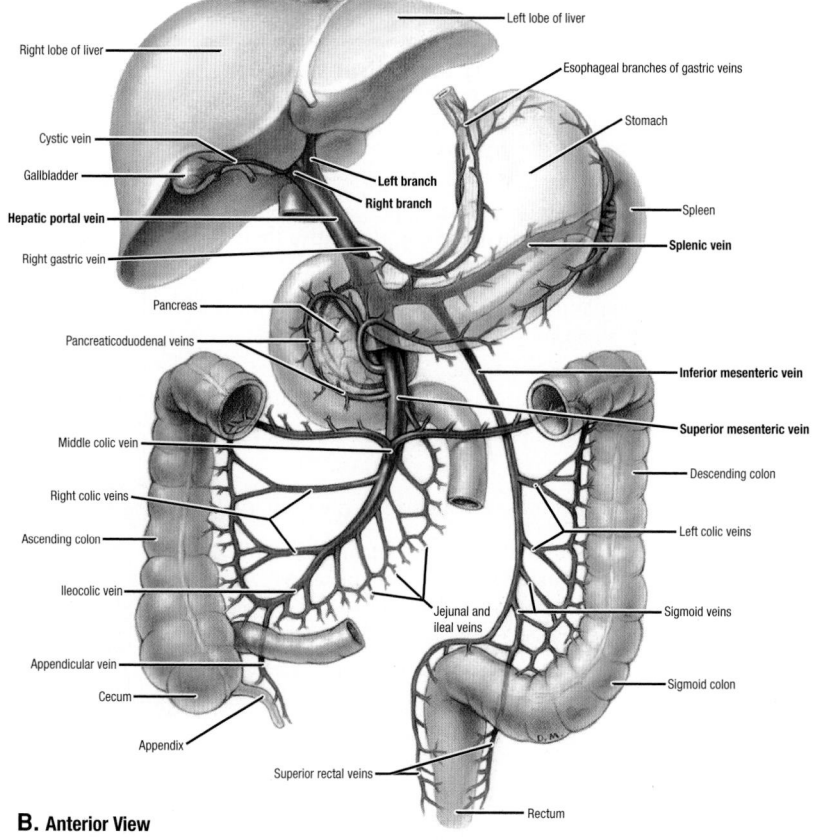

B. Anterior View

Figure 29.6 | A. N-oncoanatomy. Sentinel nodes of the colon include the pericolic nodes of the superior mesenteric (blue) and inferior mesenteric (red) nodes. Depending upon the T site colon segment of origin, the pericolic nodes adjacent are the sentinel nodes (Table 29.4). Para-aortic nodes are gray. **B. M-oncoanatomy.** The venous drainage of the colon is complex because of its length, which frames the small intestine. The right side of the colon, right hepatic flexure, and the transverse colon drain into the superior mesenteric vein, whereas the left side of the colon and splenic flexure drain into the inferior mesenteric vein and into the splenic vein, and eventually the drainage is into the portal vein, resulting predominantly in liver metastases.

STAGING WORKUP

RULES OF CLASSIFICATION AND STAGING

Clinical Staging and Imaging

Extension of diagnostic imaging to staging is gaining in popularity. Virtual colonoscopy and sigmoidoscopy are challenging endoscopic colonoscopy as to accuracy in diagnosing adenocarcinomas. Endoscopic ultrasound shows the layers of the colon and rectal wall and their penetration by cancer. Endorectal magnetic resonance imaging (MRI) is most valuable to demonstrate extracolonic and extrarectal invasion into adjacent structures. Computed tomography (CT) is preferred for detecting liver and lung metastases (Table 29.5; Fig. 29.7).

Pathologic Staging

The surgically resected colon and associated lymph nodes are assessed. Tumor extension and location of both primary and nodes should be documented. Accurate radial margins should be marked and recorded and are defined "as the surgically dissected surface adjacent to the deepest point of tumor invasion beyond the wall of the large bowel." The completeness of resection depends on the clearing of the deepest point of invasion: R0, complete; R1, microscopic; and R2, macroscopic.

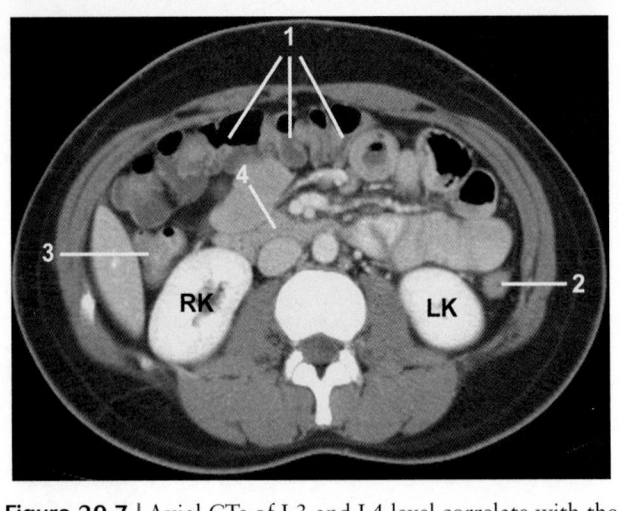

Figure 29.7 | Axial CTs of L3 and L4 level correlate with the T-oncoanatomy transverse section (Figure 29.5D). Oncoimaging with CT is commonly applied to staging cancers, often combined with PET to determine true extent of primary cancer and involved lymph nodes. 1. Transverse colon. 2. Descending colon. 3. Ascending colon. 4. Duodenum. LK, left kidney; RK, right kidney.

TABLE 29.5	Imaging Modalities for Staging for Colon Cancer	
Method	Diagnosis and Staging Capability	Recommended for Use
Primary Tumor ± Regional Nodes		
BE	Very useful in detecting and defining primary lesions in the colon; single-contrast study may be less sensitive than double-contrast in detecting polyps	Yes for diagnosis
Endoscopy	Very accurate modality for detecting and defining primary lesions; flexible sigmoidoscopy and/or colonoscopy	Yes, if used to confirm lesion detected on BE or to screen high-risk patients
Endorectal ultrasound or coil	In rectum, sigmoid (flex sigmoidoscopy), or remaining colon (colonoscopy); assess primary depth and nodes for fine needle biopsy	Yes, if preoperative chemoradiation is considered; yes, depth of wall invasion
MRI	Useful in defining depth of penetration of the primary lesion	Yes
CT	Most valuable of all modalities for determining extrarectal or extracolonic local invasion and nodal metastases	Yes
PET	Not useful for staging primary cancer; useful for suspected metastasis.	No
Metastases		
Chest film ± CT	Chest film, best for metastasis screening; CT chest, rules out multiple metastases; useful for detecting metastatic nodes, peritoneal implants, and liver metastases	Yes
CT abdomen	Most useful study to define para-aortic node enlargement or liver metastases	Yes
Liver ultrasound	Can differentiate between cystic and solid lesions	Yes

BE, barium enema; CT, computed tomography; MRI, magnetic resonance imaging; PET, positron emission tomography.

PROGNOSIS AND CANCER SURVIVAL

Oncoimaging Annotations

- Although colonoscopy is more accurate in assessment for small polyps, overall cost effectiveness is greater when double-contrast barium enema examinations are used.

- CT colonography is a recent addition to the modalities used to screen for colorectal cancer and polyps. This modality requires further refinement and testing before being more widely adopted.

- Transrectal ultrasonography and MRI can demonstrate the extent of tumor through the rectal wall and provide some assessment for lymphadenopathy.

- If there is clinical suspicion of metastasis or elevated carcinoembryonic antigen level, CT and MR scanning are useful for determining the presence and site of recurrent disease. Overall accuracy for the detection of recurrent disease with these modalities is 90% to 95%. This evaluation may require fine-needle aspiration biopsy under direct CT guidance.

- Other noninvasive means to determine the presence or absence of recurrent or metastatic tumor are nuclear medicine scanning techniques with radiolabeled monoclonal antibodies and positron emission tomography techniques using fluorodeoxyglucose. Some of these have shown great potential.

PROGNOSIS

A significant number of prognostic factors are listed in Table 29.6.

CANCER STATISTICS AND SURVIVAL

The digestive system, or gastrointestinal tract, which includes the MDG, accounts for 274,337 new patients annually, with colon and rectum responsible for >50%, or about 142,500 new diagnoses annually. Approximately half of these patients eventually die of these cancers. MDG cancers as a group are more lethal; only a handful of patients become long-term survivors. Fortunately, colon and rectal cancers are the most common, with the majority of patients becoming 5-year survivors

(63%) responding to chemoradiation programs, often with the sparing of the rectal sphincter with conservative surgery. Anal cancers are the most responsive to chemoradiation (5-fluorouracil and cisplatin), eliminating the need for surgery. The 5-year survival rate is >90%, with anal sphincter preservation. This regimen has been proven to be very effective in clinical trials and to result in more long-term survivors, which is currently reflected in the literature. Liver, bile duct, and pancreatic cancers are among the poorest in terms of survival, which is often measured in months rather than years (see Table 22.6).

Specifically, the colon accounted for 102,900 new cancer cases and 51,370 cancer deaths (50%), with a 5-year survival rate improvement over the last five decades of 22%. Currently, relative 5-year survival for all stages is 62.3%, but, when localized, it improves to 90.1% (see Table 23.8). Colon cancer (T3T4), when resected plus multinodal therapy, decreases from 70% to 80% for N0 to 50% ± 3% for N1, N2 nodal involvement (Figs. 29.8 and 29.9).

TABLE 29.6	Prognostic Factors
Required for staging	None
Clinically significant	Preoperative or pretreatment carcinoembryonic antigen (CEA) (ng/mL)
	Tumor deposits (TDs)
	Circumferential resection margin (CRM)
	Perineural invasion (PN)
	Microsatellite instability (MSI)
	Tumor regression grade (with neoadjuvant therapy)
	K-ras gene analysis

Reprinted with permission from Edge SB, Byrd DR, Compton CC, et al. *AJCC Cancer Staging Manual*, 7th ed. New York: Springer, 2010, p. 155–156.

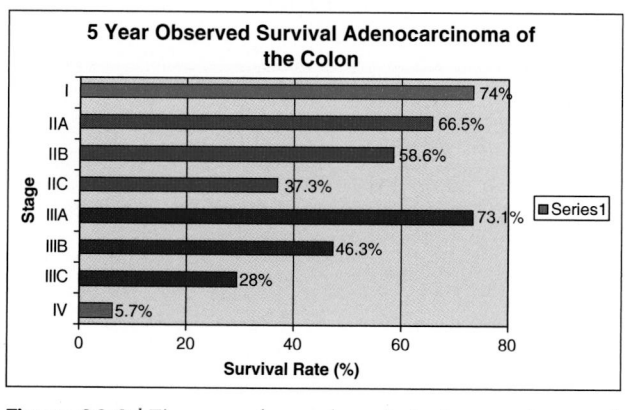

Figure 29.8 | Five-year observed survival adenocarcinoma of the colon. (Data from Edge SB, Byrd DR, Compton CC, et al., *AJCC Cancer Staging Manual, 7th edition.* New York, Springer, 2010.)

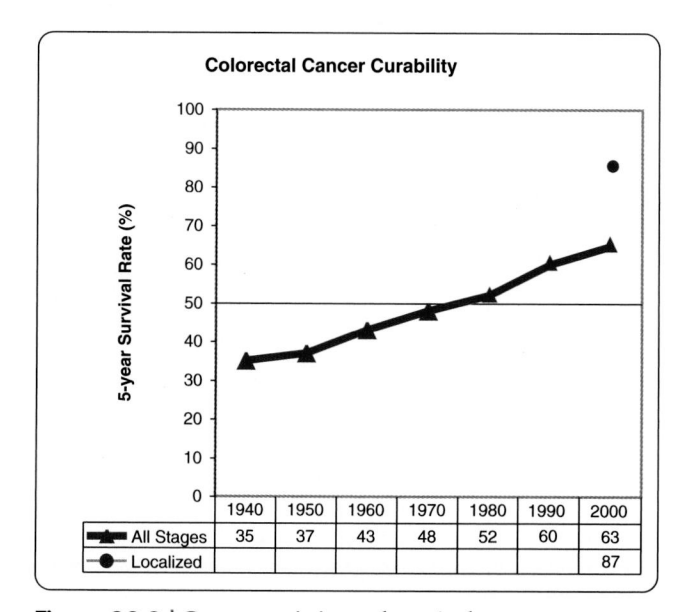

Figure 29.9 | Cancer statistics and survival rates.

Small Intestine

PERSPECTIVE, PATTERNS OF SPREAD, AND PATHOLOGY

Adenocarcinomas are more common in the duodenum, lymphomas in the jejunum, and sarcomas and carcinoids in the ileum, with the most favored site being the vermiform appendix.

beginning with hyperplasia, then dysplasia, and finally neoplasia. **The patterns of cancer spread** follow the mucosal and muscle layers of the bowel wall (Fig. 30.2; Table 30.2).

PERSPECTIVE AND PATTERN OF SPREAD

Consider the contradictory paucity of neoplasms in the small intestine in view of the extreme length of the small bowel, which exceeds in its length all other regions of the digestive system combined. It has a rich variety of metabolically active cells, with high and rapid turnover rates of regenerative cells. Its stem cells are estimated to have cell turnover times of 24 hours and travel times of 5 to 7 days from the crypt of Lieberkühn to the tip of the villus. The absence of malignancy is attributed to the rapid transport of carcinogens in luminal contents, abundant surface immunoglobulin A expression, and active enzymes. The annual rate of new cases is 6,960, with high survival rate. The surface columnar epithelial cells have brush borders for absorption of fluids and chyme, with numerous lymphoid cells, neuroendocrine cells, goblet cells, and Paneth cells with loose connective tissue filling the microvilli with its lacteal. What the small intestine lacks in number of cancers, it makes up for by their variety. Table 30.1 lists them; one notes a predilection for specific tumors in different bowel segments: Adenocarcinomas are more common in the duodenum, lymphomas in the jejunum, and sarcomas and carcinoids in the ileum, with the most favored site being the vermiform appendix (T1 histopathology versus distribution). Predisposing factors include celiac disease, Crohn disease, familial adenomatosis polyposis, Gardner syndrome, and Peutz–Jaeger syndrome, all

PATHOLOGY

Although small bowel mucosa is the most extensive cellular surface, it accounts for 1.1% to 2.4% of gastrointestinal malignancies; there are approximately 2500 cases annually, and less than half of the patients die. Adenocarcinomas (35%

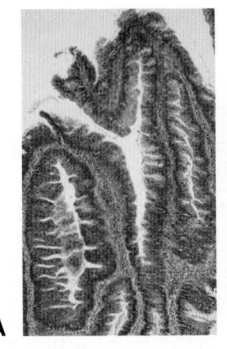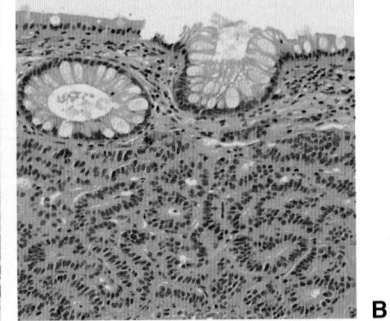

Figure 30.1 | A. Serrated adenoma. B. Neuroendocrine tumor of small intestine. B. A photomicrograph of the lesion in **A** demonstrates cords of uniform small, round cells. Neuroendocrine tumors demonstrate cords of uniform small round cells with rare mitotic figures.

TABLE 30.1	Distribution of Malignant Neoplasms in the Small Intestine[a]			
	Number and Percentage by Region			
Type of Neoplasm	Duodenum	Jejunum	Ileum	Total
Adenocarcinoma	40%	38%	22%	46%
Sarcoma	10%	36%	54%	19%
Lymphoma	16%	36%	48%	1%
Carcinoid	6%	10%	84%	34%
Total	22%	28%	50%	100%

[a]Note: Based on 2,356 cases.

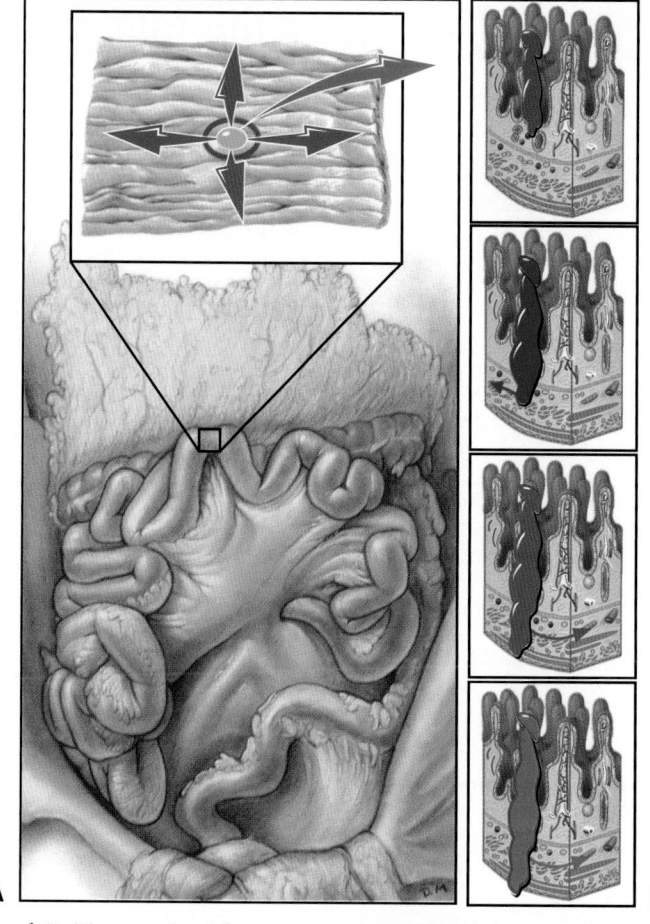

Figure 30.2 | A. Patterns of spread. B. T categories. The patterns of spread and the primary tumor classification are similarly color coded: Tis (cancer in situ of mucosa), yellow; T1 (infiltrates the submucosa), green; T2 (penetrates the muscularis externa), blue; T3 (reaches the subserosa), green; and T4 (invades through the serosa into a neighboring viscera), red. The concept of visualizing patterns of spread to appreciate the surrounding anatomy is well demonstrated by the six-directional pattern, i.e., SIMLAP Table 30.2.

to 50%) are most common, followed by carcinoids (20% to 40%). Small bowel adenomas progress to adenocarcinomas similar to what occurs in the colon. Small bowel obstruction (70%) is a common presentation, triggered by interception or volvulus. Bleeding (20% to 50%) is usually occult, but massive hemorrhage is more common with sarcomas (gastrointestinal stromal tumors).

What the small intestine lacks in numbers of cancers, it makes up for by their variety. Table 30.1 lists them succinctly and one notes a predilection for specific tumors in different bowel segments: Adenocarcinomas are more common in the duodenum, lymphomas in the jejunum and sarcomas, and carcinoids in the ileum with its most favored site being the vermiform appendix (T1 histopathology versus distribution) (Table 30.1; Fig. 30.1).

TABLE 30.2	SIMLAP		
Small Intestine (Jejunum)			
S	Duodenum	• **T2**	• T3
	Transverse colon	• T4	
I	Ileum	• T4	
M	Superior mesenteric artery	• T4	
L	Ascending, descending colon	• T4	
A	Greater omentum	• T3	
P	Mesentery, small intestine	• T3	

The six vectors of invasion are <u>S</u>uperior, <u>I</u>nferior, <u>M</u>edial, <u>L</u>ateral, <u>A</u>nterior, and <u>P</u>osterior. The color-coded dots correlate the T stage with specific anatomic structure involved.

TNM STAGING CRITERIA

CLASSIFICATION AND STAGING

TNM Staging Criteria

There has been no change or revision, with depth of wall penetration determining the stage: T1, mucosal; T2, muscularis; T3, serosa; and T4 other viscera (Fig. 30.3).

Generally, there is no overarching principle or context design for the digestive system (gastrointestinal tract) or major digestive glands (MDGs). Stages are frequently expanded to six by subdividing stages into A and B. The T and N categories are assigned to a stage grouping, specifically for division of a stage into more (a) versus less (b) favorable groupings. This occurs at different stages for different sites.

Specifically, this site is staged in the same fashion as colorectal cancers. Stages I and II are due to T progression, whereas stages III and IV are related solely to N progression: >T4 = N1.

In the seventh edition of the American Joint Committee of Cancer *AJCC Cancer Staging Manual* changes are minor and mainly involve subdividing stages I and II.

SUMMARY OF CHANGES SEVENTH EDITION AJCC

- T1 lesions have been divided into T1a (invasion of lamina propria) and T1b (invasion of submuscosa) to facilitate comparison with tumors of other gastrointestinal sites (Fig. 30.3).

- Stage II has been subdivided into Stage IIA and Stage IIB.

- The N1 category has been changed to N1 (1–3 positive lymph nodes) and N2 (four or more positive lymph nodes), leading to the division of Stage III into Stage IIIA and Stage IIIB.

The TNM Staging Matrix is color coded for identification of stage group once T and N stages are determined (Table 30.3).

TABLE 30.3	Stage Summary Matrix			
	N0	**N1**	**N2**	**M1**
T1ab	I	IIIA	IIIB	IV
T2	I	IIIA	IIIB	IV
T3	IIA	IIIA	IIIB	IV
T4	IIB	IIIA	IIIB	IV

T stage progresses and then N stage progresses in sequence determines Stage Group Progression sequential:

- $T_1T_2 = I$ then T_3, $T_4 = II$
- $N_1 = III$
- $M_1 = IV$ separate stage

SMALL INTESTINE ADENOCARCINOMA

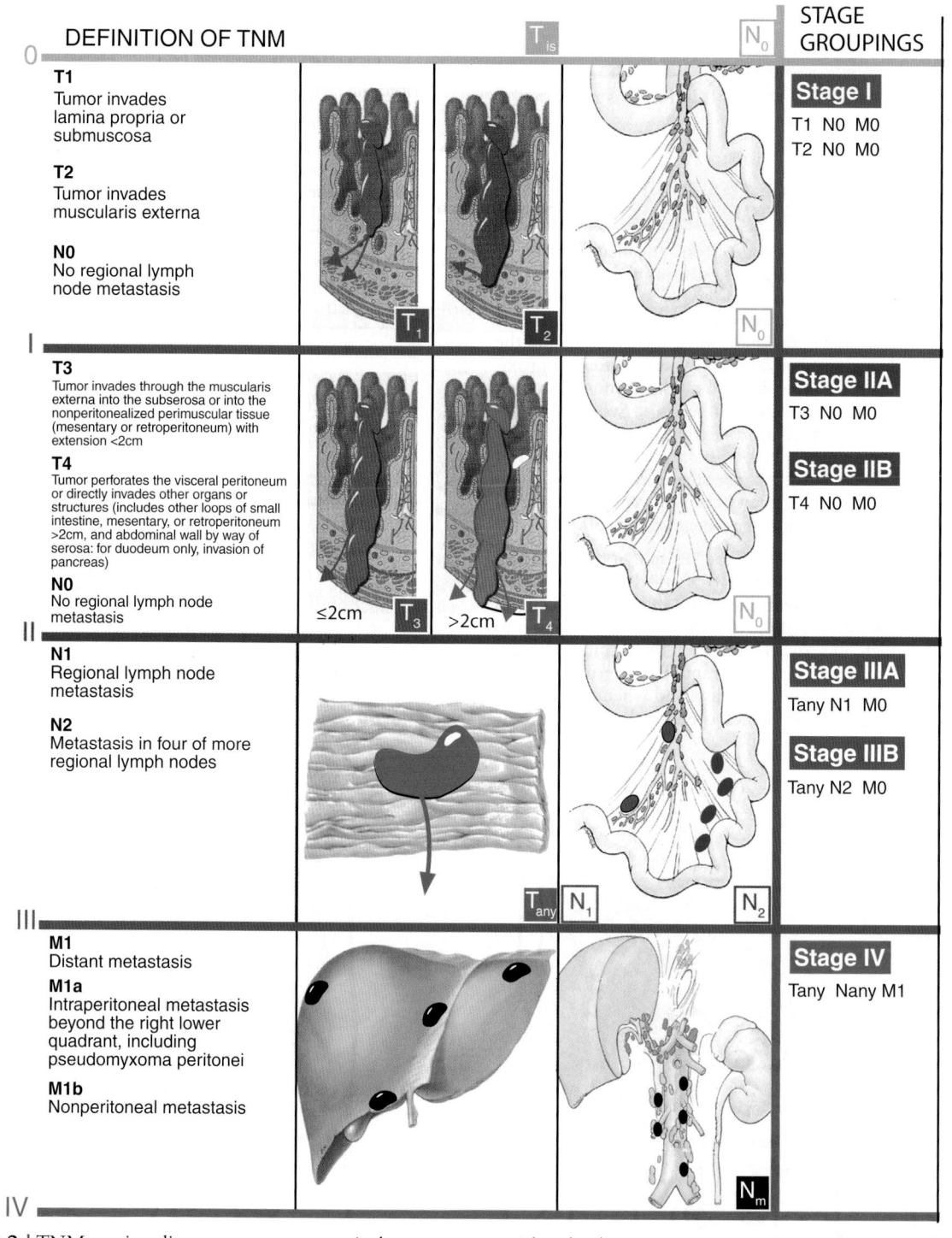

DEFINITION OF TNM

T1
Tumor invades lamina propria or submuscosa

T2
Tumor invades muscularis externa

N0
No regional lymph node metastasis

T3
Tumor invades through the muscularis externa into the subserosa or into the nonperitonealized perimuscular tissue (mesentary or retroperitoneum) with extension <2cm

T4
Tumor perforates the visceral peritoneum or directly invades other organs or structures (includes other loops of small intestine, mesentery, or retroperitoneum >2cm, and abdominal wall by way of serosa: for duodeum only, invasion of pancreas)

N0
No regional lymph node metastasis

N1
Regional lymph node metastasis

N2
Metastasis in four of more regional lymph nodes

M1
Distant metastasis

M1a
Intraperitoneal metastasis beyond the right lower quadrant, including pseudomyxoma peritonei

M1b
Nonperitoneal metastasis

STAGE GROUPINGS

Stage I
T1 N0 M0
T2 N0 M0

Stage IIA
T3 N0 M0

Stage IIB
T4 N0 M0

Stage IIIA
Tany N1 M0

Stage IIIB
Tany N2 M0

Stage IV
Tany Nany M1

Figure 30.3 | TNM staging diagram presents a vertical arrangement with color bars encompassing TN combinations showing progression. Small intestine cancers are both uncommon and unique. They are simply staged I to IV without substages, an exception for the digestive system. Stage 0, yellow; I, green; II, blue; III, purple; IV, red; and IV (metastatic), black. Definitions of TN on left and stage grouping on right.

N-ONCOANATOMY AND M-ONCOANATOMY

N-ONCOANATOMY

Despite a large variety and number of regional lymph nodes following the superior mesenteric artery and vein, the lymph node classification is simply N1, positive regional node, without qualification as to number or size of lymph nodes (Fig. 30.6A; Table 30.4).

M-ONCOANATOMY

The entire portal circulation should be considered as a unit in regard to the venous anatomy of the gastrointestinal tract below the diaphragm (see Fig. 30.6B). The two major trunks are the inferior and superior mesenteric veins. The inferior mesenteric vein drains the left colon and sigmoid colon tributaries, which cover the vascular drainage to the left of the midline originating from the superior rectal veins. On the right side, the superior mesenteric vein originates from the tributaries draining the ileum, jejunum, and the ileocolic and right and middle colic veins. The inferior mesenteric vein usually joins the splenic vein, which coalesces with the superior mesenteric

vein and forms the portal vein. The splenic vein, which is a major tributary of the portal system, also drains much of the stomach along its greater curvature and includes the short gastric veins and left and right gastroepiploic veins. The right gastroepiploic also flows into the superior mesenteric vein. The entire drainage of the lesser curvature of the stomach, including the left and right gastric veins, drains directly into the portal vein. Because the portal vein then drains directly into the liver, it is the target metastatic organ and the most commonly involved organ in hematogenous spread pattern from the venous system of the gastrointestinal tract, as compared with other parts of the body, where the drainage is directly into the lung by way of the caval system.

Venous drainage is by way of the tributaries of the superior mesenteric vein and fusion with the splenic vein to give rise to the portal vein. Liver metastases are the most common site.

The venous drainage of the small intestine is complex because of the length and its convolutions throughout the abdominal cavity. The first part of the small intestine, the duodenum, drains into the pancreaticoduodenum veins, into the portal vein, and superiorly and inferiorly into the superior mesenteric vein. The jejuneal and ileal veins drain directly into the superior mesenteric vein and then into the portal vein. Liver is the target organ.

TABLE 30.4	Lymph Nodes of Small Intestine
Sentinel Nodes Include Superior Mesenteric Nodes*	
Segment	**Regional Nodes**
Duodenum	Duodenal, hepatic, pancreaticoduodenal, infrapyloric, gastroduodenal, pyloric, superior mesenteric, pericholedochal
Ileum and jejunum	Posterior cecal (terminal ileum only), ileocolic (terminal ileum only), superior mesenteric, mesenteric
Juxtaregional nodes	
Para-aortic	
Portal	
Rectal	

*Depend on location of primary.

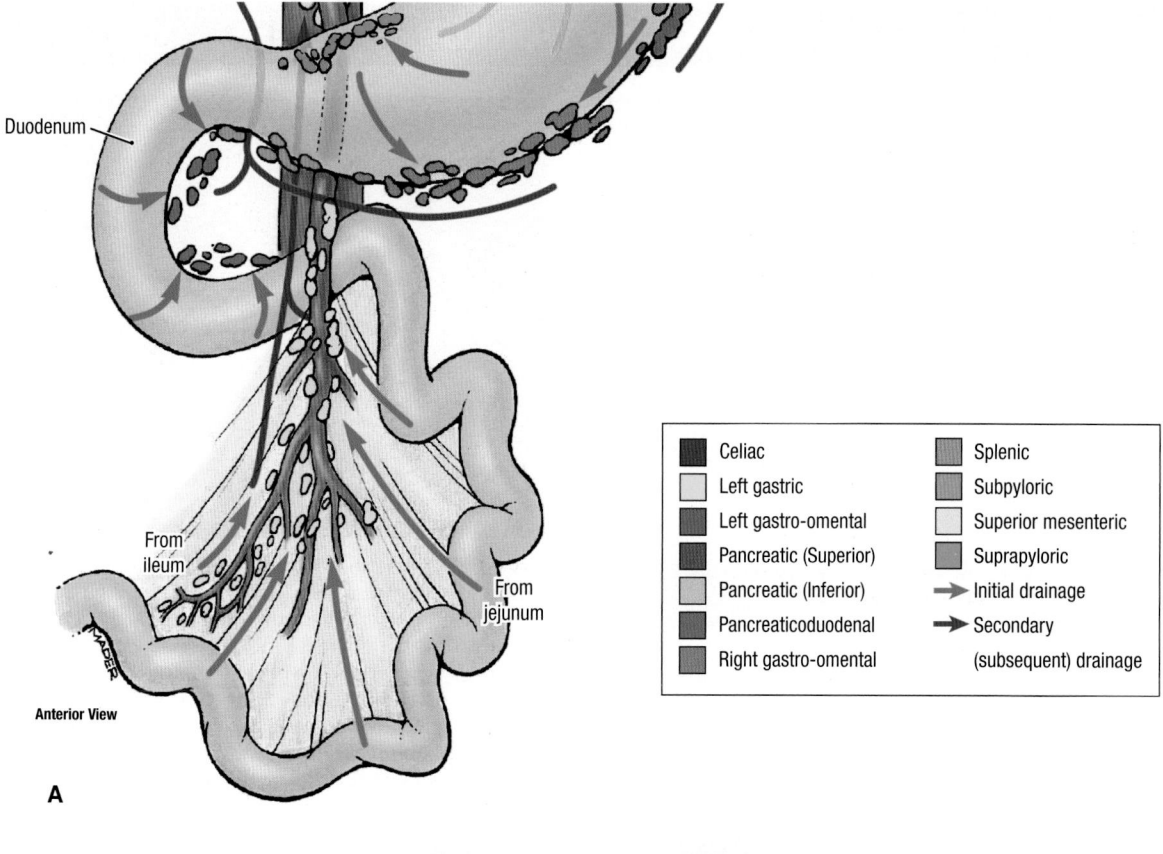

Duodenum

From ileum

From jejunum

Anterior View

A

◼ Celiac	◼ Splenic
◻ Left gastric	◼ Subpyloric
◼ Left gastro-omental	◻ Superior mesenteric
◼ Pancreatic (Superior)	◼ Suprapyloric
◻ Pancreatic (Inferior)	→ Initial drainage
◼ Pancreaticoduodenal	→ Secondary
◼ Right gastro-omental	(subsequent) drainage

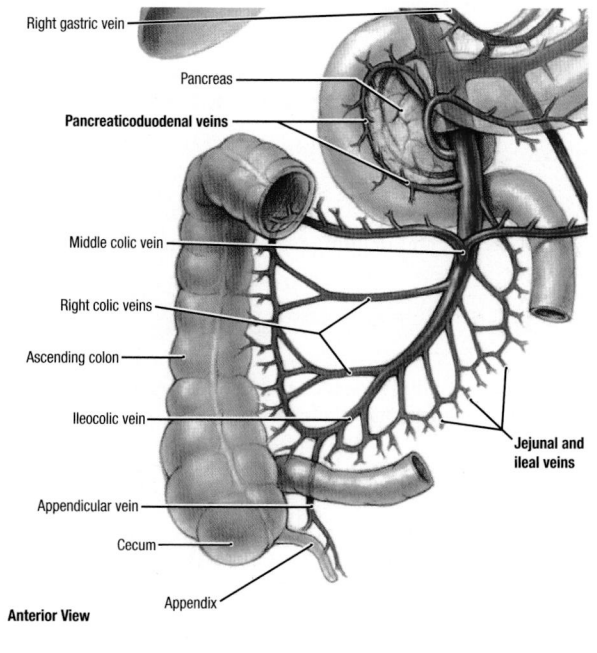

Right gastric vein

Pancreas

Pancreaticoduodenal veins

Middle colic vein

Right colic veins

Ascending colon

Ileocolic vein

Jejunal and ileal veins

Appendicular vein

Cecum

Appendix

Anterior View

B

Figure 30.6 | **A. N-oncoanatomy.** Sentinel nodes of small intestine include the mesenteric nodes. **B. M-oncoanatomy.** Along superior mesenteric artery.

STAGING WORKUP

RULES OF CLASSIFICATION AND STAGING

Clinical Staging and Imaging

Cancers of the small intestine are uncommon, and although imaging may be useful for staging, the diagnosis realistically is often uncovered at laparotomy. At the time of surgery and resection an accurate view of penetration of the bowel wall is possible. Computed tomography (CT) and magnetic resonance imaging (MRI) may be useful; however, most small bowel neoplasias are carcinoids, lymphomas, or leiomyosarcomas and are not applicable to the TNM staging system (Table 30.5; Fig. 30.7).

Pathologic Staging

The surgically resected small intestine and associated lymph nodes removed are assessed. Tumor extension and location of both primary and nodes should be documented. Accurate radial margins should be marked and recorded and are defined as the surgically dissected surface adjacent to the deepest point of tumor invasion beyond the wall of the small bowel. The completeness of resection depends on the clearing of the deepest point of invasion: R0, complete; R1, microscopic; and R2, macroscopic.

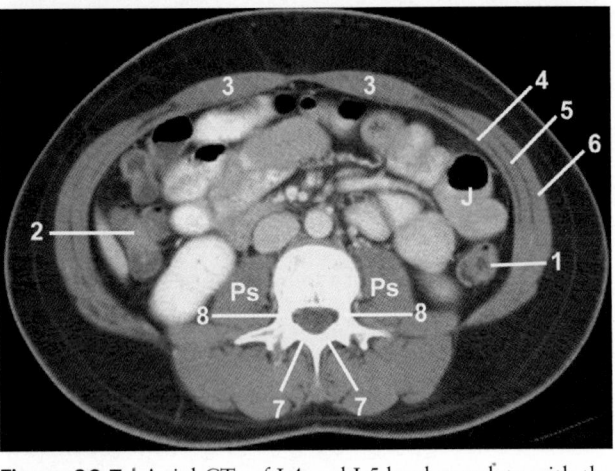

Figure 30.7 | Axial CTs of L4 and L5 level correlate with the T-oncoanatomy transverse section (Figure 30.5C). Oncoimaging with CT is commonly applied to staging cancers, often combined with PET to determine true extent of primary cancer and involved lymph nodes. 1. Descending colon. 2. Ascending colon. 3. Rectus abdominus muscles. 4. Transversus abdominus muscle. 5. Internal oblique muscle. 6. External oblique muscle. 7. Vertebral body laminae. 8. Vertebral body pedicles. J, jejunum; Ps, psoas muscles.

TABLE 30.5	Imaging Modalities for Staging for Small Intestine	
Method	**Diagnosis and Staging Capability**	**Recommended for Use**
Primary Tumor and Regional Nodes		
Single-contrast GI studies[a]	Useful in detecting and defining primary lesions in small intestine: 90%	Yes
Double-contrast GI studies[a]	Very useful in detecting early gastric cancers	Yes; should be performed along with single contrast
Endoscopy	Very accurate modality to detect and define primary lesions: ~90% confirmation rate	Yes; use to confirm lesion detected in upper GI series and to screen high-risk patients
Camera capsule endoscopy	Ideal for sites beyond routine endoscopy	Yes
CT-abdomen ± chest	Most valuable of all modalities for determining degree of extrabowel extension and distant metastases	Yes
Endoscopic ultrasound	Most accurate method of determining extension within and beyond gastric wall	Yes, if planned preoperative chemoradiation
Metastatic Tumors		
Chest films	Good for detecting metastases	Yes
Laparoscopy	May allow visualization of small serosal implants or liver metastases	Yes, if planned preoperative chemotherapy or chemoradiation
Bone film	Useful only for confirming metastases	No, unless patient has bone pain
PET: liver, brain, bone	Useful in evaluation of clinically suspected metastases; CT is better than nuclide scan for liver and brain	No, unless suspected metastases

CT, computed tomography; GI, gastrointestinal; PET, positron emission tomography.
[a]Enteroclysis.

PROGNOSIS AND CANCER SURVIVAL

Oncoimaging Annotations

- Adenocarcinomas occur in the duodenum, decreasing in frequency in the jejunum and ileum.

- Enteroclysis has a 90% success rate in imaging small bowel tumors, although it is included in 30% to 40% of small bowel followthrough studies.

- CT is best for determining penetration of the bowel into surrounding viscera; MRI is useful for detecting liver metastases.

- CT is reported to have an accuracy of detection rate between 70% and 80%. CT misses tumors <2 cm. Mucosal detail is absent. CT is best for staging and follow-up.

- At present, the role of MRI is limited to the search for liver metastases, but enthusiasm for MRI enteroclysis is increasing.

- Camera capsule endoscopy is ideal for sites beyond routine endoscopy and can identify obstructing and bleeding foci of polypoid and ulcerating lesions.

PROGNOSIS

The limited number of prognostic factors are listed in Table 30.6.

TABLE 30.6	Prognostic Factors
Required for staging	None
Clinically significant	Presurgical carcinoembryonic antigen (CEA)
	Microsatellite instability (MSI)
	Presence of Crohn disease

Reprinted with permission from Edge SB, Byrd DR, Compton CC, et al. *AJCC Cancer Staging Manual*, 7th ed. New York: Springer, 2010, p. 132.

CANCER STATISTICS AND SURVIVAL

The digestive system, or gastrointestinal tract, which includes MDGs, accounts for 275,000 new patients annually, with colon and rectum responsible for >50%, or about 140,000 new diagnoses annually. Approximately half of these patients eventually die of these cancers. MDG cancers as a group are more lethal; only a handful of patients become long-term survivors. Fortunately, colon and rectal cancers are the most common, with the majority of patients becoming 5-year survivors (63%) responding to chemoradiation programs, often with the sparing of the rectal sphincter with conservative surgery. Anal cancers are the most responsive to chemoradiation (5-fluorouracil and cisplatin), eliminating the need for surgery. The 5-year survival rate is >90%, with anal sphincter preservation. This regimen has been proven to be very effective in clinical trials and to result in more long-term survivors, which is currently reflected in the literature. Liver, bile duct, and pancreatic cancers are among the poorest in the terms of survival, which is often measured in months rather than years (Fig.30.8).

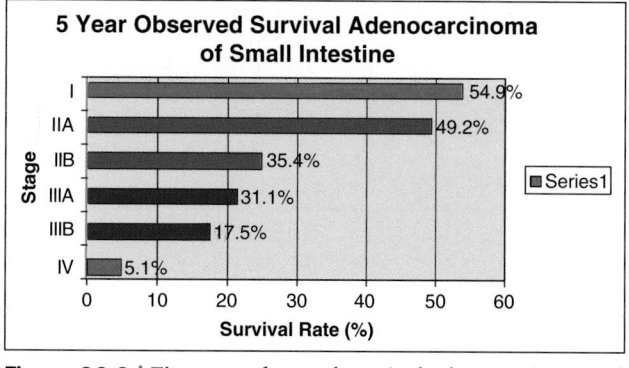

Figure 30.8 | Five-year observed survival adenocarcinoma of small intestine. (Data from Edge SB, Byrd DR, and Compton CC, et al., *AJCC Cancer Staging Manual, 7th edition.* New York, Springer, 2010, p. 129.)

Appendix Adenocarcinoma and Carcinoids

PERSPECTIVE, PATTERNS OF SPREAD, AND PATHOLOGY

The appendix is a finger-like outpouching from the cecum containing numerous lymphatic nodules similar to Peyer's patches in its wall.

PERSPECTIVE AND PATTERNS OF SPREAD

The appendix has come of age in the seventh edition of the American Joint Committee on Cancer *AJCC Cancer Staging Manual*, in which it has its own distinct staging system. The introduction of carcinoids has also been emphasized at this site, although it can occur throughout the digestive system. It may be equivalent to the bursa of Fabricius in mammals, where potential B lymphocytes acquire their immunocompetence. It is prone to infection as a blind-ended pouch.

- *Appendiceal adenocarcinomas* are grouped with mucinous adenocarcinomas, which constitute 50% versus 10% of colon carcinomas and have better survival outcomes. *Appendix carcinoids* will be considered and contrasted with adenocarcinomas at this site.

- *Appendiceal adenocarcinomas* tend to ulcerate and perforate, presenting as appendicitis with right lower quadrant pain. Their dissemination is into the peritoneal cavity.

- *Appendiceal carcinoids* produce a carcinoid syndrome. Carcinoid tumors have the capacity to produce serotonin, histamine, and bradykinin. These compounds cause a clinical syndrome manifested by attacks of watery diarrhea, cutaneous flushing, and asthmatic-type respiratory distress. Lesions of tricuspid and pulmonic valves also occur. This syndrome does not occur in all instances of carcinoid tumor. The syndrome is most frequently associated with carcinoids of the ileum or extensive hepatic metastases. Carcinoids most commonly occur on the appendix but rarely produce carcinoid syndrome from this site. Their dis-

semination is to the liver, and their hepatic multinodular spread and growth triggers the endocrine syndrome.

PATHOLOGY

Carcinoids that arise from cells of the neuroendocrine system are more in the gastrointestinal tract. The small intestine, especially the ileum, accounts for 30% of all carcinoids, but because small intestine neoplasia is uncommon, it accounts for one third of small bowel cancers. In a similar fashion, Surveillance, Epidemiology and End Results data show that appendiceal carcinoids account for less than 3% of all carcinoids, but as a percentage of appendiceal cancers, their incidence is high and similar to that in the small intestine. Therefore, carcinoid neuroendocrine tumors are covered in this chapter, recognizing the clinical manifestations are similar, independent of origin site (Tables 31.1A and B; Fig. 31.1).

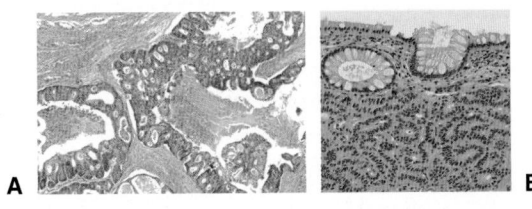

A   B

Figure 31.1 | A. Adenocarcinoma. Microscopically, this adenocarcinoma consists of moderately differentiated glands with a prominent cribriform pattern and frequent central necrosis. **B. Carcinoid tumors** are neuroendocrine tumors (NETs). The appendix and ileum are often cited as the most frequent sites, although they can and do occur throughout the digestive system. Microscopically, NETs appear as nests or rosettes of uniform round cells. Mitosis is rare, and nuclei are often regular. Goblet cells imply more aggressive behavior.

TABLE 31.1A Histopathology (MUC) Carcinoma

This staging classification applies to carcinomas that arise in the appendix. The histologic types include the following:

Adenocarcinoma in situ (the term "high-grade dysplasia" may be used as a synonym for in situ carcinoma; these cases should be assigned pTis)

Adenocarcinoma

Medullary carcinoma

Mucinous carcinoma (colloid type) (>50% mucinous carcinoma)

Signet ring cell carcinoma (>50% signet ring cell)

From Edge SB, Byrd DR, and Compton CC, et al., *AJCC Cancer Staging Manual, 7th edition.* New York, Springer, 2010, pp. 137–138.

TABLE 31.1B Histopathology Carcinoid

This staging classification applies to carcinoids that arise in the appendix. The histologic types include the following:

Carcinoid tumor

Well-differentiated neuroendocrine tumor

Tubular carcinoid

Goblet cell carcinoid

Adenocarcinoid

Atypical carcinoid

Well-differentiated neuroendocrine carcinoma after resection (relevant to resection margins that are macroscopically involved by tumor)

From Edge SB, Byrd DR, and Compton CC, et al., *AJCC Cancer Staging Manual, 7th edition.* New York, Springer, 2010, pp. 137–138.

TABLE 31.2 SIMLAP

Appendix		Carcinoids	Cancers
S	Cecum	• T2	• T4b
I	Abdominal wall	• T4b	• T4b
M	Ileum, mesoappendix	• T3	• T3
L	Abdominal wall	• T4b	• T4b
A	Urinary bladder	• T4b	• T4b
P	Rectum	• T4b	• T4b

The six vectors of invasion are Superior, Inferior, Medial, Lateral, Anterior, and Posterior. The color-coded dots correlate the T stage with specific anatomic structure involved.

The patterns of spread are limited and illustrated for cancers (Fig. 31.2B) and carcinoids (Fig. 31.2A). Both are summarized in Table 31.2.

The average age of presentation is in the 60s, and all tumors express serotonin. Small bowel carcinoids present with vague abdominal pain, related to intermittent obstruction; bleeding is rare. Appendiceal carcinoids often lead to appendicitis, with early detection and more favorable outcome, with an overall survival of 71%. Appendiceal carcinoids tend to be small, <2 cm, and appendectomy is often adequate. With lymph node invasion or penetration of serosa, or mesoappendix, a wider ileocolectomy is performed.

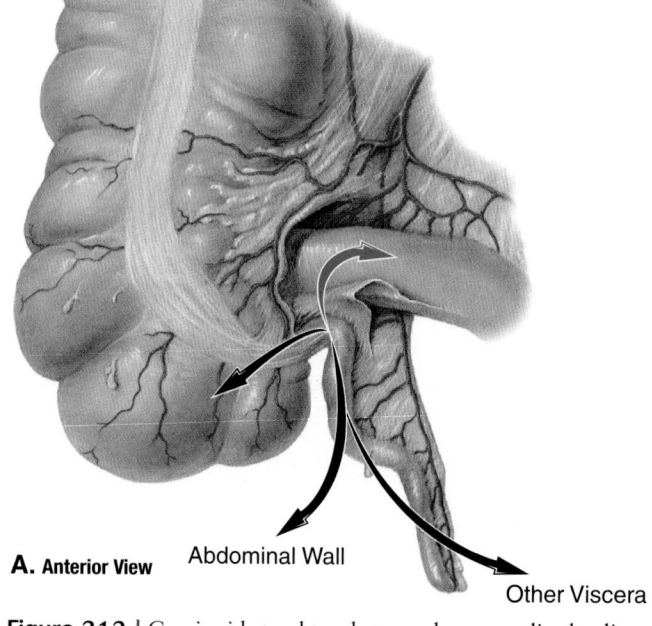

Carcinoid

A. Anterior View Abdominal Wall Other Viscera

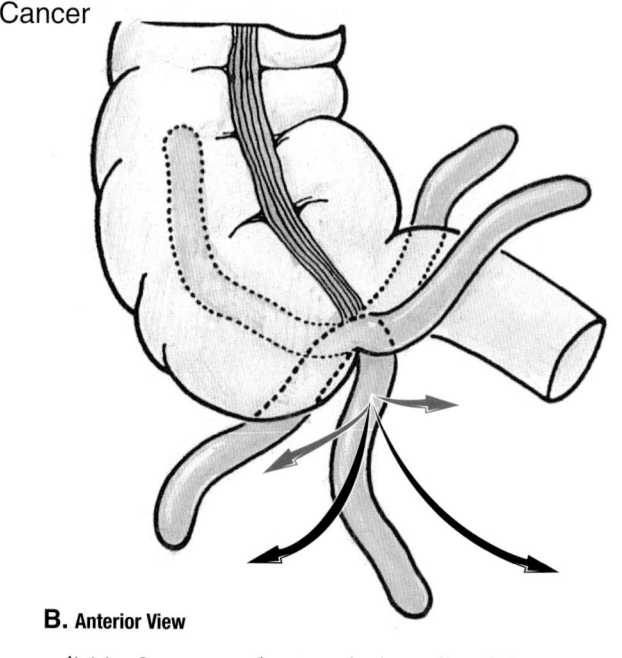

Cancer

B. Anterior View

Figure 31.2 | Carcinoids tend to obstruct the appendix, leading to appendicitis. Cancers tend to invade the wall and their patterns of spread is to adjacent viscera, i.e., secum, ileum, and depending on location, small intestine, and abdominal wall (Fig. 31.2; Table 31.2). The concept of visualizing patterns of spread to appreciate the surrounding anatomy is well demonstrated by the six-directional pattern i.e., SIMLAP Table 31.2.

TNM STAGING CRITERIA

APPENDICEAL CARCINOMAS

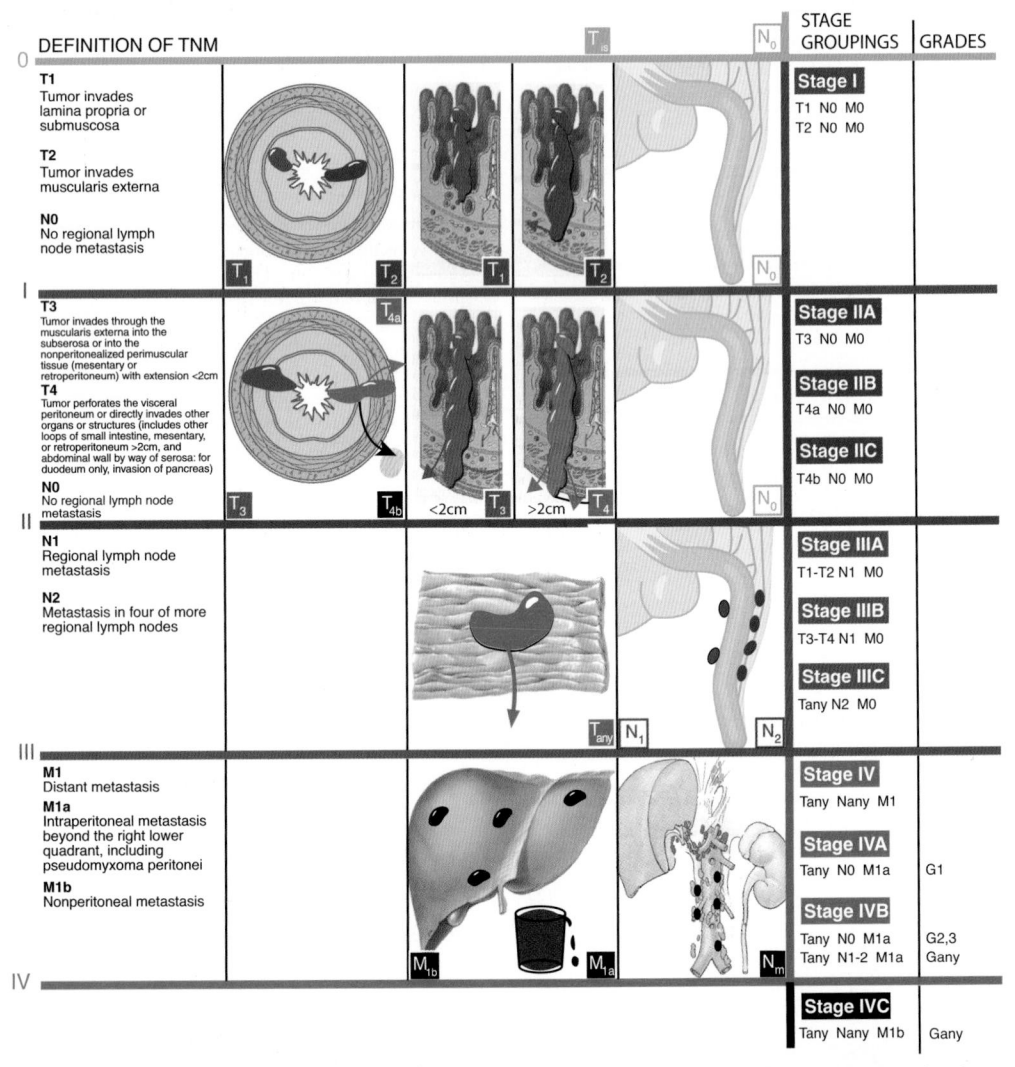

Figure 31.3A | TNM staging criteria for appendiceal carcinomas. These are separately classified in the seventh edition of the *AJCC Cancer Staging Manual*. The appendiceal adenocarcinoma staging follows the colorectal categories, in that the primary cancer invades the wall, each layer advances T stage, then N stage progresses. Mucus that has spread beyond the right lower quadrant carries a poor prognosis, as does presence of epithelial cells in the peritoneal cavity. Pseudomyxoma peritonea carries M1a designation.

TNM Staging Criteria

The appendiceal carcinomas are separately classified in the seventh edition. The appendiceal adenocarcinoma staging follow the colorectal categories in that the primary cancers invade the wall, each layer advances T stage, Then N stage progresses. Mucous that has spread beyond the RLQ as is presence of epithelial cells in peritoneal cavity carry a poor prognosis. Pseudomyxoma peritonea carries M1a designation (Fig. 31.3A).

SUMMARY OF CHANGES SEVENTH EDITION AJCC

- In the seventh edition, appendiceal carcinomas are separately classified. In the sixth edition, appendiceal carcinomas were classified according to the definitions for colorectal tumors.

- Appendiceal carcinomas are now separated into mucinous and nonmucinous types. Histologic grading is considered of particular importance for mucinous tumors. This is reflected in the staging considerations for metastatic tumors. The change is based on published data and analysis of NCDB data.

- In the seventh edition, the T4 category is divided into T4a and T4b as in the colon and is reflected in the subdivision of Stage II.

- M1 is divided into M1a and M1b where pseudomyxoma peritonei, M1a, is separated from nonperitoneal metastasis, M1b.

- In the seventh edition, Stage IV is subdivided on the basis of N, M, and G status, unlike colorectal carcinomas.

APPENDIX CARCINOID

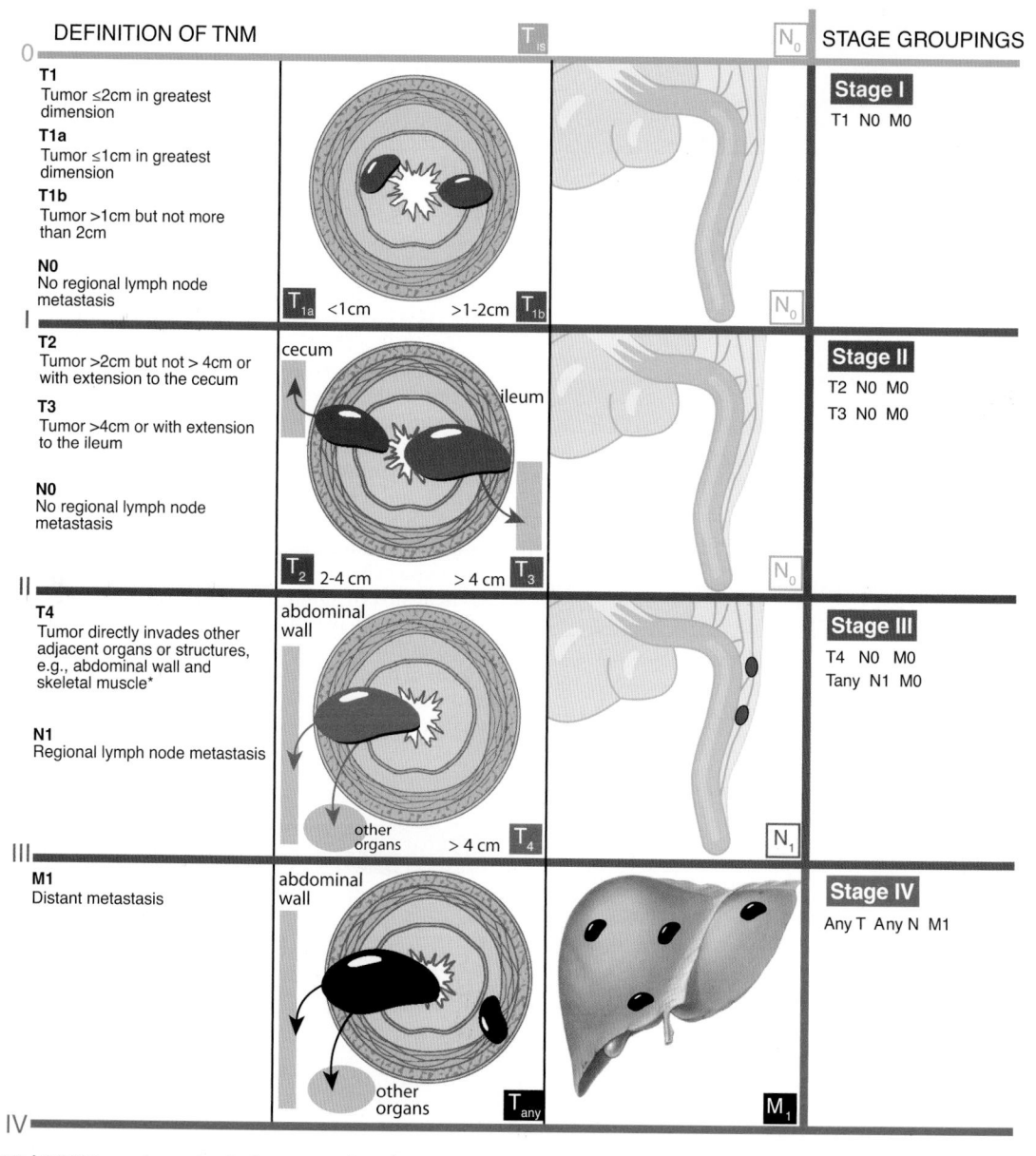

Figure 31.3B | TNM staging criteria for appendiceal carcinoids. These are new in the seventh edition of the *AJCC Cancer Staging Manual*. Staging of the appendiceal carcinoid is largely based on size. T1a, ≤1 cm, and T1b, 1 to 2 cm, tend to be localized. T2, T3, and T4 increment size and metastatic potential.

TNM STAGING CRITERIA

- The Appendiceal carcinoids are new in the seventh edition. The appendiceal carcinoid is largely based on size. T1a ≤ 1 cm and T1b 1 – 2 cm tend to be localized. T2, T3, T4 increment size and metastatic potential (Fig. 31.1B).

SUMMARY OF CHANGES SEVENTH EDITION AJCC

- A new classification is added for carcinoid tumors that were not classified previously by TNM. This is a new classifica-

tion. There are substantial differences between the classification schemes of appendiceal carcinomas and carcinoids and between appendiceal carcinoids and other well-differentiated gastrointestinal neuroendocrine tumors (carcinoids) (see chapters of the digestive system for staging of other gastrointestinal carcinoids).

- Serum chromogranin A is identified as a significant prognostic factor.

T-ONCOANATOMY

ORIENTATION OF TNM ONCOANATOMY

T-oncoanatomy

The appendix is a tubular structure that is 3 to 13 cm in length and is located 2 to 3 cm inferior to the ileocecal valve. It adjoins the cecum medially and is attached to a mesoappendix that contains its blood supply, that is, the appendicular artery. Its position can vary, and although typically it hangs inferiorly, less commonly it can be retrocecal (Figure 31.5A,B).

N-oncoanatomy

The appendiceal lymph nodes drain into ileocecal lymph nodes. Then the superior mesenteric artery lymph node drains into the para-aortic lymph nodes (Fig. 31.6A).

M-oncoanatomy

The drainage of the appendiceal vein is into the ileocolic vein, then midcolic into the superior mesenteric vein, which drains into the portal circulation. Hence, liver metastasis leads to the carcinoid syndrome. Goblet cell carcinoid tends to metastasize to the ovaries. Seeding and spreading directly into peritoneal surfaces can lead to a mucinous ascites.

The metastatic capability of carcinoid tumors is a function of size. Once tumors exceed 1.0 cm their risk for metastasizing dramatically increases (Table 31.3; Fig. 31.6B).

The typical pattern of carcinoid syndrome (CS) is triggered by liver metastases by release of tryptophan, which is converted to 5-hydroxytryptophane and then rapidly to serotonin. The serotonin then forms 5-hydroxyindoleacetic acid (5HIAA), which is excreted in the urine. The diagnosis of CS is through elevated plasma serotonin and 5HIAA in the urine (Fig. 31.4).

Typically, there is diarrhea, and flushing occurs. The appearance of red-to-purple discoloration of the face may spread to the entire torso—an erythematous rash that is pruritic with central clearing. Diarrhea also occurs with multiple loose stools. Additional symptoms include abdominal pain, cardiac symptoms, and bronchospasm. Tricuspid valvular lesions and pulmonary valve are most at risk. Carcinoid crisis can be precipitated by anesthetic and surgical intervention to establish the diagnosis. Fortunately, somatostatin analogs can counteract the CS.

Ileal diverticulum is a congenital anomaly that occurs in 1% to 2% of persons. It is a pouchlike remnant (3 to 6 cm long) of the proximal part of the yolk stalk, typically within 50 cm of the ileocecal junction. It sometimes becomes inflamed and produces pain that may mimic that produced by appendicitis.

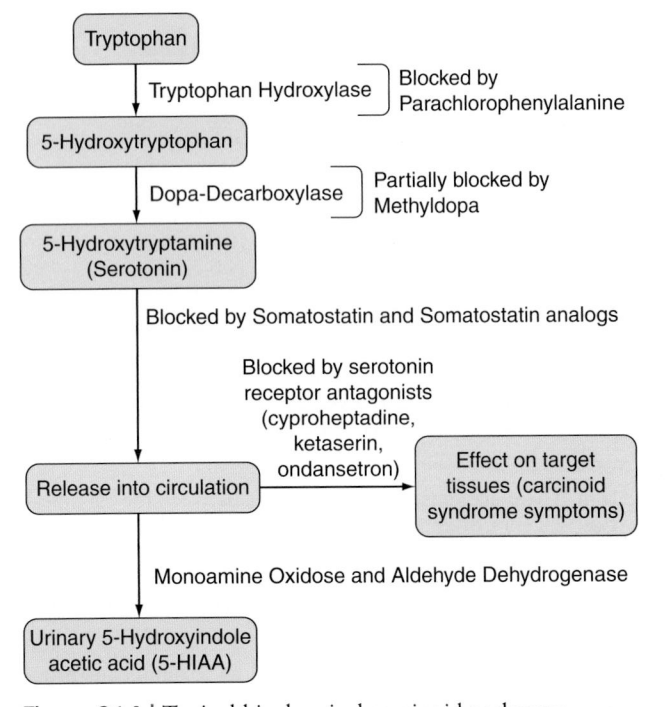

Figure 31.4 | Typical biochemical carcinoid pathways.

TABLE 31.3	Risk of Metastases from Carcinoid Tumors Arising in the Small Intestine

Size of Primary Tumor (mm)	Risk of Metastases (%)
<6	15
6–10	31
>10	73

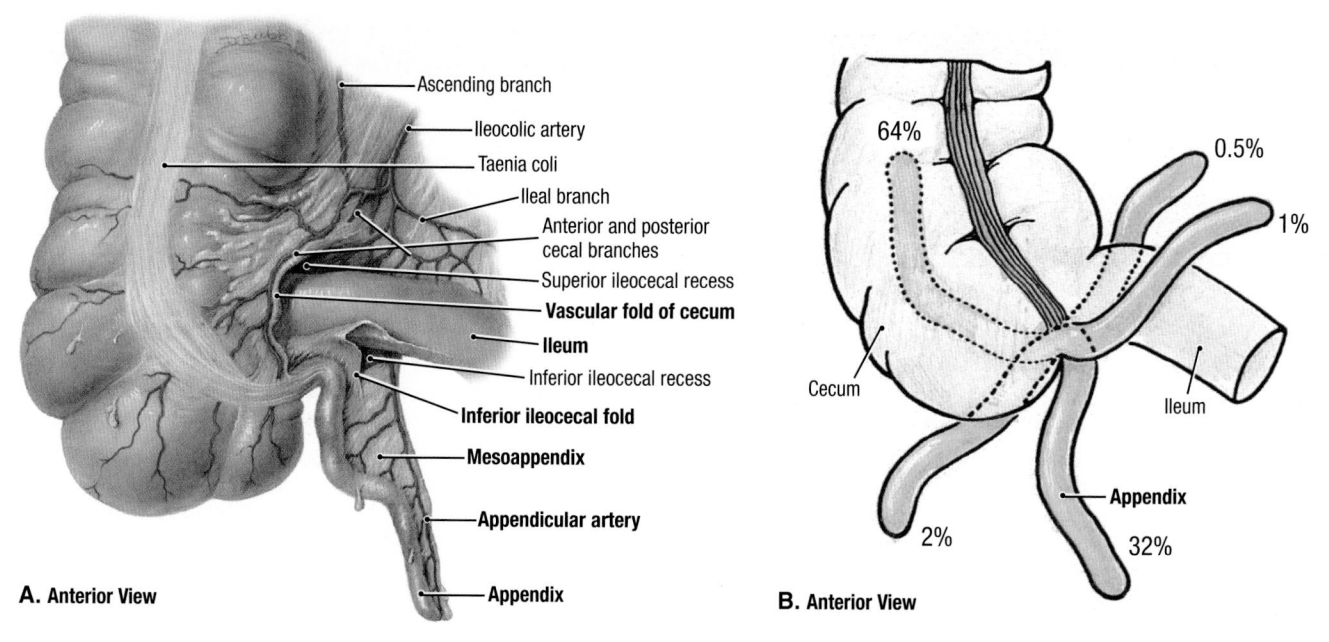

Figure 31.5 | T-oncoanatomy. **A.** Blood supply. The appendicular artery is located in the free edge of the mesoappendix. The inferior ileocecal fold is bloodless, whereas the superior ileocecal fold is called the vascular fold of the cecum. **B.** The approximate incidence at various locations of the appendix.

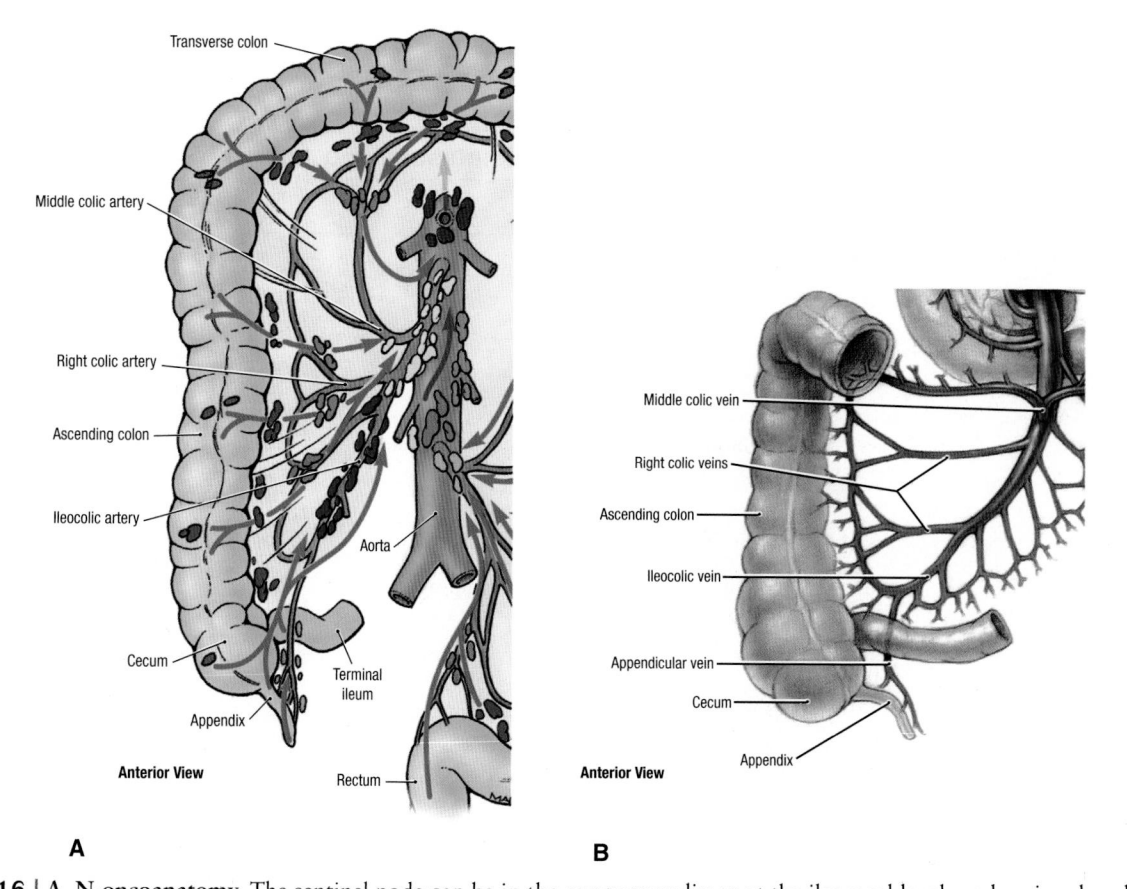

Figure 31.6 | **A.** N-oncoanatomy. The sentinel node can be in the mesoappendix or at the ileocecal level, and regional nodes are ileocolic. **B.** M-oncoanatomy. Appendiceal vein into the ileocolic vein into the superior mesenteric vein, then the portal vein; therefore liver is the target organ for metastases.

STAGING WORKUP

RULES OF CLASSIFICATION AND STAGING

Clinical Staging and Imaging

CT is essential to identify extrabowel invasion, ascites and liver metastases (Fig. 31.7, Table 31.4).

ONCOIMAGING ANNOTATIONS

Adenocarcinoma

- Search for extensions and metastatic disease once the diagnosis is made.
- Staging is based on surgical pathologic criteria, and lymphadenectomy should take account of 12 or more nodes.
- Presence of peritoneal implants and ascites is considered M1a.
- Satellite peritumoral nodule or tumor deposit in periappendiceal adipose tissue without histologic evidence of residual lymph node may be discontinuous spread (T3), venous invasion with extravascular spread (T3 V1/2), or replaced lymph node (N1/2).

Carcinoids

- 5HIAA elevation or carcinoid syndrome triggers staging workup.
- Computed tomography (CT) scans are abnormal 78% when HIAA is elevated.
- Magnetic resonance imaging (MRI) scans are similar to CTs and detect metastases.
- Positron emission tomography scans may not be useful since carcinoids are slow growing.
- Single photon emission computed tomography using ^{111}In-labeled pentetreotide is positive 80% to 90% and more accurate than CT or MRI in identifying primary, tumor deposits, and metastases.
- Radiolabeled somatostatin is effective in localizing occult tumors >1 cm in size, clarifying equivocal CT/MR findings, and predicting response to treatment.
- Gastrointestinal contrast enteroclysis can detect intraluminal primaries.
- CT can detect primary tumor and mesenteric lymph nodes with a desmoplastic "spokewheel" pattern (Fig. 31.7).

TABLE 31.4	Imaging Modalities for Staging for Small Intestine and Appendix	
Method	Diagnosis and Staging Capability	Recommended for Use
Primary Tumor and Regional Nodes		
Single-contrast GI studies[a]	Useful in detecting and defining primary lesions in small intestine: 90%	Yes
Double-contrast GI studies[a]	Very useful in detecting early gastric cancers	Yes; should be performed along with single contrast
Endoscopy	Very accurate modality to detect and define primary lesions: ~90% confirmation rate	Yes; use to confirm lesion detected in upper GI series and to screen high-risk patients
Camera capsule endoscopy	Ideal for sites beyond routine endoscopy	Yes
CT-abdomen ± chest	Most valuable of all modalities for determining degree of extrabowel extension and distant metastases	Yes
Endoscopic ultrasound	Most accurate method of determining extension within and beyond gastric wall	Yes, if planned preoperative chemoradiation
Metastatic Tumors		
Chest films	Good for detecting metastases	Yes
Laparoscopy	May allow visualization of small serosal implants or liver metastases	Yes, if planned preoperative chemotherapy or chemoradiation
Bone film	Useful only for confirming metastases	No, unless patient has bone pain
PET: liver, brain, bone	Useful in evaluation of clinically suspected metastases; CT is better than nuclide scan for liver and brain	No, unless suspected metastases

CT, computed tomography; GI, gastrointestinal; PET, positron emission tomography.
[a]Enteroclysis.

PROGNOSIS AND CANCER SURVIVAL

PROGNOSTIC FACTORS

The limited number of prognostic factors are listed in Table 31.5. Clinically significant prognostic factors are identified for collection in cancer registries including pretreatment CEA and CA 19.9, the number of tumor deposits in the mesentery, and where available, the presence of microsatellite instability and 18q loss of heterozygosity size of primary is important for carcinoids.

TABLE 31.5	Prognostic Factors
Clinically significant	Preoperative/pretreatment carcinoembryonic antigen (CEA)
	Preoperative/pretreatment CA 19-9
	Tumor deposits (TDs)
	Microsatellite instability (MSI)
	18q Loss of heterozygosity (LOH)

From Edge SB, Byrd DR, Compton CC, et al., *AJCC Cancer Staging Manual, 7th edition.* New York, Springer, 2010, p. 141.

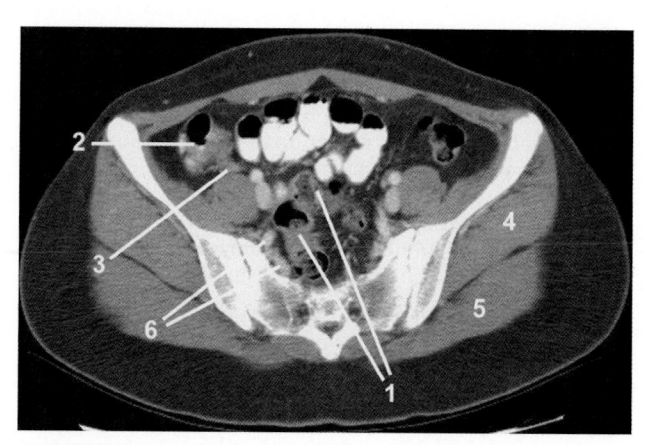

Figure 31.7 | **Portal venous phase.** 1. Sigmoid colon. 2. Cecum. 3. Vermiform appendix. 4. Gluteus medius. 5. Gluteus maximus. 6. Internal iliac art and vein.

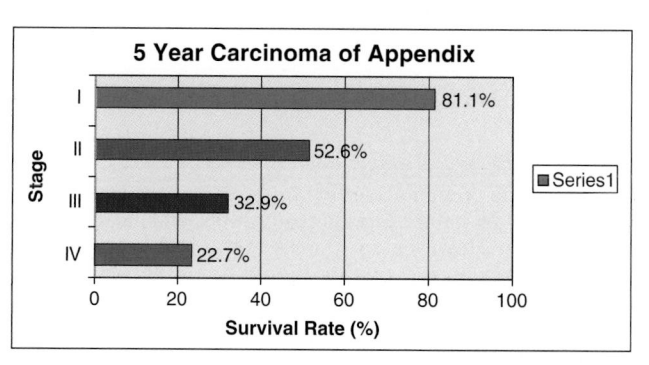

Figure 31.8 | Five-year survival for carcinoma of the appendix. (Data from Edge SB, Byrd DR, Compton CC, et al., *AJCC Cancer Staging Manual, 7th ed.* New York, Springer, 2010, p. 135).

CHAPTER
32
Rectum

PERSPECTIVE, PATTERNS OF SPREAD, AND PATHOLOGY

The rectum is the most common site for intestinal cancer, with 40,000 cases annually, equally divided by gender.

PERSPECTIVE AND PATTERN OF SPREAD

Rectal cancers present according to the early warning signs of change in bowel habits, bleeding into stools, and narrowing or pencil stools. However, such signs are not in keeping with early detection. Rectal cancers should be uncovered in their asymptomatic stage during annually performed rectal examinations and testing for hemoccult blood in the stool. The rectum is perhaps the most common site for intestinal cancer, with 40,000 cases annually, equally divided by gender. Fortunately, the vast majority of cases are controlled, and patients become cancer survivors, often with rectal sphincter preservation. More than 90% of patients become 5-year survivors, and mortality rates have been trending downward, more dramatically in females than males. The histopathology of rectal cancers is mainly adenocarcinoma, and the staging system is not applicable to lymphomas or sarcomas. Cancer spread patterns are both intraperitoneal and extraperitoneal because of its pelvic location (Fig. 32.2; Table 32.2).

The sagittal section is best to illustrate differences in males and females. Figure 32.2A-B correlates with SIMLAP Table 32.2A-B.

- Rectal lesions often present with rectal bleeding (65% to 90%), change in bowel habits (45% to 80%), and diminished stool caliber. Pain and tenesmus may occur as later symptoms. Rectal bleeding is often initially ascribed to hemorrhoids, and the lesions may go uninvestigated for long periods of time, especially in patients 40 years of age or younger. Most rectal cancers can be detected and their mobility defined by a digital rectal examination (65% to 80%). Proctosigmoidoscopy should then be performed with appropriate biopsies to establish the diagnosis.

- Rectal digital examination should be a part of every physical examination on patients older than age 40 years regardless of symptoms or physical condition. If a lesion is found, the inferior extent should be noted (relative to anal verge and coccyx), as well as its location (anterior, posterior, left, right), degree of circumference involved, and degree of mobility (mobile, tethered, fixed).

PATHOLOGY

The histopathology of rectal cancers are mainly adenocarcinomas, and the staging system is not applicable to lymphomas or sarcomas (Table 32.1; Fig. 32.1).

TABLE 32.1	Histopathologic Type: Common Cancers of the Rectum
Type	
Adenocarcinoma in situ	Squamous cell (epidermoid) carcinoma
Adenocarcinoma	Adenosquamous carcinoma
Medullary carcinoma	Small cell carcinoma
Mucinous carcinoma (colloid type; >50% mucinous carcinoma)	Undifferentiated carcinoma
Signet ring cell carcinoma (>50% signet ring cell)	Carcinoma, not otherwise specified

NOS, not otherwise specified.
Reprinted with permission from Edge SB, Byrd DR, Compton CC, et al. *AJCC Cancer Staging Manual*, 7th ed. New York: Springer, 2010, p. 156.

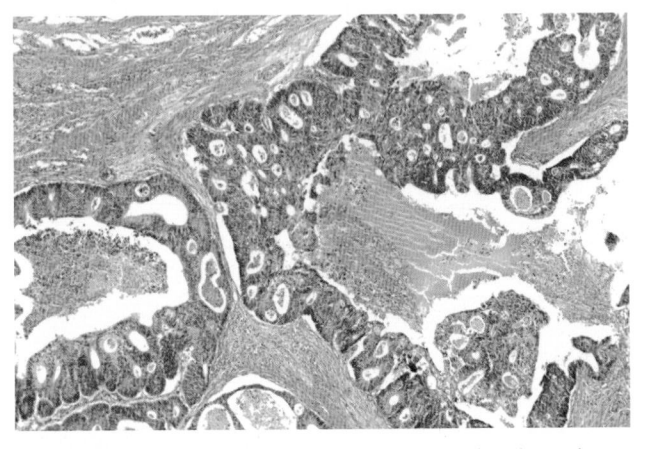

Figure 32.1 | Adenocarcinoma. Microscopically, this colon adenocarcinoma consists of moderately differentiated glands with a prominent cribriform pattern and frequent central necrosis.

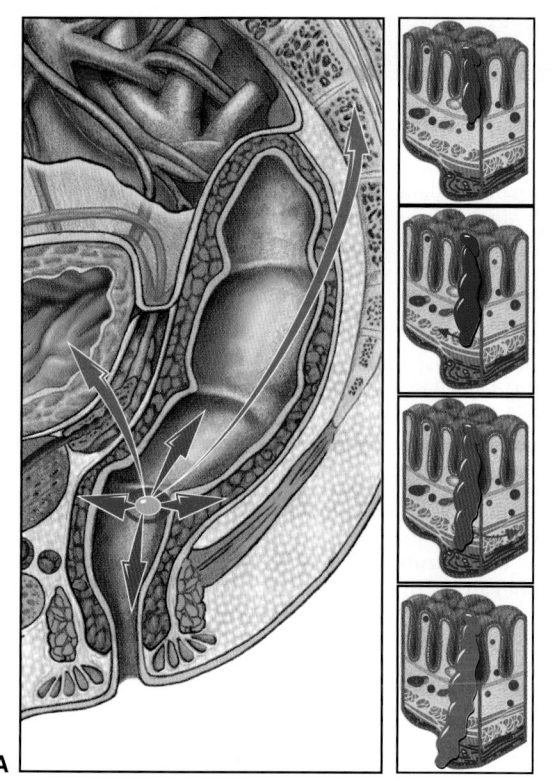
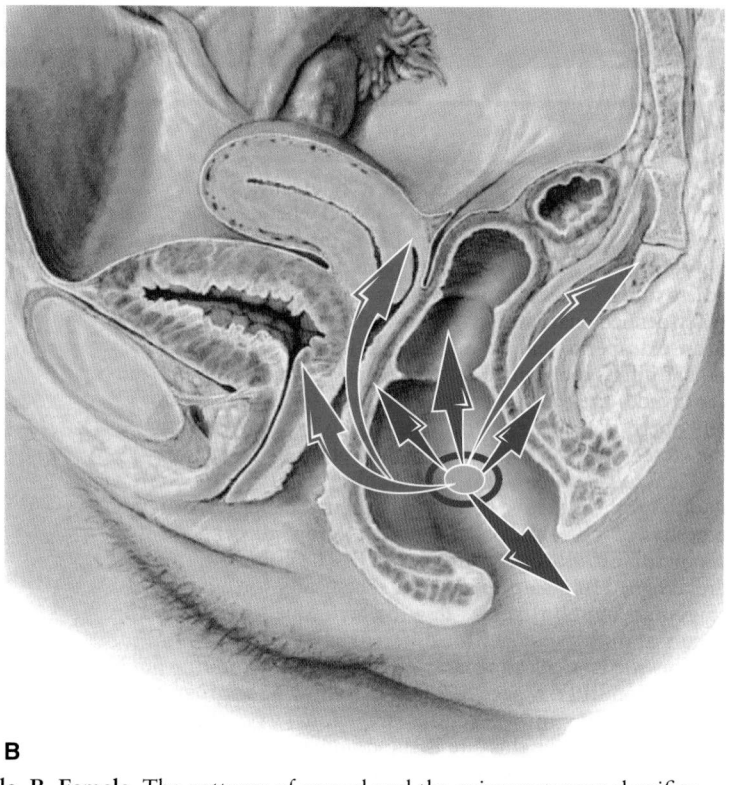

Figure 32.2 | Patterns of spread and T categories. A. Male. B. Female. The patterns of spread and the primary tumor classification are similarly color coded: Tis (cancer in situ of mucosa), yellow; T1 (infiltrates the submucosa), green; T2 (penetrates the muscularis externa), blue; T3 (reaches the subserosa), purple; and T4 (invades through the serosa into a neighboring viscera), red. The concept of visualizing patterns of spread to appreciate the surrounding anatomy is well demonstrated by the six-directional pattern, i.e., SIMLAP Table 32.2.

TABLE 32.2	SIMLAP		

Male Rectum			
S	Sigmoid	• T3	
I	Anus	• T3	
M	Rectum submucosa	• T1	
	Rectum externa	• T2	
	Rectum muscularis	• T2	
	Subserosa	• T3	
L	Levator ani muscle	N1	
	Obturator internus muscle	N1	
A	Prostate	• T4	
	Seminal vesicle	• T4	
	Urinary bladder	• T4	
P	Sacrum	• T4	N1
	Sacreal plexus	• T4	

Female Rectum			
S	Sigmoid	• T3	
	Pouch of Douglas	• T3	
I	Anus	• T3	
M	Rectum submucosa	• T1	
	Rectum externa	• T2	
	Rectum muscularis	• T2	
	Subserosa	• T3	
L	Levator ani muscle	N1	
	Obturator internus muscle	N1	
A	Cervix	• T4	
	Vagina	• T4	
	Urinary bladder	• T4	
P	Sacrum	• T4	N1
	Sacreal plexus	• T4	

The six vectors of invasion are Superior, Inferior, Medial, Lateral, Anterior, and Posterior. The color-coded dots correlate the T stage with specific anatomic structure involved.

T-ONCOANATOMY

ORIENTATION OF THREE-PLANAR ONCOANATOMY

The three-planar anatomic isocenter for the rectum occupies the sacral hollow (S1–S5) inside the true pelvis, retropubically located from an anterior view (Fig. 32.4).

T-oncoanatomy

The T-oncoanatomy is displayed in three planar views. A. Coronal, B. Sagittal, C. Transverse axial. (Fig. 32.5 Male [A,B,C]; Female [A,D,E]).

The rectum, about 12 cm long, extends from a point opposite the third sacral vertebra down to the apex of the prostate in the male and to the apex of the perineal body in the female, that is, to a point 4 cm anterior to the tip of the coccyx. It may be arbitrarily defined as the distal 10 cm of the large intestine, as measured by preoperative sigmoidoscopy from the anal verge (Fig. 32.4).

- *Coronal*: The rectum extends approximately 10 to 12 cm; the retrosigmoid area is 10 to 15 cm from this junction. The rectum has no epiploic appendages, no haustrations, and no teniae. It is covered by peritoneum in front and on both sides in its upper third and on the anterior wall only in its middle third; there is no peritoneal covering in the lower third.

- *Sagittal*: In the lower rectum, the mucosa is thrown into longitudinal folds, known as the rectal columns or the columns of Morgagni. Between them, just above the white line of Hilton, are the anal pits or sinuses. About 4 cm long, the anal canal courses downward and backward from the apex of the prostate or the perineal body. The anocutaneous line (pectinate line), or white line of Hilton, at the base of the rectal columns, marks the site of the original anal membrane that separated the endodermal gut from the ectodermal proctoderm. The transition from colon to rectum has been explicitly defined by the American Joint Committee on Cancer as marked by the fusion of the tenia of the sigmoid colon to the circumferential longitudinal muscle of the rectum. This occurs 12 to 15 cm from the dentate line. The upper third is covered anteriorly and at its sides by peritoneum, which is completely absent in its lower third.

- *Transverse*: The rectouterine cul-de-sac (pouch of Douglas) in females is the rectovesical pouch in males and inferiorly becomes the Denonvilliers fascia, separating and shielding the rectum from direct prostate cancer invasion. The rectal mucosa is smooth and is characterized by transverse folds, the valves of Houston that divide the rectum into thirds. In the three-dimensional three-planar views of the male (Fig. 32.5B,C) and female (Fig. 32.5D,E) pelvises, the axial views are most informative. Comparison of the location of the female cervix with the male prostate and their critical relationship to the rectum and bladder presents a specific challenge to radiation oncologists to avoid injuring this important organ.

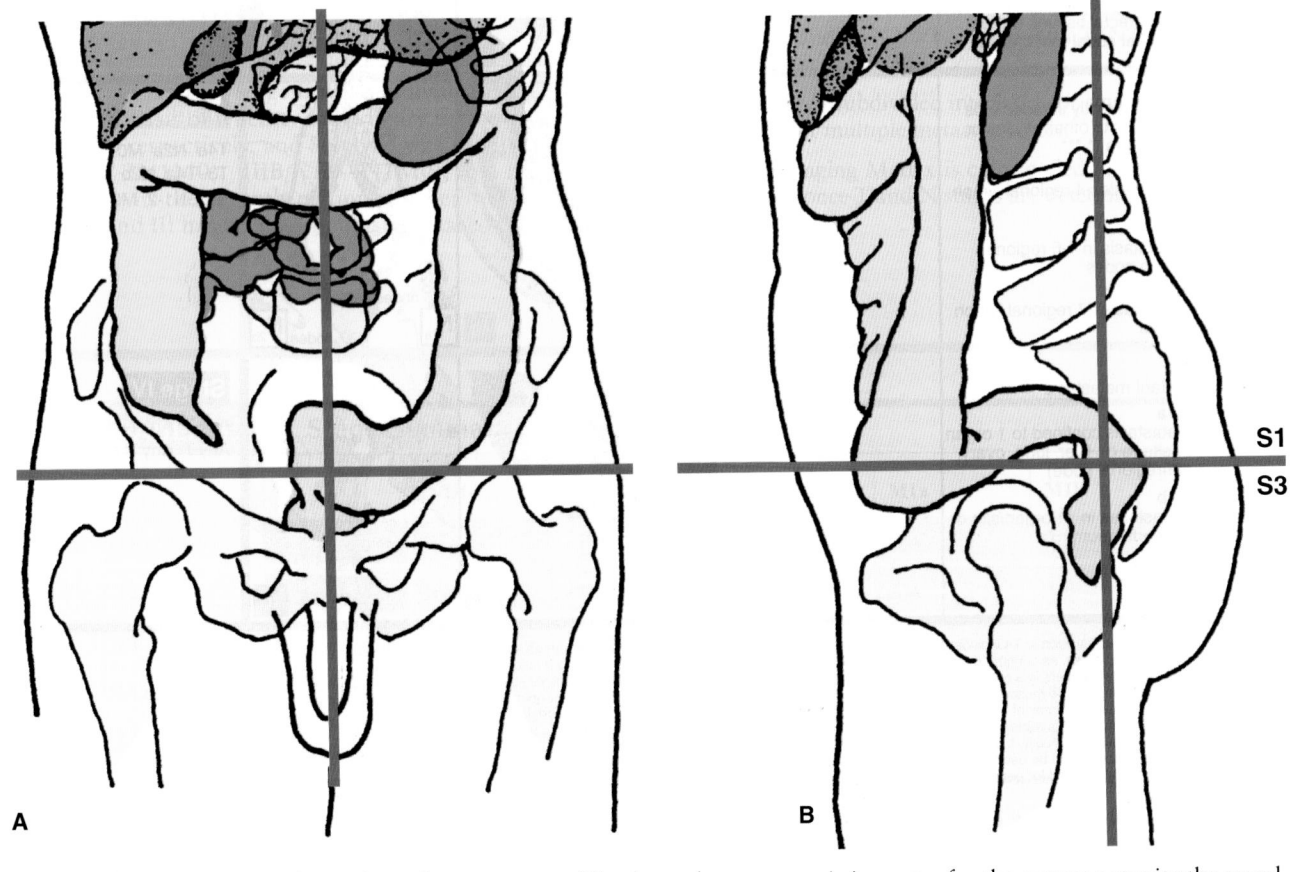

S1
S3

A

B

Figure 32.4 | Orientation and overview of oncoanatomy. The three-planar anatomic isocenter for the rectum occupies the sacral hollow (S1–S5) inside the true pelvis, retropubically located from an anterior view. **A.** Coronal. **B.** Sagittal.

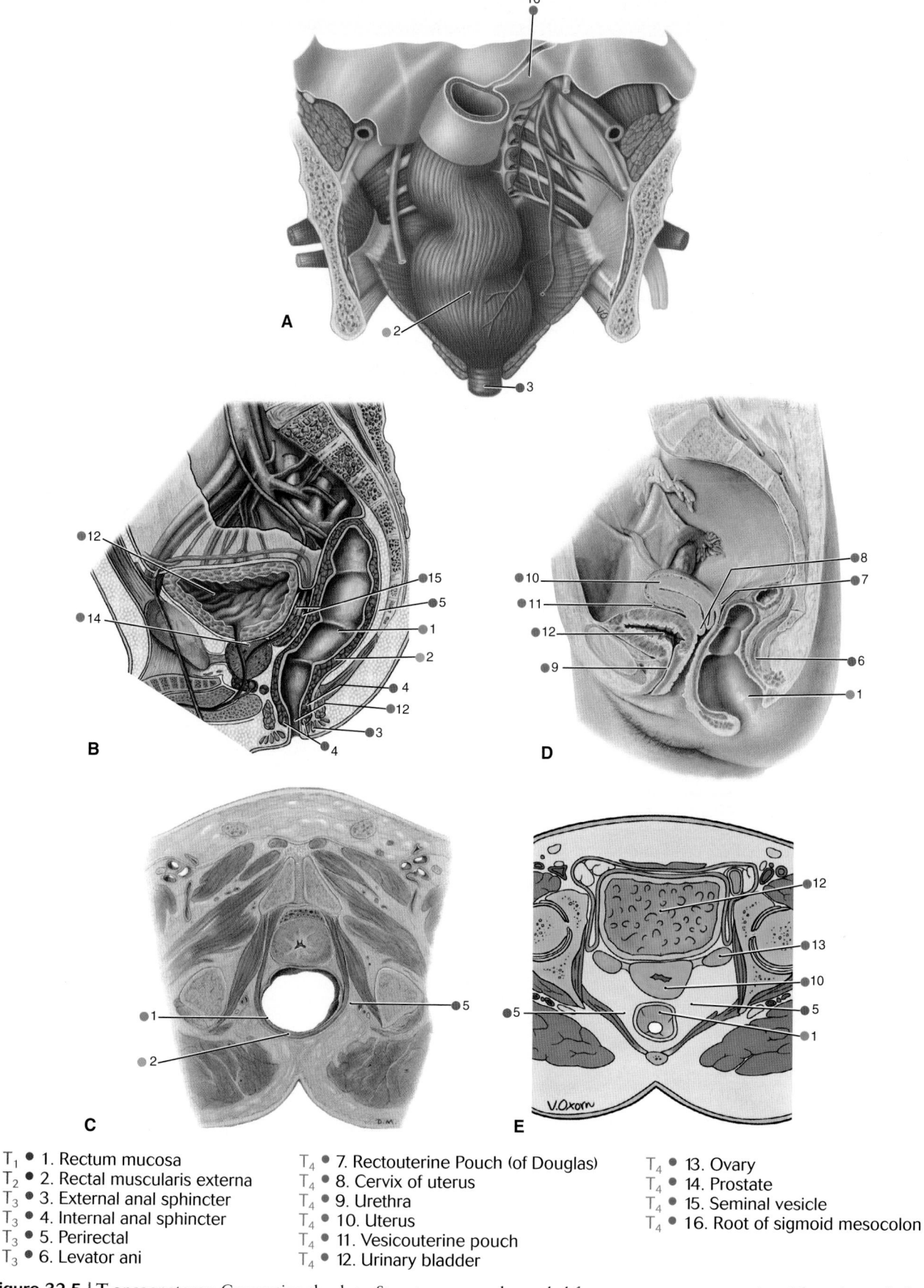

T_1 ● 1. Rectum mucosa	T_4 ● 7. Rectouterine Pouch (of Douglas)	T_4 ● 13. Ovary
T_2 ● 2. Rectal muscularis externa	T_4 ● 8. Cervix of uterus	T_4 ● 14. Prostate
T_3 ● 3. External anal sphincter	T_4 ● 9. Urethra	T_4 ● 15. Seminal vesicle
T_3 ● 4. Internal anal sphincter	T_4 ● 10. Uterus	T_4 ● 16. Root of sigmoid mesocolon
T_3 ● 5. Perirectal	T_4 ● 11. Vesicouterine pouch	
T_3 ● 6. Levator ani	T_4 ● 12. Urinary bladder	

Figure 32.5 | T-oncoanatomy. Connecting the dots. Structures are color coded for cancer stage progression. The color code for the anatomic sites correlates with the color code for the stage group (Fig. 32.3) and patterns of spread (Fig. 32.2) and SIMLAP table (Table 32.2). Connecting the dots in similar colors will provide an appreciation for the 3D oncoanatomy.

N-ONCOANATOMY AND M-ONCOANATOMY

N-ONCOANATOMY

The nodal drainage and distribution follow its blood supply, which is complicated because of its anatomy as both a pelvic and an abdominal organ. The superior third follows the superior rectal lymph nodes, which follow the inferior mesenteric node to the portal and caval nodes. The middle portion drains directly into the pelvic internal iliac nodes. The lower third drains into inguinal lymph nodes (Fig. 32.6A; Table 32.4).

Regional Lymph Nodes

Regional lymph nodes are located (i) along the course of the major vessels supplying the colon and rectum, (ii) along the vascular arcades of the marginal artery, and (iii) adjacent to the colon, that is, located along the mesocolic border of the colon. Specifically, the regional lymph nodes are the pericolic and perirectal nodes and those found along the ileocolic, right colic, middle colic, left colic, inferior mesenteric artery, superior rectal (hemorrhoidal), and internal iliac arteries.

In the assessment of pN, the number of lymph nodes sampled should be recorded. The number of nodes examined from an operative specimen has been reported to be associated with improved survival, possibly because of increased accuracy in staging. It is important to obtain at least 10 to 14 lymph nodes in radical colon and rectum resections in patients without neoadjuvant therapy, but in cases in which tumor is resected for palliation in patients who have received preoperative radiation, fewer lymph nodes may be removed or present. In all cases, however, it is essential that the total number of regional lymph nodes recovered from the resection specimen be described since that number is prognostically important. A pN0 determination is assigned when these nodes are histologically negative, even though fewer than the recommended number of nodes has been analyzed. However, when fewer than the number of nodes recommended by the College of American Pathologists have been found, it is important that pathologists report the degree of diligence of their efforts to find the lymph nodes in the specimen.

The regional lymph nodes for each segment of the large bowel are listed in Table 32.4.*

M-ONCOANATOMY

The venous drainage is different for each third of the rectum owing to its anatomic position as an abdominal and pelvic organ. Superiorly, the superior rectal vein drains into the inferior mesenteric vein and then portal vein, resulting in a high probability of liver metastases. The middle and inferior thirds drain into the internal and external iliac veins and the inferior vena cava and then to the right side of the heart and into lung. The middle rectal vein may predispose to osseous pelvic metastases because of anastomoses of perirectal veins with intervertebral veins (see Fig. 32.6B).

*Preceding passage from Edge SB, Byrd DR, Compton CC, et al., *AJCC Cancer Staging Manual, 7th edition.* New York, Springer, 2010, pp. 145–146.

TABLE 32.4	Lymph Nodes of Rectum
Sentinel Nodes Include Perirectal and Sacral Nodes	
Regional Nodes	**Juxtaregional Nodes**
Perirectal	External iliac
Sigmoid mesenteric	Common iliac
Inferior mesenteric	Para-aortic
Lateral sacral presacral	
Internal iliac	
Superior rectal (hemorrhoidal)	
Middle rectal (hemorrhoidal)	
Inferior rectal (hemorrhoidal)	

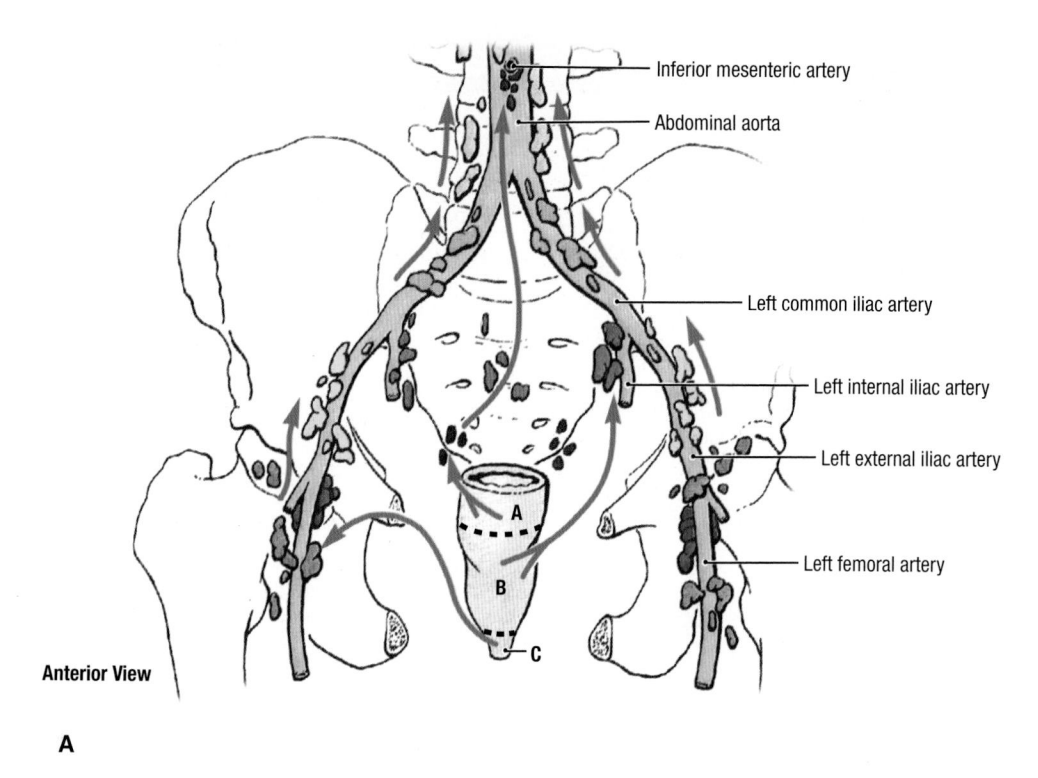

Inferior mesenteric artery

Abdominal aorta

Left common iliac artery

Left internal iliac artery

Left external iliac artery

Left femoral artery

A

B

C

Anterior View

A

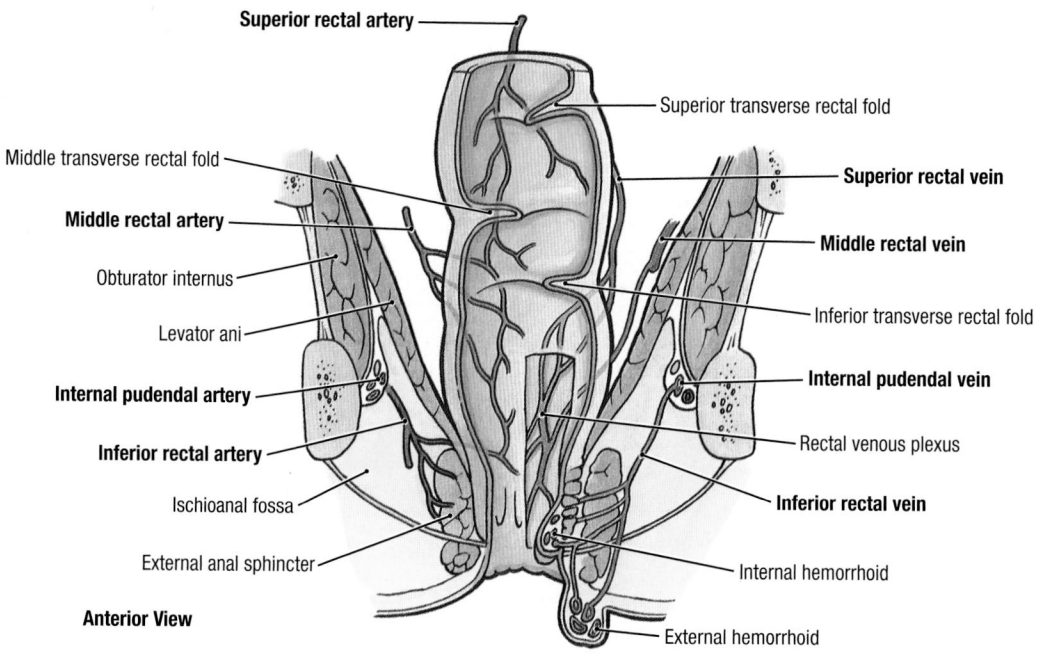

Superior rectal artery

Superior transverse rectal fold

Middle transverse rectal fold

Superior rectal vein

Middle rectal artery

Middle rectal vein

Obturator internus

Inferior transverse rectal fold

Levator ani

Internal pudendal artery

Internal pudendal vein

Inferior rectal artery

Rectal venous plexus

Ischioanal fossa

Inferior rectal vein

External anal sphincter

Internal hemorrhoid

Anterior View

External hemorrhoid

B

Figure 32.6 | A. N-oncoanatomy. Sentinel nodes of the rectum include the pelvic perirectal and sacral nodes. **B. M-oncoanatomy.**

STAGING WORKUP

RULES OF CLASSIFICATION AND STAGING

Clinical Staging and Imaging

Extension of diagnostic imaging to staging is gaining in popularity. Virtual colonoscopy and sigmoidoscopy are challenging endoscopic colonoscopy as to accuracy in diagnosing adenocarcinomas. Endoscopic ultrasound shows the layers of the colon and rectal wall and their penetration by cancer. Endorectal magnetic resonance imaging (MRI) is most valuable to demonstrate extracolonic and extrarectal invasion into adjacent structures. Computed tomography (CT) is preferred for detecting liver and lung metastases (Table 32.5).

Pathologic Staging

The surgically resected rectum and associated lymph nodes removed are assessed. Tumor extension and location of both primary and nodes should be documented. Accurate radial margins should be marked and recorded and are defined "as the surgically dissected surface adjacent to the deepest point of tumor invasion beyond the wall of the rectum." The completeness of resection depends on the clearing of the deepest point of invasion: R0, complete; R1, microscopic; and R2, macroscopic.

Oncoimaging Annotations

- Although colonoscopy is more accurate in assessment for small polyps, overall cost effectiveness is greater when double-contrast barium enema examinations are used.

- CT colonography is a recent addition to the modalities used to screen for colorectal cancer and polyps. This modality requires further refinement and testing before being more widely adopted.

- Transrectal ultrasonography and MRI are able to demonstrate the extent of tumor through the rectal wall and provide some assessment for lymphadenopathy.

- If there is clinical suspicion of metastasis or elevated carcinoembryonic antigen level, CT and MRI are useful for determining the presence and site of recurrent disease. Overall accuracy for the detection of recurrent disease with these modalities is 90% to 95%. This evaluation may require fine-needle aspiration biopsy under direct CT guidance.

- Other noninvasive means to determine the presence or absence of recurrent or metastatic tumor are nuclear medicine scanning techniques with radiolabeled monoclonal antibodies and positron emission tomography techniques using fluorodeoxyglucose. Some of these have shown great potential.

TABLE 32.5	Imaging Modalities for Staging for Rectum and Anus	
Method	Diagnosis and Staging Capability	Recommended for Use
Primary Tumor ± Regional Nodes		
BE	Very useful in detecting and defining primary lesions in the colon	Yes
Endoscopy	Single-contrast study may be less sensitive than double-contrast in detecting polyps	Yes, if used to confirm lesion detected on BE or to screen high-risk patients
Endorectal ultrasound or coil	Very accurate modality for detecting and defining primary lesions In rectum, sigmoid (flex sig), or remaining colon (colonoscopy)	Yes, if preoperative chemoradiation is considered
MRI	Useful in defining depth of penetration of the primary lesion	Yes
CT	Most valuable of all modalities for determining extrarectal or extracolonic local invasion and nodal metastases	Yes
PET	Not useful for staging primary cancer	No
Metastases		
Chest film ± CT	Chest film, best for metastasis screening; CT chest, rules out multiple metastases	Yes
CT abdomen	Most useful study to define para-aortic node enlargement or liver metastases	Yes
Liver ultrasound	Can differentiate between cystic and solid lesions	Yes

BE, barium enema; CT, computed tomography; MRI, magnetic resonance imaging; PET, positron emission tomography.

PROGNOSIS AND CANCER SURVIVAL

PROGNOSIS

The limited number of prognostic factors are listed in Table 32.6.

TABLE 32.6 | Prognostic Factors

Required for staging	None
Clinically significant	Preoperative or pretreatment carcinoembryonic antigen (CEA) (ng/mL)
	Tumor deposits (TDs)
	Circumferential resection margin (CRM)
	Perineural invasion (PN)
	Microsatellite instability (MSI)
	Tumor regression grade (with neoadjuvant therapy)
	K-ras gene analysis

Reprinted with permission from Edge SB, Byrd DR, Compton CC, et al. *AJCC Cancer Staging Manual*, 7th ed. New York: Springer, 2010. p. 155–156.

CANCER STATISTICS AND SURVIVAL

The digestive system, or gastrointestinal tract, which includes MDGs, accounts for 275,000 new patients annually, with colon and rectum responsible for >50%, or about 140,000 new diagnoses annually. Approximately half of these patients eventually die of these cancers. MDG cancers as a group are more lethal; only a handful of patients become long-term survivors. Fortunately, colon and rectal cancers are the most common, with the majority of patients becoming 5-year survivors (63%) responding to chemoradiation programs, often with the sparing of the rectal sphincter with conservative surgery (see Fig. 32.6). Anal cancers are the most responsive to chemoradiation (5-fluorouracil and cisplatin), eliminating the need for surgery. The 5-year survival rate is >90%, with anal sphincter preservation. This regimen has been proven to be very effective in clinical trials and to result in more long-term survivors, which is currently reflected in the literature. Liver, bile duct, and pancreatic cancers are among the poorest in the terms of survival, which is often measured in months rather than years.

The rectum accounted for approximately 39,670 new cancer cases, with a 5-year survival rate improvement over the last five decades of 23%. Currently, relative 5-year survival for all stages is 62.3%, but, when localized, it improves to 90.1% (see Table 23.8). Local recurrence is highly dependent on site in the rectum, that is, 18% overall for tumors <7 cm from the anal verge. Stage is a strong prognosticator for local recurrence, that is, T1, T2 38% and T3, T4 30%, but with positive node failure it doubles to 65% (Fig. 32.8).

Note the anachronism of Stage IIIA equalling Stage I = 74% 5 year survival. Stage IIIA is similar T1, T2 but N1c are tumor deposits in subserosa or mesentery without lymph node involvement. More often N1a and N1b have one or 2 to 3 nodes associated with T3, T4 primaries.

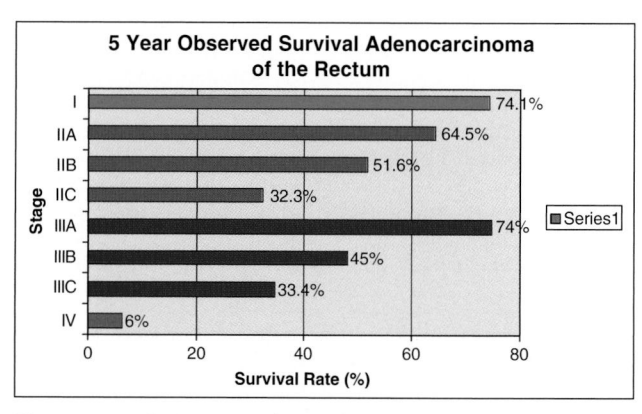

Figure 32.8 | Five-year observed survival adenocarcinoma of the rectum. (Data from Edge SB, Byrd DR, Compton CC, et al. AJCC Cancer Staging Manual, 7th ed. New York: Springer, 2010, p. 154.)

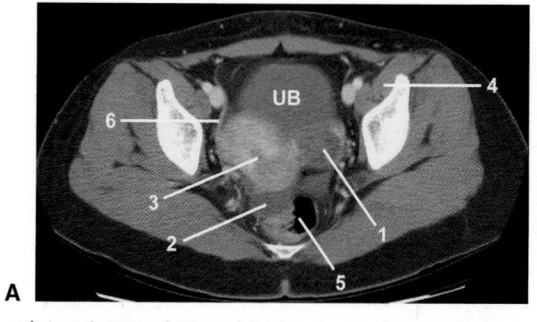
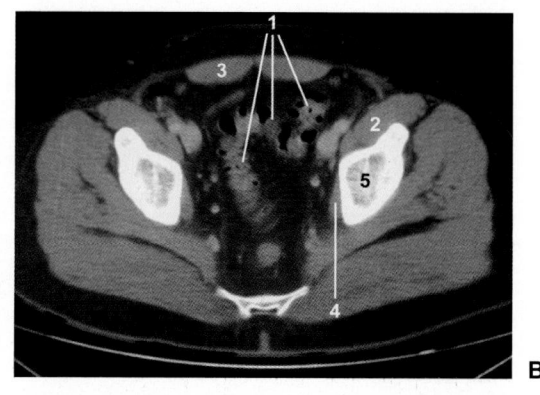

Figure 32.7 | Axial CTs of S1 and S3 level correlate with the T-oncoanatomy transverse section. Oncoimaging with CT is commonly applied to staging cancers, often combined with PET to determine true extent of primary cancer and involved lymph nodes. **A.** Female (correlates with Fig. 32.5E). 1. Left ovary. 2. Physiologic free fluid. 3. Uterus (endometrial cavity (normal in menstruating-age females). 4. Iliopsoas muscle. 5. Rectum. 6. Round ligament of uterus. UB, urinary bladder. **B.** Male (correlates with Fig. 32.5C). 1. Sigmoid colon. 2. Iliopsoas muscle. 3. Rectus abdominus muscle. 4. Obturator internus muscle. 5. Acetabular roof.

33

Anus

PERSPECTIVE, PATTERNS OF SPREAD, AND PATHOLOGY

Because of invasion and fissures, depending on location, these cancers are intersphincteric, extrasphincteric, or transphincteric, tunneling through perianal sphincter and fat to skin surface perianally (fistula-in-anus).

PERSPECTIVE AND PATTERN OF SPREAD

To understand the transformation to different malignancies in the anus and anal canal, its embryology is pivotal. The dentate line represents the junction between endoderm and ectoderm. Innervation blood supply and lymphatics vary accordingly. Proximal to the dentate line are autonomic nerves, sympathetic and parasympathetic versus somatic. Pain above the dentate line is perceived much less than that below it, where biopsies require anesthesia. The seventh edition of the American Joint Committee on Cancer (AJCC) *AJCC Cancer Staging Manual* details diagrammatically the anus and anal

TABLE 33.1	World Health Organization Classification of Carcinoma of the Anal Canal

Type
Squamous cell carcinoma
Adenocarcinoma
Rectal type
Of anal glands
Within anorectal fistula
Mucinous adenocarcinoma
Small cell carcinoma
Undifferentiated carcinoma

Used with the permission of the American Joint Committee on Cancer (AJCC) Chicago, Illinois. The original source for this material is the *AJCC Cancer Staging Manual,* Seventh edition (2010) published by Springer SBM, LLC, p 170.

canal and portrays lymphatic drainage as a function of the primary location; it is discussed in the N-oncoanatomy section. Anal cancers provide new evidence for the role of immunosuppression and viral infections in carcinogenesis. Of the 5,000 new patients expected annually, there is a bioassociation with condylomata (human papilloma virus and human immunodeficiency virus, with a higher incidence of anal cancer in homosexuals with acquired immunodeficiency syndrome). The anal canal is a transitional zone marked by the pectinate line, or mucocutaneous junction. The two predominant histologic types of anal carcinoma are variants of squamous cell cancers. Basaloid (cloacogenic) cancers arise at this junction, whereas more typical epidermoid cancers occur on the skin. The epicenter of the cancer determines its origin. According to the AJCC, cancers are anal tumors if their epicenter is ≤2 cm from the pectinate line; otherwise, they are rectal cancers with epicenters >2 cm proximal to the dentate line.

Anal sphincter preservation with radiochemotherapy is the standard of treatment for most patients with anal cancers. In fact, the application of similar treatment regimens to rectal and esophageal cancers has improved their survival outcomes with normal tissue and organ conservation. Size of tumor determines the staging categories rather than depth of invasion, similar to the skin cancer classification.

Note: It is important is to recognize the anatomic differences in males versus females as to surrounding structures. In the male, there are solid structures above the anal canal, that is, prostate, penis crura, and urethra, whereas in the female, the vaginal tube and vulva separate the urethra. Thus, different SIMLAP tables are provided (Fig. 33.1; Table 33.2).

PATHOLOGY

The anal canal is a transitional zone marked by the pectinate line, or mucocutaneous junction. The two predominant histologic types of anal carcinoma are variants of squamous cell cancers. Basaloid (cloacogenic) cancers arise at this junction, whereas more typical epidermoid cancers occur on the skin (Table 33.1).

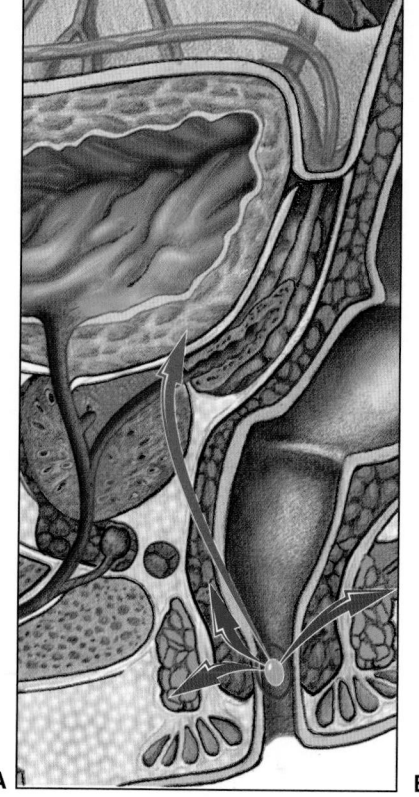 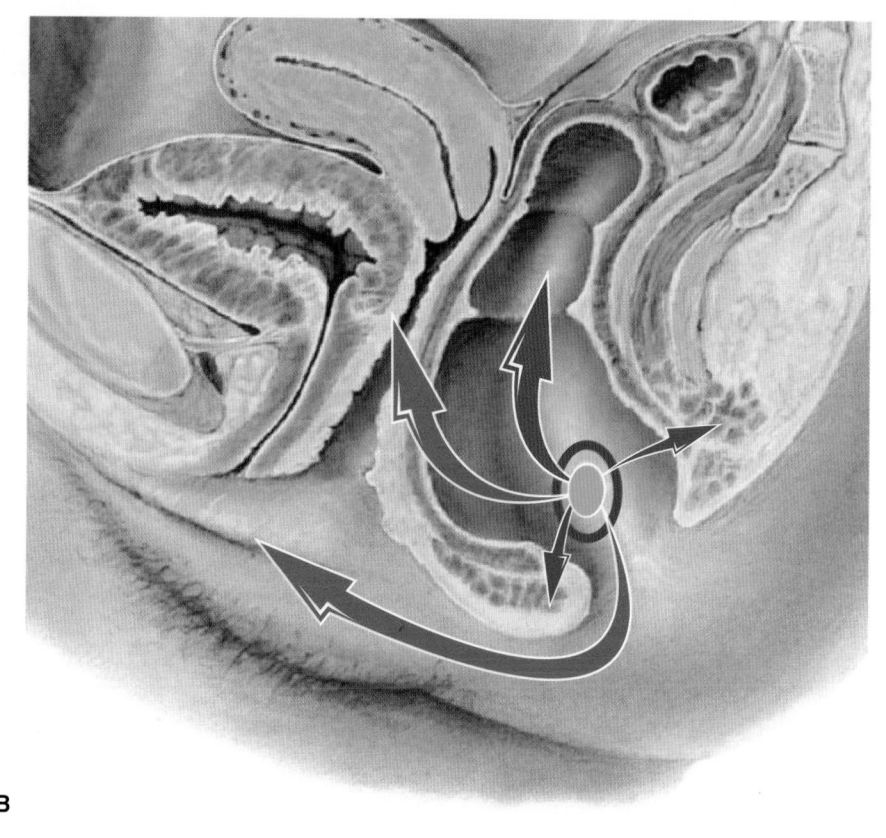

Figure 33.1 | **Patterns of spread for anal cancer are color coded for T stage. A. Male. B. Female.** Tis, yellow; T1, green; T2, blue; T3, purple; and T4, red. The concept of visualizing patterns of spread to appreciate the surrounding anatomy is well demonstrated by the six-directional pattern, i.e., SIMLAP Table 33.2A/B.

TABLE 33.2	SIMLAP

Male Anus		
S Rectum	• T3	
I Skin of anus	• T3	
Scrotum	• T4	
M Anal canal	• T1	• T2
Pectin of anal canal	• T1	• T2
L External anal sphincter	• T3	
Ischial rectal space	• T3	
A Scrotum	• T4	
Penis	• T4	
Urethra	• T4	
P Sacrum, coccyx	• T4	N1

Female Anus		
S Rectum	• T3	
I Skin of anus	• T3	
M Vulva, labia majora	• T4	
Labia majora	• T1	• T2
L External anal sphincter	• T3	
Levator ani muscle	• T3	
Ischial rectal space	• T3	
A Vagina	• T4	
Vulva, labia majora	• T4	
Urethra	• T4	
Bladder	• T4	
P Sacrum, coccyx	• T4	N1

The six vectors of invasion are Superior, Inferior, Medial, Lateral, Anterior, and Posterior. The color-coded dots correlate the T stage with specific anatomic structure involved.

TNM STAGING CRITERIA

TNM STAGING CRITERIA

The anatomy reflects the spread pattern. There is an important distinction between cancers of the anal canal (extending from the rectum to the pectinate line) and cancers on the perineal aspect of the anus to the pectinate line. Anal margin lesions are distal to the anal verge, where hair-bearing skin occurs. Cancers of the anal canal are of greater concern because they are more likely to invade the rectal sphincters and open more pathways of spread deep into the pelvis via lymphatics and hemorrhoidal veins.

The TNM staging of anal cancer has not changed. Primary anal cancers are staged based on size of the cancer rather than depth. However, it should be noted that direct invasion of the rectal wall or anal and rectal sphincter invasions are T3 and T4 cancers. Evidence of an adjacent organ, such as vagina, urethra, or bladder, is required.

Generally, there is no overarching principle or context design for the digestive system (gastrointestinal tract) or major digestive glands (MDGs). Stages are frequently expanded to six by subdividing stages into A and B. The T and N categories are assigned to a stage grouping, specifically for division of a stage into more (a) versus less (b) favorable groupings. This occurs at different stages for different sites. Specifically, this site has a similar pattern of T stage progression as N stage progression, with T3/T4 = N1; stage III is divided into A/B/C (i.e., IIIA = T3, IIIB = T4); and IIIC is N1.

SUMMARY OF CHANGES SEVENTH EDITION AJCC

- *The definitions of TNM and the stage groupings for this chapter have not changed from the sixth edition (Fig. 33.2).*
- *The descriptions of both the boundaries of the anal canal and anal carcinomas have been clarified.*
- *The collection of the reported status of the tumor for the presence of human papilloma virus is included.*

The TNM Staging Matrix is color coded for identification of Stage Group once T and N stages are determined (Table 33.3).

TABLE 33.3	Stage Summary Matrix			
	N0	**N1**	**N2**	**N3**	**M1**
T1	I	IIIA	IIIB	IIIB	IV
T2	II	IIIA	IIIB	IIIB	IV
T3	II	IIIA	IIIB	IIIB	IV
T4	IIIA	IIIB	IIIB	IIIB	IV

Progression of T stage determines stage group progression:
- *T stage T_1 = IA, T_2 = IIA, T_3 = III*
- *N stage determines substage N_1, IIB*
- *M stage is a separate stage*

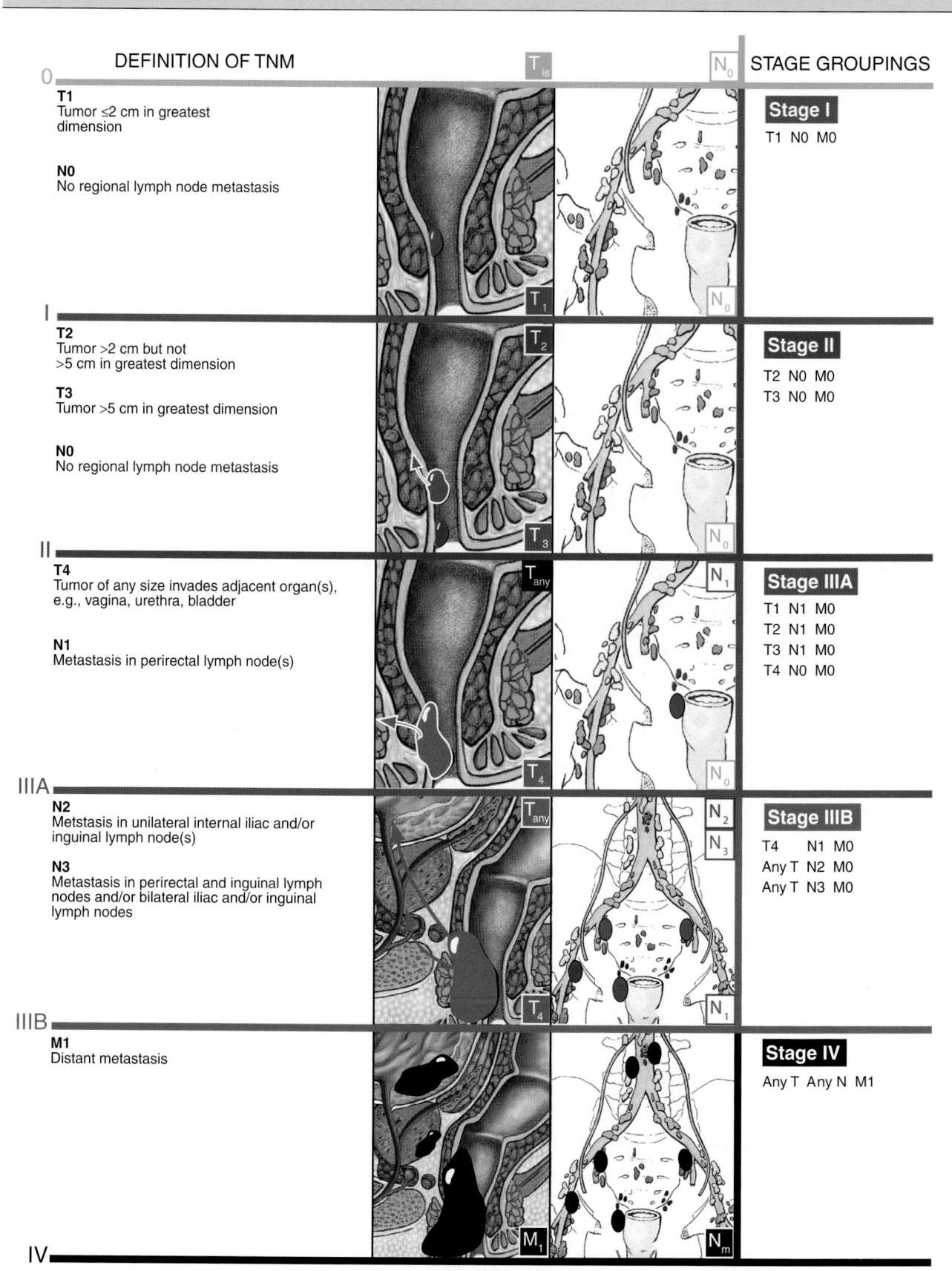

Figure 33.2 | TNM staging diagram presents a vertical arrangement with color bars encompassing TN combinations showing progression. Anal cancers are very chemoradiation sensitive, and response and survival rates are high, with anal preservation. Stage 0, yellow; I, green; II, blue; III, purple; IV, red; and IV (metastatic), black. Definitions of TN on left and stage grouping on right.

T-ONCOANATOMY

ORIENTATION OF THREE-PLANAR ONCOANATOMY

The anatomic isocenter for the anus is below the coccyx in line with the pubic bone and femoral heads and is readily identified on physical examination (Fig. 33.3).

T-oncoanatomy

Orientation views are presented in Fig. 34.3 and three-planar views in Fig. 34.4A–C. The T-oncoanatomy is displayed in three planar views. **A:** Coronal. **B:** Sagittal. **C:** Transverse axial

(Fig. 33.4 Male [A,B,C]; Female [A,B,D]). The terminal portion of the digestive system has a complex anatomy and is best viewed as follows:

- *Coronal:* Defines the anorectal line, the columns of Morgagni, and the pectinate line at the mucocutaneous junction. The anal canal extends from the dentate or pectinate line to the hair-bearing skin.

- *Sagittal:* It offers views of the various spaces of the perineopelvic region: perianal, postanal, superficial and deep, and submucosal and presacral.

- *Transverse:* Differentiates the anatomy of the female and male pelvises. The axial views relate the female and male genitalia to the anus.

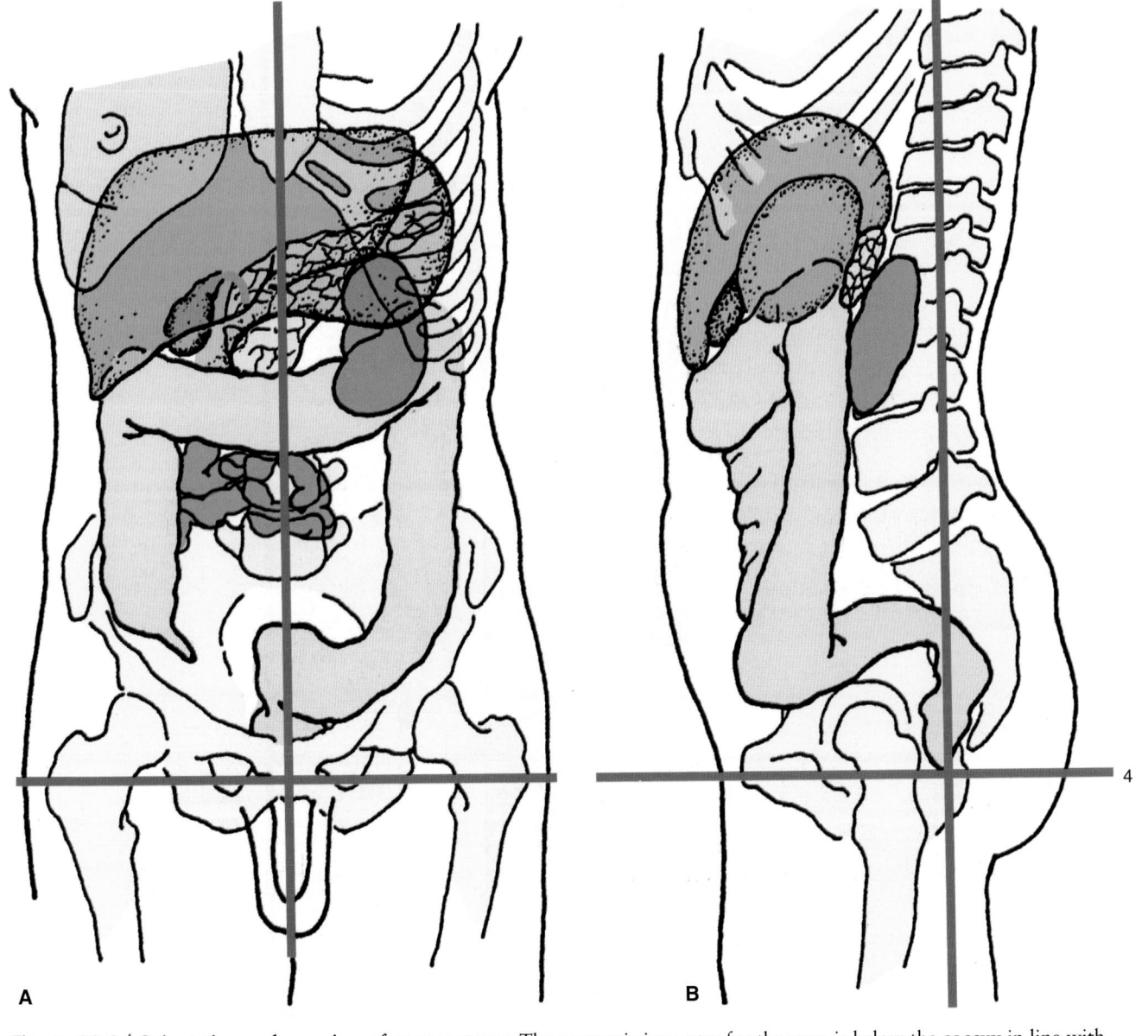

Figure 33.3 | Orientation and overview of oncoanatomy. The anatomic isocenter for the anus is below the coccyx in line with the pubic bone and femoral heads and is readily identified on physical examination. **A.** Coronal. **B.** Sagittal.

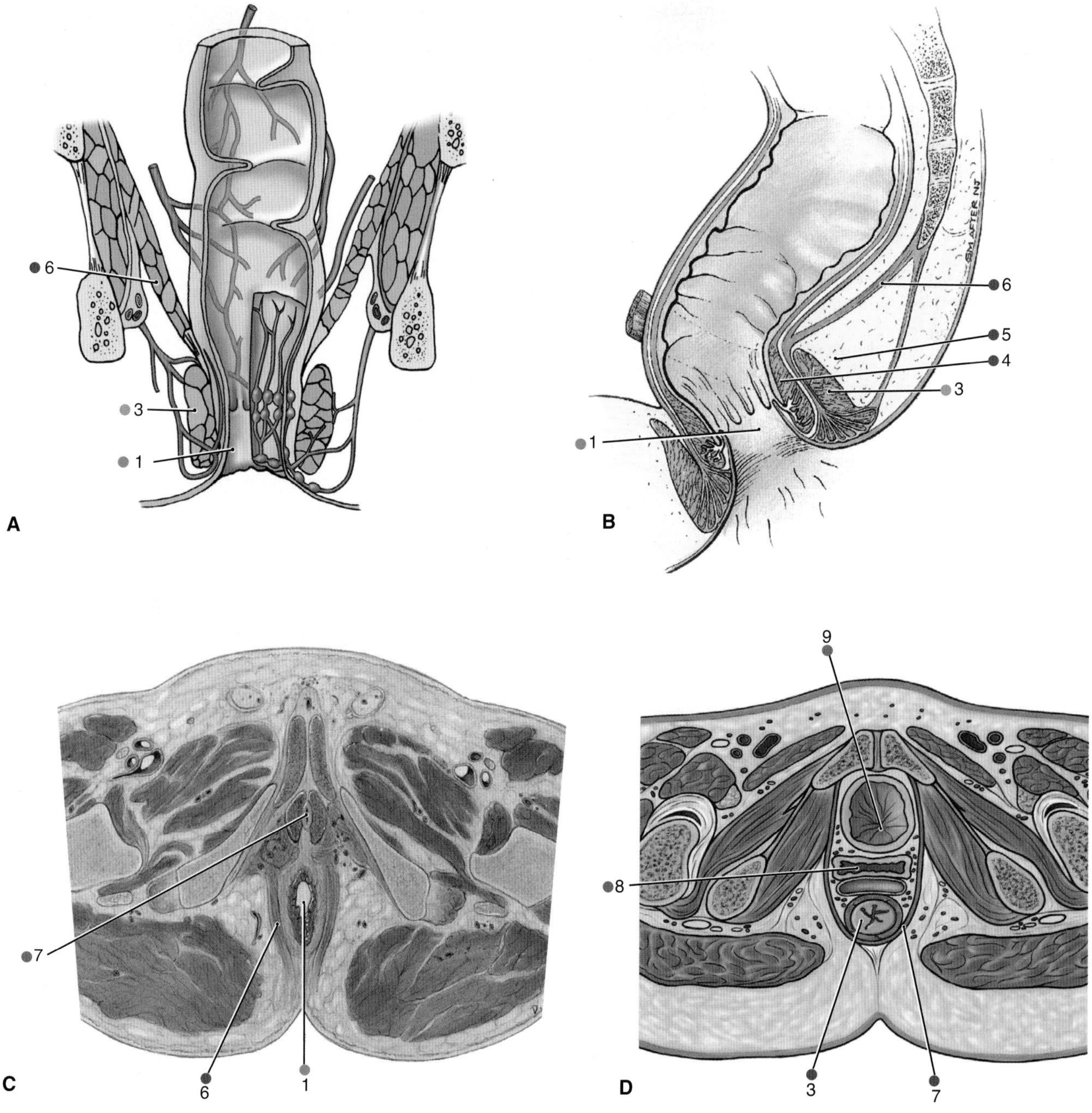

T_1 • 1. Rectum mucosa	T_3 • 4. Internal anal sphincter	T_4 • 7. Urethra
T_2 • 2. Rectal muscularis externa	T_3 • 5. Perirectal	T_4 • 8. Vagina
T_3 • 3. External anal sphincter	T_3 • 6. Levator ani	T_4 • 9. Urinary bladder

Figure 33.4 | T-oncoanatomy. Connecting the dots. Structures are color coded for cancer stage progression. The color code for the anatomic sites correlates with the color code for the stage group (Fig. 33.2) and patterns of spread (Fig. 33.1) and SIMLAP table (Table 33.2). Connecting the dots in similar colors will provide an appreciation for the 3D oncoanatomy.

N-ONCOANATOMY AND M-ONCOANATOMY

N-ONCOANATOMY

The nodal drainage again depends on which side of the pectinate line the anal cancer has its epicenter. For cancers of the anal verge, the lymphatic drainage is into inguinal nodes and then external iliac nodes. For cancers of the anal canal, particularly involving the rectum, the drainage is into internal iliac nodes. Both external and internal iliac nodes eventually drain into the common iliacs and para-aortic nodes (Fig. 33.5A; Table 33.4).

New diagrams in the seventh edition of the *AJCC Manual* portray lymph nodes at risk as a function of advancement.

N1 represents perirectal nodes in the presacral area.

N2 represents unilateral inguinal nodes with Ts below the dentate line or unilateral iliac and obturator nodes above the dentate line.

N3 can be combinations of N1 and N2 and include the following:

  A. Perirectal/inguinal unilateral nodes

  B. Bilateral internal iliac nodes

  C. Bilateral internal iliac and inguinal nodes

Regional Lymph Nodes

Lymphatic drainage and nodal involvement of anal cancers depend on the location of the primary tumor. Tumors above the dentate line spread primarily to the anorectal, perirectal, and paravertebral nodes, whereas tumors below the dentate line spread primarily to the superficial inguinal nodes.

The regional lymph nodes are as follows:

Perirectal

  Anorectal

  Perirectal

  Lateral sacral

Internal iliac (hypogastric)

Inguinal

  Superficial

All other nodal groups represent sites of distant metastasis.*

M-ONCOANATOMY

The venous drainage varies and is related to whether the primary is above or below the dentate line (DL) (Fig. 33.5B).

• Above the DL, the drainage is via the middle and superior rectal veins, placing liver metastases as the target organ.

• Below the DL, drainage is to inferior rectal vein and anastomosis to superficial inguinal/femoral vein branches and then into external iliacs; lung metastases can occur via inferior vena cava.

*Preceding passage from Edge SB, Byrd DR, Compton CC, et al., *AJCC Cancer Staging Manual, 7th edition*. New York, Springer, 2010, p. 166.

TABLE 33.4	Lymph Nodes of Anus
Sentinel Nodes Include Perirectal and Inguinal Nodes	
Regional Nodes	**Juxtaregional Nodes**
Perirectal	External iliac
Anorectal	Common iliac
Perirectal	Para-aortic
Lateral sacral	
Internal iliac (hypogastric)	
Inguinal	
Superficial	
Deep femoral	

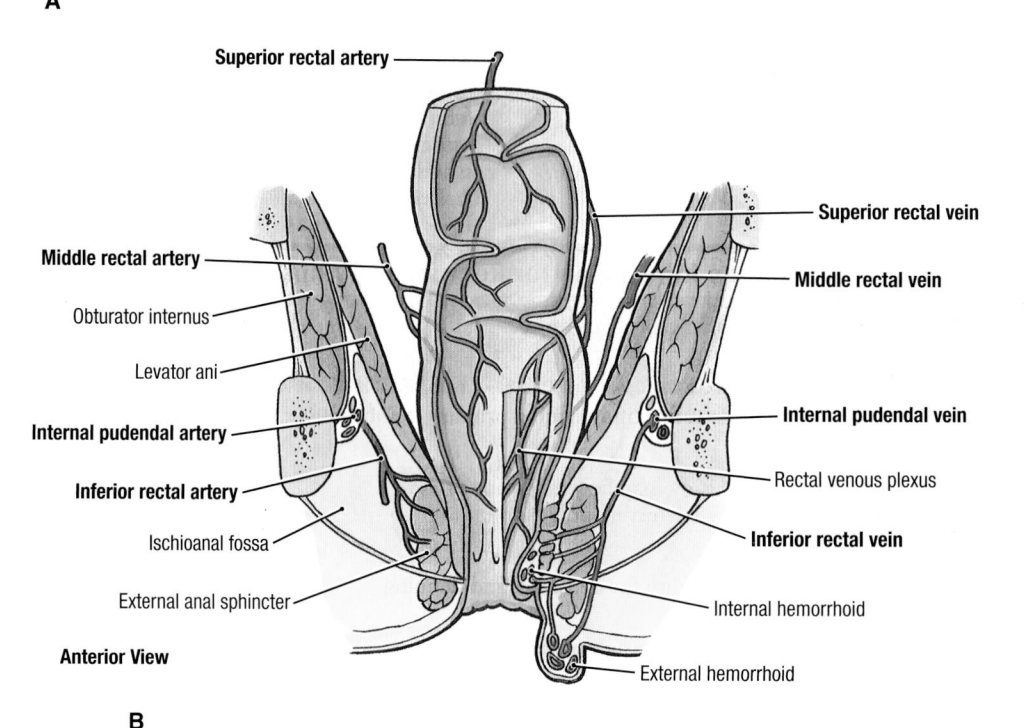

Figure 33.5 | A. N-oncoanatomy. Sentinel nodes of the anus are inguinal nodes. **B.** M-oncoanatomy. The anus and inferior portion of the rectum drain via the inferior and middle rectal veins, into the internal iliac veins, and then into the common iliacs and inferior vena cava. Thus, lung metastases are more common in this site as compared to other sites in the gastrointestinal system.

SECTION 4
Male Genital Tract and Urinary System Primary Sites

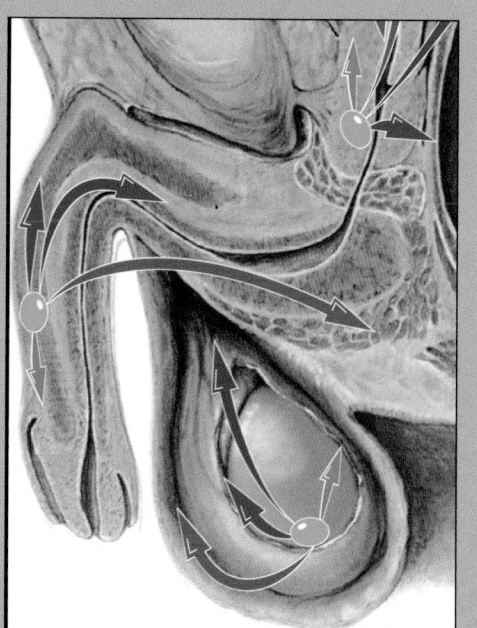

34

Introduction and Orientation

PERSPECTIVE AND PATTERNS OF SPREAD

The TNM staging system of the male genitourinary tract (MGU) depends on whether the organ oncoanatomy is solid and encapsulated or hollow and tubular.

PERSPECTIVE AND PATTERNS OF SPREAD

The urinary tract of kidney, renal pelvis and ureter, urinary bladder, and urethra can frequently be involved with carcinogenesis owing to the excretion of toxic antigenic products or proteins, which can be harmful and transform their epithelial lining. Carcinogenic field effects, cancer in situ, and seeding of the excretory urinary system are major concerns; instead of a single tumor, there can be multiple cancers. Of interest, patterns of spread are limited often to the urinary system; however, juxtaposed structures are at risk (Fig. 34.1; Table 34.1AB). Prostate cancer, which is the dominant malignancy in males, particularly among those >50 years of age, is included with cancers of the MGU. With each decade of age it increases in incidence, affecting every other male in his 80s. In contrast, testicular cancer is the most common tumor in younger males (30–50 years). Prostate and testicular cancers are among the most highly curable tumors owing to both early diagnosis and advances in multimodal treatment.

Tests for male genital cancers were among the first to incorporate the leading-edge advances in molecular biomarker prognosticators. The development of serum prostate-specific antigen (PSA) into a universal serum screening test has completely changed prostate cancer from a clinically palpable tumefaction to a nonpalpable early-stage disease for which histologic confirmation by needle biopsy is necessary to establish its existence (i.e., T1c). Serum PSA is a powerful prognosticator and is the most useful clinical biomarker for prostate cancer, which includes its rate of increase or doubling time. In testicular tumors, several serum markers exist, namely alpha fetoprotein, human chorionic gonadotropin, and lactate dehydrogenase. Staging of testicular cancers is unique because it involves the first durable instance of biomarker inclusion in the TNM staging system (Table 34.1). Furthermore, these molecular markers are useful in determining "cure" or control of the cancer and are often the first evidence of relapse if they are found to be elevated in follow-up visits.

Applying the **SIMLAP concept** to each organ in the MGU allows for understanding the anatomic interrelationships and is presented here using prostate cancer as an illustration. The prostate gland occupies a similar position to that of the cervix in the female pelvis. The prostate gland is at the anatomic isocenter in the male pelvis:

- Superior is the urinary bladder.
- Inferior is the bulb of the penis.
- Medial is the urethra.
- Lateral is the pelvic sidewall, acetebulum, and femoral head.
- Anterior is the pubic bone.
- Posterior is the rectum.

The six vectors of invasion are superior, inferior, medial, lateral, anterior, and posterior. The color-coded dots in the respective SIMLAP tables correlate the T stage with the specific anatomic structure involved.

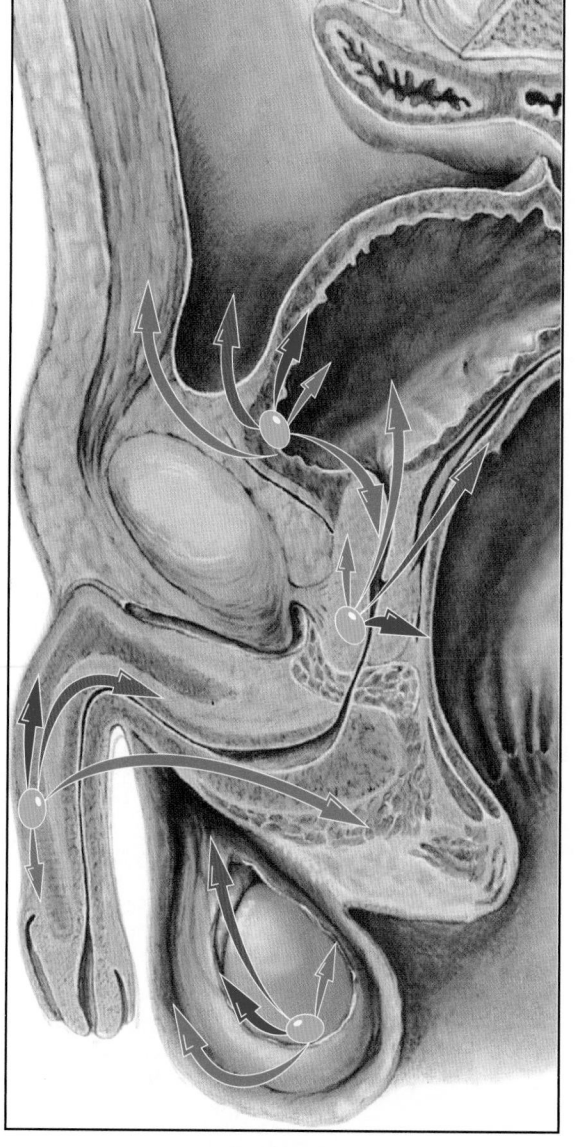

Figure 34.1 | Patterns of spread. The cancer at each primary site is presented at the different anatomic locations of the MGU, color-coded as to stage: T0, Tis, Ta, yellow; T1, green; T2, blue; T3, purple; T4, red. The primary sites shown are from superior to inferior: the urinary bladder, the prostate, the penis, and the testes.

TABLE 34.1A   SIMLAP Prostate

S	Urinary bladder	• T3a
	Ureter, unilateral	• T3b
	Ureter, bilateral	• T3b
I	External urethral sphincter	• T4
	Urethra	• T4
	Bulb of penis	• T4
M	Prostatic urethra	• T2
	Lobe (half)	• T2a
	Lobe (one)	• T2b
	Lobe (both)	• T2c
L	Seminal vesicles	• T3b
	Levator ani	• T4
	Ischiorectal fossa	• T4
A	Puboprostatic ligament	• T4
	Pubis symphysis	• T4
	Venous plexus	• T4
P	Denonvilliers' fascia	• T4
	Rectum	• T4

The six vectors of invasion are Superior, Inferior, Medial, Lateral, Anterior, and Posterior. The color-coded dots correlate the T stage with specific anatomic structure involved.

TABLE 34.1B   SIMLAP

Male Urinary Bladder

S	Peritoneum	• T4b	
	Small intestine	• T4b	
	Ureters	• T3	
	Prostate	• T4a	
	Exterior urethral		
I	Sphincter	• T4b	
	Urethra	• T4b	
	Bulb of penis	• T4b	
	Spongy urethra	• T4b	
M			
L	Levator ani muscle	• T4b	
	Obturator lymph node	N1	
	Internal iliac vein/artery/nodes	N2	
A	Retropubic space	• T4b	
	Pubis	• T4b	
	Trigone bladder		
P	Wall	• T2	• T3
	Seminal vesicles	• T3	
	Ureters	• T3	
	Rectum	• T4a	

The six vectors of invasion are Superior, Inferior, Medial, Lateral, Anterior, and Posterior. The color-coded dots correlate the T stage with specific anatomic structure involved.

TNM STAGING CRITERIA

CLASSIFICATION AND STAGING

TNM Staging Criteria

Pathology in terms of Gleason grade was added to the TNM anatomic criteria in the sixth edition of the American Joint Committee on Cancer's *AJCC Cancer Staging Manual*, and the PSA has been added in the seventh edition. Both bound and free PSA levels are useful. Thus, both the PSA and Gleason grade pathology have been incorporated into the staging system, extending criteria beyond anatomic factors.

The oncoanatomy paradigm of solid versus hollow organs is a dichotomy in organ anatomic architecture that applies to the male genitourinary system.

The staging system is based on the pattern of spread, which depends on whether the organ oncoanatomy is solid and encapsulated or hollow and tubular. With solid organs, tumor growth within the capsule has a good prognosis; however, once the capsule is breeched or penetrated, the likelihood of a successful outcome decreases (Fig. 34.2). The solid organs are kidney, prostate, and testes. Urinary tract cancers of the renal pelvis, ureters, and bladder follow the classification and staging of thin-walled, hollow organs lined with transitional epithelium over their musculature. That is, the depth of penetration of the layers in their wall determines the T stage (Fig. 34.2). The adoption of the alphabetical American Urological Association classification into the TNM language has allowed for unification of the literature. The poorly differentiated variety of cancers, especially in solid organs, can result in widespread lymphatic and hematogenous metastases. Virtually every remote and distant site can be involved. Kidney cancer has a predilection for lung, as do most testicular cancers, but bone and brain are often sites for dissemination.

An especially unique metastatic pattern is the predilection of prostate cancer to form axial vertebral metastases. The extensive osteoblastic sclerosis of bone is virtually pathognomonic when pelvis, lumbar, and thoracic vertebral bodies appear uniformly positive first on bone scans and then as white, dense bones in radiographs. This has been attributed to retrograde venous spread of prostate cancer cells from the periprostatic plexus of veins to Batson's vertebral venous plexus.

SUMMARY OF CHANGES SEVENTH EDITION AJCC

The classification of solid organs, the kidney, prostate, and testes depends on whether the tumor is confined (T1T2) or invasion through their adventitial fibrous capsule (T3) and into surrounding adjacent structures or fixation to bone (T4) has occurred (Fig. 34.2). The renal pelvis and ureter are staged similar to the bladder, and their cancers follow the same pattern for staging hollow viscera as in the digestive system: T1, mucosal; T2, submucosal muscle layer; T3, fibrous outer wall or peritoneum; and T4, invasion into adjacent tissues. The T stage determines the stage group. The N1 and M1 are considered stage IV.

The Stage Summary Matrix for Renal Cell Cancer indicates the general rule for most MGU Cancer Sites. That is, the T category determines the Stage Group whereas Testis is unique and perhaps a vision of the future in staging cancers in that serum markers are the dominant factor where the TNM paradigm is simplified. The cancer progresses in T stage then N and followed by M for Stage Group I–>II–>III respectively (Table 34.1C and Table 34.1D).

TABLE 34.1D Testes Stage Summary Matrix

	T1	T2	T3	T4	
N0	*I	I	I	I	SX
N0	IA	IB	IB	IB	S0
N0	IS	IS	IS	IS	S1-3
N1-3	II	II	II	II	SX
N1	IIA	IIA	IIA	IIA	S0-1
N2	IIB	IIB	IIB	IIB	S0-1
N3	IIC	IIC	IIC	IIC	S0-1
M1	III	III	III	III	SX
M1a	IIIA	IIIA	IIIA	IIIA	S0-1
N1-3/M0	IIIB	IIIB	IIIB	IIIB	S2
Any N/M1a	IIIB	IIIB	IIIB	IIIB	S2
N1-3/M0	IIIC	IIIC	IIIC	IIIC	S3
Any N/M1a	IIIC	IIIC	IIIC	IIIC	S3
Any N/M1b	IIIC	IIIC	IIIC	IIIC	Any S

TABLE 34.1C Kidney Stage Summary Matrix

	N0	N1	N2	M1
T1	I	III	IV	IV
T2	II	III	IV	IV
T3	III	III	IV	IV
T4	IV	IV	IV	IV

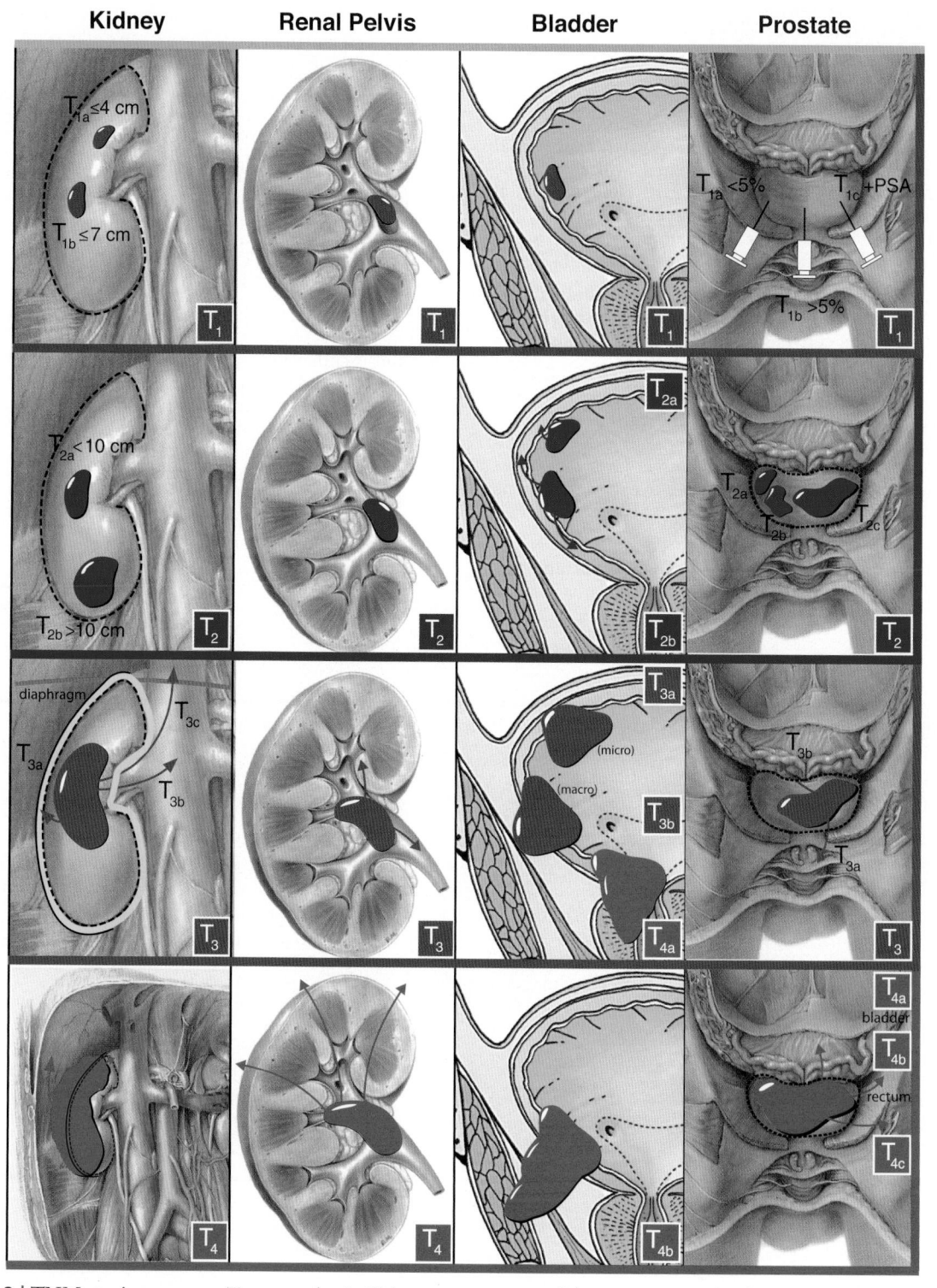

Figure 34.2 | TNM staging systems. T stage only. **A.** Kidney represents a solid organ. **B.** Renal pelvis represents a hollow organ. **C.** Urinary bladder represents a hollow organ. **D.** Prostate represents a solid organ. The T category determines the stage. Color-coded with bars: stage T0, yellow; I, green; II, blue; III, purple; and IV, red.

OVERVIEW OF THE HISTOGENESIS IN THE MALE GENITOURINARY SYSTEM

The urinary system consists of two kidneys, each with a renal pelvis that drains into two separate ureters, which enter the urinary bladder with its single urethral exit. The male genital system consists of the prostate, seminal vesicles, the testes, and the penis (Fig. 34.3). The cancer histopathology relates to the epithelium of the different sections (Fig. 34.3; Table 34.2).

- The majority of renal cancers arise in epithelium of the proximal or distal convoluted tubule. The functional unit of each kidney is the convoluted tubule, which consists of a nephron and a collecting duct (Fig. 34.3B).

- Cancers of the renal pelvis arise in the excretory portion of the urinary system, which is lined with a transitional epithelium covering a multilayered wall consisting of a submucosa, a circular and longitudinal muscle layer, and most often a fibrous adventitia or a serosa-like external covering (Fig. 34.3C).

- In the bladder, the epithelium is transitional when empty but flattened, almost squamous-like, when full and distended. Most cancers are transitional cell (Fig. 34.3C), although squamous cell cancers and adenocarcinomas can and do occur in the bladder.

- Cancers of the penis and urethra tend to be squamous cell cancers arising from stratified squamous cell mucosal lining and skin (Fig. 34.3D).

- Cancers of the prostate arise from tubuloalveolar glandular epithelium and transit into adenocarcinomas of varying grade (Fig. 34.3E).

- Cancers of the testes are highly varied owing to the testes unique genetic and gonadal function (Fig. 34.3F).

The separation of two juxtaposed abdominal and pelvic cavity systems is by a single layer of mesothelial cells. The peritoneum is sufficient to protect the genitourinary system from invasion by gastrointestinal cancers and vice versa. MGU cancers tend to spread within their system involving or complicating their function. Seeding of ureters and bladder with renal pelvis cancer is a common concern. MGU tumors never seed out into the peritoneal cavity, in contrast with gastrointestinal tract (GIT) cancers, which may. Except for the kidney and ureters, the rest of the genitourinary system is confined to the true pelvis. The two anatomic sectors are intraperitoneal and retroperitoneal.

TABLE 34.2	Orientation of Histogenesis of Primary Cancer Sites of the MGU	
Primary-Site: Normal Anatomic Structures	**Derivative Normal Cell**	**Cancer Histopathologic Type: Primary Site**
Renal parenchyma	Simple cuboidal epithelium	Clear cell renal adenocarcinoma
Renal pelvis and ureter	Transitional cell epithelium	Uroepithelial transitional cell cancer
Urinary bladder	Transitional cell epithelium	Transitional cell cancer Squamous cell cancer
Prostate	Pseudostratified columnar epithelium	Adenocarcinoma, Gleason grading
Testes	Germ cells	Seminomas, embryonal cell cancer, teratocarcinoma
Penis	Stratified squamous	Squamous cell cancer
Urethra, spongy	Pseudostratified or stratified columnar epithelium	Squamous cell cancer Transitional cell cancer

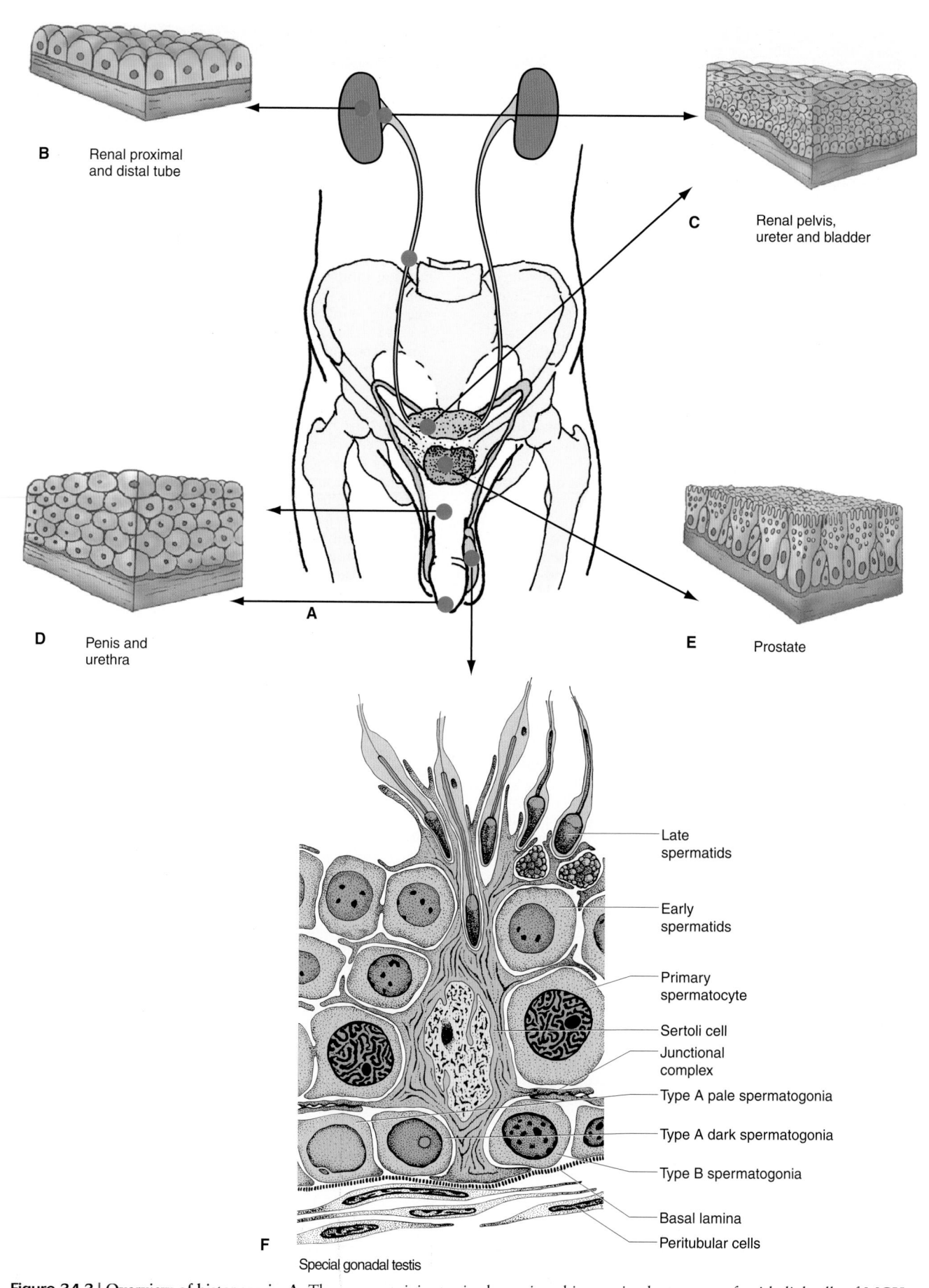

B Renal proximal and distal tube

C Renal pelvis, ureter and bladder

D Penis and urethra

E Prostate

Late spermatids

Early spermatids

Primary spermatocyte

Sertoli cell

Junctional complex

Type A pale spermatogonia

Type A dark spermatogonia

Type B spermatogonia

Basal lamina

Peritubular cells

F Special gonadal testis

Figure 34.3 | Overview of histogenesis. A. The cancer originates in the various histogenic phenotypes of epithelial cells of MGU organs. **B.** Renal. **C.** Renal pelvis, ureter, and bladder. **D.** Penis and urethra. **E.** Prostate. **F.** Special gonadal testis.

ORIENTATION OF T-ONCOANATOMY: ODYSSEY OF PRIMARY SITES

The anatomic isocenters of the seven primary sites in the male genitourinary system are presented in multiplanar orientation diagrams (Fig. 34.4A,B). Each of the primary sites is presented in three planes—coronal, sagittal, and axial—as well as their sentinel and regional lymph nodes and adjacent organs.

The odyssey of the seven MGU primary sites is presented from cephalad to caudad (Table 34.3). The tabulation aligns each primary site with associated surrounding structures and osseous landmarks when feasible. The sentinel node for each primary site is also noted. The MGU tract includes highly vascular organs, placing them at high risk for hematogenous dissemination.

The MGU are in the true pelvis in juxtaposition to the alimentary system. The orientation three-dimensional/three-planar diagram is presented from cephalad to caudad, with the kidney ranging from T12 to L3, the ureters from L3 to S4, and the urinary bladder from S3 to S5. The prostate is at the coccyx, and the penis and testes are outside the bony pelvis and are perineal structures.

In the orientation of pelvic organs it is important to view the osseous anatomy (Fig. 34.5A), the cavities in the musculoskeletal anatomy (Fig. 34.5B), and the different anatomic sectors that house the viscera and neurovasculature (Fig. 34.5C). The bony pelvis above the pelvic brim is referred to as the greater or false pelvis because it houses and contains the contents of the peritoneal cavity. The true pelvis on coronal section is below the pelvic brim, shaped like a wine glass, and houses the male and female genital organs and the urinary bladder. The floor of the true pelvis is the levator ani muscle covered with superior and inferior parietal fascia, and its roof is the peritoneal covering over the pelvic viscera. The obturator lymph nodes (green) are in the true pelvis with the obturator nerve, artery, and vein as it penetrates the levator ani. The perineum roof (levator ani muscle) is perforated by the urethra and houses the corpus cavernosum of the penis in the male and the vagina in the female.

The anatomic isocenters of the seven primary sites in the male genitourinary system are presented in multiplanar orientation diagrams (Fig. 34.4D,E). Each of the primary sites is presented in three planes—coronal, sagittal, and axial—as well as their sentinel and regional lymph nodes and adjacent organs.

The odyssey of the seven MGU primary sites is presented from cephalad to caudad (Table 34.3). The tabulation aligns each primary site with associated surrounding structures and osseous landmarks when feasible. The sentinel node for each primary site is also noted. The MGU tract includes highly vascular organs, placing them at high risk for hematogenous dissemination.

The MGU are in the true pelvis in juxtaposition to the alimentary system. The orientation three-dimensional/three-planar diagram is presented from cephalad to caudad, with the kidney ranging from T12 to L3, the ureters from L3 to S4, and the urinary bladder from S3 to S5. The prostate is at the coccyx, and the penis and testes are outside the bony pelvis and are perineal structures.

- The *kidney* is encased by a fibrous capsule and is surrounded by perirenal fat. The kidney is composed of the cortex, which includes glomeruli and convoluted tubules; and the medulla, which consists of the pyramids of converging tubules and the loops of Henle. The exterior two thirds of the kidney substance is the cortex, in contrast to the inner third, which is the medulla. The medulla contains 8 to 18 striated pyramids that send finger-like rays into the cortex and end in the minor calices. The minor calices unite and form the major calices, which drain into the renal pelvis. The hilus of the kidney has the pelvis, ureter, renal artery and veins, nerves, and lymphatics.

  There are many structures that overlie the kidney; however, they are of little concern oncologically because the peritoneal lining essentially excludes the visceral structures it contains from direct invasion. Nevertheless, it is important to recognize the intimate relationships of the stomach on the left and the duodenum on the right and the location of the hepatic and splenic flexures of the colon in relationship to the midportions of the kidneys. The lung overlies the upper poles of both kidneys due to the low insertion of the diaphragm, particularly during deep inspiration. One should be aware of the position of the pancreas, particularly of its head and tail and in regard to the right and left hila of the kidneys, respectively.

- The *renal bed* consists of renal fascia, which overlies the psoas major muscle and the quadratus lumborum musculature. The superior poles of both kidneys also lie in contact with the diaphragm. Usually, the 12th rib overlies the superior portion of the kidneys and is the only bone that is intimate anatomically. The kidney also lies opposite the transverse processes of T12 to L3.

- The course of the *ureter* is such that it is first crossed anteriorly by the renal artery and vein and then the testicular artery and vein in the male or the ovarian artery and vein in the female. In its continued descent retroperitoneally, the ureter passes anterior to the major iliac vessels. Before its insertion in the bladder, the vesical arteries and veins as well as the uterine artery and vein pass anteriorly to the ureter ("water under the bridge"). There are considerable variations in the anatomic relationships of the renal ureters with renal arteries and veins owing to normal anatomic variations of embryologic development that lead to different locations of the kidneys. In addition, anomalies in their development are common and include multiple renal arteries, fetal lobulations of the kidney, deflected and bifid ureters and pelves, and horseshoe and pelvic kidneys.

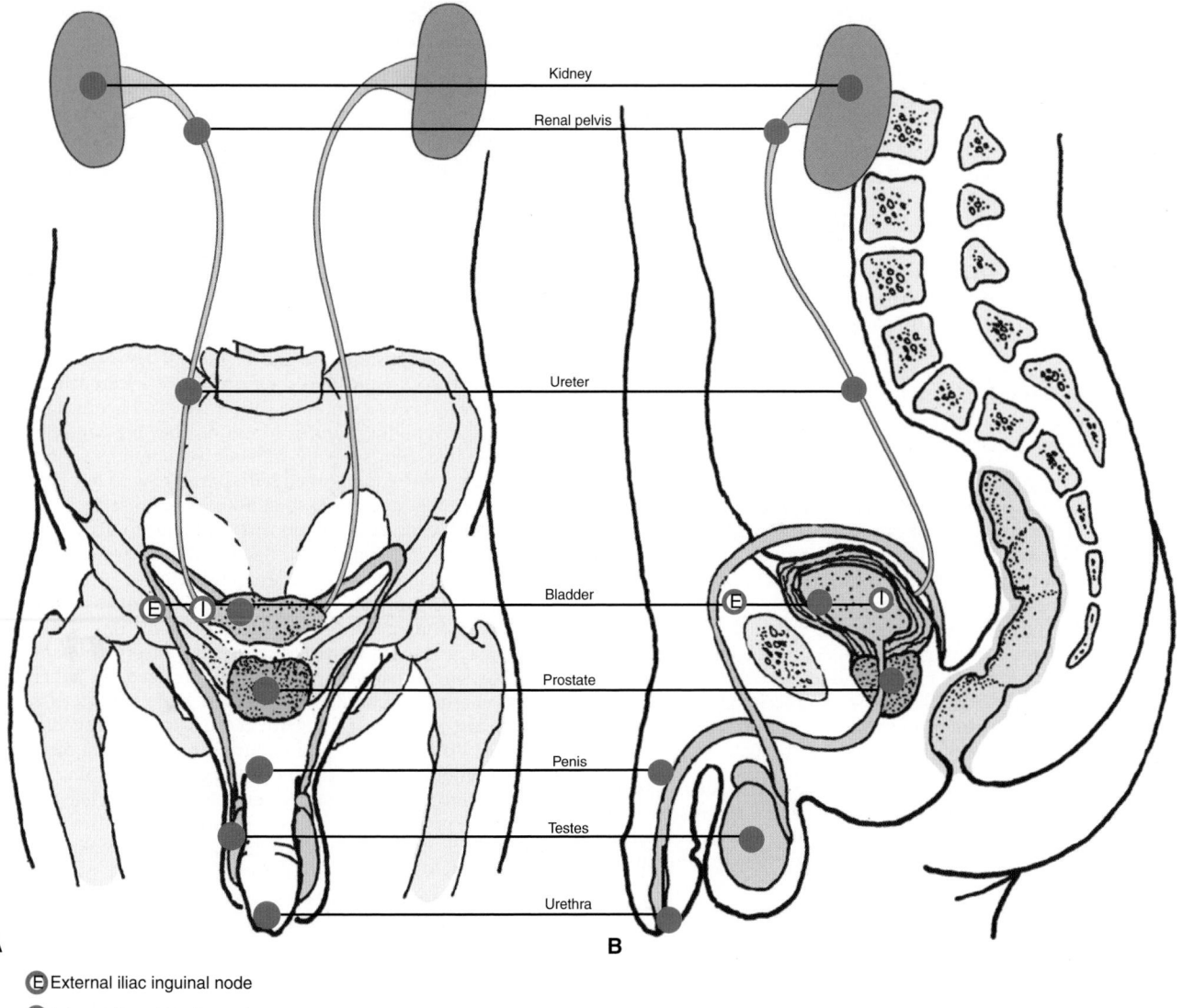

A **B**

Ⓔ External iliac inguinal node

Ⓘ Internal iliac obturator node

Figure 34.4 | Coronal (**A**) and sagittal (**B**) views with primary sites presented from cephalad to caudad at specific transverse levels related to vertebrae.

TABLE 34.3	Orientation of Three-planar T-oncoanatomy Nexi			
Primary Site	**Coronal**	**Sagittal**	**Transverse**	**Axial Level**
Renal parenchyma and renal pelvis	Renal pelvis, artery and vein	12th rib	Lesser omental sac	T12–L3
Ureter	Adrenal, liver, spleen	Major/minor calyces	Quadratus lumborum	L1–S4
Urinary bladder	Pancreas	Psoas muscle	Pubis	S3–S5
Prostate	Primary large and small intestine	Prostate, seminal vesicles, rectum	Prostatic plexus	Cx Coccyx
Testes	Prostate trigone	Bladder	Denonvilliers' fascia Hilum, epididymis	Femoral shaft
Penile	Bladder seminal vesicles, levator ani muscle Peritoneal layers within scrotum Corpus spongiosum and cavernosum	Rectum Vas deferens Inguinal canal Prostate	Corpus spongiosum and cavernosum	Pubis Femoral neck — —

ORIENTATION OF T-ONCOANATOMY: ODYSSEY OF PRIMARY SITES (CONTINUED)

The urinary bladder is the major collecting organ of urine. It is central to the anatomy and function of the urologic tract. The location of the bladder is inside the true pelvis when empty; however, it is a retroperitoneal abdominal organ when full. It relates to the pubic bone and musculature of the anterior abdominal wall and to the levator ani muscle laterally and inferiorly and to the content of the peritoneal cavity superiorly. The bladder's location requires knowledge of adjacent genital structures and disease. Symptomatology depends, in some part, on gender. The relationship of the ureters to surrounding blood vessels is important. The bladder is not a fixed structure but has considerable capacity and mobility, altering its contour contact with the colointestinal viscera as it fills with urine.

- The *urinary bladder* is a hollow viscus consisting of three layers: the mucosa and submucosa, the muscularis, and the serosa. The thickness of the wall depends on whether the bladder is expanded or contracted. In the male, the bladder is intimately related to the seminal vesicles posteriorly, the prostate inferiorly, and the pubis and peritoneum anteriorly. The seminal vesicles are situated between the bladder and the rectum. In the female, the vagina and cervix are located posteriorly to the bladder and the body of the uterus superiorly. The bladder is extraperitoneal, although the sigmoid colon and terminal portions of the ileum can be in contact with its superior peritoneal surface.

- The *prostate gland* is in the central location of the male pelvis and anatomically is positioned similar to the cervix in the female pelvis. The prostate gland—the largest accessory sex gland—is divided into several morphologic and functional zones. It consists of 30 to 50 tubuloalveolar glands arranged in three concentric layers: inner mucosal, an intermediate submucosal, and the peripheral layer containing the main prostatic glands.

- The peripheral zone corresponds to the main prostatic gland. It constitutes 70% of glandular tissue and gives rise to the majority of cancers. This is the most palpable part of the gland, which has a sulcus and feels bilobed after the major internal branching of the glands.

- The central zone contains less glandular tissue and is more resistant to both inflammation and cancer.

- The transitional zone contains the mucosal glands, and this zone has a tendency to undergo extensive division or hyperplasia, forming benign nodular masses of epithelial cells. This benign prostate hyperplasia (BPH) results in difficulty voiding but is not the site of most malignant transformations.

- The periurethral zone contains mucosal and submucosal glands and may participate in BPH.

The prostate is firmly fixed in position by a dense capsule and ligamentous attachments. The urethra courses from the base of the bladder to the bulb of the penis. The cortical structure of the prostate's apex is directed below the perineum. Its flat base touches the base of the bladder, which has no fascia separating these two sites. Thus, the bladder is prone to direct invasion by prostate cancers as they advance. Posteriorly, Denonvilliers' fascia separates the prostate gland from the rectum and acts as a major resistance to tumor invasion because it is composed of obliterated layers of the peritoneal cavity that extend downward. The ductus vas deferens and the seminal vesicles lie posterior to the bladder. They drain into the ejaculatory duct, which has the diameter of a lead pencil.

The *penis* is not a common cancer site, and neoplasms tend to locate around the glans or foreskin. They are considered to be associated with sexually transmitted papilloma virus and may frequently be manifested with partners who have cervical cancers. Penile cancers are squamous or basal cell.

Urethral cancers are more rare and tend to arise from the prostate urethral epithelium. Such malignancies can arise in females as well as males, but are quite rare.

The *testis* is a favored site for malignant disease in young adults, predominantly male, but account for only 1% of all male malignancies. Undescended testes (cryptorchidism) is a predisposing situation and is often corrected by puberty to avoid spermatogonia degeneration. A large variety of tumor types exist because of the germ cell origin and their different paths of differentiation and maturation. Two main categories are commonly noted: seminoma and nonseminoma, which include embryonal cancer and teratocarcinomas. The regional nodes are not regional, and their para-aortic location can be traced back to the gubernaculums during embryologic development when the testes are abdominal organs.

The *scrotum* also contains the vas deferens and its surrounding capsule, which includes several layers of the abdominal wall, which extend and envelope the testis. The muscular and fascial scrotal wall surrounding the testes is an extension of the anterior abdominal wall with similar layers of fascia but containing smooth muscle.

- The pelvic bony anatomy (Fig. 34.5A) houses the true pelvis which is defined by the pelvic rim.

- The coronal section (Fig. 34.5B) defines the true pelvis in blue and accounts for intestinal content overlapping (purple) into pelvis.

- The compartments (Fig. 34.5C) indicate the urinary bladder occupies the true pelvis and the prostate in the male transitions as does the cervix into the perineum.

- The location of the abturator (internal iliac node) is again presented in distinction to external iliac node.

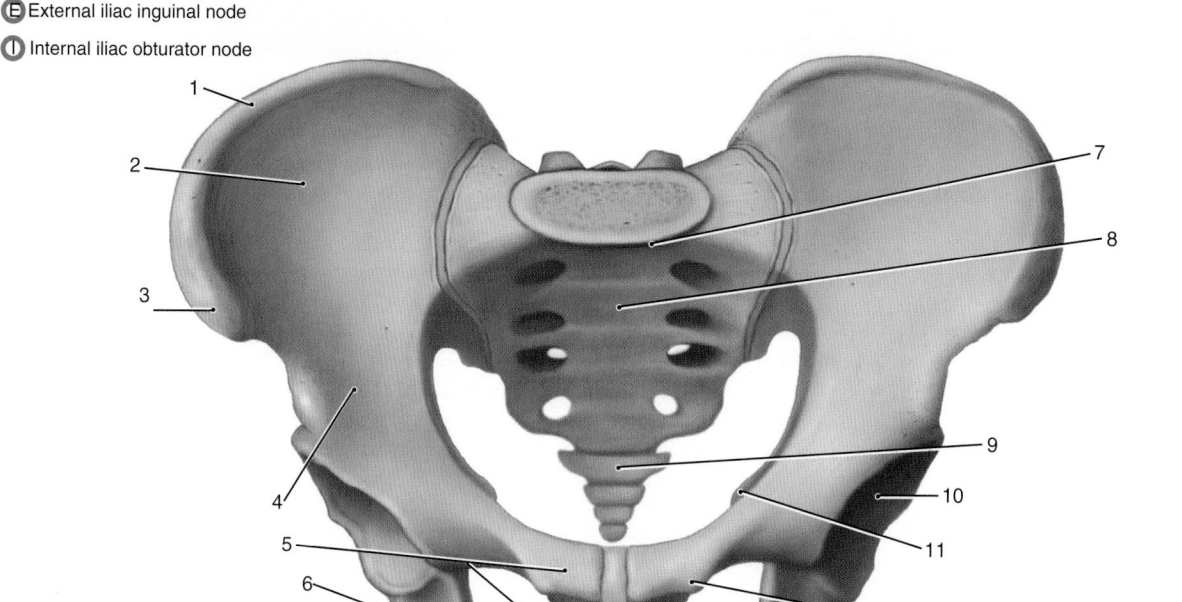

Ⓔ External iliac inguinal node

Ⓘ Internal iliac obturator node

A

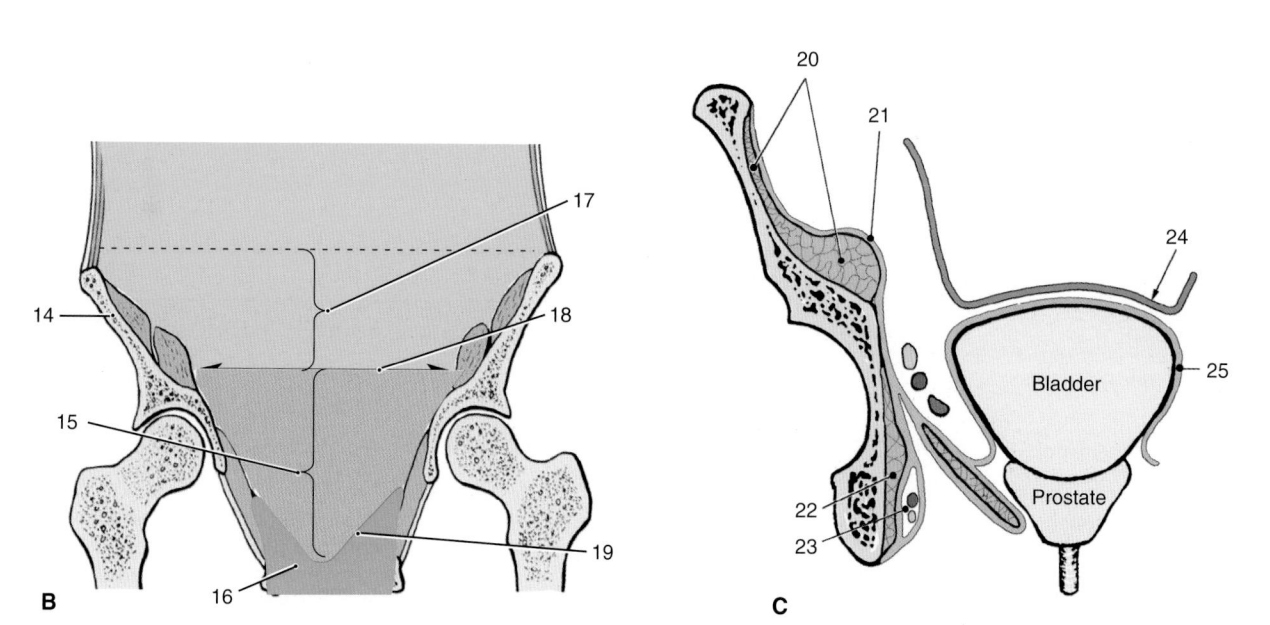

B

C

Figure 34.5 | Orientation of three-planar T-oncoanatomy. A. Three pelvic bones: The ilium holds the false pelvis or peritoneal cavity, and the pelvic inlet is framed by the ilium and the perineum by the pubic arch. **B.** Greater and lesser pelvis and perineum are color coded. **C.** Peritoneal cavity and extraperitoneal pelvic cavity and perineum with their contents. The anatomic landmarks aid in the search of the location of some MGU primary sites in the pelvis. (1) Iliac crest. (2) Iliac fossa. (3) Anterior superior iliac spine. (4) Ilium. (5) Pubis. (6) Ischium. (7) Sacral promontory. (8) Sacrum. (9) Coccyx. (10) Acetabulum. (11) Ischial spine. (12) Pubic tubercle. (13) Pubic symphysis. (14) Ala of ilium. (15) Lesser pelvis (pelvic cavity). (16) Perineum. (17) Greater brim. (18) Pelvic brim. (19) Pelvic diaphragm (levator ani and coccygeus muscles). (20) Iliopsoas muscle. (21) Parietal abdominal fascia. (22) Obturator internus muscle. (23) Pudendal canal. (24) Peritoneum. (25) Visceral pelvic fascia.

N-ONCOANATOMY

ORIENTATION OF N-ONCOANATOMY: REGIONAL LYMPH NODES

The next group of figures (Fig. 34.6A,B,C,D) provide the specific anatomic location of the regional lymph node station for each specific MGU primary site. The sentinel and regional lymph nodes for each of male pelvic organs are listed in Table 34.4. Correlating the N-oncoanatomy in Figure 34.6 A,B,C,D with Table 34.4 assisting in understanding the variation in location of sentinel lymph nodes.

- **Kidney.** The renal hilar nodes are the first involved, and the renal lymphatics then follow the renal vein and enter paracaval and para-aortic nodes. Nodes in the retroperitoneal area inferior to the kidney are considered distant metastatic. Renal pelvis and ureters are similar, except that pelvic nodes are considered regional nodes (Table 34.4; Fig. 34.6A).

- **Renal Pelvis and Ureters.** The spermatic lymphatic collecting ducts on the right side tend to follow the vascular components of the spermatic cord and drain into the paracaval lymph nodes in the area where the spermatic vein enters the inferior vena cava and the artery arises from the aorta. The spermatic lymphatic collecting ducts on the left side also tend to follow the vascular components of the cord and drain into the para-aortic nodes in the region where the spermatic and the inferior mesenteric arteries arise out of the aorta and into the nodes of the left renal hilum in the region where the left spermatic vein joins the left renal vein. Juxtaregional nodes are those of the pelvis, but mediastinal and supraclavicular nodes are metastatic (Fig. 35.6B).

- **Bladder.** The bladder's rich lymphatic network of numerous small anterior vesical lymph nodes drains into three major routes: (i) the trigone, (ii) posterior and lateral walls, and

(iii) anterior wall trunks. The regional or pelvic lymph nodes, located below the bifurcation of the common iliac arteries, include the internal iliacs, the hypogastric, the common iliac located above the pelvic basin, and the lateral, sacral, and anterior perivesicular nodes. The juxtaregional lymph nodes are the inguinal nodes, the high common iliac nodes, and the para-aortic nodes. The vessels, nerves, and lymphatics lie on the inner wall of the true pelvis, below the pelvic rim on the obturator muscle (Fig. 34.6B).

- **Prostate Gland.** The regional nodes are true pelvis nodes for the prostate gland. The lymphatic drainage of the prostate gland is to the obturator node, which is the sentinel node in the hypogastric or internal iliac chain. The obturator node is in the true pelvis, located alongside the obturator blood vessels, and is not in the medial chain of the external iliac chain in the false pelvis. The confusion is due to the projection in an anteroposterior pelvis radiograph, where the location of the obturator node appears to lie in a medial position but is actually posterior in the sagittal plane to the external iliac nodes, which are more anterior (Fig. 34.6C).

- **Testis.** The testis primary drainage on the right is to right inferior paracaval nodes and on the left to left renal hilus (Fig. 34.6C).

- **Penis and Urethra.** The lymphatic drainage is mainly to superficial inguinal and femoral nodes and then the external iliac nodes (Fig. 34.6D).

In addition, there is a rich network of lymphatics that drain into internal and external iliac nodes along the superior rectal veins and a posterior sacral trunk, which drains directly into para-aortic nodes. The nerves of the prostate are derived from the pelvic autonomic plexuses.

TABLE 34.4	**Primary Cancer Sites and Sentinel Nodes**		
Cancer Type	**Axial Level**	**Adjacent Anatomic Structure/Site**	**Sentinel Nodes (Assigned Number)**
Renal adenocarcinoma	T12–L3	Kidney, renal artery and vein, adrenal, pancreas, liver, spleen	Renal hilar (1), paracaval (2), and para-aortic (3) nodes
Renal pelvis transitional cell cancer	L1–S5	Abdominal contents	Renal hilar (1), paracaval (2), and para-aortic (3) nodes
Ureteral transitional cell cancer	L1–L5	Small and large intestine	Paracaval (2), para-aortic (3), and common iliac (4) nodes
Urinary bladder transitional cell cancers	S5	Prostate, distal, ureters	Common iliac (4) and internal iliac (6a) nodes
Prostate adenocarcinomas	Coccyx	Rectum, bladder, ureters	Internal (6) iliac, obturator (6'), and sacral (4) nodes
Penile squamous cell cancer		Scrotum, testes, dorsal vein, periprostatic venous plexus	Inguinal nodes, superficial (8) and deep (7), femoral (9) nodes
Testicular cancer		Vas deferens and inguinal canal	Left renal hilar (1) and right paracaval (2) nodes

The MGU primary cancer sites and their sentinel nodes are defined and tabulated and have a corresponding (number) in Figure 34.6A.

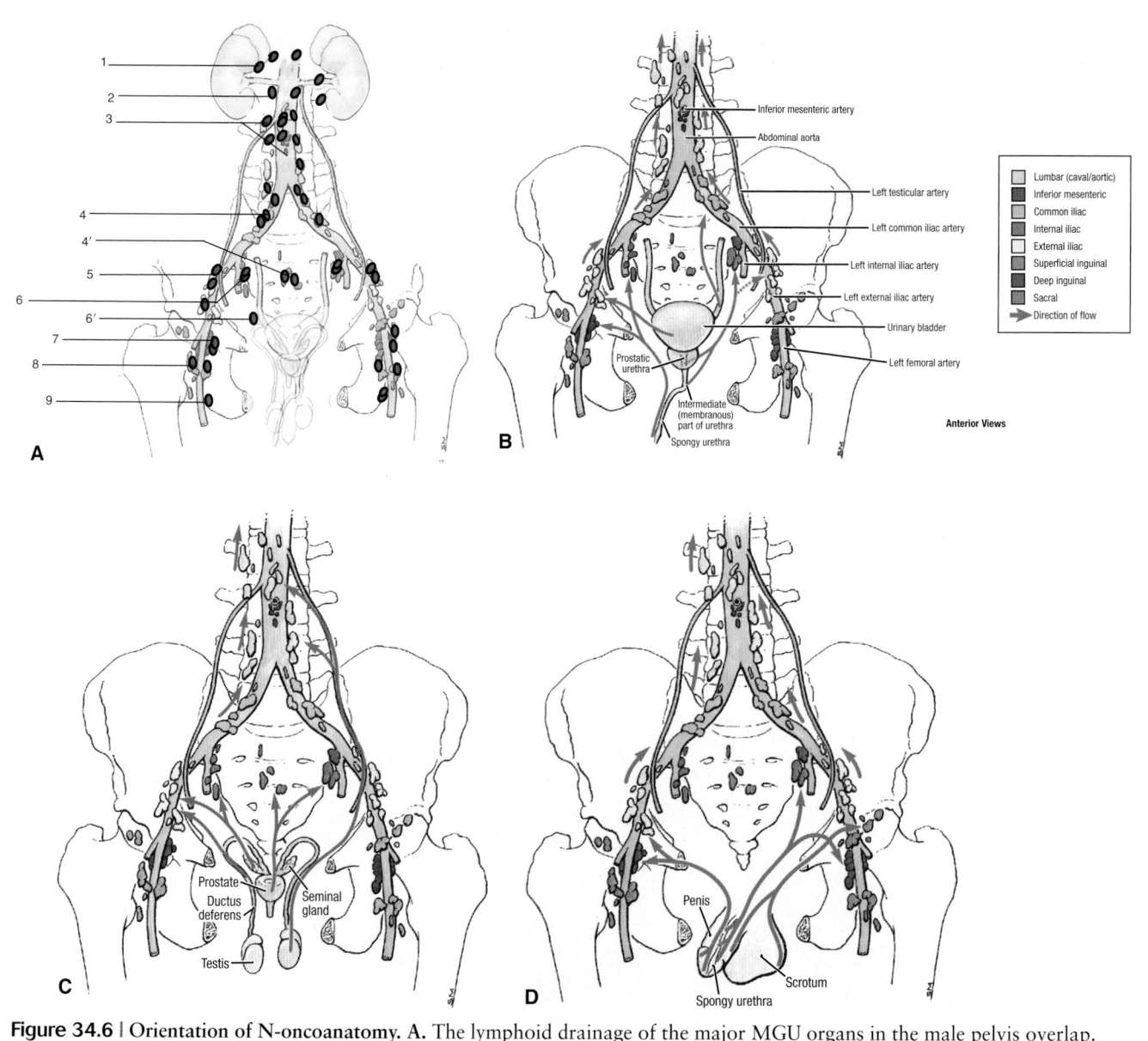

Figure 34.6 | Orientation of N-oncoanatomy. A. The lymphoid drainage of the major MGU organs in the male pelvis overlap. Lymphatic drainage of the ureters, urinary bladder, prostate, and urethra and lymphatic drainage of the testis, deferent duct, prostate, and seminal vesicles. (1) Renal hilar. (2) Renal pelvis and ureter. (3) Para-aortic and paracaval. (4) Common iliac. (4′) Presacral. (5) External iliac. (6) Internal iliac. (6′) Obturator. (7) Deep inguinal. (8) Superficial inguinal. (9) Femoral. **B-D. Lymphatic drainage of male pelvis and perineum. B.** Lymphatic drainage and station for ureter and urinary Bladder. **C.** Lymphatic drainage and station for prostate and testes. **D.** Lymphatic drainage and station for penis, urethra, and scrotum.

STAGING WORKUP

RULES OF CLASSIFICATION AND STAGING

Clinical Staging and Imaging

Clinical examination is limited and reliance on imaging is critical to properly stage cancer of the male genitourinary tract. Fortunately, modern imaging is superb and includes computed tomography (CT), magnetic resonance imaging (MRI), and selective arteriography. If the primary tumor is a renal parenchymal cancer, CT of chest for lung and mediastinal nodal metastases is advised. An intravenous pyelogram and routine laboratory studies are worthwhile. Bone scans are essential for suspected osseous metastases (Table 34.5; Fig. 34.8).

With radiologic imaging, the prostate's four compartments are visualized: the peripheral zone, the central zone, a transitional zone, and the periurethral zone. MRI allows for appreciating their relationship in axial, sagittal, and coronal views. The peripheral zone houses the majority of the branching tubuloalveolar glands and gives rise to 70% of adenocarcinomas, the submucosal glands in the central zone account for 10%, and transitional zone of mucosal glands account for 20% of cancers. The imaging procedures for the prostate gland adenocarcinoma serve as a model for the MGU because it is by far the commonest cancer.

TABLE 34.5	**Imaging Modalities for Staging Prostate Cancer**	
Method	Diagnosis and Staging Capability	Recommended for Use
Primary (T) Staging		
TRUS	Accurate for tumor localization but not for assessing T stage	Routine use for guiding biopsies of the prostate gland
CT$_e$	Not useful for stage T1–T3 disease but for evaluation of stage T4 disease (e.g., bladder, rectum invasion)	Recommended only for patients with clinically suspected stage T3–T4 disease
MRI	Probably the most accurate technique available for assessing T stage, anatomy well shown	May be cost-effective in evaluating patients at intermediate and high clinical risk of having extraprostatic disease
MRS	An adjunct to MRI for improved tumor localization and staging	Under investigation; early results useful as a helpful adjunct to MRI
Nodal (N) Staging		
CT$_e$	Excellent for detecting enlarged nodes >1 cm vs. large blood vessels	Yes, less expensive and time consuming than MRI
MRI	Excellent if node is replaced by cancer; yields positive intense signal	Yes, but more expensive and time consuming than CT$_e$
Metastases (M) Staging		
Bs-Tc	Identifies bone metastases	Recommended for patients with PSA >10 ng/mL, Gleason score >8, or clinical stage T3–T4 disease
CT-Ch	Identifies hematogenous or lymphatic metastases to chest, more sensitive than chest radiograph	May be used to confirm abnormal findings on the chest radiograph or to evaluate patients with pulmonary symptoms
CT-Ab	Identifies hematogenous metastases to liver, abdominal viscera or lymphatic metastases to para-aortic lymph nodes	Not cost-effective in the evaluation of patients with PSA <20 ng/mL because of low yield of abnormal studies
CT-Pv	Identifies invasion of adjacent organs (i.e., bladder, rectum, pelvic sidewall)	Not cost-effective in patients with PSA <20 ng/mL or clinical stage T1–T2 because of low yield of abnormal studies
PET	May increase the sensitivity for detecting lymph node and visceral metastases	Under investigation; early results show promise

BS-Tc, bone scintigraphy; CT, computed tomography; CT$_e$, CT enhanced with IV contrast; CT-Ab, abdominal CT; CT-Ch, chest CT; CT-Pv, pelvic CT; MRI, magnetic resonance imaging; MRS, magnetic resonance spectroscopic imaging; PET, positron emission tomography; TRUS, transrectal ultrasound.
Modified from Bragg DG, Rubin P, Hricak H, eds. *Oncologic Imaging.* 2nd ed. Philadelphia: Elsevier; 2002:579.

PROGNOSIS AND CANCER SURVIVAL

Pathologic Staging

Careful assessment of resected primary tumor should be done with appropriate lymph nodes. All specimens should be carefully studied for clear margins.

Oncoimaging Annotations

- Cross-sectional imaging is essential in staging and treatment guidance.

- Although the reported staging accuracy for CT and MRI is similar, CT is used as a primary imaging approach; MRI complements CT and is most useful in defining the presence and extent of intravenous tumor extension.

- Doppler ultrasonography is also recommended for the evaluation of vascular invasion.

- Pretreatment use of chest radiography versus chest CT is controversial. The use of chest CT is recommended when there is vascular tumor extension, the patient has chest symptoms, or a suspicious nodule is seen on the chest film.

CANCER STATISTICS AND SURVIVAL

Cancers of the MGU constitute almost half of all malignancies in males. Malignancies of the male genital system account for approximately 350,000 new cancers, dominated by prostate cancer at 230,000, with the urinary system accounting for the remainder. Cancer deaths have been dramatically reduced, but annually prostate cancer still claims 30,000 lives and bladder cancer 15,000.

The most dramatic gains in survival are due to multidisciplinary approaches to diagnosis and detection and a transdisciplinary attack on MGU cancer. Over the last 50 years, prostate cancer 5-year survival rates improved by 50%, testes rates by 39%, and urinary bladder, kidney, and renal pelvis rates by 30%. Even more impressive are the MGU survival rates for stage I localized cancers, which are all 90% to 100% curable according to latest Surveillance Epidemiology and End Results data: kidney, 90%; bladder, 94%; testis, 99%; and prostate, 100%. These 5-year results are plotted in Figure 34.9 and shown in Table 34.6. The pediatric Wilms tumor of the kidney was the first solid malignancy cured by combining modalities in childhood neoplasms, achieving >90% long-term survival, along with Hodgkin's disease at around 70%. The reversal of a death sentence for these pediatric tumors is strikingly demonstrated in Figure 34.9. Equally important are improvements of quality of life owing to organ function preservation of the majority of prostate cancer patients.

TABLE 34.6	Cancer Curability by Stages at Diagnosis 2010			
	5-Year Survival Rate (%)			
Site	**All Stages**	**Local**	**Regional**	**Distant**
Prostate	97	100	100	31
Testis	95	99	96	71
Urinary bladder	80	74	36	6
Kidney	68	90	60	10

Data from Ries LAG, Eisner MP, Kosary CL, et al., eds. *SEER Cancer Statistics Review, 1975–2001.* Bethesda, MD: National Cancer Institute. Available at: http://seer.cancer.gov/csr/1975_2001/, 2004; Tables XI, XXIII, XXV, XXVII.

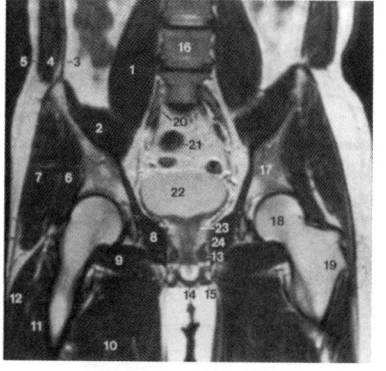

Figure 34.8 | Coronal MRI correlates with the T-oncoanatomy coronal section (Fig. 34.5). Oncoimaging with CT is commonly applied to staging cancers, often combined with PET to determine true extent of primary cancer and involved lymph nodes. 1. Psoas m. 2. Iliacus m. 3. Transverse abdominis m. 4. Internal oblique m. 5. External oblique m. 6. Gluteus minimus m. 7. Gluteus medius m. 8. Obturator internus m. 9. Obturator externus m. 10. adductor group of muscles. 11. Vastus intermedius m. 12. Vastus lateralis m. 13. Levator ani m. 14. Bulbospongiosus m. 15. Ischiocavernosus m. 16. Lumbar spine 17. Acetabulum 18. Head of the femur. 19. Greater trochanter. 20. Internal iliac vessels. 21. Sigmoid colon. 22. Urinary bladder. 23. Prostate (central zone). 24. Prostate (peripheral zone).

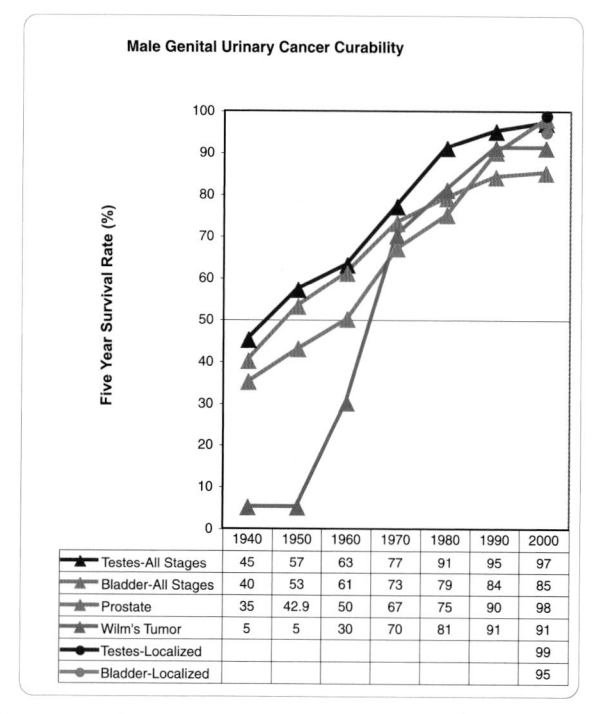

	1940	1950	1960	1970	1980	1990	2000
Testes-All Stages	45	57	63	77	91	95	97
Bladder-All Stages	40	53	61	73	79	84	85
Prostate	35	42.9	50	67	75	90	98
Wilm's Tumor	5	5	30	70	81	91	91
Testes-Localized							99
Bladder-Localized							95

Figure 34.9 | Trajectory of cancer survival for MGU organs. Prostate, bladder, testes, and Wilms' tumor.

TNM STAGING CRITERIA

The kidney has a distinct capsule separating renal parenchyma from its surrounding of perirenal fat, which in turn on its posterior surface has the perirenal fat separated by fascia (Gerota's) and lumbar quadratus muscle, 12th rib, and posterior diaphragmatic surface. Superiorly it can spread into the adrenal gland. Once the tumor penetrates the capsule it has access to regional nodes. Due to renal cancer's hypervascularization, a path of least resistance is into renal veins and the inferior vena cava. Lung metastases are very common.

Renal adenocarcinomas arise in the renal parenchyma mainly from the proximal renal tubule, in contrast to transitional cell cancers from the renal pelvis and its intrarenal collecting system. Their incidence ratio is 90% and 10%, respectively. A number of different histopathologic types of renal cancer have been identified, with subtypes clear cell and granular cell cancer or a mixture (Table 35.1; Fig. 35.1).

TNM STAGING CRITERIA

In the seventh edition of the *AJCC Cancer Staging Manual*, T2 lesions are divided into T2a (>7 to <10 cm) and T2b (>10 cm). Justification of relating cancer size to survival relates to new data from the National Cancer Data Base (Table 35.3A). Renal vein involvement is changed from T3b to T3a. Adrenal gland involvement is changed from T3a to T4 if spread is contiguous and M1 if it is not. Nodal criteria are simply N1 independent of number in the regional nodal station.

In the early stages, tumor size is the dominant criterion for renal cancer (Fig. 35.1), whereas in the more advanced stages, the staging features relate to the patterns of spread to the surrounding anatomy and, to a degree, criteria of resectability.

The TNM staging has been undergoing subtle changes reflecting the advances in imaging hypernephromas because the radiologic appearance is virtually pathognomic. Renal cancers show a supervascularity when computed tomography (CT) with contrast is used that is characteristic when compared to cysts. In the first to third editions of *AJCC Cancer Staging Manual* (1978 to 1980), T1 was distinguished from T2 by absence of deformity in the contour of pelvis calyces structures and T3 from T4 by a medial venous spread to the renal vein and/or renal pelvis invasion compared to lateral spread through the renal capsule into perirenal fat versus penetrating to Gerota's fascia. With the fourth edition in 1992, the tumor size and more specific patterns of invasion were defined to modify stage III into substages A, B, and C (Fig. 35.3A).

T2 tumors measure >7 cm and are limited to the kidney or have no renal capsule invasion. T3 cancers are subdivided according to patterns of spread. Once the renal capsule is penetrated, T3a means the cancer has spread into perirenal fat laterally or adrenal gland superiorly. T3b cancers invade medially into the renal vein and inferior vena cava, and T3c cancers extend into the vena cava above the diaphragm. T4 cancer applies to posterior and lateral invasion beyond Gerota's fascia. With a few exceptions, stage reflects the primary categories.

SUMMARY OF CHANGES SEVENTH EDITION AJCC

The following changes in the definitions of TNM and the stage grouping for kidney cancer have been made since the sixth edition (Fig. 35.3A):

- T2 lesions have been divided into T2a (greater than 7 cm but less than or equal to 10 cm) and T2b (>10 cm).

- Ipsilateral adrenal involvement is reclassified as T4 if contiguous invasion and M1 if not contiguous.

- Renal vein involvement is reclassified as T3a.

- Nodal involvement is simplified to N0 vs. N1.

The TNM Staging Matrix is color coded for identification of Stage Group once T and N stages are determined (Table 35.3B). T stage determines group stage.

TABLE 35.3A	The National Cancer Data Base Findings Regarding Impact of Size on T2 Category Cancer-Specific and Observed Survival

Size (cm)	Percent Alive at 5 Years
≤4.0	75.4
95% CI	74.6–76.1
4.1–7.0	67.9
95% CI	67.0–68.7
7.1–10.0	57.0
95% CI	55.9–58.1
>10.0	47.5
95% CI	46.1–48.9

CI, confidence interval.
Adapted from Edge SB, Byrd DR, Compton CC, et al. *AJCC Cancer Staging Manual.* 7th ed. New York: Springer, 2010, p. 480, Table 43.1.

TABLE 35.3B	Stage Summary Matrix

	N0	N1	N2	M1
T1	I	III	IV	IV
T2	II	III	IV	IV
T3	III	III	IV	IV
T4	IV	IV	IV	IV

KIDNEY

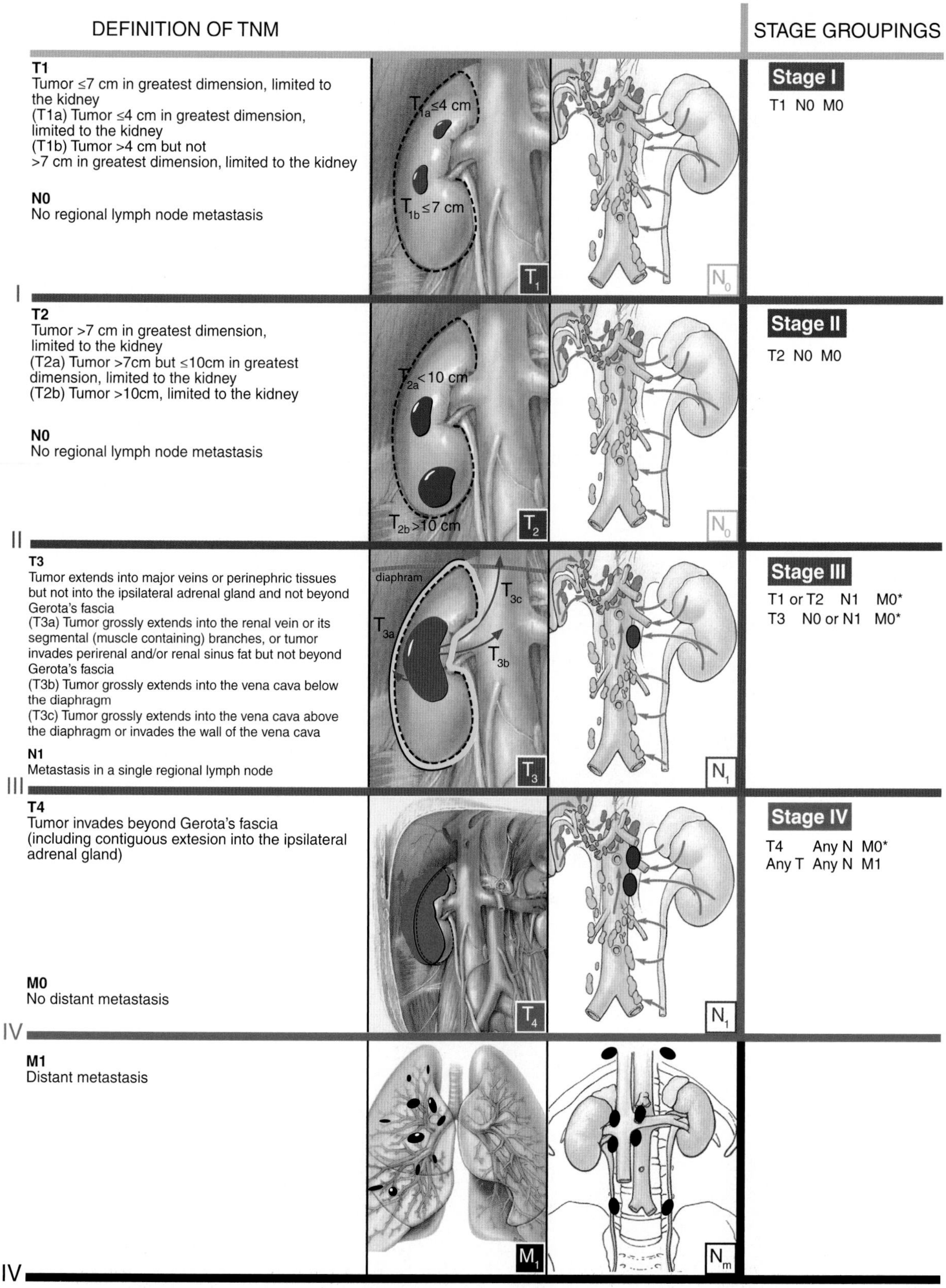

DEFINITION OF TNM

T1
Tumor ≤7 cm in greatest dimension, limited to the kidney
(T1a) Tumor ≤4 cm in greatest dimension, limited to the kidney
(T1b) Tumor >4 cm but not >7 cm in greatest dimension, limited to the kidney

N0
No regional lymph node metastasis

T2
Tumor >7 cm in greatest dimension, limited to the kidney
(T2a) Tumor >7cm but ≤10cm in greatest dimension, limited to the kidney
(T2b) Tumor >10cm, limited to the kidney

N0
No regional lymph node metastasis

T3
Tumor extends into major veins or perinephric tissues but not into the ipsilateral adrenal gland and not beyond Gerota's fascia
(T3a) Tumor grossly extends into the renal vein or its segmental (muscle containing) branches, or tumor invades perirenal and/or renal sinus fat but not beyond Gerota's fascia
(T3b) Tumor grossly extends into the vena cava below the diaphragm
(T3c) Tumor grossly extends into the vena cava above the diaphragm or invades the wall of the vena cava

N1
Metastasis in a single regional lymph node

T4
Tumor invades beyond Gerota's fascia (including contiguous extesion into the ipsilateral adrenal gland)

M0
No distant metastasis

M1
Distant metastasis

STAGE GROUPINGS

Stage I
T1 N0 M0

Stage II
T2 N0 M0

Stage III
T1 or T2 N1 M0*
T3 N0 or N1 M0*

Stage IV
T4 Any N M0*
Any T Any N M1

* not illustrated

Figure 35.3A | TNM renal cancer diagram. Renal cancers are well vascularized. When invasive, stage III, T3a, 3b, 3c (purple), they are resectable; when stage IV (red), T4, they are unresectable; and when stage IV, they are also metastatic. Vertically arranged with T definitions on the left and stage groupings on the right. Color bars are coded for stage: stage I, green; II, blue; III, purple; IV, red; and metastatic, black.

ADRENAL GLAND

The new inclusion of adrenal cell carcinoma neurologic tumors rests on its anatomic relationship to the kidney.

- **Anatomy:** The adrenal glands are located at the superior poles of the kidney and are surrounded by Gerota's fascia and separated from the renal parenchyma by the renal capsule which consists of two distinct layers of connective tissue. The outer layer of fibroblasts and collagen fibers and a cellular inner layer of myofibroblasts embryologically the cortex is derived from the mesoderm and medulla from the neural crest. Each adrenal gland consists of an outer cortex and inner medulla.

- **Histology:** The adrenal cortex exhibits 3 concentric zones (Fig. 35.4A):

  1. Zone glomerulosa (15% volume) is a thin zone inferior to the capsule and consists of cells in ovoid clumps.

  2. Zone fasciculate (80%) is the intermediate zone. The thickest and arranged in vertical columns, one-cell thick adjacent to capillaries.

  3. Zone reticularis (5%) is innermost zone arranged in cords.

- **Physiology:** Each zone produces essential hormones:

  1. Zone glomerulosa: mineral corticoids

  2. Zone fasciculate: glucocorticoids

  3. Zone reticularis: androgens

- **Pathology:** Both adrenal gland cortical adenomas and carcinomas can be functioning and produce Cushing's syndrome. Eighty percent of carcinomas are functional, occur more frequently in women, and carry a poor prognosis (Fig. 35.4B).

- **Clinical presentation:** Cushing's syndrome can vary in intensity and severity depending on the levels of corticoids and duration. Typically there is the onset of moon face, buffalo humpback, and obesity of abdomen with wasting of limbs (Fig. 35.4C).

- **Staging system** is straightforward, based on tumor size (T1<5 cm, T2>5 cm) and T3 invades perinephric fat but not Gerota's fascia, vs. T4 relates to whether there is invasion of adjacent organs i.e. kidney vs. diaphragm, great vessels, pancreas, spleen, liver. Nodal spread is to paraortic and paracaval nodes in juxtaposition to tumor. Metastatic spread is to lung and liver or distant nodes in mediastinum and retroperitoneal area (Fig. 35.3B).

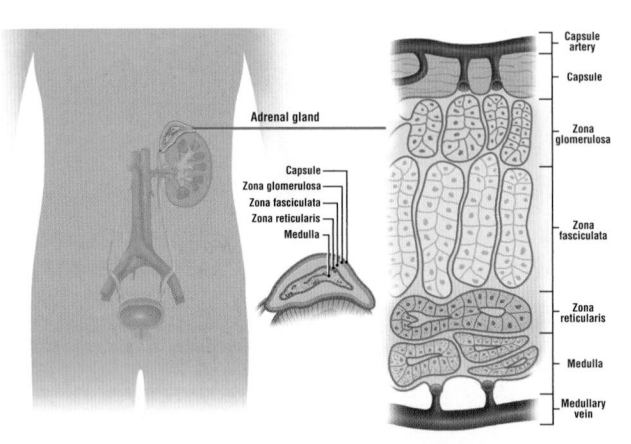

Figure 35.4A | The structural organization and general location in the body of the thyroid gland, parathyroid gland, and adrenal gland.

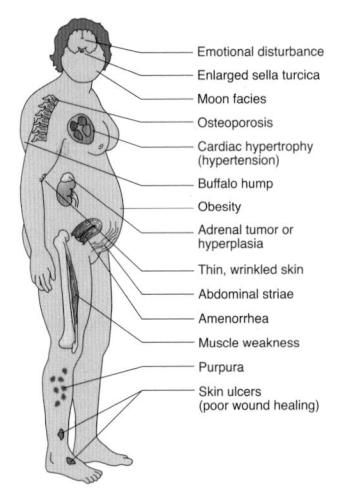

Figure 35.4C | Major clinical manifestations of Cushing's syndrome.

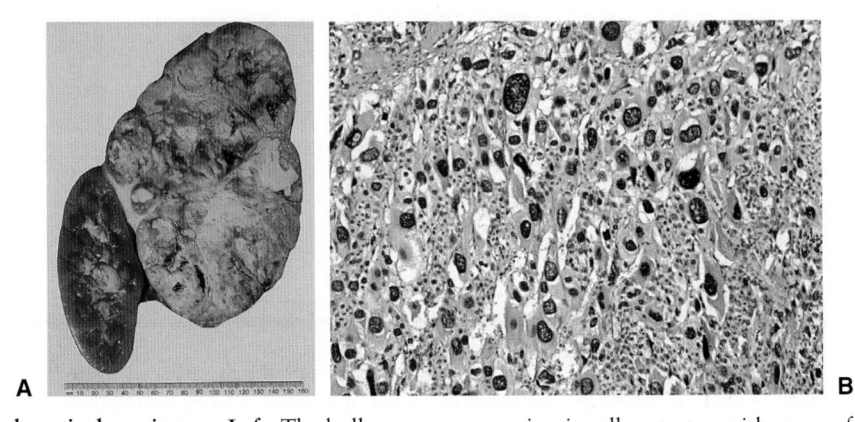

Figure 35.4B | Adrenal cortical carcinoma. Left. The bulky tumor on section is yellow to tan with areas of necrosis and cystic degeneration. **Right.** A microscopic section demonstrates marked anisocytosis and nuclear pleomorphism.

Adrenal Adenocarcinoma

DEFINITION OF TNM

STAGE GROUPINGS

T1
Tumor <5 cm in greatest dimension, limited to the adrenal gland

N0
No regional lymph node metastasis

T_1 <5 cm

T_1

N_0

Stage I
T1 N0 M0

I

T2
Tumor >5 cm in greatest dimension, limited to the adrenal gland

N0
No regional lymph node metastasis

T_2 >5 cm

T_2

N_0

Stage II
T2 N0 M0

II

T3
Tumor extends beyond the adrenal gland into perinephric fat but not beyond Gerota's fascia

N1
Metastasis in a single regional lymph node

T_3

T_3

N_1

Stage III
T1 N1 M0*
T2 N1 M0*
T3 N0 M0*
T3 N1 M0

III

T4
Tumor invades beyond Gerota's fascia into adjacent organs: kidney, pancreas, spleen, liver, and adjacent structures: diaphragm, aorta, vena cava

N2
Metastasis in >1 regional lymph node

T_4

N_2

Stage IV
T4   N0   M0*
T4   N1   M0*
Any T N2   M0
Any T Any N M1

IV

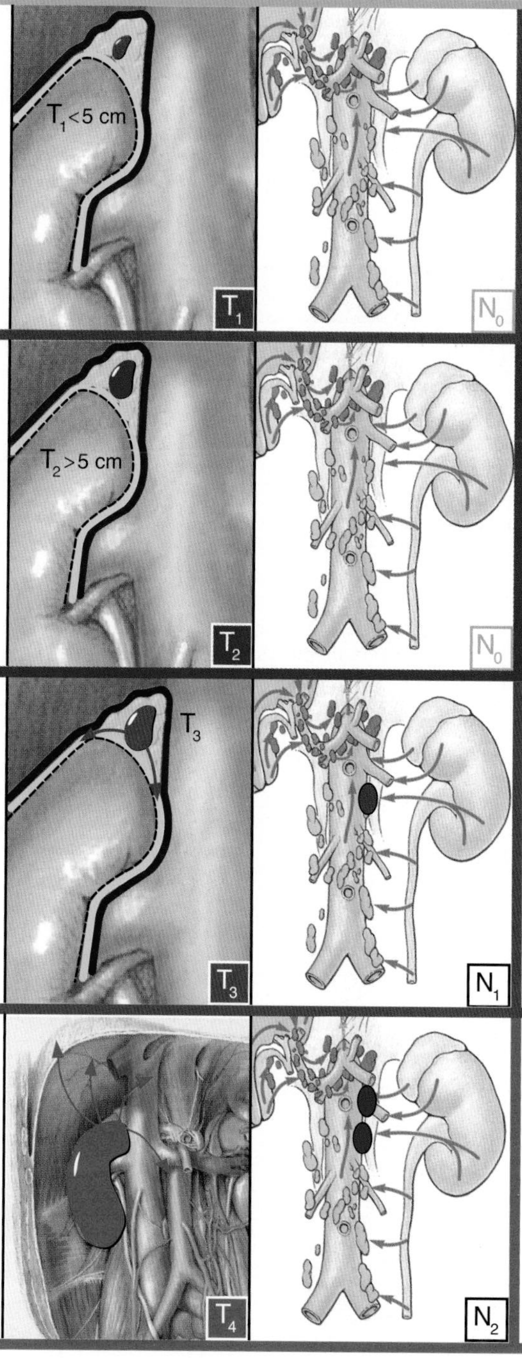

* not illustrated

— Gerota's fascia
- - - - - - renal capsule
— perinephric fat

Figure 35.3B | TNM adrenal adenocarcinoma diagram. When invasive, stage III, T3a, 3b, 3c (purple), they are resectable; when stage IV (red), T4, they are unresectable; and when stage IV, they are also metastatic. Vertically arranged with T definitions on the left and stage groupings on the right. Color bars are coded for stage: stage I, green; II, blue; III, purple; IV, red; and metastatic, black.

T-ONCOANATOMY

ORIENTATION OF THREE-PLANAR ONCOANATOMY

The isocenter of the kidney is the renal bed, which consists of Gerota's fascia and overlies the psoas major muscle and the quadratus lumborum musculature. The superior poles of both kidneys also lie in contact with the diaphragm. Usually, the 12th rib overlies the superior portion of the kidneys and is the only bone that is intimate anatomically. The kidney also lies opposite the transverse processes of T12 to L3 (Fig. 35.5).

T-oncoanatomy

The T-oncoanatomy is displayed in three planar views. A. Coronal, B. Sagittal, C. Transverse axial (Fig. 35.6).

- *Coronal:* There are many structures that overlie the kidney; however, they are of little concern oncologically because the peritoneal lining essentially excludes the visceral structures it contains from direct invasion. Nevertheless, it is important to recognize the intimate relationships of the stomach, on the left, and the duodenum, on the right, and the location of the hepatic and splenic flexures of the colon in relation to the midportions of the kidneys. The lung overlies the upper poles of both kidneys owing to the low insertion of the diaphragm, particularly during deep inspiration. One should be aware of the position of the pancreas, particularly

of its head and tail and in regard to the right and left hila of the kidneys, respectively (Fig. 35.5). The course of the ureter is such that it is first crossed anteriorly by the renal artery and vein and then the spermatic artery and vein in males or the ovarian artery and vein in females. In its continued descent retroperitoneally, the ureter passes anterior to the major iliac vessels.

- *Sagittal:* The kidney is encased by a fibrous capsule and is surrounded by perinephric fat. The kidney is composed of the cortex, which includes glomeruli; convoluted tubules; and the medulla, which consists of the pyramids of converging tubules and the loops of Henle. The exterior third of the kidney substance is the cortex, in contrast to the inner two thirds, which is the medulla. The medulla contains 8 to 18 striated pyramids that send finger-like rays into the cortex and end in the minor calices. The minor calices unite and form the major calices that drain into the renal pelvis. The hilus of the kidney has the pelvis, ureter, and renal artery and veins.

- *Transverse:* Before its insertion in the bladder, the vesical arteries and veins, as well as the uterine artery and vein, pass anteriorly to the ureter ("water under the bridge"). There are considerable variations in the anatomic relationships of the renal ureters with renal arteries and veins owing to normal anatomic variations of embryologic development that lead to different locations of the kidneys. In addition, anomalies in their development are common and include multiple renal arteries, fetal lobulations of the kidney, deflected and bifid ureters and pelves, and horseshoe and pelvic kidneys.

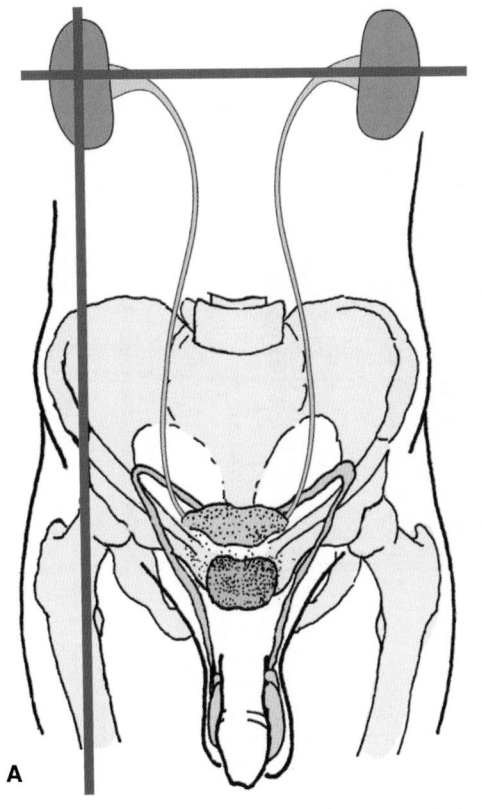 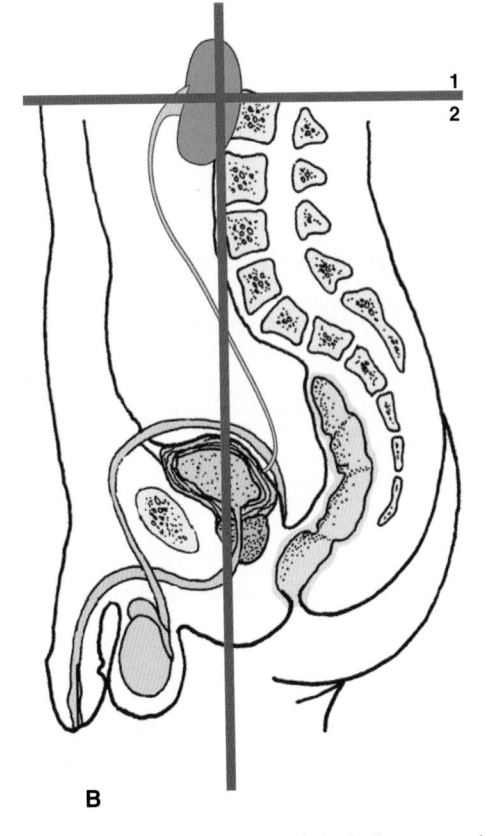

Figure 35.5 | Orientation of T-oncoanatomy. The anatomic isocenter for three-planar anatomy of the kidney is at the T12 to L3 level. **A.** Coronal. **B.** Sagittal.

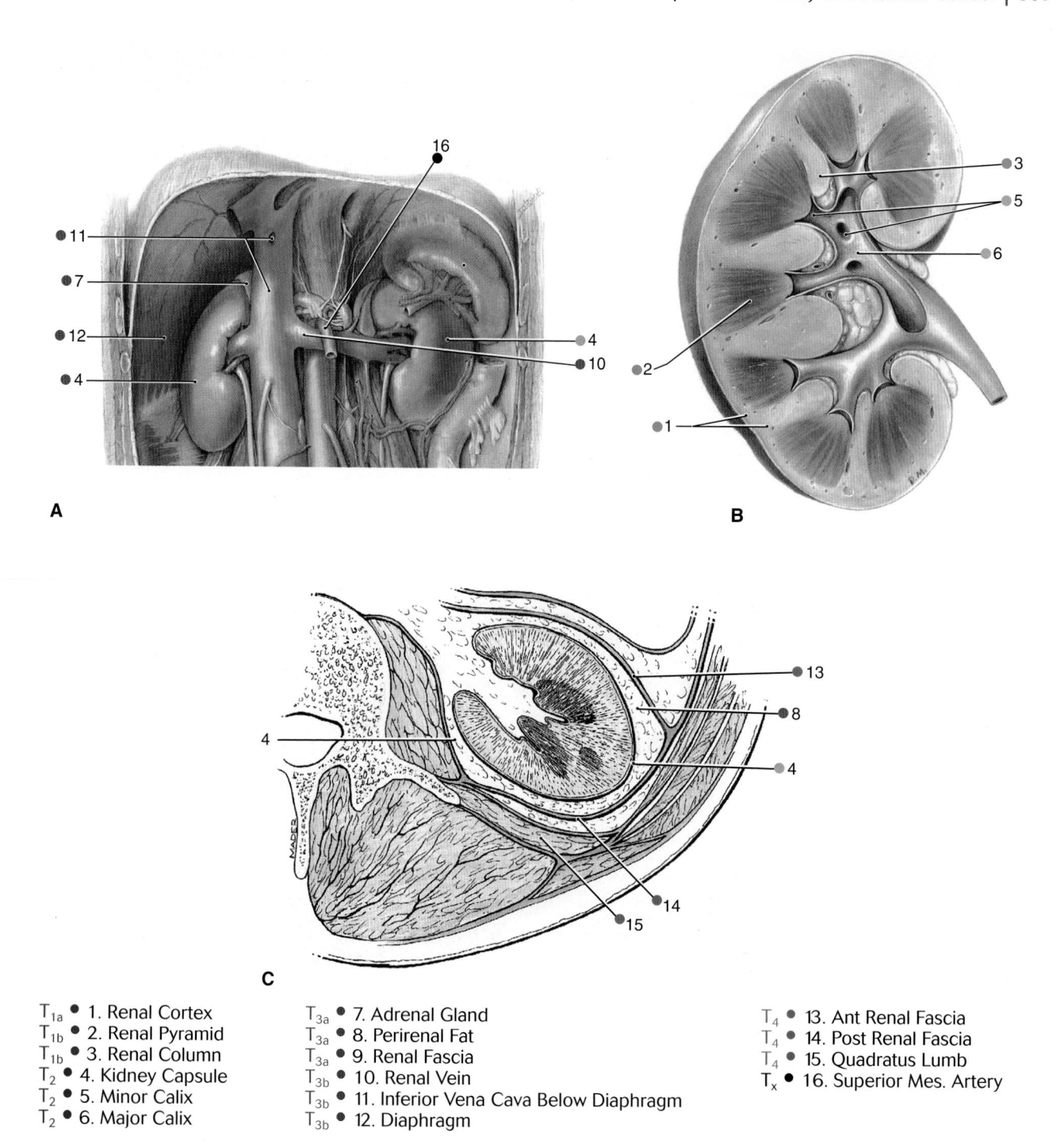

Figure 35.6 | T-oncoanatomy. Connecting the dots: Structures are color coded for cancer stage progression. The color code for the anatomic sites correlates with the color code for the stage group (Figs. 35.3A and 35.3B) and patterns of spread (Fig. 35.2) and the SIMLAP table (Table 35.2). Connecting the dots in similar colors will provide an appreciation for the three-dimensional oncoanatomy.

N-ONCOANATOMY AND M-ONCOANATOMY

N-ONCOANATOMY

The regional nodes are anterior to and surround the renal artery and vein and at the midline, para-aortic and paracaval in location. It is important to note the left testis drains to the left hilar area of the kidney and the right testis drains to paracaval nodes at the lower pole on the right. The cisterna chyli is located on the right side near the upper pole.

There are considerable variations in the anatomic relationships of the renal ureters with renal arteries and veins owing to normal anatomic variations of embryologic development that lead to different locations of the kidneys. In addition, anomalies in their development are common and include multiple renal arteries, fetal lobulations of the kidney, deflected and bifid ureters and pelves, and horseshoe and pelvic kidneys (Fig. 35.7A; Table 35.4A). For the adrenal gland lymph node drainage, see Table 35.4B.

M-ONCOANATOMY

Common metastatic sites reflect the vascular drainage of the kidney. As noted in the patterns of spread, invasion in the renal vein and inferior vena cava is common. Pulmonary spread is very common. With continued circulation of tumor cells through the left heart, metastases to bone, brain, and liver become possible. Unfortunately, remote metastases frequently occur with this tumor owing to the rich neovascularization. The T3 stage is divided according to the venous drainage of the kidney: T3a invasion into renal vein, T3b invasion into inferior vena cava infradiaphragmatic, T3a is supradiaphragmatic.

Renal pelvis transitional cell cancers are characterized similarly to transitional cell cancers of uroepithelium of bladder in their ability to "seed" throughout the urinary tract. Endoscopic assessment is important to determine when renal pelvis cancer is a primary or part of a disseminated urological cancer (Fig. 35.7B).

REGIONAL LYMPH NODES

The regional lymph nodes, illustrated in Figure 35.7A, are as follows:

Renal hilar

Caval (paracaval, precaval, and retrocaval)

Interaortocaval

Aortic (para-aortic, preaortic, and retroaortic)

The primary landing zone for right-sided tumors is the interaortocaval zone and for left-sided tumors is the aortic region. The more extended landing zone for RCC are analogous to those for right and left testicular tumors, respectively, although patterns of spread are somewhat more unpredictable. Lymph nodes outside of these templates should be considered distal (metastatic) rather than regional.*

*Preceding passage from Edge SB, Byrd DR, and Compton CC, et al. *AJCC Cancer Staging Manual*, 7th edition. New York: Springer, 2010, p. 480.

TABLE 35.4A	Lymph Nodes of Kidney	
Sentinel Nodes	**Juxtaregional Nodes**
Renal hilar	Common iliac
Paracaval	External iliac
Para-aortic	
Regional Nodes	**Metastatic Nodes**
Renal vein (left)	Mediastinal
Para-aortic (high infrarenal artery)	Left supraclavicular
Para-aortic (high suprarenal artery)	
Para-aortic low	
Lateral caval (right)	

TABLE 35.4B	Lymph Nodes of Adrenal Gland	
Sentinel Nodes	**Regional Nodes**
Renal hilar	Paracaval
	Paraortic

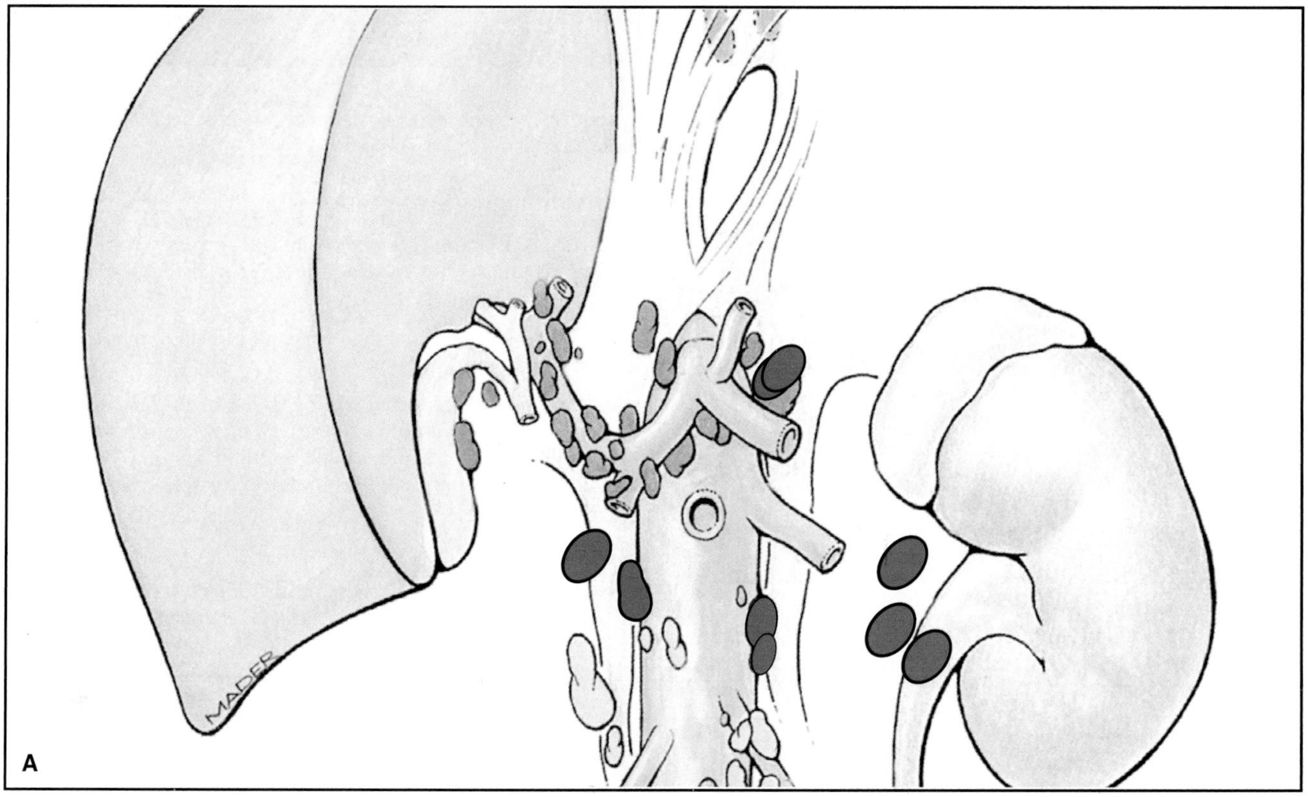

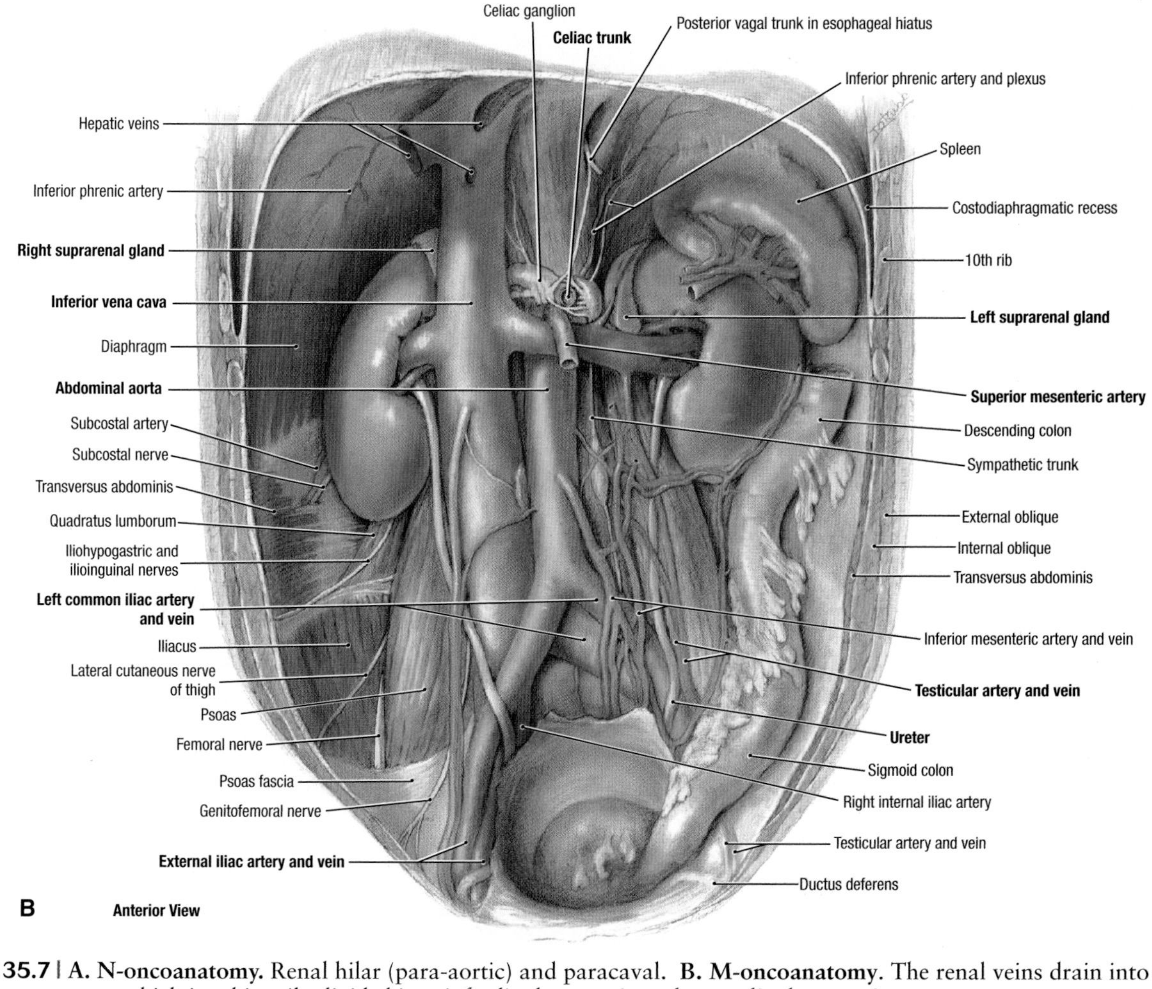

A

Celiac ganglion
Celiac trunk
Posterior vagal trunk in esophageal hiatus
Inferior phrenic artery and plexus
Hepatic veins
Spleen
Inferior phrenic artery
Costodiaphragmatic recess
Right suprarenal gland
10th rib
Inferior vena cava
Left suprarenal gland
Diaphragm
Abdominal aorta
Superior mesenteric artery
Subcostal artery
Descending colon
Subcostal nerve
Sympathetic trunk
Transversus abdominis
Quadratus lumborum
External oblique
Internal oblique
Iliohypogastric and ilioinguinal nerves
Transversus abdominis
Left common iliac artery and vein
Iliacus
Inferior mesenteric artery and vein
Lateral cutaneous nerve of thigh
Testicular artery and vein
Psoas
Ureter
Femoral nerve
Sigmoid colon
Psoas fascia
Right internal iliac artery
Genitofemoral nerve
Testicular artery and vein
External iliac artery and vein
Ductus deferens

B   Anterior View

Figure 35.7 | **A. N-oncoanatomy.** Renal hilar (para-aortic) and paracaval. **B. M-oncoanatomy.** The renal veins drain into the inferior vena cava, which is arbitrarily divided into infradiaphragmatic and supradiaphragmatic.

STAGING WORKUP

RULES OF CLASSIFICATION AND STAGING

Clinical Staging and Imaging

Clinical examination is limited, and reliance on imaging is critical. Fortunately, modern imaging is superb and includes CT, magnetic resonance imaging (MRI), and selective arteriography. If the primary tumor is advanced, CT of chest for lung and mediastinal nodal metastases is advised. An intravenous pyelogram and routine laboratory studies are worthwhile (Table 35.5; Fig. 35.8).

Pathologic Staging

Careful assessment of resected primary, which includes primary tumor, kidney, appropriate lymph nodes contained within the renal (Gerota's) fascia, perirenal fat, and renal vein/artery, is needed. Partial nephrectomy needs careful study for margins.

Oncoimaging Annotations

- Renal carcinomas are more conspicuous in the CT nephrogram phase than in the early arterial or corticomedullary phase of imaging.

- Cross-sectional imaging is essential in staging and in guiding treatment.

- Although the reported staging accuracy for CT and MRI is similar, CT is used as a primary imaging approach; MRI complements CT and is most useful in defining the presence and extent of intravenous tumor extension.

- Doppler ultrasonography is also recommended for the evaluation of vascular invasion.

- Pretreatment use of chest radiography versus chest CT is controversial. The use of chest CT is recommended when there is renal-vascular tumor extension, the patient has chest symptoms, or a suspicious nodule is seen on the chest film.

TABLE 35.5	Imaging Modalities for Staging Renal Cancer	
Method	Diagnosis and Staging Capability	Recommended for Use
Primary (T) Staging		
CT$_e$	Most accurate cross-sectional imaging; with intravenous contrast during vascular phase appears as a hypervascular lesion and a decrease in attenuation in nephrogram and excretory phase	Yes, advantage is detecting renal cancer neovascularization
MRI	Plays a complementary role to CT; with gadolinium hypernephromas appear hyperintense on T1 and T2	Yes
TAUS	Renal cancers appear as large hypoechoic masses and can guide biopsy	No
Nodal (N) Staging		
CT$_e$	Identifies nodal metastases at hilum of kidney	Yes, recommended only for patients with clinically suspected stage T3–T4 disease
MRI	Better for detecting gross vascular invasion than nodes	Yes, may be cost-effective in evaluating patients at intermediate and high clinical risk of having extrarenal disease
Metastases (M) Staging		
CT-Ch	Identifies hematogenous or lymphatic metastases to chest, more sensitive than chest radiograph; liver metastases can also often be evaluated	Yes, may be used to confirm abnormal findings on the chest radiograph or to evaluate patients with pulmonary symptoms
PET	May increase the sensitivity for detecting lymph node and visceral metastases	No, under investigation; early results show promise

CT, computed tomography; CT$_e$, CT enhanced with intravenous contrast; CT-Ch, chest CT; MRI, magnetic resonance imaging; PET, positron emission tomography; TAUS, transabdominal ultrasound.

PROGNOSIS AND CANCER SURVIVAL

PROGNOSIS

The limited number of prognostic factors are listed in Table 35.6.

CANCER STATISTICS AND SURVIVAL

When considered together, the genital and urinary systems in males are the major sites of malignancy. Prostate cancer alone accounts for 200,000 new patients annually. There are 100,000 new urinary tract cancers and 2.5-fold more male genital cancers: 250,000 cases annually (see Tables 35.7 and 35.8).

The dramatic gains in survival are due to multidisciplinary achievements in screening, early detection, precise diagnoses, and effective multimodal therapies. The cancer statistics reveal perhaps the greatest gains in survival in oncology over the last five decades. In local stage I, male genitourinary tumors are 90% to 100% curable according to the latest Surveillance Epidemiology and End Results data: kidney, 90%; bladder, 94%; testes, 99%; and prostate, 100% (Table 35.7). Death and mortality rates are declining. Pediatric Wilms' tumor was the first malignancy in childhood to be cured, achieving >90% long-term survival and heralding the success of multimodal treatment that would be achieved in adult tumors in urology (see Fig. 35.9).

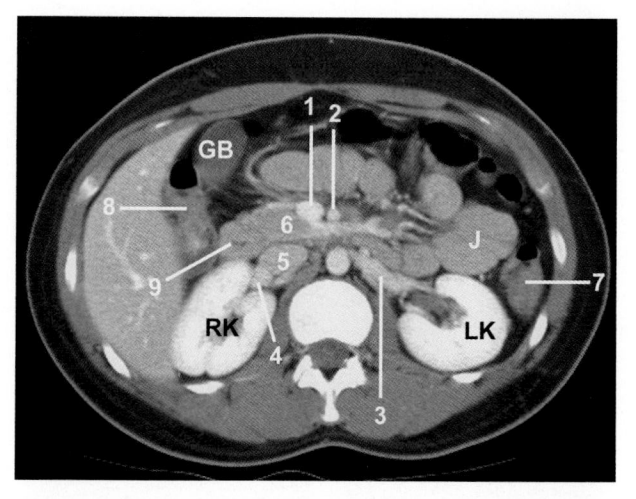

Figure 35.8 | Axial CTs of L1 and L2 level correlate with the T-oncoanatomy transverse section (Fig. 35.6C). Oncoimaging with CT is commonly applied to staging cancers, often combined with PET to determine true extent of primary cancer and involved lymph nodes. 1. Superior mesenteric vein. 2. Superior mesenteric artery. 3. Left renal artery 4. Right renal vein. 5. Inferior vena cava. 6. Pancreas. 7. Descending colon. 8. Ascending colon. 9. Duodenum. GB, gallbladder; J, jejunum; LK, left kidney; RK, right kidney.

TABLE 35.6	Prognostic Factors
Required for Staging	None
Clinically significant	Invasion beyond capsule into fat of peri-sinus tissues
	Venous involvement
	Adrenal extension
	Fuhrman grade
	Sarcomatoid features
	Histologic tumor necrosis
	Extranodal extension
	Size of metastasis in lymph nodes
	Presence or absence of extranodal extension
	Size of the largest tumor deposit in the lymph node

Edge SB, Byrd DR, Compton CC, et al. *AJCC Cancer Staging Manual.* 7th ed. New York, Springer, 2010, p. 485.

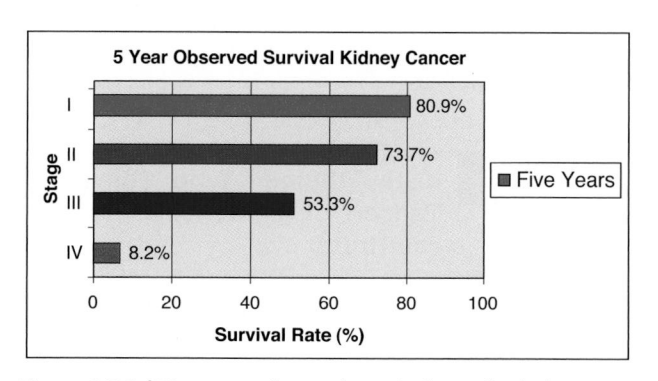

Figure 35.9 | Five-year observed survival rate for kidney cancer. (Data from Edge SB, Byrd DR, Compton CC, et al., *AJCC Cancer Staging Manual, 7th edition.* New York, Springer, 2010, p. 480.)

36

Renal Pelvis and Ureters

PERSPECTIVE, PATTERNS OF SPREAD, AND PATHOLOGY

Multifocality is a significant attribute of cancers of the renal pelvis and ureter.

PERSPECTIVE AND PATTERNS OF SPREAD

Multifocality is a significant attribute of cancers of the renal pelvis and ureter. Once a cancer appears and progresses, the issue of seeding versus field cancerization is a concern. The probability of an associated bladder cancer reaches 75% if both the renal pelvis and ureter have lesions versus half that with single cancers. Smokers and analgesic abusers (phenacetin) are at risk. Gross hematuria is the presenting sign in most patients (75%–90%), with the associated triad of flank mass, pain, and hematuria occurring in fewer than one fifth (20%) of patients. The diagnosis is readily made with either intravenous or retrograde urography, and the absence of the usual abundant tumor neovascularization suggests renal pelvic cancer.

TABLE 36.1	Histopathologic Type: Common Cancers of the Renal Pelvis and Ureter
Type	
Urothelial (transitional cell) carcinoma	Epidermoid carcinoma
Squamous cell carcinoma	Adenocarcinoma
Urothelial (transitional cell) carcinoma	
In situ	
Papillary	
Flat	
With squamous differentiation	
With glandular differentiation	
With squamous and glandular differentiation	
Squamous cell carcinoma	
Adenocarcinoma	
Undifferentiated carcinoma	

The predominant cancer is urothelial (transitional cell) carcinoma. Histologic variants include micropapillary and nested subtypes.

Edge SB, Byrd DR, Compton CC, et al. *AJCC Cancer Staging Manual*, 7th ed. New York, Springer, 2010, p. 493.

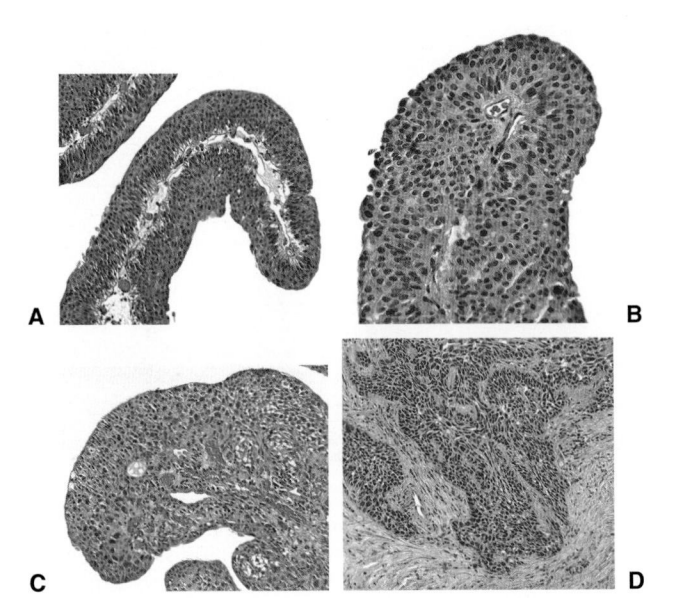

Figure 36.1 | **Urothelial tumors of the renal pelvis are similar to bladder. A.** Low-grade papillary urothelial carcinoma consists of exophytic papillae that have a central connective tissue core and are lined by slightly disorganized transitional epithelium. **B.** Low-grade papillary urothelial carcinoma at higher magnification shows mild architectural and cytologic atypia. **C.** High-grade papillary urothelial carcinoma shows prominent architectural disorganization of the epithelium which contains cells with pleomorphic hyperchromatic nuclei. **D.** Invasive high-grade papillary urothelial carcinoma consists of irregular nests of hyperchromatic cells invading into the muscularis.

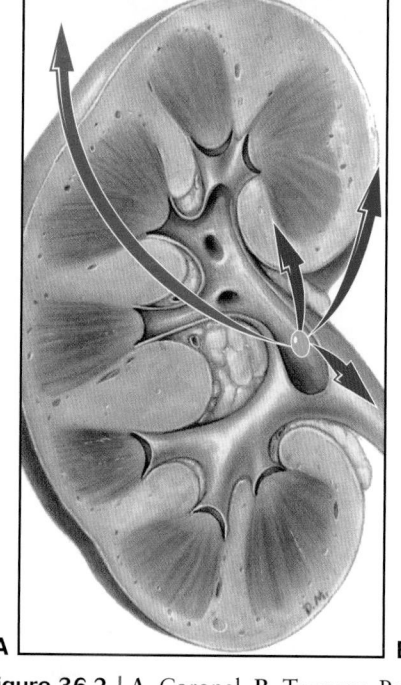
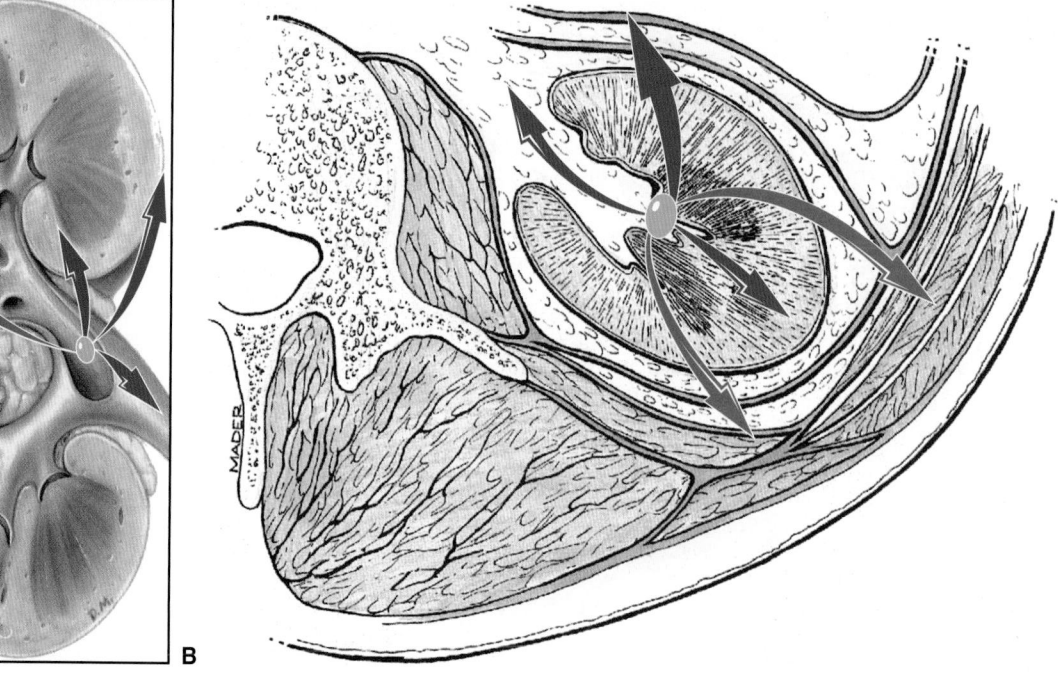

Figure 36.2 | A. Coronal. **B.** Traverse. Patterns of spread (cancer crab) of renal pelvis and ureter cancer color coded for stage: Tis or Ta, yellow; T1, green; T2, blue; T3, purple; and T4, red. The concept of visualizing patterns of spread to appreciate the surrounding anatomy is well demonstrated by the six-directional pattern (SIMLAP, Table 36.2).

TABLE 36.2	SIMLAP	
Renal Pelvis		
S	Adrenal gland	• T3a
	Inferior vena cava	• T4
I	Seed ureter	• M1
	Seed ureter bladder	• M1
M	Renal calyx minor	• T1
	Renal calyx major	
	Renal vein	• T4
	Hilar lymph nodes	• N1
	Paraortic/paracaval nodes	• N2
L	Quadratus lumborum muscle	• T4
	Renal parenchyma	• T3
	Perinephric fat	• T3
A	**Peritoneum**	
	Pancreas	• T4
	Duodenum	• T4
P	Perinephric fat	• T3
	Renal fascia (Gerota's)	• T4
	Transversus abdominis muscle	• T4
	Quadratus lumborum muscle	• T4
	Subcostal nerve	• T4

The six vectors of invasion are S̲uperior, I̲nferior, M̲edial, L̲ateral, A̲nterior, and P̲osterior. The color-coded dots correlate the T stage with specific anatomic structure involved.

The issue of multifocal disease is addressed on surgical resection—that is, nephrectomy with total ureterectomy including a cuff of the urinary bladder. Isolated ureteral cancers are rare (1%) and predominate in males (2:1).

The renal pelvises are akin to a hollow structure with a thin wall. The pattern of spread is into the muscle wall and then through the wall into the peripelvic fat and periureteral junction. As it advances, the renal parenchyma may be invaded. Seeding into the ureters and bladder is quite common (Fig. 36.2; Table 36.2).

PATHOLOGY

The majority of cancers are transitional cell (90%); the rest are squamous cell cancers often associated with chronic inflammation or infection of the renal pelvis. Adenocarcinomas are extremely rare. As it advances, the renal parenchyma may be invaded. Seeding into the ureters and bladder are quite common (Fig. 36.1; Table 36.1).

TNM STAGING CRITERIA

TNM STAGING CRITERIA

Cancers of the renal pelvis and ureters were distinguished in the fourth edition of the *AJCC Cancer Staging Manual* and have followed the tradition of staging hollow organs, similar to the digestive system (Fig. 36.3), that is, based on the depth of renal pelvis wall invasion rather than size.

Stage T1 cancer invades into subepithelial connective tissue and stage T2 cancer into the muscular layer. Stage T3 cancer invades into perirenal fat through the renal pelvis wall, and T4 cancer invades into adjacent organs (Fig. 36.3).

The regional nodes are the same for renal cancers and renal pelvis cancers. However, their definitions are different in the fourth edition of the *AJCC Cancer Staging Manual*. In renal cancers, the major criterion is node number: N1 is single and N2 is multiple nodes. In contrast, in renal pelvis cancers, size of the nodes is the critical criterion: N1, ≤2 cm; N2, 2 to 5 cm; and N3, >5 cm. Although lymph node stages defined in the fourth edition were the same, they have diverged as noted for renal parenchymal versus renal pelvis cancers.

SUMMARY OF CHANGES SEVENTH EDITION AJCC

- The definitions of TNM and the Stage Grouping for this chapter have not changed from the Sixth Edition (Fig. 26.3).

- Grading: A low- and high-grade designation will replace previous four-grade system to match current World Health Organization/International Society of Urologic Pathology (WHO/ISUP) recommended grading system.

The TNM Staging Matrix allows for identification of Stage Group once T and N stages are determined (Table 36.3). T stage determines stage group.

| TABLE 36.3 | Stage Summary Matrix |

	N0	N1	N2	N3	M1
T1	I	IV	IV	IV	IV
T2	II	IV	IV	IV	IV
T3	III	IV	IV	IV	IV
T4	IV	IV	IV	IV	IV

RENAL PELVIS

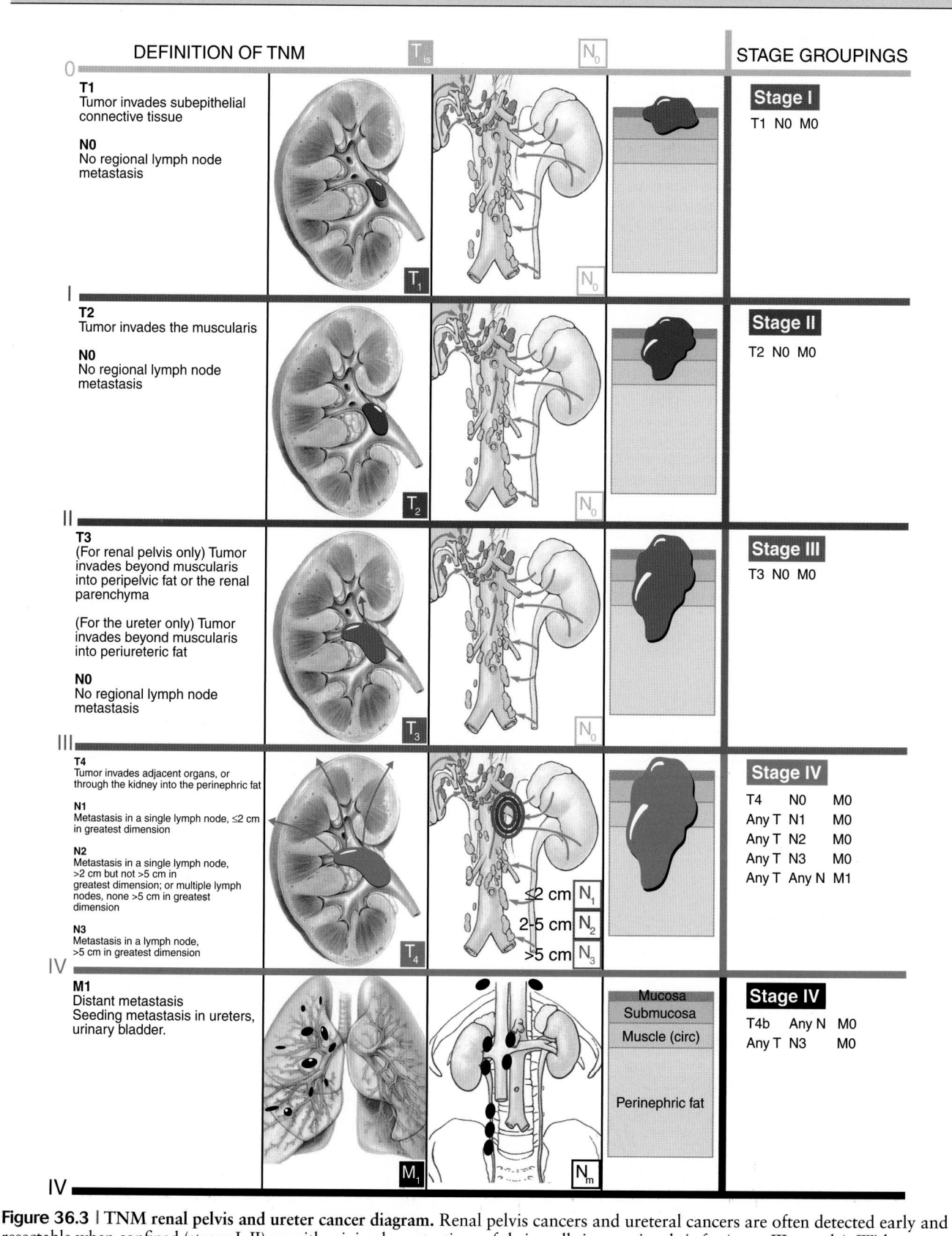

Figure 36.3 | TNM renal pelvis and ureter cancer diagram. Renal pelvis cancers and ureteral cancers are often detected early and resectable when confined (stages I, II) or with minimal penetrations of their walls into perinephric fat (stage III; purple). With extensive invasion (stage IV; red) they become unresectable, as well as become metastatic by seeding out. Vertically arranged with T definitions on the left and stage groupings on the right. Color bars are coded for stage: stage Tis or Ta, yellow; I, green; II, blue; III, purple; IV, red; and metastatic, black.

T-ONCOANATOMY

ORIENTATION OF THREE-PLANAR ONCOANATOMY

The isocenter of renal cancer is the renal bed, which consists of renal (Gerota's) fascia, which overlies the psoas major muscle and the quadratus lumborum musculature. The superior poles of both kidneys also lie in contact with the diaphragm. Usually, the 12th rib overlies the superior portion of the kidneys and is the only bone that is intimate anatomically. The kidney also lies opposite the transverse processes of T12 to L3 (Fig. 36.4).

T-oncoanatomy

The T-oncoanatomy is displayed in three planar views. A. Coronal, B. Sagittal, C. Transverse axial (Fig. 36.5).

- *Coronal:* There are many structures that overlie the kidney; however, they are of little concern oncologically because the peritoneal lining essentially excludes the visceral structures it contains from direct invasion. Nevertheless, it is important to recognize the intimate relationships of the stomach, on the left, and the duodenum, on the right, and the location of the hepatic and splenic flexures of the colon in relation to the midportions of the kidneys. The lung overlies the upper poles of both kidneys owing to the low insertion of the diaphragm, particularly during deep inspiration. One should be aware of the position of the pancreas, particularly of its head and tail and in regard to the right and left hila of the kidneys, respectively (Fig. 36.4).

- *Sagittal:* The kidney is encased by a fibrous capsule and is surrounded by perinephric fat. The kidney is composed of the cortex, which includes glomeruli; convoluted tubules; and the medulla, which consists of the pyramids of converging tubules and the loops of Henle. The exterior third of the kidney substance is the cortex, in contrast to the inner two thirds, which is the medulla. The medulla contains 8 to 18 striated pyramids that send finger-like rays into the cortex and end in the minor calices. The minor calices unite and form the major calices that drain into the renal pelvis. The hilus of the kidney has the pelvis, ureter, renal artery, and veins.

- *Transverse:* The ureteropelvic interface serves as the variable junction between pelvis and ureter, which courses inferiorly into the pelvis. The course of the ureter is such that it is first crossed anteriorly by the renal artery and vein and then the spermatic artery and vein in the male or the ovarian artery and vein in the female. In its continued descent retroperitoneally, the ureter passes anterior to the major iliac vessels. Before its insertion in the bladder, the vesical arteries and veins, as well as the uterine artery and vein, pass anteriorly ("water under the bridge") to the ureter. There are considerable variations in the anatomic relationships of the renal ureters with renal arteries and veins owing to normal anatomic variations of embryologic development that lead to different locations of the kidneys. In addition, anomalies in their development are common and include multiple renal arteries, fetal lobulations of the kidney, deflected and bifid ureters and pelves, and horseshoe and pelvic kidneys.

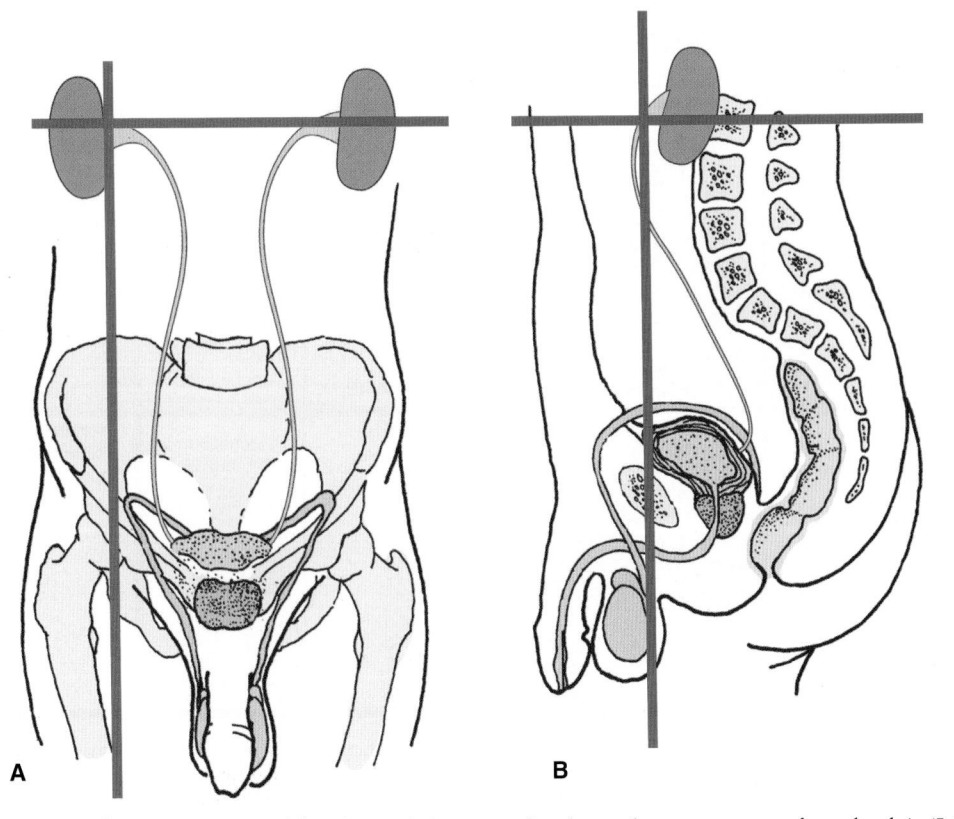

A   **B**

Figure 36.4 | Orientation of T-oncoanatomy. The anatomic isocenter for three-planar anatomy of renal pelvis (L1, L2) and ureter is at the L1 to S5 level. **A.** Coronal. **B.** Sagittal.

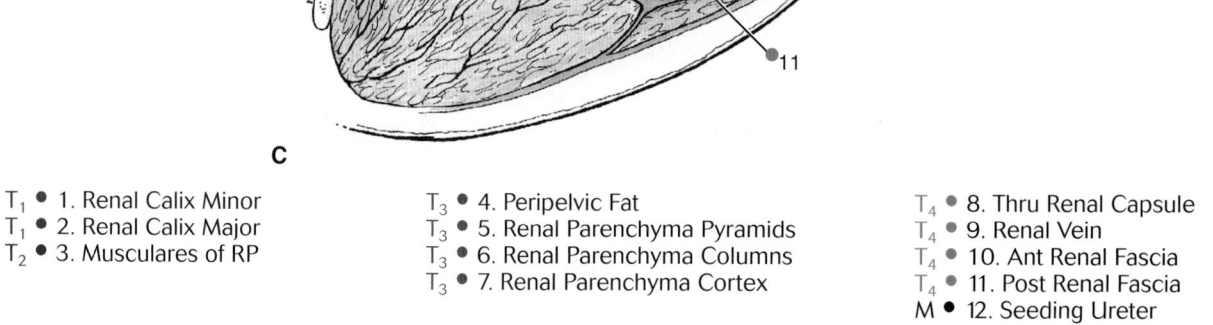

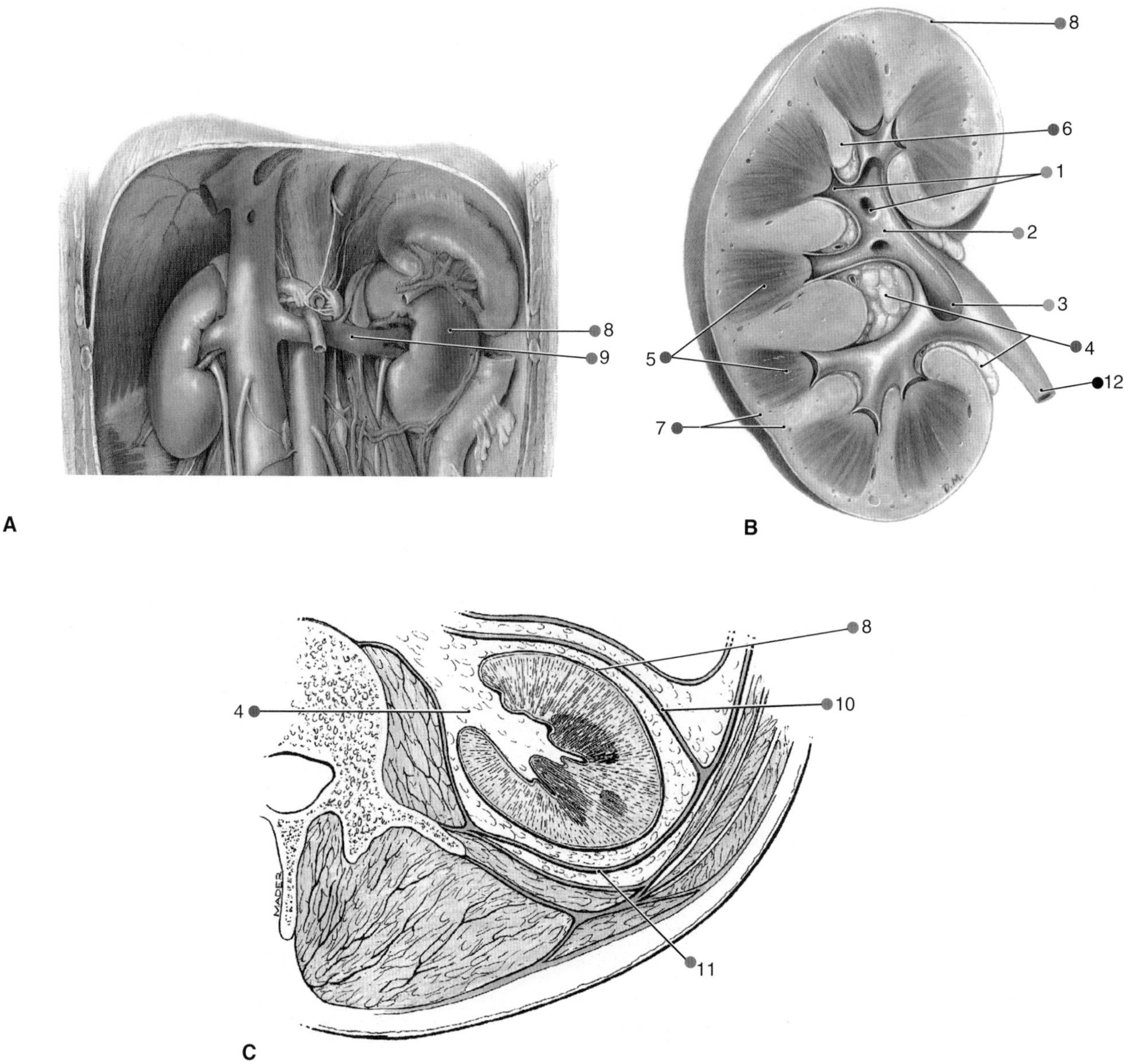

Figure 36.5 | T-oncoanatomy. The Color Code for the anatomic sites correlates with the color code for the stage group (Fig. 36.3) and patterns of spread (Fig. 36.2) and SIMLAP tables (Table 36.2). Connecting the dots in similar colors will provide an appreciation for the 3D Oncoanatomy.

T_1 • 1. Renal Calix Minor
T_1 • 2. Renal Calix Major
T_2 • 3. Musculares of RP

T_3 • 4. Peripelvic Fat
T_3 • 5. Renal Parenchyma Pyramids
T_3 • 6. Renal Parenchyma Columns
T_3 • 7. Renal Parenchyma Cortex

T_4 • 8. Thru Renal Capsule
T_4 • 9. Renal Vein
T_4 • 10. Ant Renal Fascia
T_4 • 11. Post Renal Fascia
M • 12. Seeding Ureter

N-ONCOANATOMY AND M-ONCOANATOMY

N-ONCOANATOMY

The regional nodes are anterior to and surround the renal artery and vein and at the midline, para-aortic and paracaval in location. It is important to note the left testis drains to the left hilar area of the kidney and the right testis drains to para-caval nodes at the lower pole on the right. The cisterna chyli is located on the right side near the upper pole.

There are considerable variations in the anatomic relation-ships of the renal ureters with renal arteries and veins because of normal anatomic variations of embryologic development that lead to different locations of the kidneys. In addition, anomalies in their development are common and include mul-tiple renal arteries, fetal lobulations of the kidney, deflected and bifid ureters and pelves, and horseshoe and pelvic kidneys (Fig. 36.6A; Table 36.4).

TABLE 36.4	Lymph Nodes of Renal Pelvis and Ureters
Pelvis and Ureters	
Sentinel Nodes	**Juxtaregional Nodes**
Renal hilar	External iliac
Paracaval	Mediastinal
Para-aortic nodes	
Regional Nodes	**Metastatic Nodes**
Renal hilar	Supraclavicular
Para-aortic	
Periureteral	
Common iliac	
Internal iliac	

M-ONCOANATOMY

Common metastatic sites reflect the vascular drainage of the kidney. As noted in the patterns of spread, invasion in the renal vein and inferior vena cava is common. Pulmonary spread is very common. With continued circulation of tumor cells through the left heart, metastases to bone, brain, and liver become possible. Unfortunately, remote metastases frequently occur with this tumor because of its rich neovascularization.

Renal pelvis transitional cell cancers are characterized sim-ilarly to transitional cell cancers of uroepithelium of bladder in their ability to "seed" throughout the urinary tract. Endoscopic assessment is important to determine when renal pelvis cancer is a primary or part of a disseminated urological cancer (see Fig. 36.6B).

REGIONAL LYMPH NODES

Any amount of regional lymph node metastasis is a poor prog-nostic finding, and outcome is minimally influenced by the number, size, or location of the regional nodes that are involved.*

*Preceding passage from Edge SB, Byrd DR, and Compton CC, et al. *AJCC Cancer Staging Manual, 7th edition.* New York, Springer, 2010, p. 492.

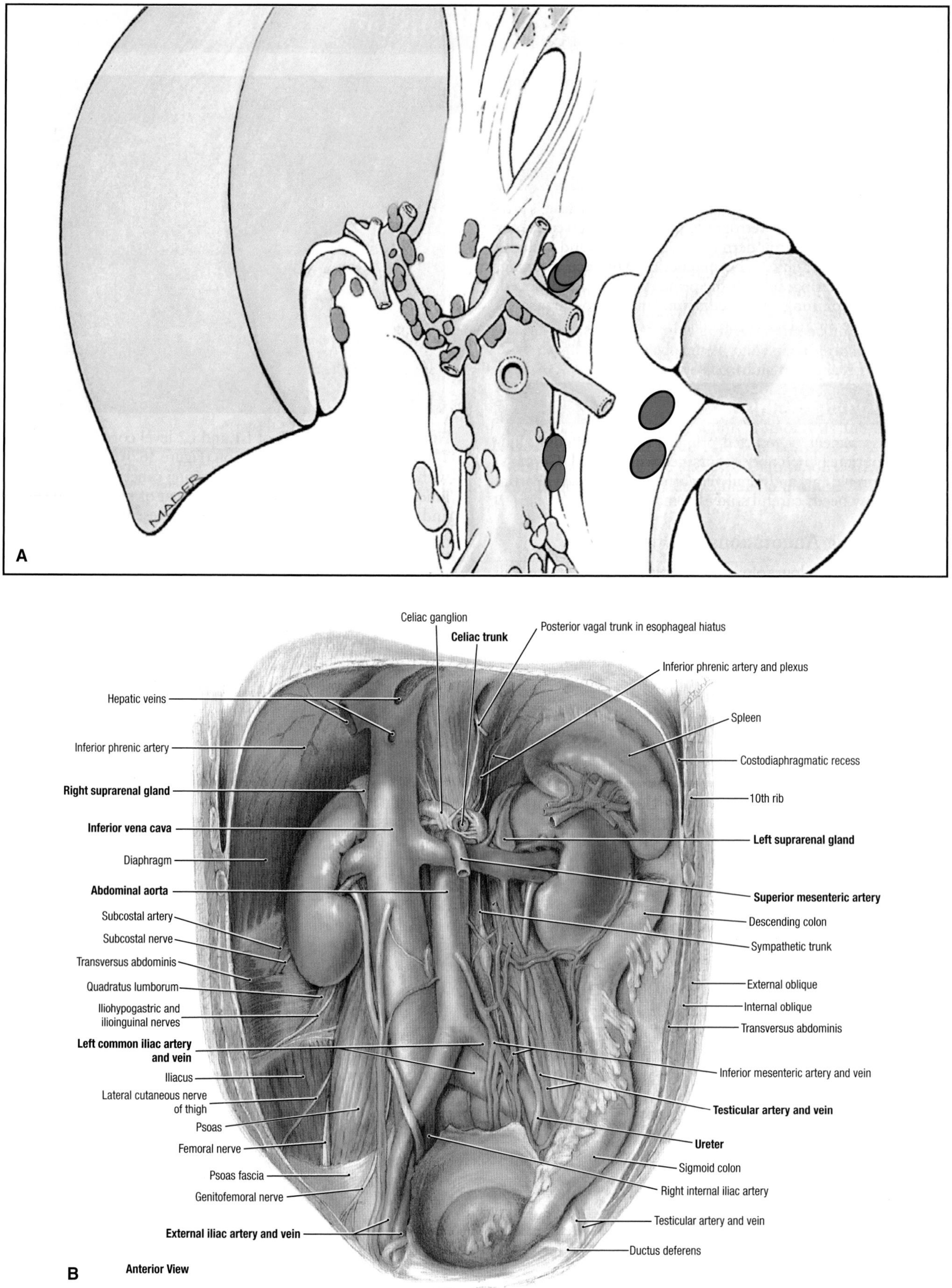

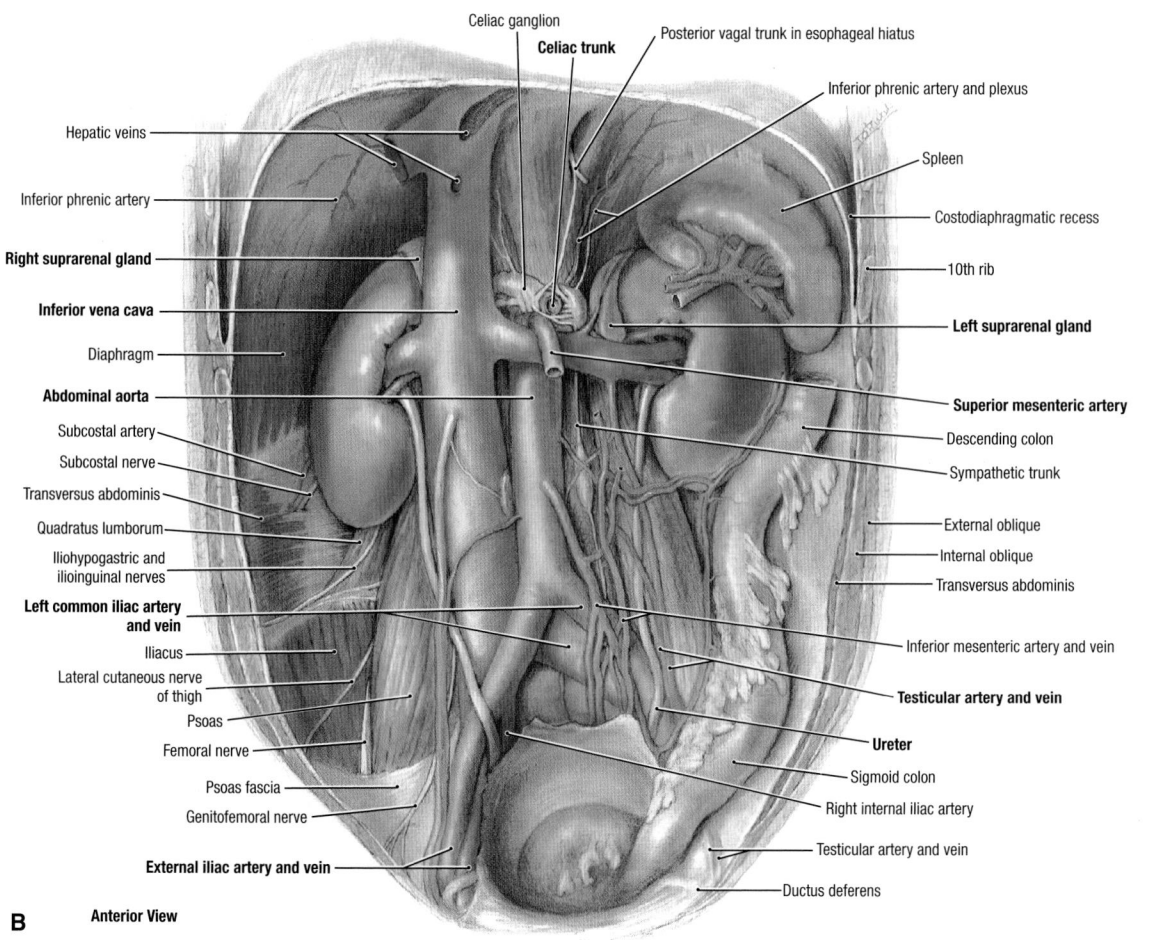

Figure 36.6 | A. N-oncoanatomy. Renal (para-aortic) and renal pelvis and ureter. B. M-oncoanatomy. Great vessels, kidneys, and suprarenal glands.

37

Urinary Bladder

PERSPECTIVE, PATTERNS OF SPREAD, AND PATHOLOGY

The uroepithelium is subject to numerous excretory products and responds with a proliferative process, often as a benign papilloma, which can become multiple, covering most of the bladder epithelium and representing a field carcinogenesis.

PERSPECTIVE AND PATTERNS OF SPREAD

Bladder cancer is a neoplasm of the elderly, peaking at 60 to 80 years of age. Despite its highly varied gross appearance in the bladder, intermittent hematuria, either macroscopic or microscopic, is the major manifestation. Occasionally, it presents as a bladder infection with irritability and dysuria, particularly recurrent in character, that suggests some underlying pathology or tumor. This is the most frequent cancer of the urinary tract, with an estimated 60,000 new cases reported annually. Bladder cancer accounts for 2.5% of all tumors, or 13,000 cancer deaths annually. Although aniline dyes have been implicated, as well as other industrial agents or some carcinogenic metabolite secreted in urine, no true cause of

TABLE 37.1 Histopathologic Type: Common Cancers of the Bladder

Type
Urothelial (transitional cell) carcinoma
In situ
Papillary
Flat
With squamous metaplasia
With glandular metaplasia
With squamous and glandular metaplasia
Squamous cell carcinoma
Adenocarcinoma
Undifferentiated carcinoma

Reprinted with permission from Edge SB, Byrd DR, Compton CC, et al. *AJCC Cancer Staging Manual.* 7th ed. New York, Springer, 2010:501.

bladder cancer is known. Some infectious agents, however, such as *Schistosoma haematobium*, have been implicated in Egypt, where the more commonly squamous cell cancer results (Table 37.1).

Worldwide, bladder cancer is among the most common malignancies, in 11th place. North Africa and western Asia are considered high-risk areas. Males predominate in a 3:1 ratio to females.

The pattern of spread is into its wall and then its surrounding structures (Fig. 37.2; Table 37.2).

Cancers of the urinary bladder typically begin as papillomas, a benign proliferative process that can become multiple papillomatosis, covering the bladder surface. Transformation into an invasive cancer results in penetration into the muscular layer, and, as depth increases, the muscle contractility increases its circumferential spread. Inferiorly in males, the prostate can be invaded since there is no capsule to separate it from the bladder. Superior spread is less likely due to its peritoneal covering. Bladder perforation leads to subcutaneous spread of urine along the anterior abdominal wall. Posteriorly the trigone of the bladder, once invaded, can obstruct the ureter(s). Lateral extension to the sidewalls can occur. In the female, invasion of the anterior lip of the cervix is possible, but more usual is the opposite invasion of cervix cancer into the bladder wall posteriorly.

PATHOLOGY

The uroepithelium is subject to numerous excretory products and responds with a proliferative process, often as a benign papilloma, which can become multiple, covering most of the bladder epithelium and representing a field carcinogenesis. The transformation to cancer depends on three criteria: cell type, pattern of growth, and grading. The majority are transitional cell carcinomas that change from mucosal exophytic lesions (grade I) to endophytic, invading into muscle (grades II and III). The patterns of spread are determined by muscular contraction of the bladder; as the tumor penetrates the wall, it spreads circumferentially. Squamous cell cancers are mainly associated with schistosomiasis. Primary adenocarcinomas tend to develop in the dome of the bladder, often from urachal epithelium rests. The various cancers of the urinary bladder are tabulated and their grading is noted (Table 37.1; Figure 37.1).

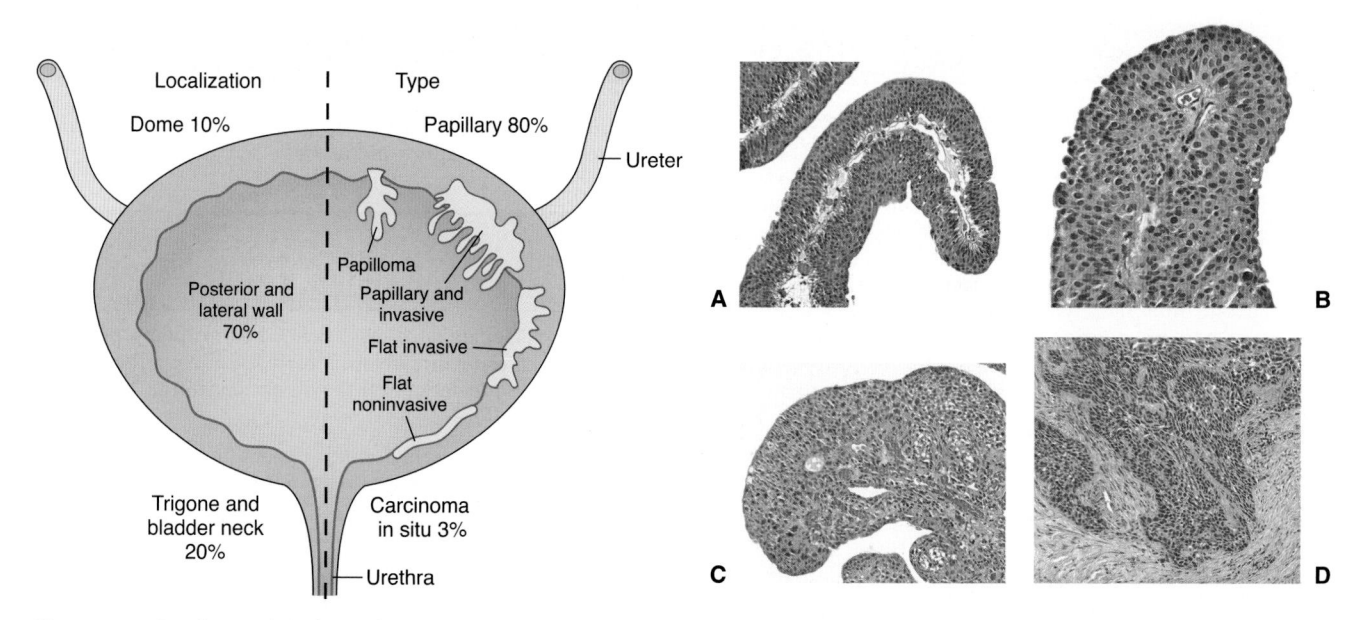

Figure 37.1 | Left. Urothelial neoplasms. Most tumors occur in the urinary bladder and are classified histologically as urothelial (transitional cell) carcinomas (TCCs). Ureters and the posterior urethra are also lined by transitional epithelium and can give rise to TCCs. TCCs can be flat, papillary, papillary and invasive, or simply invasive. Benign transitional cell papillomas are rare. **Right. Urothelial tumors of the urinary bladder. A.** Low-grade papillary urothelial carcinoma consists of exophytic papillae that have a central connective tissue core and are lined by slightly disorganized transitional epithelium. **B.** Low-grade papillary urothelial carcinoma at higher magnification shows mild architectural and cytologic atypia. **C.** High-grade papillary urothelial carcinoma shows prominent architectural disorganization of the epithelium, which contains cells with pleomorphic hyperchromatic nuclei. **D.** Invasive high-grade papillary urothelial carcinoma consists of irregular nests of hyperchromatic cells invading into the muscularis.

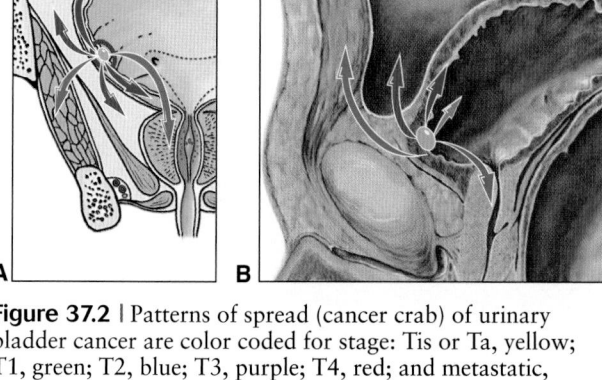

Figure 37.2 | Patterns of spread (cancer crab) of urinary bladder cancer are color coded for stage: Tis or Ta, yellow; T1, green; T2, blue; T3, purple; T4, red; and metastatic, black. Correlate patterns of spread with the SIMLAP Table 37.2. The anatomic site invaded is color coded for T stage of advancement.

TABLE 37.2	SIMLAP		
Male Urinary Bladder			
S	Peritoneum	• T4b	
	Small intestine	• T4b	
	Ureters	• T3	
	Prostate	• T4a	
	Exterior urethral		
I	Sphincter	• T4b	
	Urethra	• T4b	
	Bulb of penis	• T4b	
	Spongy urethra	• T4b	
M			
L	Levator ani muscle	• T4b	
	Obturator lymph node	N1	
	Internal iliac vein/artery/nodes	N2	
A	Retropubic space	• T4b	
	Pubis	• T4b	
	Trigone bladder		
P	Wall	• T2	• T3
	Seminal vesicles	• T3	
	Ureters	• T3	
	Rectum	• T4a	

The six vectors of invasion are Superior, Inferior, Medial, Lateral, Anterior, and Posterior. The color-coded dots correlate the T stage with specific anatomic structure involved.

TNM STAGING CRITERIA

TNM STAGING CRITERIA

In their initial phase, bladder cancers tend to be multiple, superficial mucosal and submucosal lesions (stage T1; Fig. 37.3). With invasion into the muscular wall (T2), the tumor spreads, first in depth and then circumferentially in the submucosal and muscular lymphatics. There is a relationship between depth of invasion and circumferential spread; the tumor infiltration in the wall is massaged due to the contractility of this viscus. The capacity of the bladder to expand and contract is altered somewhat as the tumor invades its walls. When circumferential spread is extensive (T2B), akin to linitis plastica of the stomach, a permanently contracted bladder results with little capacity.

Once the tumor reaches the serosal surface, invasion of perivesical fat (T3) and adjacent structures occurs (T4). Anteriorly, it can become fixed to, but rarely destroys, the bony pubis; laterally, the cancer can extend to the pelvic wall and invades lymphatics, and enlarged pelvic lymph nodes can compress the iliac vessels. Direct posterior invasion into the rectum rarely occurs in males; the same is true of direct invasion of posterior gynecological structures in females. This pattern of invasion is more representative of late or recurrent disease.

Tumors of the trigone usually result in ureteral obstruction owing to the entry of the ureters at this juncture. If secondary infection and edema cause the obstruction, it may be reversible. Once unilateral obstruction of the ureter occurs, hydronephrosis results; if unrelieved, the kidney stops functioning and atrophies. Secondary infection may lead to an ascending pyelonephritis and septicemia. Bilateral obstruction can result in renal failure and uremia.

SUMMARY OF CHANGES SEVENTH EDITION AJCC

- Primary staging: T4 disease defined as including prostatic stromal invasion directly from bladder cancer. Subepithelial invasion of prostatic urethra will not constitute T4 staging status (Fig. 37.3).

- Grading: a low-and high-grade designation will replace previous four grade system to match current World Health Organization/International Society of Urologic Pathology (WHO/ISUP) recommended grading system.

- Nodal Classification
  - Common iliac nodes defined as secondary drainage region as regional nodes and not as metastatic disease
  - N staging system change
    - N1: single positive node in primary drainage regions
    - N2: multiple positive nodes in primary drainage regions
    - N3: common iliac node involvement

The TNM Staging Matrix is color coded for identification of stage group once T and N stages are determined (Table 37.3). The T stage determines stage group.

TABLE 37.3 Stage Summary Matrix

	N0	N1	N2	N3	M1
T1	I	IV	IV	IV	IV
T2	II	IV	IV	IV	IV
T3	III	IV	IV	IV	IV
T4	IV	IV	IV	IV	IV

T stage determines stage group.

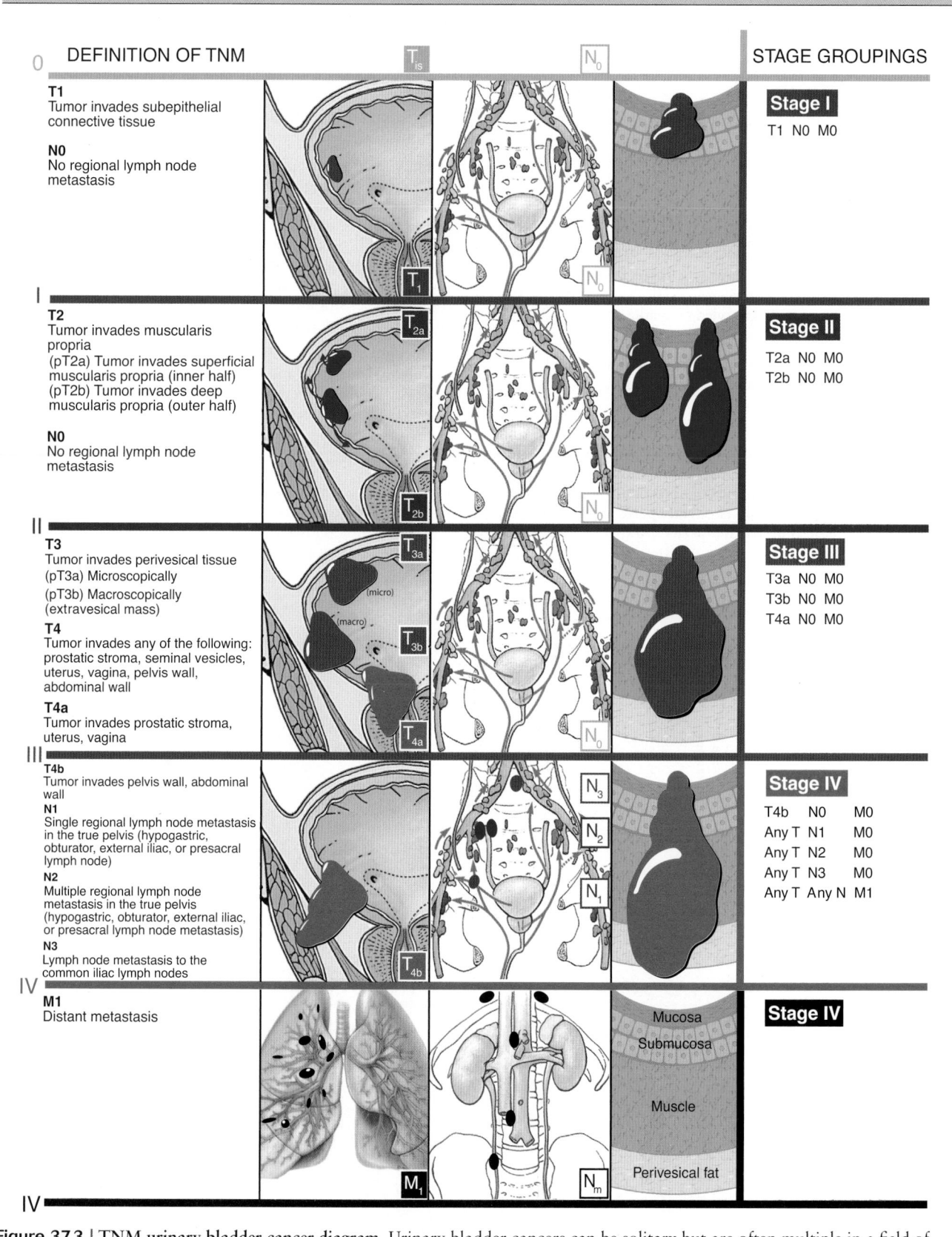

Figure 37.3 | TNM urinary bladder cancer diagram. Urinary bladder cancers can be solitary but are often multiple in a field of epithelial carcinogenesis. Stage I (*green*) papillomas are conservatively resected transurethrally, stage II (*blue*) with partial cystectomies, stage III (*purple*) require total cystectomy and urethral diversion, and stage IV (*red*) are no longer completely resectable. Vertically arranged with T definitions on the left and stage groupings on the right. Color bars are coded for stage: stages 0is and 0a, yellow; I, green; II, blue; III, purple; IV, red; and metastatic, black.

T-ONCOANATOMY

ORIENTATION OF THREE-PLANAR ONCOANATOMY

The isocenter for the urinary bladder varies depending on its fullness or whether it is empty. Most often it is depicted empty and as a pelvic organ at the S4/S5 level (Fig. 37.4).

T-oncoanatomy

The T-oncoanatomy is displayed in three planar views. A. Coronal, B. Sagittal, C. Transverse Axial. (Fig. 37.5A/B). The bladder's location requires knowledge of adjacent genital structures and disease. Symptomatology depends, in part, on gender.

- *Coronal:* In the male, the bladder is intimately related to the seminal vesicles posteriorly, the prostate inferiorly, and the pubis and peritoneum anteriorly.

- *Sagittal:* The relationship of the ureters to surrounding blood vessels is important. The bladder is not a fixed structure but has considerable capacity and mobility, altering its contour and contact with the colointestinal viscera as it fills with urine. The bladder is a retroperitoneal structure, whereas the gastrointestinal tract is intraperitoneal except for the rectum.

- *Transverse:* The seminal vesicles are situated between the bladder and rectum. In the female, the vagina and cervix are located posterior to the bladder and the body of the uterus, superiorly. The bladder is extraperitoneal, although the sigmoid colon and terminal portions of the ileum can be in contact with its superior surface.

In the female, the bladder is intimately related to the uterus and vagina. The trigone of the bladder is in direct contact on its posterior surface with the anterior lip of the cervix and anterior fornix of the vagina. The urethra is located in the anterior wall of the vagina. Cancers of the bladder rarely invade the female genital tract, but cancers of the cervix infiltrate and invade the bladder. The ureters, which have a horizontal course, straddle the cervix and are commonly strapped and obstructed by parametrial invasion.

- *Coronal view:* The opened bladder is situated above the pubis. The trigone and ureteral orifices are noted in the corners, with the ureter coursing superiorly alongside the cervix. The uterus is anteflexed and rests on the bladder.

- *Sagittal view:* The bladder is anterior and the rectum posterior to the female genital organs.

- *Axial view:* The superior axial section shows the intimate relationship of the cervix to the bladder wall. The inferior axial section shows the relationship of the urethra in the anterior wall of the vagina.

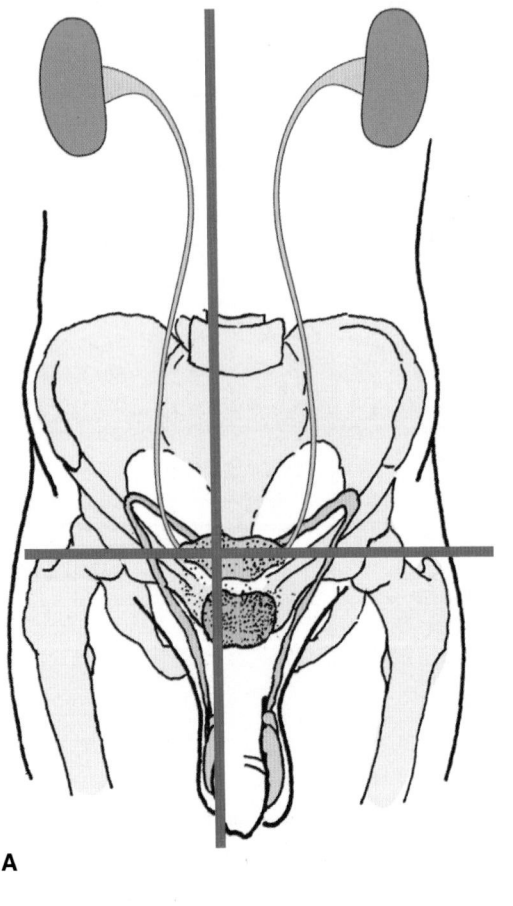

A

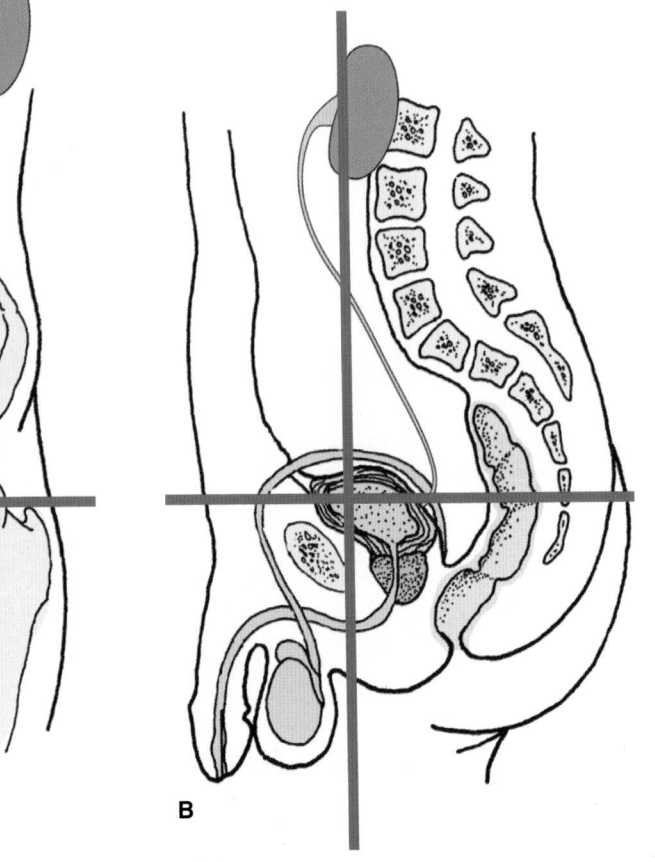

B

Figure 37.4 | Orientation of T-oncoanatomy. The anatomic isocenter for three-planar anatomy of renal pelvis and ureter is at the S1 to S5 level. **A.** Coronal. **B.** Sagittal.

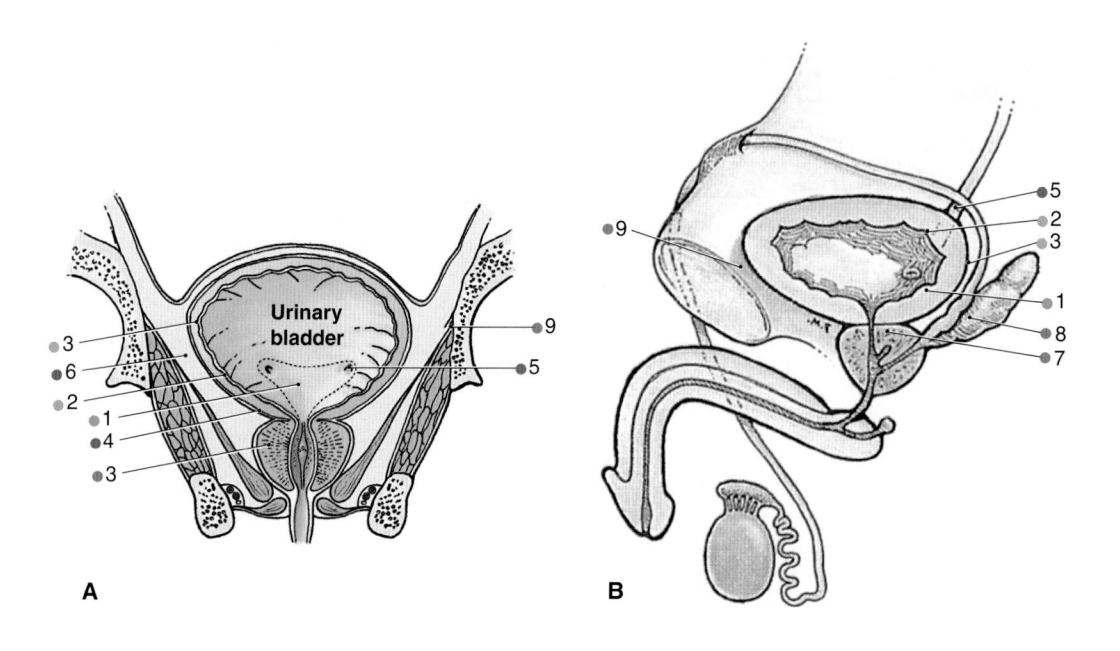

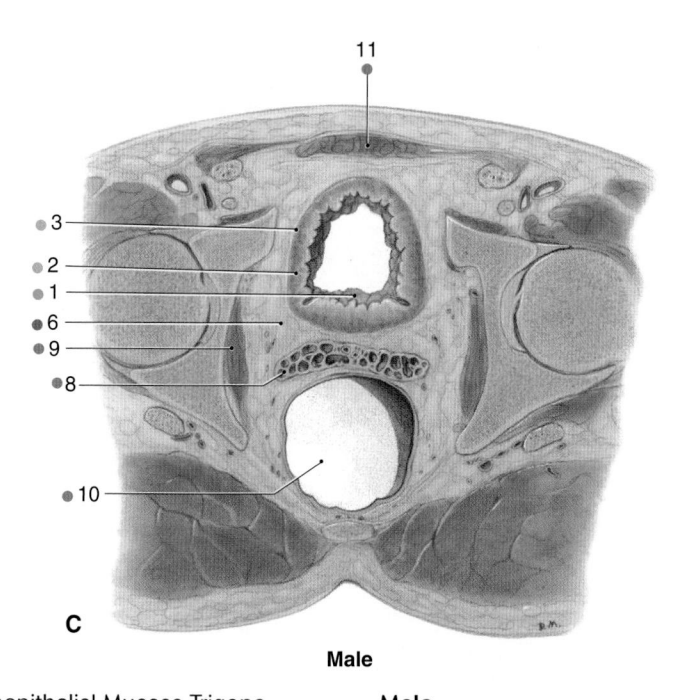

T$_1$ ● 1. Subepithelial Mucosa Trigone	**Male**
T$_{2a}$ ● 2. Superficial Muscle	T$_{4a}$ ● 7. Prostate Prostatic Urethra
T$_{2b}$ ● 3. Deep Muscle	T$_{4a}$ ● 8. Seminal Vesicle
T$_{3a}$ ● 4. Perivesical	T$_{4b}$ ● 9. Pelvic Wall
T$_{3a}$ ● 5. Ureter	T$_{4b}$ ● 10. Rectum
T$_{3b}$ ● 6. Extravesical Vesicouterine	T$_{4b}$ ● 11. Abdominal Wall

Figure 37.5 | The color code for the anatomic sites correlates with the color code for the stage group (Fig. 37.3) and patterns of spread (Fig. 37.2) and SIMLAP table (Table 37.2). Connecting the dots in similar colors provides an appreciation for the three-dimensional oncoanatomy.

N-ONCOANATOMY AND M-ONCOANATOMY

N-ONCOANATOMY

Lymph node invasion is common once the tumor has penetrated into the deep muscular layer and the serosa. The lymph nodes most commonly involved are the obturator or hypogastric nodes and the internal iliacs on the pelvic wall. All of these first station nodes are bilateral; however, the node at risk depends on the location of the primary tumor in the bladder. Eventually, invasion of the common iliac and para-aortic retroperitoneal nodes occurs, and drainage into the thoracic duct could naturally progress to supraclavicular node metastases; this is a rare presentation for a metastatic neck node with obscure etiology (Fig. 37.6A; Table 37.4A, and 4B).

The regional or pelvic lymph nodes, located below the bifurcation of the common iliac arteries, include the internal iliacs, the hypogastric, the common iliac located above the pelvic basin, and the posterior, presacral, and anterior perivesical nodes. The juxtaregional lymph nodes are the inguinal nodes, the high common iliac, and the para-aortic nodes. The vessels, nerves, and lymphatics lie on the inner wall of the true pelvis, below the pelvis basin on the obturator internus muscle.

In the female as in the male, the lymphatic drainage is to perivesical channels into the internal iliacs and to common iliac and then para-aortic nodes.

The incidence of lymph node metastases increases with stage of primary cancer (Table 37.4B).

M-ONCOANATOMY

Vascular spread, although uncommon, is usually a late event. Dissemination follows the vesical veins into the internal iliac veins and inferior vena cava. Tumor cells could reach the right side of the heart and then manifest as pulmonary metastases. Once the left heart is reached, the tumor cells could target to any other distant remote site (Fig. 37.6B).

REGIONAL LYMPH NODES

The regional lymph nodes draining the bladder include primary and secondary nodal drainage regions. Primary lymph nodes include the external iliac, hypogastric, and obturator basins. The presacral lymph nodes are classified as a primary drainage region; however, mapping studies have found this area to be a less frequent site of primary regional metastases. Primary nodal regions drain into the common iliac nodes, which constitute a secondary drainage region. Regional lymph node staging is of significant prognostic importance, given the negative impact on recurrence after treatment and long-term survival. The relevant information from regional lymph node staging is obtained from the extent of disease within the nodes (number of positive nodes, extranodal extension), not from whether metastases are unilateral or contralateral. Overall 5-year survival in node-positive bladder cancer following definitive local therapy is approximately 33%; however, patients with a greater node burden may be expected to do significantly worse.*

*Preceding passage from Edge SB, Byrd DR and Compton CC, et al. *AJCC Cancer Staging Manual*, 7th edition. New York, Springer, 2010, p. 498.

TABLE 37.4A Lymph Nodes of Urinary Bladder

Sentinel Nodes	Juxtaregional Nodes
Common iliac	Para-aortic
Internal iliac nodes	
Regional nodes	Metastatic
Common iliac	Inguinal
Internal iliac	
Anterior paravesical (obturator)	
External iliac	
Presacral	

TABLE 37.4B Incidence of Lymph Node Metastasis Following Radical Cystectomy, Correlation to Primary Tumor

Authors	Period (years)	Number of Patients	LN Met[a] No. (%)	Bladder Tumor Stage[a] No. (%)				
				P0, Pis, Pa, P1	P2a	P2b	P3	P4
Poulsen et al.	1990–1997	191	50 (26)	2 (4)	4 (18)	7 (25)	33 (51)	4 (43)
Vieweg et al.	1980–1990	686	193 (28)	10 (10)	12 (9)	22 (23)	97 (42)	52 (41)
Leissner	1999–2002	290	81 (28)	1 (3)	5 (13)	12 (22)	53 (43)	10 (50)
Stein et al.	1971–1997	1,054	246 (24)	19 (5)	21 (18)	35 (27)	113 (44)	58 (42)
Vazina et al.	1992–2002	176	43 (24)	1 (215)	10 (16)	—	20 (236)	12 (50)
Abdel-Latif et al.	1997–1999	418	110 (26)	3 (215)	4 (7)	29 (25)	59 (48)	15 (65)
Madersbacher et al.	1985–2000	507	124 (24)	2 (3)	26 (17)	—	64 (34)	32 (41)
Hautmann et al.	1986–2003	788	142 (18)	2 (2)	31 (10)	—	73 (41)	36 (43)
Total		4,110	989 (24)					

From Halperin EC, Perez CA, Brady LW, et al. *Perez and Brady's Principles and Practice of Radiation Oncology*. 5th ed. Philadelphia: Lippincott Williams & Wilkins, 2008:1419.

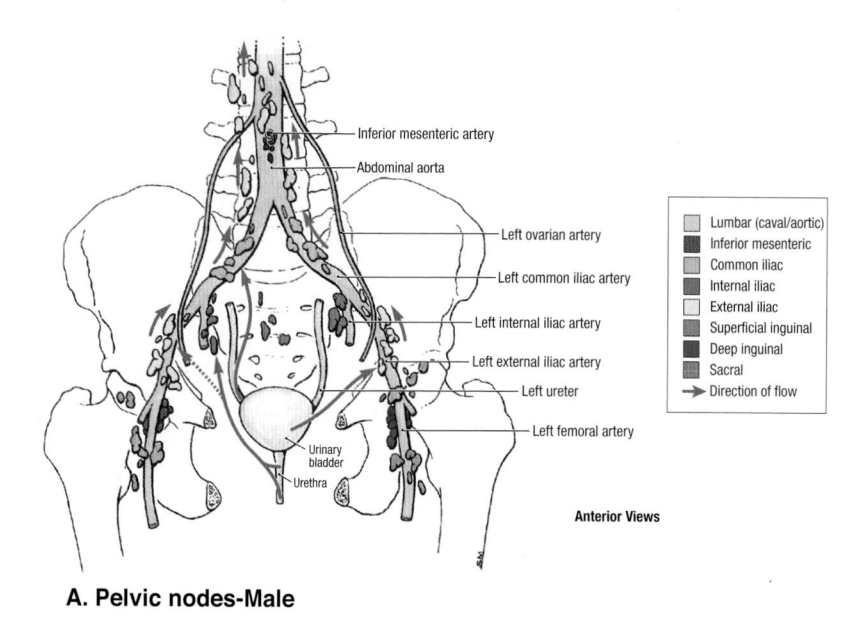

Inferior mesenteric artery

Abdominal aorta

Left ovarian artery

Left common iliac artery

Left internal iliac artery

Left external iliac artery

Left ureter

Left femoral artery

Urinary bladder

Urethra

Lumbar (caval/aortic)
Inferior mesenteric
Common iliac
Internal iliac
External iliac
Superficial inguinal
Deep inguinal
Sacral
Direction of flow

Anterior Views

A. Pelvic nodes-Male

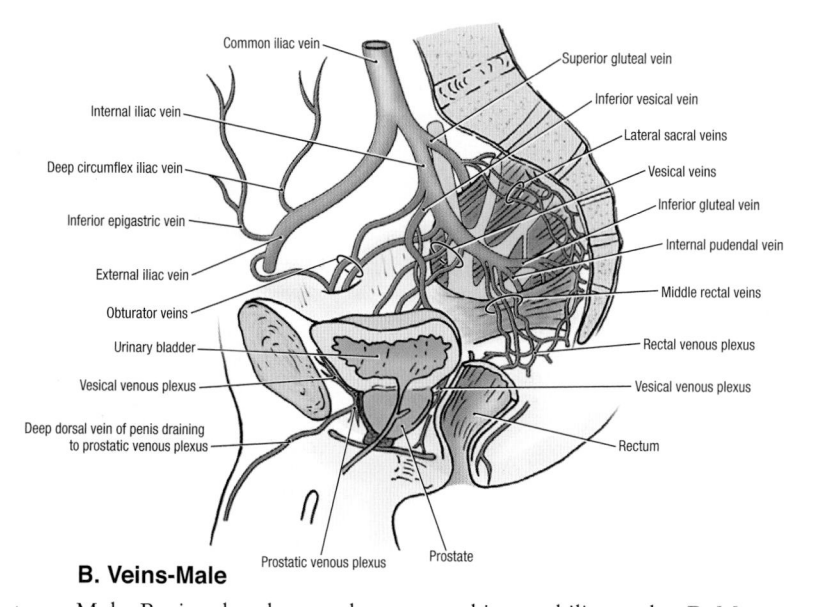

Common iliac vein

Superior gluteal vein

Internal iliac vein

Inferior vesical vein

Deep circumflex iliac vein

Lateral sacral veins

Vesical veins

Inferior epigastric vein

Inferior gluteal vein

Internal pudendal vein

External iliac vein

Middle rectal veins

Obturator veins

Urinary bladder

Rectal venous plexus

Vesical venous plexus

Vesical venous plexus

Deep dorsal vein of penis draining
to prostatic venous plexus

Rectum

Prostatic venous plexus

Prostate

B. Veins-Male

Figure 37.6 | **A.** N-oncoanatomy. Male: Regional nodes are obturator and internal iliac nodes. **B.** M-oncoanatomy. Medial view.

STAGING WORKUP

RULES OF CLASSIFICATION AND STAGING

Clinical Staging and Imaging

Primary evaluation is done preferentially under anesthesia before and after endoscopic surgery, providing histologic verification of depth of invasion. After transurethral resection, the bladder is palpated against the endoscope. No thickening in the wall suggests T1; some induration, T2. A thickened wall or mass suggests T3, and, if fixed or massive, T4. Modern modalities or enhanced computed tomography (CT) and magnetic resonance imaging (MRI) are most useful (Fig. 37.7); positron emission tomography is more investigational. Multiple biopsies are advised for field effect and presence of Tis. The entire urinary tract should be fully evaluated to exclude renal pelvis and ureters as sites of disease. Metastases workup should be considered for advanced-stage bladder cancer (Table 37.5).

Pathologic Staging

Following total cystectomy and pelvic node dissection, pathologic assessment of primary and nodes is feasible.

Oncoimaging Annotations

- Transabdominal ultrasonography can be used for bladder cancer surveillance, detecting 80% to 90% of tumors >5 mm in size.
- Virtual CT and MRI cystoscopy are being evaluated.
- Superficial bladder cancer (i.e., that which has not extended into the muscular layer of the bladder, stages T1 and below) is treated by transurethral resection.
- Muscle invasive bladder cancer, either alone (T2 or T3A) or with spread to the perivesical fat (T3B), to contiguous organs (T4), or to regional lymph nodes, requires radical surgical resection, often with radiotherapy.

- The critical distinction between superficial and muscle-invasive bladder cancer is established by transurethral resection and not by imaging. Clinical staging is not accurate for advanced disease.
- Cross-sectional imaging using either CT or MRI aids in the preoperative evaluation of locally advanced bladder cancer by demonstrating involvement of perivesical fat, invasion of contiguous organs, spread to the pelvic sidewall or anterior abdominal wall, or locoregional adenopathy.
- CT or MRI staging should be performed either before or 2 weeks after cystoscopy to minimize diagnostic errors and avoid misinterpretation.
- Both CT and MRI have a tendency to overestimate muscle and perivesical extension; both have excellent negative predictive value in excluding extravesical extension. MRI is superior to CT and transurethral ultrasonography in the evaluation of lesions located at the base or dome of the bladder.
- Differentiation of granulation tissue from persistent tumor after transurethral resection is better with MRI than CT, but limitations persist for both modalities.

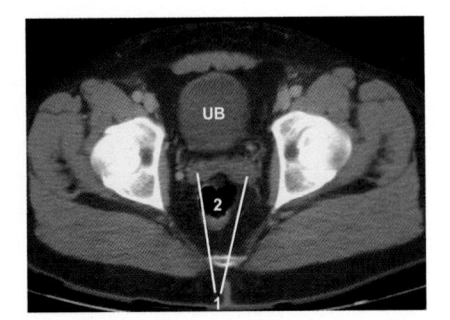

Figure 37.7 | CT level of the inferior aspect of the actabulum correlates with Fig. 37.5C. Male UB = urinary bladder. 1. Seminal vesicles. 2. Rectum.

TABLE 37.5	Imaging Modalities for Staging Urinary Bladder Cancer	
Method	**Diagnosis and Staging Capability**	**Recommended for Use**
Primary (T) Staging		
TAUS	More useful for detection than staging	No
CT$_e$	Accurate for staging advanced T3, T4 invasion beyond bladder wall	Yes, cost-effective
MRI	Provides most anatomic detail of cancer invasion into and beyond wall of urinary bladder	Yes, more accurate
Nodal (N) Staging		
CT$_e$	Valuable in assessing pelvic and para-aortic nodal enlargements	Yes, cost-effective
MRI	More valuable in distinguishing adenopathy secondary to inflammation versus cancer	Yes, more cost-effective
Metastases (M) Staging		
Chest film	Can detect gross pulmonary or mediastinal metastases	Yes, cost-effective

CT, computed tomography; CT$_e$, CT enhanced with intravenous contrast; MRI, magnetic resonance imaging; TAUS, transabdominal ultrasound.

PROGNOSIS AND CANCER SURVIVAL

PROGNOSIS

The limited number of prognostic factors are listed in Table 37.6.

CANCER STATISTICS AND SURVIVAL

When considered together, the male genital and urinary systems are major sites of malignancy. Prostate cancer alone accounts for 200,000 new patients annually. There are 100,000 new urinary tract cancers and 2.5-fold more male genital cancers: 250,000 cases annually.

The dramatic gains in survival are due to multidisciplinary achievements in screening, early detection, precise diagnoses, and effective multimodal therapies. The cancer statistics reveal perhaps the greatest gains in survival in oncology over the last five decades. In local stage I, male genitourinary tumors, all are 90% to 100% curable according to the latest Surveillance Epidemiology and End Results data: kidney, 90%; bladder, 94%; testes, 99%; and prostate, 100%. Mortality rates are declining. The pediatric Wilms' tumor was the first malignancy in childhood to be cured, achieving >90% long-term survival and heralding the success of multimodal treatment that would be achieved in adult tumors in urology (Table 37.7; Fig. 37.8).

TABLE 37.6	Prognostic Factors
Required for Staging	None
Clinically significant	Presence or absence of extra-nodal extension
	Size of the largest tumor deposit in the lymph nodes
	World Health Organization/International Society of Urologic Pathology (WHO/ISUP) grade

Reprinted with permission from Edge SB, Byrd DR, Compton CC, et al. *AJCC Cancer Staging Manual.* 7th ed. New York, Springer, 2010:504.

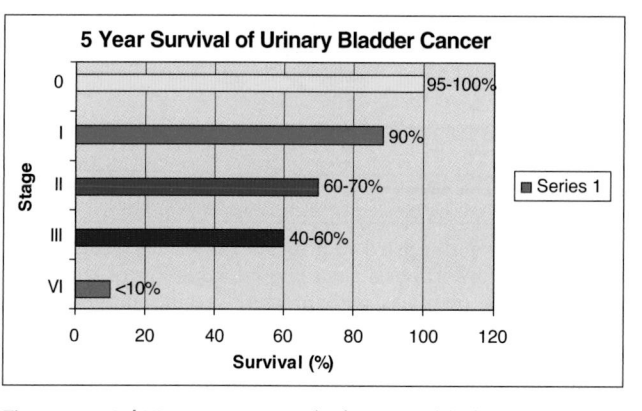

Figure 37.8 | Five-year survival of urinary bladder cancer. (Data from Edge SB, Byrd DR, and Compton CC, et al. *AJCC Cancer Staging Manual*, 7th edition, New York, Springer, 2010.)

T-ONCOANATOMY

ORIENTATION OF THREE-PLANAR ONCOANATOMY

The isocenter of the prostate is the central position in male pelvis oncoanatomy (Fig. 38.4). The prostate is positioned at the bladder neck. It is traversed by the proximal portion of the urethra, which is subject to compression and direct invasion. Once the cancer invades through the capsule, the common spread patterns are posterior, lateral, and/or superior. Lateral extension into the sulcus may lead to fixation of the gland to the lateral wall of the pelvis.

As the tumor extends superiorly, it invades into the seminal vesicle and it can block the ejaculatory ducts that traverses the substance of the gland. In its superior or anterior direction, a cancer can invade into the bladder because the capsular wall of the prostate thins and is in direct contact with its vesical muscular wall and lymphatics.

T-oncoanatomy

The prostate is both a glandular and a muscular organ that consists of four zones. It is firmly fixed in position by a dense capsule and ligamentous attachments. The zonal anatomy is defined in Fig. 38.5A legend. The urethra courses from the base of the bladder to the bulb of the penis. The cortical structure of the prostate's apex is directed below the perineum. Its flat base

touches the base of the bladder. The lateral surfaces are convex, resting against the fascia of the levator ani muscles (Fig. 38.5).

- *Coronal:* The prostate sits at the pelvic inlet and is surrounded by a number of distinct ligamentous structures as it rests along the levator ani muscles and on the sphincter urethrae muscle and its superior fascia. The urogenital diaphragm along with the central tendon of the perineum (perineal body) and the deep perineal space act as a distinct floor.

- *Sagittal:* This diaphragm separates the prostate gland from the bulb of the penis. Posteriorly, Denonvilliers' fascia separates the prostate gland from the rectum and acts as a major resistance to tumor invasion because it is composed of obliterated layers of the peritoneal cavity that extend downward.

- *Transverse:* The prostate gland lies anterior to the rectum and is readily palpable. Transrectal imaging with ultrasound and biopsy is possible because of this anatomy. Note that the prostatic venous plexus is rich anteriorly and communicates with the dorsal vein of the penis.

The ductus vas deferens and the seminal vesicles lie posterior to the bladder. They drain into the ejaculatory duct, which has the diameter of a lead pencil. The nerves of the prostate are derived from the pelvic sympathetic plexuses.

The color code for the anatomic sites correlates with the color code for the stage group (Fig. 38.3) and patterns of spread (Fig. 38.2) and the SIMLAP table (Table 38.2). Connecting the dots in similar colors provides an appreciation for the three-dimensional oncoanatomy.

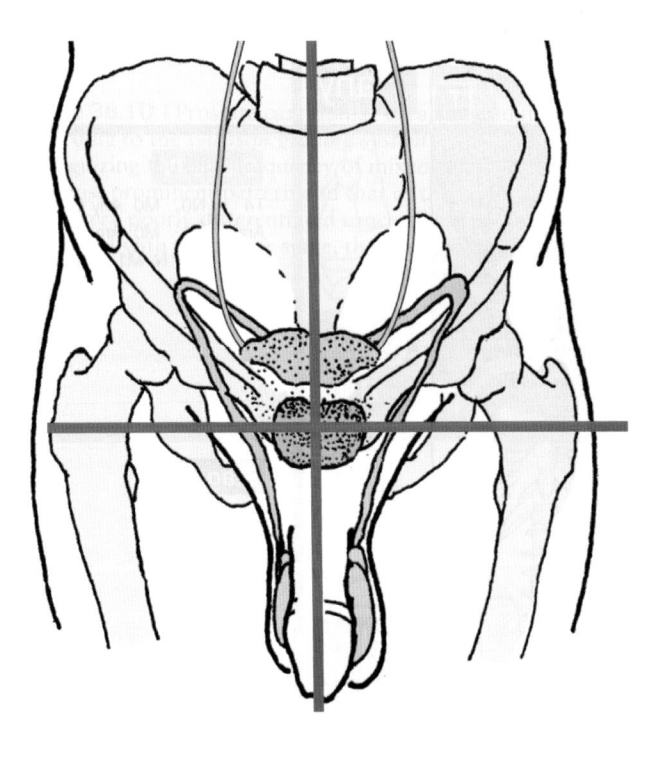 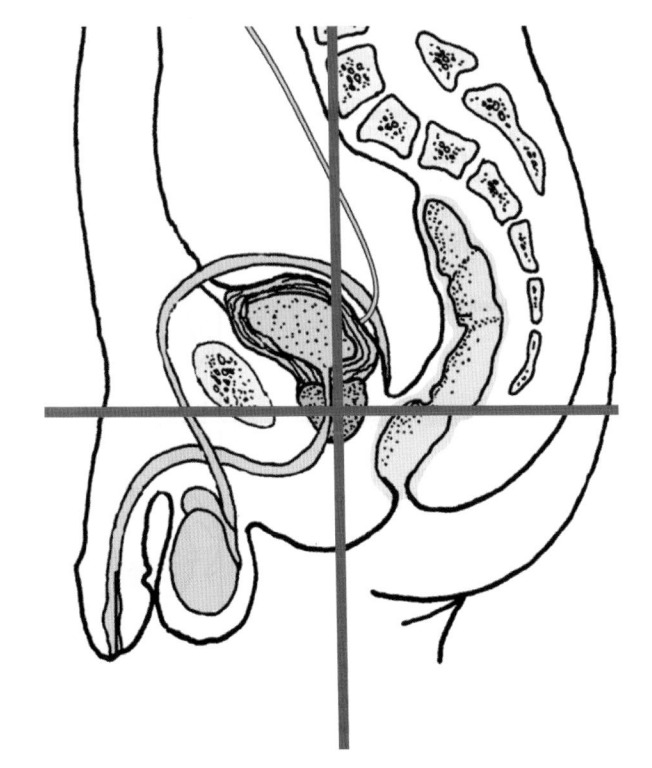

Figure 38.4 | Orientation of T-oncoanatomy. The anatomic isocenter for three-planar anatomy of the prostate is at the coccyx level. **Left.** Coronal. **Right.** Sagittal.

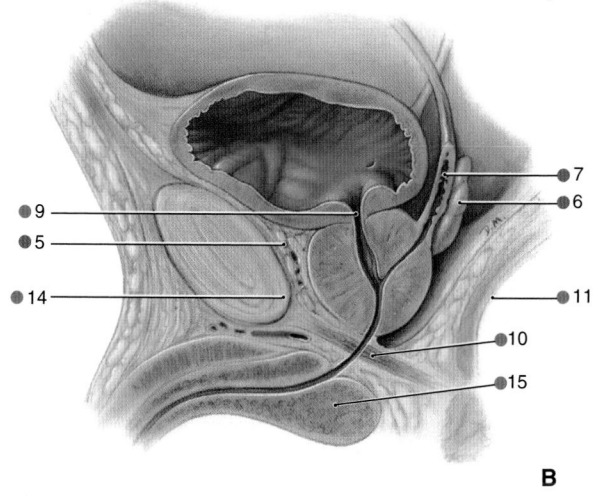

Figure 38.5A | Zonal anatomy of the prostate. On the left, a young man with minimal transition zone (TZ) hypertrophy. Note that preprostatic sphincter (internal urethral sphincter) and periejaculatory duct zone (central zone of McLean) (CZ) are clearly defined. On the right, an older man with TZ hypertrophy, which effaces the preprostatic sphincter and compresses the periejaculatory duct zone. AFS, anterior fibromuscular stroma; CZ, central zone; PZ, peripheral zone; SV, seminal vesicle.

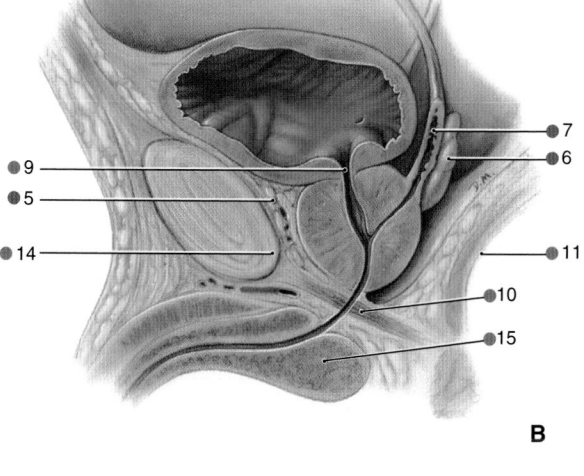

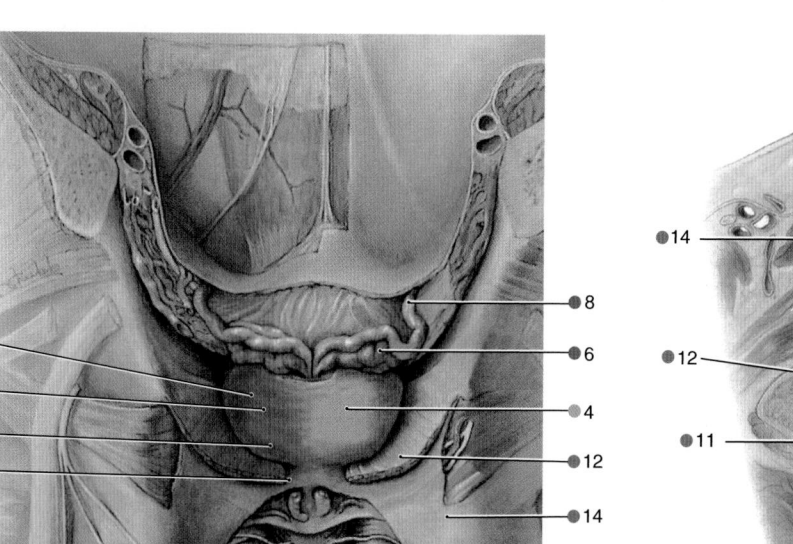

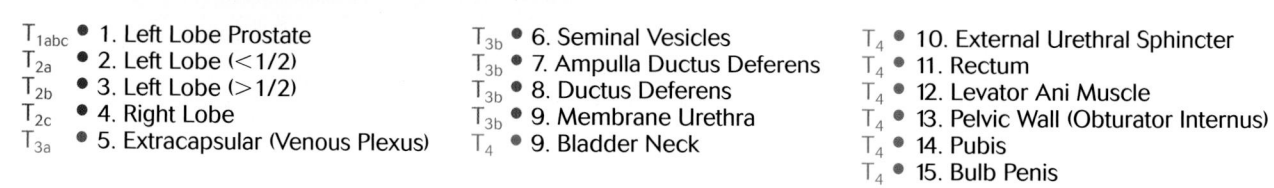

T_{1abc} • 1. Left Lobe Prostate		T_{3b} • 6. Seminal Vesicles		T₄ • 10. External Urethral Sphincter	
T_{2a} • 2. Left Lobe (<1/2)		T_{3b} • 7. Ampulla Ductus Deferens		T₄ • 11. Rectum	
T_{2b} • 3. Left Lobe (>1/2)		T_{3b} • 8. Ductus Deferens		T₄ • 12. Levator Ani Muscle	
T_{2c} • 4. Right Lobe		T_{3b} • 9. Membrane Urethra		T₄ • 13. Pelvic Wall (Obturator Internus)	
T_{3a} • 5. Extracapsular (Venous Plexus)		T₄ • 9. Bladder Neck		T₄ • 14. Pubis	
				T₄ • 15. Bulb Penis	

Figure 38.5B–D | T-oncoanatomy. Connecting the dots. Structures are color coded for cancer stage progression.

N-ONCOANATOMY AND M-ONCOANATOMY

N-ONCOANATOMY

A rich lymphatic network exists with lateral drainage and posterior sacral trunk. In addition to the internal and external iliac lymph nodes, it is possible, because of the latter trunk, for prostate cancers to bypass pelvic lymph nodes and spread directly to retroperitoneal lymph nodes in the para-aortic region first. The most commonly involved lymph node is the obturator node. In addition, there is a rich network of lymphatics that drain into internal and external iliac nodes and along the superior hemorrhoidal veins and a posterior sacral trunk directly into para-aortic nodes (Fig. 38.6A; Table 38.4A). The incidence for lymph node involvement is based on the part in nomogram for prediction of final pathologic stage based on the PSA, the Gleason score, and clinical stage of the primary cancer (Table 38.4B).

M-ONCOANATOMY

The arteries are branches of the rectal (hemorrhoidal) and inferior vesical arteries. The thin-walled veins are set inside and outside the prostatic capsule, forming a plexus of prostatic-vesical veins. This rich plexus of veins surrounds the prostate and interconnects with the blood in the dorsal vein of the penis. These veins drain into another rich plexus of veins in addition to the internal iliac vein. A rich anastomosis of intervertebral veins ascends from the internal iliac veins. This is referred to as the Batson's circulation. This venous pathway accounts for the distribution and frequency of osseous metastases; it also connects with ventral venous plexus (Fig. 38.6B).

| TABLE 38.4A | Lymph Nodes of the Prostate |

Regional lymph nodes. The regional lymph nodes are the nodes of the true pelvis, which essentially are the pelvic nodes below the bifurcation of the common iliac arteries. They include the following groups:

Pelvis, NOS

Hypogastric

Obturator

Iliac (internal, external, or NOS)

Sacral (lateral, presacral, promontory [Gerota's], or NOS)

Laterality does not affect the N classification

Reprinted with permission from Edge SB, Byrd DR, Compton CC, et al. *AJCC Cancer Staging Manual.* 7th ed. New York: Springer, 2010:458.

| TABLE 38.4B | Incidence of Lymph Node Metastases |

	PSA (ng/mL)																							
	0.0–4.0						**>4.0–10**						**>10–20**						**>20**					
Score	*Clinical Stage*						*Clinical Stage*						*Clinical Stage*						*Clinical Stage*					
	T1a	T1b	T2a	T2b	T2c	T3a	T1a	T1b	T2a	T2b	T2c	T3a	T1a	T1b	T2a	T2b	T2c	T3a	T1a	T1b	T2a	T2b	T2c	T3a
	Prediction of lymph node involvement (%)																							
2–4	0	2	1	2	4	—	0	2	1	2	5	—	0	—	1	3	—	—	—	—	2	7	—	—
5	0	4	2	4	8	—	0	4	2	5	10	8	0	5	2	6	13	11	—	—	3	—	29	—
6	0	8	3	9	17	15	0	9	4	11	19	16	—	11	5	13	22	20	—	—	9	18	53	31
7	—	15	7	18	31	—	0	18	8	20	34	28	—	21	9	24	39*	35	—	—	11	44	62	55
8–10	—	—	13	32	—	—	—	30	15	35	53	50	—	41	17	40	59	54	—	—	35	76	73	65

Dash represents lack of sufficient data to calculate probability.
From Partin AW, Yoo J, Carter B, et al: The use of prostate specific antigen, clinical stage and Gleason score to predict pathological stage in men with localized prostate cancer. *J Urol* 1993;150:110–114, with permission.

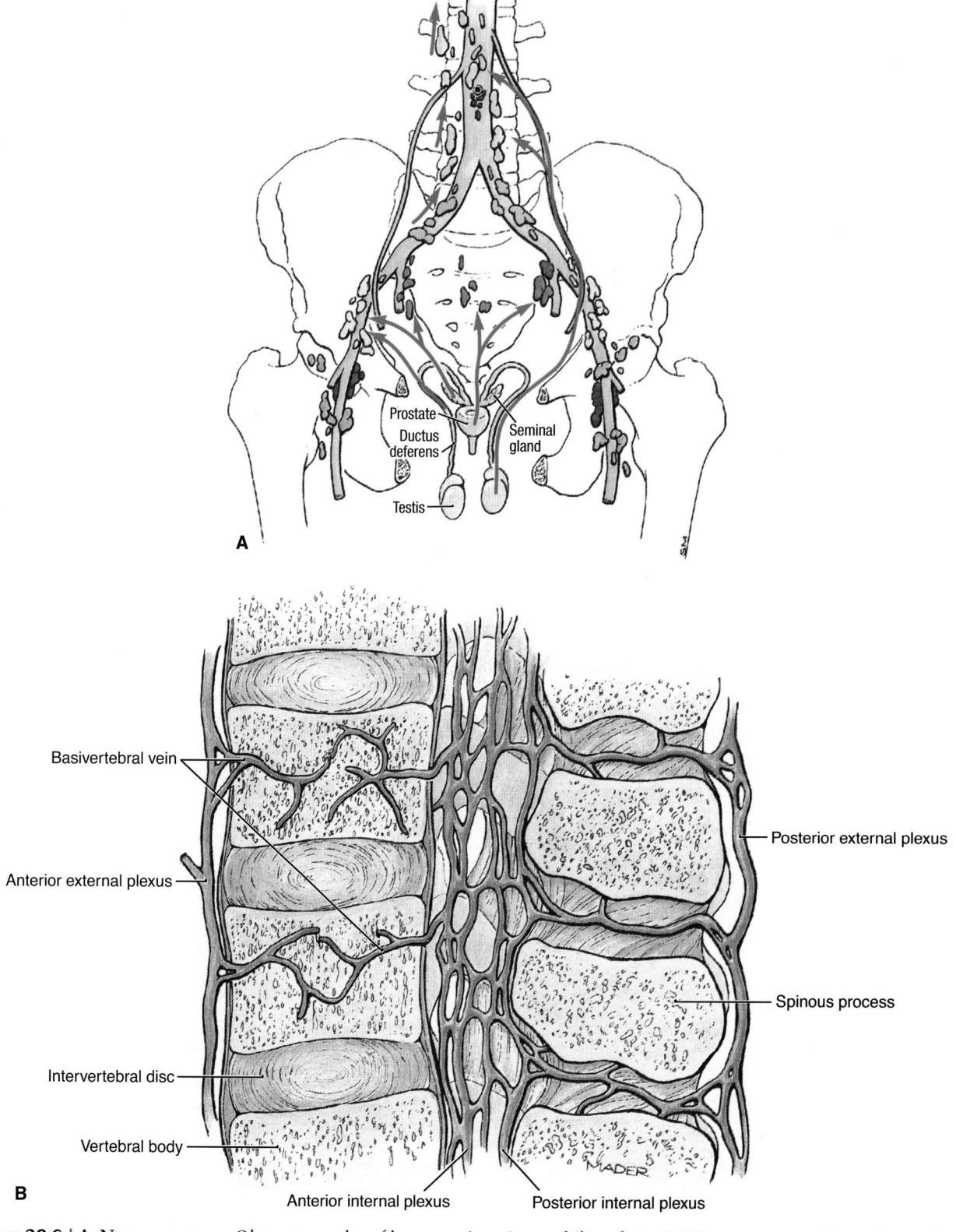

Figure 38.6 | **A. N-oncoanatomy.** Obturator nodes of hypogastric or internal iliac chain. **B. M-oncoanatomy.** Batson's vertebral venous plexus.

STAGING WORKUP

RULES OF CLASSIFICATION AND STAGING

Clinical Staging and Imaging

Clinical assessment before treatment includes a digital rectal examination and needle biopsy guided by TRUS. For nonpalpable disease, imaging with endorectal magnetic resonance imaging (MRI) is superior to computed tomography (CT). Enhanced CT is valuable for assessing lymph nodes, but if PSA is low (<20 mg/mL) and the Gleason grade is favorable (<7), sophisticated imaging is discouraged because of a high false-positive rate with imaging. Stages T2A, 2B, and 2C of the fourth edition have returned because the recurrence-free survival rate was significantly different for definitions in the fifth edition (Table 38.5; Fig. 38.7).

Pathologic Staging

With a total prostatectomy seminal vesiculectomy, regional nodes are carefully examined for surgical margins by descriptors: R1, microscopic; R2, macroscopic. A positive rectal biopsy permits pT4 and a positive biopsy of extraprostatic soft tissue justifies pT3, as does a positive biopsy of seminal vesicles.

TABLE 38.5	Imaging Modalities for Staging Prostate Cancer	
Method	**Diagnosis and Staging Capability**	**Recommended for Use**
Primary (T) Staging		
TRUS	Accurate for tumor localization but not for assessing T stage	Routine use for guiding biopsies of the prostate gland
CT_e	Not useful for stage T1–T3 disease but for evaluation of stage T4 disease (e.g., bladder, rectum invasion)	Recommended only for patients with clinically suspected stage T3–T4 disease
MRI	Probably the most accurate technique available for assessing T stage; anatomy well shown	May be cost-effective in evaluating patients at intermediate and high clinical risk of having extraprostatic disease
MRS	An adjunct to MRI for improved tumor localization and staging	Under investigation; early results useful as an adjunct to MRI
Nodal (N) Staging		
CT_e	Excellent for detecting enlarged nodes >1 cm versus large blood vessels	Yes, less expensive and time consuming than MRI
MRI	Excellent if node is replaced by cancer; yields positive intense signal	Yes, but more expensive and time consuming than CT_e
Metastases (M) Staging		
Bs-Tc	Identifies bone metastases	Recommended for patients with PSA >10 ng/mL, Gleason score >8, or clinical stage T3–T4 disease
CT-Ch	Identifies hematogenous or lymphatic metastases to chest, more sensitive than chest radiograph	May be used to confirm abnormal findings on the chest radiograph or to evaluate patients with pulmonary symptoms
CT-Ab	Identifies hematogenous metastases to liver, abdominal viscera, or lymphatic metastases to para-aortic lymph nodes	Not cost-effective in the evaluation of patients with PSA <20 ng/mL because of low yield of abnormal studies
CT-Pv	Identifies invasion of adjacent organs (i.e., bladder, rectum, pelvic sidewall)	Not cost-effective in patients with PSA <20 ng/mL or clinical stage T1–T2 because of low yield of abnormal studies
PET	May increase the sensitivity for detecting lymph node and visceral metastases	Under investigation; early results show promise

Bs-Tc, bone scintigraphy; CT, computed tomography; CT_e, CT enhanced with intravenous contrast; CT-Ab, abdominal CT; CT-Ch, chest CT; CT-Pv, pelvic CT; MRI, magnetic resonance imaging; MRS, magnetic resonance spectroscopic imaging; PET, positron emission tomography; PSA, prostate-specific antigen; TRUS, transrectal ultrasound.
Modified from Bragg DG, Rubin P, Hricak H, eds. *Oncologic Imaging*. 2nd ed. Philadelphia: Elsevier; 2002:579.

PROGNOSIS AND CANCER SURVIVAL

Oncoimaging Annotations

- TRUS is recommended if either digital rectal exam or PSA is abnormal.
- The main role of TRUS is in ultrasound-guided biopsy.
- The role of CT is detection of lymph node or other distant metastases.
- Endorectal MRI (eMRI) is superior to the use of body coil.
- eMRI renders the highest detection of extracapsular extension or seminal vesicle invasion, but variations in image quality and interpretation are among the main reasons for the slow dissemination of this technique.
- Early results on the use of spectroscopic MRI are promising, but the modality is still considered a research tool.
- Treatment follow-up is limited by imaging; either TRUS (with biopsy) or eMRI is most commonly used.

PROGNOSIS

The limited number of prognostic factors are listed in Table 38.6.

CANCER STATISTICS AND SURVIVAL

When considered together, the male genital and urinary systems are the major sites of malignancy. Prostate cancer alone accounts for 200,000 new patients annually. There are 100,000 new urinary tract cancers and 2.5-more male genital cancers, or 250,000 cases annually.

Between 1988 and 1992, the incidence rate of prostate cancers tripled from 75,000 new cases annually to 225,000. Prostate cancer in men is similar to breast cancer in women,

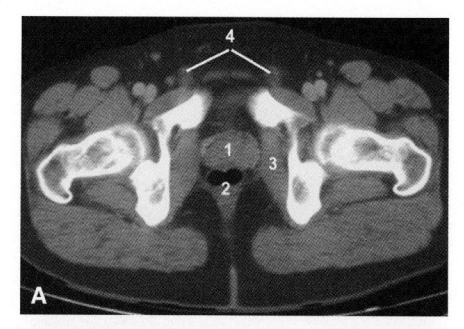

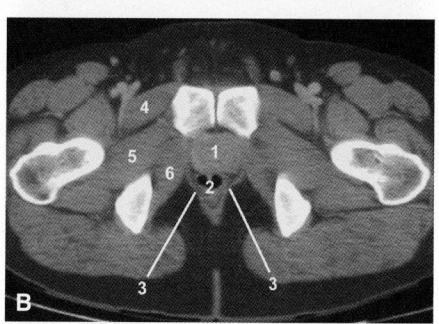

Figure 38.7 | **A.** 1. Prostate. 2. Rectum. 3. Obturator internus muscle. 4. Spermatic cords. **B.** 1. Prostate. 2. Rectum. 3. Levator ani muscle. 4. Pectineus muscle. 5. Obturator externus muscle. 6. Obturator internus muscle. Correlates with Fig. 38.5D.

TABLE 38.6	Prognostic Factors
Required for Staging	Prostate-specific Antigen
Clinically significant	Gleason score
	Gleason primary and secondary patterns
	Gleason tertiary pattern
	Clinical staging procedures performed
	Number of biopsy cores examined
	Number of biopsy cores positive for cancer

Reprinted with permission from Edge SB, Byrd DR, Compton CC, et al. *AJCC Cancer Staging Manual.* 7th ed. New York: Springer; 2010:466.

accounting for 33% of all cancers and outdistancing lung cancer (13%) and colon and rectum cancers (11%) combined. The 5-year survival is best of all cancers at 98.5%, but this cancer still causes 30,000 deaths yearly and is the second-leading cause of cancer death among men in the United States. Despite declining death rates in whites, African American men are dying of prostate cancer at twice the rate. Significant geographic variation has been observed; it is highest among blacks in the United States, followed by whites in Scandinavia and the United States. The lowest rates are in Asia.

The dramatic gains in survival are due to multidisciplinary achievements in screening, early detection, precise diagnoses, and effective multimodal therapies. The cancer statistics reveal perhaps the greatest gains in survival in oncology over the last five decades. For local stage I, male genitourinary tumors are all 90% to 100% curable according to the latest Surveillance Epidemiology and End Results data: kidney, 90%; bladder, 94%; testes, 99%; and prostate, 100%. Mortality rates are declining. The pediatric Wilms' tumor was the first malignancy in childhood to be cured, achieving >90% long-term survival, heralding the success of multimodal treatment that would be achieved in adult tumors in urology (see Table 38.7).

TABLE 38.7	Estimated 12-Year Disease-Specific Survival (DSS) After Radical Prostatectomy
High-Risk Definition	**12-Year DSS (95% CI)**
Biopsy Gleason 8–10	80 (69, 91)
Preoperative PSA ≥20	86 (76, 96)
1992 TNM stage T3	78 (69, 89)
PSA ≥20 or ≥T2c or GS ≥8	93 (89, 97)
Nomogram 5-y PFP ≤50%	90 (84, 96)
PSA ≥20 or ≥T3 or GS ≥8	91 (86, 96)
PSA ≥15 or ≥T2b or GS ≥8	94 (92, 96)
PSA velocity >2 ng/mL/y	94 (90, 98)

CI, confidence interval; PSA, prostate-specific antigen; GS, Gleason score; PFP, progression-free probability.
Yossepowitch O, Eggener SE, Bianco FJ, et al. Radical prostatectomy for clinically localized, high risk prostate cancer: critical analysis of risk assessment methods. *J Urol* 2007;178(2):493.

39

Penis

PERSPECTIVE, PATTERNS OF SPREAD, AND PATHOLOGY

Cross-sectional anatomy of the penis reflects the staging system of penile and urethral cancers.

PERSPECTIVE AND PATTERNS OF SPREAD

Penile and urethral cancers are uncommon in the United States, accounting for 1% of all malignancies in men. Circumcision has been shown to be effective in decreasing and preventing such cancers in Jewish, Nigerian, and Ugandan men who practice circumcision. Phimosis and smegma correlate with penile cancers. A relationship to sexually transmitted diseases, chronic infection, and trauma has been implicated in urethral cancers. The age group most afflicted are men in their 50s and 60s. Presenting symptoms are superficial nodular lesions, ulcerative sores, pain and itching, bleeding, and urinary burning. Palpable inguinal nodes are often present but may be ignored. If ignored, adenopathy may be present in 30% to 45% of cases; fortunately, at least half are due to associated infection rather than cancer.

The skin continues distal to the glans penis to form a smooth, retractable sheath, the prepuce, which is lined by mucous membrane and has a moist, stratified squamous epithelium. The prepuce is most often the site of premalignant in situ lesions, followed by the glans. Bowen disease is squamous cell cancer in situ that may involve the skin of the shaft. It often appears as a dull-red plaque with crusting and oozing. Erythroplasia of Queyrat is an epidermoid cancer in situ that involves the mucosal or mucocutaneous junction at the prepuce or glans.

The patterns of spread vary with location. Cancers of the skin and mucous membrane of the glans invade superficially and then penetrate into the corpus spongiosum and cavernosum (Fig. 39.2; Table 39.2).

There are a variety of presentations, as an ulcer, to a friable mass, or an exophytic papillary tumor. Once erosion into the urethra occurs, multiple fistulas lead to a "watering can" perineum. A curious differential diagnosis is that of mass lesion due to condyloma acuminatum, which is benign.

PATHOLOGY

The predominant cancer is squamous cell carcinoma, as expected with mucous membranes. Basal cell cancers account for only 1% to 2% of penile cancers. The glans (60%) and the prepuce (30%) are most often the sites of origin of cancer. Skin of the shaft accounts for <10% (Table 39.1; Fig. 39.1).

Condyloma acuminata of the penis is an important differential diagnosis, showing benign epidermal hyperkeratosis, parakerotosis, acanthosis, and papillomatosis.

TABLE 39.1	Histopathologic Type: Common Cancers of the Penis

Type
Cell types are limited to carcinomas
Squamous cell carcinoma, not otherwise specified
Verrucous carcinoma
Papillary squamous carcinoma
Warty squamous carcinoma
Basaloid carcinoma

From Edge SB, Byrd DR, Compton CC, et al., eds. *AJCC Cancer Staging Manual*. 7th ed. New York: Springer; 2010:450.

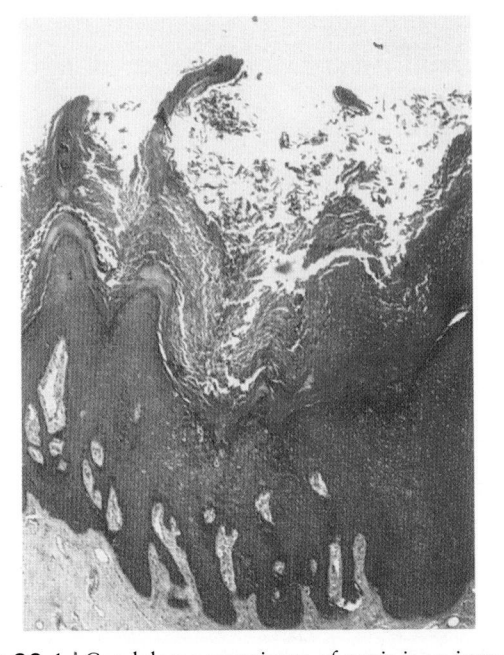

Figure 39.1 | Condyloma acuminata of penis is an important differential diagnosis showing benign epidermal hyperkeratosis, parakerotosis, acenthosis, and pappilomatosis.

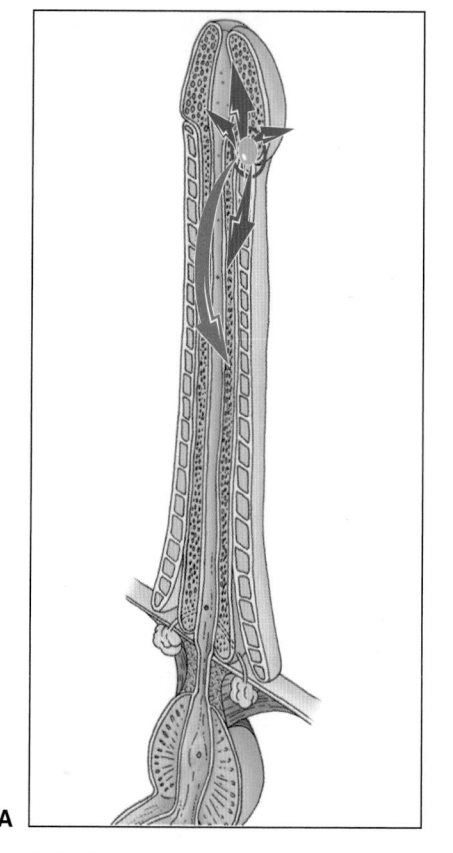
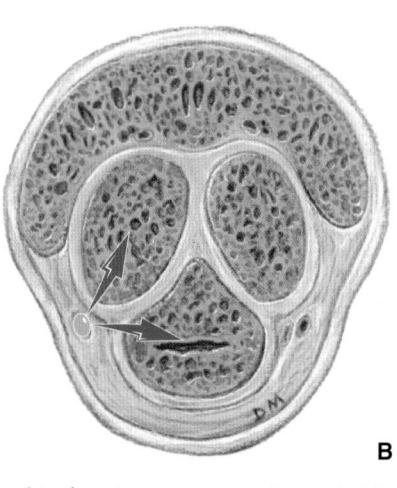

Figure 39.2 | A. Coronal. B. Transverse. Patterns of spread (cancer crab) of penis cancer are color coded for stage: Tis or Ta, yellow; T1, green; T2, blue; T3, purple; and T4, red. The patterns of spread of penis assumes erect position as in diagram. The concept of visualizing patterns of spread to appreciate the surrounding anatomy is well demonstrated by the six-directional pattern (SIMLAP, Table 39.2).

TABLE 39.2	SIMLAP	
Penis (erect)		
S	Prepuce primary	• T1
	Glans	• T1
I	Skin of penis	• T1
	Corpus cavernosum	• T2
	Corpus spongiosum	• T2
	Bulb of penis	• T3
M	Urethra	• T3
	Corpus spongiosum	• T2
L	Corpus spongiosum	• T2
A	Corona of glans	• T2
P	Corpus spongiosum	• T2
	Prostate	• T3
	Anus	• T4
	Scrotum/testis	• T4
	Urinary bladder	• T4

The six vectors of invasion are Superior, Inferior, Medial, Lateral, Anterior, and Posterior. The color-coded dots correlate the T stage with specific anatomic structure involved.

TNM STAGING CRITERIA

TNM STAGING CRITERIA

The staging of penile cancers and urethral cancers has been based on depth of invasion rather than size. In the early versions of the International Union Against Cancer classification, it was classified similarly to other skin cancers. There have been no changes in penile cancer staging since the third edition; urethral cancers are noted separately. Cross-sectional anatomy of the penis reflects the staging system of penile and urethral cancers.

Initial superficial stage Tis is cancer in situ, and Ta is verrucal, noninvasive lesion. Subepithelial or subcutaneous spread is T1. Once invasion occurs through the deep (Buck's) fascia, the corpus spongiosum or cavernosum is invaded (stage T2). Invasion into urethra is T3 and into adjacent structures is T4 (Fig. 39.3).

SUMMARY OF CHANGES SEVENTH EDITION AJCC

The following changes in the definition of TNM and the Stage Grouping for this chapter have been made since the Sixth Edition (Fig. 39.3).

- T1 has been subdivided into T1a and T1b based on the presence or absence of lymphovascular invasion or poorly differentiated cancers.
- T3 category is limited to urethral invasion, and prostatic invasion is now considered T4.
- Nodal staging is divided into both clinical and pathologic categories.

- The distinction between superficial and deep inguinal lymph nodes has been eliminated.
- Stage II grouping includes T1b N0M0 as well as T2-3 N0M0.

With the Seventh Edition, lymph node staging is divided into a clinical vs. pathologic stage definition, reflecting the importance and impact of node positive spread. Location and mobility of inguinal nodes is the key clinical criteria, whereas spread to deep pelvic external iliac nodes is a most important determinant of survival.

Lymphatic and vascular embolizations are independent predictive variables of inguinal lymph node involvement in patients with squamous cell carcinoma of the penis (Table 39.3A).

The TNM staging matrix is color coded for identification of stage group once T and N stages are determined (Table 39.3B). T stage determines stage group, and N1 can occur with early cancers T1, T2, as well as with advanced T3 lesions.

TABLE 39.3B | **Stage Summary Matrix**

	N0	N1	N2	N3	M1
T1a	I*	IIIA	IIIB	IV	IV
T1b	II	IIIA	IIIB	IV	IV
T2	II	IIIA	IIIB	IV	IV
T3	II	IIIA	IIIB	IV	IV
T4	IV	IV	IV	IV	IV

TABLE 39.3A | **Predictive Variables of Inguinal Node Involvement**

Variable	Hazard Ratio	95% Confidence Interval	P value
Tumor thickness (5 vs. >5 mm)	1.435	0.538–3.833	0.47
Pathologic tumor classification (pTa/pT1 vs. pT2 vs. >pT2)	2.288	1.118–4.684	0.02
Histologic grade (grade 1 vs. grades 2–3)	4.268	1.278–14.364	0.01
Venous embolization (absent vs. present)	5.240	1.139–24.101	0.03
Lymphatic embolization (absent vs. present)	6.941	1.967–24.498	0.003

From Ficarra V, Zattoni F, et al. *Cancer* 2005;103:2507.

PENIS

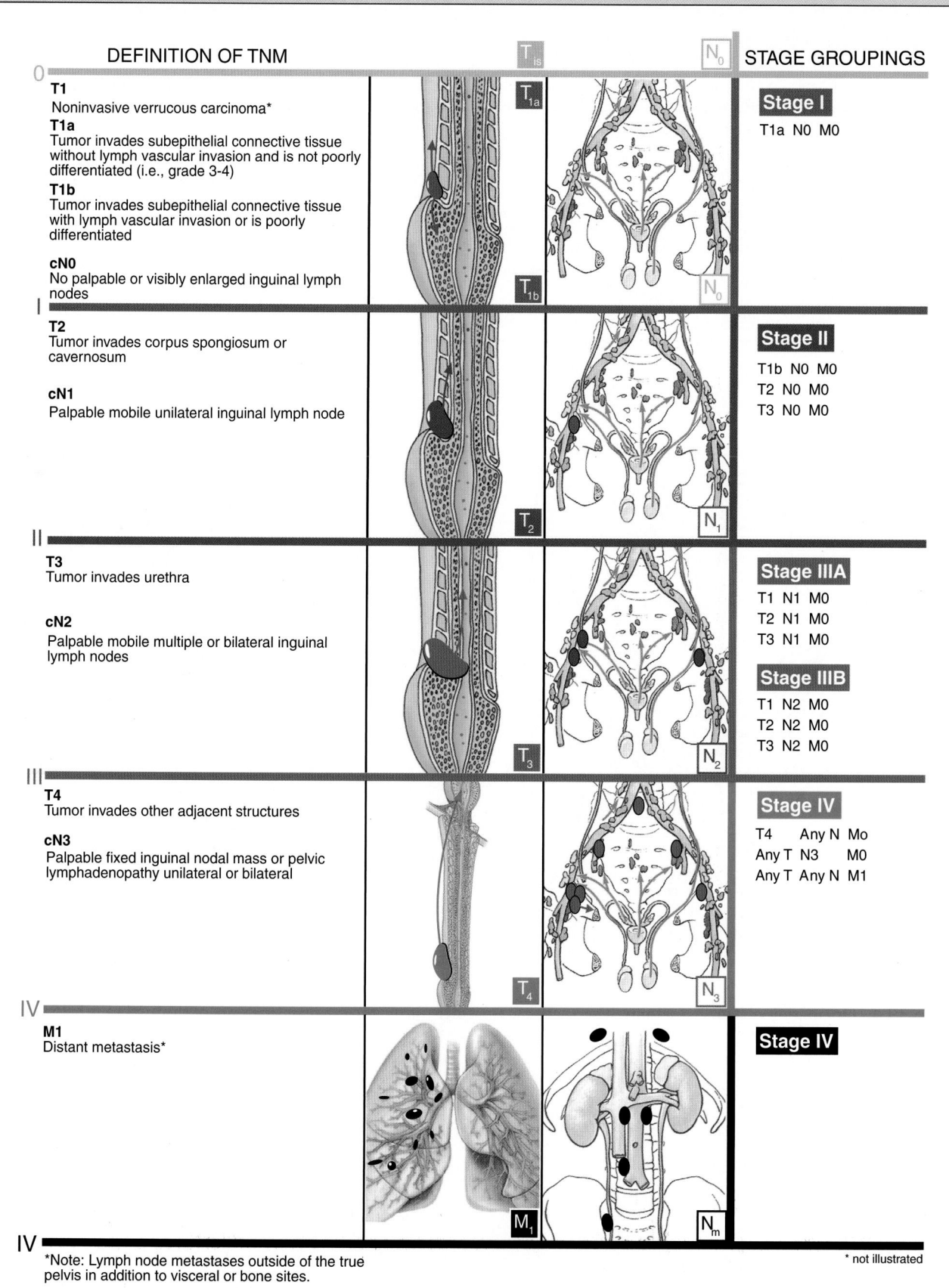

DEFINITION OF TNM

T1
Noninvasive verrucous carcinoma*
T1a
Tumor invades subepithelial connective tissue without lymph vascular invasion and is not poorly differentiated (i.e., grade 3-4)
T1b
Tumor invades subepithelial connective tissue with lymph vascular invasion or is poorly differentiated

cN0
No palpable or visibly enlarged inguinal lymph nodes

T2
Tumor invades corpus spongiosum or cavernosum

cN1
Palpable mobile unilateral inguinal lymph node

T3
Tumor invades urethra

cN2
Palpable mobile multiple or bilateral inguinal lymph nodes

T4
Tumor invades other adjacent structures

cN3
Palpable fixed inguinal nodal mass or pelvic lymphadenopathy unilateral or bilateral

M1
Distant metastasis*

STAGE GROUPINGS

Stage I
T1a N0 M0

Stage II
T1b N0 M0
T2 N0 M0
T3 N0 M0

Stage IIIA
T1 N1 M0
T2 N1 M0
T3 N1 M0

Stage IIIB
T1 N2 M0
T2 N2 M0
T3 N2 M0

Stage IV
T4   Any N Mo
Any T N3   M0
Any T Any N M1

Stage IV

*Note: Lymph node metastases outside of the true pelvis in addition to visceral or bone sites.

* not illustrated

Figure 39.3 | TNM penis cancer diagram. Vertically arranged with T definitions on the left and stage groupings on the right. Color bars are coded for stage: stage 0, yellow; I, green; II, blue; III, purple; IV, red; and metastatic, black.

T-ONCOANATOMY

ORIENTATION OF THREE-PLANAR ONCOANATOMY

The isocenter is taken at the penile base inferior to the bony pelvis (Fig. 39.4).

T-oncoanatomy

The T-oncoanatomy is displayed in three planar views in Fig. 39.5:

• *Coronal:* The penis and urethra have an anterior projectile portion and a posterior anchoring part into the prostate in males.

• *Sagittal:* These are surrounded by a deep penile fascia (Buck's fascia), which is separated from skin by a layer of connective tissue. Penile and urethral cancers mirror image their patterns of invasion and advancement as to depth of tissue penetration.

• *Transverse:* The axial cross section identifies the major anatomic features: The urethra is embedded in the corpus spongiosum and the main erectile corpora cavernosum.

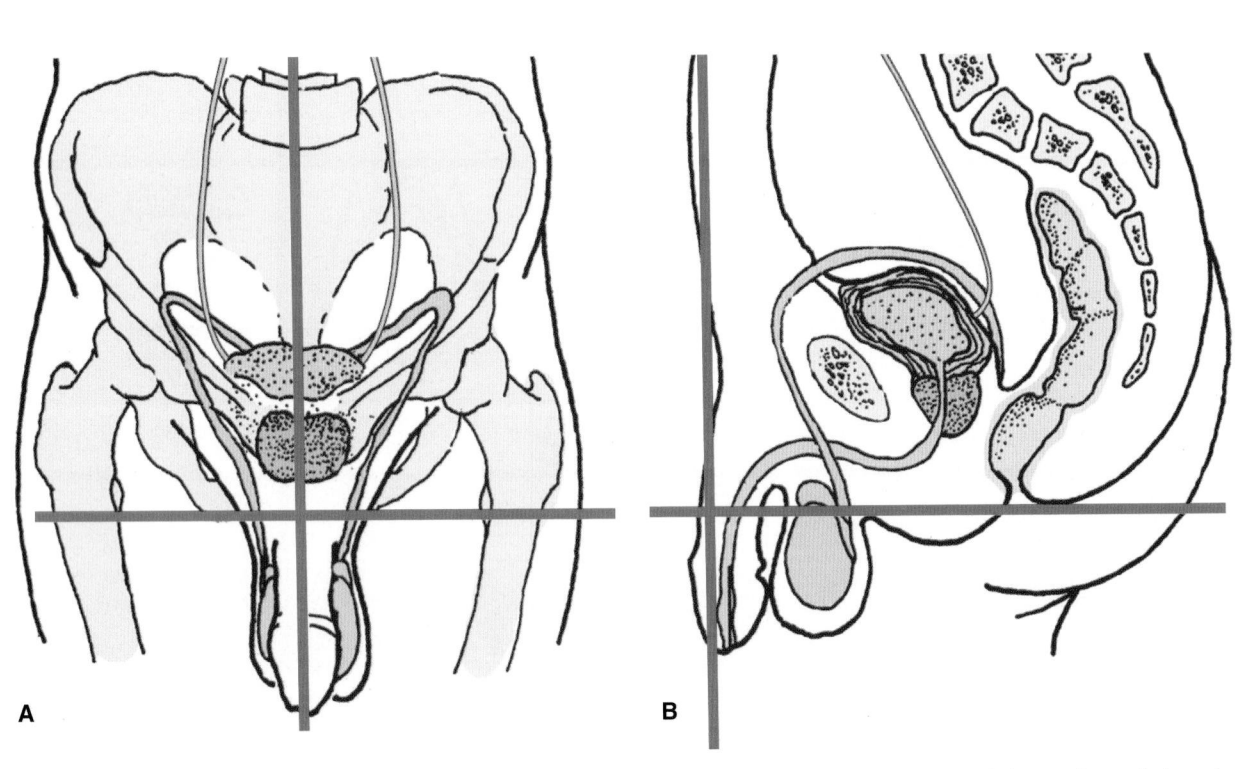

A

B

Figure 39.4 | Orientation of T-oncoanatomy. The anatomic isocenter for the three-planar anatomy of the urethra is below the pelvis. **A.** Coronal. **B.** Sagittal.

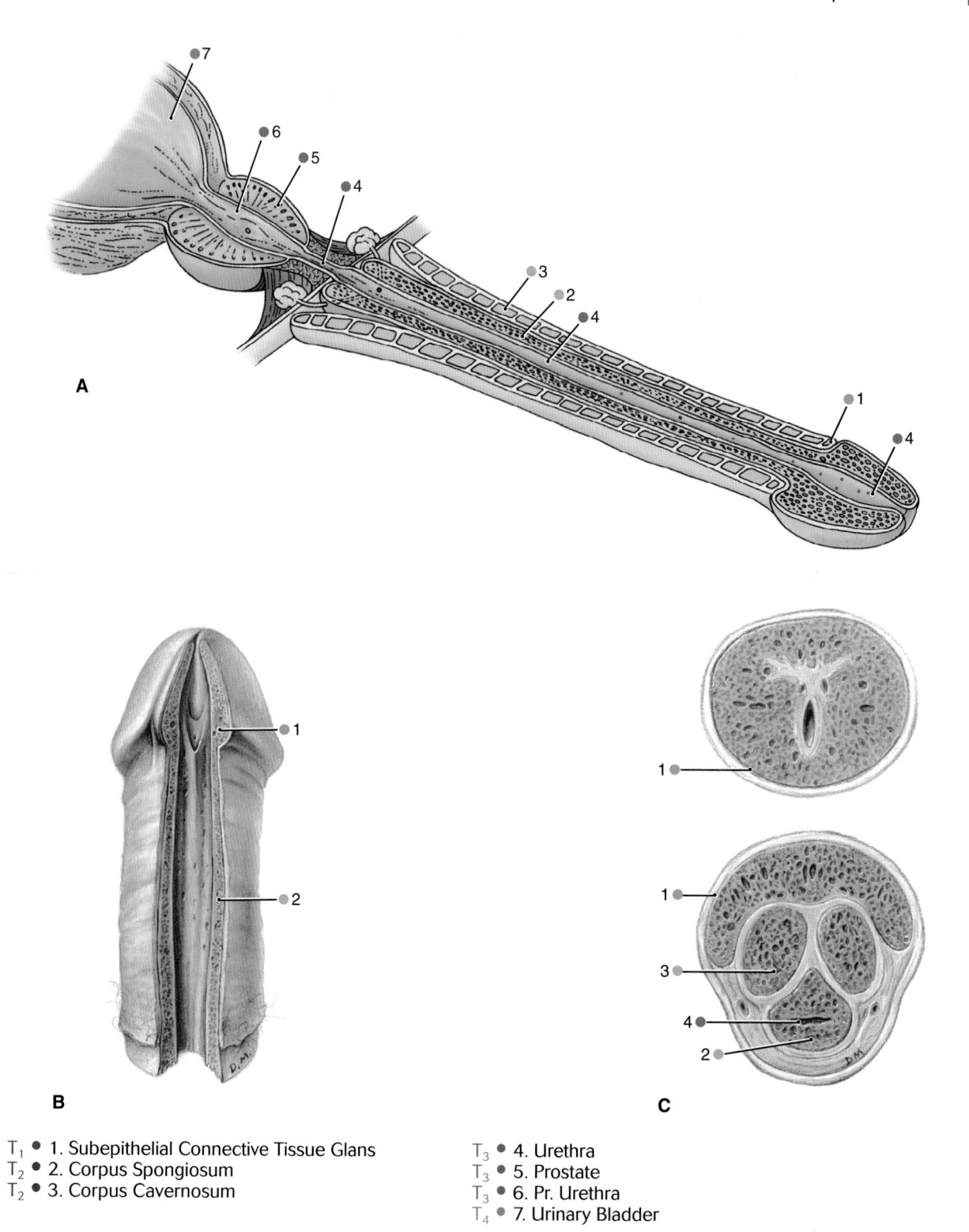

A

B

C

T_1	● 1. Subepithelial Connective Tissue Glans		T_3	● 4. Urethra
T_2	● 2. Corpus Spongiosum		T_3	● 5. Prostate
T_2	● 3. Corpus Cavernosum		T_3	● 6. Pr. Urethra
			T_4	● 7. Urinary Bladder

Figure 39.5 | T-oncoanatomy. Connecting the dots. Structures are color coded for cancer stage progression. The color code for the anatomic sites correlates with the color code for the stage group (Fig. 39.3) and patterns of spread (Fig. 39.2) and SIMLAP table (Table 39.2). Connecting the dots in similar colors will provide an appreciation for the three-dimensional oncoanatomy.

N-ONCOANATOMY AND M-ONCOANATOMY

N-ONCOANATOMY

The lymphatic channels of the prepuce and penis are rich, and the shaft skin drains into inguinal nodes. The rich anastomoses at the base of the penis result in bilateral drainage into superficial and deep inguinal nodes. Sentinel nodes are often located at the junction of saphenous and superficial epigastric veins. The lymphatics of the bulbomembranous and prostatic urethra follow three routes: external iliac nodes, obturator and internal iliac nodes, and presacral nodes. Pelvic external iliac nodes are seldom involved without inguinal node involvement first (Fig. 39.6A,B; Table 39.4).

An important observation is the extensions of due extranodal invasion. Mobility of nodes versus matting, fixation and ulceration of inguinal nodes. Once there is evidence of nodal invasion, the 5-year survival drops to 5% to 15%, an ominous outcome.

A very interesting set of nomograms were published by Ficarra et al.* relating a variety of primary characteristics that predict for lymph node involvement:

- Tumor thickness
- Growth pattern
- Grade
- Embolization
- Corpus cavernosum
- Corpus spongiosum
- Urethral infiltration

REGIONAL LYMPH NODES

- The regional lymph nodes are as follows:
- Superficial and deep inguinal (femoral)

*Ficarra V, Zattoni F, Artibani W, et al. *J Urol* 2006;175(5): 1700–1704; discussion 1704–1705.

- External iliac
- Internal iliac
- Pelvic nodes, NOS

Clinical examination by palpation of the inguinal region is required. Computed tomography is a useful adjunct to palpation in patients with palpable inguinal adenopathy or those in whom palpation is unreliable (i.e., obese, prior inguinal surgery).

M-ONCOANATOMY

Distant metastases are uncommon, except in advanced disease at the base of the penis, despite the rich vascular anastomoses and penile blood supply, which drains into the dorsal vein of the penis and then into the periprostatic and perivesical venous plexus (Fig. 39.6C).

TABLE 39.4	Lymph Nodes of the Penis	
Sentinel Nodes		
Superficial inguinal		
Femoral		
Regional Nodes		**Metastatic Nodes**
Deep inguinal (Cloquet's node)		Right para-aortic
Bilateral inguinal		Left para-aortic
		Mediastinal
		Left supraclavicular
Juxtaregional Nodes		
Common iliac		
Internal iliac		
External iliac		

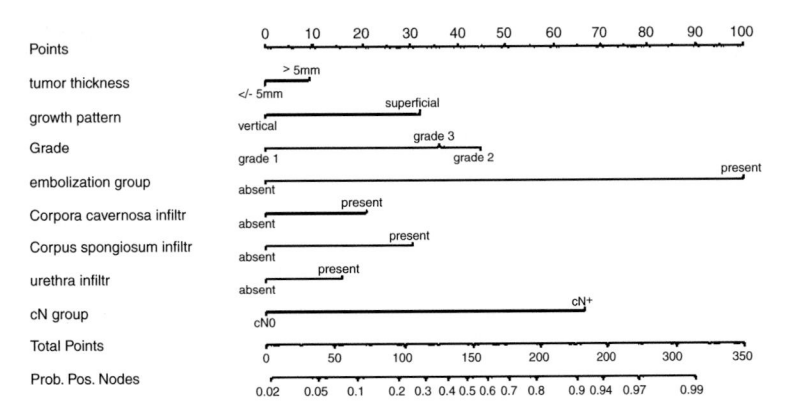

Instructions for Physicians: Locate the tumor thickness on its axis. Draw a line straight upwards to the Points axis to determine how many points received for his tumor thickness. Repeat this process for the remaining axes, each time drawing straight upward to the Point axis. Sum the points achieved for each predictor and locate the sum on the Total Points axis. Draw a line straight down to find the probability of positive inguinal lymph nodes.

Instructions for Patient: "Mr. X, if we had 100 men exactly like you, we would expect <probability from nomogram x100> to have positive lymph nodes.

A

Figure 39.6 | A. Nomogram to predict lymph node involvement for squamous cell carcinoma of the penis. (From Ficarra V, Zattoni F, Artibani W, et al. Nomogram predictive of pathological inguinal lymphnode involvement in patients with squamous cell carcinoma of the penis. *J Urol* 2006;175:1700.)

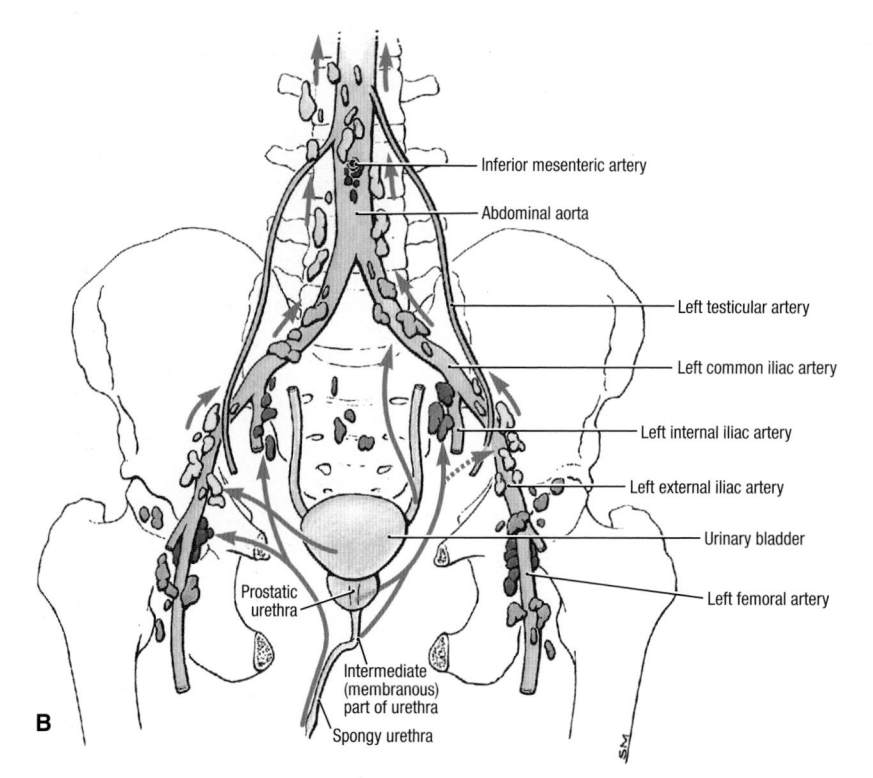

Figure 39.6 | B. N-oncoanatomy. Obturator nodes of hypogastric or internal iliac chain.

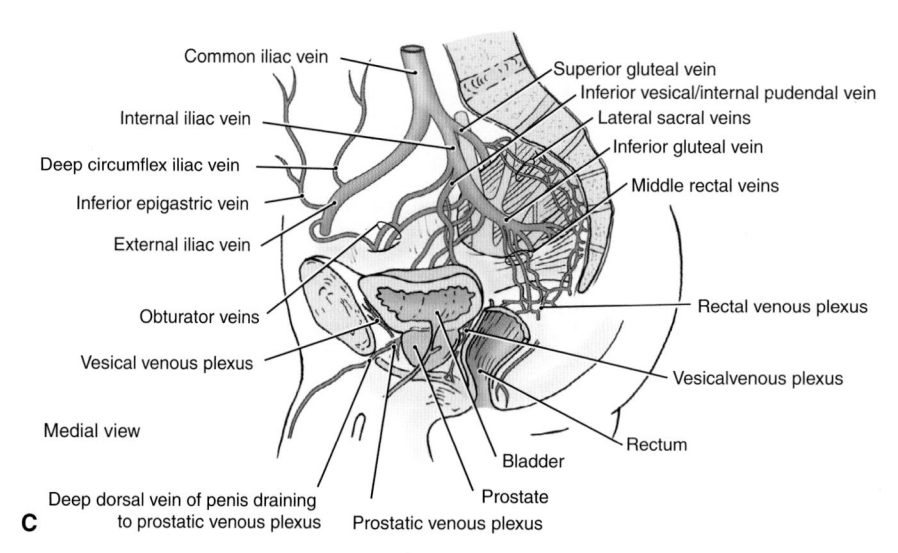

Figure 39.6 | C. M-oncoanatomy.

STAGING WORKUP

RULES OF CLASSIFICATION AND STAGING

Clinical Staging and Imaging

Careful physical examination and endoscopy are adequate to determine primary extension and nodal involvement. Imaging is reserved for determining metastatic pelvic nodal involvement and remote metastases when stage is advanced. Computed tomography is preferred to magnetic resonance imaging because it is more cost-effective (Table 39.5; Fig. 39.7).

Pathologic Staging

Complete resection of the primary and of part of the penis requires determination of the appropriate clearance of surgical margins. Lymphadenectomy specimens should note number, size, and extranodal extensions.

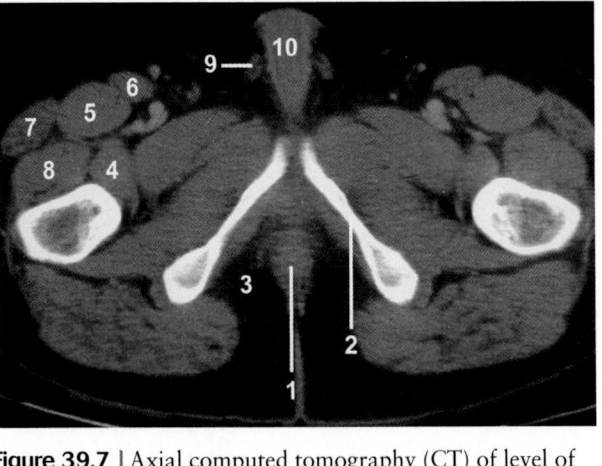

Figure 39.7 | Axial computed tomography (CT) of level of corpora cavernosa of penis. Oncoimaging with CT is commonly applied to staging cancers, often combined with positron emission tomography to determine the true extent of primary cancer and involved lymph nodes. 1. Rectum. 2. Inferior pubic ramus. 3. Ischiorectal fossa. 4. Iliopsoas muscle. 5. Rectus femoris muscle. 6. Sartorius muscle. 7. Tensor fasciae latae muscle. 8. Vastus lateralis muscle. 9. Spermatic cord. 10. Corpora cavernosa of penis.

TABLE 39.5	**Imaging Modalities for Staging Penile Cancer**	
Method	Diagnosis and Staging Capability	Recommended for Use
Primary (T) Staging		
TAUS	More useful for detection than staging	No
Ct_e	Accurate for staging advanced T3, T4 invasion beyond the bladder wall	Yes, cost-effective
MRI	Provides most anatomic detail of cancer invasion into and beyond the wall of the urinary bladder	Yes, more accurate
Nodal (N) Staging		
Ct_e	Valuable in assessing pelvic and para-aortic nodal enlargements	Yes, cost-effective
MRI	More valuable in distinguishing adenopathy secondary to inflammation versus cancer	Yes, more cost-effective
Metastases (M) Staging		
Chest film	Can detect gross pulmonary or mediastinal metastases	Yes, cost-effective

CT, computed tomography; Ct_e, CT enhanced with intravenous contrast; MRI, magnetic resonance imaging; TAUS, transabdominal ultrasound.

PROGNOSIS AND CANCER SURVIVAL

PROGNOSIS

The limited number of prognostic factors are listed in Table 39.6.

CANCER STATISTICS AND SURVIVAL

Again, Ficarra et al. have developed nomograms for both clinical and pathologic staging of lymph nodes, predicting cancer-specific survival based on mainly the inguinal lymph node status in addition to primary tumor characteristics (Fig. 39.8). Note the impact of cNo versus cN+ with the drop in survival. If this were updated using current American Joint Committee on Cancer path N+ criteria, the horizontal line would extend to between 5% and 15% as mentioned earlier.

TABLE 39.6	Prognostic Factors
Required for staging	None
Clinically significant	Involvement of corpus spongiosum
	Involvement of corpus cavernosum
	Percent of tumor that is poorly differentiated
	Verrucous carcinoma depth of invasion
	Size of largest lymph node metastasis
	Extranodal/extracapsular extension
	Human papilloma virus status

Edge SB, Byrd DR, Compton CC, et al., eds. *AJCC Cancer Staging Manual.* 7th ed. New York: Springer; 2009:454.

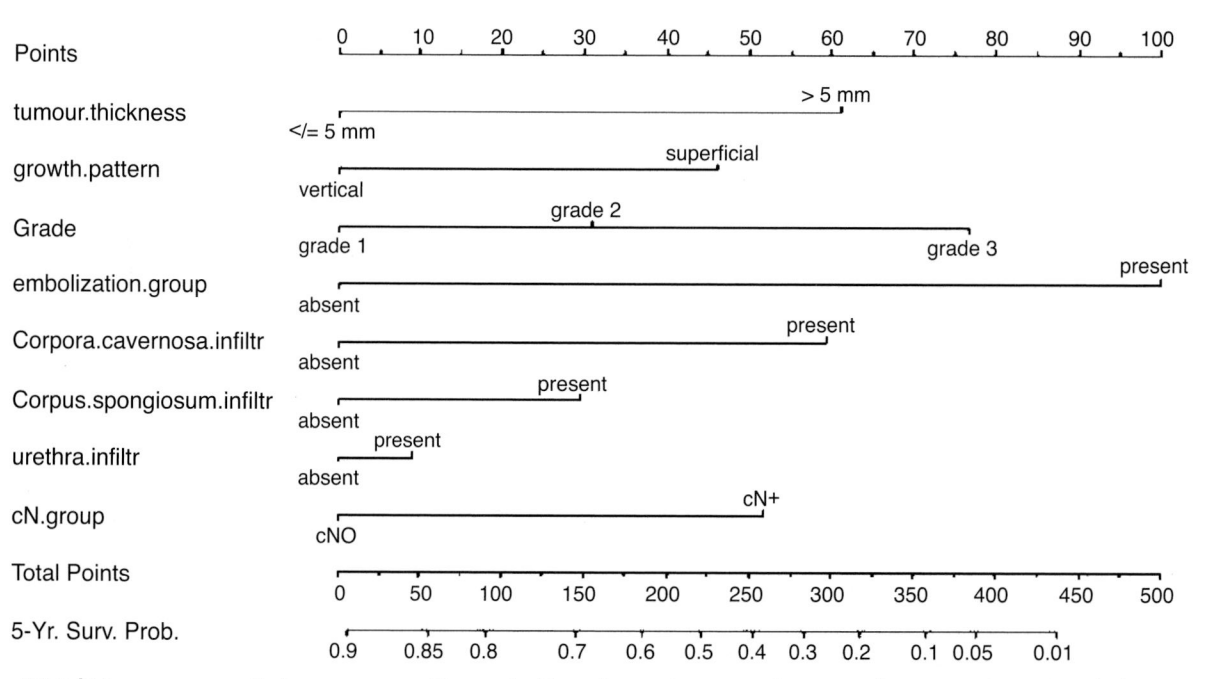

Figure 39.8 I Nomogram predicting cancer-specific survival based on primary penile tumor characteristics and pathologic stage of inguinal lymph nodes. (From Ficarra V, Zattoni F, Artibani W, et al. Nomogram predictive of pathological inguinal lymphnode involvement in patients with squamous cell carcinoma of the penis. *J Urol* 2006;175:1700.)

Urethra

PERSPECTIVE, PATTERNS OF SPREAD, AND PATHOLOGY

Urethral cancers vary in their clinical expression as a function of anatomic location in both the male and female urethra.

PERSPECTIVE AND PATTERNS OF SPREAD

Cancers of the urethra are quite uncommon. They occur more often among females. Common presentation is a structure interfering with urination in males; in females, urinary frequency, hesitancy, and a palpable urethral mass are often noted. Bleeding without a history of trauma or venereal disease should raise suspicion of an underlying malignancy. On examination, a palpable urethral mass especially in females is present in the majority of cases (75%) and can appear as papillary growths, soft, fungating lesions, or ulcerations with a foul-smelling discharge. Obstructive symptoms and incomplete voiding (66%) also lead patients to seek medical evaluation, as well as relief of symptoms.

The patterns of cancer spread relate to surrounding anatomy in males and females. In the male, it advances and eventually may invade the penis, prostate, or urinary bladder whereas, in the female, vaginal invasion along the anterior wall of the vagina is more frequent. The labia can be involved if it spreads inferiorly or into the bladder if it progresses superiorly (Fig. 40.2; Table 40.2).

Cancer of the urethra is the only genitourinary cancer that is more common in women than men. Predisposing factors are repeated infections; human papilloma virus (HPV) may be a factor. Urethrorrhagia is often the early symptom, then stricture or mass in anterior vaginal wall.

Cancer of the urethra in males, in contrast, usually is initiated as noted with a stricture and occurs in 25% to 75% of cases, most often in the bulbomembranous urethra, associated with HPV.

PATHOLOGY

The histopathology differs in incidence in males versus females: squamous cell carcinoma (80% vs. 60%), transitional cell (15% vs. 20%), and adenocarcinoma (5% vs. 10%) (Table 40.1; Figure 40.1).

TABLE 40.1	Histopathic Type: Tumors of Urinary Bladder

Urothelial cell papilloma

    Exophytic papilloma

    Inverted papilloma

Urothelial carcinoma in situ

Papillary urothelial carcinoma, low grade or high grade

Squamous cell carcinoma

Adenocarcinoma

Neuroendocrine (small cell) carcinoma

Carcinosarcoma

Sarcoma

From Edge SB, Byrd DR, Compton CC, et al., *AJCC Cancer Staging Manual*, *7th edition*. New York: Springer, 2010, p. 501.

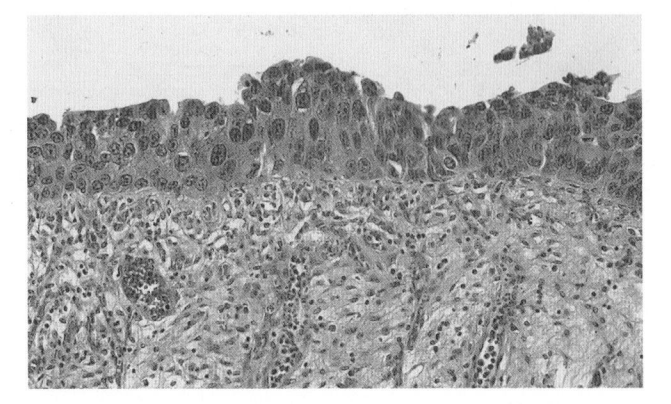

Figure 40.1 | Urothelial carcinoma in situ. The urothelial mucosa shows nuclear pleomorphism and lack of polarity from the basal layer to the surface, without evidence of maturation.

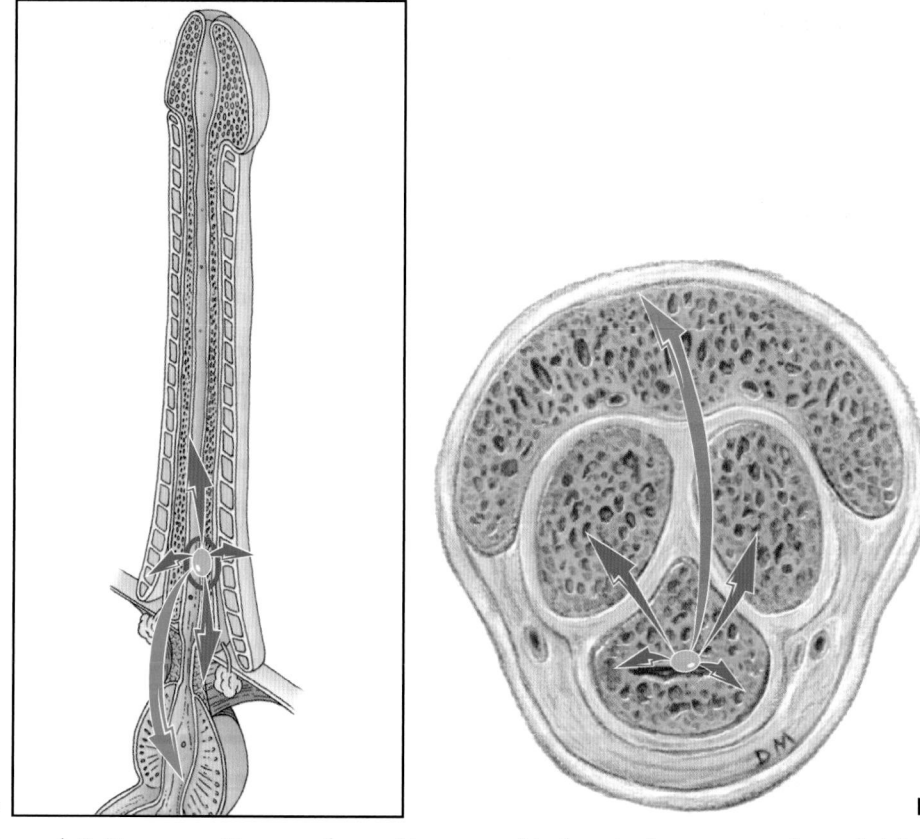

Figure 40.2 | A. Coronal. **B.** Transverse. Patterns of spread (cancer crab) of urethral cancer are color coded for stage: Tis or Ta, yellow; T1, green; T2, blue; T3, purple; and T4, red. The concept of visualizing patterns of spread to appreciate the surrounding anatomy is well demonstrated by the six-directional pattern (SIMLAP, Table 40.2).

TABLE 40.2	SIMLAP	
Urethra		
S	Corpus cavernosum	• T3
	Prostate gland	• T2
I	Corpus spongiosum	• T2
M	Urethra	• T1
L	Crura penis	• T3
	Bulb of penis	• T3
A	Shaft of penis	• T3
P	Perineal membrane	• T3
	Urinary bladder neck	• T3
	Bladder wall	• T4
	Anus	• T4
	Scrotum/testis	• T4

The six vectors of invasion are Superior, Inferior, Medial, Lateral, Anterior, and Posterior. The color-coded dots correlate the T stage with specific anatomic structure involved.

STAGING WORKUP

RULES OF CLASSIFICATION AND STAGING

Clinical Staging and Imaging

Imaging is reserved for determining metastatic pelvic nodal involvement and remote metastases when stage is advanced. The primary site is assessed by physical examination—inspection and palpation followed by cystourethroscopy with biopsy and cytology. Contrast filling of bladder and voiding cystometrogram are worthwhile (Table 40.5, Fig. 40.7).

Pathologic Staging

Complete resection of the primary and part of the penis requires determination of appropriate clearance of surgical margins. Lymphadenectomy specimens should note number, size, and extranodal extensions. Assignment of stage following resection allows depth of invasion to be determined. In males, urethral neoplasms can arise in prostate epithelium or ducts and are classified as prostate urethral cancer.

Oncoimaging Annotations

- Diagnosis of urethral cancer is by cystoscopy and biopsy.
- Magnetic resonance imaging is superior to computed tomography in the evaluation of local tumor extent.

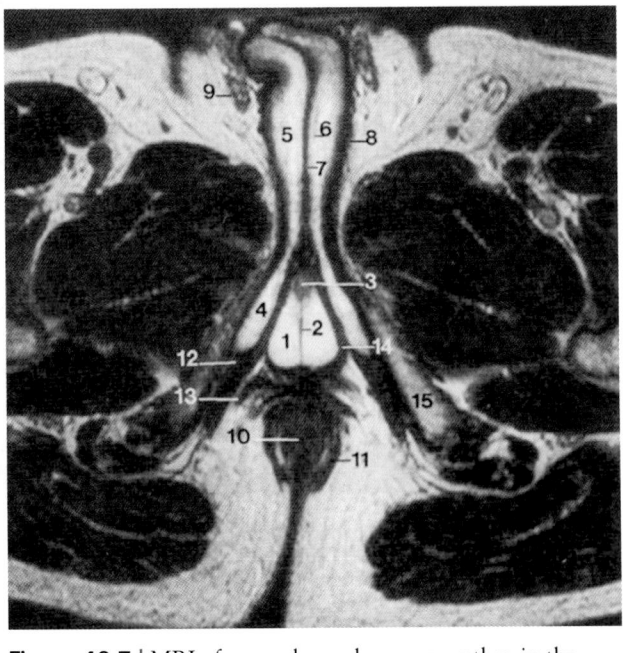

Figure 40.7 | MRI of normal membranous urethra in the transverse plane. 1. corpus spongiosum (bulb of the penis) 2. septum of the corpus spongiosum 3. bulbous urethra 4. crus of the corpus cavernosum 5. corpus cavernosum 6. deep cavernous a. 7. septum of the corpus cavernosum 8. Buck's fascia and tunica albuginea 9. spermatic cord 10. anal canal 11. sphincter ani externus m. 12. ischiocavernosus m. 13. transversus perinei superficialis m. 14. bulbospongiosus m. 15. ischium

TABLE 40.5	Imaging Modalities for Staging Urethra Cancer	
Method	**Diagnosis and Staging Capability**	**Recommended for Use**
Primary (T) Staging		
TAUS	More useful for detection than staging	No
Ct$_e$	Accurate for staging advanced T3, T4 invasion beyond the bladder wall	Yes, cost-effective
MRI	Provides most anatomic detail of cancer invasion into and beyond the wall of the urinary bladder	Yes, more accurate
Nodal (N) Staging		
Ct$_e$	Valuable in assessing pelvic and para-aortic nodal enlargements	Yes, cost-effective
MRI	More valuable in distinguishing adenopathy secondary to inflammation versus cancer	Yes, more cost-effective
Metastases (M) Staging		
Chest film	Can detect gross pulmonary or mediastinal metastases	Yes, cost-effective

CT, computed tomography; Ct$_e$, CT enhanced with intravenous contrast; MRI, magnetic resonance imaging; TAUS, transabdominal ultrasound.

PROGNOSIS AND CANCER SURVIVAL

PROGNOSIS

The limited number of prognostic factors are listed in Table 40.6.

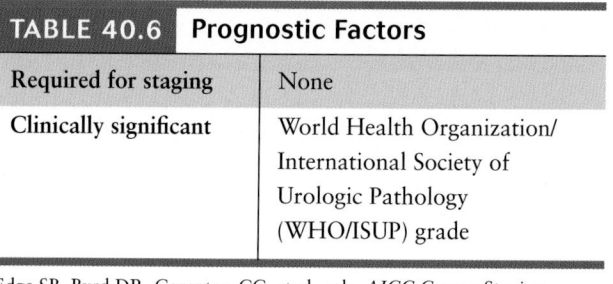

TABLE 40.6	Prognostic Factors
Required for staging	None
Clinically significant	World Health Organization/ International Society of Urologic Pathology (WHO/ISUP) grade

Edge SB, Byrd DR, Compton CC, et al., eds. *AJCC Cancer Staging Manual.* 7th ed. New York: Springer; 2009:512.

CANCER STATISTICS AND SURVIVAL

When considered together, the male genital and urinary systems are the major sites of malignancy. Prostate cancer alone accounts for 200,000 new patients annually. There are 100,000 new urinary tract cancers and 2.5-fold more male genital cancers, or 250,000 cases annually.

The dramatic gains in survival are due to multidisciplinary achievements in screening, early detection, precise diagnoses, and effective multimodal therapies. The cancer statistics reveal perhaps the greatest gains in survival in oncology over the last five decades. In local stage I, male genitourinary tumors are 90% to 100% curable according to the latest Surveillance Epidemiology and End Results data: kidney, 90%; bladder, 94%; testes, 99%; and prostate, 100%. Mortality rates are declining. The pediatric Wilms' tumor was the first malignancy in childhood to be cured, achieving >90% long-term survival, heralding the success of multimodal treatment that would be achieved in adult tumors in urology (Fig. 40.8).

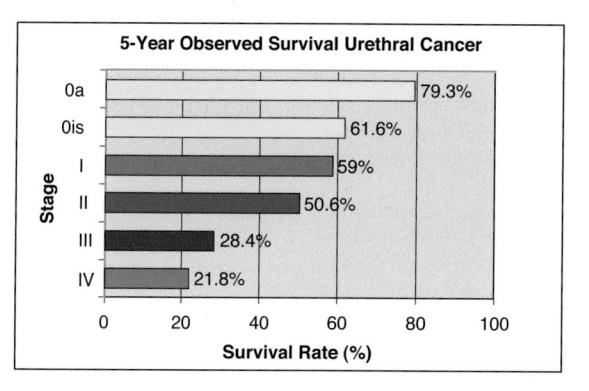

Figure 40.8 | Observed and overall survival rates for 1,278 patients with urethral cancer classified by the current American Joint Committee on Cancer staging classification. Data taken from the National Cancer Data Base (Commission on Cancer of the American College of Surgeons and the American Cancer Society) for the years 1998 to 2002. Stage 0a includes 129 patients; stage 0is, 170; stage I, 243; stage II, 193; stage III, 250; and stage IV, 293. (Data from Edge SB, Byrd DR, and Compton CC, et al., *AJCC Cancer Staging Manual, 7th edition.* New York, Springer, 2010, p. 509.)

Testes

PERSPECTIVE, PATTERNS OF SPREAD, AND PATHOLOGY

The staging criteria are based on conceiving of the testes as an abdominal organ.

PERSPECTIVE AND PATTERNS OF SPREAD

An enlarged or swollen testes is common in young men. It is usually due to a benign event such as an epididymitis or a swelling indicative of some trauma. Despite the infrequent occurrence of testicular tumors, which only account for 1% of all cancers in males, it is the most common tumor in young men between 20 and 40 years of age. However, the benign appearance of hydroceles and varicoceles may disguise a testicular tumor. Thus, increased size of the testes, whether it is sudden or slow in onset, painless or tender, requires careful investigation and consideration before a course of treatment can be decided upon.

The remarkable aspect of all testicular tumors is their high curability. Seminomas traditionally treated with radical orchidectomy followed by para-aortic radiation have yielded cure rates of ≥95%. One of the first malignancies controlled by multiagent chemotherapy were the nonseminomatous cancers (NSCs) of the testes. Stages I and II NSC have 95% long-term survivals; even disseminated metastatic disease can be eradicated the majority of times (50% to 60%). The best example of success is Lance Armstrong, the record-setting cycling champion and seven-time winner of the Tour de France.

Seminomas, embryonal tumors, and teratocarcinomas tend to be confined to the testes. Direct extension through the capsule of the testis into the fascia and muscle of the scrotal wall is an uncommon pattern of spread (Fig. 41.2; Table 41.2). Occasionally, the epididymis is invaded early. Involvement of the rete testis without evidence of further extension is considered an early lesion in behavior if the involvement is contained within the epididymis.

PATHOLOGY

Testicular tumors are divided into seminomas, embryonal cancers, teratocarcinomas or teratomas, and choriocarcinomas (Table 41.1; Fig. 41.1A,B). There are two hypotheses for the generation of this large variety of tumors. The most popular thesis is that a single germ cell gives rise to seminomas and to the multipotential cells that form the other tumor types; the second thesis is that totipotent cells exist that can give rise to the nonseminomatous tumors only (Fig. 41.1C).

TABLE 41.1 | World Health Organization Histologic Classification of Tumors of the Testis

Type
Seminomatous germ cell tumor
Classic type
With syncytiotrophoblasts
Nonseminomatous
Pure
Embryonal carcinoma
Yolk sac tumor
Teratoma
Choriocarcinoma
Mixed

Modified from Edge SB, Byrd DR, Compton CC, et al., eds. *AJCC Cancer Staging Manual.* 7th ed. New York: Springer, 2010:473.

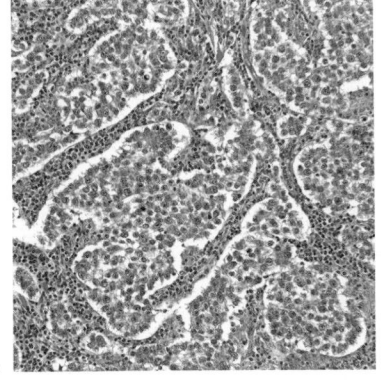

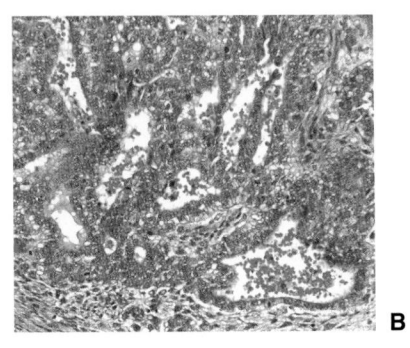

A

B

Figure 41.1 | A. Seminoma. Groups of tumor cells are surrounded by fibrous septa infiltrated with lymphocytes. Tumor cells have vesicular nuclei that are much larger than the small, round nuclei of the lymphocytes.
B. Embryonal. Embryonal carcinoma component of a nonseminoma germ cell tumor. Because these undifferentiated cells have scant cytoplasm, their hyperchromatic nuclei impart a bluish color to the tumor. The nuclei appear crowded and seem to overlap each other. The cells form cords and sheets surrounding dilated vascular channels filled with red blood cells. (*continued*)

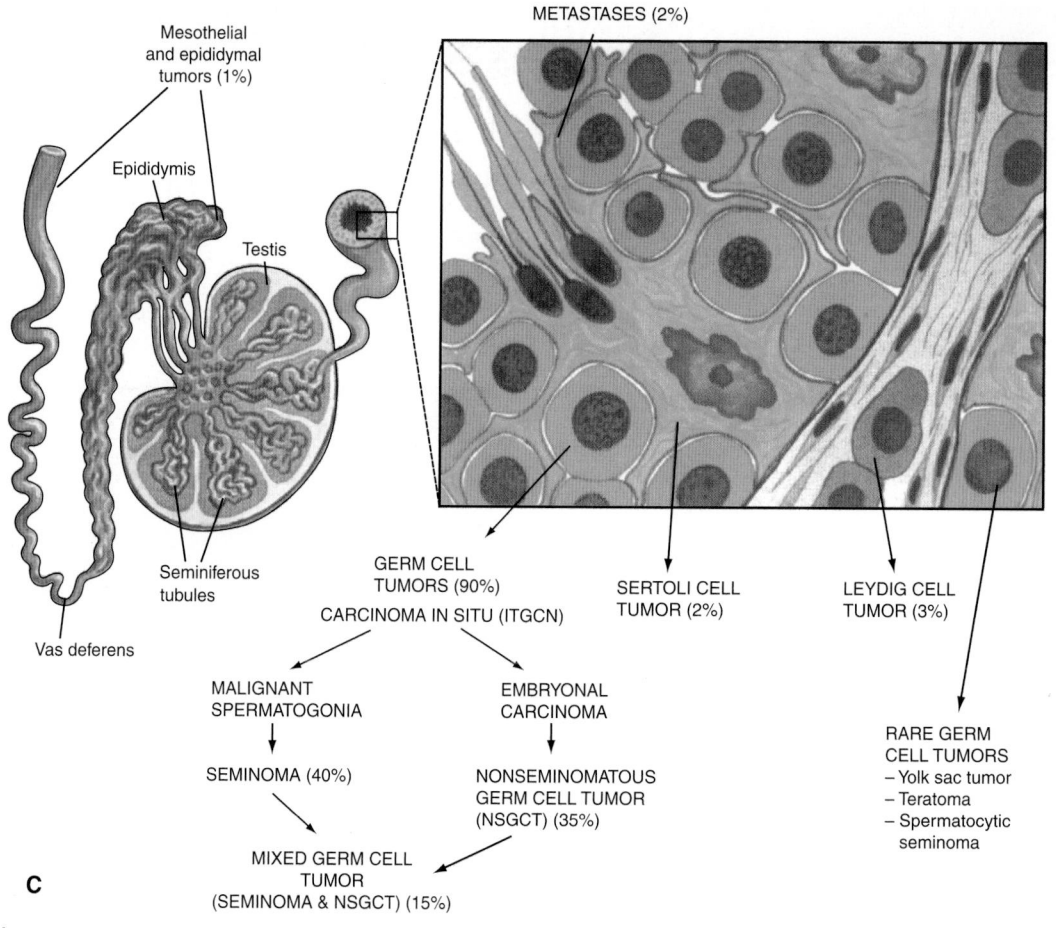

Figure 41.1 | (*Continued*) **C.** Tumors of the testis, epididymis, and related structures.

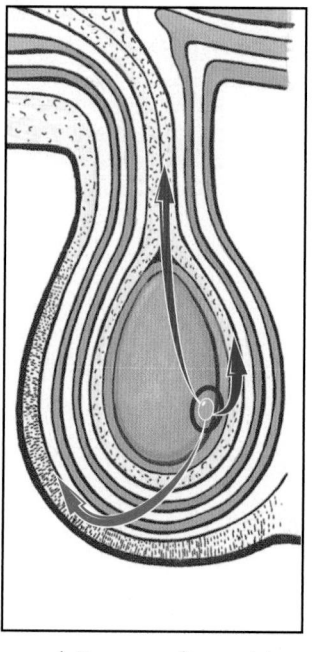

Figure 41.2 | Coronal. Patterns of spread (cancer crab) of testes cancer are color coded for stage: T0, yellow; T1, green; T2, blue; T3, purple. The concept of visualizing patterns of spread to appreciate the surrounding anatomy is well demonstrated by the six-directional pattern (SIMLAP, Table 41.2).

TABLE 41.2	SIMLAP	
Testis		
S	Epididymis	• T1
	Pampiniform plexus	• T3
	Spermatic cord	• T3
	Inguinal canal	• T4
I	Tunica albuginea	• T1
	Tunica vaginalis, visceral layer	• T2
	Tunica vaginalis, cavity	• T2
	Tunica vaginalis, parietal layer	• T2
	Cremaster muscle and fascia	• T4
	Dartos fascia	• T4
	Scrotal skin	• T4
M	Same as above inferior	
L	Same as above inferior	
A	Same as above inferior	
P	Ductus deferens inferior	• T3

The six vectors of invasion are <u>S</u>uperior, <u>I</u>nferior, <u>M</u>edial, <u>L</u>ateral, <u>A</u>nterior, and <u>P</u>osterior. The color-coded dots correlate the T stage with specific anatomic structure involved.

TNM STAGING CRITERIA

TNM STAGING CRITERIA

The staging criteria are based on conceiving of the testes as an abdominal organ. The tunica albuginea is the equivalent of the first wrap of the serosa and, once penetrated by cancer, is T1. If the tunica vaginalis is penetrated, it is equivalent to the peritoneum and is T2. The tunica vaginalis has a visceral and a parietal layer and both need to be penetrated for the cancer to invade the scrotal wall (T4; Fig. 41.3).

The major route for local extension is through the lymphatic channels of the testes that emerge from the mediastinum of the testis and continue along the spermatic cord. The major lymphatic drainage of the testes is different on the left and right. The lymphatics of the testes follow the spermatic vessels and are very commonly the major route of spread of testicular tumors.

Cancer from the germ cells of the testis usually develops during the years of greatest sexual activity. The undescended testis has a greater tendency to undergo carcinomatous change, even after an orchiopexy has been performed. The associated hormonal secretions and the amount of the hormone may produce endocrine effects, including gynecomastia and altered laboratory determinations (human chorionic gonadotropin). In addition, because of their embryonal origin, testicular tumors may produce the tumor-associated antigen alpha fetoprotein. A third serum marker is lactic acid dehydrogenase. Collectively, these three serum biomarkers are incorporated into the staging system as S1, S2, or S3, depending on their level of elevation. Particularly noteworthy is this is the first and only staging system that incorporates serum biomarkers into its progression.

SUMMARY OF CHANGES SEVENTH EDITION AJCC

The definition of TNM and the Stage Grouping for this chapter have not changed from the Sixth Edition (Fig. 41.3). T stage determines stage group (Table 41.3).

GENESIS AND EVOLUTION

Testes cancers are indicative of the robustness and the impact that molecular markers can have in determining stage groups. Including them in the staging system has altered the 4 stages into 13 stage subgroupings. Stage IS is a unique stage with no visible tumor in the TNM compartments. Detection of a serum marker category S1, S2, or S3 depends on titer levels.

TABLE 41.3 Stage Summary Matrix

	T1	T2	T3	T4	
N0	*I	I	I	I	SX
N0	IA	IB	IB	IB	S0
N0	IS	IS	IS	IS	S1-3
N1-3	II	II	II	II	SX
N1	IIA	IIA	IIA	IIA	S0-1
N2	IIB	IIB	IIB	IIB	S0-1
N3	IIC	IIC	IIC	IIC	S0-1
M1	III	III	III	III	SX
M1a	IIIA	IIIA	IIIA	IIIA	S0-1
N1-3/M0	IIIB	IIIB	IIIB	IIIB	S2
Any N/M1a	IIIB	IIIB	IIIB	IIIB	S2
N1-3/M0	IIIC	IIIC	IIIC	IIIC	S3
Any N/M1a	IIIC	IIIC	IIIC	IIIC	S3
Any N/M1b	IIIC	IIIC	IIIC	IIIC	Any S

TESTES

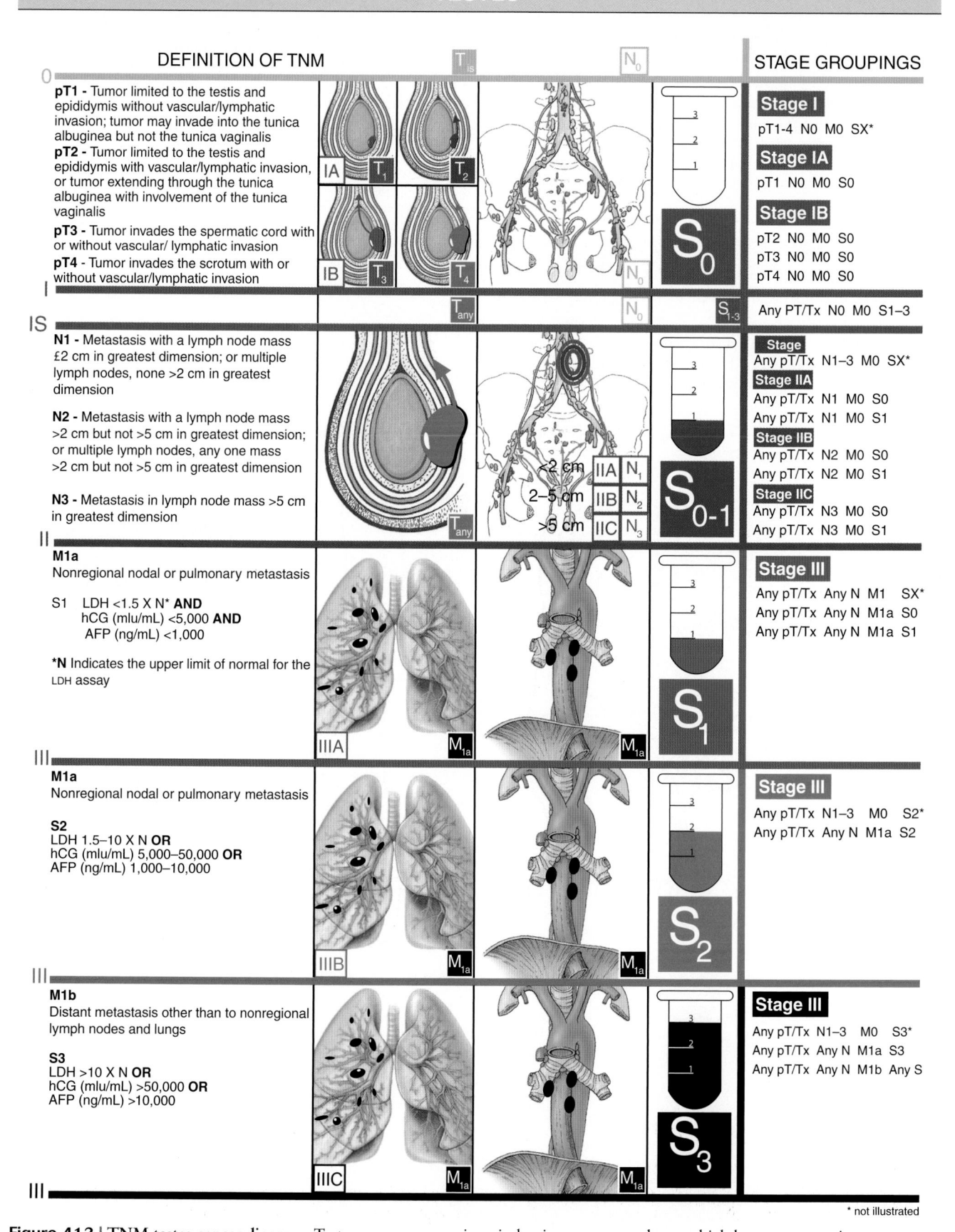

DEFINITION OF TNM

pT1 - Tumor limited to the testis and epididymis without vascular/lymphatic invasion; tumor may invade into the tunica albuginea but not the tunica vaginalis

pT2 - Tumor limited to the testis and epididymis with vascular/lymphatic invasion, or tumor extending through the tunica albuginea with involvement of the tunica vaginalis

pT3 - Tumor invades the spermatic cord with or without vascular/ lymphatic invasion

pT4 - Tumor invades the scrotum with or without vascular/lymphatic invasion

N1 - Metastasis with a lymph node mass £2 cm in greatest dimension; or multiple lymph nodes, none >2 cm in greatest dimension

N2 - Metastasis with a lymph node mass >2 cm but not >5 cm in greatest dimension; or multiple lymph nodes, any one mass >2 cm but not >5 cm in greatest dimension

N3 - Metastasis in lymph node mass >5 cm in greatest dimension

M1a
Nonregional nodal or pulmonary metastasis

S1   LDH <1.5 X N* **AND**
hCG (mIu/mL) <5,000 **AND**
AFP (ng/mL) <1,000

***N** Indicates the upper limit of normal for the LDH assay

M1a
Nonregional nodal or pulmonary metastasis

S2
LDH 1.5–10 X N **OR**
hCG (mIu/mL) 5,000–50,000 **OR**
AFP (ng/mL) 1,000–10,000

M1b
Distant metastasis other than to nonregional lymph nodes and lungs

S3
LDH >10 X N **OR**
hCG (mIu/mL) >50,000 **OR**
AFP (ng/mL) >10,000

<2 cm   IIA   N1
2–5 cm   IIB   N2
>5 cm   IIC   N3

STAGE GROUPINGS

Stage I
pT1-4   N0   M0   SX*

Stage IA
pT1   N0   M0   S0

Stage IB
pT2   N0   M0   S0
pT3   N0   M0   S0
pT4   N0   M0   S0

Any PT/Tx   N0   M0   S1–3

Stage
Any pT/Tx   N1–3   M0   SX*

Stage IIA
Any pT/Tx   N1   M0   S0
Any pT/Tx   N1   M0   S1

Stage IIB
Any pT/Tx   N2   M0   S0
Any pT/Tx   N2   M0   S1

Stage IIC
Any pT/Tx   N3   M0   S0
Any pT/Tx   N3   M0   S1

Stage III
Any pT/Tx   Any N   M1   SX*
Any pT/Tx   Any N   M1a   S0
Any pT/Tx   Any N   M1a   S1

Stage III
Any pT/Tx   N1–3   M0   S2*
Any pT/Tx   Any N   M1a   S2

Stage III
Any pT/Tx   N1–3   M0   S3*
Any pT/Tx   Any N   M1a   S3
Any pT/Tx   Any N   M1b   Any S

* not illustrated

Figure 41.3 | TNM testes cancer diagram. Testes cancers are unique in having serum markers, which have a greater impact on stage groupings and substages than anatomic extent. Vertically arranged with T definitions on the left and stage groupings on the right. Color bars are coded for stage: stage 0, yellow; I, green; II, blue; III, purple; IV, red; and metastatic, black.

T-ONCOANATOMY

ORIENTATION OF THREE-PLANAR ONCOANATOMY

The isocenter is taken at the center of the scrotum inferior to the bony pelvis (Fig. 41.4).

The testes are composed of convoluted seminiferous tubules with a stroma containing functional endocrine interstitial cells.

T-oncoanatomy

The T-oncoanatomy is displayed in three planar views in Fig. 41.5:

- *Coronal:* Both are encased in a dense barrier capsule, the tunica albuginea, with fibrous septa extending into and separating the testes into lobules.

- *Transverse:* The testis is surrounded by a remnant of the peritoneum, the tunica vaginalis, which explains the occurrence of hydroceles, which account for approximately 10% of testicular tumors.

- *Sagittal:* The tubules converge and exit at the mediastinum of the testis into the rete testis and efferent ducts, which join a single tubule. This tubule, the epididymis, is coiled outside the upper and lower poles of the testicle, then joins the muscular vas deferens conduit that accompanies the vessels and lymphatic channels of the spermatic cord.

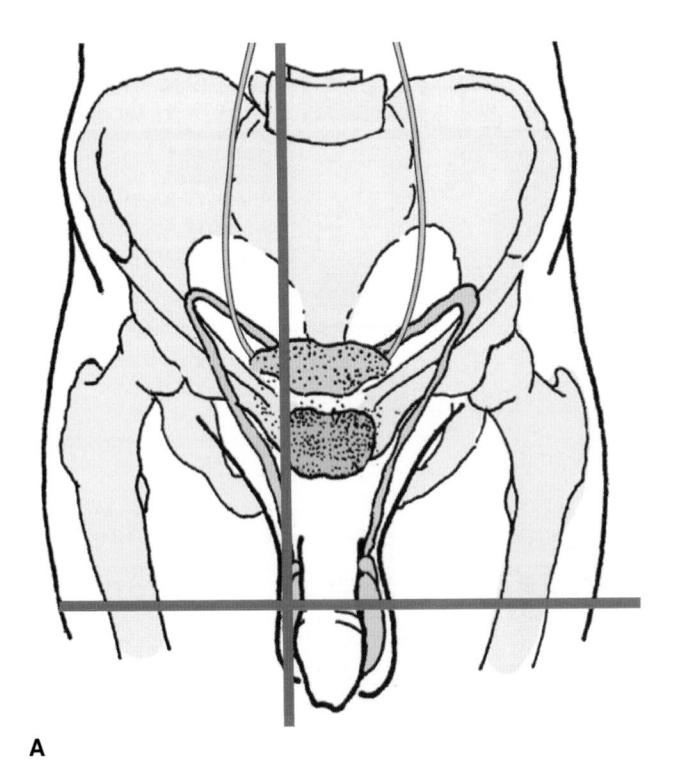

A

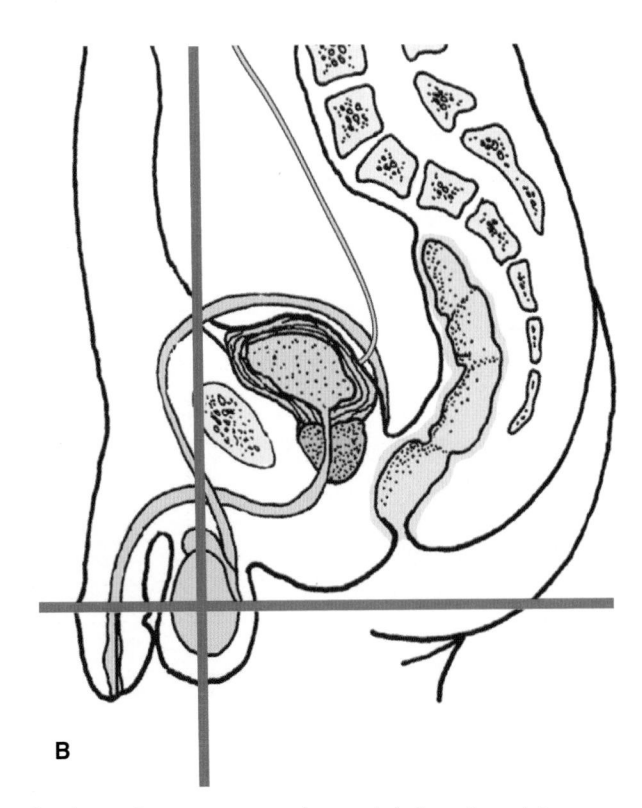

B

Figure 41.4 | Orientation of T-oncoanatomy. The anatomic isocenter for three-planar anatomy of testes is below the pelvis. **A.** Coronal. **B.** Sagittal.

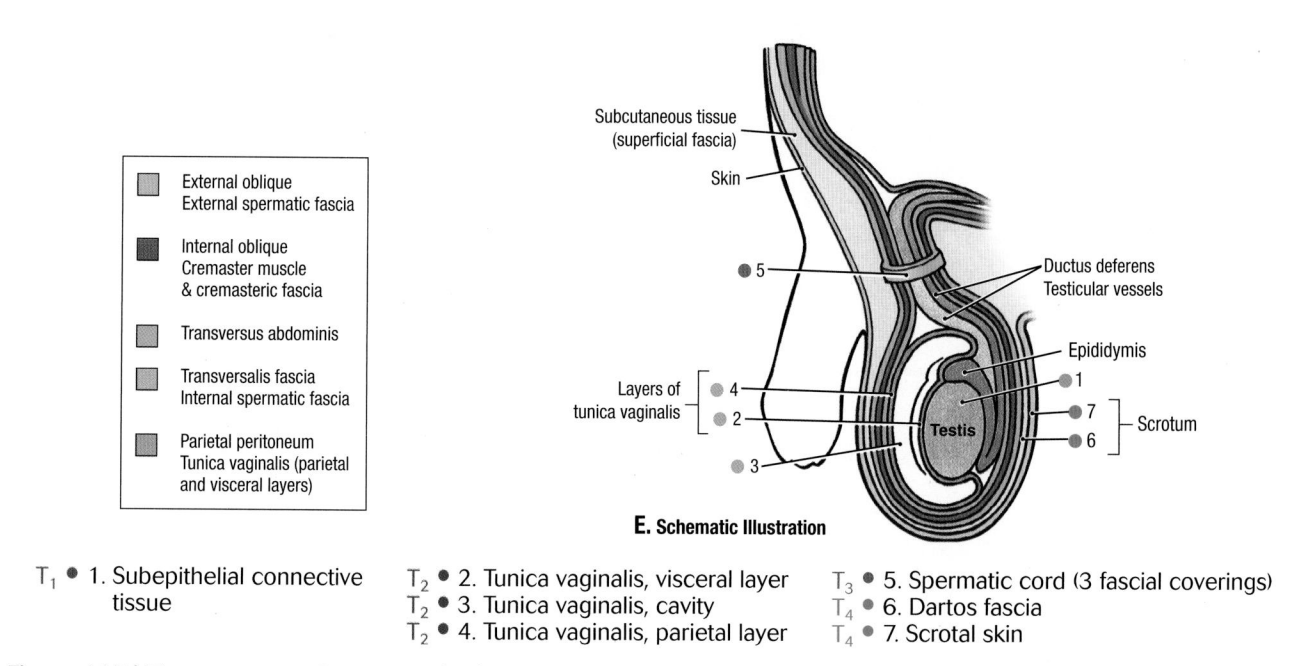

C. Lateral View

- 5
- Internal spermatic fascia
- Cremaster (muscle) within cremasteric fascia
- External spermatic fascia
- Lobules of epididymis
- Efferent ductules of testis
- Tunica vaginalis (parietal layer)
- Tunica vaginalis (visceral layer) covering testis

D. Anterior View

- Testicular veins
- Testicular artery
- Ductus deferens
- 5
- Testicular artery
- Pampiniform plexus of veins
- Ductus deferens
- Epididymis
- External spermatic fascia
- Cremaster and fascia
- Internal spermatic fascia
- 7

Legend:
- External oblique / External spermatic fascia
- Internal oblique / Cremaster muscle & cremasteric fascia
- Transversus abdominis
- Transversalis fascia / Internal spermatic fascia
- Parietal peritoneum / Tunica vaginalis (parietal and visceral layers)

E. Schematic Illustration

- Subcutaneous tissue (superficial fascia)
- Skin
- 5
- Ductus deferens / Testicular vessels
- Epididymis
- Layers of tunica vaginalis — 4, 2
- 1
- 7
- Scrotum
- Testis
- 6
- 3

T₁ • 1. Subepithelial connective tissue
T₂ • 2. Tunica vaginalis, visceral layer
T₂ • 3. Tunica vaginalis, cavity
T₂ • 4. Tunica vaginalis, parietal layer
T₃ • 5. Spermatic cord (3 fascial coverings)
T₄ • 6. Dartos fascia
T₄ • 7. Scrotal skin

Figure 41.5 | T-oncoanatomy. Connecting the dots. Structures are color coded for cancer stage progression. The color code for the anatomic sites correlates with the color code for the stage group (Fig. 41.3) and the patterns of spread (Fig. 41.2) and SIMLAP table (Table 41.2). Connecting the dots in similar colors will provide an appreciation for the three-dimensional oncoanatomy.

N-ONCOANATOMY AND M-ONCOANATOMY

N-ONCOANATOMY

The spermatic lymphatic collecting ducts on the right side tend to follow the vascular components of the cord and drain into the paracaval lymph nodes in the area where the spermatic vein enters the inferior vena cava and the artery arises from the aorta. The spermatic lymphatic collecting ducts on the left side also tend to follow the vascular components of the cord and drain into the para-aortic nodes in the region where the spermatic and the inferior mesenteric arteries arise out of the aorta and also into the nodes of the left renal hilum in the region where the left spermatic vein joins the left renal vein. Juxtaregional or second station nodes are those of the pelvis and mediastinal and supraclavicular regions (Fig. 41.6A; Table 41.4).

TABLE 41.4	Lymph Nodes of Testes	
Sentinel Nodes	
Left renal hilar	
Right paracaval nodes	
Regional Nodes	**Metastatic Nodes**
Right para-aortic	Mediastinal
Left para-aortic	Left supraclavicular
Left renal vein	Hilar
Juxtaregional nodes	
Common iliac	
External iliac	
Inguinal	

The left and right testicles demonstrate different patterns of primary drainage that mirror the differences in venous drainage. The left testicle primarily drains to the para-aortic lymph nodes and the right testicle primarily drains to the interaortocaval lymph nodes. The intrapelvic, external iliac, and inguinal nodes are considered regional only after scrotal or inguinal surgery prior to the presentation of the testis tumor. All nodes outside the regional nodes are distant. Nodes along the spermatic vein are considered regional. A varicoel can result from the left renal vein being compressed by metastatic renal hilar and para aortic lymph nodes.

M-ONCOANATOMY

The spermatic vein on the right side drains directly into the inferior vena cava. On the left side, it drains into and through the renal vein. This causes a higher pressure gradient in the left spermatic vein, which leads to slight dilation of the pampiniform venous plexus that accounts for the lower-lying position of the left testicle as compared to the right (Fig. 41.6B).

Venous drainage of the spermatic veins is into the systemic circulation by way of the inferior vena cava, placing the lungs as the major metastatic target organ. The lung is the major target organ for nonseminoma testicular cancers. Seminomas tend to follow lymphatic progression, giving rise to transdiaphragmatic nodes if retroperitoneal nodes are involved. Either mediastinal nodes or a left supraclavicular node can be involved if the thoracic duct is infiltrated.

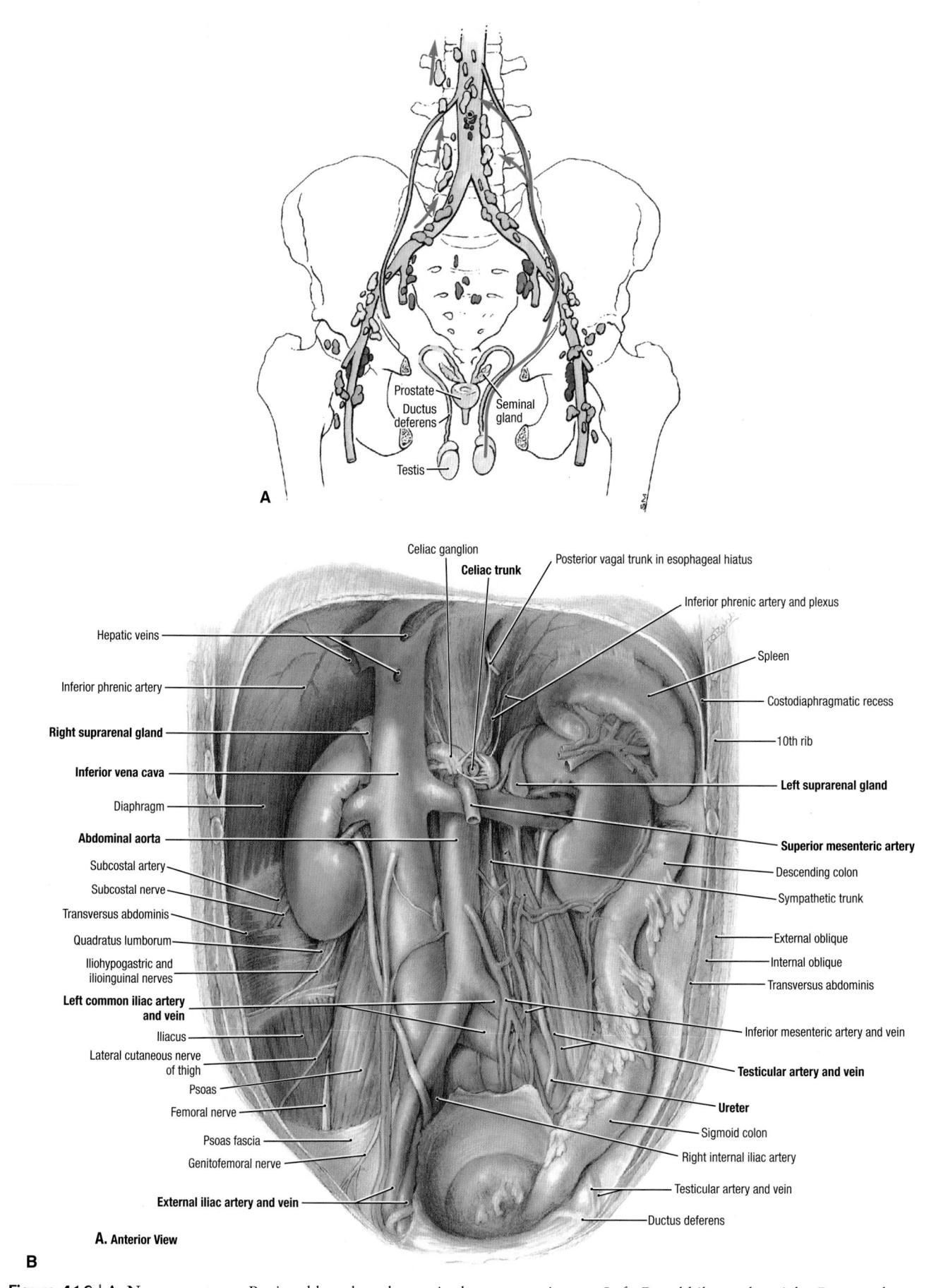

A. Anterior View

B

Figure 41.6 | A. N-oncoanatomy. Regional lymph nodes are in the para-aortic area. Left: Renal hilar nodes; right: Paracaval nodes. **B. M-oncoanatomy:** Great vessels, kidneys, and suprarenal glands.

RULES OF CLASSIFICATION AND STAGING

Clinical Staging and Imaging

Clinical examination of primary can be enhanced by sonograms, computed tomography (CT), and magnetic resonance imaging (MRI)/coil examination. In addition, nodal assessment entails CT of abdomen and pelvis for para-aortic and renal hilar nodes and chest for mediastinal nodes and lung. Serum for marker should be collected before treatment (Table 41.5; Fig. 41.7).

Pathologic Staging

Full assessment of radical orchidectomy specimen for spread, that is, intratesticular or extratesticular, is worth noting, as is invasion of epididymis and for spermatic cord. Multiple tissue sections include one distant from the tumor to determine whether tubular germ cell neoplasia (cancer in situ) is present. Careful evaluation for vascular invasion in multiple sections should be noted. If a retroperitoneal node is evaluated, location, size, and extranodal soft tissue extension should be recorded.

Oncoimaging Annotations

- Scrotal ultrasonographic scanning is an extension of the physical examination. It should be used in most patients with a scrotal mass, especially when the physical examination is difficult or inconclusive.

- MRI is considered an adjunct to ultrasonography for indeterminate testicular lesions or in patients with a discrepancy between ultrasonographic findings and the physical examination. Cross-sectional imaging (CT preferred over MRI) is helpful in the evaluation of nodal disease and metastatic spread.

- The finding of the nodal location (regional nodes), nodal size (>10 mm), and number of detected nodes all play a role in CT/MRI diagnosis of nodal disease.

- Neither CT nor MRI can differentiate benign from malignant nodal involvement, and both understage the early metastatic disease in up to 30% of patients.

- Neither CT nor MRI can differentiate between active tumor and posttreatment fibrosis.

TABLE 41.5	Imaging Modalities for Staging Testis Cancer	
Method	Diagnosis and Staging Capability	Recommended for Use
Primary (T) Staging		
Scrotal US	More useful for differential diagnosis (tumor vs. cyst)	No
Scrotal MRI	Only if physical examination and US show a discrepancy	No
Nodal (N) Staging		
CT$_e$-Abd	Most helpful for detecting the number and size of abdominal para-aortic lymph nodes	Yes, most cost-effective
MRI	Less valuable for determining adenopathy in abdomen	No
Metastases (M) Staging		
Chest film	Can detect metastases >2 cm in size	Yes
Ct$_e$-Ch	Effective for detecting suspected pulmonary or mediastinal nodes	Yes, if chest film is suspicious
CT$_e$-Abd	Can detect liver and visceral metastases	Yes
PET	Identifies bone metastases	No, investigational
BS-Tc Bone scan		

CT, computed tomography; CT-Ch, chest CT; CT$_e$, CT enhanced with intravenous contrast; CT$_e$-Abd, abdominal CT$_e$; MRI, magnetic resonance imaging; PET, positron emission tomography; TAUS, transabdominal US; US, ultrasound.
Modified from Bragg DG, Rubin P, Hricak H, eds. *Oncologic Imaging*. 2nd ed. Philadelphia: Elsevier; 2002:605.

PROGNOSIS AND CANCER SURVIVAL

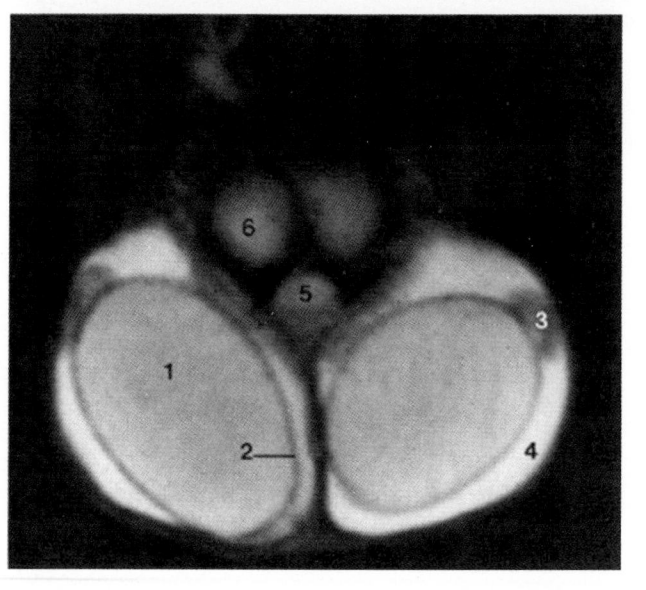

Figure 41.7 | 1. testis 2. tunica albuginea 3. epididymis 4. hydrocele 5. corpus spongiosum 6. corpus cavernosum

PROGNOSIS

The limited number of prognostic factors are listed in Table 41.6.

TABLE 41.6	Prognostic Factors
Required for staging	Serum tumor markers (S)[a,b]
	SX: Marker studies not available or not performed
	S0: Marker study levels within normal limits
	S1: LDH <1.5 × N, hCG <5,000 mIU/mL, and AFP <1,000 ng/mL
	S2: LDH 1.5–10 × N or hCG 5,000–50,000 mIU/mL or AFP 1,000–10,000 ng/mL
	S3: LDH >10 × N or hCG >50,000 mIU/mL or AFP >10,000 ng/mL
Clinically significant	Size of largest metastases in lymph nodes
	Radical orchiectomy performed

[a]Serum tumor marker levels should be measured prior to orchiectomy for assignment of the S category. The only exception is for stage grouping classification of stage IS, in which persistent elevation of serum tumor markers following orchiectomy is required. The serum tumor markers (S) category comprises alpha fetoprotein (AFP), human chorionic gonadotropin (hCG), and lactate dehydrogenase (LDH).
[b]N indicates the upper limit of normal for the LDH assay.
Edge SB, Byrd DR, Compton CC, et al., eds. *AJCC Cancer Staging Manual.* 7th ed. New York: Springer; 2010:476.

CANCER STATISTICS AND SURVIVAL

When considered together, the male genital and urinary systems are the major sites of malignancy. Prostate cancer alone accounts for 200,000 new patients annually. There are 100,000 new urinary tract cancers and 2.5-fold more of male genital cancers, or 250,000 cases annually.

The dramatic gains in survival are due to multidisciplinary achievements in screening, early detection, precise diagnoses, and effective multimodal therapies. The cancer statistics reveal perhaps the greatest gains in survival in oncology over the last five decades. In local stage I, male genitourinary tumors are 90% to 100% curable according to the latest Surveillance Epidemiology and End Results data: kidney, 90%; bladder, 94%; testes, 99%; and prostate, 100%. Death and mortality rates are declining. The pediatric Wilms' tumor was the first malignancy in childhood to be cured, achieving >90% long-term survival, heralding the success of multimodal treatment that would be achieved in adult tumors in urology.

SECTION 5
Gynecologic Primary Sites

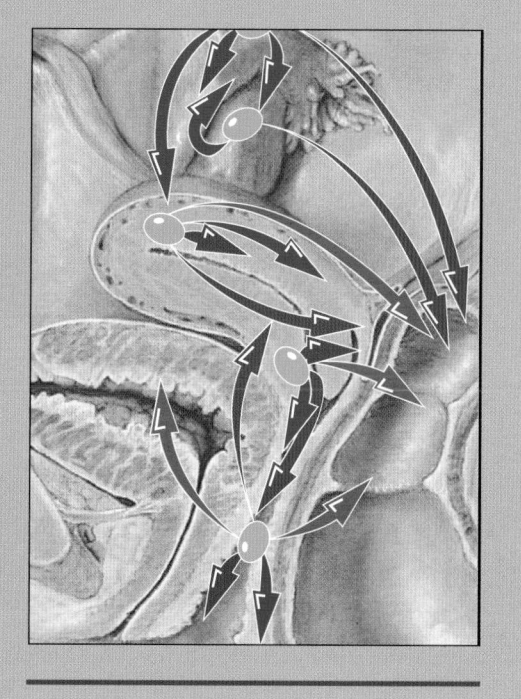

42

Introduction and Orientation

PERSPECTIVE AND PATTERNS OF SPREAD

The staging criteria for gynecologic cancers reflect their oncoanatomy, which can be characterized as variants of both hollow and solid organs.

PERSPECTIVE AND PATTERNS OF SPREAD

The cervix uteri is the anatomic isocenter and an excellent starting point.

Although the incidence of gynecologic cancers is highest during the reproductive years, it does not become a significant killer until menarche. In developing countries, carcinoma of the cervix remains a leading cause of death, often following multiple pregnancies. By contrast, in the Western world, with the introduction of the Papanicolaou smear cytology tests, the cancer can be detected in its early stages. Its incidence remains high; it is the third-most-common gynecologic cancer, largely owing to increases in sexual activity as a result of better contraception, especially among women who have begun at an early age and have multiple sexual partners. According to the most recent Surveillance Epidemiology and End Results figures, uterine cervix, uterine corpus, and ovary account for 10% of all new cases and the same percentage of deaths. This translates into approximately 83,000 diagnoses and 28,000 deaths annually.

Ovarian and uterine cancers often occur during menopause. Although death rates have dramatically declined for cervical and uterine cancers, ovarian cancer survival rates remain the same. Most ovarian cancers are advanced on detection and spread widely. In contrast, uterine cancers usually remain contained within the uterus, and are clinically more evident, as they produce postmenopausal bleeding.

Three of the six sites that give rise to a large variety of neoplasms are discussed in this chapter. The ovary, the fallopian (uterine) tubes, uterus, cervix, vagina, and vulva are each afflicted with neoplastic disease. Adenocarcinomas predominate in the ovary, fallopian tube, and uterus. Squamous cell cancers occur in the cervix, vagina, and vulva. Special germ cell tumors or dysgerminomas, teratomas, and granulosa cell cancers are unique to the ovary. Gestational trophoblastic neoplasms and sarcomas are aggressive malignancies that invade deeply into the uterus. Uterine sarcomas have been emphasized in the seventh edition of the *AJCC Cancer Staging Manual* and expanded to include four different types, each with its own unique staging system. The patterns of spread of each malignancy

TABLE 42.1	SIMLAP*	
Uterine Cervix		
S	Uterus fundus	Tx
	Ovary	Tx
	Fallopian tube	Tx
I	Vagina furnix	• T2a
	Vagina tube	• T3a
	Vulva	• T3a
M	Exocervix	• T1a
	Endocervix	• T1b
L	Broad ligament	• T2a
	Ureter	• T3b
	Levator ANI	• T3b
	Pelvic bone wall	• T3b
A	Urinary bladder	• T4a
	Vesicourinary pouch	• T4a
P	Rectovalinal pouch	• T4b
	Posterior fornix	• T2a
	Rectum	• T4b
	Rectal vaginal septum	• T4b
	Vagina	• T4b
	Uterosacran ligament	• T2a

*The six vectors of invasion are Superior, Inferior, Medial, Lateral, Anterior, and Posterior. The color-coded dots correlate the T stage with specific anatomic structure involved.

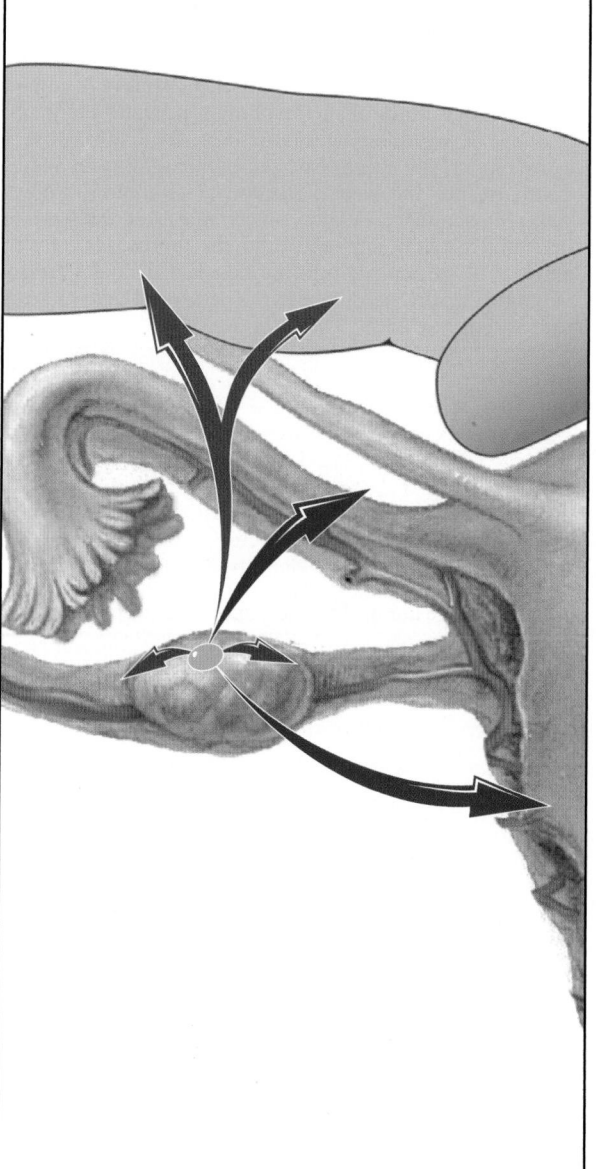 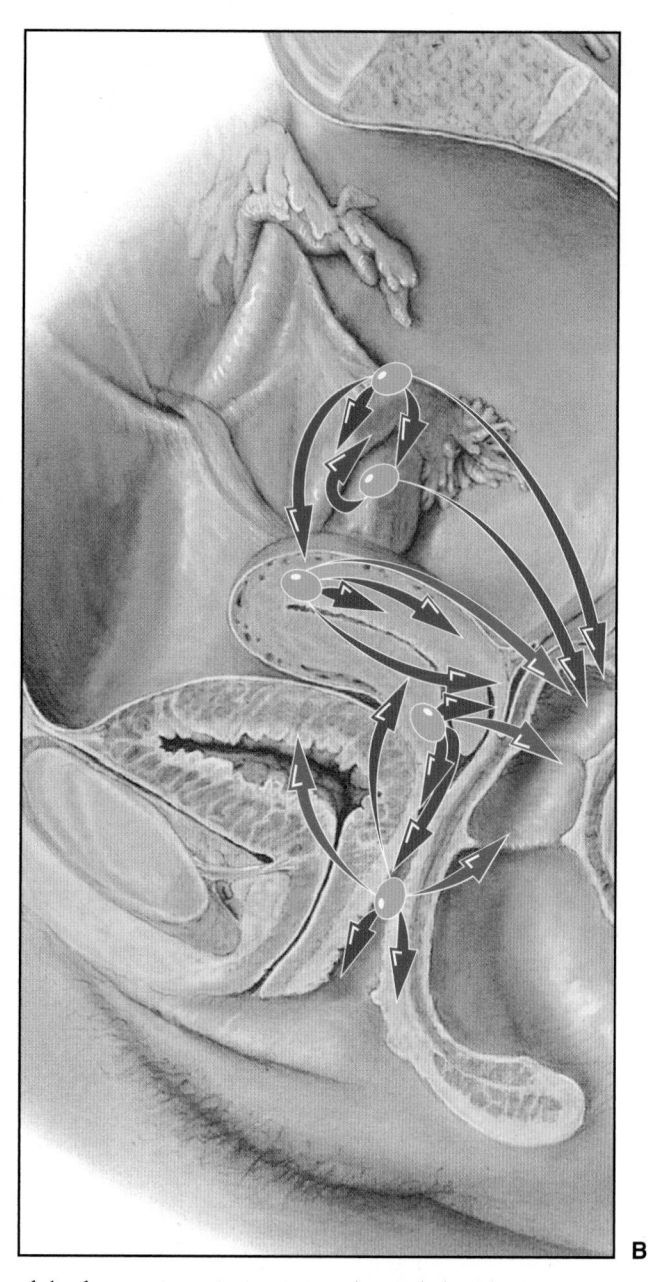

Figure 42.1 | Patterns of spread. A. Coronal. **B.** Sagittal. Collage of the four major primary sites color coded to demonstrate T0 (yellow), T1 (green), T2 (blue), T3 (purple), and T4 (red). The concept of visualizing patterns of spread to appreciate the surrounding anatomy is well demonstrated by the six-directional pattern, SIMLAP (Table 42.1).

determine the outcome: some are invasive; others grow slowly (Fig. 42.1). Each has a different tendency to metastasize.

In summary, the patterns of spread in cervical cancer can act as a compass to female pelvic anatomy (Table 42.1). SIMLAP:

- <u>S</u>uperiorly into the uterine fundus

- <u>I</u>nferiorly into the vaginal walls

- <u>M</u>edially into the ureters that run along the floor of the pelvis

- <u>L</u>aterally further into the parametrium via the broad ligament to the sidewalls of the boney pelvis

- <u>A</u>nteriorly into the trigone of the bladder

- <u>P</u>osteriorly into the rectum via the posterior vaginal wall

TNM STAGING CRITERIA

TNM STAGING CRITERIA

At gynecologic sites, the TNM staging criteria have been relatively stable and developed in conjunction with the Fédération Internationale de Gynécologie et d'Obstétrique (FIGO). A variety of primary of cancer sites are illustrated in Fig. 42.2 to provide an overview of gynecologic cancers.

The cervix uteri cancer is a good starting point for comprehension of the oncoanatomy of the female pelvis by understanding spread patterns of cancer of the cervix. Cervical cancers are most often detected by Papanicolaou smear tests when they are localized to the cervix in their in situ phase. The concept of microinvasion was first defined in the cervix as 5.0 mm depth and then 3.0 mm. Once a cancer forms, it can spread in numerous directions as it invades deeper into the stroma and then adjacent structures. Superficial spread involves the uterus superiorly and the vagina inferiorly. The common infiltration pattern is laterally into the parametrial ligaments, where the ureter and the uterine branches of the hypogastric or internal iliac artery and veins are present. Surgical dissections require isolation of the uterine artery to avoid ligation of the ureter. As the tumor extends laterally into the cardinal or broad ligaments, it becomes fixed to the sidewall of the pelvis. When this occurs, the prognosis becomes grave, and leg edema and pelvis pain occur (stage T3). With anteroposterior spread, the bladder and the rectum are invaded, and fistula formation can occur.

Pelvic pain can have many different patterns. It can even be referred to the extremities. As invasion occurs in the sacral and coccygeal plexus areas, zones of hyperesthesia, hypoesthesia, and even anesthesia can occur in and around the perineum, radiating into the thigh and lower limb. Eventually, muscle invasion and bone destruction can be seen in uncontrolled, advanced, and, particularly, recurrent tumors when standard treatment procedures have failed. The borderline between the false and true pelvis is particularly vulnerable because this is the attachment of the lateral cervical ligaments. Erosion of the medial inner cortex of the true pelvis occurs. In the anterior direction, cervical cancer invades into the bladder and can cause bullous edema and eventually erosion of the mucosa, which leads to urinary bleeding and fistula formation. Posteriorly, rectal invasion can lead to bleeding and fistula formation. This complication is rarely found in fundal uterine cancer.

The uterine fundus usually contains the malignant process within itself. This may relate to the fact that the uterus is normally invaded by a more naturally occurring neoplastic process, namely, the placenta of pregnancy. Thus, the first pathways of cancer spread are superficial: inferiorly into the cervix and superiorly and laterally into the fallopian tubes. When deep invasion occurs, it is usually into the myometrium, toward the serosal surface. With cervical invasion, the spread pattern is similar to that of cervical cancer that invades laterally into the parametrium. Vaginal metastases commonly follow lymphatic channels, skip into the distal vagina, and occur as suburethral nodules. In summary, the major tumor spread patterns at this site are into the (i) myometrium, (ii) serosa and peritoneal cavity, (iii) cervix, (iv) vagina, and (v) fallopian tube and ovary.

The ovary is as much a structure of the whole peritoneal cavity as it is of the pelvis. This is particularly true once it has become subject to malignant transformation. The ovary is positioned essentially at the bottom of the peritoneal cavity. Its blood supply reflects its abdominal origin. When cancer forms in the ovary, it invades through its capsule and forms excrescences. Tumor cells are released and seed the peritoneal surface, often invading the gynecologic tract in the manner of ovulation and/or filling the cul-de-sac. Because there is no true separation between the pelvic and abdominal cavities, this cancer often seeds the omentum, mesentery, and intestine serosal surface. The inferior surface of the diaphragm provides the lymphatic drainage of the abdominal cavity. Thus, the diaphragm may act as a "blotter" for these dispersed tumor cells in the peritoneal cavity. Ascites and pleural effusion are common in advanced stages. In summary, ovarian cancer spread patterns are inferiorly and medially into and onto the uterus, laterally to the pelvic wall, posteriorly into the pouch of Douglas (rectouterine), or superiorly seeding into the peritoneal cavity.

TNM STAGING OF UTERINE CERVIX

Uterine cervix cancer is the archetype and prototype for cancer staging (Fig. 42.2C). The League of Nations introduced the concept of cancer classification and staging more than 70 years ago in 1937 in accord with the FIGO. Pierre Denoix in the 1950s introduced the TNM staging system. In the 1970s, the American Joint Cancer Committee (AJCC) and the Union Internationale Contre le Cancer (UICC) developed an active collaboration and became the first to jointly elaborate the TNM system to encompass all gynecologic cancers. For most decades in the twentieth century FIGO published gynecologic cancer survival results from a selected number of institutions that stringently followed the basic ground rules:

- *Clinical staging* excluded surgical pathologic staging.
- *Joint pelvic examination* by a gynecologist and radiation oncologist *under anesthesia* allowed for speculum and coloscopy observation and rectal/vaginal palpation to determine extent of cancer progression. Radiologic procedures were not admissible, to avoid exclusion of hospitals with limited resources.
- *Biopsy specimens* were eventually required as Papanicolaou smears shifted advanced disease to earlier stages at the time of detection. Surgically resected specimens could not alter the initial clinical stage.
- *Microinvasion of cancer* in the first site, which introduced the criteria for Tis (in situ) stages.
- *Bladder and rectal invasion*: T4 could not rely on endoscopic viewing alone but required biopsy confirmation.

*When there is doubt, the lesser stage should be assigned to make survival results appear worse and avoid stage migration.

The TNM Staging Matrix is color coded for identification of Stage Group once T and N stages are determined (Table 42.2).

TABLE 42.2 Stage Summary Matrix

	N0	N1	M1
T1a1	IA1	IIIB	IVB
T1a2	IA2	IIIB	IVB
T1b	IB	IIIB	IVB
T2a	IIA	IIIB	IVB
T2b	IIB	IIIB	IVB
T3a	IIIA	IIIB	IVB
T3b	IIIB	IIIB	IVB
T4	IVA	IVA	IVB

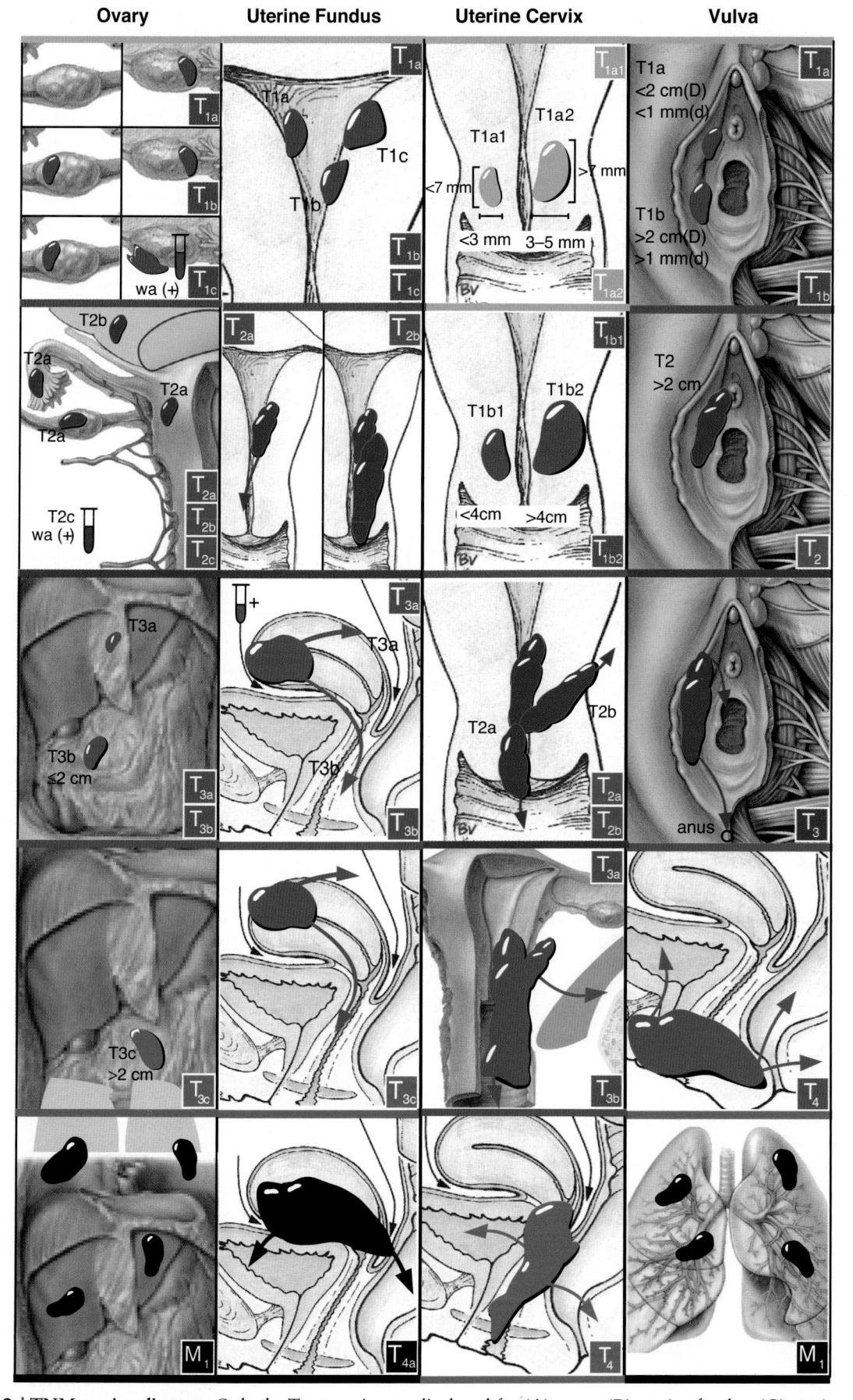

Figure 42.2 | TNM staging diagram. Only the T categories are displayed for (**A**) ovary, (**B**) uterine fundus, (**C**) uterine cervix, and (**D**) vulva. Color bars are coded for stage: stages 0 and IA, yellow; IB, green; II, blue; III, purple; IV, red; and metastatic disease to viscera and nodes, black.

OVERVIEW OF HISTOGENESIS

The specific normal epithelial cell is paired with the derivative cancer histopathologic type (Table 42.3). The overview of histogenesis is presented for the six potential sites that constitute the female reproductive organs (Fig. 42.3). The female reproductive system consists of paired ovaries, paired uterine fallopian tubes, and a single uterus, which is pear shaped with thick muscular walls terminating into cervix. The cervix is at the apex of the vagina with its vestibule centered in the vulva. The specialized gonadal cells of the ovary are in sharp contrast to the epithelial surface of the fallopian tube, which is lined by simple columnar ciliated cells projecting into its lumen as folds, and the endometrial lining of the uterus, which has simple columnar cells over a spongy functionalis layer, which is shed during menses. All of these structures give rise to adenocarcinomas. The cervix is the transitional organ, with an endocervical canal rich in mucous secretion and a surface of squamous cells that blend into the vagina as a stratified squamous cell epithelium. The vulva labia mucosa is a mucosal surface that becomes skin in the labia majora, again lined by stratified squamous cells. Squamous cell cancers are the predominant cancer in the lower female genital tract (cervix, vagina, and vulva).

Referring to Fig. 42.3, we can see that there are six gynecologic sites with distinct cytohistologic features; each can give rise to malignancies:

A *Ovaries* are encapsulated by a simple cuboidal epithelium similar to peritoneal lining cells, which, with repeated microtrauma of oocyte ejection monthly in the adult, can lead to adenocarcinomas that are histologically varied—serous, mucinous, and endometroid.

B *Ovary germ cells* are highly carried and have the potential to transition into granulosa cell cancers, dysgerminomas, and so on.

C *Fallopian tubes* are lined by ciliated simple columnar cells and peg cells, preferably giving rise to serous adenocarcinomas.

D *Uterine fundus* epithelial lining is hormonally activated at puberty, rapidly divides and proliferates monthly, and then sheds during menses. This glandular lining consists of simple columnar cells. These cells at menopause can transition from hyperplasia due to hormonal excess stimuli into neoplasia, leading to adenocarcinomas, which undergo metaplasia into adenosquamous cell mixtures, each of which can become malignant, giving rise to both squamous cell cancers and adenocarcinomas. Endometriosis is a benign proliferative phase in which foci can disseminate into the peritoneal cavity, as well as in other parts of the female gynecologic system. These deposits can transition into endometroid cancers. The *fibrocytes* and *smooth muscle* lieomyocytes commonly give rise to fibromas referred to as fibroids and to leiomyomas, respectively. These mesenchymal cells each can morph into malignant sarcomas, that is, endometrial stromal sarcomas and leiomyosarcomas. In addition, mixed cellular components can both be malignant, giving rise to adenosarcomas intermeshed with adenocarcinomas. The seventh edition of the *AJCC Cancer Staging Manual* offers separate staging systems for sarcomas, and these are discussed in more detail in Chapter 44.

E *Uterine placenta*, with its actively mitosing chorionic villi, can be genetically altered to evolve into hydatiform moles and less frequently transform into choriocarcinomas, which are highly invasive and aggressive, resulting in their rapid metastatic dissemination to distant sites.

F *Uterine cervix* both has a simple columnar epithelium lining the endocervical canal and transitions into a squamous cell lining of the exocervix as it extends to the vaginal fornix. Each cell type can transform into cancers, that is, mucinous adenocarcinomas and squamous cell cancers in varying degrees of differentiation. Cancer in situ is most often discovered at this site.

G *Vagina* is lined by stratified squamous cells, which can give rise to squamous cell cancer. The exception to this rule can occur in young women exposed to hormones, which can lead to a distinct vaginal adenocarcinoma.

H *Vulva*, because of its distinct organization of various lining tissues and glandular elements, can give rise to both squamous cell cancers from the mucosal surface of the labia minora and squamous cell cancer from the skin surface of both the labia majora and minora covered by stratified squamous epithelium. Basal cell cancers can occur on its skin surface. The Bartholin glands can transform into adenocarcinomas.

TABLE 42.3	Overview of Histogenesis of Primary Cancer Sites of the Gynecologic Pelvis	
Primary-Site: Normal Anatomic Structures	**Derivative: Normal Cell Epithelium**	**Cancer: Histopathologic Type, Primary Site**
Ovary	Peritoneal lining Germ cells	Serous, mucinous, and endometrioid adenocarcinomas Special cancers: granulosa cell dysgerminoma
Fallopian tubes	Ciliated simple columnar cells and peg cells	Serous adenocarcinoma
Uterine fundus	Simple columnar Deep glands	Endometrioid adenocarcinoma Adenosquamous cancer mixed Note differentiation and grading
Uterine placenta	Chorionic villi	Choriocarcinoma
Uterine cervix	Stratified squamous Mucous secretory columnar epithelium	Squamous cell cancers Mucinous adenocarcinoma
Vagina	Stratified squamous cell	Squamous cell cancer
Vulva	Stratified squamous epithelium Bartholin gland	Basal cell cancer Squamous cell cancer Adenocarcinoma

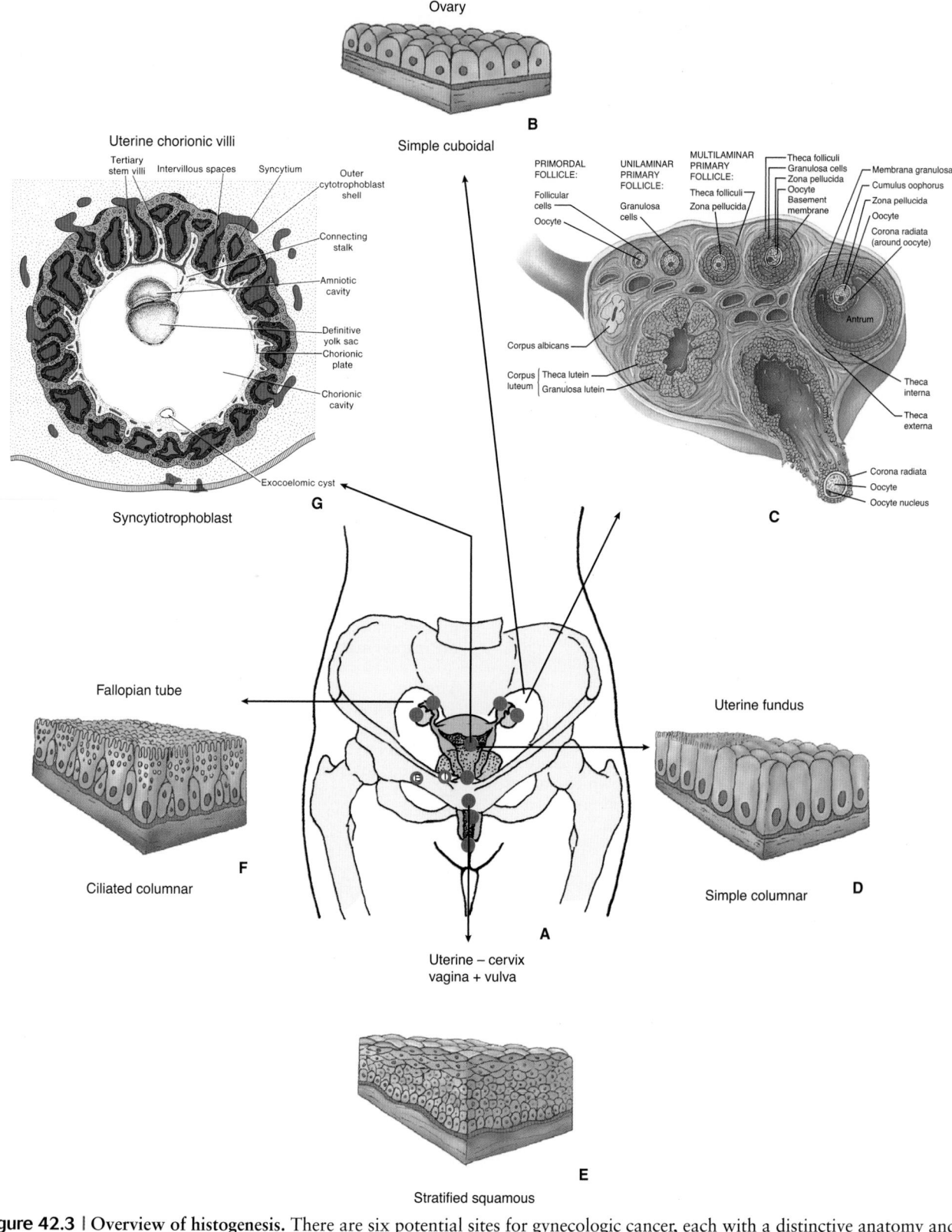

Figure 42.3 | Overview of histogenesis. There are six potential sites for gynecologic cancer, each with a distinctive anatomy and histology. The cancer can be traced to a derivative cell. **A.** Schematic of female internal sex organs. The anatomic isocenters are displayed for gynecologic primary cancer sites. **B.** Ovary epithelial neoplasms include the common varieties of adenocarcinoma (serosa, endometrioid, mucinous), **(C)** Ovary also gives rise to a rich variety of cells leading to germ cell neoplasms. **D.** The uterine wall undergoes dramatic proliferative change monthly in its glandular epithelium during the menstrual cycle and gives rise to adenocarcinomas. **E.** The cervix has a simple columnar epithelium and changes to a stratified squamous epithelium, which gives rise to squamous cell cancers. **F.** The fallopian tube is lined by ciliated columnar epithelium and tends to give rise mainly to serous adenocarcinomas. **G.** Syncytiotrophoblast gives rise to choriocarcinoma and gestational trophoblast tumors.

T-ONCOANATOMY

ORIENTATION OF THREE-PLANAR ONCOANATOMY

Overview of T-oncoanatomy

The juxtaposition of pelvic and abdominal viscera obscures the fact of their separation by the peritoneum. The entire gynecologic tract is retroperitoneal except for the ovary; the digestive system is intraperitoneal. The isocenters of the six primary gynecologic cancers are shown in their pelvic location and range from S2 to the coccyx (Fig. 42.4).

Table 42.4 lists the six primary sites with their surrounding anatomic structures and viscera, their sentinel lymph nodes, and osseous landmarks. The presentation is in a cephalad-to-caudad fashion and includes relationships to the urinary bladder, urethra, rectum, and anus, which are also extraperitoneal in the true pelvis.

Ovary

The ovaries are a pair of solid, flattened ovoids 2.0 to 4.0 cm in diameter. They are connected by a peritoneal fold to the broad ligament and by the suspensory ligament of ovary to the lateral wall of the pelvis. Cancers arise from the mesothelial covering of the ovary rather than its germ cells.

The lymphatic drainage occurs via the ovarian and round ligament trunks and an external iliac accessory route into the following regional nodes: The para-aortic nodes are the major regional nodes, followed by the external iliac, common iliac, hypogastric, lateral sacral, and, rarely, the inguinal nodes. Although the ovary is pelvic in location, its lymphatic drainage recapitulates its abdominal or homologous origin, namely, the para-aortic lymph nodes. Its vestigial relationship via the round ligament to the labia majora reaffirms its similarity to the testes in its intimate scrotal location, which makes drainage to inguinal nodes possible. Ovarian cancers seed and invade the uterus, which drains into pelvic nodes.

Uterus and Fallopian Tubes

Oviducts are paired organs with fimbrae designed to catch an oocyte. The ampulla is characterized by a virtual labyrinth maze of primary, secondary, and tertiary longitudinal folds that narrow at the isthmus as it joins the uterine fundus. The mucosa consists of simple columnar epithelium, which can be ciliated and nonciliated. This can give rise to adenocarcinomas, usually of serous cell variety. The upper two thirds of the uterus above the level of the internal cervical os is called the corpus uteri. The fallopian tubes enter at the upper lateral corners of its pear-shaped body. That portion of the muscular organ positioned above the line joining the tubouterine orifices is called the fundus. Cancers arise mainly from its epithelial columnar lining cells. The relationship of the uterus to other pelvic tissues is important, particularly to the rectum and bladder. The body of the uterus sits in the peritoneal cavity. Although it is juxtaposed to these structures, it is separated by the peritoneal lining, making direct invasion rare.

Cervix

The cervix comprises the lower one third of the uterus. It is roughly cylindrical in shape, projecting into the upper anterior vaginal fornix. It communicates with the vagina through an orifice, namely, the cervical os. Cancer of the cervix may originate on the vaginal surface or in the cervical canal and be either squamous cell or adenocarcinoma. The mesometrium, or broad ligament of the uterus, contains a number of very important structures that determine the course of events in a number of oncologic presentations and complications. The course of the ureter, which is the critical structure, passes from its lateral position in the abdomen to its medial location in the pelvis by moving horizontally to insert into the bladder. It is crossed superiorly and medially by the uterine artery. The long, transverse course of the ureter makes it particularly vulnerable to entrapment by cancer spread from the cervix because it lies juxtaposed to the cervix before its entry to the bladder. Along the sidewall of the pelvis, the obturator nerve and vessel enter into the obturator canal. Cervical cancer tends to invade these structures instead of the body of the uterus; when the rectovaginal or vesicovaginal septum is invaded, the juxtaposition of the vaginal wall directly to the bladder and the rectum makes these organs directly accessible.

Vagina

The vagina is the external os, and the cervix is the internal os. The vagina itself is a fibromuscular tube that extends from the cervix to the vestibule of the external genitalia. It consists of numerous folds of an inner mucosa, a middle muscle layer, and an outer fibrous adventitia. The vagina has no glands and is lubricated by the cervical mucous glands. It is lined by stratified squamous epithelium and has a loose fibroelastic connective tissue and rich vasculature, which comprise the lamina propria, then a smooth muscle layer. The urethra runs anteriorly. The predominant cancer is squamous cell.

Vulva

The vestibule of the vagina is the region between the labia minora and hymen. The labia majora are external and fuse into the mons pubis. The prepuce of the clitoris is like a hood over the clitoris. The underlying musculature consists of three muscles: the bulbospongiosus, the ischiocavernosus, and the transverse perineal superficialis. Deep to this is the perineal membrane and the "urogenital diaphragm" or urethral sphincter.

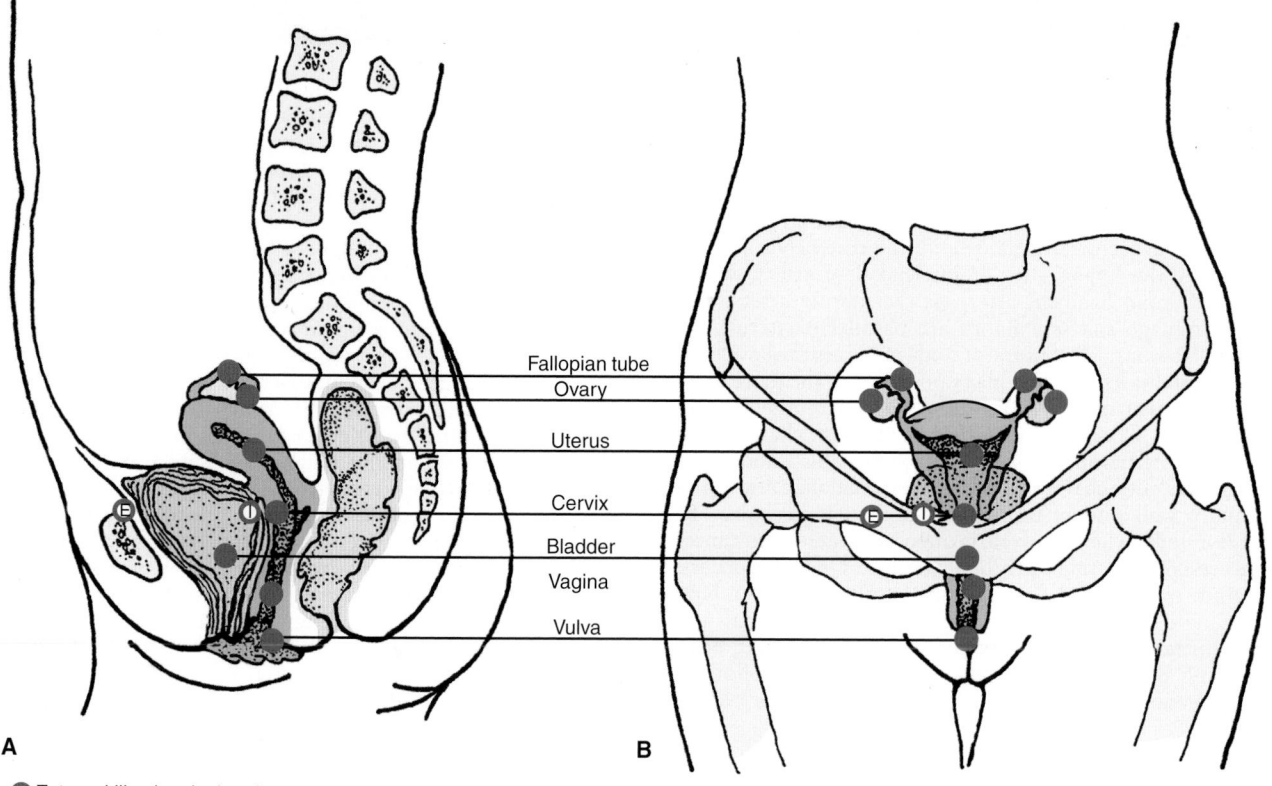

Ⓔ External iliac inguinal node

Ⓘ Internal iliac obturator node

Figure 42.4 | Orientation of T-oncoanatomy of the female pelvis, which houses all the internal female genital organs. From a cephalad-to-caudad fashion each is presented at a different vertebral level. (**A**) Coronal and (**B**) sagittal views with primary sites presented from cephalad to caudad at specific transverse levels related to vertebrae.

TABLE 42.4	Orientation of T-oncoanatomy of Gynecologic Primary Sites			
Primary Site	**Coronal**	**Sagittal**	**Transverse**	**Axial Level**
Ovary	Lateral/apical parametrium	Intimacy with fallopian tubes	Positioned in both peritoneal and pelvic cavities	S3
Fallopian tube	Lateral/apical parametrium	Intimacy with fallopian tubes	Positioned in both peritoneal and pelvic cavities	S2, S3
Uterine fundus	Superior portion of uterus	Antiflexed superior to cervix	Rests on urinary bladder	S2
Cervix	Inferior portion of uterus	Intimate contact of anterior lip of cervix to urinary bladder	Urinary bladder anteriorly and rectum posteriorly	Femoral head
Vagina	Urethra in anterior wall	Urethra in anterior wall and rectum next to posterior wall	Intimate to urethra and anus	Coccyx
Vulva	Perineum showing muscle anatomy and compartment	Relationship to urinary tract and urethra and anus	Intimate to urethral meatus and anus	Femoral trochanter

N-ONCOANATOMY AND M-ONCOANATOMY

N-ONCOANATOMY

To avoid confusion with regard to lymph node drainage and each pelvic site at which a cancer arises, see Table 42.5A for the sentinel nodes as a key to the N-oncoanatomy (Fig. 42.5A). The gynecologic organs lie in the true pelvis and are supplied by the hypogastric or internal iliac artery, which enters the broad ligament artery as the uterine artery. The venous drainage and lymphatics are parallel reentering the internal iliac veins. The obturator node is the sentinel node for the cervix and is located in a plane posterior to the more anterior external iliac nodes (Table 42.5A). This lymph node is in the true pelvis. Occasionally, there is an aberrant channel connecting an internal iliac node to an external iliac node. The external iliac node chain runs with the external iliac artery and vein and is well anterior to the internal iliac node chain. The obturator node, when involved, is often associated with cancer of the cervix infiltrating the broad ligament. Once this occurs, retrograde or abnormal flow patterns alter the course of lymphatics, and collateral channels can connect internal and external iliac nodes. The cervix is drained by preuteral, postuteral, and uterosacral lymphatic routes into the following first station nodes: parametrial, hypogastric (obturator), external iliac, presacral, and common iliac. Para-aortic nodes are second station and juxtaregional nodes.

The lymphatic drainage of gynecologic primary sites is displayed in Fig. 42.5B and Table 42.5B. The fundus of the uterus and fallopian tubes may follow lymphatic channels related to the ovarian artery and vein. The major lymphatic trunks are the utero-ovarian (infundibulopelvic), parametrial, and presacral and drain into the hypogastric, external iliac, common iliac, presacral, and para-aortic nodes. The ovaries descend from their retroperitoneal para-aortic location in the fetus by the gubernaculums. Thus, ovarian cancer can spread to nonregional as well as regional nodes, that is, the para-aortic, pelvic, and even inguinal nodes, owing to attachment of the round ligament. The sentinel nodes depend on location of the cancer in the vagina: In the superior portico, it is similar to the cervix; inferiorly, it is similar to the vulva. The distal vagina and vulva can drain into the inguinal and femoral nodes, as well as into the pelvic iliac lymph nodes. The vaginal drainage depends on the location of the primary. Proximal cancers juxtaposed to the cervix will drain into obturator nodes first, then internal and external iliac nodes. Distal cancers will drain to inguinal nodes. The sentinel nodes will vary with location and can be either femoral or inguinal nodes.

TABLE 42.5A	Orientation of Gynecologic Primary Sites and Sentinel Lymph Nodes		
Cancer Type	**Axial Level Structure/Site**	**Anatomic Adjacent Structure/Site**	**Sentinel Nodes**
Adenocarcinoma of ovary	S3	Small intestine, mesentery omentum, uterus	Para-aortic nodes
Adenocarcinoma of fallopian tubes	S2/3	Large intestine, mesentery omentum, uterus	Para-aortic nodes
Adenocarcinoma of uterine fundus*	S2	Small intestine, sigmoid, bladder, rectum	Para-aortic and obturator nodes
Squamous cell cancer of the cervix	S1	Bladder, rectum, uterus, vagina	Obturator and internal iliac nodes
Squamous cell of the vagina	Coccyx, axial level, ischium	Cervix, bladder, rectum, pouch of Douglas	Obturator, internal and external iliac nodes
Basaloid cancer of vulva	Femur	Anus, urethra, vagina	Inguinal and femoral nodes

*Trophoblastic gestational cancers are uterine in location but placental in origin.

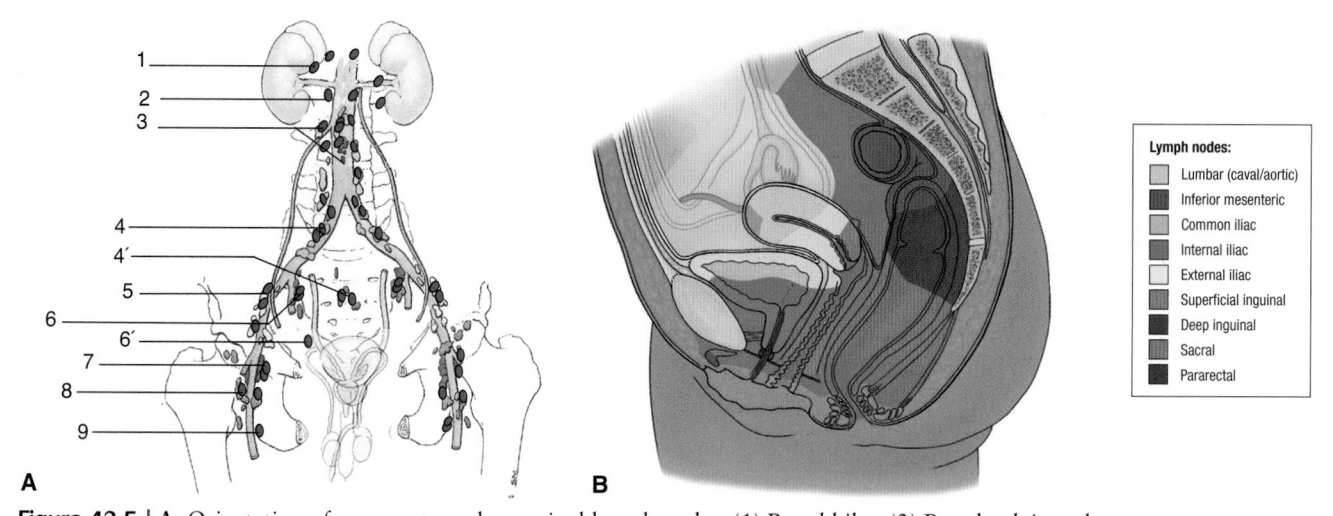

Figure 42.5 | **A.** Orientation of oncoanatomy by sentinal lymph nodes. (1) Renal hilar. (2) Renal pelvis and ureter. (3) Para-aortic and paracaval. (4) Common iliac. (4′) Presacral. (5) External iliac. (6) Internal iliac. (6′) Obturator. (7) Deep inguinal. (8) Superficial inguinal. (9) Femoral. **B:** Orientation of oncoanatomy by lymphatic drainage of primary site.

TABLE 42.5B	Lymphatic Drainage of the Structures of the Female Pelvis and Perineum
Lymph Node Group	**Structures Typically Draining to Lymph Node Group**
Lumbar	Gonads and associated structures (along ovarian vessels), ovary, uterine tube (except isthmus and intrauterine parts), fundus of uterus, common iliac nodes
Inferior mesenteric	Superiormost rectum, sigmoid colon, descending colon, pararectal nodes
Common iliac	External and internal iliac lymph nodes
Internal iliac	Inferior pelvic structures, deep perineal structures, sacral nodes, base of bladder, inferior pelvic ureter, anal canal (above pectinate line), inferior rectum, middle and upper vagina, cervix, body of uterus, sacral nodes
External iliac	Anterosuperior pelvic structures, deep inguinal nodes, superior bladder, superior pelvic ureter, upper vagina, cervix, lower body of uterus
Superficial inguinal	Lower limb, superficial drainage of inferolateral quadrant of trunk, including anterior abdominal wall inferior to umbilicus, gluteal region, superolateral uterus (near attachment of round ligament), skin of perineum including vulva, ostium of vagina (inferior to hymen), prepuce of clitoris, perianal skin, anal canal inferior to pectinate line
Deep inguinal	Glans of clitoris, superficial inguinal nodes
Sacral	Posteroinferior pelvic structures, inferior rectum, inferior vagina
Pararectal	Superior rectum

M-ONCOANATOMY

The internal and external iliac veins drain the female reproductive organs, and metastatic dissemination is via the inferior vena cava to the lung, which is the favored target organ (Fig. 42.6A,B).

- *Ovarian cancers* arise from the epithelial surface, which during embryogenesis is derived from the coelomic cavity lined by mesothelial cells that became specialized to form a serosal covering of the gonadal ridge. As ovarian cancers shed their cells into the peritoneal cavity, they behave as peritoneal mesotheliomas, studding the omentum, the intestinal tissues, liver, and diaphragm, resulting in ascites.

- *Uterine cancers* illustrate the difference between circulating cancer cells that are released as a result of the curettage of endometrial cancer to establish the diagnosis compared to the incidence of metastases. The presence of circulating cancer cells is a universal phenomenon compared to the low incidence of pulmonary and other metastases. Unique to uterine cancers is the occurrence of vaginal metastases, which can be synchronous or metachronous. A nodule in the vaginal wall that is an adenocarcinoma in an adult should be considered a signal that there may be a uterine fundal cancer.

- *Cervical cancers* target the lungs or can present as mediastinal adenopathy if para-aortic nodes are present. Unique to cancer of the cervix is the aggressiveness of bone invasion as a result of extension in broad ligament to obturator nodes located at the lateral brim of the true pelvis wall. In addition, common iliac nodes and para-aortic nodes can massively erode vertebras as well as intervertebral disc, leading to curvature of the lumbar spine.

- *Vaginal and vulvar cancers* tend to be diagnosed in their localized stages, and lymph node metastases predominate in hematogenous spread to lung.

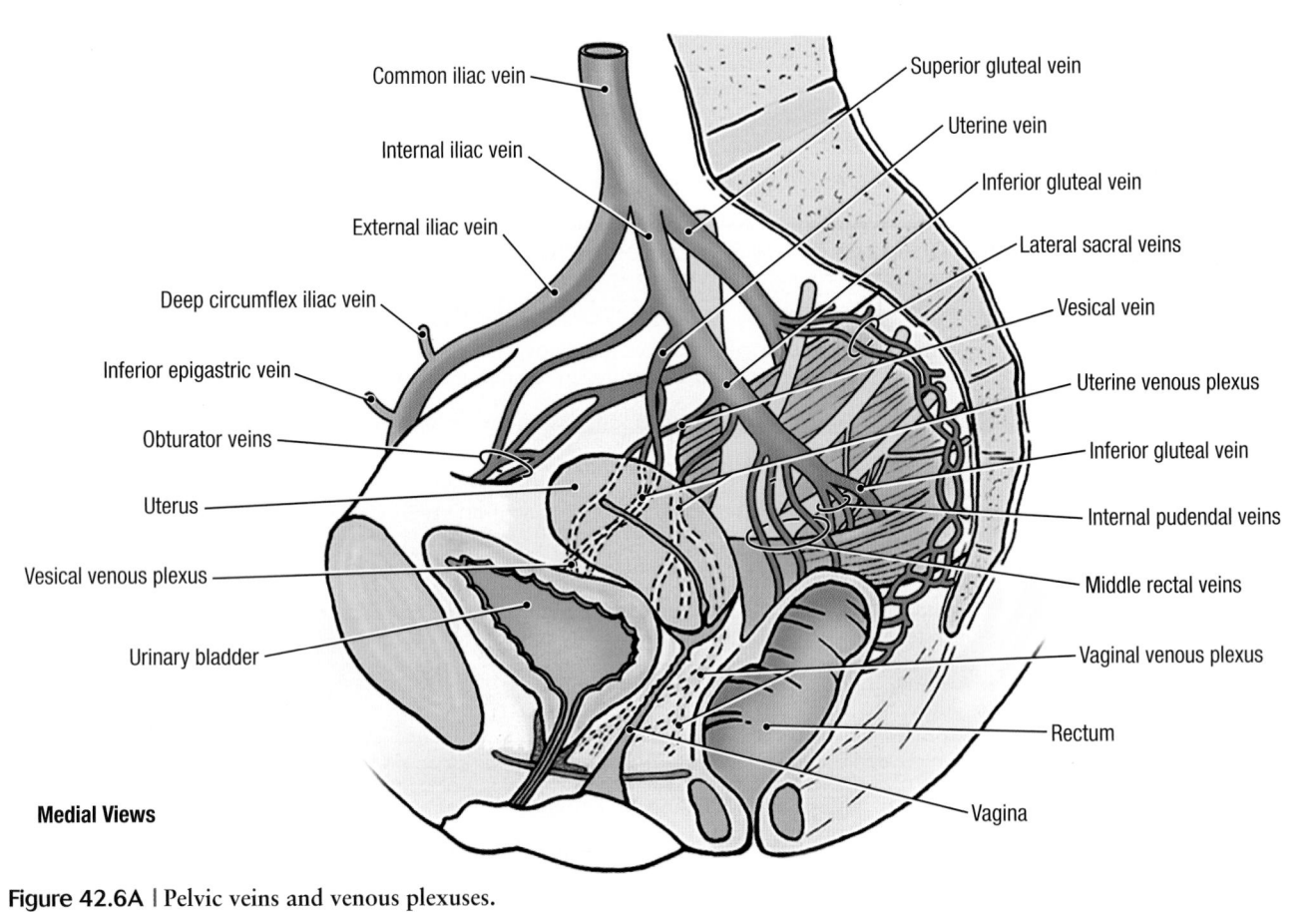

Medial Views

Figure 42.6A | Pelvic veins and venous plexuses.

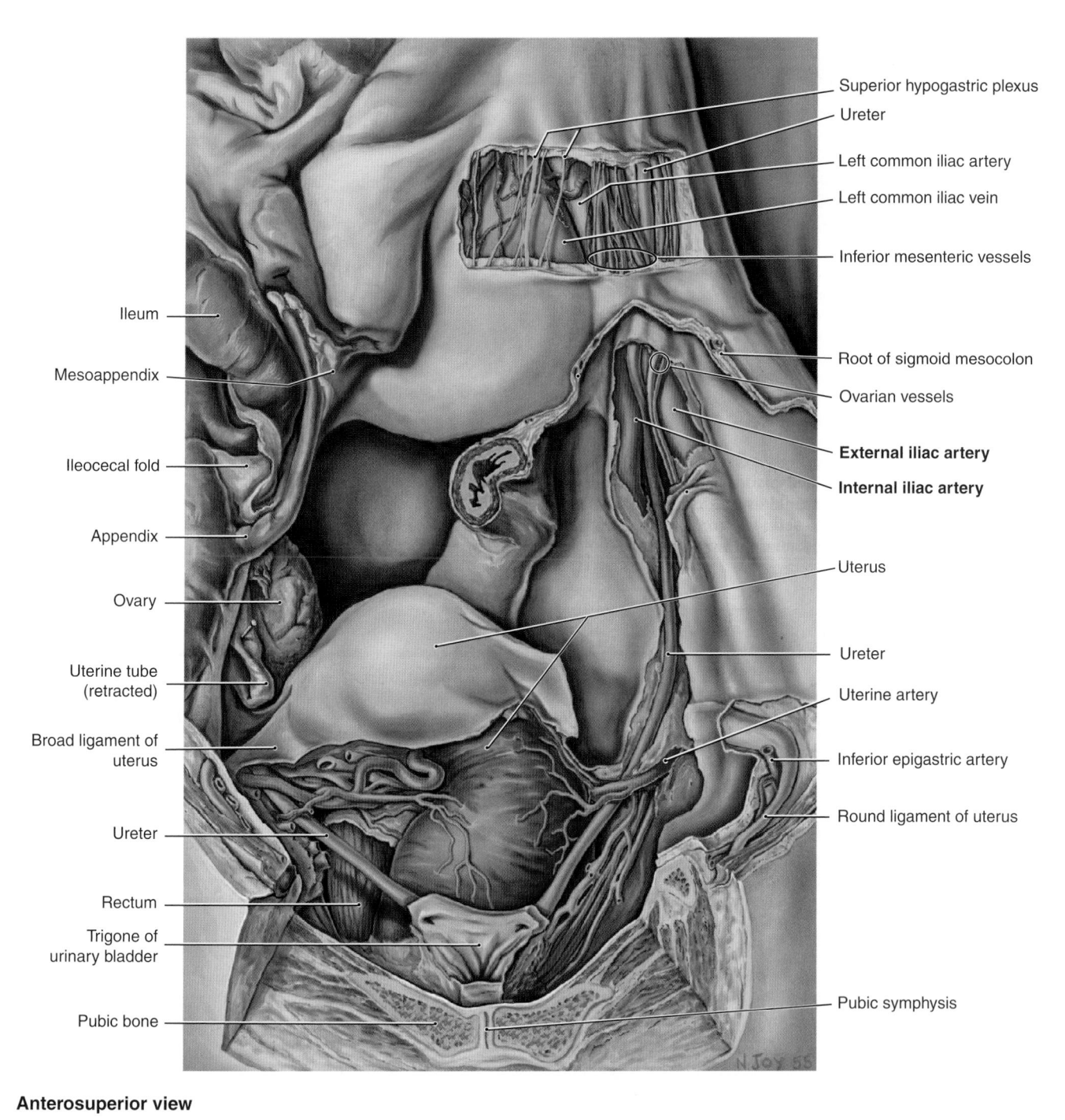

Anterosuperior view

Figure 42.6B | Orientation of M-oncoanatomy.

PROGNOSIS AND CANCER SURVIVAL

CANCER STATISTICS AND SURVIVAL

Female genital system cancers collectively account for 80,000 new cases annually, with uterine corpus exceeding cervix cancer by a factor of four. Both cervical and uterine cancers are highly curable, and deaths are relatively low. The major gynecologic killer is ovarian cancer, with 16,000 annual deaths, which exceeds the other six primary sites combined.

The survival rate gains in both cervix uteri and fundus uteri have been incremental. Given that invasive cancers of the gynecologic tract have had a higher baseline—greater than 50% in the 1950s—the gains for all stages are only 15%, or 2% to 3% per decade. As noted, mortality rates have plummeted owing to early detection, especially of cervical cancer because it is most often detected in its noninvasive stage. Localized uterine cancers are more than 90% curable.

The cancer survival rates indicate the gain in survival for uterine corpus and cervix cancer have been modest (14%) over the last five decades. However, most uterine cervix cancers are detected as cancer in situ, and this is not reflected in the figures. Ovarian cancer survival has improved by 22% and, as stated, remains lethal because most cases are detected late owing to its insidious onset and the inaccessibility of ovarian cysts and nodules to early diagnosis. On the bright side is the high cure and 5-year survival rates for stage I patients with cervical cancer (92%), uterine corpus cancer (96%), and ovarian cancer (95%) (Fig. 42.8).

The most recent survival rate data is provided in the AJCC 7th Edition for most common gynecologic cancers. As observed survival curves over five years based on large patient populations. In Figures 42.9, the five year observed survival is shown as a series of bar graphs. Note that early localized stages yield very high survival rates. These survival statistics are confirmed in the most recent ACS facts and figures (Table 42.7).

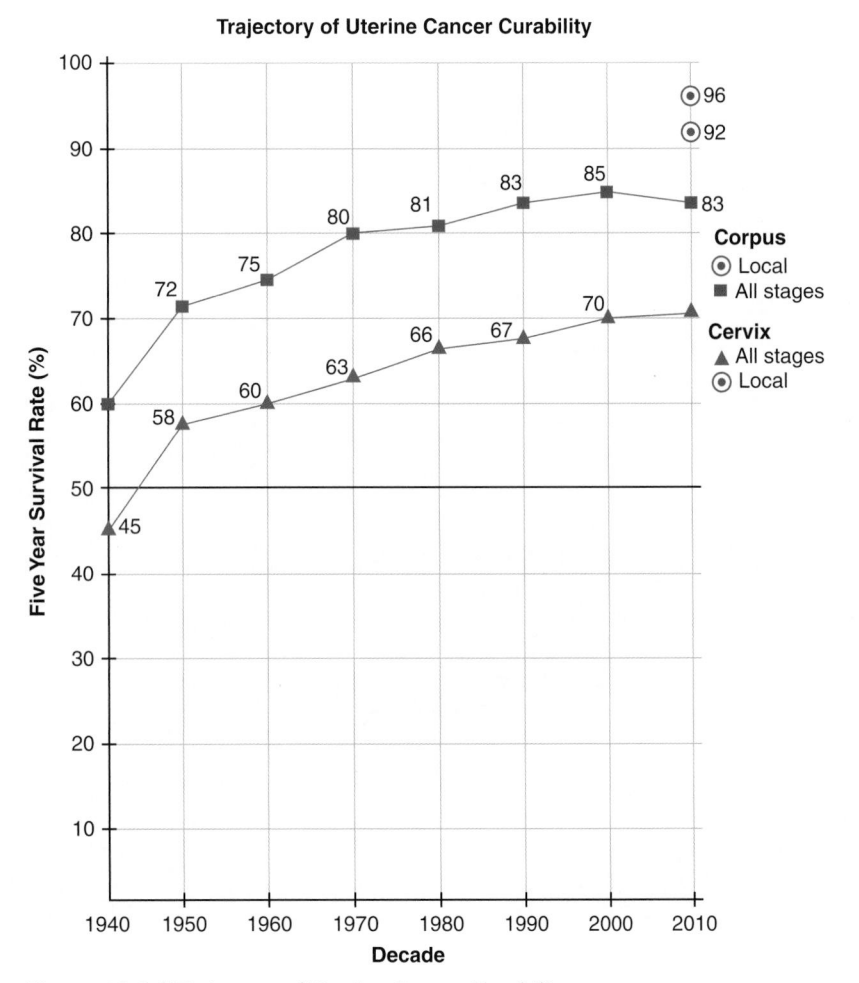

Figure 42.8 | Trajectory of Uterine Cancer Curability.

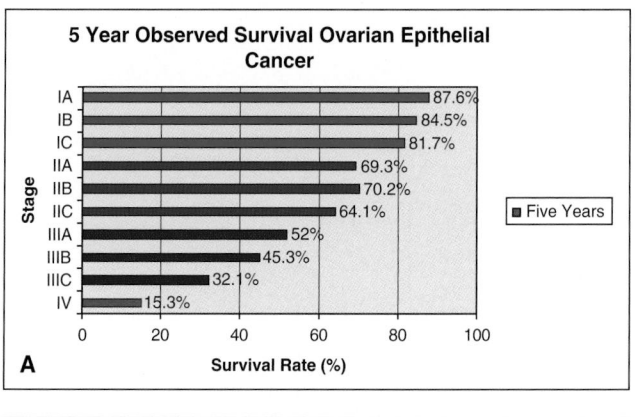

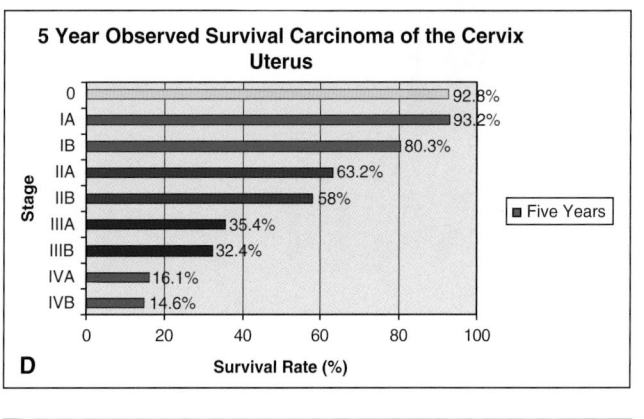

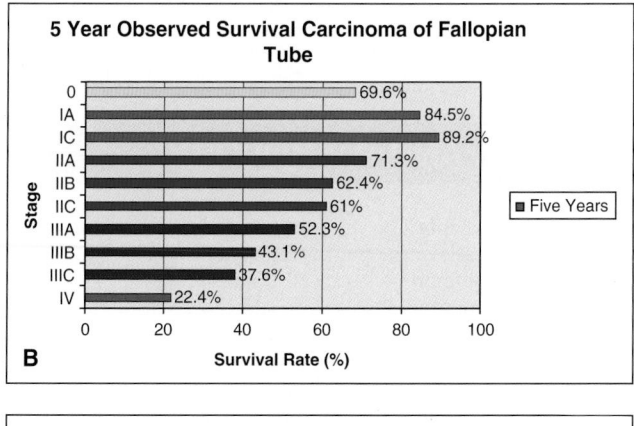

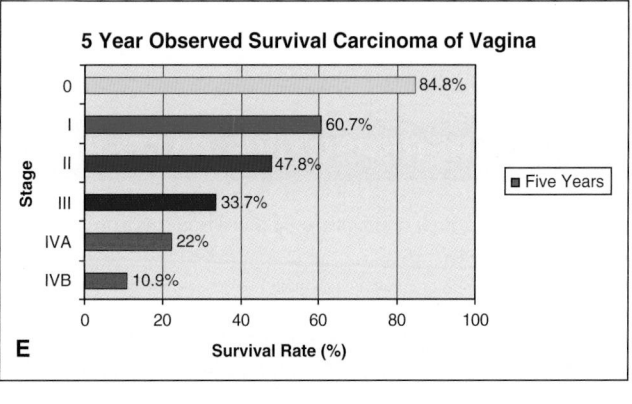

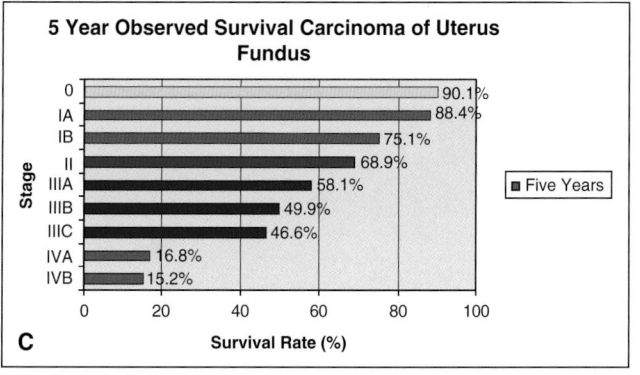

Figure 42.9 | Five-year observed survival rates for the most common gynecologic cancers. **A.** Ovary. **B.** Fallopian tube. **C.** Uterine fundus. **D.** Cervix. **E.** Vagina. (Data from Edge SB, Byrd DR, and Compton CC, et al., *AJCC Cancer Staging Manual*, 7th edition, New York: Springer; 2010.)

TABLE 42.7	Five-year Relative Survival Rates (%) by Stage at Diagnosis, 1999–2005			
SITE	All Stages	Local	Regional	Distant
Uterine Fundus	83	96	67	17
Uterine Cervix	71	92	58	17
Ovary	46	94	73	28

Data from Horner MJ, Ries LAG, Krapcho M, et al. (eds) *SEER Cancer Statistics Review, 1975–2006*, National Cancer Institute, Bethesda, MD. From American Cancer Society. Cancer Facts and Figures 2010. http://www.cancer.org/Research/CancerFactsFigures/CancerFactsFigures/cancer-facts-and-figures-2010. Accessed July 31, 2011.

CHAPTER

43

Ovary and Fallopian Tube

PERSPECTIVE, PATTERNS OR SPREAD, AND PATHOLOGY

The ovary is as much a structure of the whole peritoneal cavity as it is of the pelvis.

OVARY

PERSPECTIVE AND PATTERNS OF SPREAD

Ovarian cancer is the most lethal cancer of the female genital tract. Deaths from this cancer surpass deaths attributed to gynecologic cancers at all other sites combined. The total loss of life in 2010 was 21,880, compared with 13,000 for all other gynecologic sites. The estimated incidence is 25,000 new cases annually. The common symptom and sign is the insidious accumulation of ascitic fluid masquerading as weight gain and increase in abdominal girth. Unlike the other common gynecologic cancers, in this case vaginal bleeding is rare. Clinical detection is most often due to routine physical and pelvic examination coupled with pursuit of imaging and serum markers in high-risk patients with familial histories or those testing positive for both BRCA-1 and -2 oncogene mutations.

The staging of these cancers demands surgical laparotomy exploration of both the pelvic and peritoneal cavity, including the omentum, the mesentery, the liver, and the diaphragm, because abdominal seeding is the dominant pattern of spread (Fig. 43.1, Table 43.1). The ovary is as much a structure of the whole peritoneal cavity as it is of the pelvis. This is particularly true once it has become subject to malignant transformation. The ovary is positioned essentially at the bottom of the peritoneal cavity. Its blood supply reflects its abdominal origin; that is, ovarian arteries arise from the aorta, and ovarian veins drain directly to the inferior vena cava, unlike uterine vessels that arise from the pelvic internal iliac artery and drain into pelvic internal iliac veins.

When cancer forms in the ovary, it invades through its capsule and forms excrescences. Tumor cells are released and seed the peritoneal surface, often invading the gynecologic tract in the manner of an ovum or filling the cul-de-sac. Because there is no true separation between the pelvic and abdominal cavities, this cancer often seeds the omentum, mesentery, and

intestine. The diaphragm may act as a "blotter" for these dispersed tumor cells in the peritoneal cavity. Ascites and pleural effusion are common in advanced stages.

Molecular markers such as CA-125 can be elevated at diagnosis and are useful for following response versus relapse. Germ cell tumors can have elevated serum markers, such as α-fetoprotein (AFP) and human chorionic gonadotropin (β-HCG), which can be used to assess treatment.

TABLE 43.1	SIMLAP*	
Ovary and Fallopian Tube		
S	Fallopian tube	• T2a
	Peritoneal cavity cell	• T1c
	Small intestine	• T3abc
	Colon	• T3abc
	Broad ligament	• T2b
I	Vagina	• T2b
	Uterine fundus	• T2a
M	Uterus	• T2c
	Opposite ovary	• T1b
	Uterine artery	• T2b
	Ligament ovary	• T2b
	Levator ani muscles	• T2b
L	Ovarian artery	• T2b
	Urinary bladder	• T2b
A	Vesicouterine pouch	• T2b
	Pouch of Douglas	• T2b
P	Rectum	• T2b

*The six vectors of invasion are Superior, Inferior, Medial, Lateral, Anterior, and Posterior. The color-coded dots correlate the T stage with the specific anatomic structure involved.

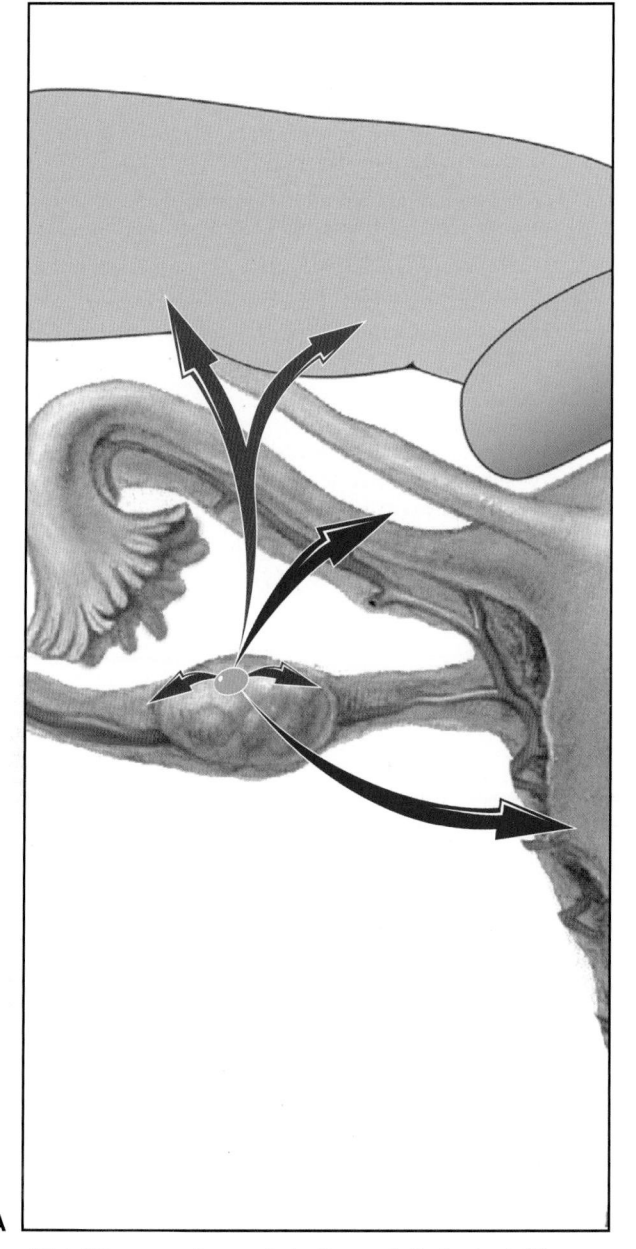

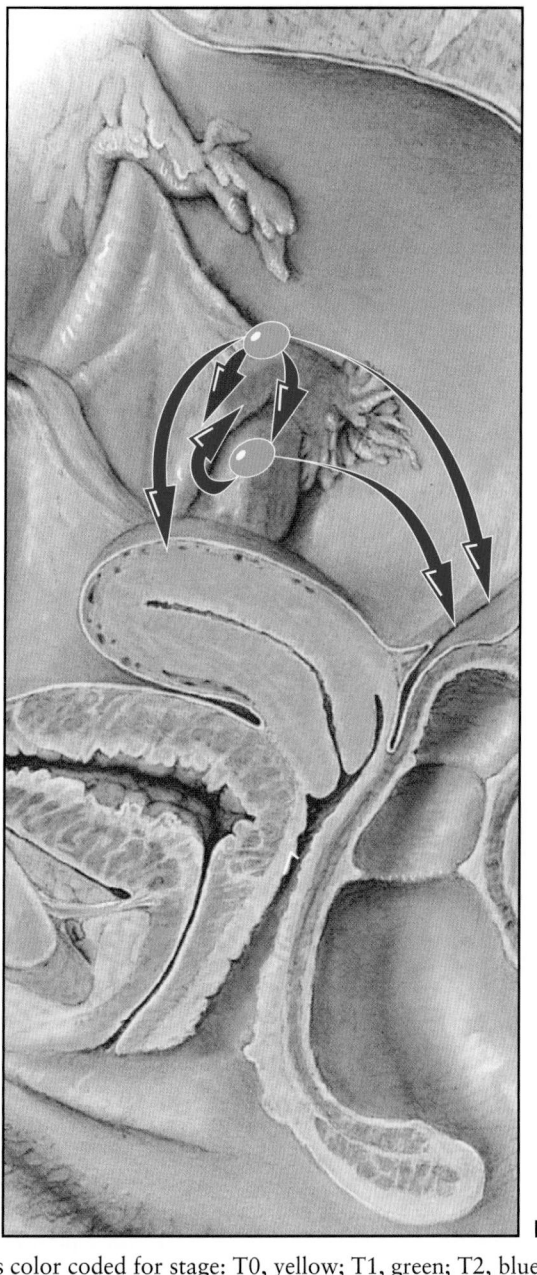

Figure 43.1 | **Patterns of spread. A.** Coronal. **B.** Sagittal. The cancer is color coded for stage: T0, yellow; T1, green; T2, blue; T3, purple. The concept of visualizing patterns of spread to appreciate the surrounding anatomy is well demonstrated by the six-directional pattern, i.e., SIMLAP Table 43.1.

Histopathology

The coelomic cavity mesothelial lining specializes when it encapsulates the ovary, forming a simple cuboidal epithelial cell wrap. With repetitive oocyte ejection and rupture of this layer, transformation of the epithelium-stroma into a benign proliferation, then borderline changes, and finally into malignant carcinoma occurs. The dedifferentiation into serous, endometroid, mucinous histologies relates to the Müllerian epithelial anlage. The World Health Organization list of histopathologies is endorsed by the American Joint Committee on Cancer/International Union Against Cancer (Table 43.2). Between 80% and 90% are epithelial cancers; 5% to 10% are bilateral. Serous carcinomas are the most common subtype, microscopically containing papillary and glandular elements. To understand the full range of diversity of histopathologic types of ovarian tumors, one must recapitulate the embryogenesis of the ovary and its unique relationship to the peritoneal cavity (Table 43.2, Fig. 43.2).

- *Serous cancers* are similar to fallopian tube epithelia (Fig. 43.2A).
- *Mucinous cancers* are similar to endocervix epithelia (Fig. 43.2B).
- *Endometroid cancers* are similar to endometrial epithelia (Fig. 43.2C).

The specialized tumors of the ovary are derived from germ cells and their supporting cells, which, during their differentiation, can result in a genetic error and mutate into a variety of cancers unique to the ovary.

- *Dysgerminomas* resemble oogonia of the fetal ovary and are the female counterpart of seminomas (Fig. 43.2D).
- *Endodermal sinus* (yolk sac) tumors resemble the mesenchyme of primitive yolk sac (Fig. 43.2E).
- *Granulosa cell tumors* occur in adults, often in menopause (Fig. 43.2F).
- *Krukenberg tumors are metastatic cancers* from gastrointestinal primaries—mainly stomach and colon—that can seed and grow into bilateral symmetric ovarian masses, which is the converse of ovarian cancers seeding into the peritoneal cavity (Fig. 43.2G).
- *Peritoneal mesotheliomas* that minimally involve the ovary are considered primary peritoneal carcinomas (Fig. 43.2H).

TABLE 43.2	Histopathologic Type: Common Cancers of the Ovary

Epithelial tumors

A. Serous tumors (Fig. 43.2A)
   1. Benign serous cystadenoma
   2. Of borderline malignancy: serous cystadenoma with proliferating activity of the epithelial cells and nuclear abnormalities but with no infiltrative destructive growth (carcinomas of low potential malignancy)
   3. Serous cystadenocarcinoma

B. Mucinous tumors (Fig. 43.2B)
   1. Benign mucinous cystadenoma
   2. Of borderline malignancy: mucinous cystadenoma with proliferating activity of the epithelial cells and nuclear abnormalities but with no infiltrative destructive growth (carcinomas of low potential malignancy)
   3. Mucinous cystadenocarcinoma

C. Endometrioid tumors (Fig. 43.2C).
   1. Benign endometrioid cystadenoma
   2. Endometrioid tumors with proliferating activity of the epithelial cells and nuclear abnormalities but with no infiltrative destructive growth (carcinomas of low potential malignancy)
   3. Endometrioid adenocarcinoma

D. Clear cell tumors
   1. Benign clear cell tumors
   2. Clear cell tumors with proliferating activity of the epithelial cells and nuclear abnormalities but with no infiltrative destructive growth (low potential malignancy)
   3. Clear cell cystadenocarcinoma

E. Brenner (transitional cell tumor)
   1. Benign Brenner
   2. Borderline malignancy
   3. Malignant
   4. Transitional cell

F. Squamous cell tumor

G. Undifferentiated carcinoma
   1. A malignant tumor of epithelial structure that is too poorly differentiated to be placed in any other group

H. Mixed epithelial tumor (Fig. 43.2H)
   1. Tumors composed of two or more of the five major cell types of common epithelial tumors (types should be specified)

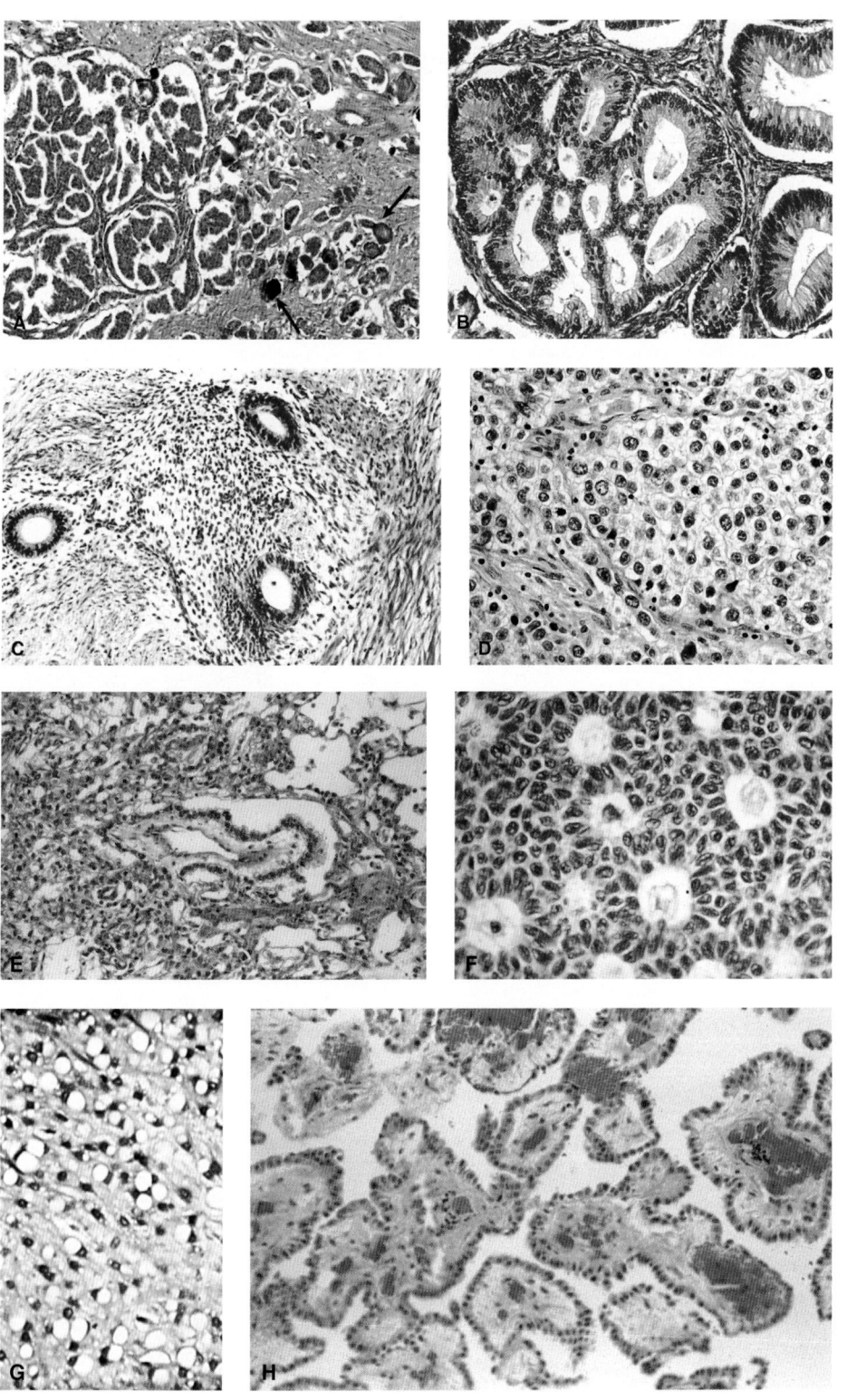

Figure 43.2 | A. Serous cystadenocarcinoma. (1) The ovary is enlarged by a solid tumor that exhibits extensive necrosis (N).
(2) Microscopic examination shows a papillary cancer invading the ovarian stroma. Several psammoma bodies are present
(arrows). **(3)** A higher-power view shows the laminated structure of a psammoma body. **B. Mucinous cystadenocarcinoma.** The
malignant glands are arranged in a cribriform pattern and are composed of mucin-producing columnar cells. **C. Endometriod
tumors. D. Dysgerminoma.** The neoplastic germ cells have clear, glycogen-filled cytoplasm and central nuclei. Fibrous septa containing lymphocytes traverse the tumor. **E. Yolk sac carcinoma of ovary.** The tumor cells are arrayed in a reticular pattern. A
Schiller-Duval body **(center)** resembles the endodermal sinuses of the rodent placenta and consists of a papilla protruding into a
space lined by tumor cells. **F. Granulosa cell tumor of the ovary. (1)** Cross section of the enlarged ovary shows a variegated solid
tumor with focal hemorrhages. The yellow areas represent collections of lipid-laden luteinized granulosa cells. **(2)** The orientation
of tumor cells about central spaces results in the characteristic follicular pattern (Call-Exner bodies). **G. Krukenberg tumor. (1)**
The ovary is enlarged and partially hemorrhagic. **(2)** A microscopic section of panel (1) reveals mucinous (signet-ring) cells infiltrating the ovary. **H. Well-differentiated peritoneal mesothelioma.** Cuboidal epithelium lines papilla.

TNM STAGING CRITERIA

TNM STAGING CRITERIA

The evolution of ovarian cancer staging criteria has rested on careful exploratory laparotomy and gradually required multiple sampling of a variety of peritoneal sites such as omentum, mesentery, liver, and the diaphragm. By the fourth edition, the three stages of each had three subcategories. The pattern of spread in the earliest stages is limited to the ovary (stage T1a); if both ovaries are involved, stage is T1b, and with positive washings or ascites it is T1c. Once extension occurs to pelvic organs or implants on uterus or tubes, it is T2a; onto pelvic wall or bladder, T2b; and with positive washings or ascites, T2c. Once peritoneal metastatic seeding occurs into the abdominal peritoneal cavity but is microscopic tumor, it is stage T3a; macroscopic tumor <2 cm, T3b; and macroscopic tumor >2 cm, T3c (Fig. 43.3A).

Important clarifications include the following: Only malignant ascites affect staging, and liver capsule metastases are T3, but liver parenchyma metastases are M1. Pleural effusion must have positive cytology to be M1 stage. Patients with only intraperitoneal carcinoma without ovarian involvement or minimally involved should be labeled as having "extraovarian" peritoneal carcinoma and by definition are stage T3 or M1.

SUMMARY OF CHANGES SEVENTH EDITION AJCC

- The definition of TNM and the Stage Grouping for this chapter have not changed from the Sixth Edition (Fig. 43.3A).

- Primary peritoneal carcinoma has been included in this chapter.

The TNM staging matrix allows for identification of stage group once T and N stages are determined (Table 43.3).

TABLE 43.3 Stage Summary Matrix

	N0	N1	M1
T1	I	IV	IV
T2	II	IV	IV
T3	III	IV	IV
T4	IV	IV	IV

*Same for fallopian tube.

Cancer of the ovary has three major stages (I, II, III), and each stage is divided into A, B, or C reflecting the T stage, with T_3 reflecting peritoneal spread and N_1 being stages IIIC and IV for M_1. There is a total of 11 stage groups.

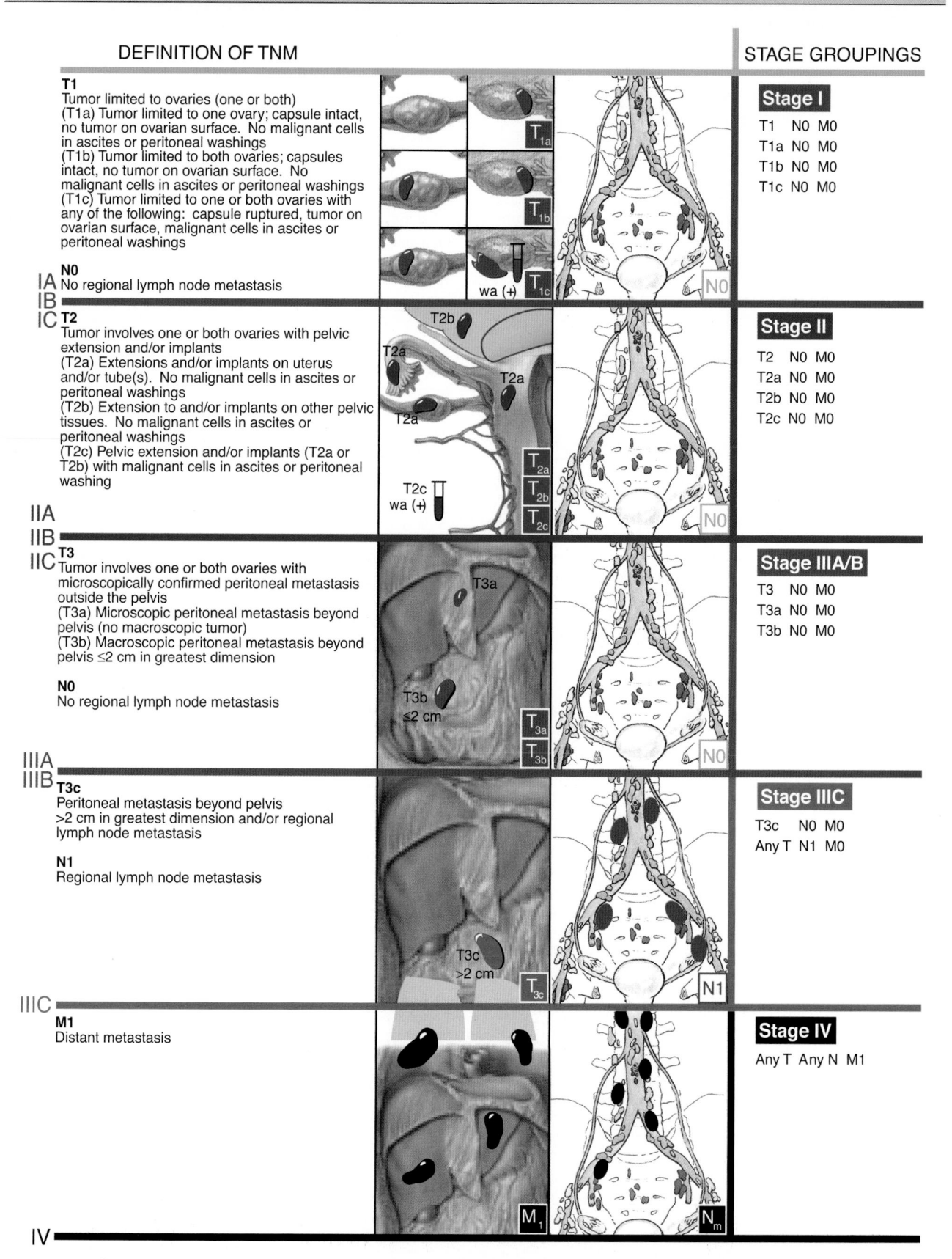

OVARY

DEFINITION OF TNM

T1
Tumor limited to ovaries (one or both)
(T1a) Tumor limited to one ovary; capsule intact, no tumor on ovarian surface. No malignant cells in ascites or peritoneal washings
(T1b) Tumor limited to both ovaries; capsules intact, no tumor on ovarian surface. No malignant cells in ascites or peritoneal washings
(T1c) Tumor limited to one or both ovaries with any of the following: capsule ruptured, tumor on ovarian surface, malignant cells in ascites or peritoneal washings

N0
No regional lymph node metastasis

IA
IB
IC

T2
Tumor involves one or both ovaries with pelvic extension and/or implants
(T2a) Extensions and/or implants on uterus and/or tube(s). No malignant cells in ascites or peritoneal washings
(T2b) Extension to and/or implants on other pelvic tissues. No malignant cells in ascites or peritoneal washings
(T2c) Pelvic extension and/or implants (T2a or T2b) with malignant cells in ascites or peritoneal washing

IIA
IIB
IIC

T3
Tumor involves one or both ovaries with microscopically confirmed peritoneal metastasis outside the pelvis
(T3a) Microscopic peritoneal metastasis beyond pelvis (no macroscopic tumor)
(T3b) Macroscopic peritoneal metastasis beyond pelvis ≤2 cm in greatest dimension

N0
No regional lymph node metastasis

IIIA
IIIB

T3c
Peritoneal metastasis beyond pelvis >2 cm in greatest dimension and/or regional lymph node metastasis

N1
Regional lymph node metastasis

IIIC

M1
Distant metastasis

IV

STAGE GROUPINGS

Stage I

T1	N0	M0
T1a	N0	M0
T1b	N0	M0
T1c	N0	M0

Stage II

T2	N0	M0
T2a	N0	M0
T2b	N0	M0
T2c	N0	M0

Stage IIIA/B

T3	N0	M0
T3a	N0	M0
T3b	N0	M0

Stage IIIC

T3c	N0	M0
Any T	N1	M0

Stage IV

Any T	Any N	M1

Figure 43.3A | TNM staging diagram arranged vertically with T definitions on the left and stage groupings on the right. Ovarian cancers are cancers of the pelvis and peritoneal cavity. Resectability depends on the number and size of peritoneal implants. Color bars are coded for stage: stage I, green; II, blue; III, purple; IV, red; and metastatic disease to viscera and nodes, black.

FALLOPIAN TUBES

The basis for staging carcinomas of the fallopian tube clearly parallels that for ovarian cancer.

PERSPECTIVE AND PATTERNS OF SPREAD

Carcinoma of the fallopian tube (FT) is rare and most often simulates ovarian cancers in presentation as an adnexal mass (Fig. 43.2G). Often, FT cancers are associated with two symptoms: vaginal bleeding and abdominal pelvic pain, often spasmodic in nature. This is an uncommon female malignant cancer, representing <1% of all female cancers.

Histopathologically, FT cancers are serous adenocarcinomas. The majority are identified at surgery, and the basis of this staging system is surgical-pathologic. The histopathology is similar to that of ovarian cancers (Table 43.2).

EPIDEMIOLOGY AND ETIOLOGY*

Carcinoma of the fallopian tube is an uncommon malignancy that accounts for 0.3% to 1.1% of all female genital tract cancers. The most common form of this cancer is a papillary serous carcinoma, but only about 300 cases of this are reported each year in the United States. The paucity of information makes its natural history and management unfamiliar. In most series, the median patient age at diagnosis is between 55 and 60 years. The clinical course of fallopian tube carcinoma is often similar to that of epithelial ovarian carcinoma, although there are several significant differences.

DETECTION AND DIAGNOSIS

Unlike epithelial ovarian carcinoma, fallopian tube carcinoma is often symptomatic. The three most common symptoms and signs are abnormal vaginal bleeding, a pelvic mass, and abdominal or pelvic pain. Pelvic pain is more common in tubal carcinoma than in ovarian carcinoma; as the tumor in the fallopian tube enlarges, pain results from the peristaltic contractions of a hollow viscus. The lack of specificity of these findings and the rarity of tubal carcinoma make accurate preoperative diagnosis very difficult.

Fallopian tube carcinoma often may be mistaken for an ovarian neoplasm, uterine leiomyomata, hydrosalpinx, or a tubo-ovarian abscess—all of which are more common than tubal carcinoma. Therefore, the diagnosis of fallopian tube carcinoma is considered before surgery in only 0% to 15% of patients. The majority are identified during surgery or by pathologic examination.

- Rarely, fallopian tube carcinoma is detected on Pap smear, but in general the positivity of this method is only 25% to 50%. Cytologic findings play the greatest role in staging.

- Pelvic ultrasound may demonstrate tubal carcinoma, but it is often mistaken for an ovarian tumor because tubal carcinoma appears frequently as a complex fusiform mass on ultrasound. A number of studies have shown that contrast-enhanced magnetic resonance imaging (MRI) demonstrates superior characterization and differentiation compared to ultrasound.

- Although laparotomy is necessary for definitive diagnosis of primary tubal carcinoma, there still can be uncertainty on gross examination.*

HISTOPATHOLOGY

Histopathology is similar to ovarian cancer but largely to serous cytadenocarcinoma (refer to Fig. 43.2A).

TNM STAGING CRITERIA

The basis for staging carcinomas of the FT clearly parallels that for ovarian cancer. The patterns of spread are similar, with invasion into the uterus and female genital tract versus seeding into the peritoneal cavity. The American Joint Committee on Cancer introduced the TNM staging in the fifth edition and left it unchanged in the sixth edition (Fig. 43.3B). Laparotomy and resection of tubal masses, as well as hysterectomy and suspicious sites, require biopsy and histology for confirmation.

SUMMARY OF CHANGES SEVENTH EDITION AJCC

The definitions of TNM and the Stage Groupings for this chapter have not changed from the Sixth Edition.

Oncoimaging Annotations

- Hydrosalpinx with solid nodulation suggests FT carcinoma.

- Computed tomography (CT) is the recommended imaging modality for staging. MRI is reserved for patients with contraindications to iodinated contrast media (essential for diagnostic CT study) and for questions unanswered by CT.

- CT with intravenous contrast, helical technique, provides excellent cross-sectional imaging for detecting signs of malignancy such as varied morphology of cystic/solid walls or internal septa, lobulated papillary mass, implants 1 to 3 cm in size, and coarse calcifications.

- MRI is highly accurate in determining the origin of an adnexal mass and in characterizing ovarian masses as benign, malignant, or nonneoplastic. Intravenous gadolinium should be used because it improves lesion characterization.

- CT is useful for detecting small or large bowel invasion, mesenteric and omental "cake" masses, adenopathy, liver involvement, and ascites.

*Rubin P, Williams J, eds. *Clinical Oncology: A Multidisciplinary Approach for Physicians and Students*. 8th ed. Philadelphia: Elsevier, 2001:489.

FALLOPIAN TUBE

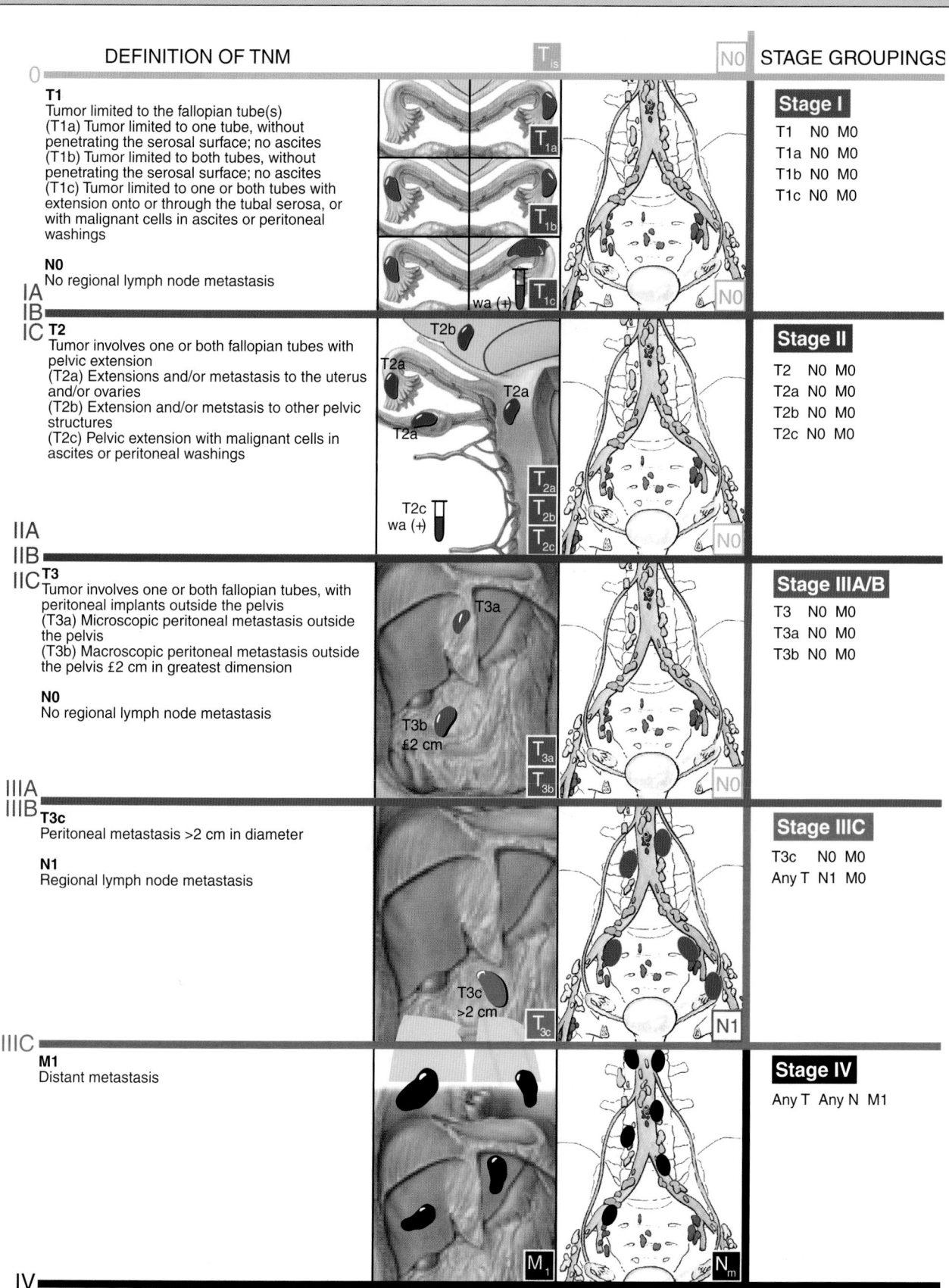

DEFINITION OF TNM

0

T1
Tumor limited to the fallopian tube(s)
(T1a) Tumor limited to one tube, without penetrating the serosal surface; no ascites
(T1b) Tumor limited to both tubes, without penetrating the serosal surface; no ascites
(T1c) Tumor limited to one or both tubes with extension onto or through the tubal serosa, or with malignant cells in ascites or peritoneal washings

N0
No regional lymph node metastasis

IA
IB
IC

T2
Tumor involves one or both fallopian tubes with pelvic extension
(T2a) Extensions and/or metastasis to the uterus and/or ovaries
(T2b) Extension and/or metstasis to other pelvic structures
(T2c) Pelvic extension with malignant cells in ascites or peritoneal washings

IIA
IIB
IIC

T3
Tumor involves one or both fallopian tubes, with peritoneal implants outside the pelvis
(T3a) Microscopic peritoneal metastasis outside the pelvis
(T3b) Macroscopic peritoneal metastasis outside the pelvis £2 cm in greatest dimension

N0
No regional lymph node metastasis

IIIA
IIIB

T3c
Peritoneal metastasis >2 cm in diameter

N1
Regional lymph node metastasis

IIIC

M1
Distant metastasis

IV

STAGE GROUPINGS

Stage I
T1   N0 M0
T1a N0 M0
T1b N0 M0
T1c N0 M0

Stage II
T2   N0 M0
T2a N0 M0
T2b N0 M0
T2c N0 M0

Stage IIIA/B
T3   N0 M0
T3a N0 M0
T3b N0 M0

Stage IIIC
T3c   N0 M0
Any T   N1 M0

Stage IV
Any T Any N M1

Figure 43.3B ⏐ TNM staging diagram arranged vertically with T definitions on the left and stage groupings on the right. Fallopian tube cancers are quite rare and are resectable as stage II (*blue*) and are borderline resectable in stage IIIA. Color bars are coded for stage: stage 0, yellow; I, green; II, blue; III, purple; IV, red; and metastatic disease to viscera and nodes, black.

N-ONCOANATOMY AND M-ONCOANATOMY

N-ONCOANATOMY

Ovarian cancers, by the nature of their peritoneal dissemination, alter normal lymphatic drainage of the ovary to that of the entire abdominal cavity and its contents.

The lymphatic drainage occurs via the ovarian ligament and round ligament trunks and an external iliac accessory route into the following regional nodes: The para-aortic nodes are the major regional nodes followed by the external iliac, common iliac, hypogastric, lateral sacral, and, rarely, to the inguinal nodes (Fig. 43.6A, Tables 43.4A, 43.4B). Although the ovary is pelvic in location, its lymphatic drainage recapitulates its abdominal or homologous origin—the para-aortic lymph nodes. Its vestigial relationship via the round ligament to the labia reaffirms its similarity to the testes in its intimate scrotal location, which makes drainage to inguinal nodes possible. Although an inguinal node can be considered a first station node, most oncologists regard an extrapelvic node as metastatic.

M-ONCOANATOMY

The ovarian veins drain into the inferior vena cava and targets the right side of the heart and then the lungs (see Fig. 43.6B, Table 43.4C). However, peritoneal seeding, as mentioned, is a predominant metastatic pattern involving the abdominal cavity, liver, and diaphragm. Malignant ascites is the predominant death pattern.

The internal and external iliac veins drain the female reproductive organs, and metastatic dissemination is via the inferior vena cava to lung, which is the favored target organ.

- *Ovarian cancers* arise from the epithelial surface, which, during embryogenesis, is derived from the coelomic cavity lined by mesothelial cells, which become specialized to form a serosal covering of the gonadal ridge. As ovarian cancers shed their cells into the peritoneal cavity, they behave like peritoneal mesotheliomas, studding the omentum, the intestinal tissues, liver, and diaphragm, resulting in ascites.

- Distant metastases ultimately occur in 38% of patients who were originally limited to the peritoneal cavity and their length of survival.

- Significant risk factors for developing metastases are malignant ascites, peritoneal implants, paraortic lymph nodes, and aneuploid tumors.

TABLE 43.4B | **Incidence of Lymph Node Metastases by Stage**

Stage	% Positive
I	18%
II	20%
III	42%
IV	67%

TABLE 43.4A | **Lymph Nodes of Ovary**

Sentinel Nodes	Juxtaregional Nodes
Obturator	Common iliac
Internal iliac	Hypogastric Lateral sacral
Regional Nodes	
Left: renal hilar Right: paracaval Para-aortic Inguinal External iliac	

TABLE 43.4C | **Distribution of Distant Metastases**

Metastatic Cite	Median Survival
Lung 71.1%	9 months
Subcutaneous nodules 3.5%	12 months
Pericardial effusion 2.4%	2.3 months
Brain 2%	1.3 months
Bone 1.6%	4 months

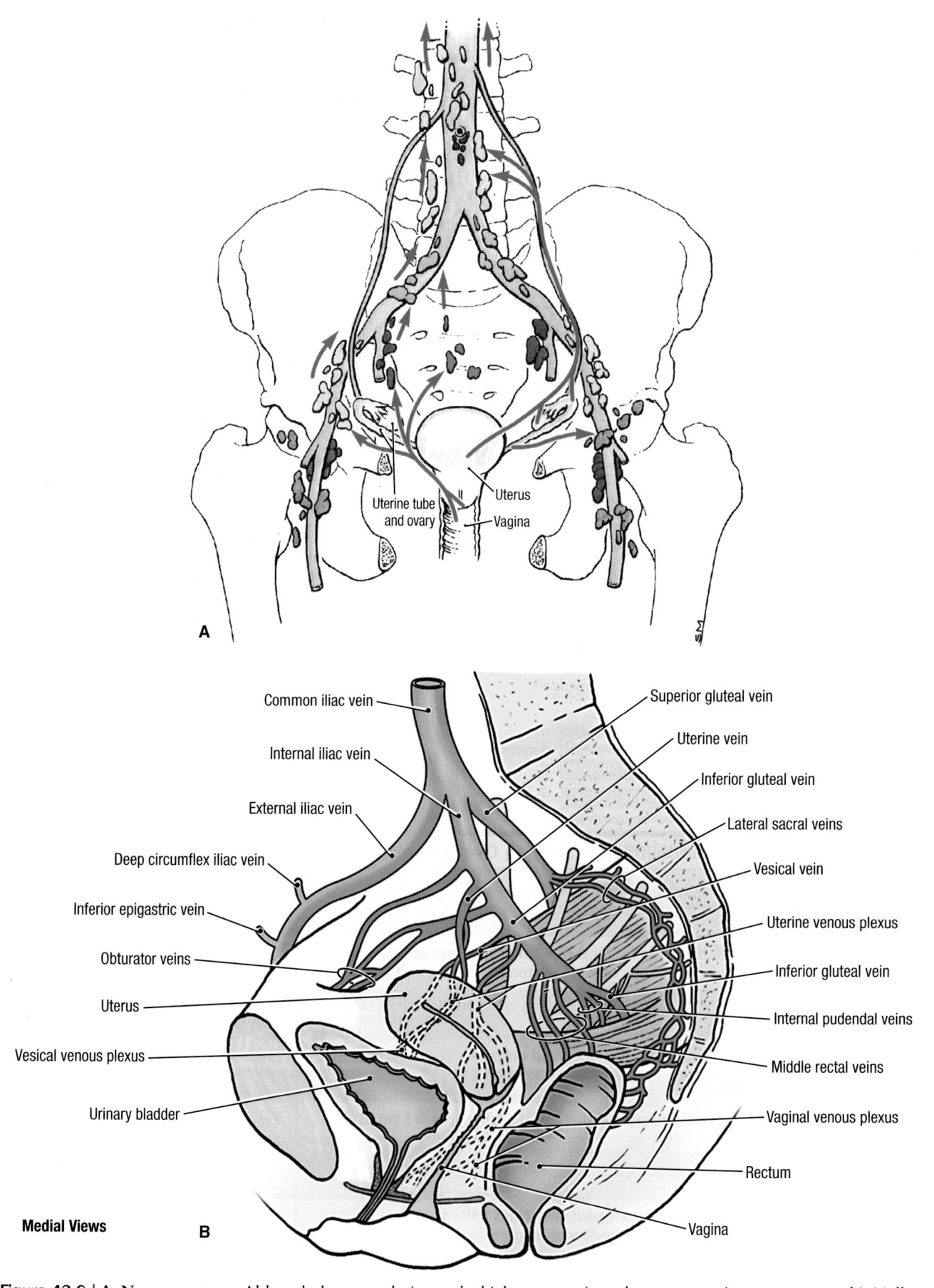

Figure 43.6 | A. N-oncoanatomy. Although the ovary drains to the high para-aortic nodes, most ovarian cancers spread initially in the pelvis, placing both the internal and external iliac nodes at risk. **B. M-oncoanatomy.**

Fundus Uteri

PERSPECTIVE, PATTERNS OF SPREAD, AND PATHOLOGY

The uterine cancers and sarcomas are related to the essential components of the uterus—a pear-shaped organ lined by simple columnar epithelium and tubular glands that extend to the myometrium.

PERSPECTIVE AND PATTERNS OF SPREAD

Endometrial cancers are among the most curable gynecologic cancers and may relate to the normal physiologic functions of menstruation and pregnancy with shedding of the lining and the placenta. In addition, pregnancy, with its invasive placenta, is limited to myometrial extensions. With the continual stimulus of hormones, it is not surprising that these are the most common gynecologic cancers in the United States and Western Europe. With approximately 43,470 cases, deaths are limited to 18%, or 2% of all cancer deaths in women. The postmenopausal woman presenting with unexpected menstruation or vaginal bleeding should have early referral. Diagnosis is readily made on histologic examination of the fractional dilation and curettage. Risk factors include obesity, diabetes mellitus, and hypertension. Unopposed estrogen replacement and tamoxifen therapy have been cited as reasons to abandon such treatment for postmenopausal women owing to increased risk of inducing endometrial cancers.

The pattern of spread is reflected in the basic anatomy of the uterine fundus (Table 44.2, Fig. 44.2), anteriorly or posteriorly into its muscle wall. Inferiorly, it invades the cervix and vagina. With further advance, it can enter rectum and/or bladder once the cervix is invaded. The serosa, once penetrated, allows for speed into the peritoneal cavity and bowel. The

uterus is a pear-shaped organ lined by simple columnar epithelium and tubular glands that extend to the myometrium. The endometrium consists of two layers—the functionalis, a superficial layer sloughed with menstruation; and the basalis, which is a deep, narrow layer whose glands regenerate the functionalis. The uterine cancers and sarcomas are related to the essential components of the uterus (Fig. 44.1A–C). The dominant malignancy is endometrial carcinoma (90%), mesenchymal tumors (stromal sarcomas and leiomyosarcomas [5%]), and mixed tumors (carcino sarcoma & adenocarcinoma [3%]).

TABLE 44.1	Histopathologic Type
Endometrioid carcinomas
Villoglandular adenocarcinoma
Adenocarcinoma with benign squamous elements, squamous metaplasia, or squamous differentiation (adenoacanthoma)
Adenosquamous carcinoma (mixed adenocarcinoma and squamous cell carcinoma)
Mucinous adenocarcinoma
Serous adenocarcinoma (papillary serous)
Clear cell adenocarcinoma
Squamous cell carcinoma

Edge SB, Byrd DR, Compton CC, et al., eds. *AJCC Cancer Staging Manual.* 7th ed. New York: Springer, 2010:408.

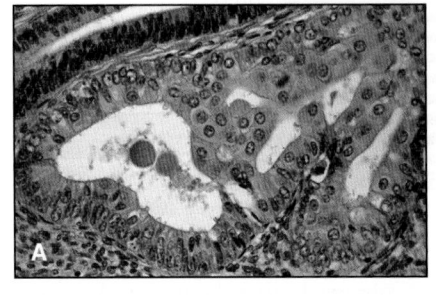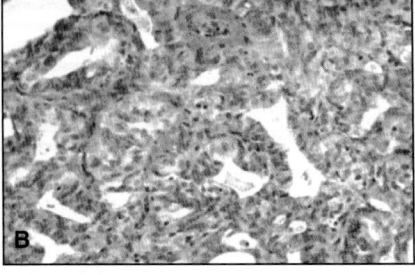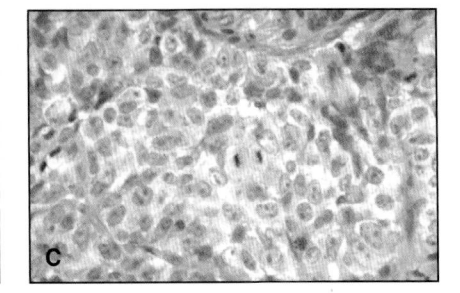

Figure 44.1A–C | Grading of endometrial adenocarcinoma. The grade depends primarily on the architectural pattern, but significant nuclear atypia changes a grade 1 tumor to grade 2, and a grade 2 tumor to grade 3. Nuclear atypia is characterized by round nuclei; variation in shape, size, and staining; hyperchromasia; coarsely clumped chromatin; prominent nucleoli; and frequent and abnormal mitoses. Significant nuclear atypia, if present, increases the tumor grade. **Gland percentage: A.** Greater than 5%. **B.** Greater than 50%. **C.** Less than or equal to 50%. **Solid growth percentage: A.** Less than or equal to 5% **B.** Less than or euqal to 50%. **C.** Greater than 50%.

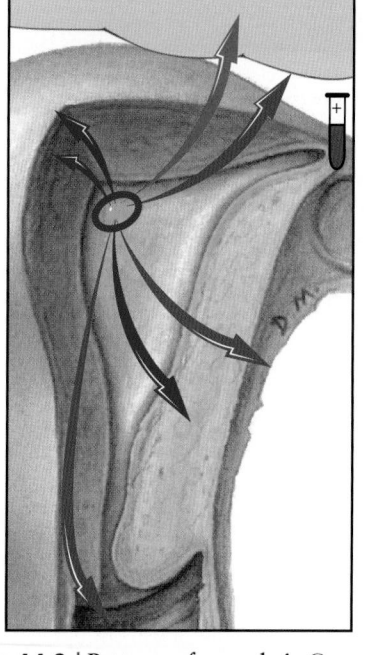
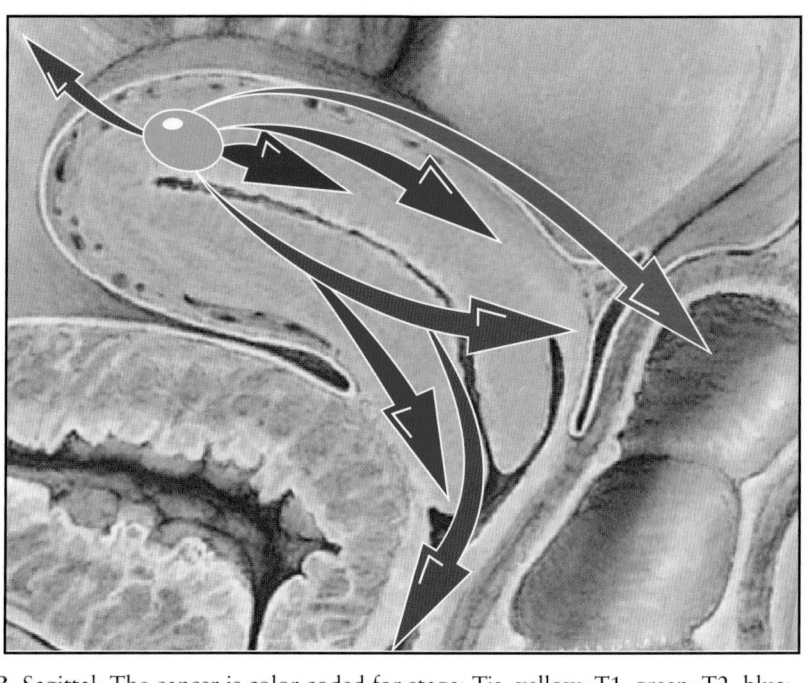

Figure 44.2 | Patterns of spread. A. Coronal. **B.** Sagittal. The cancer is color coded for stage: Tis, yellow; T1, green; T2, blue; T3, purple; and T4, red. The concept of visualizing patterns of spread to appreciate the surrounding anatomy is well demonstrated by the six-directional pattern, i.e., SIMLAP, Table 44.2.

PATHOLOGY

These cancers are predominantly adenocarcinomas; however, they can be serous, endometrioid, or mucinous, similar to the ovarian cancers. This reflects the embryonic mesonephros anlage. The current, seventh edition of the *AJCC Cancer Staging Manual* expands the histopathologic malignancies to be classified and staged. The most common form remains endometrial carcinoma, which is induced by estrogen excess exposure exogenously or due to diabetes and obesity. Increased risk occurs with granulosa cell carcinoma (Table 44.1, Fig. 44.1A).

TABLE 44.2	SIMLAP*	
Uterine Fundus		
S	Peritoneus (serosa)	• T3a
	Ovary	• T3a
	Fallopian tube	• T3a
	Peritoneal cavity washings	• T3a
I	Exocervix epithelium	• **T2a**
	Endocervix	• **T2b**
	Vagina	• **T3b**
	Vesicouterine pouch	• **T3**
	Urinary bladder	• **T4**
M	Uterine wall, endometrium	• **T1a**
	Uterine wall, surface muscle	• **T1b**
	Uterine wall, deep muscle	• **T1c**
L	Ovary	• **T3a**
	Fallopian tube	• **T3a**
	Levator ani	• **T4**
	Broad ligament	• **T3a**
A	Urinary bladder	• **T4**
	Broad ligament	• **T4**
P	Rectum	• T4
	Pouch of Douglas	• T4

*The six vectors of invasion are Superior, Inferior, Medial, Lateral, Anterior, and Posterior. The color-code dots correlate the T stage with the specific anatomic structure involved.

TNM STAGING CRITERIA

TNM STAGING CRITERIA

The T staging criteria are similar to those for a hollow organ, with minor modification (Fig. 44.3A). The criteria for corpus uteri have remained the same; however, the clinical examination has been supplanted by surgical pathologic assessment. In the early editions, stage I was confined to the corpus and classified according to its enlargement: stage IA, ≥8 cm, and stage IB, ≥8 cm in greatest length. With the fourth edition, stage I was limited to endometrium (IA); with myometrial invasion, stage IB penetrates less than half the thickness of the myometrium, and IC, more than half the thickness. In earlier editions, stage II was gross clinical involvement of the cervix, but this was changed and now requires specific histopathologic verification. Stage IIA is surface endocervical involvement; deeper stomal invasions signify stage IIB. Stage III is extension beyond the uterus, spreading into serosa or adnexa. Stage IIIA is vaginal involvement; IIIB is invasion of other genital sites but remaining in the true pelvis. Stage IV was divided into IVA, which is similar to the cervix with invasion of the rectum and bladder, and stage IVB, metastatic spread to distant organs. These criteria did not change in the sixth edition. Lymph node invasion was relegated to stage III, and more recently advanced and categorized to stage IIIC.

The rules for classification were noted in the fourth edition. Uterine enlargement could be due to fibroids and other disorders, such as adenomyosis. These argued for dilation and curettage to establish the diagnosis, with emphasis on fractional curettage beginning with scraping the cervix. In the sixth edition, that **fractional curettage requires histopathologic evidence** of stromal invasion or hysterectomy with microscopic verification.

The importance of surgical-pathologic evaluation applies to regional lymph nodes, as well as to the primary sites.

Adenocarcinomas include three more histopathologies:

- *Endometroid Carcinomas* arising in endometriosis. Simultaneous cancers of uterine corpus and ovary in association with pelvic endometriosis are classified as separate, independent primaries.

- *Squamous Cell Cancers* mixed with Adenocarcinomas are due and arise in islands of squamous cell metaplasia.

- *Carcinosarcomas* in which both elements are malignant.

SUMMARY OF CHANGES SEVENTH EDITION AJCC

- The definition of TNM and the Stage Grouping for this chapter have changed from the Sixth Edition and reflect new staging adopted by the International Federation of Gynecology and Obstetrics (FIGO) (2008).

- Three new separate staging schemas for uterine sarcomas adopted by FIGO have been added.

The TNM Staging Matrix allows for identification of stage group once the T and N stages are determined (Table 44.3).

TABLE 44.3	Stage Summary Matrix			
	N0	**N1**	**N2**	**M1**
T1a	IA	IIIC1	IIIC2	IVB
T1b	IB	IIIC1	IIIC2	IVB
T2	II	IIIC1	IIIC2	IVB
T3a	IIIA	IIIC1	IIIC2	IVB
T3b	IIIB	IIIC1	IIIC2	IVB
T4	IVA	IVA	IVA	IVB

Stage III is further divided into A, B, or C, and stage IV into A or B.

FUNDUS UTERI ADENOCARCINOMA: ENDOMETROID CARCINOMA, MIXED SQUAMOUS CELL AND ADENOCARCINOMA, AND CARCINOSARCOMA

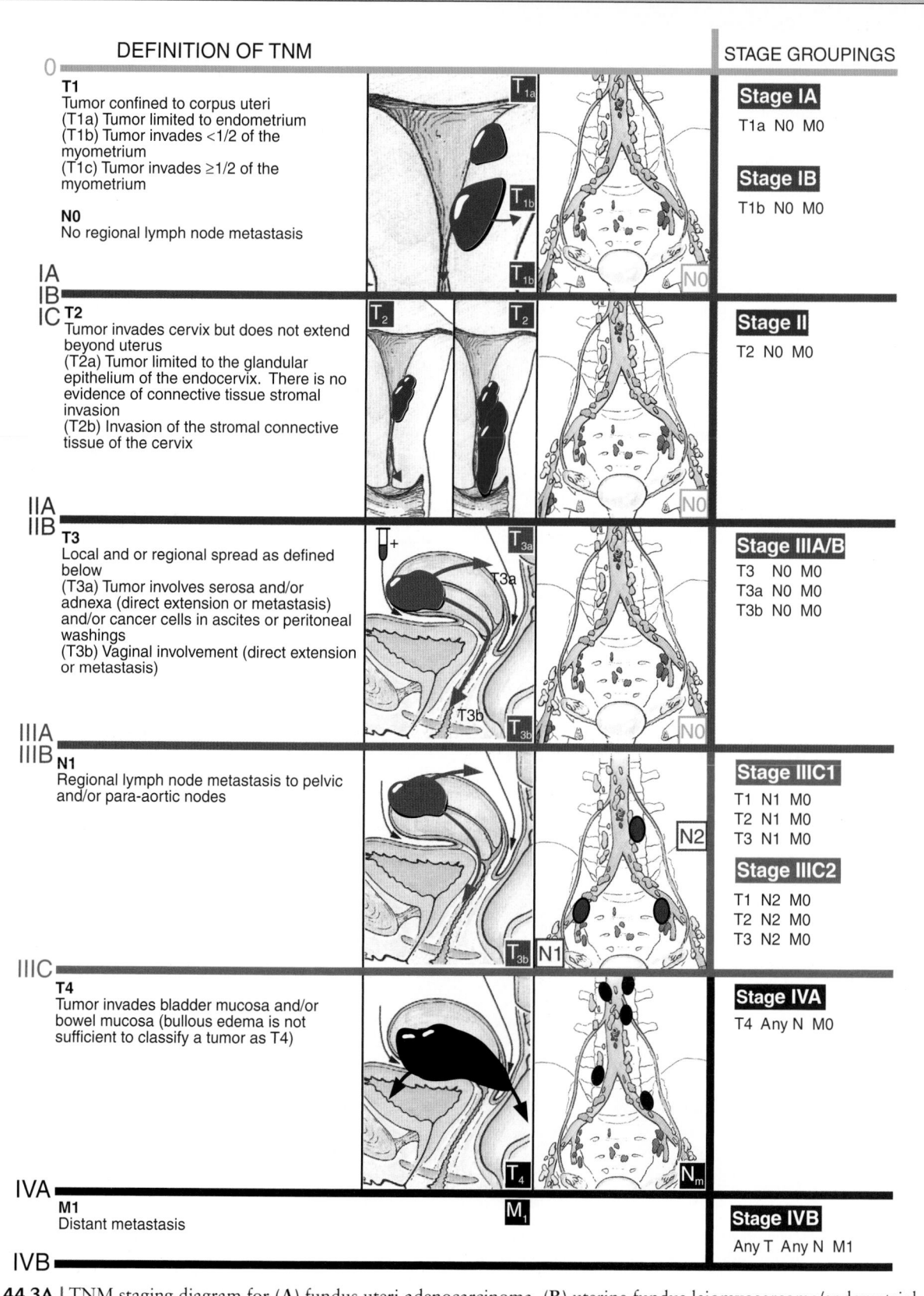

DEFINITION OF TNM

T1
Tumor confined to corpus uteri
(T1a) Tumor limited to endometrium
(T1b) Tumor invades <1/2 of the myometrium
(T1c) Tumor invades ≥1/2 of the myometrium

N0
No regional lymph node metastasis

T2
Tumor invades cervix but does not extend beyond uterus
(T2a) Tumor limited to the glandular epithelium of the endocervix. There is no evidence of connective tissue stromal invasion
(T2b) Invasion of the stromal connective tissue of the cervix

T3
Local and or regional spread as defined below
(T3a) Tumor involves serosa and/or adnexa (direct extension or metastasis) and/or cancer cells in ascites or peritoneal washings
(T3b) Vaginal involvement (direct extension or metastasis)

N1
Regional lymph node metastasis to pelvic and/or para-aortic nodes

T4
Tumor invades bladder mucosa and/or bowel mucosa (bullous edema is not sufficient to classify a tumor as T4)

M1
Distant metastasis

STAGE GROUPINGS

Stage IA
T1a N0 M0

Stage IB
T1b N0 M0

Stage II
T2 N0 M0

Stage IIIA/B
T3 N0 M0
T3a N0 M0
T3b N0 M0

Stage IIIC1
T1 N1 M0
T2 N1 M0
T3 N1 M0

Stage IIIC2
T1 N2 M0
T2 N2 M0
T3 N2 M0

Stage IVA
T4 Any N M0

Stage IVB
Any T Any N M1

Figure 44.3A I TNM staging diagram for (**A**) fundus uteri adenocarcinoma, (**B**) uterine fundus leiomyosarcoma/endometrial stromal sarcoma, and (**C**) uterine fundus adenosarcoma arranged vertically with T definitions on the left and stage groupings on the right. Uterine fundus cancers are most often detected early and are readily resectable at stage I and II with excellent cure rates. There are four main stages, each with two or three substages. Color bars are coded for stage: Stage 0, yellow; I, green; II, blue; III, purple; IV, red; and metastatic disease to viscera and nodes, black.

UTERINE FUNDUS LEIOMYOSARCOMA/ENDOMETRIAL STROMAL SARCOMA

STAGING HISTOPATHOLOGY

Uterine sarcomas constitute less than 1% of gynecologic malignancies and only 1% to 3% of malignant tumors of the uterus. The TNM staging is new and is illustrated in Fig. 44.3B. Size and extensions are the key criteria. To understand the new staging systems proposed, reference to the Uterine Sarcoma Classification of the Gynecologic Oncology Group is helpful, which divides sarcomas into two major groups as the basis for the new staging systems:

- **Mesenchymal tumors** having an overlapping benign epithelial lining, where the malignant element is the underlying fibrous stroma.

- **Mixed epithelial–stromal** elements combining adenocarcinoma and stromal sarcoma.

These are discussed later.

Histology is an important prognostic factor in uterine sarcoma, and mitotic activity and grade strongly influence the natural history of the tumor (Fig. 44.1D–F). The histologic classification used most often is that of the Gynecologic Oncology Group. Note that the uterine neoplasm classification of the International Society of Gynecologic Pathologists uses the term *carcinoma* for all primary uterine neoplasms containing malignant elements of both epithelial and stromal light-microscopic appearance, regardless of whether malignant heterologous elements are present.

- **Pure leiomyosarcomas** constitute about 20% to 50% of uterine sarcomas. These tumors often occur in premenopausal women and are not associated with prior pelvic irradiation. The leiomyosarcoma frequently is diagnosed after a hysterectomy is performed for a presumed leiomyomatous uterus. Histologically, the smooth muscle cells have increased atypia, pleomorphism, and cellularity. The degree of atypia and mitotic activity are used to differentiate leiomyosarcomas from benign smooth muscle tumors. Leiomyosarcomas that have more than 10 mitoses per 10 high-power fields are classified as malignant.

- **Mixed mesodermal tumors** represent about 30% to 50% of all uterine sarcomas. These tumors are composed of an admixture of a sarcomatous stromal component and malignant epithelium. The epithelial component frequently is adenocarcinoma; however, squamous carcinoma also may be present. The mesenchymal component may be fibrosarcoma, rhabdomyosarcoma, or an endometrial stromal sarcoma component. Carcinosarcoma (malignant mixed Müllerian tumor, homologous type) is the most common type.

- **Endometrial stromal sarcoma** occurs in about 15% to 20% of patients with uterine sarcomas. Histologically, increased numbers of endometrial stromal cells are seen with varying degrees of atypia and pleomorphism. High-grade stromal sarcomas have 10 or more mitotic figures per 10 high-power fields, whereas low-grade stromal sarcomas have fewer than 10. Low-grade tumors were formerly termed *endolymphatic stromal myosis*, which is descriptive of their predilection to extend into lymphatic or vascular channels within the uterus. These low-grade sarcomas have a protracted natural history and may recur many years after the initial diagnosis. High-grade tumors have a poor prognosis.

SUMMARY OF CHANGES SEVENTH EDITION AJCC

- The definition of TNM and the Stage Grouping for this are new in the seventh edition and reflect new staging adopted by the International Federation of Gynecology and Obstetrics (FIGO) (2008).

- A separate staging schema adopted by FIGO for uterine sarcoma has been added.

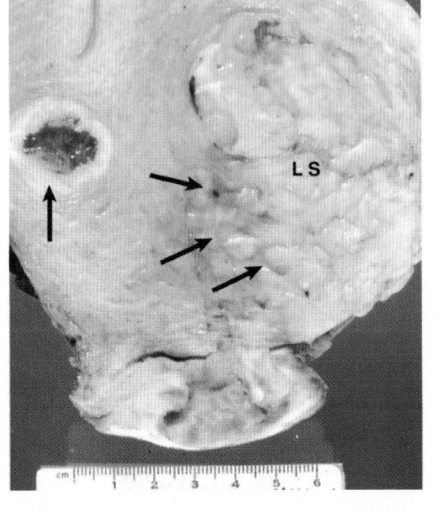 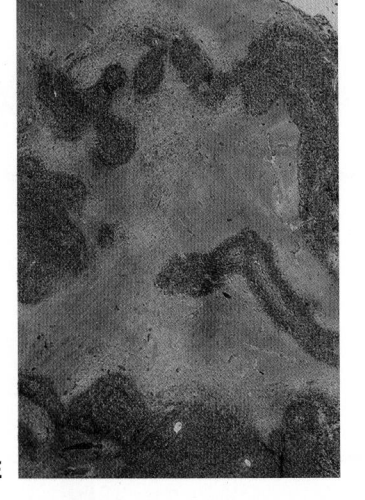 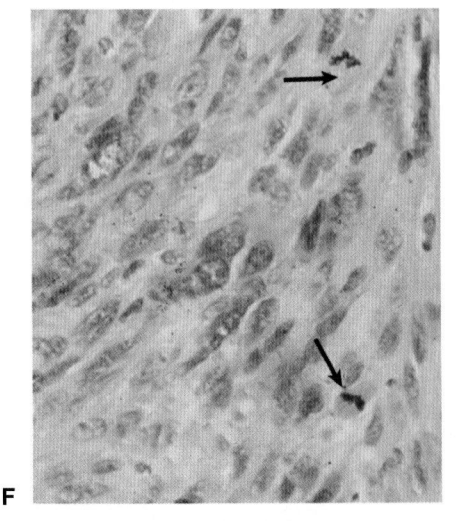

Figure 44.1D–F | D. The uterus has been opened to reveal a large, soft leiomyosarcoma (LS) that has irregular borders *(horizontal arrows)* and invades the surrounding myometrium. By comparison, a small, firm leiomyoma *(vertical arrow)* with a hemorrhagic center is sharply demarcated. **E.** At low magnification, areas of necrosis are sharply demarcated from the viable tumor. **F.** The malignant cells are moderately disorganized in arrangement; they are irregular in shape and display numerous mitoses *(arrows)*.

UTERINE FUNDUS LEIOMYOSARCOMA AND ENDOMETRIAL STROMAL SARCOMA

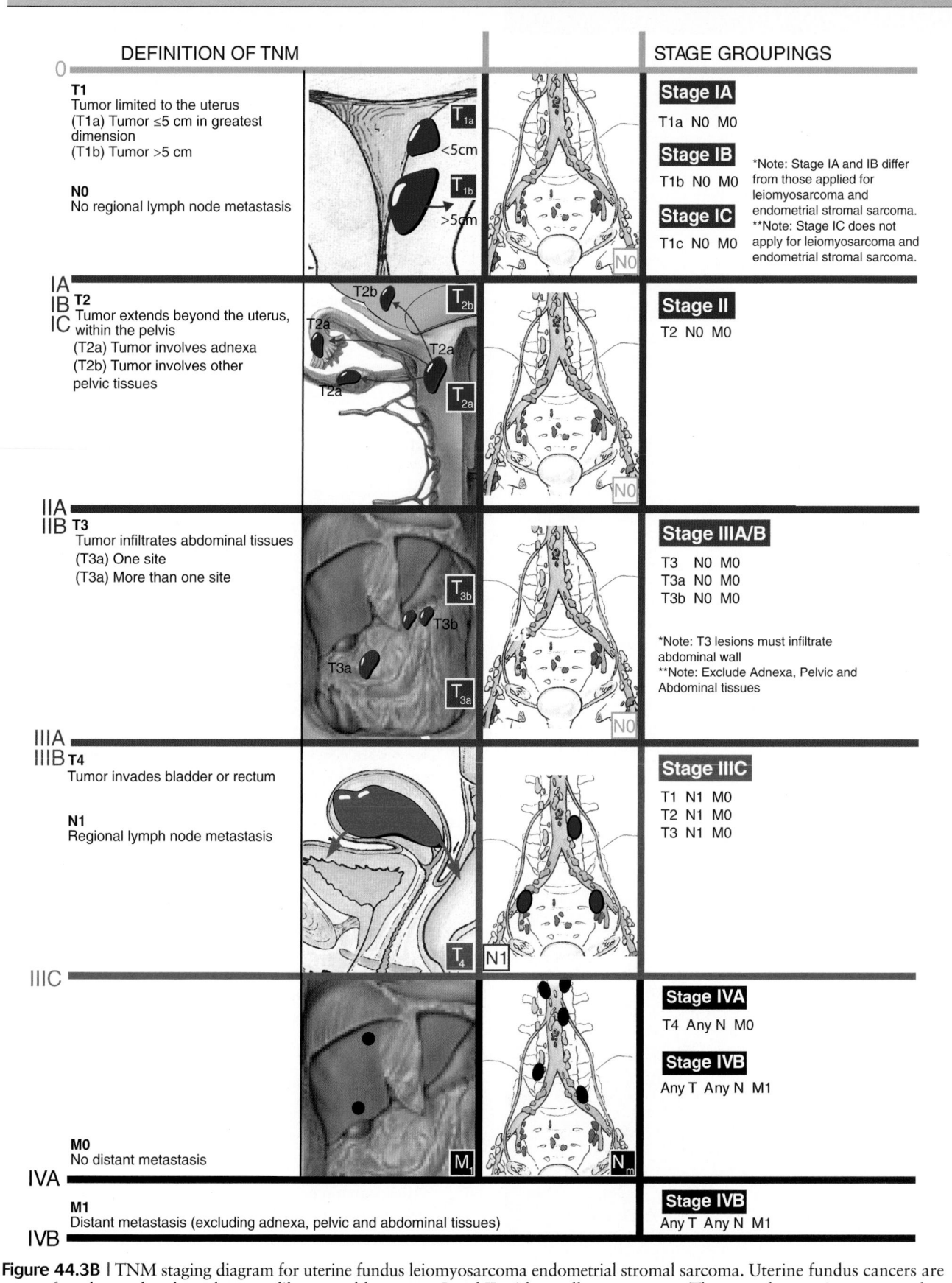

DEFINITION OF TNM

T1
Tumor limited to the uterus
(T1a) Tumor ≤5 cm in greatest dimension
(T1b) Tumor >5 cm

N0
No regional lymph node metastasis

T2
Tumor extends beyond the uterus, within the pelvis
(T2a) Tumor involves adnexa
(T2b) Tumor involves other pelvic tissues

T3
Tumor infiltrates abdominal tissues
(T3a) One site
(T3a) More than one site

T4
Tumor invades bladder or rectum

N1
Regional lymph node metastasis

M0
No distant metastasis

M1
Distant metastasis (excluding adnexa, pelvic and abdominal tissues)

STAGE GROUPINGS

Stage IA
T1a N0 M0

Stage IB
T1b N0 M0

Stage IC
T1c N0 M0

*Note: Stage IA and IB differ from those applied for leiomyosarcoma and endometrial stromal sarcoma.
**Note: Stage IC does not apply for leiomyosarcoma and endometrial stromal sarcoma.

Stage II
T2 N0 M0

Stage IIIA/B
T3 N0 M0
T3a N0 M0
T3b N0 M0

*Note: T3 lesions must infiltrate abdominal wall
**Note: Exclude Adnexa, Pelvic and Abdominal tissues

Stage IIIC
T1 N1 M0
T2 N1 M0
T3 N1 M0

Stage IVA
T4 Any N M0

Stage IVB
Any T Any N M1

Stage IVB
Any T Any N M1

Figure 44.3B | TNM staging diagram for uterine fundus leiomyosarcoma endometrial stromal sarcoma. Uterine fundus cancers are most often detected early and are readily resectable at stage I and II with excellent cure rates. There are four main stages, each with two or three substages. Color bars are coded for stage: Stage 0, yellow; I, green; II, blue; III, purple; IV, red; and metastatic disease to viscera and nodes, black.

UTERINE FUNDUS ADENOSARCOMA

STAGING AND PATTERNS OF SPREAD

Carcinosarcomas need to be distinguished from adenosarcomas (Fig. 44.1G). The latter sarcomas have an overlying benign epithelial lining and a malignant fibrous stroma, whereas carcinosarcomas have both carcinoma and sarcomatous elements.

SARCOMAS OF THE UTERUS

Sarcomas constitute less than 1% of gynecologic malignancies and represent about 1% to 3% of all malignant tumors of the uterus. These tumors are derived from pure mesenchymal tissue or mixtures of epithelial and mesenchymal tissue (Table 44.4). The mean patient age at diagnosis is about 60 years; women with endometrial stromal sarcomas and leiomyosarcomas tend to be younger than those with mixed mesodermal tumors. Some studies also have demonstrated the possibility of a racial component.

The etiology of uterine sarcomas is often attributed to previous pelvic irradiation:

- Previous pelvic irradiation, often administered for benign uterine bleeding 5 to 25 years earlier, is one of the few known etiologic factors for uterine sarcomas; about 2.4% to 17% of women with uterine sarcomas have a history of previous pelvic irradiation. Of the different types of uterine sarcomas, mixed mesodermal tumors are most often associated with previous irradiation.

- As with endometrial carcinomas, at least one study has shown an association between uterine sarcomas and endogenous estrogen use and marital status, but it is not known to be associated with nulliparity or obesity.

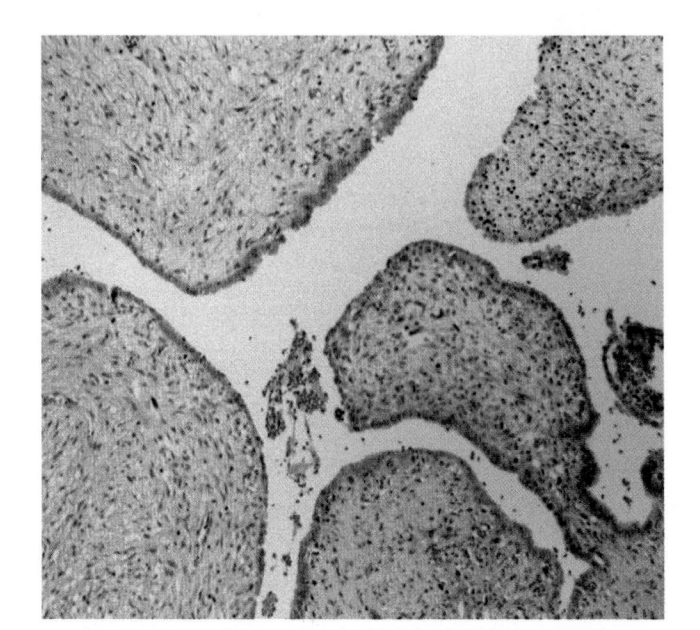

Figure 44.1G | A benign epithelial lining covers a malignant stroma.

DETECTION AND DIAGNOSIS

- Common presenting symptoms and signs are abnormal uterine bleeding, abdominal pain, tumor prolapse through the cervical ox, or a pelvis mass; the diagnostic evaluation of patients for uterine sarcomas is the same as that for endometrial carcinoma.

- The Pap smear is rarely diagnostic, and an endometrial biopsy or dilation and curettage is performed for diagnosis.

- It is not uncommon for the dilation and curettage to reveal copious amounts of tissue from the endometrial cavity, and this material is often diagnostic. When small amounts of tissue are obtained or only an endometrial biopsy is performed, only 4% of stromal sarcomas and leiomyosarcomas are identified correctly, compared with 91% of mixed mesodermal tumors.

STAGING

Uterine adenosarcomas are a new TNM system. Depth of invasion and extensions are key criteria (Fig. 44.3C). A thorough abdominal exploration, including inspection of peritoneal surfaces and pelvic and para-aortic lymph node sampling, is an important determinant of the exact disease extent. In stage I and II disease, lymph node metastases occur in 15% to 45%; tumor extent at initial diagnosis is the most important predictor of prognosis, and patients with lymph node metastases have a poor outlook.

SUMMARY OF CHANGES SEVENTH EDITION AJCC

- The definition of TNM and the Stage Grouping for this chapter are new in the seventh edition and reflect new staging adopted by the International Federation of Gynecology and Obstetrics (FIGO) (2008).

- A separate staging schema adopted by FIGO for uterine sarcoma has been added.

TABLE 44.4	Uterine Sarcoma Classification Proposed by the Gynecologic Oncology Group

Mesenchymal
    Leiomyosarcoma
    Endometrial stromal sarcoma: low and high grade
    Mixed differentiated sarcomas with epithelial elements
    Other uterine sarcomas

Mixed epithelial–stromal
    Adenocarcinoma with heterologous elements
    Carcinosarcoma with heterologous elements

Modified from Rubin P, Williams J, eds. *Clinical Oncology: A Multidisciplinary Approach for Physicians and Students.* 8th ed. Philadelphia: Elsevier, 2001:484.

UTERINE FUNDUS ADENOSARCOMA

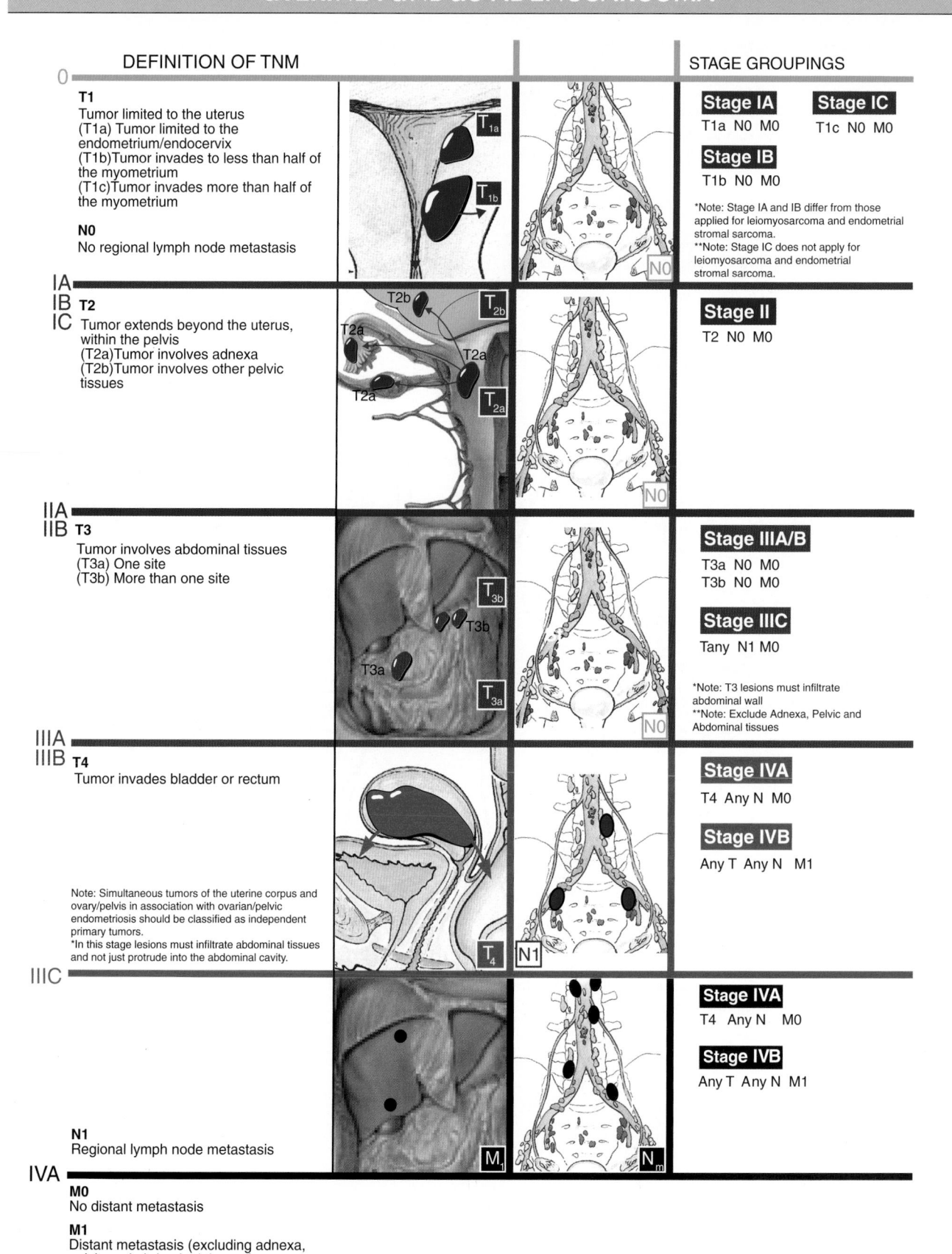

Figure 44.3C | TNM staging diagram for uterine fundus adenosarcoma. Uterine fundus cancers are most often detected early and are readily resectable at stage I and II with excellent cure rates. There are four main stages, each with two or three substages. Color bars are coded for stage: Stage 0, yellow; I, green; II, blue; III, purple; IV, red; and metastatic disease to viscera and nodes, black.

T-ONCOANATOMY

ORIENTATION OF THREE-PLANAR T-ONCOANATOMY

The isocenter for the uterus is at the S4 level but can vary from S2 to S5, depending on the degree of anteflexion or retroflexion (Fig. 44.4).

T-oncoanatomy

The T-oncoanatomy is displayed in three planar views in Fig. 44.5:

* *Coronal*: The upper two thirds of the uterus above the level of the internal cervical os is called the "corpus uteri." The fallopian tubes enter at the upper lateral corners of its pear-shaped body. The portion of the muscular organ positioned above the line joining the tubouterine orifices is called the "fundus."

* *Sagittal*: The body of the uterus sits in the peritoneal cavity. Although it is juxtaposed to these structures, it is separated by the peritoneal lining, making direct invasion rare.

* *Transverse*: The relationship of the uterus to other pelvic tissues is important, particularly to the rectum and bladder. The rectouterine or the vesicouterine septum becomes invaded. Note that the juxtaposition of the vaginal wall directly to the bladder and the rectum makes these organs directly accessible (Fig. 44.5).

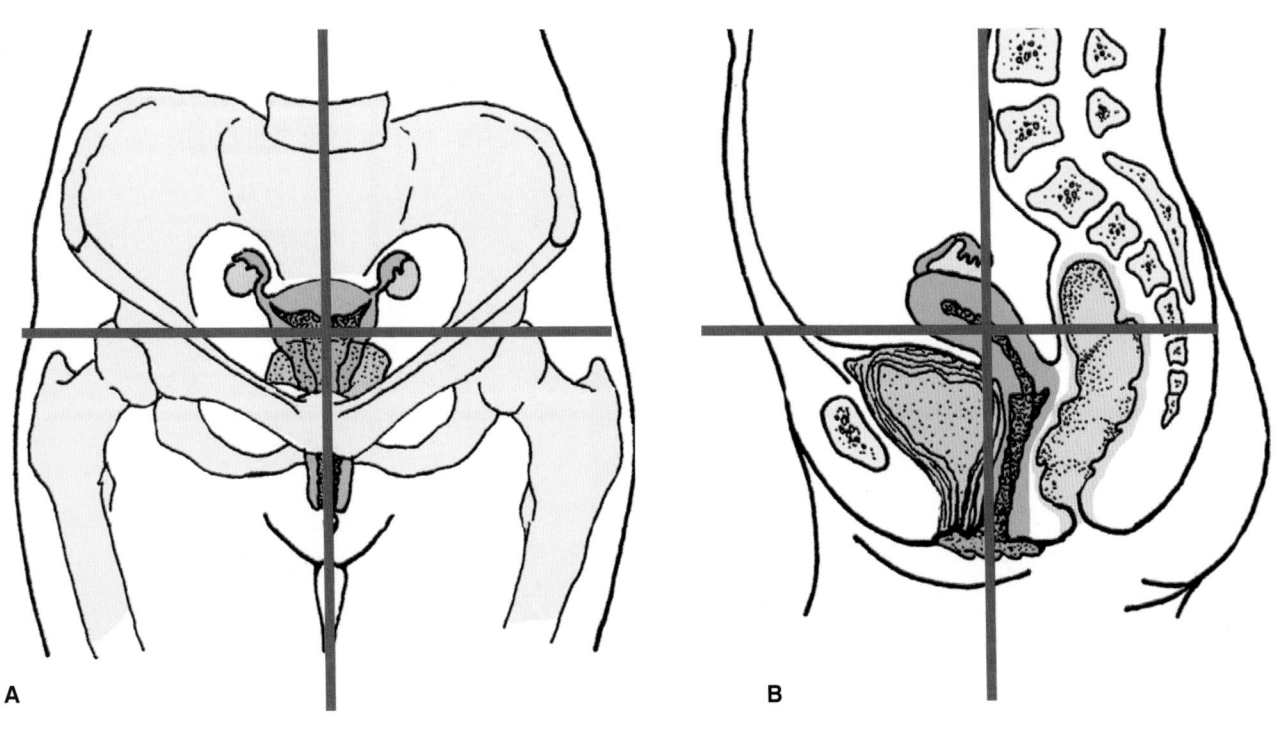

Figure 44.4 | **Orientation of oncoanatomy of uterine fundus.** The anatomic isocenter is at the midline and at the S3 to S4 level inside the true pelvis. **A.** Coronal. **B.** Sagittal.

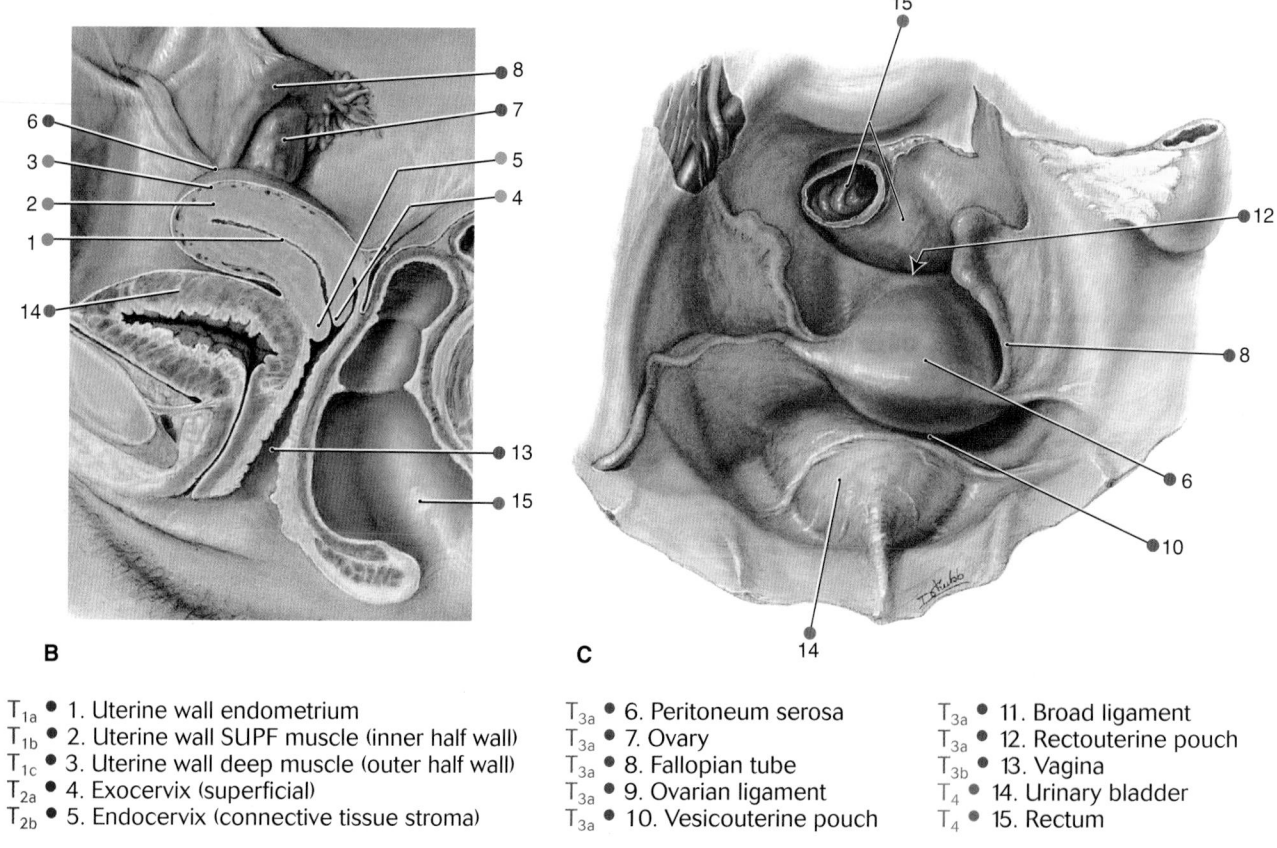

Figure 44.5 | T-oncoanatomy. A. Coronal. **B.** Sagittal. **C.** Transverse axial. The color code for the anatomic sites correlates with the color code for the stage group (Fig. 44.3), patterns of spread (Fig. 44.2), and SIMLAP table (Table 44.2). Connecting the dots in similar colors will provide an appreciation for the three-dimensional oncoanatomy.

Note: The foregoing applies only to adenocarcinomas, not sarcomas.

STAGING WORKUP

RULES OF CLASSIFICATION AND STAGING

Clinical Staging

With few exceptions, hysterectomy and bilateral salpingo-oophorectomy are performed for both staging and diagnosis. Uterine enlargement can be assessed, but myometrial and serosal invasion is difficult to determine on pelvic examination. FIGO mandates surgical staging, cautioning that aggressive wide lymph node sampling may be too risky because pelvic and para-aortic nodes are at risk. Imaging is utilized when available, especially for high-grade cancer and enlarged uteri preoperatively (Table 44.6). Both computed tomography and magnetic resonance imaging are useful for defining tumor invasion and extension (Fig. 44.7).

Surgical-pathologic Staging

The completely resected specimen, including the primary site and regional lymph nodes, must be thoroughly analyzed and are pTNM designated. Radical hysterectomy and bilateral salpingo-oophorectomy with pelvic lymph node resection is the usual procedure for pathologic evaluation.

Although the staging has remained unchanged at most gynecologic primary sites, the rules for classification still do not allow for sophisticated imaging, which includes computed tomography, magnetic resonance imaging, and ultrasonography to alter staging. The multidisciplinary approach to decision making is truly interdisciplinary, most often involving a gynecologic oncologist and a dedicated radiation oncologist. Over the decades, diagnostic and therapeutic protocols in national cooperative groups have provided a scientific basis for introducing combined modalities and introducing innovations into clinical practice.

Oncoimaging with computed tomography is commonly applied to staging cancers, often combined with positron emission tomography to determine the true extent of primary cancer and involved lymph nodes.

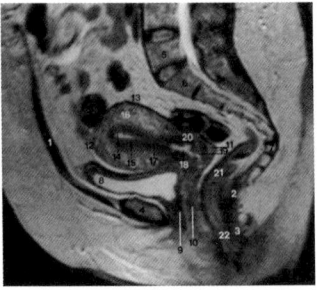

B

Figure 44.7 | MRI Sagittal section of female pelvis. 1. Rectus abdominis m. 2. Levator ani (pubococcygeus) m. 3. Sphincter ani externus m. 4. Pubis 5. Vertebral body (L5) 6. Sacrum (S1) 7. Coccyx 8. Urinary bladder 9. Urethra 10. Vagina 11. Posterior fornix of the vagina 12. Fundus uterus 13. Corpus uterus 14. Endometrium 15. Junctional zone 16. Myometrium 17. Internal os cervix 18. Endocervical canal 19. External os cervix 20. Cervical stroma 21. Rectum 22. Anal canal

TABLE 44.6	Imaging Modalities for Staging Uterine Corpus Cancer	
Method	Diagnosis and Staging Capability	Recommended for Use
Primary (T) Staging		
CTe	Reliable for defining adnexal ovarian masses, extension to gynecologic organs, peritoneal seeding and ascites	Yes, contrast to visualize vessels and intestines
MRI	Role of MRI is emerging as the criteria for malignancy are defined	Yes, but supplemental to CT for soft tissue
TVUS	Excellent for screening and diagnosis	No, not reliable to define invasion
PET	High activity suggests malignancy versus benign status of solid or cystic pelvic masses	No
Nodal (N) Staging		
CTe	Excellent for detecting nodal adenopathy >1 cm in size	Yes, cost effective
MRI	Available for supplementing CT	Yes, if cancer is high grade
Needle biopsy	Confirms lesions detected by radionuclide scan, CT scans, or lymphangiogram	Patients with suspicious lesions, image-guided aspirations
Metastases (M) Staging		
Barium enema		Yes, for patients with suspicious lesions
Urography	Detects ureteral obstruction, bladder invasion; screens for unsuspected renal anomaly	All operative candidates
Bone scan	Useful to assess omental and liver metastases	Yes, if suspected
CT		Yes, if suspected

CT, computed tomography; CTe, CT enhanced with intravenous contrast; MRI, magnetic resonance imaging; PET, positron emission tomography; TVUS, transvaginal ultrasound.

PROGNOSIS AND CANCER SURVIVAL

Oncoimaging Annotations

- Magnetic resonance imaging (MRI) is preferred for detecting tumors that are hyperintense on T2-weighted and gadolinium-enhanced images and helps to distinguish between lesions versus fluid and necrosis in heterogeneous uterine masses.

- MRI after gadolinium is best for determining myometrial invasion.

- MRI best demonstrates cervical stromal invasion on sagittal gadolinium-enhanced views but still needs pathologic confirmation.

- MRI is a useful adjunct to clinical staging and is between 84% and 94% accurate overall.

- Computed tomography is useful for guiding needle biopsies.

- Ultrasonography has its advocates for determining the depth of myometrial invasion and is recommended for screening postmenopausal bleeders: An endometrial stripe of ≤7 mm is within normal range, and ≤4 mm virtually excludes carcinoma.

- MRI for staging: Sagittal and axial images assess spread to uterus, bladder, rectum, and pelvic sidewall.

- Positron emission tomography with ^{18}F-fluorodeoxyglucose can detect 1-cm nodules with 80% accuracy for peritoneal metastases.

- Ultrasonography has been used to evaluate depth of myometrial invasion.

- Gadolinium is useful for differentiating tumor infiltrate (enhanced) versus debris (nonenhanced) in enlarged uterus.

PROGNOSIS

The majority of the identified prognostic factors are related to histologic features (Table 44.7).

- In a large study of 310 cases of uterine sarcomas of mixed pathology, survival was found to be best in those patients with either leiomyosarcomas or endometrial stromal sarcomas and worst with carcinosarcomas or mixed mesodermal sarcomas.

- Larson and coworkers studied 143 patients with uterine leiomyosarcomas and demonstrated that the 5-year survival rate was 65% for cases with a low mitotic rate (>10 mitotic figures per 10 high-power fields), compared with 17% for those with a higher mitotic rate. (Fig. 44.1F).

- Major and coworkers evaluated 453 cases of stage I and stage II uterine sarcomas and demonstrated that the recurrence rates were 53% for mixed Müllerian tumors and 71% for leiomyosarcomas.

Other reported factors are similar to those identified with endometrial carcinomas (i.e., deep myometrial invasion, lymphatic or vascular space invasion, involvement of the isthmus or cervix, and high-grade, serous, and clear cell carcinomatous components).

CANCER STATISTICS AND SURVIVAL

Survival rates have been excellent for uterine fundus, improving over five decades from 78% to 86%, an increase of 14%. For stage IA, the 5-year results are outstanding, rising to almost 90% (Fig. 44.8).

Then decrement to 50% survival as stage progresses from stage II to stage III.

TABLE 44.7A	Prognostic Factors (Site-Specific Factors) (Recommended for Collection for Carcinomas and Sarcomas)
Required for Staging	None
Clinically significant	FIGO stage
	Peritoneal cytology results
	Pelvic nodal dissection with number of nodes positive/examined is most important
	Para-aortic nodal dissection with number of nodes positive/examined
	Percentage of glandular cell type in mixed histology tumors is more valuable
	Omentectomy performed
	Value of positive peritoneal washings that are positive and metastatic foci in adnexal structures is equivocal

Edge SB, Byrd DR, Compton CC, et al., *AJCC Cancer Staging Manual, 7th edition.* New York, Springer, 2010, p. 406.

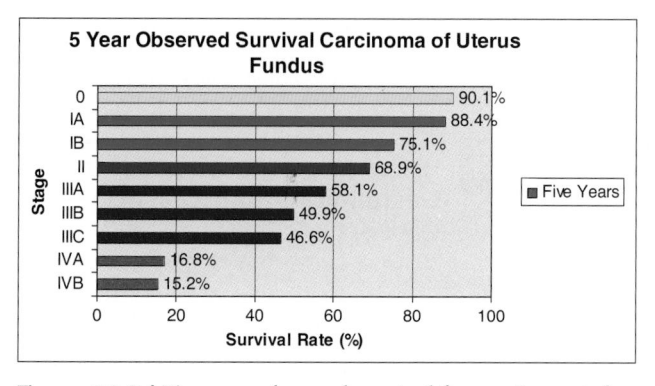

Figure 44.8 | Five-year observed survival for carcinoma of the uterus fundus. (Data from Edge SB, Byrd DR, Compton CC, et al., *AJCC Cancer Staging Manual, 7th edition.* New York, Springer, 2010, p. 408.)

Gestational Trophoblastic Tumors of the Uterus

PERSPECTIVE, PATTERNS OF SPREAD, AND PATHOLOGY

In addition to an anatomic stage, a substage—A (low risk) or B (high risk)—is assigned based on nonanatomic factors.

PERSPECTIVE AND PATTERNS OF SPREAD

The spectrum of gestational trophoblastic tumors (GTTs) can include molar pregnancy, invasive hydatiform mole to the neoplastic placental-derived trophoblastic tumor, and the very aggressive choriocarcinoma (Table 45.1; Fig. 45.1A,B). A history of molar gestation is a major risk factor that is somewhat higher among black women. At one time GTTs were incurable, but with chemotherapy complete regression and ablation are readily achievable. In fact, the eradication of GTTs was among the first chemotherapeutic successes and provided a major stimulus to pursue other malignancies with drug therapy. Human chorionic gonadotropin (hCG) is a marker for persistent tumor. If hCG levels remain elevated after delivery of a molar pregnancy with dilation and curettage, then persistent disease remains to be treated. Methotrexate is effective as single-agent therapy.

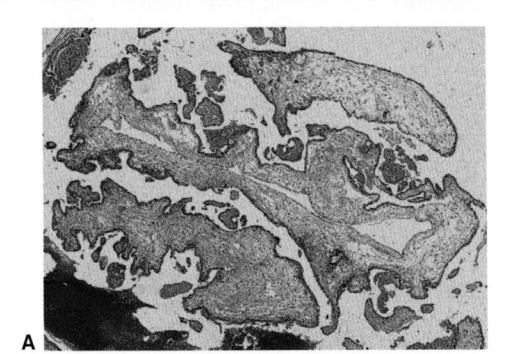

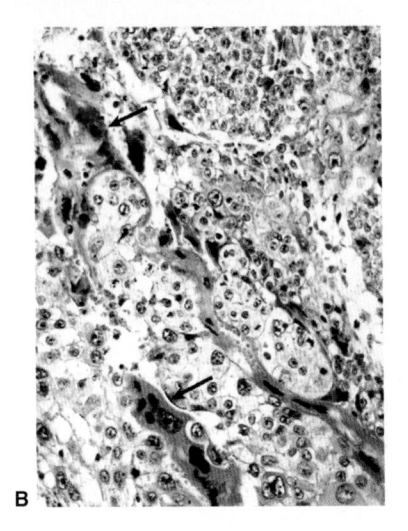

TABLE 45.1	Histopathologic Type: Common Gestational Trophoblastic Cancers
Hydatidiform mole	
Complete	
Partial	
Invasive hydatidiform mole	
Choriocarcinoma	
Placental site trophoblastic tumors	

Modified from Edge SB, Byrd DR, Compton CC, et al., *AJCC Cancer Staging Manual*. 7th ed. New York, Springer, 2010, p. 439.

Figure 45.1 | A. Partial hydatidiform mole. Two populations of chorionic villi are evident. Some are normal; others are conspicuously swollen. Trophoblastic proliferation is focal and less conspicuous than in a complete mole. **B: Choriocarcinoma.** Malignant cytotrophoblast and syncytiotrophoblast *(arrows)* are present.

The staging system has evolved over time, recognizing that anatomic extent and histopathology were elegant but limited in their ability to prognosticate. In the 1990s, the International Federation of Gynecology and Obstetrics introduced a Prognosis Scoring Index, which includes age, antecedent pregnancy, interval months from index pregnancy, largest tumor size, size of metastases, number of metastases identified, and response to chemotherapy. In addition to an anatomic stage, a substage—A (low risk) or B (high risk)—is assigned based on nonanatomic factors. The prognostic scores are ≥0, 1, 2, or 4 for individual risk factors. A score of ≤7 is A (low risk) and one of ≥8 is B (high risk).

PATHOLOGY

This highly invasive malignancy is illustrated by the patterns of spread in Fig. 45.2 and Table 45.2. Once this cancer spreads to extrauterine sites (Fig. 45.2B) it behaves aggressively, invading surrounding tissues. Common sites invaded include cervix, vagina, and ovary; these cancers behave similar to primary cancers at these sites.

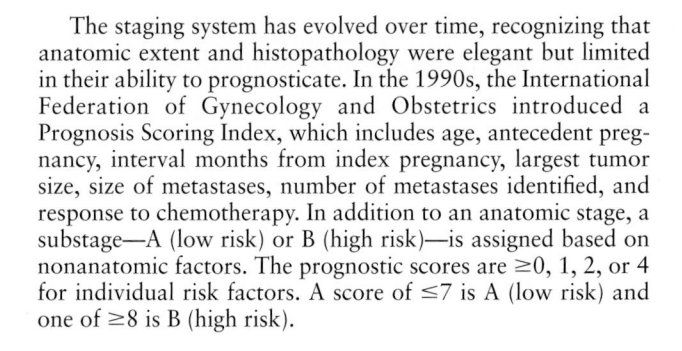

TABLE 45.2	SIMLAP*	
Gestational Trophoblast		
S	Peritoneum (serosa)	• M1b
	Ovary	• T2
	Fallopian tube	• T2
I	Cervix	• T1
	Vagina	• T2
	Vesicouterine pouch	• M1b
	Urinary bladder	• M1b
M	Uterine wall endometrium	• T1
	Uterine wall surface muscle	• T1
	Uterine wall deep muscle	• T1
L	Ovary	• T2
	Fallopian tube	• T2
	Levator ani	• M1b
	Broad ligament	• T2
A	Urinary bladder	• M1b
	Broad ligament	• T2
P	Rectum	• M1b

*The six vectors of invasion are Superior, Inferior, Medial, Lateral, Anterior, and Posterior. The color-coded dots correlate the T stage with the specific anatomic structure involved.

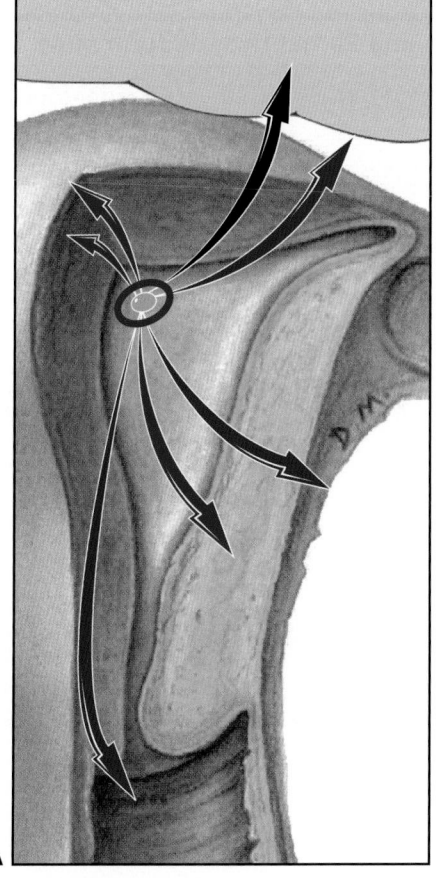

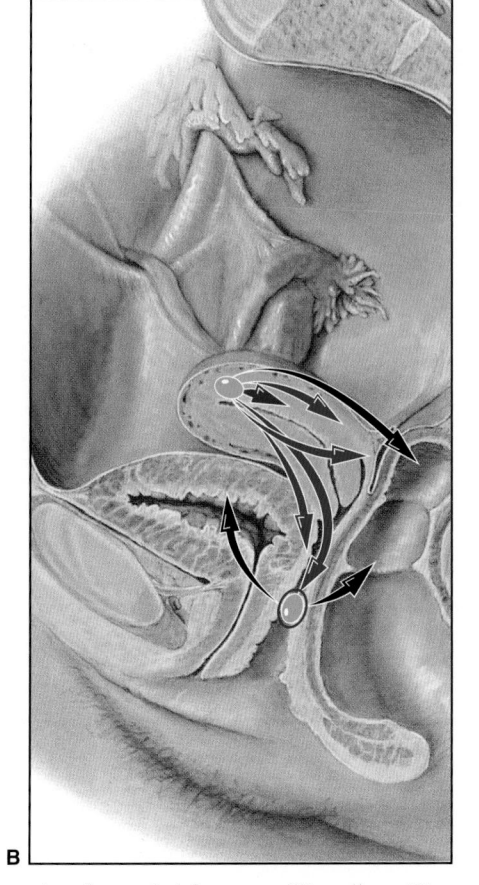

Figure 45.2 | Patterns of spread. **A.** Coronal. **B.** Sagittal. The cancer is color coded for stage: T0, yellow; T1, green; T2, blue. The concept of visualizing patterns of spread to appreciate the surrounding anatomy is well demonstrated by the six-directional pattern, i.e., SIMLAP, Table 45.2.

TNM STAGING CRITERIA

TNM STAGING CRITERIA

The highly malignant choriocarcinoma has access to the rich vascular blood supply of a failed placenta and can rapidly invade hematogenously. Presentations of metastatic disease may be encountered before recognition of the local regional manifestations of GTT. As noted, the serum tumor marker β-hCG is an important diagnostic as well as a staging prognostic aid.

After surgical removal by dilation and curettage or hysterectomy, myometrial invasion may be evident (T1). Nodal metastases are uncommon. Local spread to cervix, ovary, or vagina (stage T2) is common, and lung is a favored metastatic site. Dissemination to liver often occurs, but such remote sites as the kidney, gastrointestinal tract, spleen, bone, and brain also may be involved.

SUMMARY OF CHANGES SEVENTH EDITION AJCC

The definitions of TNM and the Stage Grouping for this chapter have not changed from the Sixth Edition (Fig. 45.3).

The "Risk Factors" (7) portion of the stage groups has been revised as Table 45.3A into A Low Risk (score 7 or less); B High Risk (score 8 or more).

The TNM Staging Matrix allows for identification of stage group once T and N stages are determined (Table 45.3A).

TABLE 45.3A Stage Summary Matrix

	N0	M1a	M1b*	M1b**
T1	I	IIIA	IVA	IVB
T2	II	IIIA	IVA	IVB

*Low risk, **High risk.

TABLE 45.3B Comparative Features of Complete and Partial Hydatidiform Mole

Features	Complete Mole	Partial Mole
Karyotype	46,XX	47,XXY or 47,XXX
Parental origin of haploid genome sets	Both paternal	One maternal, two paternal
Preoperative diagnosis	Mole	Missed abortion
Marked vaginal bleeding	3+	1+
Uterus	Large	Small
Serum hCG	High	Less elevated
Hydropic villi	All	Some
Trophoblastic proliferation	Diffuse	Focal
Atypia	Diffuse	Minimal
hCG in tissue	3+	1+
Embryo present	No	Some
Blood vessels	No	Common
Nucleated erythrocytes	No	Sometimes
Persists after initial therapy	20%	7%
Choriocarcinoma	2% after mole	No choriocarcinoma

hCG, human chorionic gonadotropin.

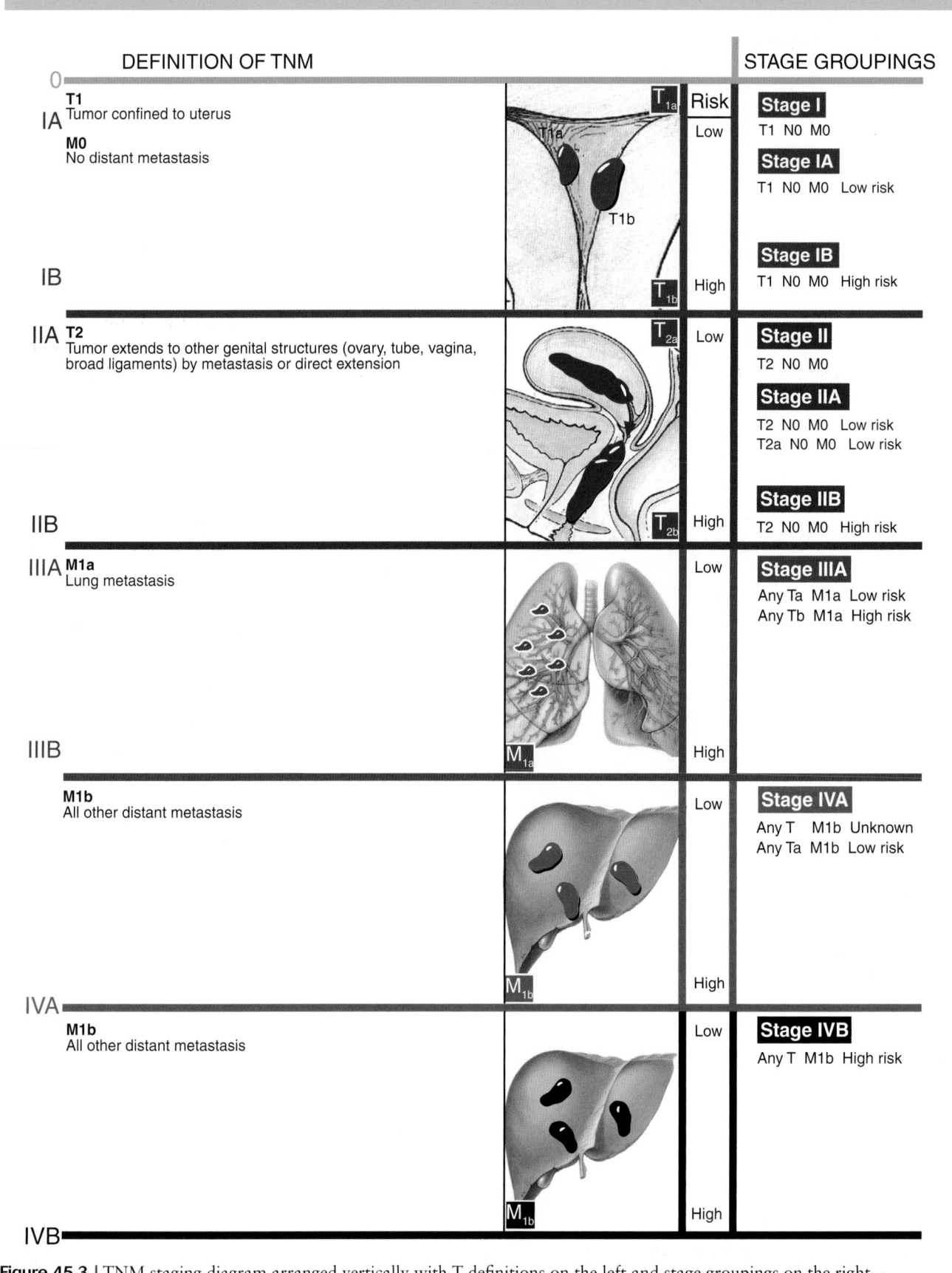

Figure 45.3 | TNM staging diagram arranged vertically with T definitions on the left trond stage groupings on the right. Gestational trophoblastic tumors are highly metastatic but highly curable with chemotherapy. There are four main stages, each with two or three substages. Color bars are coded for stage: stage 0, yellow; I, green; II, blue; III, purple; IV, red; metastatic disease to viscera and nodes, black.

T-ONCOANATOMY

ORIENTATION OF THREE-PLANAR T-ONCOANATOMY

The isocenter for the uterus is at the S4 level but can vary from S2 to S5, depending on the degree of anteflexion or retroflexion (Fig. 45.4).

T-oncoanatomy

The T-oncoanatomy is displayed in three planar views in Fig. 45.5:

- *Coronal*: The upper two thirds of the uterus above the level of the internal cervical os is called the "corpus uteri." The fallopian tubes enter at the upper lateral corners of its pear-shaped body. The portion of the muscular organ positioned above the line joining the tubouterine orifices is called the "fundus."

- *Sagittal*: The body of the uterus sits in the peritoneal cavity. Although it is juxtaposed to these structures, it is separated by the peritoneal lining, making direct invasion rare.

- *Transverse*: The relationship of the uterus to other pelvic tissues is important, particularly to the rectum and bladder. The rectovaginal or the vesicovaginal septum can be invaded. Note that the juxtaposition of the vaginal wall directly to the bladder and the rectum makes these organs directly accessible.

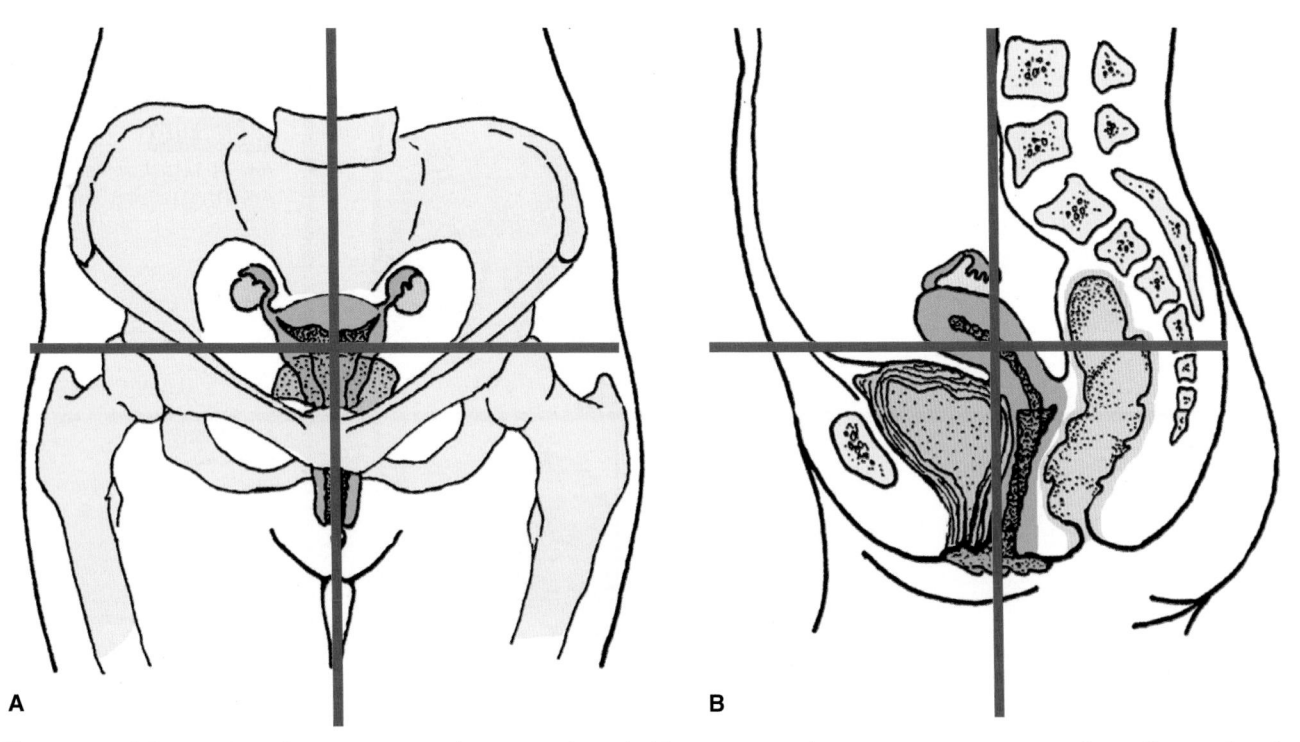

A

B

Figure 45.4 | Orientation of oncoanatomy of gestational trophoblastic tumor. The anatomic isocenter is at the midline and at the S3 to S4 level inside the true pelvis. **A.** Coronal. **B.** Sagittal.

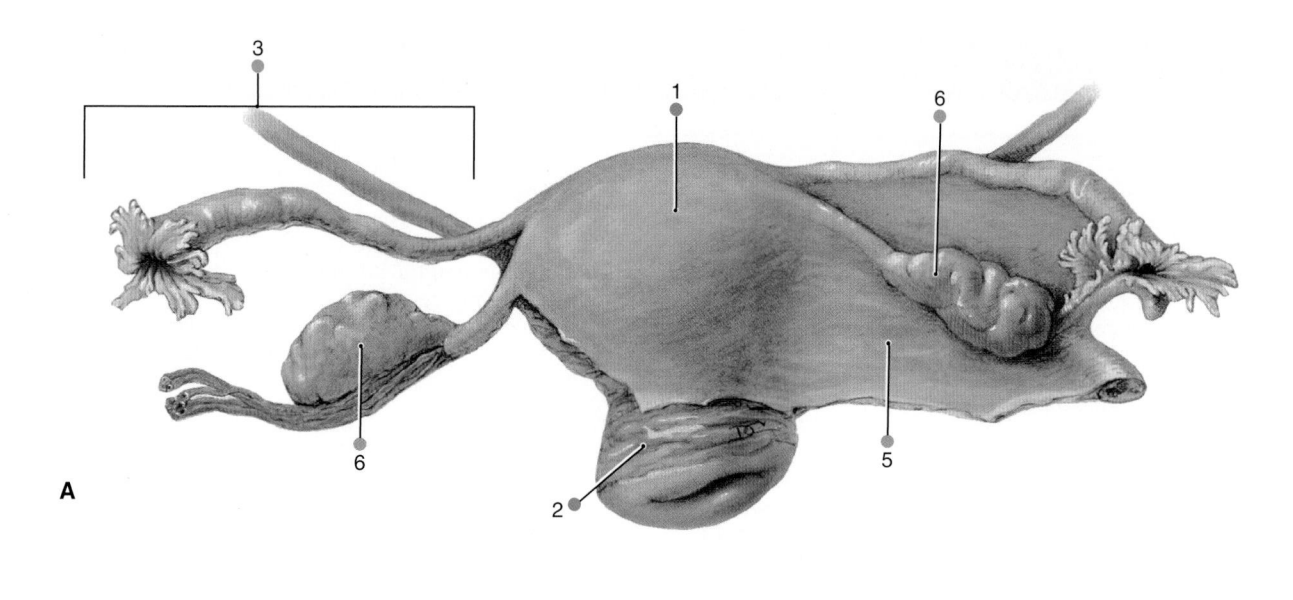

A

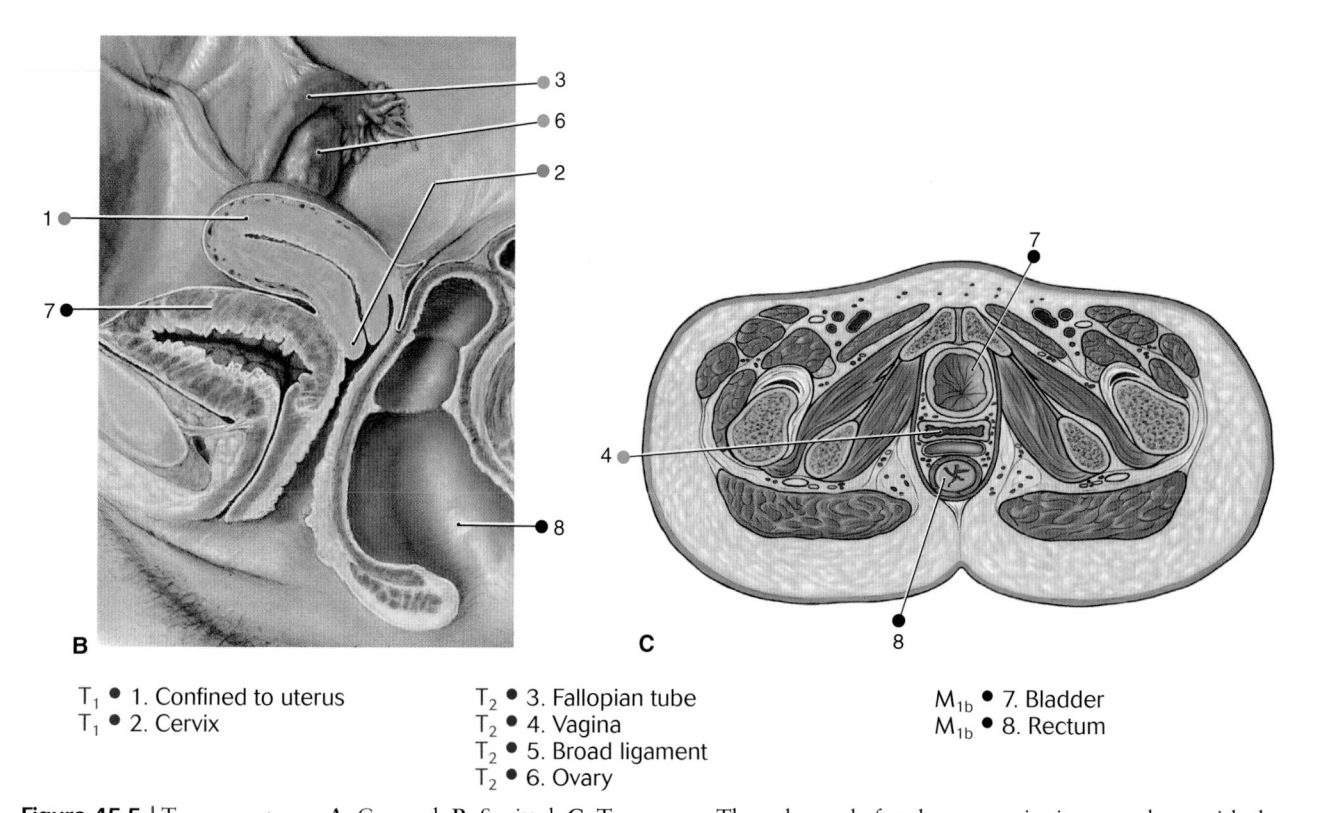

B

C

T_1 • 1. Confined to uterus	T_2 • 3. Fallopian tube	M_{1b} • 7. Bladder
T_1 • 2. Cervix	T_2 • 4. Vagina	M_{1b} • 8. Rectum
	T_2 • 5. Broad ligament	
	T_2 • 6. Ovary	

Figure 45.5 | T-oncoanatomy. **A.** Coronal. **B.** Sagittal. **C.** Transverse. The color code for the anatomic sites correlates with the color code for the stage group (Fig. 45.3), patterns of spread (Fig. 45.2), and SIMLAP table (Table 45.2). Connecting the dots in similar colors will provide an appreciation for the 3D oncoanatomy.

N-ONCOANATOMY AND M-ONCOANATOMY

N-ONCOANATOMY

Lymphatic invasion is uncommon. When the cervix is invaded, extension into bladder and rectum can be due to the major lymphatic trunks, the utero-ovarian (infundibulopelvic), parametrial, and presacral nodes that drain into the hypogastric, external iliac, common iliac, presacral, and para-aortic nodes. However, the fundus also drains via ovarian lymphatics to retroperitoneal lymph nodes. The sentinel node could be either an obturator node or a para-aortic lymph node (Fig. 45.6A, Table 45.4).

TABLE 45.4	Lymph Nodes of Gestational Trophoblastic Tumors

Sentinel Nodes	Juxtaregional Nodes
Internal iliac	Common iliac
Para-aortic	Hypogastric
	Lateral sacral
Regional Nodes	
Renal hilar	
Para-aortic	
External iliac	
Inguinal	

M-ONCOANATOMY

The major venous drainage is via uterine veins or ovarian veins into the vena cava (see Fig. 45.6B). Pulmonary metastases are more common (90%), followed by liver, which is reflected in the staging system. Choriocarcinoma invades primarily through venous sinuses in the myometrium. It metastasizes widely by the hematogenous route, especially lungs (>90%), brain, and gastrointestinal tract, liver, and vagina (Table 45.3B).

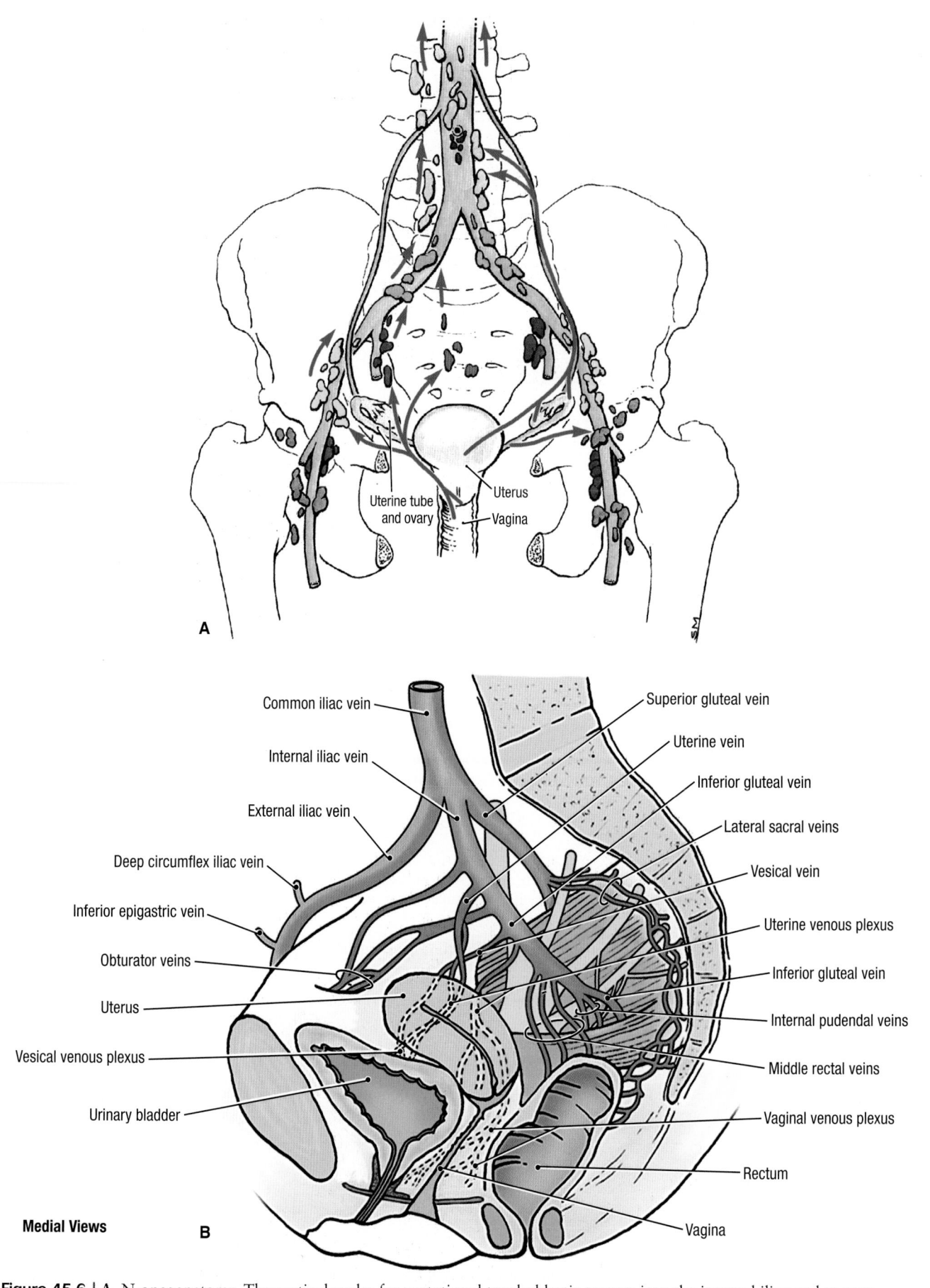

Figure 45.6 | A. N-oncoanatomy. The sentinel nodes for gestational trophoblastic tumors into the internal iliac and to para-aortic nodes. With invasion of the cervix (T2) the cancer behaves like cancer of the cervix and can spread to hypogastric or obturator nodes. **B.** M-oncoanatomy.

STAGING WORKUP

RULES OF CLASSIFICATION AND STAGING

The initial diagnostic procedures are the staging criteria. Both clinical and pathologic criteria establish the primary tumor anatomic extent; however, specific criteria suggest persistent and/or metastatic GTT and require chemotherapy.

Imaging recommendations apply to the metastatic workup, and are similar to those for the uterine fundus as to primary site and pelvic nodes (Table 45.6, Fig. 45.7).

Clinical Staging

With few exceptions, hysterectomy and bilateral salpingo-oophorectomy are performed for both staging and diagnosis. Uterine enlargement can be assessed, but myometrial and serosal invasion is difficult to determine on pelvic examination. The International Federation of Gynecology and Obstetrics mandates surgical staging, cautioning that aggressive and wide lymph node sampling may be too risky because pelvic and para-aortic nodes are at risk. Imaging is utilized when available, especially for high-grade cancer and enlarged uteri preoperatively.

Surgical-pathologic Staging

The completely resected specimen, including the primary site and regional lymph nodes, which must be thoroughly ana-lyzed, are pTNM designated. Radical hysterectomy and bilateral salpingo-oophorectomy with pelvic lymph node resection is the usual procedure for pathologic evaluation.

Although the staging has remained unchanged at most gynecologic primary sites, the rules for classification still do not allow for sophisticated imaging, which includes computed tomography (CT), magnetic resonance imaging (MRI), and ultrasonography (US) to alter staging. The multidisciplinary approach to decision making is truly interdisciplinary, most often involving a gynecologic oncologist and a dedicated radiation oncologist. Over the decades, diagnostic and therapeutic protocols in national cooperative groups have provided a scientific basis for introducing combined modalities and innovations into clinical practice.

Oncoimaging with CT is commonly applied to staging cancers, often combined with positron emission tomography to determine the true extent of primary cancer and involved lymph nodes.

Oncoimaging Annotations

- Chest CT with helical techniques allow for detection of pulmonary metastases of 5 to 10 mm.
- CT is preferred over US for pathologic confirmation of liver metastases.
- MRI is superior to CT for detecting peritoneal metastases.

TABLE 45.5	Imaging Modalities for Staging Gestational Trophoblastic Cancer	
Method	Diagnosis and Staging Capability	Recommended for Use
Primary (T) Staging		
CTe	Defines cervical involvement, tumor size, and vaginal extension; myometrial invasion may suggest cervix invasion	Yes, has displaced barium enema and IVP; need histologic confirmation
MRI	Preferred for cross-sectional anatomy tumor size, depth of myometrial invasion	Yes, for high-grade cancers
EUUS	Can detect widening of echogenic endometrial stripe and myometrial invasion	No, more for detection; accuracy not high
Nodal (N) Staging		
CTe	Excellent for detecting nodal adenopathy >1 cm in size	Yes, cost effective
MRI	Available for supplementing CT	Yes, if cancer is high grade
Metastases (M) Staging		
Barium enema		Yes, for patients with suspicious lesions
Bone scan	Useful to assess omental and liver metastases	Yes, if suspected
CT		Yes, if suspected

CT, computed tomography; CTe, CT enhanced with intravenous contrast; EUUS, endouterine ultrasound; IVP, intravenous pyelography; MRI, magnetic resonance imaging.

PROGNOSIS AND CANCER SURVIVAL

PROGNOSIS

Patients with molar gestations can be stratified into low- and high-risk categories on the basis of clinical and laboratory parameters. Those who have large-for-dates uteri or a pre-evacuation serum hCG level higher than 100,000 mIU/mL (high-risk molar pregnancy) have about a 50% risk of developing invasive mole. Patients without these and other high-risk features have less than a 5% risk.

Follow-up

Surveillance of patients treated for gestational trophoblastic disease is mandatory. Fortunately, these tumors produce large amounts of hCG (with the exception of placental-site tumors), which can be measured accurately in the serum and is close to an ideal tumor marker. Patients with either a complete or partial mole should undergo weekly serum β-hCG measurement until a normal level is reached. After three normal levels, serum hCG measurements may be obtained at longer intervals. The follow-up for patients with invasive mole or choriocarcinoma is similar to that for patients with molar pregnancy. However, in cases in which remission was difficult to achieve (requiring more than three or four courses of chemotherapy), the period of serum hCG follow-up should be extended to 2 years because late recurrences are possible.

Survival

Currently, patients undergoing evacuation of a molar pregnancy have an excellent prognosis, both in terms of their outlook for future fertility and with respect to the available treatment should an invasive mole or choriocarcinoma develop. Most patients (80%) with a molar pregnancy have no further sequelae after evacuation of the mole; the remaining 20%

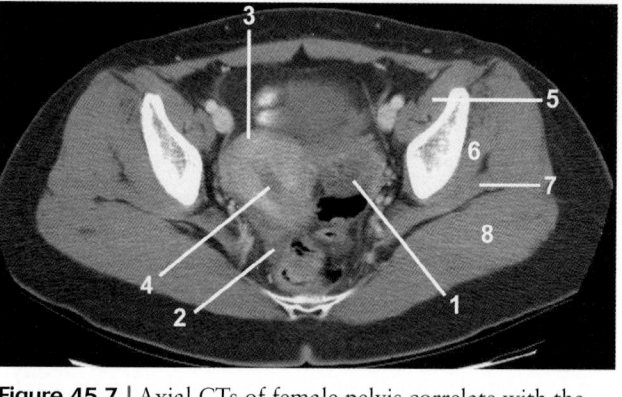

Figure 45.7 | Axial CTs of female pelvis correlate with the T-oncoanatomy transverse section (Fig. 45.5C). (1) Left ovary. (2) Physiologic fluid in pelvis (normal in menstruating-age female). (3) Uterine fundus. (4) Endometrial cavity. (5) Iliopsoas muscle. (6) Gluteus minimus muscle. (7) Gluteus medius muscle. (8) Gluteus maximus muscle.

develop either nonmetastatic or metastatic gestational trophoblastic neoplasia (GTN) that requires chemotherapy. However, virtually all patients with nonmetastatic disease are cured, although some (<5%) may require hysterectomy or uterine resection to remove a focus of resistant tumor. Patients with low-risk metastatic GTN also have an excellent prognosis.

Currently, about 5% of patients with high-risk metastatic GTN die of the disease. Poor prognostic factors have been identified, such as the presence of liver or brain metastases, or both, an interval of more than 24 months since the antecedent pregnancy, patient age, and previous inadequate chemotherapy. In patients with two or more poor prognostic factors, the survival rates are 82% and 43%, respectively. Of some concern, a small but significant increase in the risk of secondary malignant tumors has been reported following treatment with sequential or combination therapy.

TABLE 45.6	Prognostic Scoring Index			
	Risk Score			
Prognostic Factor	**0**	**1**	**2**	**4**
Age (years)	<40	≥40		
Antecedent pregnancy	Hydatidiform mole	Abortion	Term pregnancy	
Interval months from index pregnancy	<4	4 to <7	7–12	>12
Pretreatment hCG (IU/mL)	$<10^3$	$\geq10^3-<10^4$	$10^4-<10^5$	$\geq10^5$
Largest tumor size, including uterus (cm)	<3	3 to <5	≥5	
Site of metastases	Lung	Spleen, kidney	Gastrointestinal tract	Brain, liver
Number of metastases identified		1–4	5–8	>8
Previous failed chemotherapy			Single drug	Two or more drugs
Total score				

Low risk is a score of ≤7. High risk is a score of ≥8.
Reprinted from Edge SB, Byrd DR, Compton CC, et al., eds. *AJCC Cancer Staging Manual.* 7th ed. New York: Springer, 2010, p. 438.

46

Uterine Cervix

PERSPECTIVE, PATTERNS OF SPREAD, AND PATHOLOGY

The patterns of cancer spread are determined by the anatomy and the central position of the cervix in the female genital system.

PERSPECTIVE AND PATTERNS OF SPREAD

The success in conquering cancer of the uterine cervix is due to widespread and highly effective screening using the Papanicolaou (Pap) smear of exfoliative cytology. There are 65,000 cases new cases each year of noninvasive carcinoma in situ, compared with 13,000 new cases of invasive cancer, usually early stages. There are fewer than 5,000 deaths annually. Most are of elderly, postmenopausal women who are less active sexually and are not being screened, or women in low socioeconomic groups, Latinos, and African Americans. The low incidence among Jewish women suggests that male circumcision may be a factor.

The patterns of cancer spread are determined by the anatomy and the central position of the cervix in the female genital system: First, within the cervix, then (i) inferiorly into the vagina, (ii) laterally into the parametrium, or (iii) anteriorly into the bladder or posteriorly into the rectum (Fig. 46.2; Table 46.2).

PATHOLOGY

The cervix is the terminal end of the uterus that protrudes into the vagina, and its lumen is lined with a mucus-secreting, simple columnar epithelium. However, when the cervix protrudes into the vagina, the epithelium is stratified squamous and is nonkeratinized (Fig. 46.1A–D). It is not surprising that of the several histopathologic types, 80% to 90% are squamous cell cancers and only 5% to 10% are adenocarcinomas. Table 46.1 lists the variations and subtypes, as well as the grading of cervical cancers.

TABLE 46.1	Histopathologic Type: Common Cancers of the Cervix
Squamous carcinoma	Mixed epithelial carcinoma
Large cell nonkeratinizing	Adenosquamous
Large cell keratinizing	Glassy cell
Small cell nonkeratinizing	
Adenocarcinoma	Neuroendocrine
Endocervical	Carcinoid
Endometrioid	Small cell
Clear cell	
Others	

From Edge SB, Byrd DR, Compton CC, et al., *AJCC Cancer Staging Manual, 7th edition.* New York, Springer, 2010, p. 398.

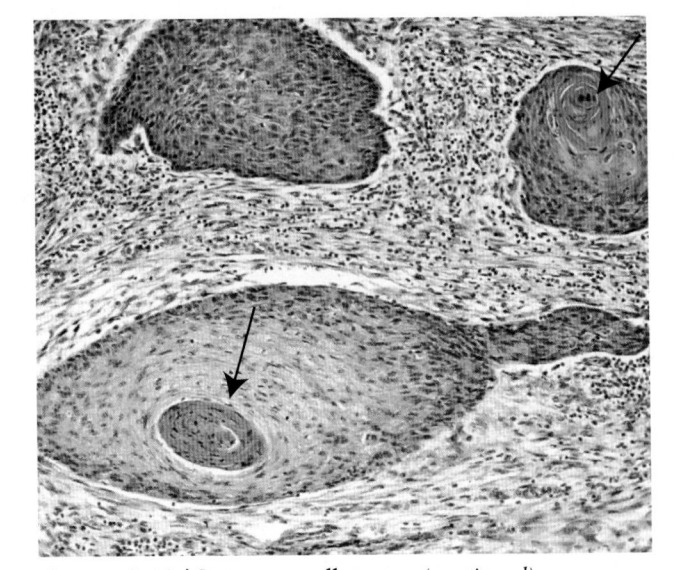

Figure 46.1A | Squamous cell cancer. *(continued)*

Interrelations of naming systems in Premalignant Cervical Cancer interepithelial neoplasia (CIN) is a spectrum of cellular changes that begins as atypia and then progresses to invasive cancer. The grades progress to cancer have corresponding cytologic changes that are shed and graded as squamous intraepithelial lesions (SIL).

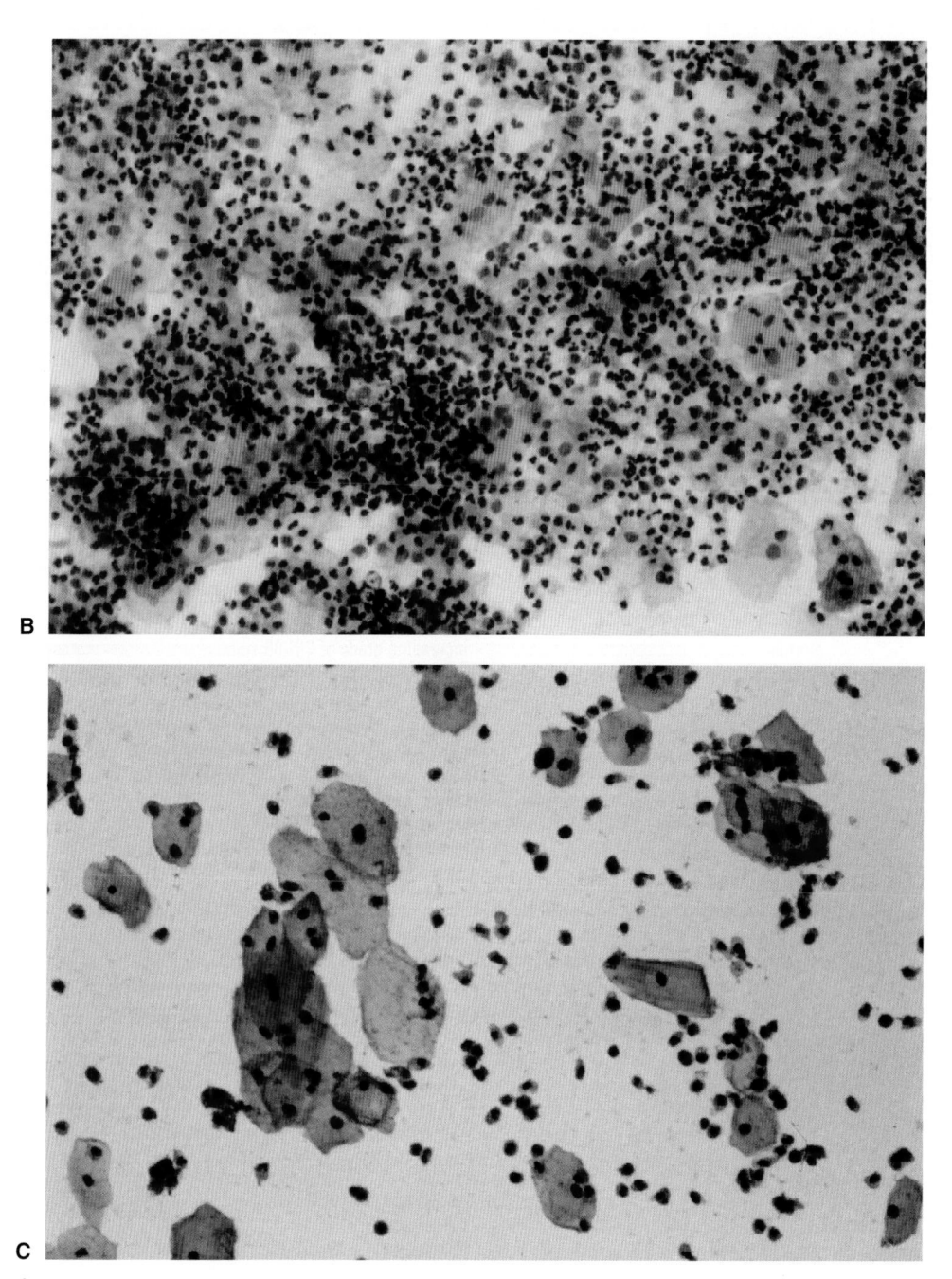

B

C

Figure 46.1B–C | *(Continued)* **Comparison of (B) standard Papanicolaou smear with (C) mono-layer preparation.** There has been rapid adoption of liquid based cytology (LBC) for cervical screening over the past decade. Most cervical smears in the United States are taken into solution despite the lack of large randomized studies. Recent technological improvements in automation of processing and assessment of LBC specimens, particularly the use of an automated imager, are likely to increase this utilization. The ability to test LBC specimens for HPV DNA and other sexually transmitted organisms further enhances the clinical appeal of this technology.

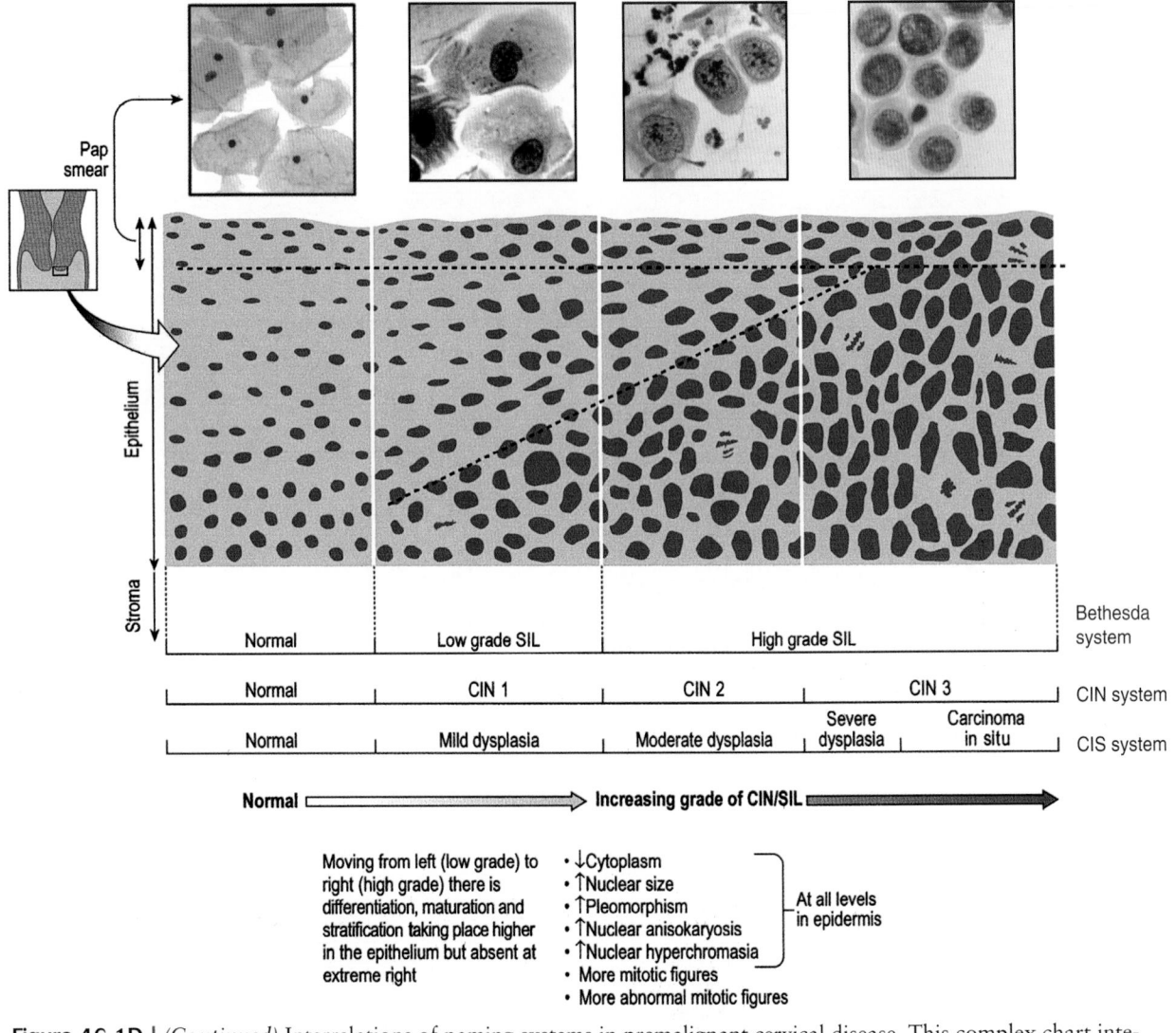

Pap
smear

Epithelium

Stroma

| Normal | Low grade SIL | High grade SIL | Bethesda system |

| Normal | CIN 1 | CIN 2 | CIN 3 | CIN system |

| Normal | Mild dysplasia | Moderate dysplasia | Severe dysplasia | Carcinoma in situ | CIS system |

Normal ⟹ Increasing grade of CIN/SIL ⟹

Moving from left (low grade) to right (high grade) there is differentiation, maturation and stratification taking place higher in the epithelium but absent at extreme right

- ↓Cytoplasm
- ↑Nuclear size
- ↑Pleomorphism
- ↑Nuclear anisokaryosis
- ↑Nuclear hyperchromasia
- More mitotic figures
- More abnormal mitotic figures

At all levels in epidermis

Figure 46.1D | *(Continued)* Interrelations of naming systems in premalignant cervical disease. This complex chart integrates multiple aspects of the disease complex. It lists the qualitative and quantitative features that become increasingly abnormal as the premalignant disease advances in severity. It also illustrates the changes in progressively more abnormal disease states and provides translation nomenclature for the dysplasia/carcinoma in situ (CIS) system, cervical intraepithelial neoplasia (CIN) system, and Bethesda system. Finally, the scheme illustrates the corresponding cytologic smear resulting from exfoliation of the most superficial cells, indicating that even in the mildest disease state, abnormal cells reach the surface and are shed. SIL = squamous intraepithelial lesion.

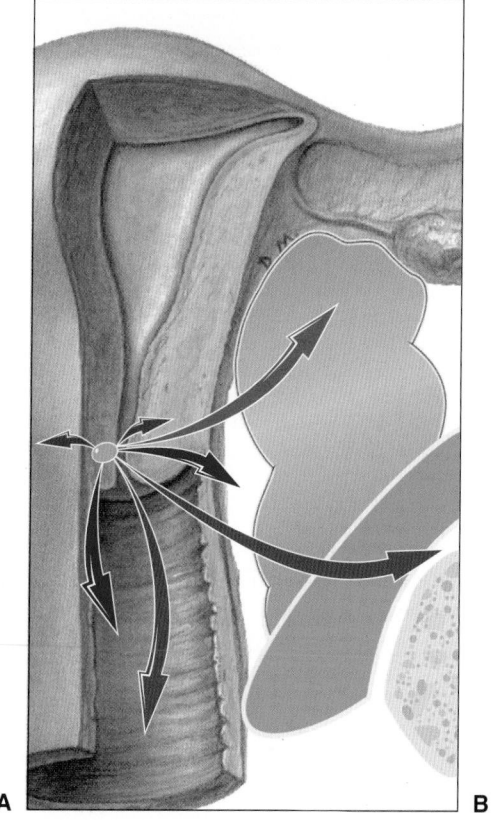

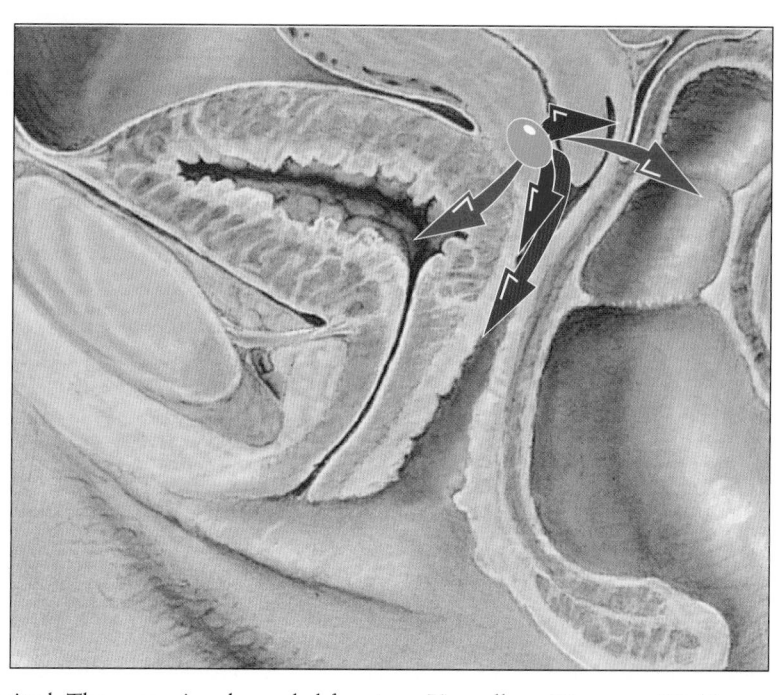

Figure 46.2 | Patterns of spread. **A.** Coronal. **B.** Sagittal. The cancer is color coded for stage: Tis, yellow; T1, green; T2, blue; T3, purple; and T4, red. The concept of visualizing patterns of spread to appreciate the surrounding anatomy is well demonstrated by the six-directional pattern, i.e., SIMLAP, Table 46.2.

TABLE 46.2	SIMLAP*	
Uterine Cervix		
S	Uterus fundus	Tx
	Ovary	Tx
	Fallopian tube	Tx
I	Vagina fornix	• T2a
	Vagina upper ⅓	• T3a
	Lower ⅓	• T3b
M	Exocervix	• T1a
	Endocervix	• T1b
L	Broad ligament	• T2b
	Ureter	• T3b
	Levator ani	• T3b
	Pelvic bone wall	• T3b
A	Urinary bladder	• T4a
	Vesicourinary pouch	• T4a
P	Rectovaginal pouch	• T4b
	Posterior fornix	• T2a
	Rectum	• T4b
	Rectal vaginal septum	• T4b
	Uterosacral ligament	• T2a

*The six vectors of invasion are Superior, Inferior, Medial, Lateral, Anterior, and Posterior. The color-coded dots correlate the T stage with the specific anatomic structure involved.

TNM STAGING CRITERIA

TNM STAGING CRITERIA

Cancer of the cervix is the archetype for staging cancer. Review of the first six editions of the *AJCC Cancer Staging Manual* shows that the main stages I, II, III, and IV have consistently reflected the progression of the primary cancer. As cervical cancer was detected earlier due to the Pap smear being applied universally, microinvasion was defined and T1 was divided into multiple subgroups, but stage I remained confined to the cervix. Other stages also have been divided into A and B to reflect different vectors and degrees of spread. These eight substages encompass the numerous T, N, and M combinations and subgroups; with stage 0 added for T_{is}, the total becomes 9.

The cervix is at the anatomic isocenter of the female pelvis. The TNM staging criteria have been established and reflect cancer spread patterns. Cervical cancer is the archetype as the first cancer staged more than 70 years ago. Since 1937, the International Federation of Gynecology and Obstetrics (FIGO) has collected data on cervical cancer survival and outcomes from numerous institutions. The pooled results have become the international gold standard on reporting cancer survival results.

The TNM introduced by Pierre Denoix simply adapted their categories to fit the FIGO stages. Although the basic definitions have been stable, the increasing success of finding preinvasive cancers has led to expanding the subcategories of stage I because of conization techniques. Thus, in early versions of the American Joint Committee on Cancer/International Union Against Cancer system, stage I was simply a cancer confined to the cervix, without any size or specific measurement requirements. The staging preferably was a bimanual examination under anesthesia. With the fourth edition (1992), microscopic sizing of invasion was introduced as subcategory IA and further defined in the fifth edition with the subcategory

IB, with ≤4.0 cm designated as IB1 and >4.0 cm as IB2. The stage IA microinvasive lesions are defined as a maximum depth of 5.0 mm for the favorable category, which implies that there will be few instances of lymphatic or capillary infiltration, which, even if present, does not change this criterion. Stage IB are visible lesions or microinvasion beyond 5.0 mm. As noted, 4.0 cm divides stage IB1 and IB2 cancers (Fig. 46.3).

Spread patterns beyond the cervix lead to stage II. Superior invasion into the uterus is ignored for staging. Inferior invasion into the vagina is T2a, and lateral spread into the parametrium is T2b. Stage III cancers extend to the pelvic wall (T3b) or lower third of the vagina (T3a), which alters lymph nodes at risk. Stage T4a is designated for anterior spread into the bladder, which requires biopsy proof; T4b is rectal invasion, which occurs only from vaginal extension because the posterior lip of the cervix is separated from the rectum by the rectouterine pouch of Douglas.

SUMMARY OF CHANGES SEVENTH EDITION AJCC

The definitions of TNM and the Stage Grouping for this chapter have changed from the Sixth Edition and reflect new staging adopted by the International Federation of Gynecology and Obstetrics (FIGO) (2008) (Fig. 46.3).

The 2008 FIGO staging classification has adopted T subclassifications based on tumor size ≤4 cm (T2a1) and >4 cm (T2a2) for cervical carcinoma spreading beyond the cervix but not to the pelvic side wall or lower one third of the vagina (T2 lesions).

The TNM Staging Matrix allows for identification of stage group once T and N stages are determined (Table 46.3).

TABLE 46.3	Stage Summary Matrix		
	N0	**N1**	**M1**
T1a1	IA1	IIIB	IVB
T1a2	IA2	IIIB	IVB
T1b	IB	IIIB	IVB
T2a	IIA	IIIB	IVB
T2b	IIB	IIIB	IVB
T3a	IIIA	IIIB	IVB
T3b	IIIB	IIIB	IVB
T4	IVA	IVA	IVB

UTERINE CERVIX

DEFINITION OF TNM

T1
Cervical carcinoma confined to uterus
(T1a) Invasive carcinoma diagnosed only by microscopy. Stromal invasion with a maximum depth of 5 mm measured from the base of the epithelium and a horizontal spread of ≤7 mm. Vascular space involvement, venous or lymphatic, does not affect classification.
(T1a1) Measured stromal invasion ≤3 mm in depth and ≤7 mm in horizontal spread
(T1a2) Measured stromal invasion >3 mm and not >5 mm with a horizontal spread ≤7 mm

T1b
Clinically visible lesion confined to the cervix or microscopic lesion greater than T1a/IA2
(T1b1) Clinically visible lesion ≤4 cm in greatest dimension
(T1b2) Clinically visible lesion >4 cm in greatest dimension

N0
No regional lymph node metastasis

T2
Cervical carcinoma invades beyond uterus but not to pelvic wall or to lower third of vagina
(T2a) Tumor without parametrial invasion
(T2a1) Clinically visible lesion ≤4 cm in greatest dimension
(T2a2) Clinically visible lesion >4 cm in greatest dimension
(T2b) Tumor with parametrial invasion

T3
Tumor extends to pelvic wall and/or involves lower third of vagina, and/or causes hydronephrosis or nonfunctioning kidney
(T3a) Tumor involves lower third of vagina, no extension to pelvic wall
(T3b) Tumor extends to pelvic wall and/or causes hydronephrosis or nonfunctioning kidney

N1
Regional lymph node metastasis

T4
Tumor invades mucosa of bladder or rectum, and/or extends beyond true pelvis (bullous edema is not sufficient to classify a tumor as T4)

M0
No distant metastasis

M1
Distant metastasis (including peritoneal spread, involvement of supraclavicular, mediastinal, or paraaortic lymph nodes, lung, liver, or bone)

STAGE GROUPINGS

Stage IA

T1	N0	M0
T1a	N0	M0
T1a1	N0	M0
T1a2	N0	M0

Stage IB

T1b	N0	M0
T1b1	N0	M0
T1b2	N0	M0

Stage II

T2	N0	M0
T2a	N0	M0
T2b	N0	M0

Stage III

T3	N0	M0
T3a	N0	M0

Stage IIIB

T1	N1	M0
T2	N1	M0
T3a	N1	M0
T3b	Any N	M0

Stage IVA

T4	Any N	M0

Stage IVB

Any T	Any N	M1

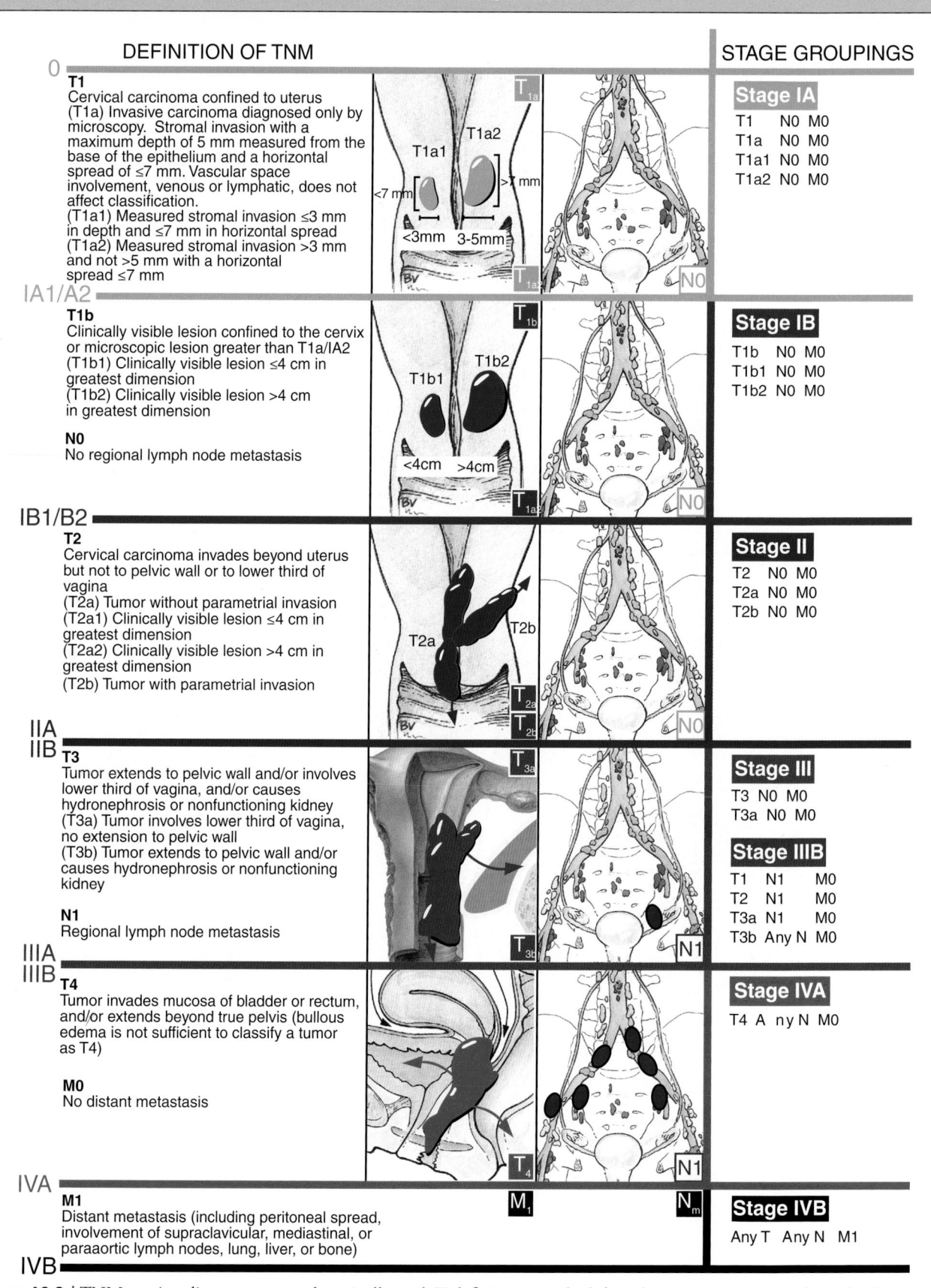

Figure 46.3 | TNM staging diagram arranged vertically with T definitions on the left and stage groupings on the right. Uterine cervix cancers are often detected in microinvasive stages and are most resectable in stage IA or IB cancers. With further invasion, chemoradiation treatment is effective. There are four main stages, each with two or three substages. Color bars are coded for stage: stage 0 and IA, yellow; IB, green; II, blue; III, purple; IV, red; and metastatic disease to viscera and nodes, black.

T-ONCOANATOMY

ORIENTATION OF THREE-PLANAR ONCOANATOMY

The isocenter of the cervix is the central structure in the female pelvis. It is retropubic at the level of the coccyx and midway between the ovaries and vulva (Fig. 46.4).

T-oncoanatomy

The T-oncoanatomy is displayed in three planar views in Fig. 46.5:

* *Coronal*: The cervix comprises the lower third of the uterus. It is roughly cylindrical in shape, projecting through the upper vaginal wall. It communicates with the vagina through an orifice called the "external os." Cancer of the cervix may originate on the vaginal surface or in the cervical canal.

* *Sagittal*: There is invasion of the bladder trigone from a cancer in the anterior lip of the cervix and fornix of the vagina. Vaginal extension into its posterior fornix and wall precedes rectal wall invasion.

* *Transverse*: The mesometrium or the broad ligament of the uterus contains a number of very important structures that determine the course of events in a number of oncologic presentations and complications. The course of the ureter, which is a critical normal structure, passes from its lateral position in the abdomen to its medial location in the pelvis by moving horizontally to insert into the bladder. It is crossed superiorly and medially by the uterine artery. The long transverse course of the ureter makes it particularly vulnerable to entrapment by cancer spread from the cervix because it lies juxtaposed to the cervix before its entry to the bladder. Uncontrolled stage IV cancer blocks both ureters, resulting in hydronephrosis and renal failure, leading to uremic death. Along the sidewall of the pelvis, the obturator nerve and vessel enter into the obturator foramen.

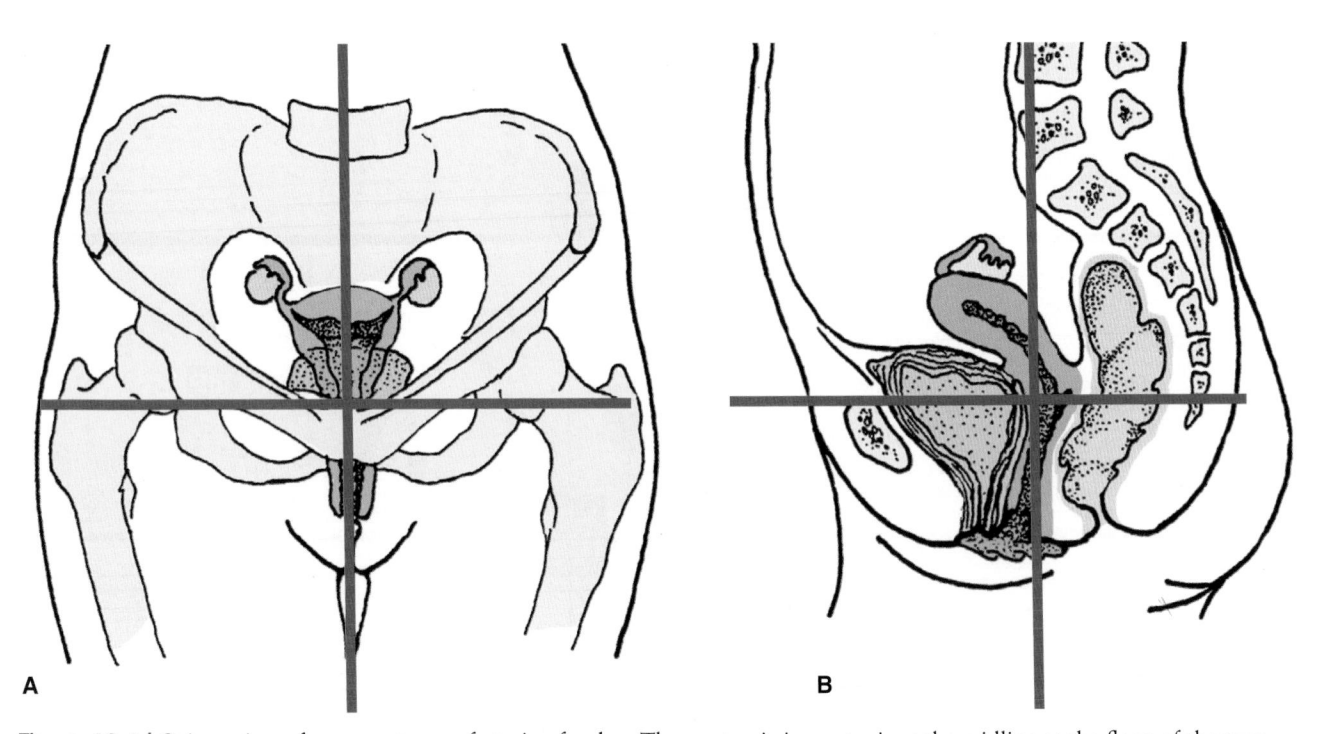

A   **B**

Figure 46.4 | Orientation of oncoanatomy of uterine fundus. The anatomic isocenter is at the midline at the floor of the true pelvis at the S4/S5 level. **A.** Coronal. **B.** Sagittal.

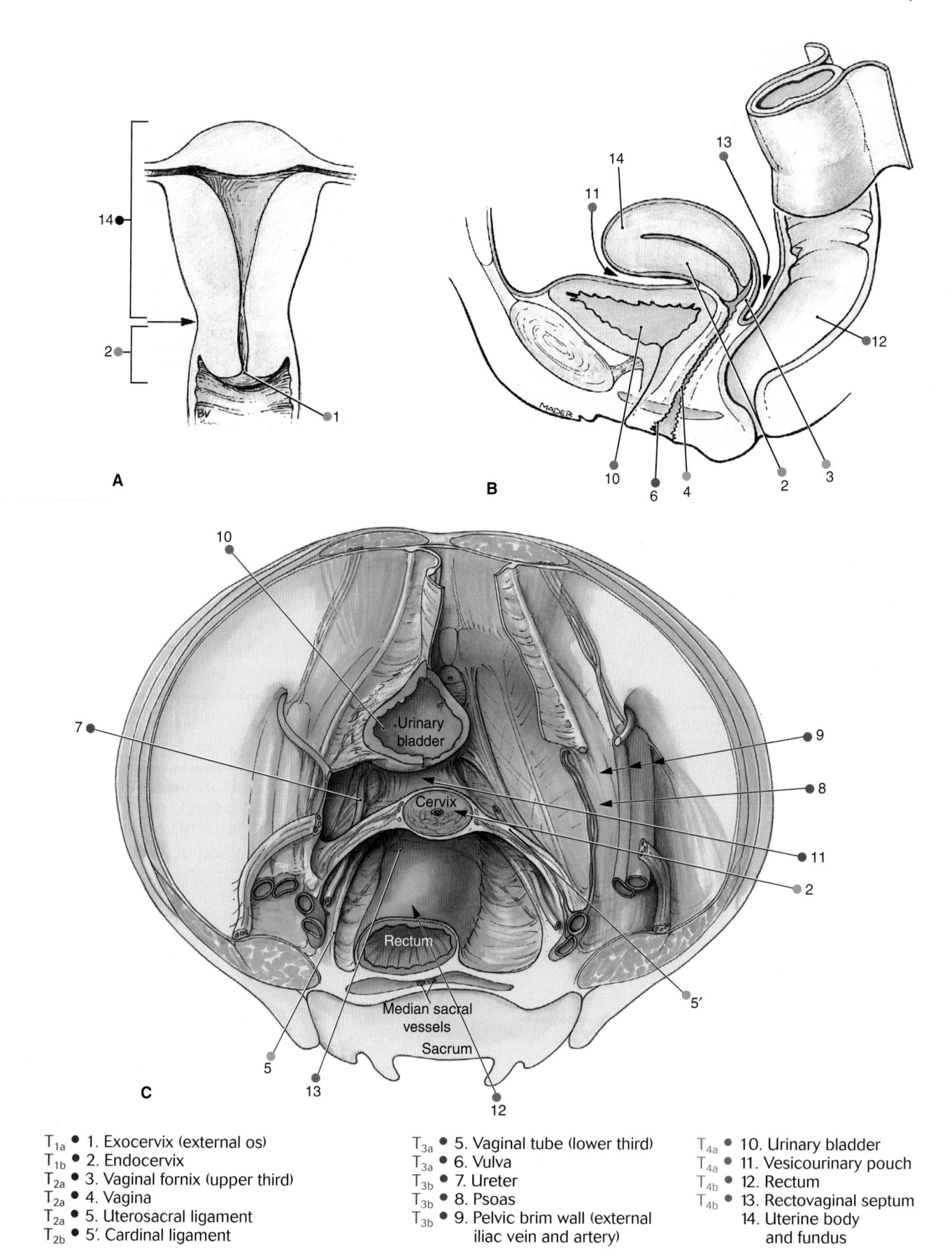

A

B

C

T₁ₐ ● 1. Exocervix (external os)	T₃ₐ ● 5. Vaginal tube (lower third)	T₄ₐ ● 10. Urinary bladder
T₁ᵦ ● 2. Endocervix	T₃ₐ ● 6. Vulva	T₄ₐ ● 11. Vesicourinary pouch
T₂ₐ ● 3. Vaginal fornix (upper third)	T₃ᵦ ● 7. Ureter	T₄ᵦ ● 12. Rectum
T₂ₐ ● 4. Vagina	T₃ᵦ ● 8. Psoas	T₄ᵦ ● 13. Rectovaginal septum
T₂ₐ ● 5. Uterosacral ligament	T₃ᵦ ● 9. Pelvic brim wall (external	14. Uterine body
T₂ᵦ ● 5′. Cardinal ligament	iliac vein and artery)	and fundus

Figure 46.5 | T-oncoanatomy. **A.** Coronal, **B.** Sagittal, **C.** Transverse axial. The color code for the anatomic sites correlates with the color code for the stage group (Fig. 46.3), patterns of spread (Fig. 46.2), and SIMLAP table (Table 46.2). Connecting the dots in similar colors will provide an appreciation for the three-dimensional oncoanatomy.

N-ONCOANATOMY AND M-ONCOANATOMY

N-ONCOANATOMY

The cervix is drained by preureteral, postureteral, and uterosacral lymphatics. Cancers confined to the cervix drain first to obturator nodes, then to hypogastric or internal iliac nodes. These are the first station lymph nodes and are on the lateral wall of the true pelvis, where the internal obturator artery and vein penetrate the levator ani muscle. The lymphatics follow the uterine vein, which drains into the internal and not the external iliac (Fig. 46.6A; Table 46.4A). As the cancer invades more deeply and extensively, the lymph nodes beyond the true pelvis are at risk. When the cancer invades the parametrium and is fixed to the sidewall of the pelvis, lymphatic anastomoses to the external iliac nodes may lead to their involvement. With vaginal invasions up to its lower third, inguinal nodes are at risk. Rectal invasions may lead to the inferior mesenteric nodes being at risk.

The cervical cancer sentinel node is the obturator node, placing the internal iliac chain at risk when the cancer is stage I or II. With more extensive infiltration of the cancer, second and third stations or echelons of nodes are at risk.

The distribution and incidence of pelvic lymph node metastases is illustrated for early stage cervical cancer (stage I and IIA) (Fig. 46.7A).

As the stage advances the incidence increases but can be modified and decreases with both radiation and neoadjuvant chemotherapy prior to lymph adenectomy (Fig. 46.7B).

Para-ortic lymph nodes generally increase with stage advancement (Table 46.4B).

M-ONCOANATOMY

The arterial and venous blood supply and drainage are via the uterine vessels, and hematogenous spread is via the internal iliac to the common iliacs and inferior vena cava (Fig. 46.6B). The lung is the target metastatic organ. Skeletal invasion of the lateral cortex of the true pelvis or vertebrae is due to lymphatic and lymph node metastatic cancer penetrating the nodal capsule and directly invading the juxtaposed bone. Once this occurs, the cancer spreads beyond the confines of the lymph nodes, and it often savagely destroys the pelvic bone and/or vertebrae crossing and eradicating intervertebral discs.

The incidence and distribution of distant metastases by anatomic site of first metastases is shown in table 46.4C.

TABLE 46.4B Metastases to Para-aortic Lymph Nodes in Carcinoma of the Uterine Cervix

Stage	Positive Nodes %
IB	8%
IIA	18%
IIB	20–33%
IIIB	31–46%
IV	57%

TABLE 46.4A Lymph Nodes of Cervix

Sentinel Nodes	Juxtaregional Nodes
Obturator nodes of the internal iliac chain	Para-aortic
Regional Nodes	
Left: renal hilar Right: paracaval External iliac Hypogastric Lateral sacral Common iliac	

TABLE 46.4C Carcinoma of the Uterine Cervix (Mallinckrodt Institute of Radiology 1959–1986): Anatomic Site of First Metastasis

Site	No. of Patients with Distant Metastases (*n* = 322)
Lung	69 (21%)
Para-aortic nodes	37 (11%)
Abdominal cavity	26 (8%)
Supraclavicular nodes	21 (7%)
Spine	21 (7%)
Gastrointestinal tract	14 (4%)
Liver	13 (4%)
Inguinal nodes	10 (3%)
Miscellaneous	111 (35%)

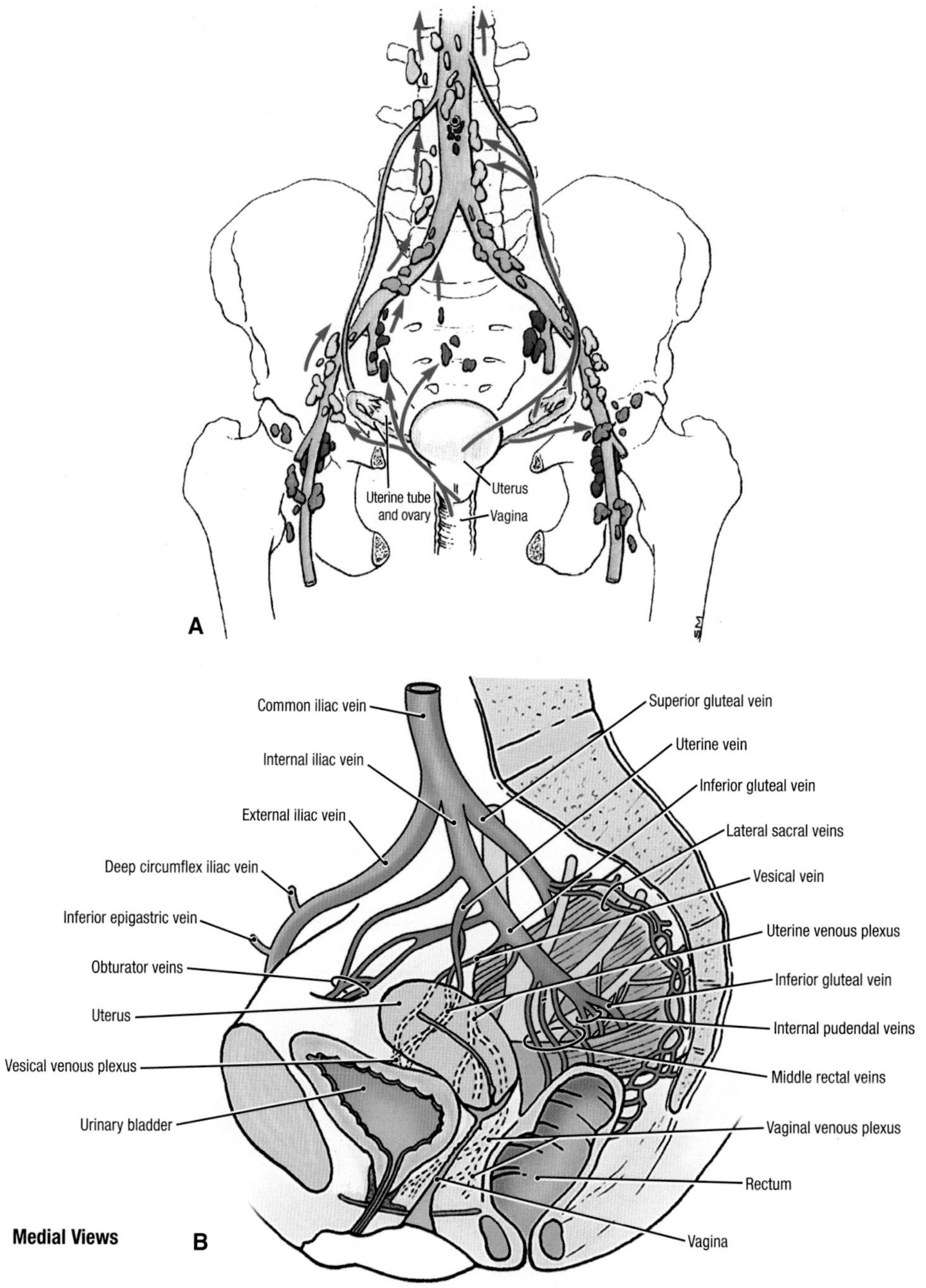

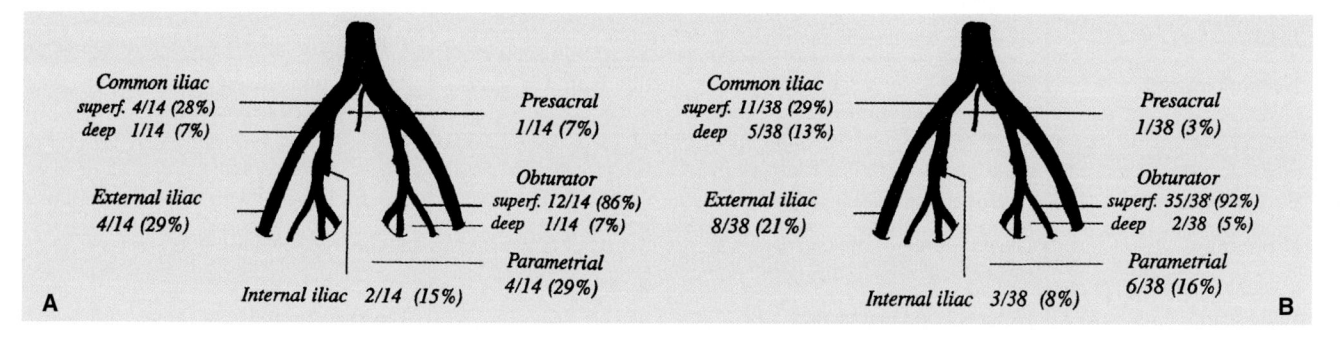

Figure 46.6 | A. N-oncoanatomy. The sentinel nodes are the obturator nodes of the internal iliac chain. Para-aortic nodes are juxtaregional. **B.** M-oncoanatomy.

Figure 46.7 | A. Distribution of pelvic node metastases in 14 patients with stage IB to IIA cervical cancer, tumor size <4 cm, and (**B**) 38 patients with locally advanced cervical cancer treated with neoadjuvant chemotherapy. (From Benedetti-Panici P, Maneschi F, Scambia G, et al. Lymphatic spread of cervical cancer: an anatomical and pathological study based on 225 radical hysterectomies with systematic pelvic and aortic lymphadenectomy. *Gynecol Oncol* 1996;62:19–24, with permission.)

STAGING WORKUP

RULES OF CLASSIFICATION AND STAGING

Clinical Staging and Imaging

The sine qua non of clinical staging occurs before treatment, preferably performed by a multidisciplinary team consisting of a gynecologic oncologist and a radiation oncologist with the patient under anesthesia. Imaging is advisable but cannot be used to alter staging; however, there is little doubt that newer modalities such as computed tomography (CT), magnetic resonance imaging (MRI), ultrasonography (US), and positron emission tomography are more accurate than clinical palpation, inspection, colposcopy, endocervical curettage, hysteroscopy, or cystoscopy. Suspected bladder and rectal invasion must be confirmed on biopsy. Fine-needle aspiration should be used to determine enlarged node status (Table 46.5; Fig. 46.8).

Surgical-pathologic Staging

The completely resected specimen, including the primary site and regional lymph nodes, which must be thoroughly analyzed, are pTNM designated. Radical hysterectomy and bilateral salpingo-oophorectomy with pelvic lymph node resection is the usual procedure for pathologic evaluation.

Although the staging has remained unchanged at most gynecologic primary sites, the rules for classification still do not allow for sophisticated imaging, which includes CT, MRI, and US, to alter staging. The multidisciplinary approach to decision making is truly interdisciplinary, most often involving a gynecologic oncologist and a dedicated radiation oncologist. Over the decades, diagnostic and therapeutic protocols in national cooperative groups have provided a scientific basis for introducing combined modalities and innovations into clinical practice.

Oncoimaging Annotations

- CT is most useful for advanced stages greater than stage III and is worthwhile in assessing cervix size. Because cancers are isodense on CT, cervical cancer dimensions are not as accurate but are excellent for staging purposes.

- CT is not reliable for early parametrial invasion but is accurate in determining advanced disease with pelvic sidewall fixation.

- CT suggests parametrial, bladder, and rectal invasion when fat planes exist between cervix and structure or they show irregular thickening.

- MRI identifies cancer on T2-weighted images as an intense signal, increasing its accuracy to detect cancer size and lymph nodes involved.

- Gadolinium-enhanced MRI allows for identification of soft tissue invasion in vagina and parametria.

- CT: Early parametrial invasion is not as reliably predicted as advanced parametrial extension to the pelvic wall.

- MRI: More accurate for assessing parametrial invasion and tumor size.

TABLE 46.5	Imaging Modalities for Staging Cervix Cancer	
Method	Diagnosis and Staging Capability	Recommended for Use
Primary (T) Staging		
CTe	Reliable for defining adnexal ovarian masses, extension to gynecologic organs, peritoneal seeding, and ascites	Yes; contrast helps to visualize vessels and intestines
MRI	Role of MRI is emerging as criteria for malignancy defined	Yes, but supplemental to CT for soft tissues
TVUS	Excellent for screening and diagnosis	No, not reliable to define invasion
PET	High activity suggests malignancy versus benign status of solid or cystic pelvic masses	No
Nodal (N) Staging		
CTe	Excellent for detecting nodal adenopathy >1 cm in size	Yes, cost effective
MRI	Available for supplementing CT	Yes, if cancer is high grade
Needle biopsy	Confirms lesions detected by radionuclide scan, CT scans, or lymphangiogram	Patients with suspicious lesions, image-guided aspirations
Metastases (M) Staging		
Barium enema	Rectovaginal wall invasion	Yes, for patients with suspicious lesions
Urography	Detects ureteral obstruction, bladder invasion; screens for unsuspected renal anomaly	All operative candidates
Bone scan	Detects bone metastases	Yes, if suspected
CT	Useful to assess omental and liver metastases	Yes, if suspected

CT, computed tomography; CTe, CT enhanced with intravenous contrast; MRI, magnetic resonance imaging; PET, positron emission tomography; TVUS, transvaginal ultrasound.

PROGNOSIS AND CANCER SURVIVAL

- MRI can demonstrate intact normal fibrous rim around cervix cancer and has high negative predictive value (95%) for parametrial invasion.

- MRI provides a more accurate assessment of cancer infiltration of rectum and bladder.

PROGNOSIS

The limited number of prognostic factors are listed in Table 46.6.

CANCER STATISTICS AND SURVIVAL

Female genital system cancers collectively account for 80,000 new cases a year, with uterine corpus exceeding cervix cancer by a factor of four. Both are highly curable, and deaths are relatively low. The major gynecologic killer is ovarian cancer, with 16,000 deaths annually, which exceeds the other six primary sites combined.

Survival Rates

The survival rate gains in both cervix uteri and fundus uteri cancer have been incremental. Given that invasive cancers of the gynecologic tract have had a higher baseline—greater than 50% in the 1950s—the gains for all stages are only 15%, or 2% to 3% per decade. As noted, mortality rates have plummeted owing to early detection, especially of cancer of the cervix because it is most often detected in its noninvasive stage. Localized uterine cancers are >90% curable.

TABLE 46.6	Prognostic Factors
Required for Staging	None
Clinically Significant	International Federation of Gynecology and Obstetrics stage
	Pelvic nodal status and method of assessment
	Distant (para-aortic) nodal status and method of assessment
	Distant (mediastinal, scalene) nodal status and method of assessment

From Edge SB, Byrd DR, Compton CC, et al., *AJCC Cancer Staging Manual*, 7th edition. New York: Springer, 2010, p. 400.

The cancer survival rates indicate that the gain in survival for uterine corpus and cervix cancer have been modest (14%) over the last five decades. However, most uterine cervix cancers are detected as cancer in situ, and this is not reflected in the figures. Ovarian cancer survival has improved by 22% and, as stated, remains lethal because most cases are detected late owing to its insidious onset and the inaccessibility of ovarian nodules to early diagnosis. Brighter notes are the high cure and 5-year survival rates for stage I patients with cervical cancer (92%), uterine corpus cancer (96%), and ovarian cancer (95%) (Fig. 46.9).

Survival rates for cancer of the cervix have improved from 1950 to 2000 for all stages, rising from 59% to 67%, an increment of 18%. For stage I localized cancers, the cure rate exceeds 90% (Fig. 46.9).

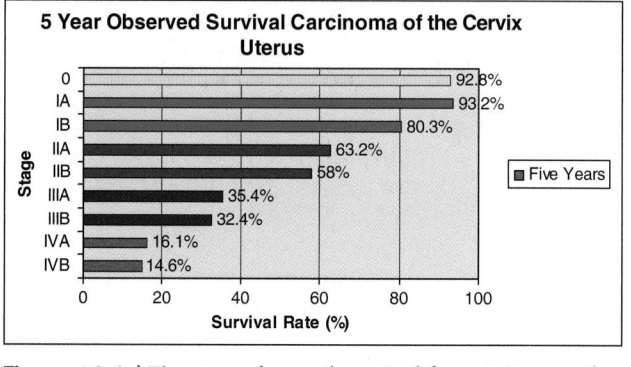

Figure 46.9 | Five-year observed survival for carcinoma of the cervix. (Edge SB, Byrd DR, and Compton CC, et al., *AJCC Cancer Staging Manual*, 7th edition. New York: Springer, 2010, p. 398.)

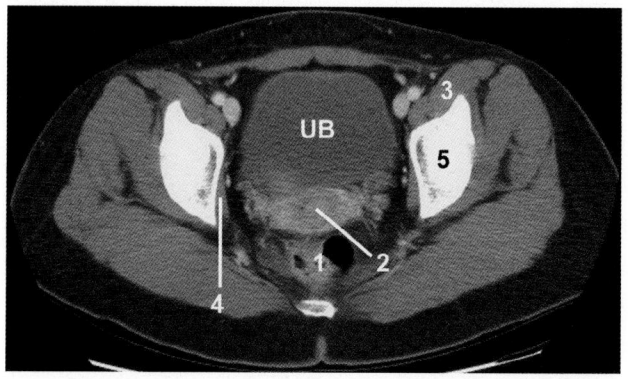

Figure 46.8 | Axial CTs of uterine cervix correlate with the T-oncoanatomy transverse section (Fig. 46.5C). Oncoimaging with CT is commonly applied to staging cancers, often combined with positron emission tomography to determine the true extent of primary cancer and involved lymph nodes. (1) Rectum. (2) Uterine cervix. (3) Iliopsoas muscle. (4) Obturator internus muscle. (5) Acetabular roof. UB, urinary bladder.

CHAPTER
47
Vagina

PERSPECTIVE, PATTERNS OF SPREAD, AND PATHOLOGY

The pattern of spread relates to paravaginal invasion into lateral soft tissues and follows the same criteria as the staging system of cervix uteri (Fig. 47.2; Table 47.2).

PERSPECTIVE AND PATTERNS OF SPREAD

The vagina is a fibromuscular tubular structure about 8 and 10 cm long connecting the uterus to the external female genitals. Vaginal cancer is a rare gynecologic malignancy, constituting only 1% of malignant neoplasms of the female genital tract. Indeed, metastatic involvement of the vagina, particularly by cervical or vulvar carcinoma, occurs much more frequently than primary vaginal cancer. This fact has led to the International Federation of Gynecology and Obstetrics staging system requiring that tumors involving both the vagina and cervix or the vagina and vulva be classified as primary cervical or vulvar carcinoma, respectively.

In the past 30 years, interest has focused on an increased incidence of clear cell adenocarcinoma of the vagina in young women, which, in 1971, was found to be related to the administration of diethylstilbestrol (DES) to their mothers during pregnancy. The incidence of clear cell adenocarcinoma in women exposed prenatally to DES is estimated to be about 1 per 10,000; it has been observed that the risk was greatest for those exposed during the first 18 weeks in utero.

PATHOLOGY

Although, classically, squamous cell cancer arises from its stratified squamous epithelium, it is second in incidence to adenocarcinoma. This is because most common isolated vaginal cancers are most often adenocarcinomas, metastatic often from endometrial malignancies. Of special interest are adenocarcinomas in young women, attributed to the administration of DES to their mothers during pregnancy, particularly in the first 18 weeks in utero. Fortunately, once suspected, these clear cell cancers can be diagnosed in early stages (I and II). A large variety of malignancies can occur and are given in Table 47.1. Sarcoma botryoides occurs mainly in children younger than 5 years of age and is characterized as grape-like clusters (Fig. 47.1). Patterns of spread are given in Fig. 47.2.

- Squamous cell carcinoma accounts for 85% of primary vaginal cancers (most nonkeratinizing), with adenocarcinoma, melanoma, and other histologic subtypes making up the remainder (Table 47.1).

- The majority of nonsquamous vaginal cancers are adenocarcinomas and comprise approximately 5% of primary vaginal tumors; endometrioid, mucinous, papillary, and clear cell variants have been reported. Vaginal

TABLE 47.1	Histopathologic Classification of Malignant Tumors of the Vagina	
Metastatic (e.g., cervical , endometrial, ovarian)	—
Squamous cell carcinoma	82%
Adenocarcinoma clear cell	9.6%
Endodermal sinus tumor	—
Malignant melanoma	3.3%
Sarcoma botryoides	—
Lymphomas	0.3%
Carcinoid	0.1%
Rhabdomyosarcoma	3.1%

Rubin P, Williams J, eds. *Clinical Oncology: A Multidisciplinary Approach for Physicians and Students.* 8th ed. Philadelphia: Elsevier; 2001:499.

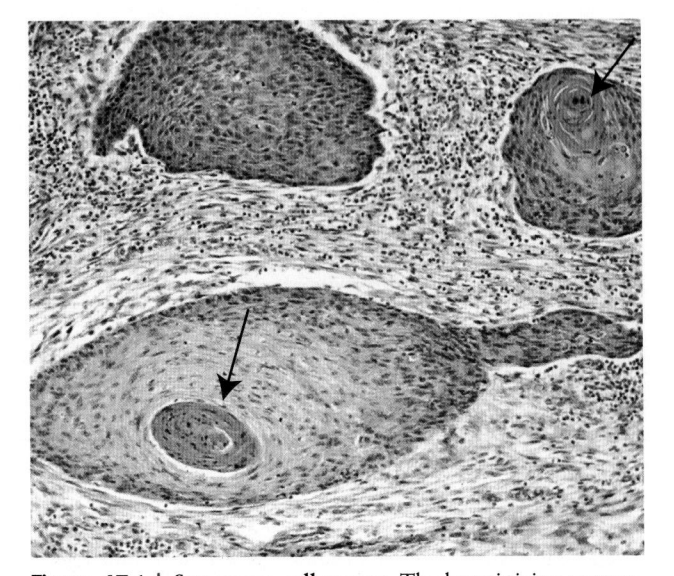

Figure 47.1 | Squamous cell cancer. The keratinizing pattern of the tumor is manifested as whorls of keratinized cells ("keratin pearls") (*arrows*).

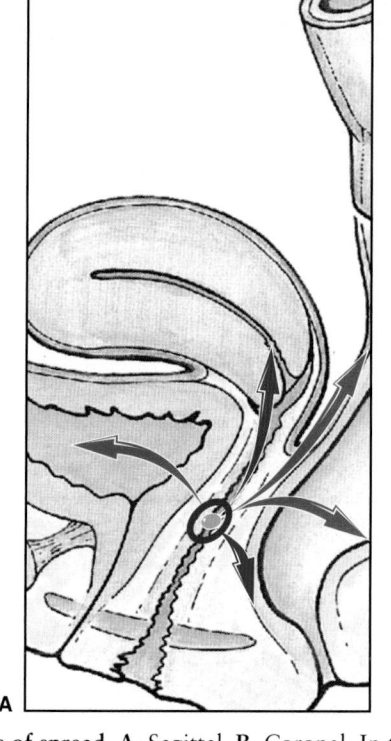 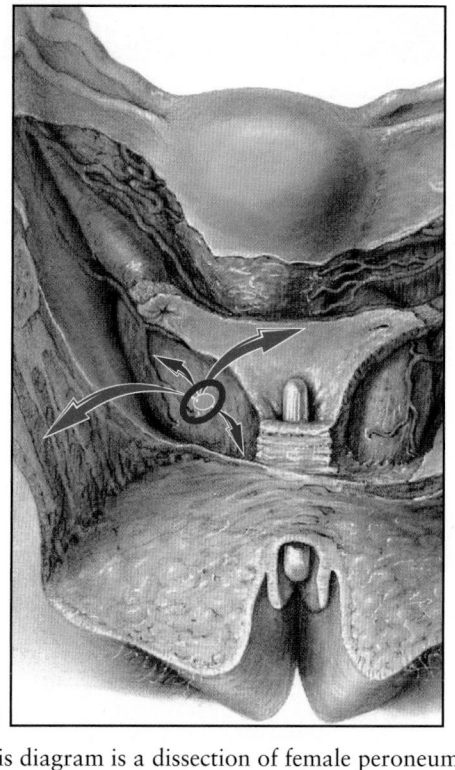

Figure 47.2 | Patterns of spread. A. Sagittal. **B.** Coronal. In this diagram is a dissection of female peroneum. The vagina is a muscular tumor posterior to trigone of urinary bladder and urethra with rod insert (see also Fig. 47.5A). The cancer is color coded for stage: Tis, yellow; T1, green; T2, blue; T3, purple; and T4, red. The concept of visualizing patterns of spread to appreciate the surrounding anatomy is well demonstrated by the six-directional pattern SIMLAP, Table 47.2.

adenocarcinomas occur in younger patients than do squamous cell carcinomas, and they usually arise from the Bartholin or Skene submucosal glandular epithelium. Most of these tumors are polypoid or nodular.

- Adenoid cystic carcinoma of the vagina is extremely rare. Until 1996, only 45 cases of adenoid cystic carcinoma of Bartholin's gland had been reported in the world literature.

- Neuroendocrine small cell carcinoma may occur in the vagina, either in pure form or associated with squamous or glandular elements. A high proportion show ultrastructural or immunohistochemical evidence of neuroendocrine differentiation. The tumor tends to be aggressive, with a propensity for early spread.

- Sarcoma botryoides occurs primarily in children younger than 5 years old, and it is characterized grossly by a polypoid mass resembling a bunch of grapes and microscopically by crowded rhabdomyoblasts in a distinct subepithelial cambium layer.

- Melanoma accounts for only 3% of vaginal malignancies; it is usually located in the distal third of the vagina. Microscopy demonstrates pleomorphic cells laden with melanin, although pigmentation may be absent in the amelanotic variety. Progression of preexisting melanosis to malignant melanoma of the vagina has been reported.

- Endodermal sinus tumor of the vagina is similar histologically to its ovarian counterpart, with typical Schiller-Duval bodies.

- Most primary malignant lymphomas involving the vagina are the diffuse large cell type, but nodular lymphomas also occur. Characteristically, the mucosa is intact; a submucosal mass is frequently seen. Marker studies are useful in equivocal cases of lymphoma-like lesions.*

*Rubin P, Williams J, eds. *Clinical Oncology: A Multidisciplinary Approach for Physicians and Students.* 8th ed. Philadelphia: Elsevier, 2001:499–500.

TABLE 47.2	Vagina SIMLAP	
S	Cervix	Tx†
	Uterus	Tx†
I	Vulva	Tx
	Labia minora	Tx
	Labia majora	Tx
M	Urethra	• T2
	Vaginal wall	• T1
L	Levator ani muscle	• T2
	Obturator internus muscle	• T3
	Pudendal canal	• T2
A	Urinary bladder	• T4
	Urethra	• T2
P	Rectouterine pouch	• T4
	Rectum	• T4

The six vectors of invasion are <u>S</u>uperior, <u>I</u>nferior, <u>M</u>edial, <u>L</u>ateral, <u>A</u>nterior, and <u>P</u>osterior. The color-coded dots correlate the T stage with the specific anatomic structure involved.
†Tx if involved, the cancer is designated to have originated in that site.

TNM STAGING CRITERIA

TNM STAGING CRITERIA

The pattern of spread relates to paravaginal invasion and in lateral soft tissues is stage T2; it follows the same criteria as the staging system of cervix uteri. Thus extension to the pelvic sidewall laterally (stage T3) and anteriorly into the urethra can occur or into the urinary bladder or posteriorly into the rectum (stage T4). Most cancers are squamous cell carcinomas arising from the vaginal mucosa of stratified squamous epithelium (Fig. 47.3).

SUMMARY OF CHANGES SEVENTH EDITION AJCC

The definitions of TNM and the Stage Groupings for this chapter have not changed from the Sixth Edition (Fig. 47.3).

The TNM Staging Matrix allows for identification of Stage Group once T and N stages are determined (Table 47.3).

Cancer of the vagina has four main stages, I to IV, following the T category, and stage IV is divided into IVA (N_1) and IVB (M_1). There are seven stage groups in total.

TABLE 47.3A	Stage Summary Matrix		
	N0	**N1**	**M1**
T1	I	III	IV
T2	II	III	IV
T3	III	III	IV
T4	IV	IV	IV

TABLE 47.3B	Primary Vaginal Cancer % Distribution by Stage
Stage	**% Distribution**
I	28.4%
II	36.6%
III	21.7%
IV	13.3%

*Based on collating approximately 2000 cases in literature.

VAGINA

DEFINITION OF TNM

T1
Tumor confined to vagina

N0
No regional lymph node metastasis

T2
Tumor invades paravaginal tissues but not to pelvic wall

N0
No regional lymph node metastasis

T3
Tumor extends to pelvic wall

N1
Pelvic or inguinal lymph node metastasis

T4
Tumor invades mucosa of the bladder or rectum and/or extends beyond the true pelvis (bullous edema is not sufficient evidence to classify a tumor as T4)

M1
Distant metastasis

STAGE GROUPINGS

Stage I
T1 N0 M0

Stage II
T2 N0 M0

Stage III
T1-3 N1 M0
T3   N0 M0

Stage IVA
T4 Any N M0

Stage IVB
Any T Any N M1

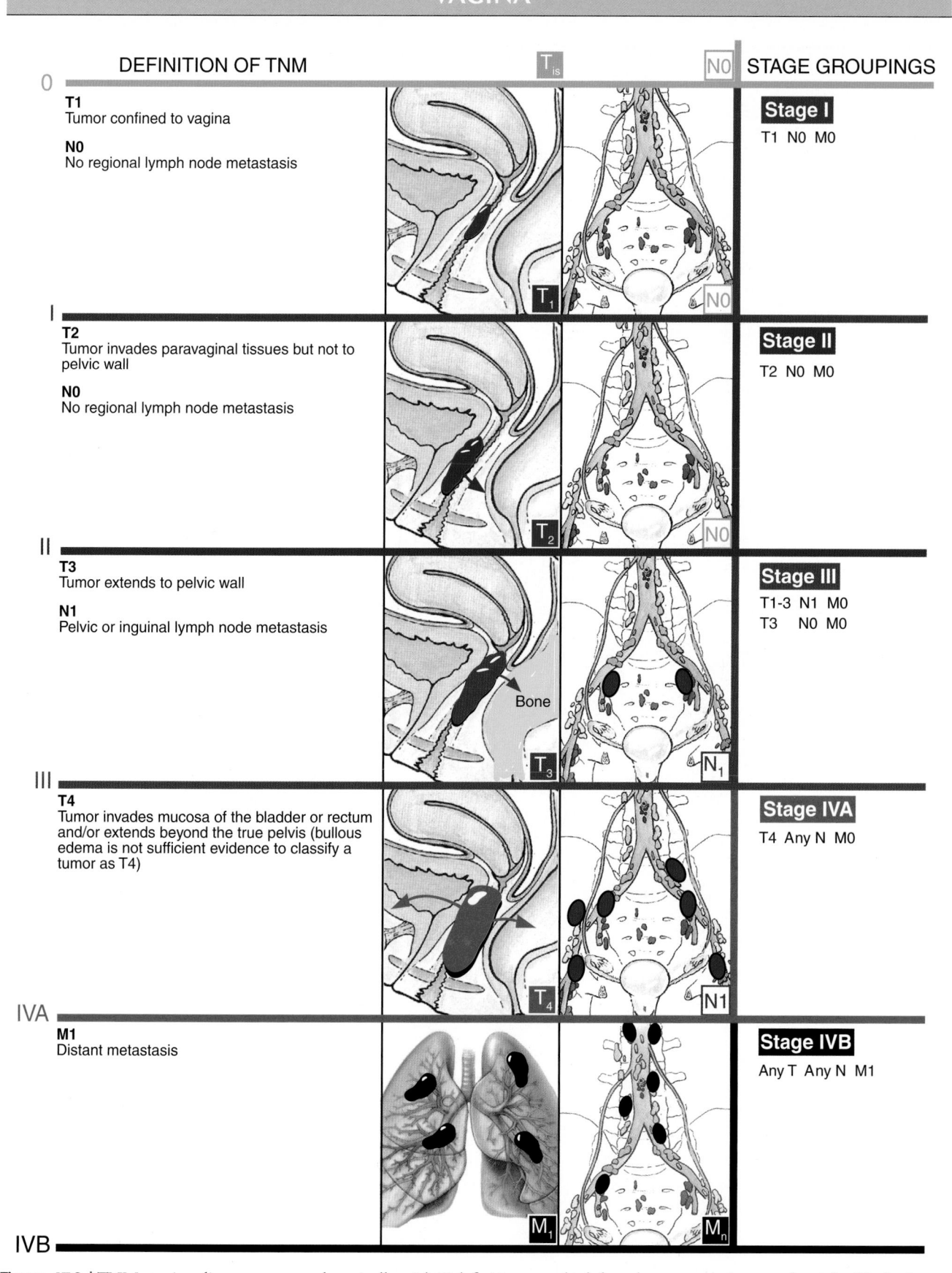

Figure 47.3 | TNM staging diagram arranged vertically with T definitions on the left and stage groupings on the right. Vaginal cancers are not common, and if the diagnosis is adenocarcinoma, metastatic uterine cancer should be considered in older women and a search for history of DES administration in younger women. There are four main stages, each with two or three substages. Color bars are coded for stage: stage 0, yellow; I, green; II, blue; III, purple; IV, red; and metastatic disease to viscera and nodes, black.

T-ONCOANATOMY

ORIENTATION OF THREE-PLANAR ONCOANATOMY

The isocenter of the vagina is retropubic with inferior extension and is well below the level of the coccyx to the inferior aspect of the pubic bone (Fig. 47.4).

T-oncoanatomy

The T-oncoanatomy is displayed in three planar views in Fig. 47.5. The vagina is a fibromuscular sheath composed of three layers: mucosa, muscle, and adventitia.

- *Coronal*: The intimate relationship of the urethra in the anterior wall of the vagina is noted.
- *Sagittal*: The muscle layer is composed of smooth muscle arranged in a circular, then longitudinal direction. The sphincter muscle urethrovaginalis composed of skeletal muscle is at its terminal end, the vestibule.
- *Transverse*: The pelvic wall is closer to the vagina than at the cervical level, and vaginal cancer becomes fixed earlier.

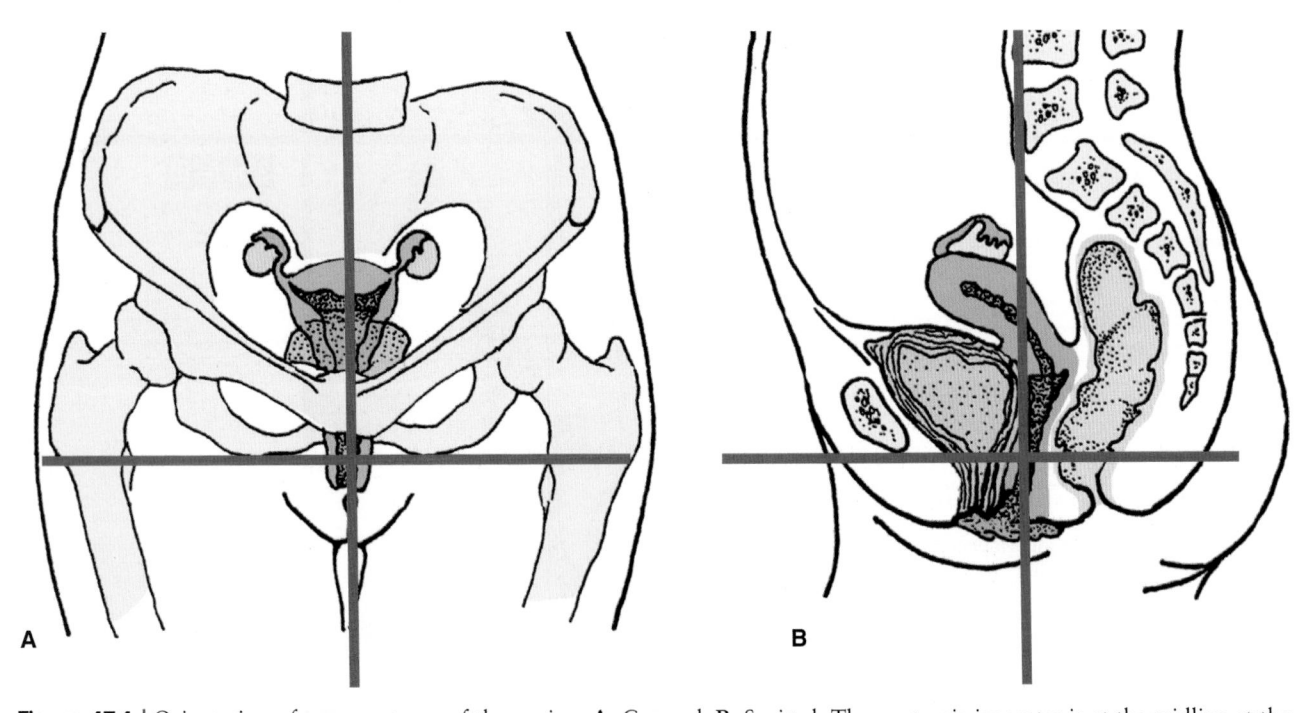

Figure 47.4 | Orientation of oncoanatomy of the vagina. **A.** Coronal. **B.** Sagittal. The anatomic isocenter is at the midline at the floor of the true pelvis at the S4/S5 level.

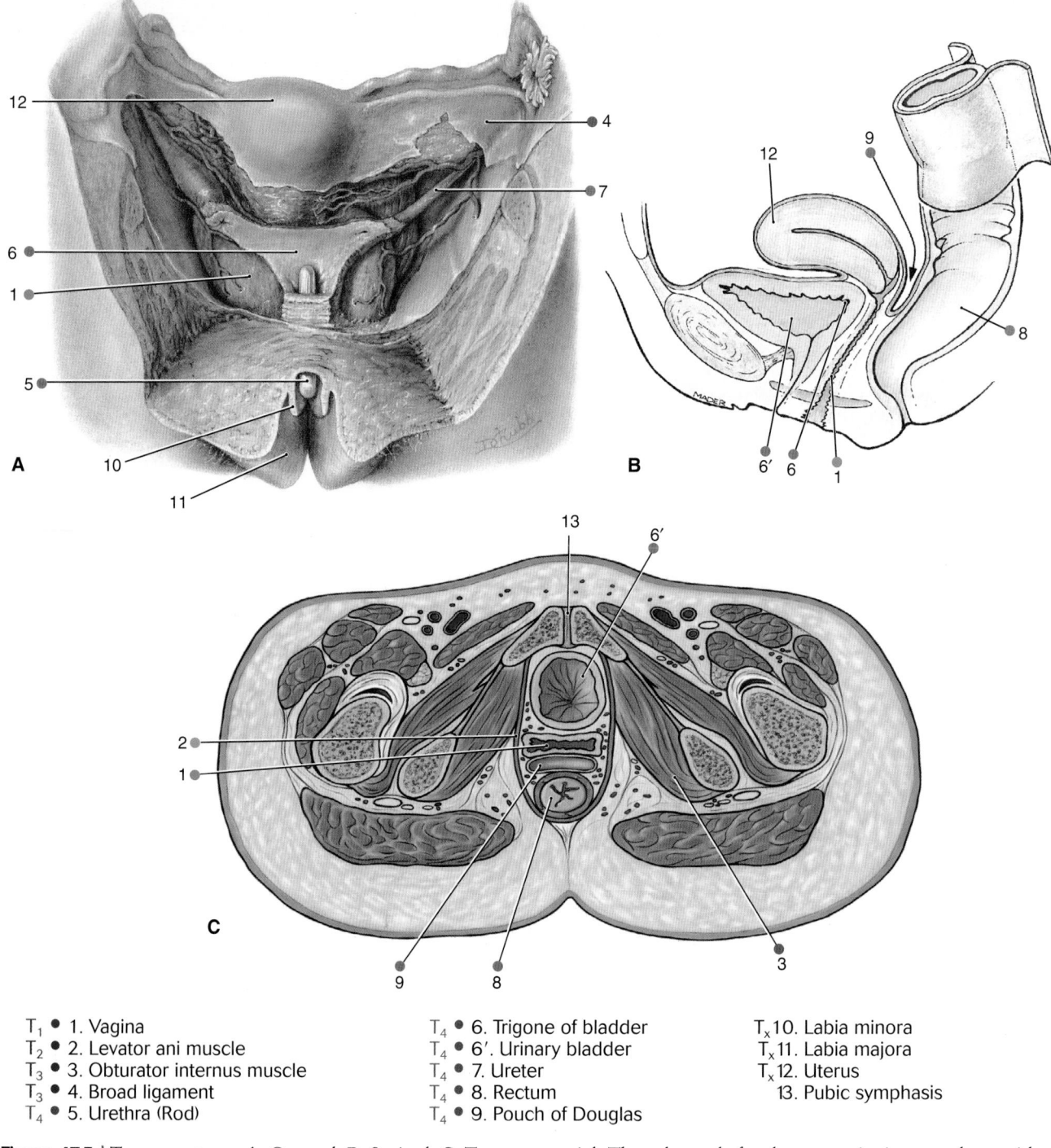

Figure 47.5 | T-oncoanatomy. **A.** Coronal. **B.** Sagittal. **C.** Transverse axial. The color code for the anatomic sites correlates with the color code for the stage group (Fig. 47.3), patterns of spread (Fig. 47.2), and SIMLAP table (Table 47.2). Connecting the dots of similar colors will provide an appreciation for the 3D oncoanatomy.

T_1 ● 1. Vagina
T_2 ● 2. Levator ani muscle
T_3 ● 3. Obturator internus muscle
T_3 ● 4. Broad ligament
T_4 ● 5. Urethra (Rod)

T_4 ● 6. Trigone of bladder
T_4 ● 6'. Urinary bladder
T_4 ● 7. Ureter
T_4 ● 8. Rectum
T_4 ● 9. Pouch of Douglas

T_x10. Labia minora
T_x11. Labia majora
T_x12. Uterus
13. Pubic symphasis

N-ONCOANATOMY AND M-ONCOANATOMY

N-ONCOANATOMY

The upper two thirds of the vaginal tube lymphatics drains into the obturator and hypogastric nodes in the true pelvis. In its lower third, it drains into inguinal nodes and then the external iliac node (Fig. 47.6A; Table 47.4).

The incidence of positive lymph nodes varies with the procedure to identify them: PET (35%), lymph angiograms (42.1%), lymph node dissections (28.6%), bilateral pelvic lymph node dissections (34.5%), and para-aortic lymph node dissection (12.5%).

M-ONCOANATOMY

The adventitia has a rich vascular venous plexus, which attracts metastatic deposits. It is anastomosed to the vesical veins and drains into the internal iliacs similar to the cervix. However, at its inferior vestibule it follows pudendal vessels into the internal iliacs and femorals into the external iliacs (see Fig. 47.6B).

Hematogenis dissemination to distant organs is to lung, then liver and bone. This is a late phenomenon since vaginal cancer usually remains confined to pelvis.

TABLE 47.4	Lymph Nodes of Vagina	
Sentinel Nodes	**Juxtaregional Node**
Obturator	Para-aortic
Internal iliac (proximal)	
Inguinal (distal)	
Regional Nodes	
Hypogastric	
External iliac	
Deep inguinal	
Common iliac	
Lateral sacral	
Paracaval	

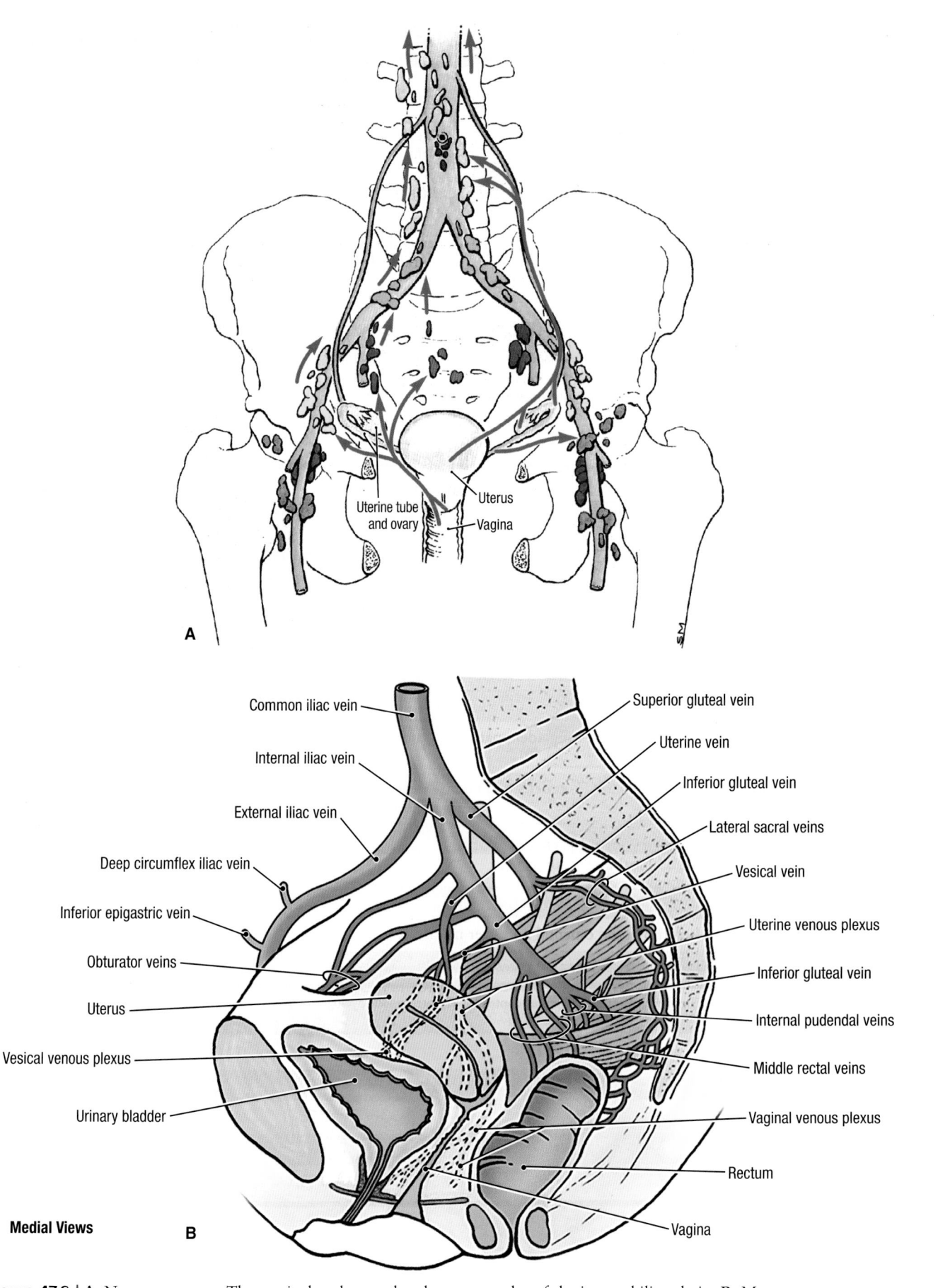

Medial Views

Figure 47.6 | A. N-oncoanatomy. The sentinel nodes are the obturator nodes of the internal iliac chain. **B.** M-oncoanatomy.

48

Vulva

PERSPECTIVES, PATTERNS OF SPREAD, AND PATHOLOGY

The staging is similar to that for most skin cancers; both size and depth of invasion are the critical criteria.

PERSPECTIVE AND PATTERNS OF SPREAD

Cancers of external female genitalia arise in a variety of anatomic sites and are difficult to recognize and identify because of their location. A predisposing factor is human papilloma virus (HPV); HPV16 is the most common variety and requires cofactors such as herpes simplex virus to complete the induction neoplastic process. Vulval cancers are uncommon—slightly greater than 1% of all gynecologic cancers, with approximately 4,000 new cases a year, 20% of which may result in death. The majority occur in the labia majora and minora (70%) and 10% to 15% in the clitoris, with other sites being infrequent. Ten percent of vulvar cancers are too extensive to determine site of origin, and 5% are multifocal. The most common symptoms are vulval pruritus and bleeding or spotting, but otherwise these are asymptomatic.

The spread patterns are similar to those of other skin cancers, appearing as surface lesions that fail to heal and gradually spread superficially and then in depth (Fig. 48.2, Table 48.2). The rich lymphatics of the perineum result in lymph node enlargement in the groin, which can be unilateral or bilateral.

PATHOLOGY

The external genitalia are lined by stratified squamous epithelium and lead to squamous cell carcinomas (90%). In addition, there are numerous secretory glands (Skene's and Bartholin's) that may give rise to adenocarcinomas. Preinvasive changes such as Bowen's disease or Paget's disease with erythroplasia or leukoplasia may be the earliest sign of disease. Melanomas account for a few percent of most series (Table 48.1; Fig. 48.1).

TABLE 48.1	Histopathologic Type: Common Cancers of the Vulva
Squamous cell carcinoma in situ	Adenocarcinoma, NOS
Squamous cell carcinoma (not in FIGO)	Basal cell carcinoma, NOS
Verrucous carcinoma	Bartholin's gland carcinoma
Paget's Disease of Vulva	

NOS, not otherwise specified.
From Edge SB, Byrd DR, and Compton CC, et al., eds. *AJCC Cancer Staging Manual.* 7th ed. New York: Springer, 2010, p. 381.

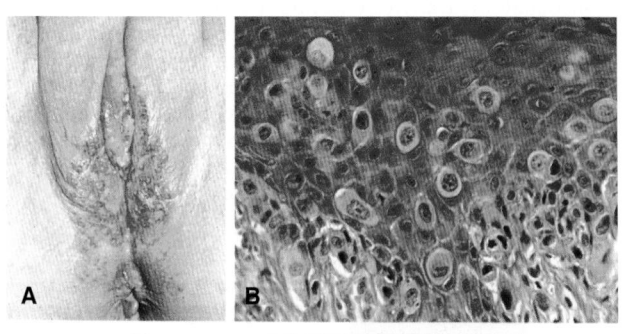

Figure 48.1 | Squamous cell carcinoma of vulva. **A.** The tumor is situated in an extensive area of lichen sclerosus (*white*). **B.** Small nests of neoplastic squamous cells, some with keratin pearls, are evident in this well-differentiated tumor.

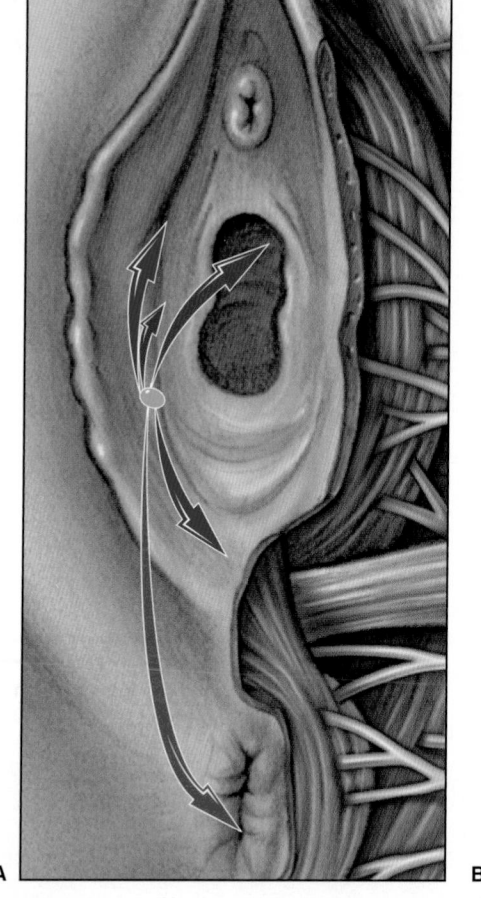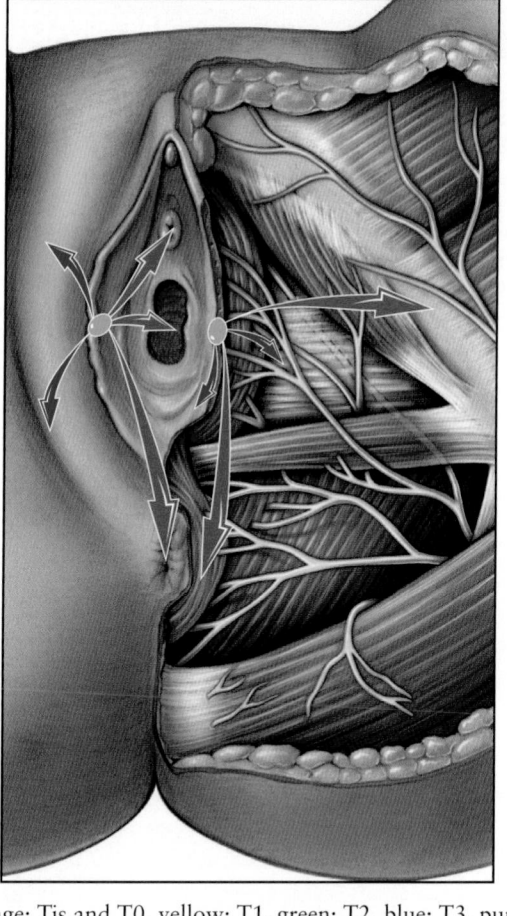

Figure 48.2 | Patterns of spread. The cancer is color coded for stage: Tis and T0, yellow; T1, green; T2, blue; T3, purple; and T4, red. The concept of visualizing patterns of spread to appreciate the surrounding anatomy is well demonstrated by the six-directional pattern, i.e., SIMLAP, Table 48.2.

TABLE 48.2	SIMLAP*	
Vulva		
S	Urethral orifice	• T3
	Clitoris glans	• T2
I	Perineum skin	• T1b
	Anus	• T2
M	Labia minora	• T1a
	Vestibule	• T1a
	Vagina orifice	• T2
	Vagina	• T3
L	Labia majora	• T2
A	Urethra distal ⅓	• T2
	Urethra upper	• T4**
	Bladder	• T4**
P	Rectum	• T4**

*The six vectors of invasion are Superior, Inferior, Medial, Lateral, Anterior, and Posterior. The color-coded dots correlate the T stage with the specific anatomic structure involved.
**FIGO T4 in the TNM is T3.

TNM STAGING CRITERIA

TNM STAGING CRITERIA

The staging is similar to that for most skin cancers; both size and depth of invasion are the critical criteria: T1, <2 cm; and T2, >2 cm; with modification in stage I for depth of invasion: 1a, <1 mm; and 1b, >1 mm. T3 has superior spread into the vagina or urethra, and T4 has reached more deeply to the bladder or rectum. Lymph nodes are simply categorized as N1, unilateral, or N2, bilateral. When extensive, cancerous infiltration of the entire perineum may occur with recurrent cancers that are incompletely treated.

The staging criteria have remained stable (Fig. 48.3).

SUMMARY OF CHANGES SEVENTH EDITION AJCC

The definition of TNM and the Stage Grouping for this chapter have changed for the Seventh Edition and reflect new staging criteria adopted by the International Federation of Gynecology and Obstetrics (FIGO) (2008) (Fig. 48.3).

FIGO uses the classification T2/T3. This is defined as T2 in TNM.

FIGO uses the classification T4. This is defined as T3 in TNM.

The TNM staging matrix allows for identification of stage group once T and N stages are determined (Table 48.3).

TABLE 48.3	Stage Group Matrix						
	N0	N1	N2a	N2b	N2c	N3	M1
T1a	IA	IIIA	IIIB	IIIB	IIIC	IVA	IVB
T1b	IB	IIIA	IIIB	IIIB	IIIC	IVA	IVB
T2	II	IIIA	IIIB	IIIB	IIIC	IVA	IVB
T3	IVA	IVA	IVA	IVA	IVA	IVA	IVB

Staging of cancer of the vulva follows the primary tumor T mainly, and results in eight stage groups (I to IV, each A or B).

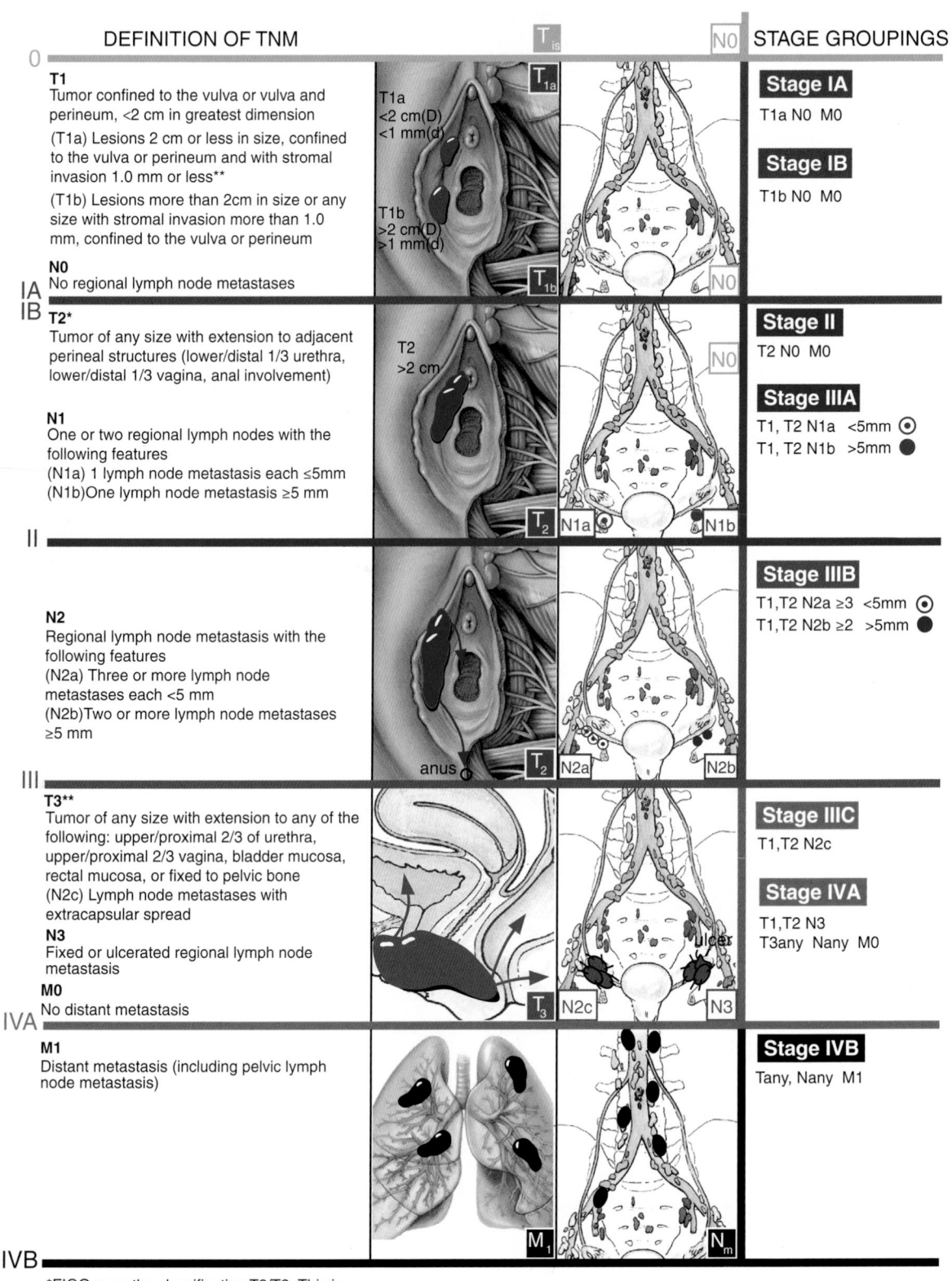

VULVA

DEFINITION OF TNM

T1
Tumor confined to the vulva or vulva and perineum, <2 cm in greatest dimension

(T1a) Lesions 2 cm or less in size, confined to the vulva or perineum and with stromal invasion 1.0 mm or less**

(T1b) Lesions more than 2cm in size or any size with stromal invasion more than 1.0 mm, confined to the vulva or perineum

N0
No regional lymph node metastases

T2*
Tumor of any size with extension to adjacent perineal structures (lower/distal 1/3 urethra, lower/distal 1/3 vagina, anal involvement)

N1
One or two regional lymph nodes with the following features
(N1a) 1 lymph node metastasis each ≤5mm
(N1b)One lymph node metastasis ≥5 mm

N2
Regional lymph node metastasis with the following features
(N2a) Three or more lymph node metastases each <5 mm
(N2b)Two or more lymph node metastases ≥5 mm

T3**
Tumor of any size with extension to any of the following: upper/proximal 2/3 of urethra, upper/proximal 2/3 vagina, bladder mucosa, rectal mucosa, or fixed to pelvic bone
(N2c) Lymph node metastases with extracapsular spread
N3
Fixed or ulcerated regional lymph node metastasis
M0
No distant metastasis

M1
Distant metastasis (including pelvic lymph node metastasis)

STAGE GROUPINGS

Stage IA
T1a N0 M0

Stage IB
T1b N0 M0

Stage II
T2 N0 M0

Stage IIIA
T1, T2 N1a <5mm ◉
T1, T2 N1b >5mm ●

Stage IIIB
T1,T2 N2a ≥3 <5mm ◉
T1,T2 N2b ≥2 >5mm ●

Stage IIIC
T1,T2 N2c

Stage IVA
T1,T2 N3
T3any Nany M0

Stage IVB
Tany, Nany M1

*FIGO uses the classification T2/T3. This is defined as T2 in TNM.

**FIGO uses the classification T4. This is defined as T3 in TNM.

Figure 48.3 | TNM staging diagram arranged vertically with T definitions on the left and stage groupings on the right. Vulva cancers are most resectable when detected as stage I or II lesions; stage III requires radical vulvectomy with inguinal node dissection, often bilaterally. There are four main stages, with two substages for stages II and IV. Color bars are coded for stage: stage 0, yellow; I, green; II, blue; III, purple; IV, red; and metastatic disease to viscera and nodes, black.

T-ONCOANATOMY

ORIENTATION THREE-PLANAR ONCOANATOMY

The orientation three-planar anatomy shows the vulvar isocenter is at the level of the perineum (Fig. 48.4).

T-oncoanatomy

The T-oncoanatomy is displayed in three planar views in Fig. 48.5:

- *Coronal*: The labia majora and labia minora are folds of skin with varying degrees of fat covered by stratified squa-

mous epithelium, and covered with hair on the external surface labia majora but devoid of hair on the inner, smooth surface. The male homolog for the labia majora is the scrotum.

- *Sagittal*: The vestibule is the space surrounded by the labia minora. The clitoris is located between the labia minora and is the homolog to the erectile bodies of the male penis containing numerous capillaries and autonomic nerve fibers.

- *Transverse*: The urethra and crus of the clitoris are shown anteriorly at the vestibule of the vagina.

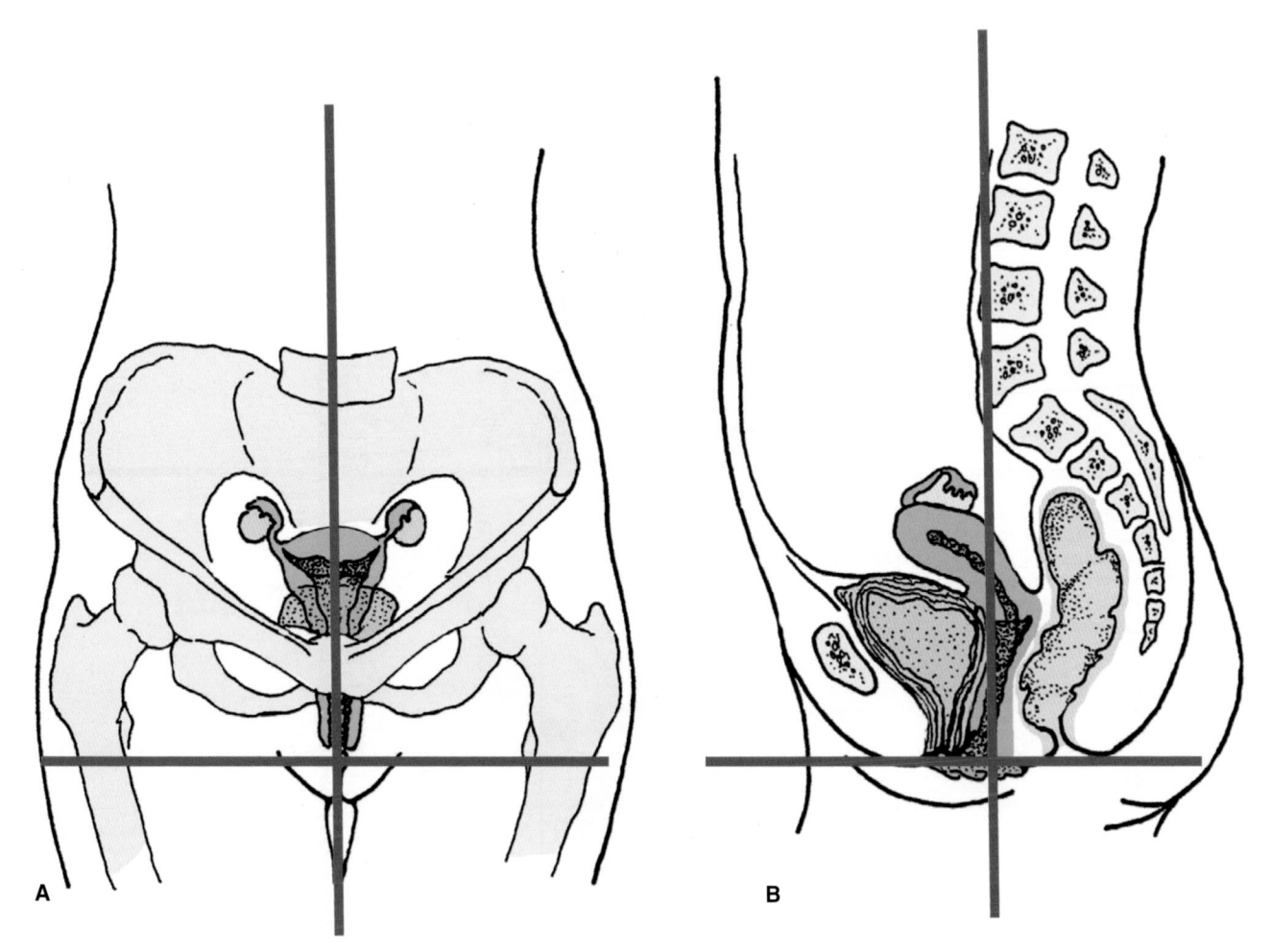

Figure 48.4 | Orientation of oncoanatomy of the vulva. The anatomic isocenter is at the midline at the vestibule of the vulva. **A.** Coronal. **B.** Sagittal.

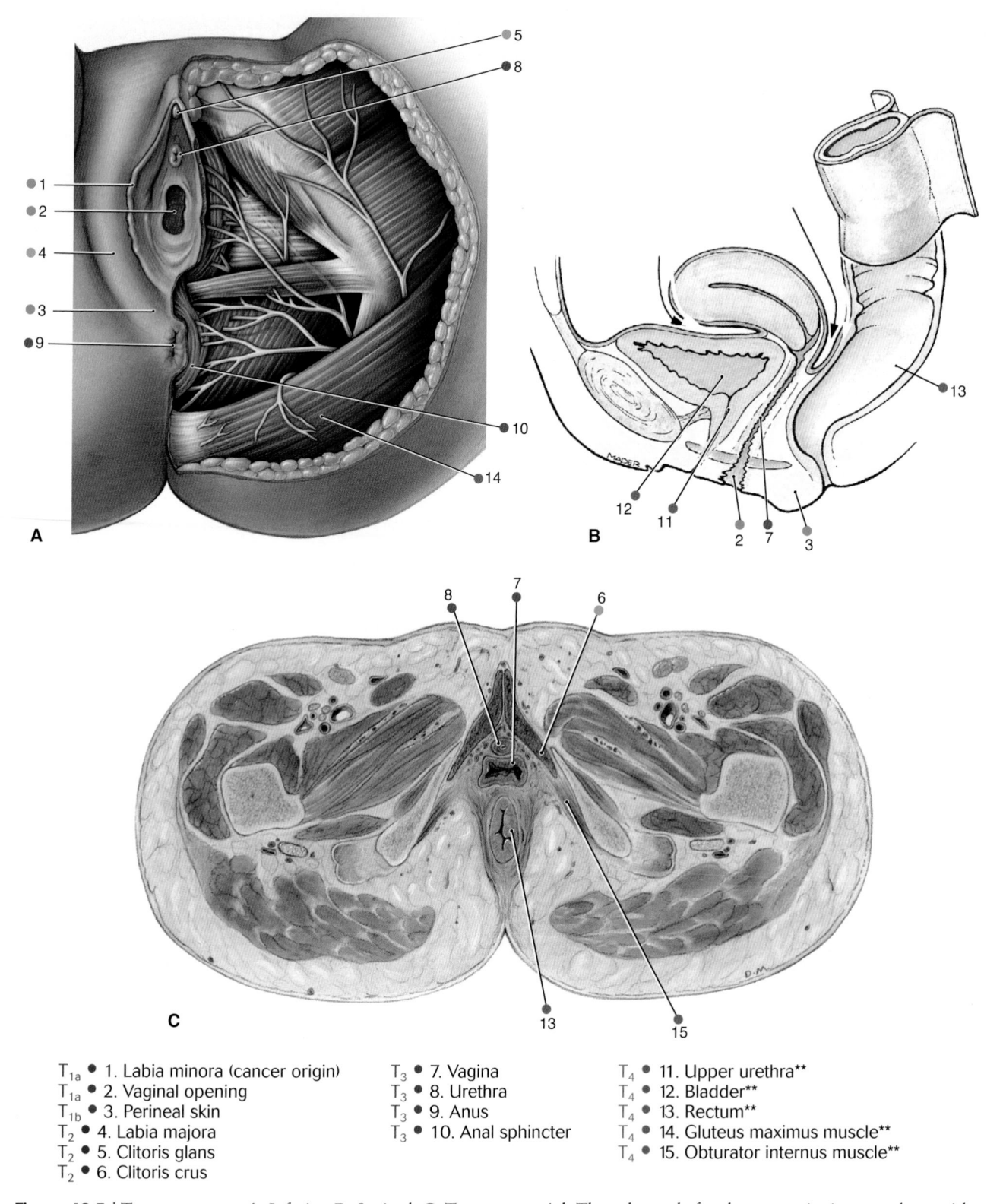

T_{1a} •	1. Labia minora (cancer origin)	T_3 •	7. Vagina	T_4 •	11. Upper urethra**
T_{1a} •	2. Vaginal opening	T_3 •	8. Urethra	T_4 •	12. Bladder**
T_{1b} •	3. Perineal skin	T_3 •	9. Anus	T_4 •	13. Rectum**
T_2 •	4. Labia majora	T_3 •	10. Anal sphincter	T_4 •	14. Gluteus maximus muscle**
T_2 •	5. Clitoris glans			T_4 •	15. Obturator internus muscle**
T_2 •	6. Clitoris crus				

Figure 48.5 | T-oncoanatomy. **A.** Inferior. **B.** Sagittal. **C.** Transverse axial. The color code for the anatomic sites correlates with the color code for the stage group (Fig. 48.3), patterns of spread (Fig. 48.2), and SIMLAP table (Table 48.2). Connecting the dots in similar colors will provide an appreciation for the three-dimensional oncoanatomy. **FIGO T_4 in the TNM is T_3.

N-ONCOANATOMY AND M-ONCOANATOMY

N-ONCOANATOMY

The femoral and inguinal nodes are the first station sentinel nodes, and spread into the external iliac pelvic nodes follows. If the cancer invades the vagina or bladder, the obturator and internal iliac nodes are at risk (Fig. 48.6A; Table 48.4).

TABLE 48.4A   Lymph Nodes of Vulva

Sentinel Nodes	Juxtaregional Nodes
Superficial femoral	External iliac
Inguinal	Contralateral inguinal
	Common iliac
	Para-aortic
Regional Nodes	
Superficial femoral	
Superficial inguinal	
Node of Cloquet	
Deep inguinal	

Since 1970, the overall incidence of lymph node metastases is approximately 30%. The relationship of clinical stage to the incidence of positive lymph nodes is shown in Table 48.4B. Based on an extensive review of the literature from 1975–1989, from 10 different sources, the depth of stromal invasion is a robust determinant of lymph node involvement (Table 48.4C).

Metastases to pelvic nodes are uncommon, the overall frequency is approximately 9%; approximately 20% of vulvar cancers with positive inguinal nodes have positive pelvic nodes. Clinical evaluation of inguinal/femoral lymph nodes prove to be inaccurate in 25–30% of patients.

Compared with surgical staging, the percentage of error in clinical staging increases from 18% in stage I to 44% in stage IV. Generally patients with negative lymph nodes have an excellent prognosis, regardless of the size of the primary tumor. Survival depends on the number of positive nodes, therefore stage IIIABC and stage IVA are a very heterogeneous group of patients.

M-ONCOANATOMY

The perineal veins drain into the femoral/inguinal, then the external iliac veins to inferior vena cava or internal pudendal veins into internal iliac veins to inferior vena cava (Fig. 48.6B). Lung is the target organ for metastases.

TABLE 48.4B   Incidence of Lymph Node Metastases in Relation to Clinical Stage of Disease

Stage	No. of Cases	Positive Nodes	Percent
I	140	15	10.7
II	145	38	26.2
III	137	88	64.2
IV	18	16	88.9

TABLE 48.4C   Nodal Status in T_1 Squamous Cell Carcinoma of the Vulva Versus Depth of Stromal Invasion

Depth of Invasion	No.	Positive Nodes	Nodes
<1 mm	163	0	0
1.1–2 mm	145	11	7.6
2.1–3 mm	131	11	8.4
3.1–5 mm	101	27	26.7
>5 mm	38	13	34.2
Total	578	62	10.7

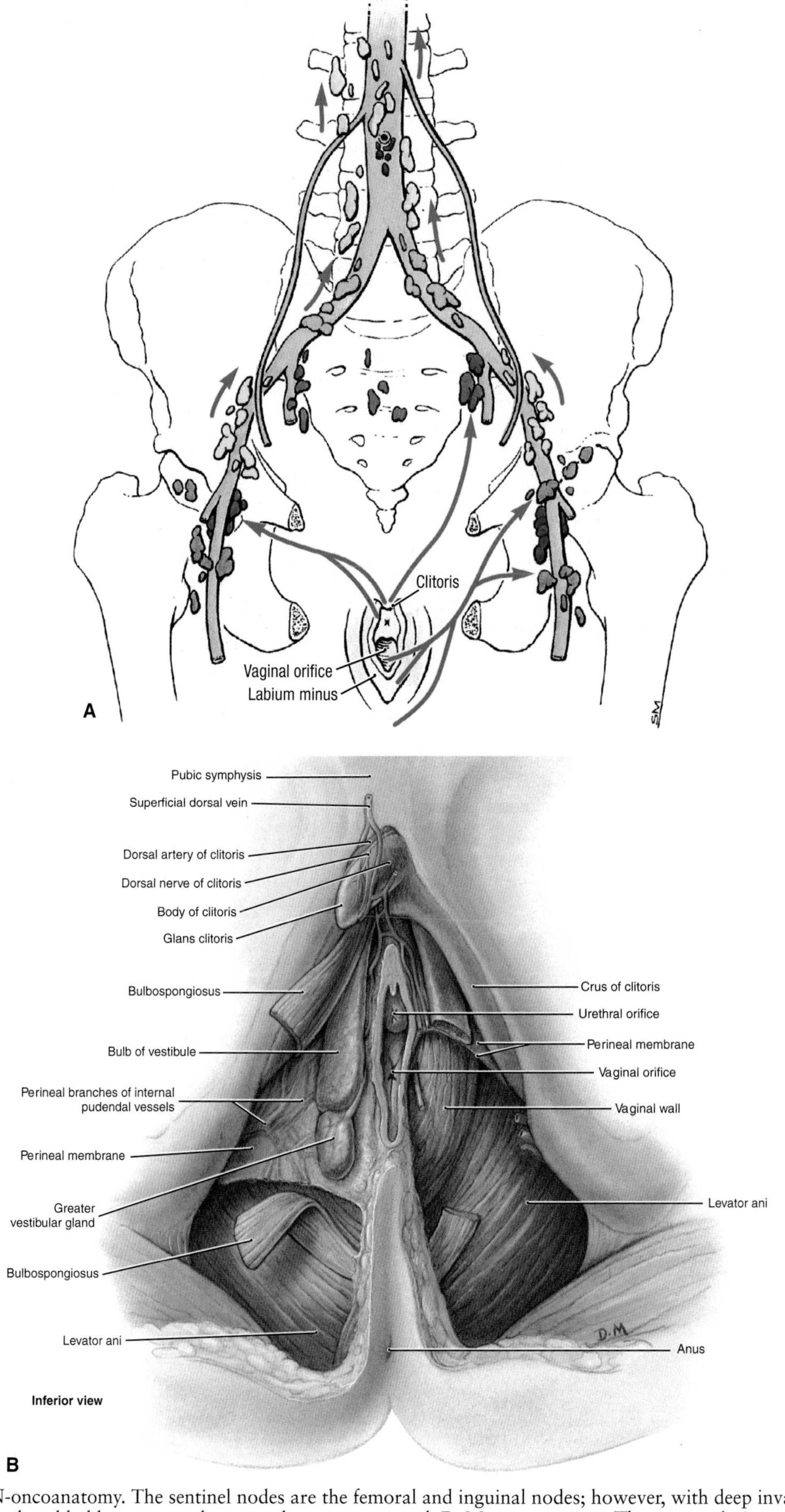

Figure 48.6 I **A.** N-oncoanatomy. The sentinel nodes are the femoral and inguinal nodes; however, with deep invasion of vagina or pelvic organs, such as bladder or anus, deeper pathways are opened. **B.** M-oncoanatomy. The venous drainage is via internal pudendal vein into the internal iliac veins to the vena cava and right heart.

STAGING WORKUP

RULES OF CLASSIFICATION AND STAGING

Clinical Staging

Clinical staging involves careful scrutiny and inspection, palpation, and speculum evaluation for vaginal and urethral extension. (If the cervix is involved, the staging is assigned similar to that for cervical carcinoma (Table 48.5; Fig. 48.7).

Surgical–pathologic Staging

Staging can be made if the resection is performed before radiation or chemotherapy. The International Federation of Gynecology and Obstetrics/American Joint Committee on Cancer/International Union Against Cancer criteria are similar to those for other skin cancers, emphasizing the 2-cm size criterion.

Oncoimaging Annotations

Imaging recommendations apply only to adnexal unresectable stage III or IV presentations that involve the vagina.

TABLE 48.5	Imaging Modalities for Staging Vulva Cancer with Vaginal Invasion	
Method	Diagnosis and Staging Capability	Recommended for Use
Primary (T) Staging		
CTe	Defines cervical involvement and tumor size, also vaginal extension	Yes, has displaced barium enema and IVP
MRI	Preferred for cross-sectional anatomy of pelvis to assess by the high signal intensity of the cancer invasion	Yes, gadolinium enhances signal intensity of cancer; recommended for TIb and higher
Nodal (N) Staging		
CTe	Excellent for assessing adenopathy and tumor necrosis in nodes	Yes, cost effective
MRI	Comparable to CT in detecting nodal disease	Yes, T and N can be simultaneously assessed
Metastases (M) Staging		
Barium enema		Yes, for patients with suspicious lesions
Bone scan		Yes, if suspected
CT	Useful to assess omental and liver metastases	Yes, if suspected
PET	Useful body scan for metastases	No, investigational

CT, computed tomography; CTe, CT enhanced with intravenous contrast; IVP, intravenous pyelography; MRI, magnetic resonance imaging; PET, positron emission tomography.

PROGNOSIS AND CANCER SURVIVAL

CANCER STATISTICS AND SURVIVAL

Female genital system cancers collectively account for 80,000 new cases per year, with uterine corpus exceeding cervix cancer by a factor of four. Both are highly curable, and deaths are relatively low. The major gynecologic killer is ovarian cancer, with 16,000 deaths annually, which exceeds that from the other six primary sites combined. Vulvar cancers are detected in early localized stages I-II yielding excellent survival rates of 98% and 85%, respectively (Fig. 48.8). As aforementioned survival decreases as lymph nodes become involved. Patients with negative lymph nodes have survival rates of approximately 81% which decrements to 13% when four or more nodes are positive. In Table 48.6, the five year survival rate, as a function of lymph node status is presented.

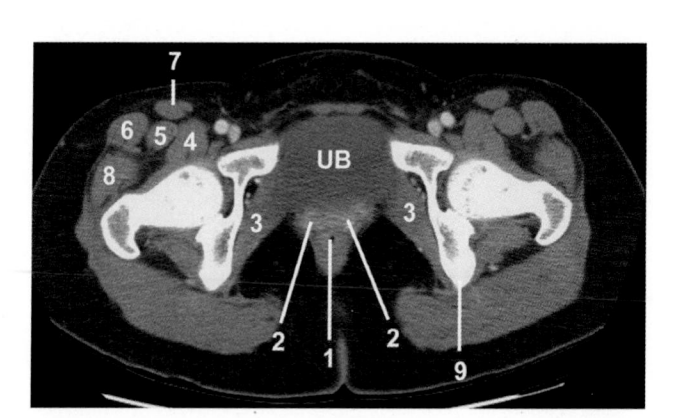

Figure 48.7 | Axial CTs of female pelvis correlate with the T-oncoanatomy transverse section (Fig. 48.5C). Oncoimaging with CT is commonly applied to staging cancers, often combined with positron emission tomography to determine the true extent of primary cancer and involved lymph nodes. (1) Anus. (2) Vagina. (3) Obturator internus muscle. (4) Iliopsoas muscle. (5) Rectus femoris muscle. (6) Tensor fasciae latae muscle. (7) Sartorius muscle. (8) Vastus lateralis muscle. (9) Ischium. UB, urinary bladder.

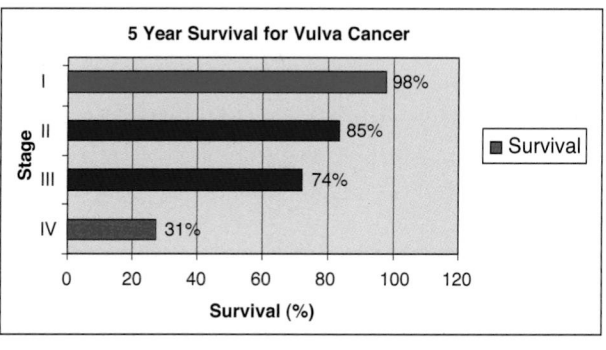

Figure 48.8 | Five-year survival rates for vulva cancer. (Edge SB, Byrd DR, and Compton CC, et al. *AJCC Cancer Staging Manual*, 7th edition. New York: Springer, 2010.)

TABLE 48.6	Five-Year Survival Versus Lymph Node Status for Squamous Cell Carcinoma of the Vulva		
Lymph Node Status	**Patients**	**5-Year Survival (%)**	**Hazard Ratio (95% CI)**
Negative	302	80.7	Reference
1 positive	66	62.9	2.1 (1.2–3.4)
2 positive	43	30.4	6.0 (3.7–9.8)
3 positive	24	19.2	5.3 (3.0–9.5)
4+ positive	62	13.3	2.6 (1.9–3.7)

Beller U, Quinn MA, Benedet JL, et al., Carcinoma of the vulva. FIGO 26th Annual Report on the Results of Treatment in Gynecological Cancer. *Int J Gynaecol Obstet* 2006; 95 Suppl 1;S7–S27.

SECTION 6
Generalized Anatomic Primary Sites

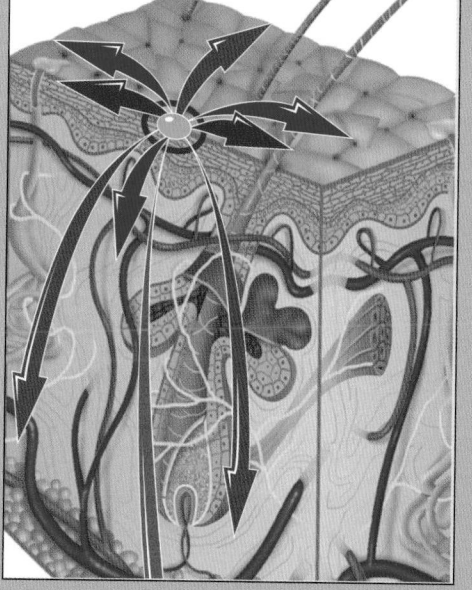

Introduction and Orientation

There is a need to view generalized systems from their embryogenesis to their histogenesis in addition to their ubiquitous anatomy to provide insights into the malignancies that arise within them.

PERSPECTIVES AND PATTERNS OF SPREAD

The generalized sites can give rise to primary tumors (T)—sarcomas rather than carcinomas—in many different anatomic sites but in addition, the lymphoid system and the circulatory system are intimately related to N and M categories, respectively. In contrast to carcinomas, sarcomas can arise in a large variety of anatomic sites because the tissues are located in the many different regions that constitute the human body architecture. Their patterns of spread depend on the exact site of tumor origin. The anatomy that will be portrayed will largely be the extremities.

Each generalized anatomic site (GAS) will be concisely reviewed in this introduction.

The GASs are the ectoderm integument system and mesodermal systems, that is, connective tissues, musculoskeletal and lymphoid, with a wide spectrum of cell types.

Thus, the GAS's TNM staging is complex conceptually; in addition there are an infinite number of potential geographic loci in a GAS tissue. Each GAS normal tissue consists of a variety of cell types, which results in a wide array of histopathologic classifications. The complexity is in applying one TNM staging system when the tumor can be located in numerous and varied geographic anatomic regions. Each major generalized system will be presented more from the histogenic than the anatomic perspective.

The spread of lymphatic and hematogenous metastases varies with body anatomy site.

In embryogenesis, the vertebrate body plan is established by the HOX genes and forms a surface ectoderm, a mesoderm, and an endoderm. Each somite differentiates into a dermatome, a myotome, and a sclerotome with a section of the splanchnopleura, the primordium of the visceral organs (Fig. 49.1).

- The *ectoderm* forms the integument, composed of a keratinized epithelial layer with glands and invagination with a large variety of cells that can transform into tumors.

- The *mesoderm* is a dense cellular tissue surrounded by mesenchyme and gives rise to the musculoskeletal system, soft connective tissue of dermis, gastrointestinal (GI) tract connective tissue stroma, and the cardiac mesoderm. The embryonic cardinal system of the veins will develop an extensive network of arteries and veins postnatally. The formation of endothelium and primitive blood cells comes from condensation of mesenchyme. Capillaries of vessels and lymphatics form in the base mesenchyme of each organ. The mesenchyme forms the lymphatic system as part of other organs such as tonsils, vermiform appendix, gut-associated tissues, the respiratory system with its bronchus-associated lymphatic system (BALT), and various mucous membranes (MALTs). The ability to detect antigens that are self versus foreign is inherent to three major types of lymphocytes: B cells, T cells, and NK cells. These immunocompetent cells each has its specific identity and functions, giving rise to a highly varied list of lymphomas. *T lymphocytes* account for the majority of circulating lymphocytes and differentiate in the thymus. B lymphocytes differentiate in bursa of Fabricius–like organs from γ-interferon–inducible lysosomal thiol reductase and bone marrow.

- *Endoderm* or gut tube provides the epithelial lining of various viscera and systems, including the respiratory and digestive systems, and some of the parenchyma of organs such as liver, pancreas, urinary bladder, urethra, thyroid, and parathyroid glands. This germ layer gives rise to a large variety of cancers.

To recapitulate: The anatomic odyssey through 60 anatomic sites is based largely on carcinomas and on concepts of regional anatomy and TNM cancer staging. Three-dimensional oncoanatomy is conceived on patterns of cancer spread. That is, each cancer is assigned to a designated anatomic isocenter in which the major common cancers arise. The primary tumor (T) pattern of spread is then presented in six basic directions: superior–inferior, medial–lateral, and anterior–posterior (SIMLAP). Each cancer site has specific sentinel and regional lymphatic and nodal drainage (N) and venous drainage to a target organ (M).

- *The segmented human body plan* consists of somites arranged along three axes: caudiocranial or superior inferior and medial lateral and anterior posterior (Fig. 49.1).

- Each segment consists of annealed trigeminal layers.

- These trigeminal somites provide specific landmarks that can serve as references.

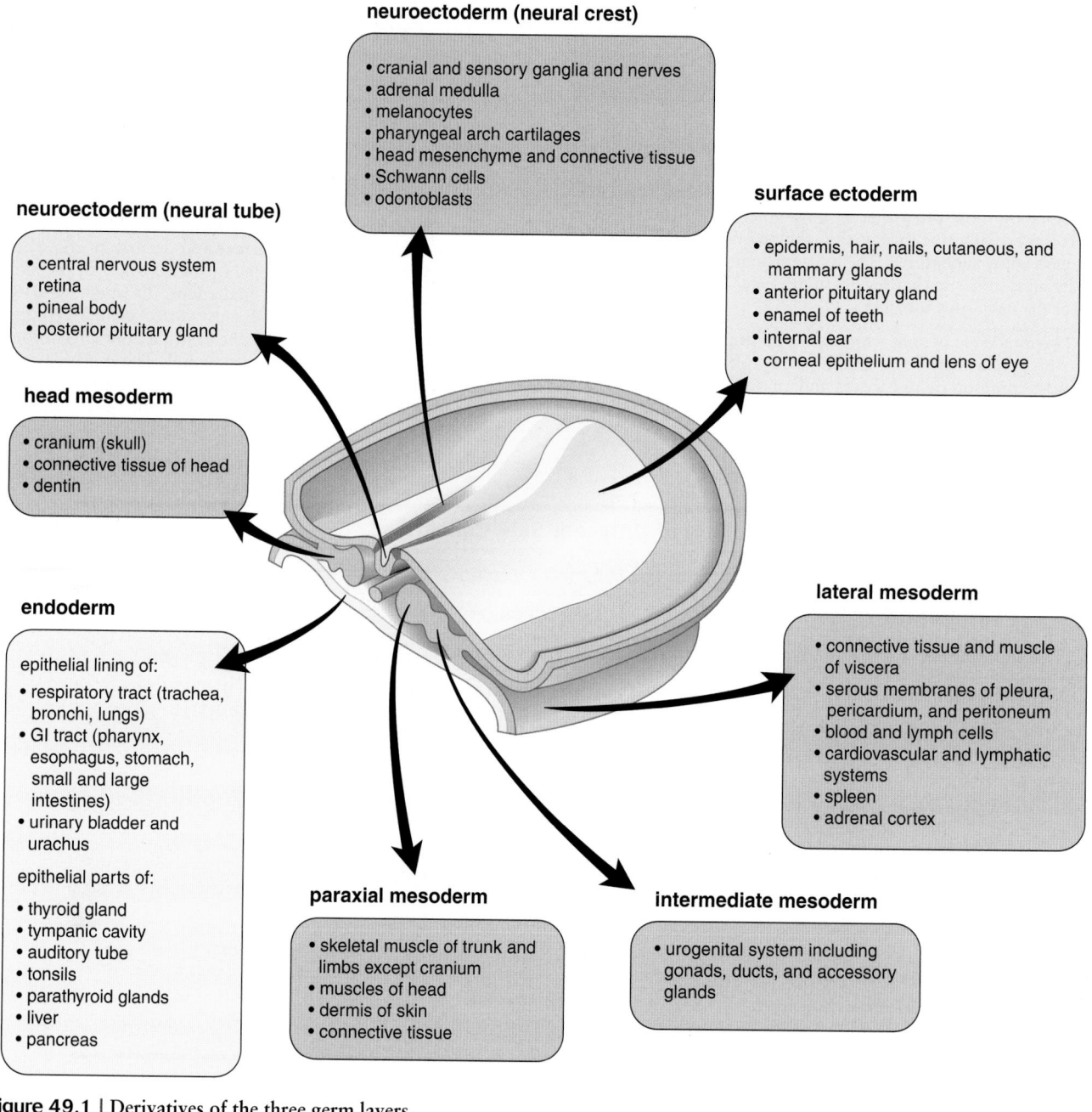

neuroectoderm (neural crest)
- cranial and sensory ganglia and nerves
- adrenal medulla
- melanocytes
- pharyngeal arch cartilages
- head mesenchyme and connective tissue
- Schwann cells
- odontoblasts

surface ectoderm
- epidermis, hair, nails, cutaneous, and mammary glands
- anterior pituitary gland
- enamel of teeth
- internal ear
- corneal epithelium and lens of eye

neuroectoderm (neural tube)
- central nervous system
- retina
- pineal body
- posterior pituitary gland

head mesoderm
- cranium (skull)
- connective tissue of head
- dentin

endoderm

epithelial lining of:
- respiratory tract (trachea, bronchi, lungs)
- GI tract (pharynx, esophagus, stomach, small and large intestines)
- urinary bladder and urachus

epithelial parts of:
- thyroid gland
- tympanic cavity
- auditory tube
- tonsils
- parathyroid glands
- liver
- pancreas

lateral mesoderm
- connective tissue and muscle of viscera
- serous membranes of pleura, pericardium, and peritoneum
- blood and lymph cells
- cardiovascular and lymphatic systems
- spleen
- adrenal cortex

paraxial mesoderm
- skeletal muscle of trunk and limbs except cranium
- muscles of head
- dermis of skin
- connective tissue

intermediate mesoderm
- urogenital system including gonads, ducts, and accessory glands

Figure 49.1 | Derivatives of the three germ layers.

The anatomic neoplastic odyssey, in addition to the 60 specific primary sites, includes six generalized anatomic systems: the integumentary system, the musculoskeletal systems, and the lymphoid and hematopoietic systems. The sixth system, the cardiovascular system, is low in incidence for primary tumors, but is the major distribution and transport means of circulating cancer cells to distant and remote sites. Unlike specific site cancers, these malignancies can arise in a large variety of locations, making them a true challenge to diagnose, stage, and manage.

INTEGUMENT SYSTEM

Perspective

The skin and its derivative cellular elements consist largely of keratinized squamous epithelial cells with numerous distinct cell types resting on connective tissue dermis, each of which can result in a tumor. The integument can be transformed into malignancy most often due to ultraviolet rays from the sun. This is especially true for fair skin-skinned people and individuals who enjoy sunbathing. The integumentary system (Fig. 49.2) is the anatomic site that results in more cancers than all of the other primary sites together.

- *The incidence of skin cancers* has continued to rise rapidly over the last 30 years (Table 49.1). Skin cancers are the most common of all cancers and among the most preventable. In the United States alone, 900,000 to 1,200,000 new cases are predicted each year. The high curability of basal and squamous cell skin cancers reduces the threat to life, but disfigurement can occur in individuals who are predisposed genetically (xeroderma pigmentosa), children irradiated for acne treatment, or sun worshippers, owing to the multiplicity of lesions. Basal cell cancers rarely spread.

- *Melanomas* are the antithesis to ordinary skin cancers, in that widespread metastases can occur with these malignancies, which are measured in millimeters. Essential to understanding the TNM staging system is the need to study the cellular complexity of epidermal and dermal layers. There are a myriad of different cells, up to 20 to 25 in the skin, each of which can become malignant. To understand the biologic behavior of these highly varied cellular components, an understanding of the cellular and physiologic activities of the integument is essential. The melanocyte at the epidermal–dermal interface is a cell with long dendritic processes that extend between cells into the basal stratum.

TABLE 49.1	Histopathology of Different Skin Cancers
Normal Cell	**Cancer Derivative**
Stratum basal	Basal cell cancer
Keratinocyte	Squamous cell cancer
Stratum spinosum	Intraepithelial cancer (Bowen's disease)
Stratum granulosum	Kerotoacanthoma
Merkel cell	Merkel cell cancer
Melanocyte	Melanoma
Adnexal merocrine gland	Adenocarcinoma
Langerhans cell	Histiocytosis X
T cell	Mycosis fungoides
B cell	Cutaneous lymphomas
Endothelial cell	Kaposi sarcoma
Fibroblast	Fibrosarcoma

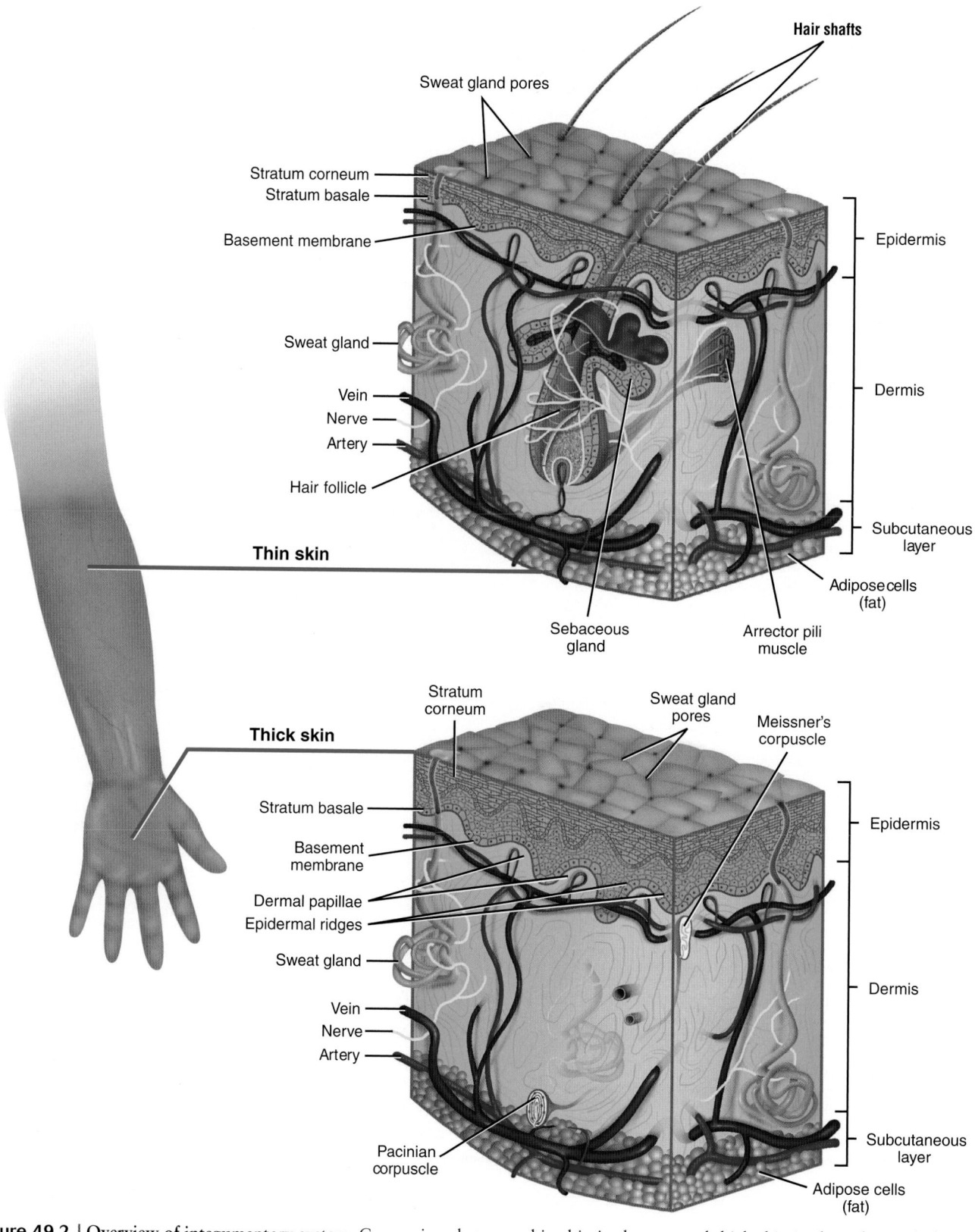

Figure 49.2 | Overview of integumentary system. Comparison between thin skin in the arm and thick skin in the palm, including contents of the connective tissue dermis.

SOFT TISSUE SYSTEMS

Perspective

Musculoskeletal systems consist of soft tissues as connective tissue (Fig. 49.3A) and muscle (Fig. 49.3B), each of which can give rise to malignancies that are referred to as sarcomas rather than carcinomas.

- *Soft tissue sarcomas* are a unique class of tumors, distinct from skin cancers. As a class, soft tissue tumors are highly varied despite their origin from the omnipresent mesenchymal cell. The mesenchymal cell, through a derepression process, can proliferate and dedifferentiate, yielding multiple histopathologic subtypes (Table 49.2). The degree of malignancy is based more on the tumor grade than on the tissue type and in fact dominates in TNM staging and classification over anatomic extent of the malignant infiltration. There are many nuances and clinical challenges for the same tumor types in different parts of the anatomy. Soft tissue tumors arising in the extremity are more manageable and favorable than those in truncal and axial locations. Of particular note is the predominance of soft tissue sarcomas in children and the relative rarity of epithelial cancers, which is the reverse of the situation with regard to adult malignancies. Muscle per se can give rise to a variety of sarcomas, reflecting the type of muscle cell. Most rhabdosarcomas are embryonal and occur in childhood. An element of gene deletions and overexpression is often associated, with both benign and malignant growth abnormalities being present in pediatric populations. Proto-oncogenes can be expressed in these circumstances, providing genetic and chromosomal biomarkers that may be useful in the future for staging.

The mesenchymal soft tissue and muscle compartments contain a highly variegated population of cell types. Each derivative normal cell can yield a malignancy. The pediatric population is prone to develop sarcomas rather than carcinomas in view of accelerated musculoskeletal growth early in childhood (1 to 6 years) and in adolescence (12 to 18 years).

TABLE 49.2	Histopathologic Types of Soft Tissue Sarcomas
Type	**Derivative Normal Cell**
Alveolar soft-part sarcoma	Neuromyogenic cell
Desmoplastic small round-cell tumor	Epithelioid endothelial
Epithelioid sarcoma	Fascial tendon fibrocyte
Clear cell sarcoma	Primitive mesenchymal
Chondrosarcoma, extraskeletal	Chondroblast
Osteosarcoma, extraskeletal	Osteoblast
Gastrointestinal stromal tumor	Leiomyoblast
Ewing's sarcoma/primitive neuroectodermal tumor	Primitive mesenchymal
Fibrosarcoma	Fibroblast
Leiomyosarcoma	Smooth myocyte
Liposarcoma	Adipolyte
Malignant fibrous histiocytoma	Fibroblast/histiocyte
Malignant hemangiopericytoma	Pericytes
Malignant peripheral nerve sheath tumor	Neurilemma (Schwann)
Rhabdomyosarcoma	Myofibroblast
Synovial sarcoma	Biphasic synovial epithelial cell
Sarcoma, not otherwise specified	Mesenchymal cell

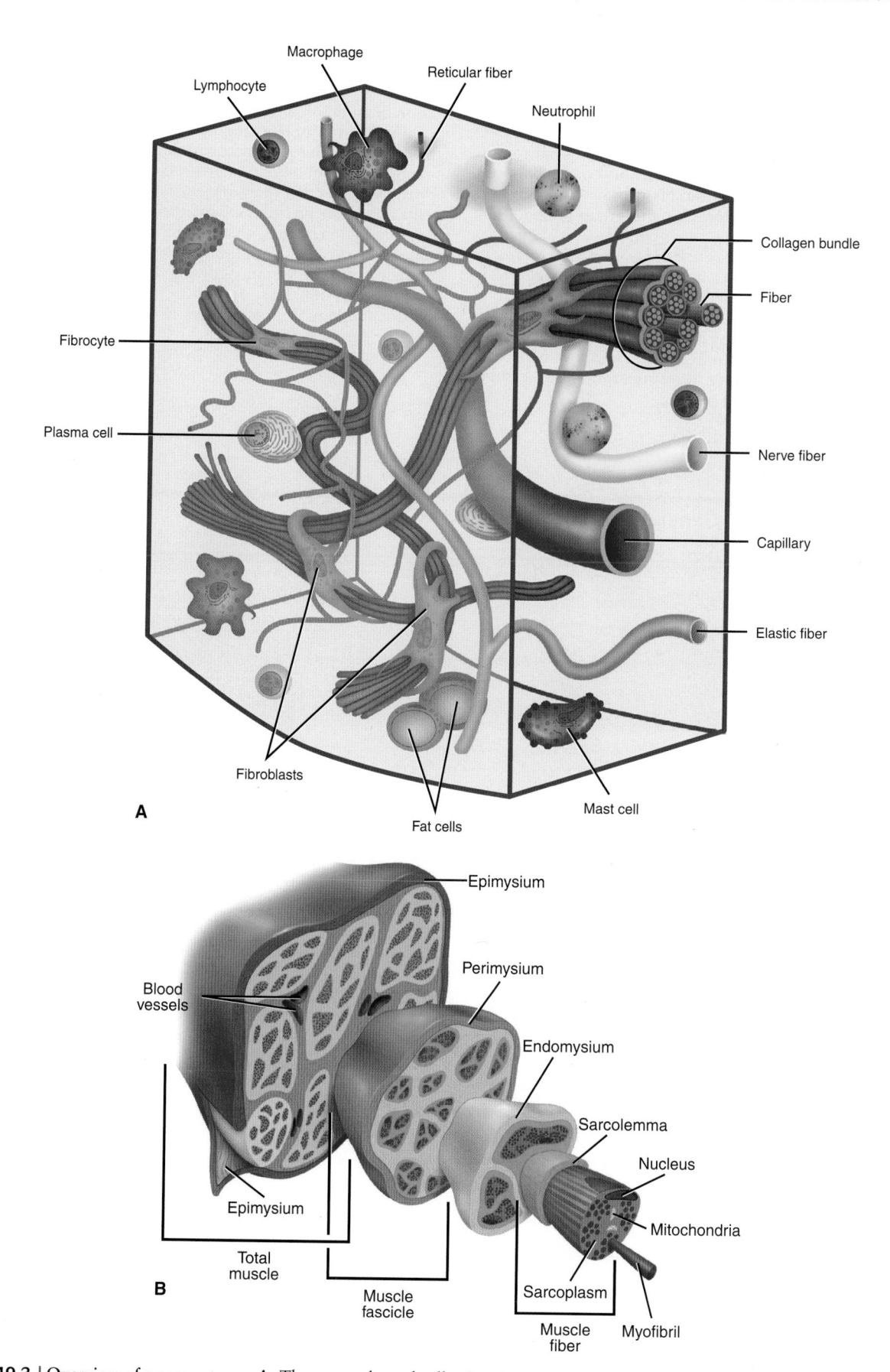

Figure 49.3 | **Overview of oncoanatomy. A.** The mesenchymal cells give rise to a variety of loose connective tissue (LCT) elements and include fibrocytes, fibroblasts, adipocytes, macrophages, and mast cells, which include both collagen and reticular and elastic fibers. **B.** Muscle compartments are composed of muscle cells and, in addition, cardiac muscle. Muscle cells are multinucleated and tend to hypertrophy rather than undergo hyperplasia.

OSSEOUS SYSTEMS

Perspective

- *Bone tumors*: The classification and staging of bone tumors has been as varied as their malignant histopathologic typing, which often requires supplementary radiographic images to ascertain their location and origin (Table 49.3). Again, as in other sarcomas, the grade impacts staging, as does anatomic extent, but to a lesser degree than anatomic size. Rules for classification allow for the use of imaging technologies ranging from magnetic resonance imaging (MRI) to computed tomography (CT) and, to some extent, radioisotope ^{99m}Tc scanning. Biopsy is an essential aspect of staging and needs to be thoughtfully located to allow for subsequent en bloc bone tumor resection for more accurate histopathology typing and grading.

The anatomic aspects of skeletal growth are essential to understanding biologic behavior and patterns of spread of osseous malignancies (Fig. 49.4). The fundamental organization of bone formation as endochondral or intramembranous is the key to appreciating how the skeleton grows, models, and remodels into compact and cancellous bone. Each bone—long, short, cuboid, and flat—is organized and grows differently as a function of age. Malignant tumors tend to occur in sites of major growth activity, that is, the distal or proximal physis of long bone, that is, the distal femur or proximal humeral physis. Neoplasms are more likely to occur at puberty and in young, growing adults than in the elderly because of the loss of mitotic potential with age. The histopathology of bone tumors is highly varied and depends on the derivative normal cell.

TABLE 49.3	**General Classification of Bone Tumors**	
Histologic Type[a]	**Benign**	**Malignant**
Hematopoietic (41.4%)	—	Myeloma
	—	Reticulum cell sarcoma
Chondrogenic (20.9%)	Osteochondroma	Primary chondrosarcoma
	Chondroma	Secondary chondrosarcoma
	Chondroblastoma	Dedifferentiated chondrosarcoma
	Chondromyxoid fibroma	Mesenchymal chondrosarcoma
Osteogenic (19.3%)	Osteoid osteoma	Osteosarcoma
	Benign osteoblastoma	Parosteal osteogenic sarcoma
Unknown origin (9.8%)	Giant cell tumor	Ewing's tumor
	—	Malignant giant cell tumor
	—	Adamantinoma
	(Fibrous) histiocytoma	(Fibrous) histiocytoma
Fibrogenic (3.8%)	Fibroma	Fibrosarcoma
	Desmoplastic fibroma	—
Notochordal (3.1%)	—	Chordoma
Vascular (1.6%)	Hemangioma	Hemangioendothelioma
	—	Hemangiopericytoma
Lipogenic (<0.5%)	Lipoma	—
Neurogenic (<0.5%)	Neurilemmoma	—

[a]Distribution based on Mayo Clinic experience.
From Malawer MM, Helman LJ, and O'Sullivan, B. Sarcomas of Bone in DeVita, Jr. VT, Lawrence TS, and Rosenberg SA (eds). *DeVita, Hellman, and Rosenberg's Cancer: Principles and Practice of Oncology, 9th edition.* Philadelphia, Lippincott Williams & Wilkins, 2011. Table 116.1, p. 1580.
Adapted from Dahlin DC. *Bone Tumors: General Aspects and Data on 6,221 Cases.* 3rd ed. Springfield, IL: Charles C Thomas, 1978, with permission.

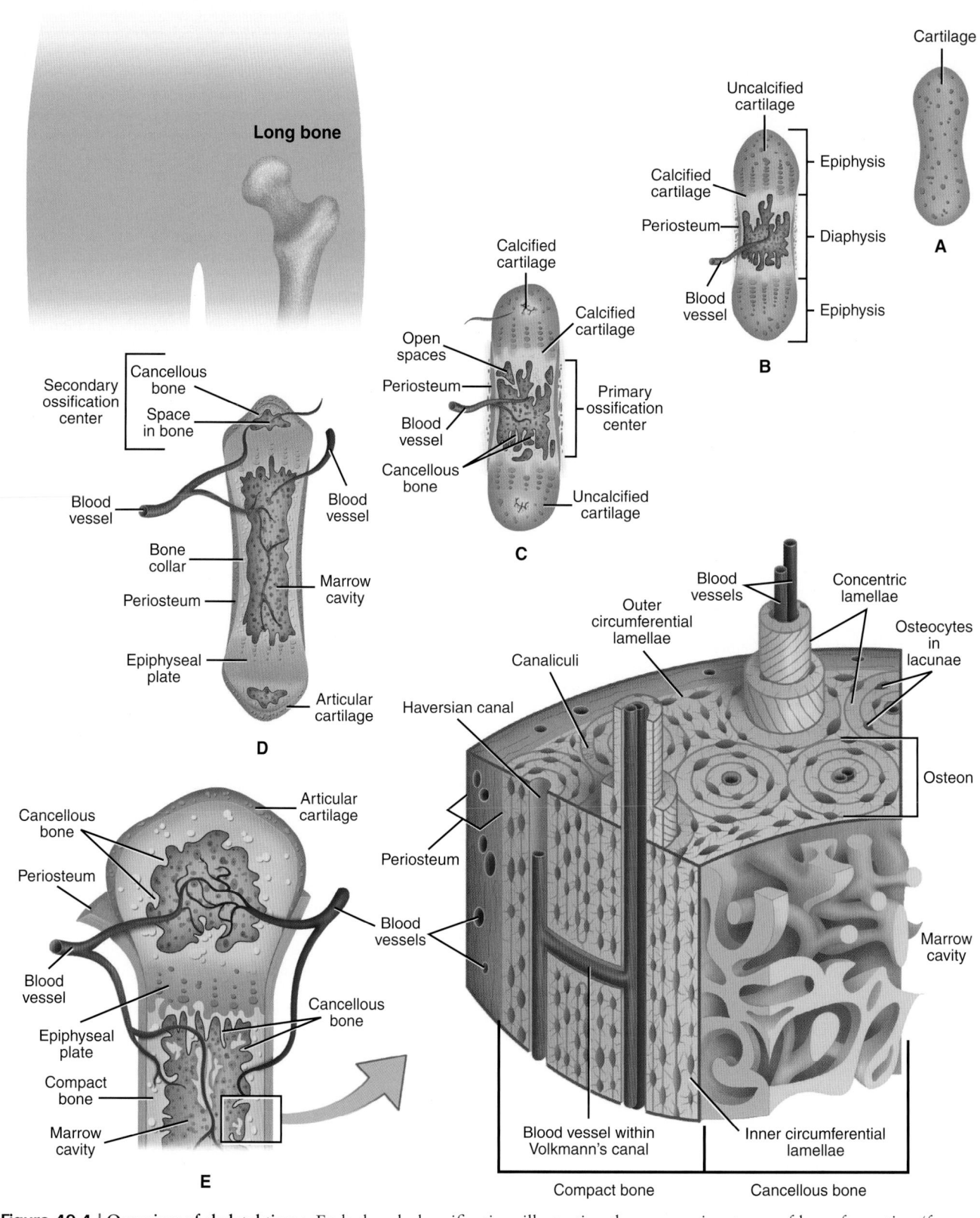

Figure 49.4 | Overview of skeletal tissue. Endochondral ossification, illustrating the progressive stages of bone formation (from cartilage model to bone) and including the histology of a section of formed bone.

LYMPHOID SYSTEM

Perspective

The lymphoid system (Fig. 49.5) is ubiquitously distributed, and lymphomas affect all age groups. The lymphoid system consists of an elaborate fine network of channels that drain into a lymphatic chain of nodes, eventually emptying into the right lymphatic duct or thoracic duct. In addition to regional lymph nodes, there are numerous extranodal collections of lymphoid tissue. The lymphoid system, although generally associated with the nodal category of cancer spread, has a large variety of B cell and T cell lymphomas (Table 49.4).

- *Hodgkin's disease*: The staging of anatomic extent in both Hodgkin's disease and lymphoma led to the term "lymph node regions" (LNR) defined in 1965. Although they are not based on any physiologic or natural anatomic bound-

aries, LNRs have become accepted by clinical consensus. The diaphragm acts as the great divide, with the cisterna chyli located inferior to the right diaphragmatic leaf and giving rise to the thoracic duct, which courses through the thorax, where it crosses over to the left side at T4 and terminates in the left neck. The anatomy of lymphomas in terms of "lymph node–bearing regions" needs to be reconciled with "regional first-station nodes" of normal anatomic structures that constitute organ primary sites that give rise to cancer. Extranodal sites are "E," although in some sense they are equivalent to the "T" of cancers. The concept of retrograde spread from a lymph node to a structure such as Waldeyer's ring or lung may be treated as a subgroup of stage, namely, IIE, whereas bone marrow, liver, pleura, or cerebrospinal fluid requires a stage IV disseminated designation.

- *Lymphomas* are a heterogeneous group of malignancies that often present as either limited or diffuse adenopathy.

TABLE 49.4

B Cell Neoplasms	T Cell Neoplasms
Precursor	*Precursor*
B-Lymphoblastic leukemia/lymphoma (B cell acute lymphoblastic leukemia)	T-Lymphoblastic lymphoma/leukemia (T cell acute lymphoblastic leukemia)
Mature (Peripheral) B Cell Neoplasms	*Mature (Peripheral) T/NK Cell Neoplasms*
• Chronic lymphocytic leukemia/small lymphocytic lymphoma • B cell prolymphocytic leukemia • Lymphoplasmacytic lymphoma • Splenic marginal zone B cell lymphoma (with or without villous lymphocytes) • Hairy cell diseases • Splenic lymphoma/leukemia, unclassifiable • Plasma cell myeloma/plasmacytoma • Heavy chain diseases • Extranodal marginal zone B cell lymphoma (with or without monocytoid B cells) • Follicular lymphoma • Primary cutaneous follicle center lymphoma • Mantle cell lymphoma • Diffuse large B cell lymphoma (DLBCL) • Diffuse large B cell lymphoma, not otherwise specified • T cell/histiocyte rich large B cell lymphoma • DLBCL associated with chronic inflammation • EBV-positive DLBCL of the elderly • Lymphomatoid granulomatosis • Primary mediastinal (thymic) large B cell lymphoma • Intravascular large B cell lymphoma • Primary cutaneous DLBCL, leg type • ALK-positive DLBCL • Plasmablastic lymphoma • Primary effusion lymphoma • Large B cell lymphoma arising in HHV8-associated multicentric Castleman's disease • Burkitt lymphoma/Burkitt cell leukemia • B cell lymphoma, unclassifiable, with features intermediate between those of diffuse large B cell lymphoma and Burkitt's lymphoma • B cell lymphoma, unclassifiable, with features intermediate between those of diffuse large B cell lymphoma and classical Hodgkin's lymphoma	• T cell prolymphocytic leukemia • T cell large granular lymphocytic leukemia • Aggressive NK cell leukemia • Systematic EBV-positive T cell lymphoproliferative disease of childhood (associated with chronic active EBV infection) • Hydroa vacciniforme–like lymphoma • Adult T cell lymphoma/leukemia (HTLV 1+) • Extranodal NK/T cell lymphoma, nasal type • Enteropathy-type T cell lymphoma • Hepatosplenic T cell lymphoma • Subcutaneous pannicullitis-like T cell lymphoma • Mycosis fungoides/Sézary syndrome • Primary cutaneous anaplastic large-cell lymphoma • Primary cutaneous aggressive epidermotropic CD8-positive cytotoxic T cell lymphoma • Primary cutaneous gamma-delta T cell lymphoma • Primary cutaneous small/medium CD4-positive T cell lymphoma • Peripheral T cell lymphoma, not otherwise characterized • Angioimmunoblastic T cell lymphoma • Anaplastic large-cell lymphoma, ALK-positive • Anaplastic large-cell lymphoma, ALK-negative

ALK, anaplastic lymphoma kinase; EBV, Epstein–Barr virus; HHV8, human herpes virus 8; HTLV 1, human T-cell lymphotropic virus 1.
Used with the permission of the American Joint Committee on Cancer (AJCC) Chicago, Illinois. The original source for this material is the *AJCC Cancer Staging Manual*, Seventh edition (2010) published by Springer SBM, LLC, p 602. WHO Classification of lymphoid neoplasms, 4th ed.

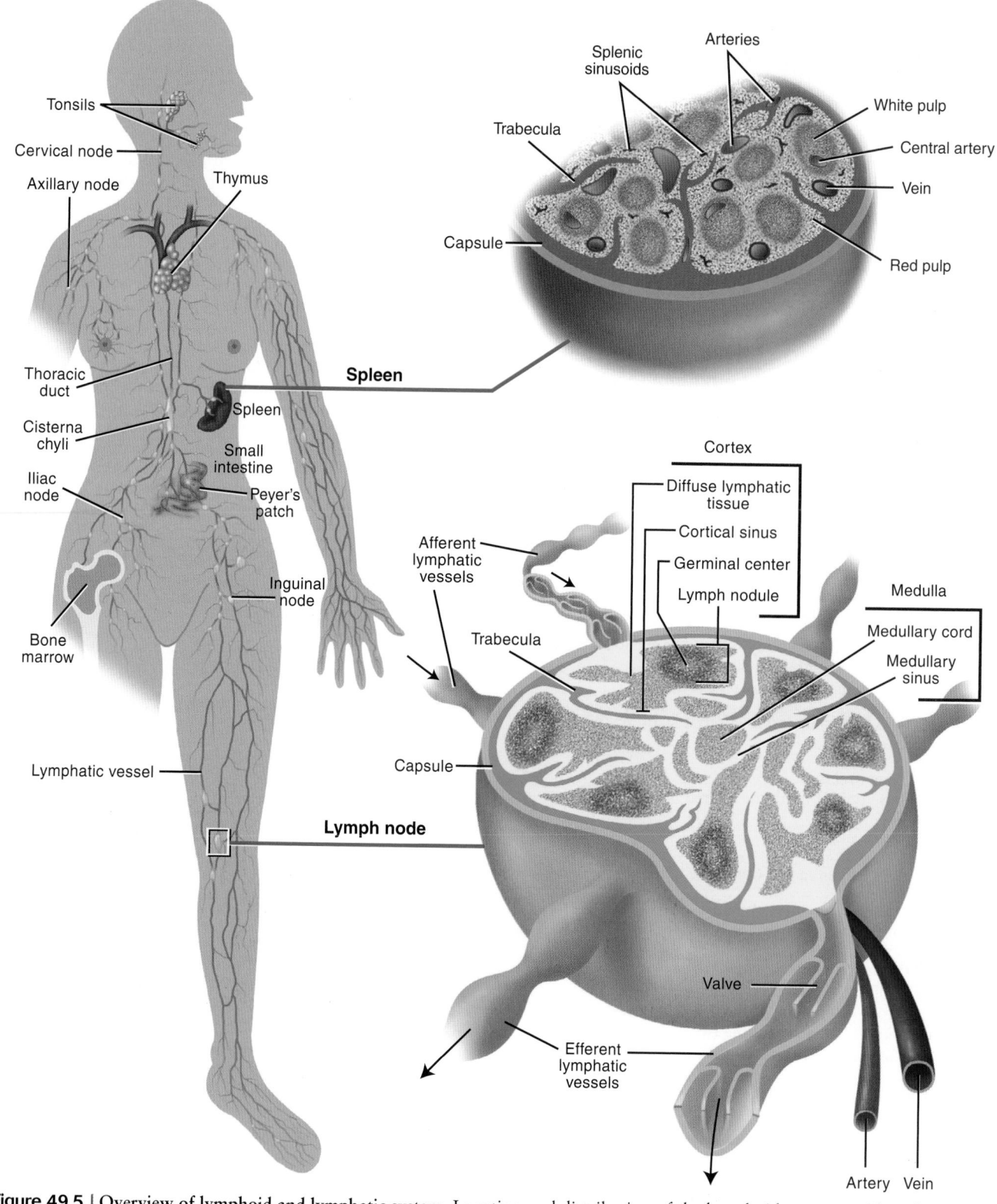

Figure 49.5 | Overview of lymphoid and lymphatic system. Location and distribution of the lymphoid organs and lymphatic channels in the body. Internal contents of the lymph node and spleen are illustrated in greater detail.

The classification of lymphoid malignancies has mutated to its present diversity because of the continual progress of immunobiology, which is superimposed on descriptive histopathology. Immunophenotyping and genetic features have resulted in 25 different categories of lymphoma, including Hodgkin's disease. The Revised European–American Classification is now the standard adopted by the World Health Organization, which has B cell and the T cell/natural killer cells as the great divide. The staging workup to determine anatomic extent is demanding because numerous ancillary procedures include sophisticated imaging, exploratory procedures, and biopsy proof of involvement.

- *Mycosis fungoides* is a primary cutaneous T cell lymphoma that involves soft tissues and regional lymph nodes and has a TNM classification that is clinically used and deserves to be maintained.

HEMATOPOIETIC SYSTEM

Perspective

The hematopoietic system (Fig. 49.6B) is constituted by the bone marrow and its cellular products in the blood. The bone marrow, although intimately related to the lymphoid system in a neoplastic sense, is integrated with bone anatomically. Fetal bone marrow at birth occupies the shaft of all long bones in their medullary cavity and then recedes at puberty and adolescence to proximal portions of the humerus and femur.

- *Multiple myelomas*: Multiple myeloma is a neoplastic disorder characterized by a single clone of plasma cells, believed to be derived from B cells. Diffuse, small, lytic bone lesions are more common than solitary plasmacytomas, which are highly curable. For the diagnosis of multiple myeloma, 10% of bone marrow cells on aspiration need to be plasma cells; the production of monoclonal (M) protein encountered in serum and urine is characteristic of this disease.

- The *leukemias* have not been included in TNM classification and are considered disseminated diseases; anatomic staging per se may not be relevant. However, these diseases of white blood cells are either myeloid or lymphoid neoplasms and provide a view of the future, in that molecular biology technology has enabled the identification of leukemia-specific cytogenetic and molecular signatures. The correlation of clinicopathologic courses and a specific cytogenetic marker can lead to the development and use of specific targeted therapy to molecular events. The ability to detect minimal residual disease provides a sharper endpoint to terminate aggressive cyclic chemotherapy and/or radiation regimens. Generally, leukemias are divided into acute or chronic, depending on whether the clonal hematopoietic stem cell disorder is characterized by arrested differentiation of stem cells leading to immature blast cells. This block in differentiation may occur in hematopoietic lineages, before lineage commitment, or during developmental stages within a lineage.

TABLE 49.5A	WHO Classification of Acute Myeloid Leukemia (AML)

Acute myeloid leukemia with recurrent genetic abnormalities

AML with t(8;21)(q22;q22);(AML 1/ETO)
AML with abnormal bone marrow eosinophils inv(16)(p13q22) or t(16;16)(p13;q22):(CBFβ/MY<H1>1)
Acute promyelocytic leukemia (AML with t(15;17)(q22;q12)(PML/RARα) and variants (M3)
AML with 11q23 (MML) abnormalities

Acute myeloid leukemia with multilineage dysplasia

Following a myelodysplastic syndrome or myelodysplastic syndrome/myeloproliferative disorder
Without antecedent myelodysplastic syndrome

Acute myeloid leukemia and myelodysplastic syndromes, therapy-related

Alkylating agent related
Topoisomerase type II inhibitor related (some may be lymphoid)
Other types

Acute myeloid leukemia not otherwise categorized

AML minimally differentiated (**M0**)
AML without maturation (**M1**)
AML with maturation (**M2**)
AML (**M4**)
Acute monoblastic and monocytic leukemia (**M5**)
Acute erythroid leukemia (**M6**)
Acute megakaryoblastic leukemia (**M7**)

MML = myelomonocytic leukemia; PML = promyelocytic leukemia; RAR = retinoic acid receptor; WHO = World Health Organization.

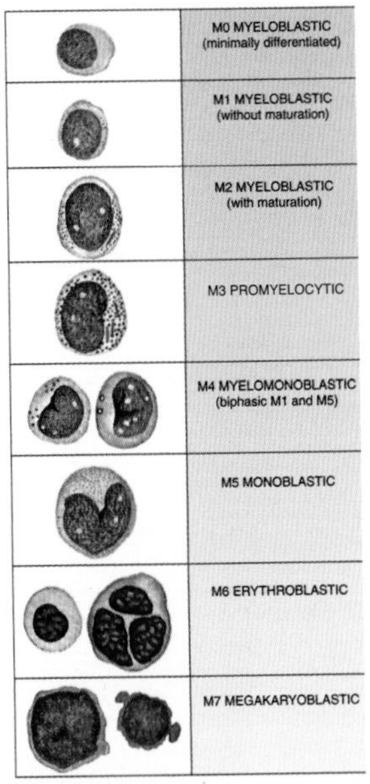

Figure 49.6A | Morphology of acute myeloid leukemia (AML) in the traditional French-American-British (FAB) classification, now within the framework of the World Health Organization (WHO) classification "AML—not otherwise categorized." *(continued)*

TABLE 49.5B	Chronic Myeloproliferative Syndromes			
	Chronic Myelogenous Leukemia	Polycynthemia Vera	Chronic Idiopathic Myelofibrosis	Essential Thrombocythemia
Acute Leukemia Conversion	80%	5–10%	5–10%	2–5%
Bone Marrow Histopathology	Panhyperplasia (predominately granulocytic)	Panhyperplasia (predominately erythroid)	Panhyperplasia with fibrosis	Large megakaryocytes in clusters
Genetics	Philadelphia chromosome: BCR/ABL gene	JAK2	JAK2	JAK2

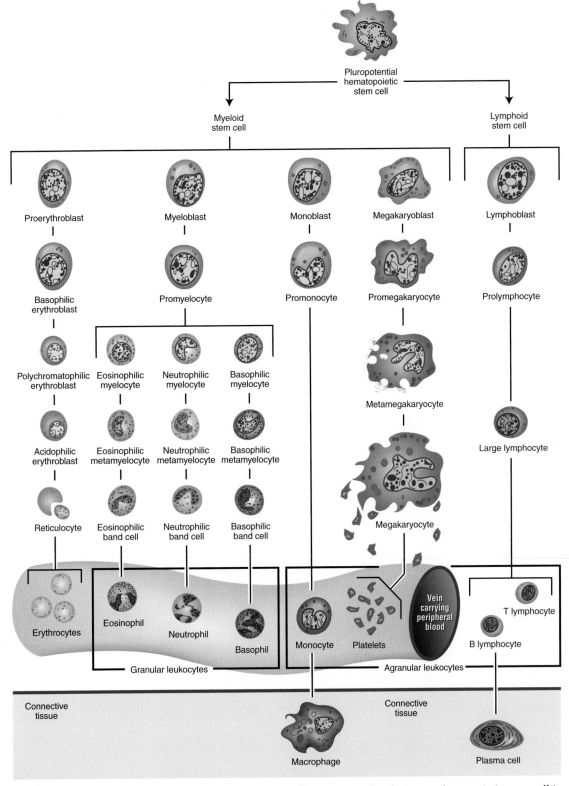

Figure 49.6B | *(Continued)* **Overview of hematopoietic system.** Differentiation of a pluripotent hemopoietic stem cell into the myeloid stem cell line and lymphoid stem cell line during hemopoiesis.

Malignant Myelodysplastic syndromes and Leukemias originate from proliferations of either leukocytes or lymphocytes. According to the WHO, a diagnosis of acute myelogenous leukemia must have 20% blasts in the bone marrow. The blasts require signatures of cytochemical or immunophenotypic traits of myeloid cells. The WHO classification of Acute Myeloid Leukemias is listed in Table 49.5A and are morpho-

logically presented in Figure 49.6A based on the French American British (FAB) classification.

The chronic Myeloproliferative syndromes usually involve proliferation of more mature myeloid lineages i.e. granulocytes, erythrocytes, or megakaryocytes. Their tabulation (Table 49.5B) emphasizes their acute leukemia conversion rate, bone marrow features, and genetic factors.

CARDIOVASCULAR SYSTEM

Perspective

The cardiovascular system (Fig. 49.7) is the major means of circulation of blood cells, nutrients, and electrolytes to all normal tissues and organs in the body. The main components are the heart and an elaborate vascular tree consisting of arteries carrying oxygenated blood, veins returning deoxygenated blood, and a vast mesh of microvascularization, which is the microcirculation of capillaries in all normal tissues and organs. Although neoplastic disease rarely affects the heart as a primary site, it is the major means of distributing neoplastic cancer and sarcoma cells to remote sites resulting in disseminated metastases. The venous system is of greater interest to explain the distribution of metastases than the arterial system.

The concept of oligometastases as the first stage of a more disseminated process is defined as a limited number or a few foci of cancer cells in one organ system. Although there are numerous circulating cells, oligometastases may be the initial phase of metastatic cancer residing in another organ system than the one in which the cancer cell originated. The argument as to a genetically programmed "seed versus soil" as the basis for metastases is not addressed. The anatomic basis for oligometastases is hypothesized on the basis of venous drainage of the primary site and the target metastatic organ being the first to receive the released cancer cells. The four most common sites for remote metastases are lung, liver, bone, and lymphoid.

- *Lung*: Pulmonary metastases are the most common because the entire venous hypoxic blood is returned to the heart via the superior and inferior vena cava. Primary cancer sites such as head and neck, lung, breast, male genitourinary, and female gynecologic cancers tend to appear initially as lung metastases. Bone and soft tissue sarcomas tend to appear in lung first as the target metastatic organ.

- *Liver*: The digestive system from the distal esophagus to the rectum drains into portal circulation; solitary or oligometastases to the liver are frequently present for gastrointestinal tract cancers.

- *Bone's* medullary cavity consists of sinusoidal sites that attract metastatic cells. Thus, the bone marrow is an optimal site to initiate metastases in bone, with the vertebrae as the most common osseous metastases, as well as the proximal portion of the femur and pelvis. The prostate is the most common primary cancer site, followed by breast and lung. The Batson circulation is a rich network of intervertebral veins that interconnects with the periprostatic plexus, the hemiazygos, and azygos veins so that a retrospread from primary sites can float malignant cells into vertebrae.

- *Lymphoid*: Because lymph node involvement is so common, one needs to note that all lymphatics drain into the cisterna chyli and then into the thoracic duct, which drains into the left neck at the junction of the internal jugular and subclavian veins. The first sign of a hidden primary is often a left supraclavicular node, so-called *Virchow's node*.

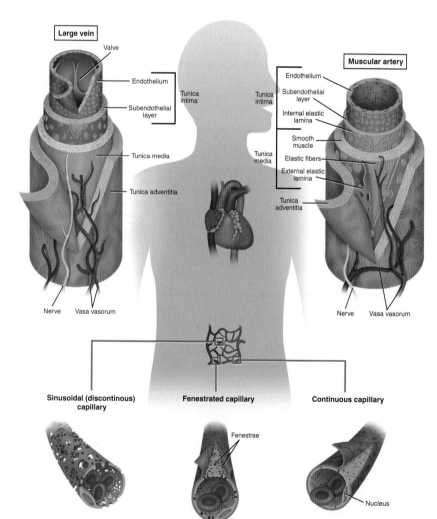

Figure 49.7 | Overview of cardiovascular system. Comparison (transverse sections) of a muscular artery, large vein, and the three types of capillaries.

TNM STAGING CRITERIA

TNM PATTERNS OF SPREAD AND STAGING CRITERIA

Each of the generalized systems has classification and staging criteria that are unique and idiosyncratic to that tissue/organ. As such, each system and its associated malignancies are presented separately.

Overview of the Oncoanatomy

The oncoanatomy of each generalized system is concisely described, with a more thorough presentation offered in the chapter dealing with the staging of its malignant tumors.

Orientation of Three-planar Oncoanatomy

Because major regional sectors—head and neck, thorax, abdomen, male and female pelvis—have been thoroughly covered in the presentation of the 50 primary cancer sites, the focus of the oncoanatomy is the appendicular anatomy, that is, lower and upper limbs.

Rules for Classification and Staging

The value and importance of cross-sectional imaging are well demonstrated and recognized when determining the anatomic extent of the malignancy involving a generalized site. CT, MRI, single-photon emission computed tomography, and positron emission tomography each have a role in both the initial staging and follow-up evaluation. Detailed oncoimaging recommendations are offered in relation to each site.

CANCER STATISTICS AND SURVIVAL

Skin cancers are the most preventable and most curable. Hodgkin's disease was the first lymphoma to become highly curable; the other lymphomas followed because of continued gains in survival with combination chemotherapy and biologic response modifiers. The leukemias are being controlled with aggressive supralethal chemoradiation therapy and bone marrow transplantation. Acute lymphoblastic leukemia in children has a very high survival rate. Soft tissue and bone sarcoma remain challenging to cure; equally important is limb preservation. Detailed statistics and survival are presented in each chapter devoted to a generalized site. Figure 49.8 illustrates the dramatic gains in survival over the last five decades and shows the trajectory of pediatric malignancies rising from incurability to curability as testimony to the multidisciplinary approach to a variety of sarcomas of these generalized anatomic systems.

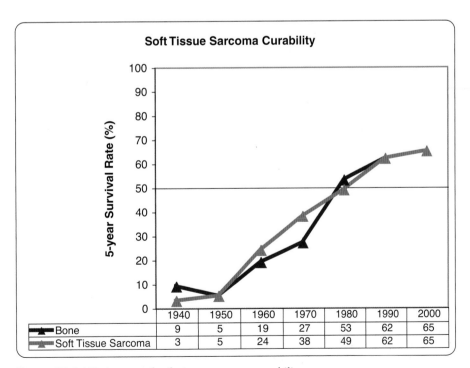

	1940	1950	1960	1970	1980	1990	2000
Bone	9	5	19	27	53	62	65
Soft Tissue Sarcoma	3	5	24	38	49	62	65

Figure 49.8 | Trajectory of soft tissue sarcoma curability.

Skin Integumentary System

PERSPECTIVE, PATTERNS OF SPREAD, AND PATHOLOGY

The T-zone around the eyes, nose, and mouth demand a curative outcome that preserves cosmesis and function.

PERSPECTIVE AND PATTERNS OF SPREAD

Nonmelanoma skin cancer (NMSC) largely consists of basal cell cancers (BCCs) and cutaneous squamous cell cancers (SCCs). A new addition is Merkel cell cancers (MCC) among the many different malignancies in the histopathologic classification (T1 histopathology skin cancers).

Patterns of spread tend to be bidirectional—horizontal or vertical—and provide the two major stage criteria: diameter measured in centimeters and depth measured in millimeters, respectively. With deeper penetration into dermis and hypodermis, invasion of underlying muscle and bone occur and prognosis becomes poor. Access to lymphatics in dermis increases risk for lymph node spread and possible perineural invasion, especially for the parotid gland region because of the widely distributed facial nerve (CNVII) and its numerous branches, which rapidly fan out in the face deep to the epidermis.

Cancers of the skin are the most common of all malignancies, with approximately 1 million new cancers annually in the Unites

States. Worldwide, its overall incidence approaches that of all noncutaneous malignancies combined. Fortunately, these lesions are readily recognized and treatment is effective, resulting in high curability. The 1,000 deaths annually indicate that a fraction of 1% are dying (0.001%), often in reclusive or neglected patients. Skin cancer is largely due to actinic exposure, and the majority of neoplastic lesions arise in preexisting lesions. Premalignant lesions include solar keratosis, epithelial hyperplasia, leukoplakia, nevi, and burn scars. The face, eyelid, and ear are the most common sites for BCCs and SCCs (Fig. 50.1A).

Although the predominant cancers are basal cell or squamous cell, virtually every component cell or adnexal structure can give rise to a malignancy. The common etiology is mainly chronic exposure to ultraviolet, especially when coupled with a genetic predisposition (fair skin). Albinism, xeroderma pigmentosa, and basal cell nevus syndrome are hereditary, and individuals with these syndromes are vulnerable. Immunosuppressed patients are prone to squamous cell cancer. Papillomavirus—an oncovirus—has been implicated as a cause for keratoacanthomas. Chronic irritation or inflammation, as with burn scars, can give rise to squamous cell cancer and contribute to its more aggressive behavior. Radiation induction of skin cancer is common, particularly in adolescents and young adults treated with moderate doses for acne. In blacks, mortality rates are disproportionately high and may be due to their more

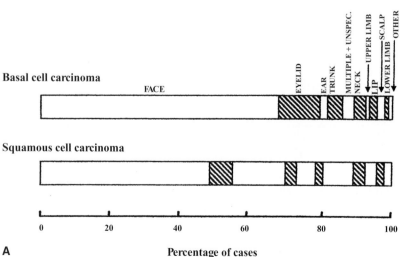

Figure 50.1 | A. Incidence rate for basal cell carcinoma and squamous cell carcinoma. *(continued)*

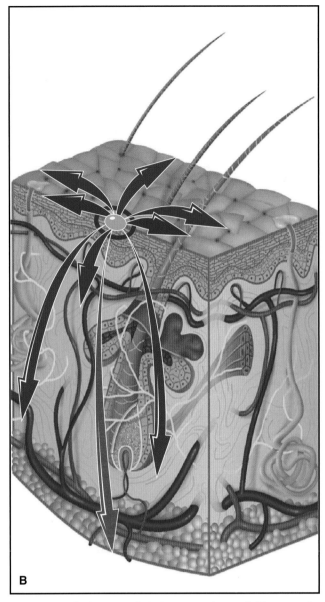

B

Figure 50.1 | *(Continued)* **B.** Patterns of spread. The spread pattern in skin is both horizontal and vertical and is color coded for stage: Tis, yellow; T1, green; T2, blue; T3, purple; and T4, red. The concept of visualizing patterns of spread to appreciate the surrounding anatomy is well demonstrated by the six-directional pattern (SIMLAP, Table 50.1).

TABLE 50.1	SIMLAP	
Skin Cancer: Cancer Originates in Basal Cell Stratum		
S	Spinosum	• T1
	Granulosum	• T1
	Lucidum stratum	• T1
I	Dermis papillary	• T2
	Reticular layers	• T2
	Appendages:	• T2
	Eccrine + apocrine glands	• T2
	Arteriole/venule	• T4
	Muscle	• T4
	Bone	• T4
	Subcutaneous fat	• T3
M	Melanocytes	
	Lymphatics/nodes	N0
L	Meissner corpuscles	• T2
	Pacinian corpuscles	• T2
	Hair follicles	

The six vectors of invasion are Superior, Inferior, Medial, Lateral, Anterior, and Posterior. The color-coded dots correlate the T stage with the specific anatomic structure involved.

advanced stage at diagnosis. Facial cosmetic destruction is due to recurrent basal cell cancer, and death follows when this superficial cancer gains access to lymph nodes and then becomes metastatic, most often to lung.

Cancers of the skin are very superficial tumors by virtue of location. The **patterns of spread** initially may be horizontal or vertical (Fig. 50.1B, Table 50.1). Once deeper invasion occurs, the exact anatomic site provides many nuances to management because the head and neck are the prime sites. The T-zone around the eyes, nose, and mouth demand an outcome for deeper invasion of skin cancers that preserves cosmesis and

function. If the underlying structures—muscle, bone, or cartilage—are involved, they play an important role in success or failure. Clinical detection is often by an annual systematic examination of the integumentary system by a dermatologist. Excisional biopsy or the Mohs technique of microscopic analysis of skin shavings is commonly used for diagnosis staging, as well as for treatment, to assure complete excision with clear margins. Careful palpation is essential in identifying the indurated cancer-infiltrated skin from normal skin and whether the lesion is fixed or freely mobile. Lymph node regions require careful clinical assessment with biopsy of suspicious nodes.

ORIENTATION OF HISTOGENESIS AND HISTOPATHOLOGY

Histogenesis

The integumentary system encompasses the entire skin surface, including its folds, openings, adnexae, derivatives, and appendages. In humans, it is the largest organ, and its derivatives include nails, hair, and sweat and sebaceous glands (Fig. 50.2A–C). The skin consists of two layers—the epidermis and the dermis. The superficial epidermis is nonvascular and consists of a stratified squamous epithelium with distinct cell types and layers referred to as stratums (Fig. 50.2A). The dermis is the vascular zone, and the epidermis is avascular. The majority of the dermis is a dense, irregular tangle of connective tissue, and below this is the hypodermis or subcutaneous tissue, which is mainly a mixture of fat and connective tissue that forms the fascial layers. The epidermis can be thick or thin in different regions of the body. Thick skin is largely keratinized and devoid of hair and glands, whereas thin skin contains hair and sweat and sebaceous glands and tends to be the site for malignancy.

This layer is loose connective tissue that has capillary loops, fibroblasts, and macrophages. The reticular layer is thicker and denser and has connective tissue without distinct boundaries. The hypodermis blends inferiorly and contains superficial fascia and fat tissues. This layer contains Pacinian corpuscles, whereas Meissner's corpuscles are at the dermal papillary level. Both provide the sensory receptors for skin. The skin appendages lie in the reticular layer, extend into the hypodermis, and include hair follicles, merocrine sweat glands, and apocrine sebaceous glands.

The layers that constitute the epidermis begin with germinal stem cells, stratum basale (Fig. 50.2B). The next layer is the stratum spinosum, which is four or five cells thick. The stratum granulosum is filled with granules of keratohyalin. When the cell loses its nucleus, it becomes the stratum lucidum. Finally, the piling of cells in the stratum corneum consists of flat, dead cells that provide the thickness to skin and account for its desquamation. There are numerous ancillary cells for different functions, such as sensory nerve endings into Merkel cells.

The dermis consists of a papillary and a reticular layer. The papillary layer is at the junction of epidermis and dermis and is irregular owing to raised projections of dermal papillae that interdigitate with epidermal ridges (Fig. 50.2C).

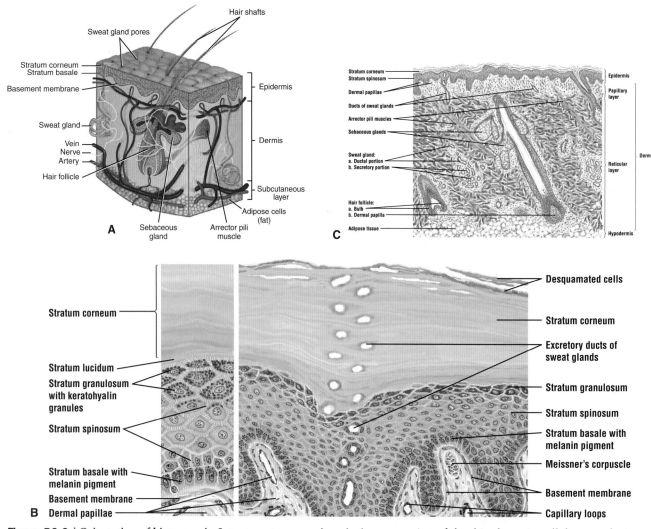

Figure 50.2 | Orientation of histogenesis. Integumentary overview. A. A cross section of the skin shows its cellular complexity and structures. There is the epidermis epithelial cover from which most skin cancers arise. This epidermal avascular layer rests on a base of subcutaneous tissue of fat and connective tissue, which is divided into a dermis of a papillary and areticular layer. **B.** Schematic diagram of keratinocytes in the epidermis consists of four layers of cells: basal cells, spinous cells, granular cells, and keratinized cells. rER, rough endoplasmic reticulum. **C.** Appendages such as eccrine gland and apocrine gland can give rise to adenocarcinomas. *(continued)*

Histopathology

The two most common cancers are basal cell cancer and squamous cell cancer, which are illustrated in Fig. 50.2D,E.

However, because of the numerous cell types present in the dermis, a large variety of cancers, lymphomas, and melanomas can originate in the skin layer. The normal cell and the derivative malignancies are given in Table 50.2.

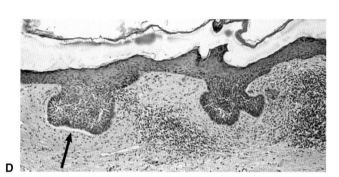

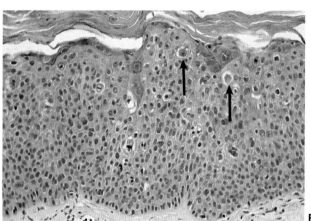

Figure 50.2 | *(Continued)* **D. Basal cell carcinoma, superficial type.** Buds of atypical basaloid keratinocytes extend from the overlying epidermis into the papillary dermis. The peripheral keratinocytes mimic the stratum basalis by palisading. The separation artifact *(arrow)* is present because of poorly formed basement membrane components and the hyaluronic acid–rich stroma that contains collagenase. **E. Squamous cell carcinoma.** A microscopic view of the periphery of the lesion shows squamous cell carcinoma in situ. The entire epidermis is replaced by atypical keratinocytes. Mitoses and multinucleation of keratinocytes are apparent, as is apoptosis *(straight arrows)*.

TABLE 50.2	Histopathology of Different Skin Cancers
Normal Cell	**Cancer Derivative**
Stratum basal	Basal cell cancer
Keratinocyte	Squamous cell cancer
Stratum spinosum	Intraepithelial cancer (Bowen's disease)
Stratum granulosum	Kerotoacanthoma
Merkel cell	Merkel cell cancer
Melanocyte	Melanoma
Adnexal merocrine gland	Adenocarcinoma
Langerhans cell	Histiocytosis X
T cell	Mycosis fungoides
B cell	Cutaneous lymphomas
Endothelial cell	Kaposi sarcoma
Fibroblast	Fibrosarcoma

TNM STAGING CRITERIA

TNM STAGING CRITERIA

For the first six stages of the TNM staging system, the main criterion for skin cancer has been size: T1, 2 cm; T2, <5 cm; T3 >5 cm; and T4, invades deep underlying extradermal structures such as cartilage, bone, and skeletal muscle. The nodal categorization is simply N1 for nodal involvement. The reason for this rather simple staging system is that the vast majority of skin cancers fall into the T1N0 stage I. On the face or head and neck region, a 2-cm cancer is a relatively large area, particularly if negative margins are required. It is not only the margin around the cancer, but the depth of excision that matters. The major concern and reason for failure is the recurrent cancer that invades perineurally or into bone. These cancers can become very erosive and destructive. Distant metastases are rare and tend to be mainly pulmonary with squamous cell cancers. Basal cancers virtually never metastasize unless they are neglected and allowed to advance. The staging generally reflects the T stage progression.

SUMMARY OF CHANGES SEVENTH EDITION AJCC

Skin, Cutaneous Squamous Cell Carcinoma, and Other Cutaneous Carcinomas

- Anatomic site of the eyelid is not included. It is staged by ophthalmic carcinoma of the Eyelid (see Chap. 48; Fig. 50.3).

- The T staging has eliminated the 5 cm size breakpoint and invasion of extradermal structures for T4. Two cm continues to differentiate T1 and 2; however, a list of clinical and histologic "high-risk features" has been created that can increase the prognosis of T staging, independent of tumor size.

- Grade has been included as one of the "high-risk features" within T category and now contributes toward the final stage grouping. Other "high-risk features" include primary anatomic site ear or hair-bearing lip, >2mm depth, Clark level ≥ IV, or perineural invasion.

- Advanced T stage is reserved for bony extension or involvement (e.g., maxilla, mandible, orbit, temporal bone, or perineural invasion of skull base or axial skeleton for T3 and T4, respectively).

- Nodal (N) staging has been completely revised to reflect published evidence-based data demonstrating that survival decreases with increasing nodal size and number of nodes involved.

- Because the majority of cSCC tumors occur on the head and neck integument, the seventh edition staging system for cSCC and other cutaneous carcinomas was made congruent with the general principles of AJCC Head and Neck staging system.

  - In the seventh edition of the TNM Staging Manual, dramatic changes have occurred. "Cutaneous Basal and Squamous Cell Carcinoma and Other Cutaneous Carcinomas" is an entirely new staging system that, for the first time, reflects a multidisciplinary effort to provide a mechanism for staging nonmelanoma skin cancers according to evidence-based medicine. In total, seven board-certified disciplines collaborated to develop this chapter: Dermatology, Otolaryngology-Head and Neck Surgery, Surgical Oncology, Dermatopathology, Oncology, Plastic Surgery, and Oral and Maxillofacial Surgery. The basis of the data is focused on squamous cell carcinoma. All other nonmelanoma skin carcinomas (except Merkel cell carcinoma) will be staged according to the cSCC staging system.

  - The Merkel Cell carcinoma staging system has also been newly designed and added.

The TNM staging matrix is color coded for identification of stage group once T and N stages are determined (Table 50.3).

TABLE 50.3A	Stage Summary Matrix			
	N0	**N1**	**N2**	**M1**
T1	*I	III	IV	IV
T2	II	III	IV	IV
T3	III	III	IV	IV
T4	IV	IV	IV	IV

The T stage progression determines the stage group progression.
- $T_{1,2,3,4}$ = stage I, II, III, IV.
- N stage = N_1 = T_3 = stage III.
- M stage is stage IV and separate.

BASAL CELL AND SQUAMOUS CELL CANCER

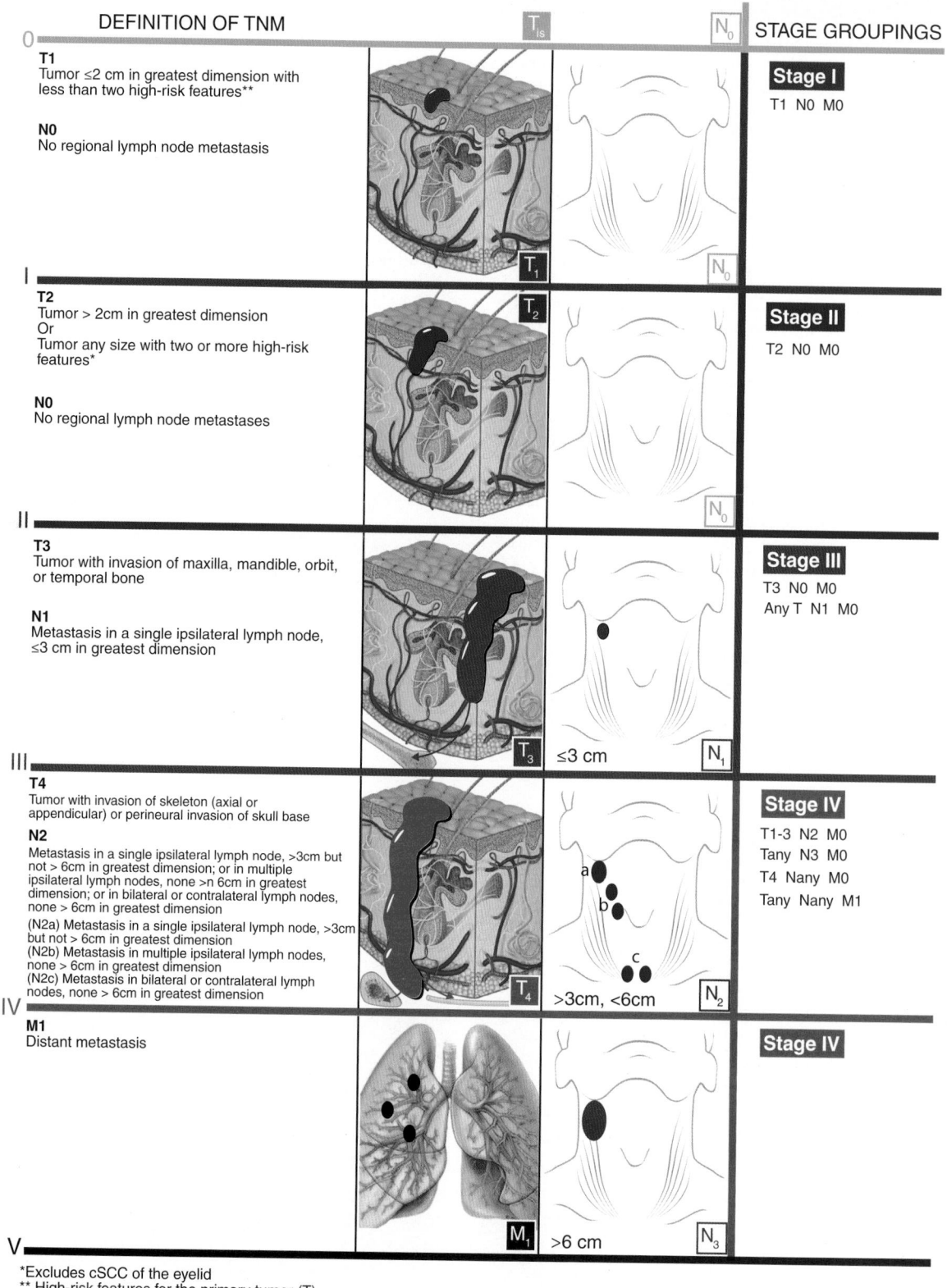

DEFINITION OF TNM

STAGE GROUPINGS

T1
Tumor ≤2 cm in greatest dimension with less than two high-risk features**

N0
No regional lymph node metastasis

Stage I
T1 N0 M0

T2
Tumor > 2cm in greatest dimension
Or
Tumor any size with two or more high-risk features*

N0
No regional lymph node metastases

Stage II
T2 N0 M0

T3
Tumor with invasion of maxilla, mandible, orbit, or temporal bone

N1
Metastasis in a single ipsilateral lymph node, ≤3 cm in greatest dimension

≤3 cm

Stage III
T3 N0 M0
Any T N1 M0

T4
Tumor with invasion of skeleton (axial or appendicular) or perineural invasion of skull base
N2
Metastasis in a single ipsilateral lymph node, >3cm but not > 6cm in greatest dimension; or in multiple ipsilateral lymph nodes, none >n 6cm in greatest dimension; or in bilateral or contralateral lymph nodes, none > 6cm in greatest dimension
(N2a) Metastasis in a single ipsilateral lymph node, >3cm but not > 6cm in greatest dimension
(N2b) Metastasis in multiple ipsilateral lymph nodes, none > 6cm in greatest dimension
(N2c) Metastasis in bilateral or contralateral lymph nodes, none > 6cm in greatest dimension

>3cm, <6cm

Stage IV
T1-3 N2 M0
Tany N3 M0
T4 Nany M0
Tany Nany M1

M1
Distant metastasis

>6 cm

Stage IV

*Excludes cSCC of the eyelid
** High-risk features for the primary tumor (T) staging

Figure 50.3 | TNM staging diagram arranged vertically with TN definitions on the left and stage groupings on the right. Skin cancers are the most common curable cancers when detected early (T1, T2) and even when advanced (T3), but resectability decreases with T4 cancers due to deep invasion of cartilage, muscle, and bone (*purple lane*). Color bars are coded for stage: stage T0, yellow; I, green; II, blue; III, purple; IV, red; and metastatic disease to viscera and nodes, black.

MERKEL CELL CARCINOMA

Perspective and Patterns of Spread

Merkel cell carcinomas (MCCs) are aggressive primary cutaneous neuroendocrine cancers resembling small-cell cancers of lung in their clinical behavior. Typically the lesion presents as a nodular, firm, red-to-violaceous papule on the exposed areas of the face, neck, and hand. Hosts tend to be fair skinned, favor sunbathing, and tend to be older (>50 years) and male. A specific virus has been identified in MCC and is termed MC polyoma virus. Other predisposing factors are immunosuppression and organ transplantation. The first sign could be a metastasis in nodes or lung in 10% to 15% of presentations.

The predominant spread pattern is to regional lymph nodes. Clinically negative lymph nodes are positive pathologically in one third of patients. Sentinel lymph node biopsies are advised and necessary to stage patients. The status of lymph node involvement affects survival.

Histopathology Classification

MCC consists of large, solid nests of undifferentiated cells that microscopically suggest small-cell lung cancers with active mitosis and nuclear fragments (Fig. 50.4A, B). Immunostaining is specific with cytokeratin 20, resulting in a "perinuclear dot" pattern, and neuroendocrine markers such as chromogranin and synaptophysin can also be positive.

TNM Staging Criteria

MCCs are staged for first time in the seventh edition of the American Joint Committee on Cancer's *AJCC Cancer Staging Manual*. According to p. 315, patients with primary Merkel cell carcinoma with no evidence of regional or distant metastases (either clinically or pathologically) are divided into two stages: stage I for primary tumors ≤2 cm in size and stage II for primary tumors >2 cm in size. Stages I and II are further divided into A and B substages based on method of nodal evaluation. Patients who have pathologically proven node-negative disease (by microscopic evaluation of their draining lymph nodes) have improved survival (substaged as A) compared with those who are only evaluated clinically (substaged as B). Stage II has an additional substage (IIC) for tumors with extracutaneous invasion (T4) and negative node status regardless of whether the negative node status was established microscopically or clinically. Stage III is also divided into A and B categories, for patients with microscopically positive and clinically occult nodes (IIIA) and macroscopic nodes (IIIB). There are no subgroups of stage IV Merkel cell carcinoma (Table 50.3B).

The T stage is similar to that for other skin cancers, but stage groups are different due to N staging, which emphasizes pathologic staging (Fig. 50.4C).

TABLE 50.3B

	pN0	cN0	N1a	N1b	N2	M1
T1	*IA	IB	IIIA	IIIB	IIIB	IV
T2	IIA	IIB	IIIA	IIIB	IIIB	IV
T3	IIA	IIB	IIIA	IIIB	IIIB	IV
T4	IIC	IIC	IIIA	IIIB	IIIB	IV

Combination of T and N determine stage group progression.

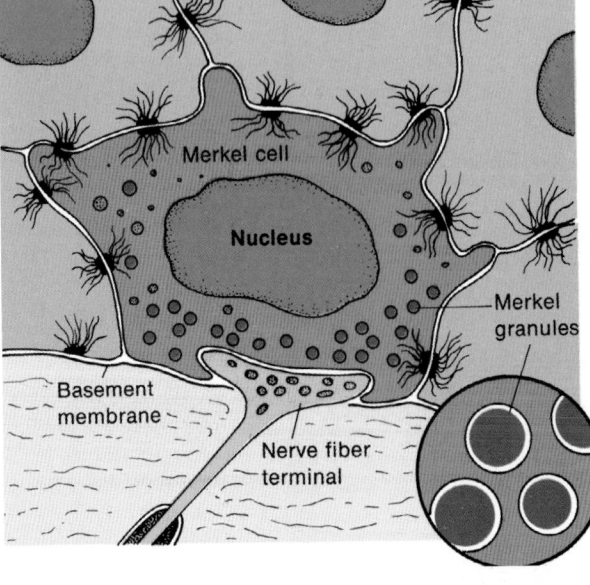

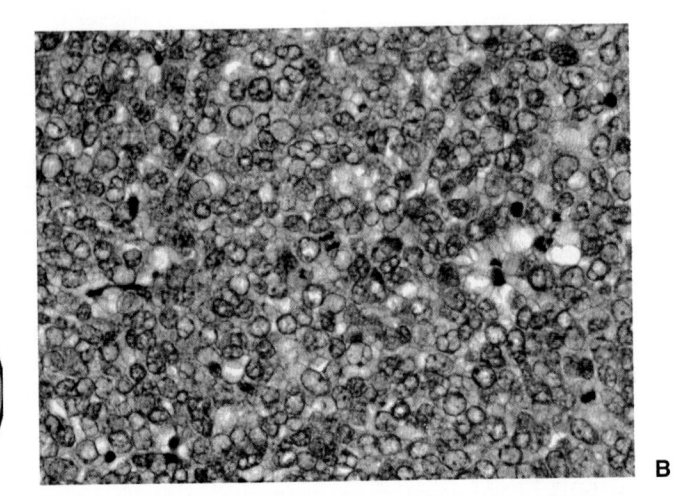

Figure 50.4 | A. The Merkel cell, which differs from other immigrant cells, forms desmosomes with keratinocytes and is attached to a small nerve plate (nerve fiber terminal). The membrane-delimited, dense core granule is distinctive (*inset*). **B. Merkel cell carcinoma.** The tumor is composed of solid nests of undifferentiated cells that resemble small-cell carcinoma of the lung. (*continued*)

MERKEL CELL CARCINOMA

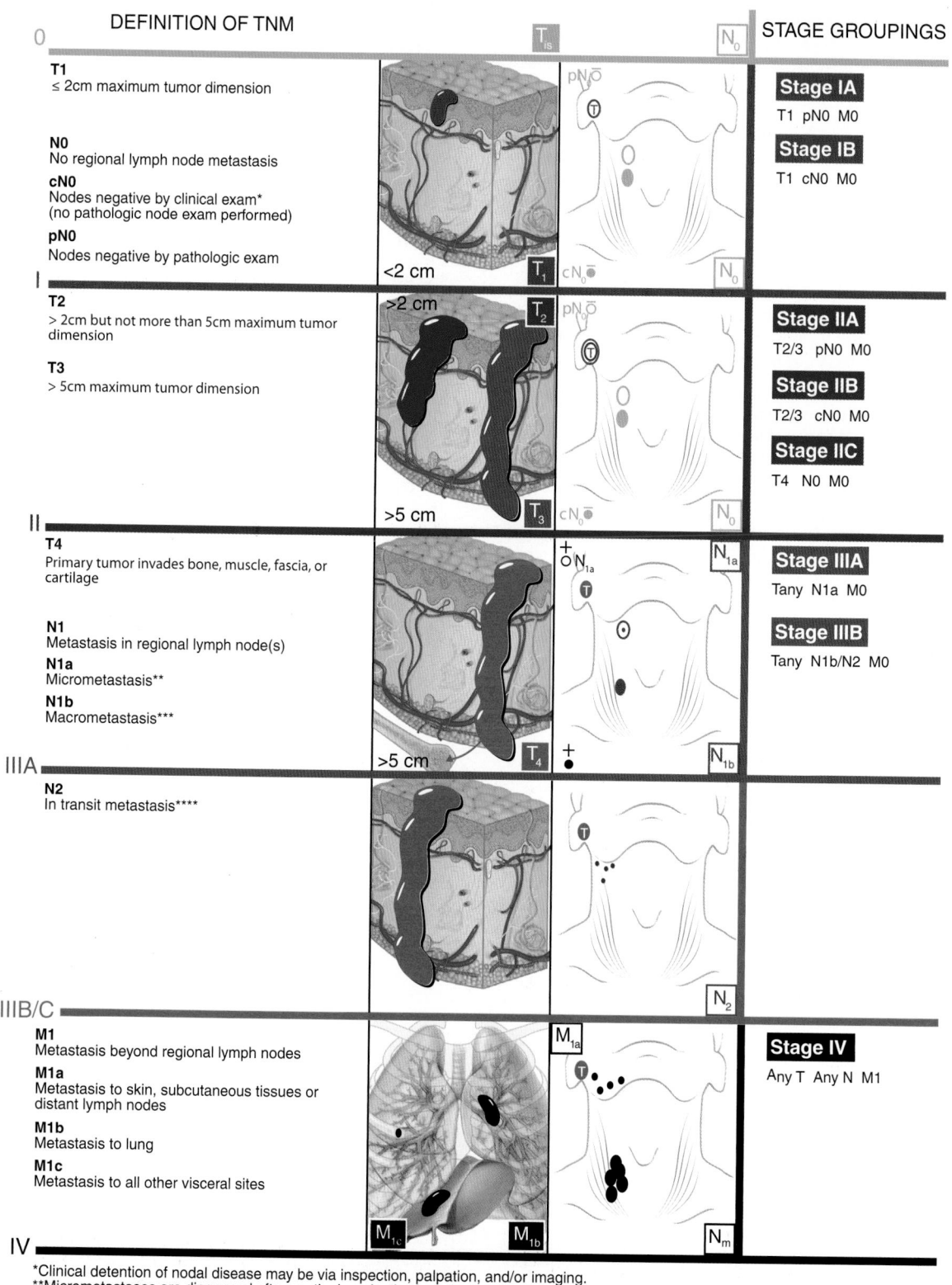

DEFINITION OF TNM

STAGE GROUPINGS

0

T1
≤ 2cm maximum tumor dimension

N0
No regional lymph node metastasis
cN0
Nodes negative by clinical exam*
(no pathologic node exam performed)
pN0
Nodes negative by pathologic exam

<2 cm

Stage IA
T1 pN0 M0

Stage IB
T1 cN0 M0

I

T2
> 2cm but not more than 5cm maximum tumor dimension

T3
> 5cm maximum tumor dimension

>2 cm

>5 cm

Stage IIA
T2/3 pN0 M0

Stage IIB
T2/3 cN0 M0

Stage IIC
T4 N0 M0

II

T4
Primary tumor invades bone, muscle, fascia, or cartilage

N1
Metastasis in regional lymph node(s)
N1a
Micrometastasis**
N1b
Macrometastasis***

>5 cm

Stage IIIA
Tany N1a M0

Stage IIIB
Tany N1b/N2 M0

IIIA

N2
In transit metastasis****

IIIB/C

M1
Metastasis beyond regional lymph nodes
M1a
Metastasis to skin, subcutaneous tissues or distant lymph nodes
M1b
Metastasis to lung
M1c
Metastasis to all other visceral sites

Stage IV
Any T Any N M1

IV

*Clinical detention of nodal disease may be via inspection, palpation, and/or imaging.
**Micrometastases are diagnosed after sentinel or elective lymphadenectomy.
***Macrometastases are defined as clinically detectable nodal metastases confirmed by therapeutic lymphadenectomy or needle biopsy.
****In transit metastasis: a tumor distinct from the primary lesion and located either (1) between the primary lesion and the draining regional lymph nodes or (2) distal to the primary lesion.

Figure 50.4 | (*Continued*) **C.** TNM staging diagram arranged vertically with TN definitions on the left and stage groupings on the right. Color bars are coded for stage: stage T0, yellow; I, green; II, blue; III, purple; IV, red; and metastatic disease to viscera and nodes, black.

T-ONCOANATOMY

T-ONCOANATOMY

The skin can be divided into its surface sectors and the lymph node region that drains a sector.

The head and neck includes the face and scalp. The vast majority of cancers arise on the skin of the face. Therefore, it is the face and scalp that demand careful attention clinically because of the complex functions, cosmesis, and special senses. All need to be preserved when resecting the cancer. The lymph node drainage of the integumentary surface differs from the upper aerorespiratory and digestive passages.

- Anterior chest wall from the clavicles to the navel in males tends to be hirsute. Lesions on the skin of the anterior thoracic wall drain to the anterior axillary nodes.

- Posterior chest wall to the same level tends to be less hirsute, is exposed more often to the sun, and is subject to forming cancers. The regional nodes are along the posterior wall of the axilla, although all axillary nodes are at risk.

- The upper extremity is an infrequent sector involved with skin cancer, but it can be a site for burn and chronic inflammation. It is notorious for radiation-induced cancer in dentists who finger-held dental films during their practice.

Serial resections occur, with loss of fingers, then the hand, and then the forearm. Involvement of epitrochlear node and then axillary nodes invariably leads to death from pulmonary metastases.

- Anterior abdominal wall drains into the femoral and inguinal nodes, but this sector of skin is rarely involved with skin cancers.

- Posterior abdominal wall or skin of the lower back is an infrequent site of malignancy and also drains to femoral and inguinal nodes anteriorly.

- The lower extremity is not a common site for skin cancers. Burns or chronic inflammation may cause lesions to evolve from hyperplasia to dysplasia and on to neoplasia. Popliteal nodes drain the foot and leg and ultimately drain into superficial femoral lymph nodes, which also drain the thigh.

Skin cancers are predominantly located on and in the face. To fully appreciate the anatomy, it is important to be aware of the surrounding structures and especially the underlying muscles and nerves. As the cancer advances and invades, the reconstruction is more than cosmesis. A particularly troublesome area is over the parotid gland because perineural invasion of the widely branching facial nerve is a major concern (Fig. 50.5A, B).

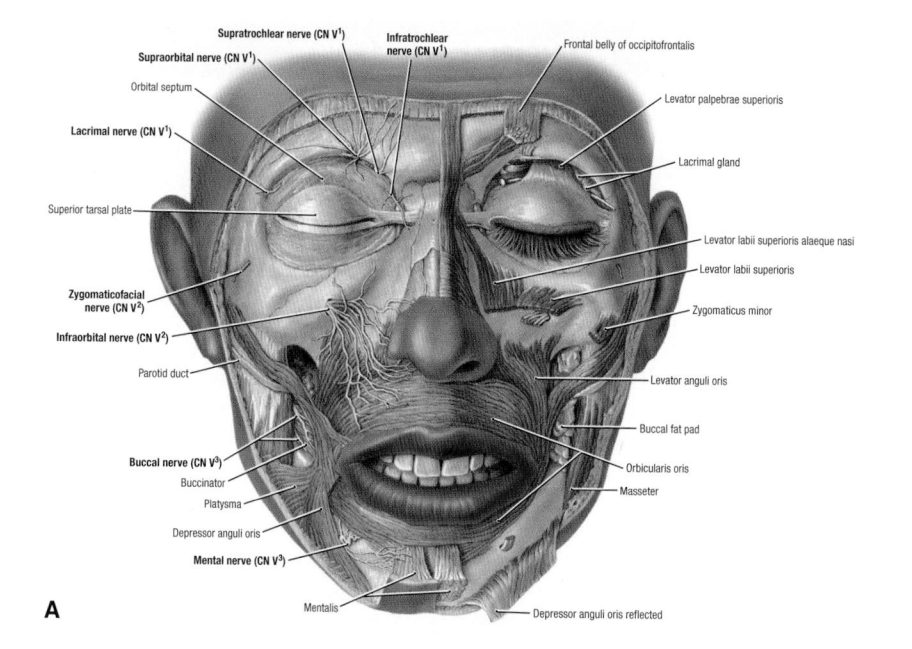

Supratrochlear nerve (CN V¹)
Supraorbital nerve (CN V¹)
Orbital septum
Lacrimal nerve (CN V¹)
Superior tarsal plate
Zygomaticofacial nerve (CN V²)
Infraorbital nerve (CN V²)
Parotid duct
Buccal nerve (CN V³)
Buccinator
Platysma
Depressor anguli oris
Mental nerve (CN V³)
Mentalis

Infratrochlear nerve (CN V¹)
Frontal belly of occipitofrontalis
Levator palpebrae superioris
Lacrimal gland
Levator labii superioris alaeque nasi
Levator labii superioris
Zygomaticus minor
Levator anguli oris
Buccal fat pad
Orbicularis oris
Masseter
Depressor anguli oris reflected

A

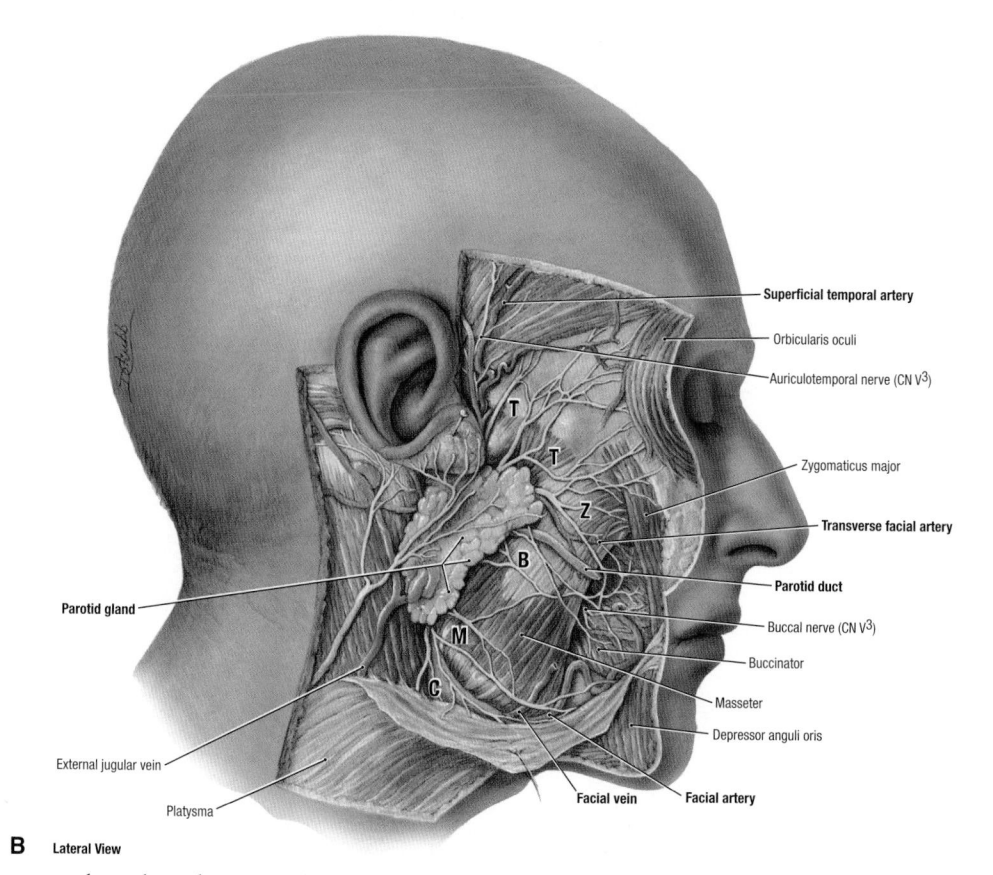

Superficial temporal artery
Orbicularis oculi
Auriculotemporal nerve (CN V³)
Zygomaticus major
Transverse facial artery
Parotid duct
Buccal nerve (CN V³)
Buccinator
Masseter
Depressor anguli oris
Facial vein
Facial artery

Parotid gland
External jugular vein
Platysma

B   Lateral View

Figure 50.5 | Cutaneous branches of trigeminal nerve, muscles of facial expression, and arteries of the face. **A.** Anterior view dissection of facial skin to reveal underlying muscles, nerves, and bones. **B.** Lateral view. Note the wide web distribution of facial nerve branches.

N-ONCOANATOMY

N-ONCOANATOMY

N-oncoanatomy of the skin surfaces emphasizes the anterior location for most if not all lymph node stations.

- The face and scalp drain into the superficial ring of high neck nodes at the junction of the mandible and neck: submental, submandibular, preauricular, mastoid, and occipital nodes. Once involved, the rest of the deep lymph nodes in the neck along the carotid sheath and internal jugular vein are at risk (Fig. 50.6A).

- The axillary nodes are the recipients of lymphatics of the upper extremity and upper half of the body, both anterior and posterior skin surfaces (Fig. 50.6A).

- The femoral and inguinal nodes drain the lower extremity and the lower half of the body, both the anterior and posterior skin surfaces (Fig. 50.6A).

The skin lymphatics of the face are different from head and neck cancers, since they drain to a ring of nodes that hang like a necklace from the occiput to below the ear and the parotid and anteriorly to the submaxillary and submandibular regions (Fig. 50.6B).

Once the cancer invades and advances, involving deeper underlying structures, the deeper cervical nodes can become at risk for involvement (Fig. 50.6C).

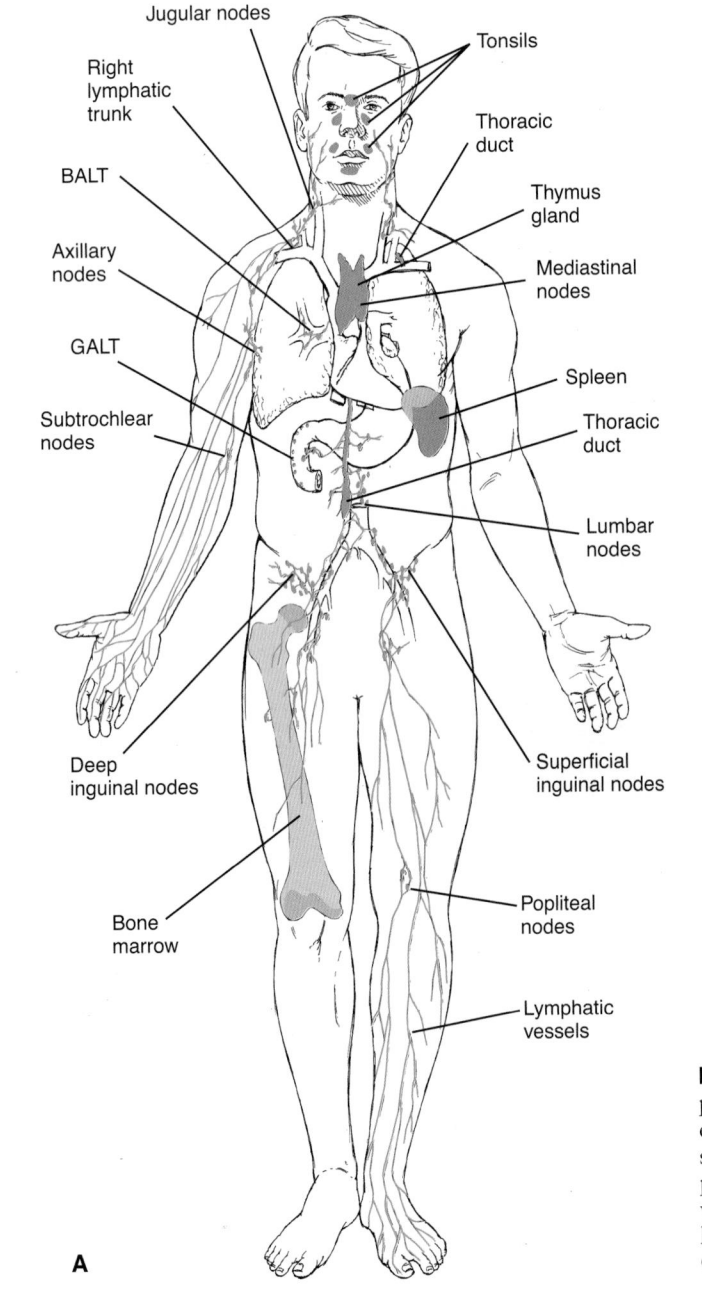

Jugular nodes

Right lymphatic trunk

BALT

Axillary nodes

GALT

Subtrochlear nodes

Deep inguinal nodes

Bone marrow

Tonsils

Thoracic duct

Thymus gland

Mediastinal nodes

Spleen

Thoracic duct

Lumbar nodes

Superficial inguinal nodes

Popliteal nodes

Lymphatic vessels

A

Figure 50.6 | A. Overview of the structures constituting the lymphatic system. Because lymphatic tissue is the main component of some organs, they are regarded as organs of the lymphatic system (spleen, thymus, and lymph nodes). Ultimately, the lymphatic vessels empty into the bloodstream by joining the large veins at the base of the neck. The thoracic duct is the largest lymphatic vessel. BALT, bronchus-associated lymphoid tissue; GALT, gut-associated lymphoid tissue. (*continued*)

M-ONCOANATOMY

M-ONCOANATOMY

There is a rich network of venous channels beneath all skin surfaces that allows for venous hematogenous spread once the dermal and hypodermal layers are penetrated by invading cancers. These venous collateral channels and plexus are rich and appear once obstruction occurs. The venous drainage of the face is shown in Fig. 50.6B, C.

Metastatic spread via superficial and deep jugular vein is to lung predominantly. With extensive recurrent and destructive basal cancers, which seldom metastasize early, aspiration into lung has been postulated but is an unlikely mechanism. Squamous cell cancers, as they invade lymph nodes, disseminate via focal veins. Merkel cell cancers are more virulent and are more prone to become metastatic.

MERKEL CELL CANCERS

These are similar to other cutaneous cancers and spread by jugular venous drainage with lung the major target organ, although remote cutaneous sites can be "in-transit" metastases distal to the primary site and between primary and regional nodes. Clinical detection of nodal disease may be via inspection, palpation, and/or imaging. Micrometastasis and macrometastasis are also possible:

- In-transit metastases: a tumor distinct from the primary lesion and located either (i) between the primary lesion and the draining regional lymph nodes or (ii) distal to the primary lesion.

- Micrometastases are diagnosed after sentinel or elective lymphadenectomy.

- Macrometastases are defined as clinically detectable nodal metastases and confirmed by therapeutic lymphadenectomy or needle biopsy.

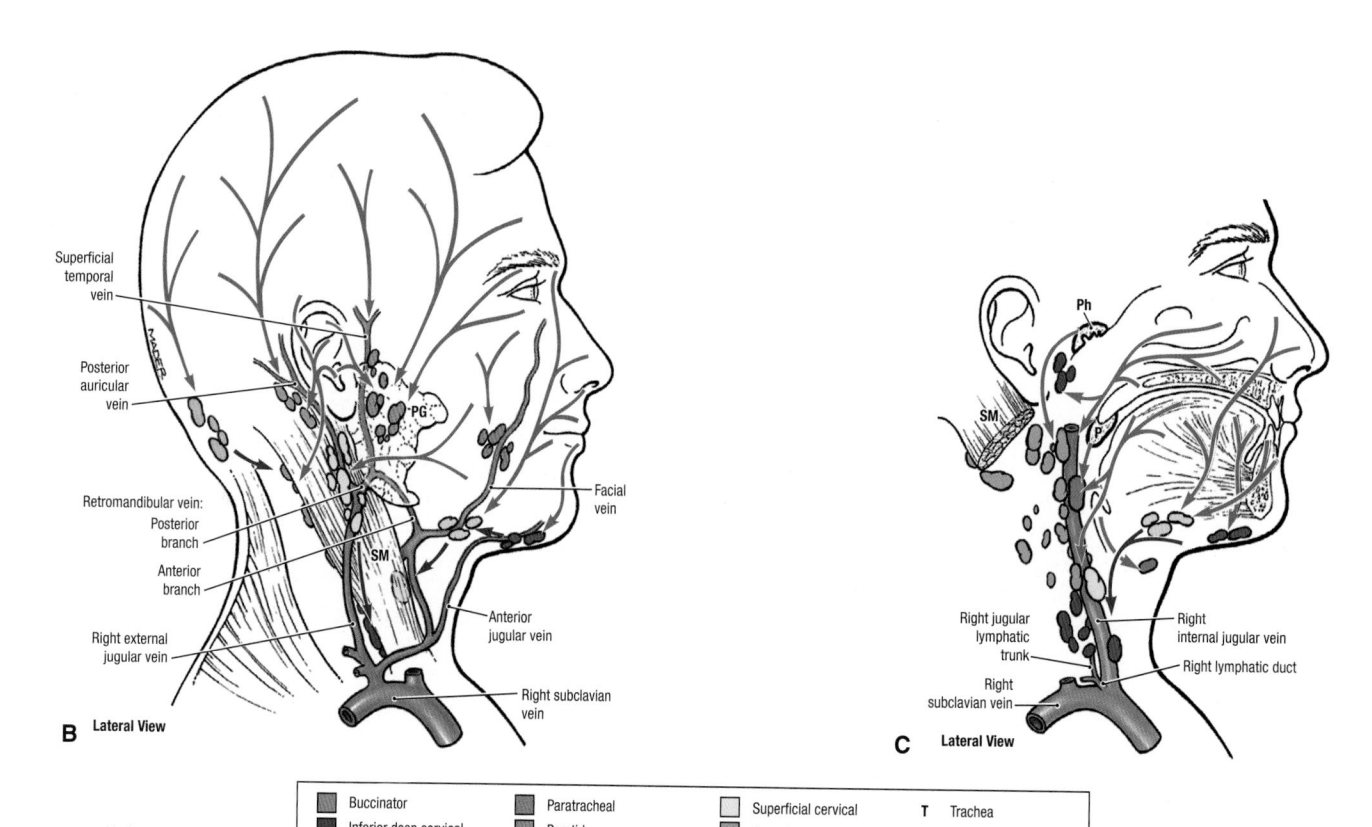

Buccinator	Paratracheal	Superficial cervical	T	Trachea
Inferior deep cervical	Parotid	Superior deep cervical	TC	Thyroid cartilage
Infrahyoid	Prelaryngeal	H Hyoid	TG	Thyroid gland
Jugulodigastric	Pretracheal	P Palatine tonsil		
Jugulo-omohyoid	Retropharyngeal	PG Parotid gland		Initial drainage
Mastoid (retroauricular)	Submandibular	Ph Pharyngeal tonsil		Secondary (subsequent) drainage
Occipital	Submental	SM Sternocleidomastoid		

Figure 50.6 | (*Continued*) **B.** Superficial lymphatic and venous drainage of the head and neck. **C.** Deep drainage.

STAGING WORKUP

Rules of Classification and Staging

The clinical and pathologic classifications are identical; excisional biopsy is often performed. Clinical staging is based on physical examination, inspection and palpation of primary sites, and draining of regional nodes. Imaging with regular radiographs is adequate, and skull films may include facial bones and mandible for deeply invading or fixed cancers beyond T1 in size. Computed tomography may be desirable for deeper invasion and to detect subtle cortical erosions and sclerosis (Table 50.4).

Pathologic Staging

Complete resection of the entire site is most often performed and must provide adequate margins to determine whether there is any residuum. An immediate frozen section is essential to assure complete excision and negative margins. Mohs microsurgery provides free margins but is a time-consuming and meticulous surgical excision technique. The major advantage is being able to know that a clean, deep margin has been obtained. Cancer grading is advised, as well as determining histopathologic type.

Rules for Staging Merkel Cell Cancers

These include the same imaging workup (T) as for advanced squamous cell cancers. Pathologic staging is emphasized especially for nodes.

TABLE 50.4	Imaging Modalities for Staging Skin Cancer	
Method	Diagnosis and Staging Capability	Recommended for Use
Primary (T) Staging		
STUS	Mainly useful for recurrent deeply invading cancers	No, unless advanced
Nodal (N) Staging		
CT	Searching for adenopathy in regional lymph node station	Yes, for recurrent disease
Metastases (M) Staging		
CT-Ch	Evaluation for pulmonary and mediastinal disease	Yes, for advanced T3, T4 invasive disease
CT-Abd	Evaluation of liver for defects compatible with metastases	Yes, for advanced T3, T4 invasive disease
Bone scan Tc	Assessment of bone for activity followed by regular radiographs if positive	Yes, for advanced T3, T4 invasive disease or symptomatic lesions
PET	Ability to find occult foci in total body scan, especially with CT	No, investigational mainly

CT, computed tomography; CT-Abd; abdominal CT; CT-Ch, chest CT; PET, positron emission tomography; STUS, soft tissue ultrasound.

PROGNOSIS AND CANCER SURVIVAL

PROGNOSIS AND SURVIVAL

Cutaneous Basal and Squamous Cell Cancers

Early stage T1 cancers <2 cm in diameter and <2 mm in depth rarely recur or metastasize. Risk of local recurrence doubles with lesions >2 cm (15% vs. 7%).

Immunosuppressed (I) patients are very prone to develop SCC; organ transplant patients are 65 times more prone than age-matched controls and have an increased risk of local recurrence; these lesions can be large, >5 cm, and prove to be lethal. The limited number of prognostic factors are listed in Table 50.5.

TABLE 50.5	Prognostic Factors for Cutaneous Basal and Squamous Cell Cancers
Required for staging	Tumor thickness (in mm)
	Clark's level
	Presence/absence of perineural invasion
	Primary site location on ear or hair-bearing lip
	Histologic grade
	Size of largest lymph node metastasis
Clinically significant	No additional factors

Edge SB, Byrd DR, and Compton CC, et al., *AJCC Cancer Staging Manual,* *7th ed.* New York, Springer, 2010, p. 312.

Cancer Statistics and Survival

New cases of skin cancer are in the 1 million range annually and are highly curable when excised completely in their first, early stage, namely, precancerous keratosis or lesions <1 cm. Fortunately, heightened awareness by the medical profession and patients has resulted in high curability rates (>95%). Once skin cancers recur in excisional scars or are neglected and invade deeply into muscle, cartilage, or bone, disfigurement and death can and do occur, with local control falling to <75%.

Merkel Cell Cancers

See Table 50.6.

TABLE 50.6	Prognostic Factors for Merkel Cell Cancers
Clinically significant	Measured thickness (depth)
	Tumor base transaction status
	Profound immune suppression
	Tumor-infiltrating lymphocytes in the primary tumor (TIL)
	Growth pattern of primary tumor
	Size of tumor nests in regional lymph nodes
	Clinical status of regional lymph nodes
	Regional lymph nodes pathologic extracapsular extension
	Isolated tumor cells in regional lymph nodes(s)

Edge SB, Byrd DR, and Compton CC, et al., *AJCC Cancer Staging Manual,* *7th edition.* New York, Springer, 2010, p. 319.

Merkel Cell Survival Statistics

The seventh edition of the *AJCC Cancer Staging Manual* has the largest pool of patients (4,700, T = 3,297, N = 4,426) and provides detailed analysis based on stage T, N, M, T size, and N status.*

*Preceding passage from Edge SB, Byrd DR, Compton CC, et al., *AJCC Cancer Staging Manual, 7th edition.* New York: Springer, 2010. p. 317–318.

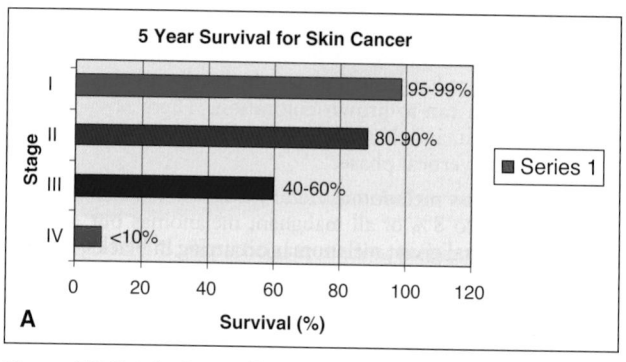

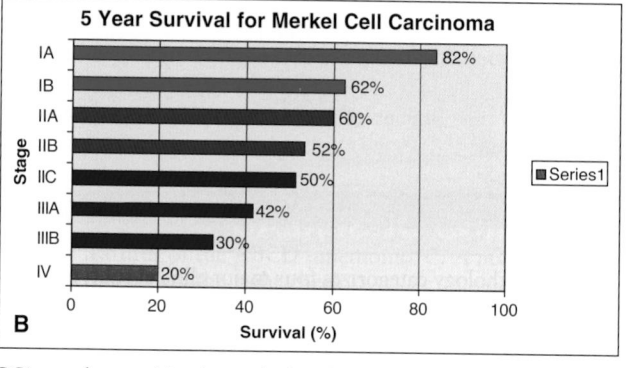

Figure 50.7 | A. Generally, early localized skin cancers (BCC and SCC) are detected in the early localized stages and are highly curable. As the cancer progresses and the stage advances, survival decreases sharply. B. There are a larger number of prognostic factors for Merkel cell cancer (MCC) listed in the accompanying table. (Data from Edge SB, Byrd DR, and Compton CC, et al, *AJCC Cancer Staging Manual, 7th edition.* New York, Springer, 2010.)

Radial Growth Phase

In the *radial growth phase* (Fig. 51.1D), cells grow in the epidermis and are present in the dermis. They grow in all directions: outward, peripherally, and downward. The net direction of growth is peripheral—along the radii of an imperfect circle. Growth, as manifested by mitotic activity, is largely in the epidermis. No cells in the dermis seem to have a growth preference over others. The nest depicted here is shown as it evolves into the vertical growth phase. The anatomic landmarks of the levels of invasion are shown. Level III is not simply the occasional impingement of a tumor cell against the reticular dermis but indicates a collection of cells that fills and widens the papillary dermis and broadly abuts the reticular dermis. Level III invasion is usually a manifestation of the vertical growth phase. Level IV invasion should be designated only when tumor cells clearly permeate between otherwise unaltered collagen bundles of the reticular dermis.

Vertical Growth Phase

The evolved *vertical growth phase* (Fig. 51.1E) in malignant melanoma of the superficial spreading type is shown, with an indication of how thickness is measured. In this illustration, the vertical growth phase has extended into the reticular dermis. Small nodules of tumor cells that clearly have a growth preference over other tumor cells may be a manifestation of the vertical growth phase. Thickness measurements (*arrows*) are taken from the outermost granular layer across the tumor in its thickest part.

There are numerous modifications in some of the criteria such as mitotic rate, metastatic volume, elevated serum LDH, and level of invasion, which has been abandoned for staging. Thickness of the melanoma and ulceration are the same key criteria for staging.

TABLE 51.1B	Changes in the Melanoma Staging System between the Sixth Edition (2002) and the Seventh Edition (2010) of the *AJCC Cancer Staging Manual*		
Factor	**Sixth Edition Criteria**	**Seventh Edition Criteria**	**Comments**
Thickness	Primary determinant of T staging; thresholds of 1.0, 2.0, 4.0 mm	Same	Correlation of metastatic risk is a continuous variable
Level of invasion	Used only for defining T1 melanomas	No longer used	Clark's levels ≥IV or V may be used in rare instances as a criterion for defining T1b melanoma *only* if mitotic rate cannot be determined in a nonulcerated T1 melanoma
Ulceration	Included as a second determinant of T and N staging	Same	Signifies a locally advanced lesion; dominant prognostic factor for grouping stage I, II, III.
Mitotic rate per mm^2	Not used	Used for categorizing T1 melanoma	Mitosis ≥1/mm^2 used as a primary determinant for defining T1b melanoma
Satellite metastases	In N category	Same	Merged with in-transit lesions
Immunohistochemical detection of nodal metastases	Not allowed	Allowed	Must include at least one melanoma-specific marker (e.g., HMB-45, Melan-A, MART 1)
0.2-mm threshold of defined node-positive	Implied	No lower threshold of staging node-positive disease	
Number of nodal metastases	Dominant determinant of N staging	Same	Thresholds of 1 vs. 2–3 vs. ≥4 nodes
Metastatic "volume"	Included as a second determinant of N staging	Same	Clinically occult ("microscopic") vs. clinically apparent ("macroscopic") nodal volume.
Lung metastases	Separate category as M1b	Same	Has a somewhat better prognosis than other visceral metastases
Elevated serum LDH	Included as a second determinant of M staging	Same	Recommend a second confirmatory LDH if elevated
Clinical vs. pathologic staging	Sentinel node results incorporated into definition of pathologic staging		Large variability in outcome between clinical and pathologic staging; sentinel node staging encouraged for standard patient care and should be required prior to entry into clinical trials.

LDH, lactate dehydrogenase.
Used with the permission of the American Joint Committee on Cancer (AJCC) Chicago, Illinois. The original source for this material is the *AJCC Cancer Staging Manual,* Seventh edition (2010) published by Springer SBM, LLC, p 327.

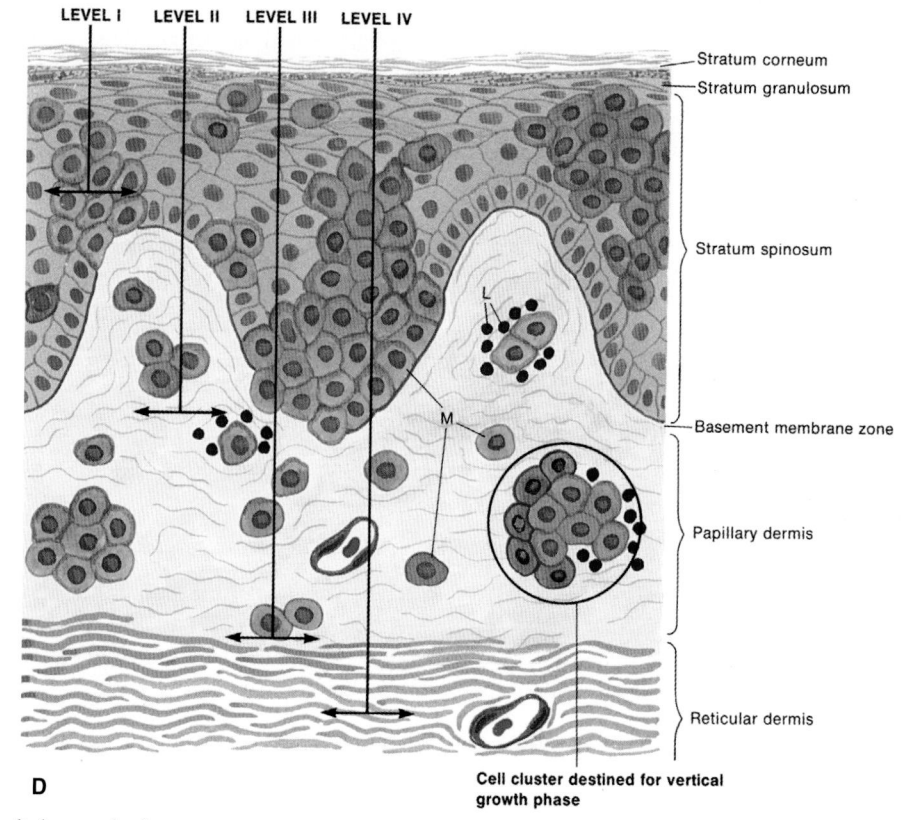

Figure 51.1 | D. Radial growth phase.

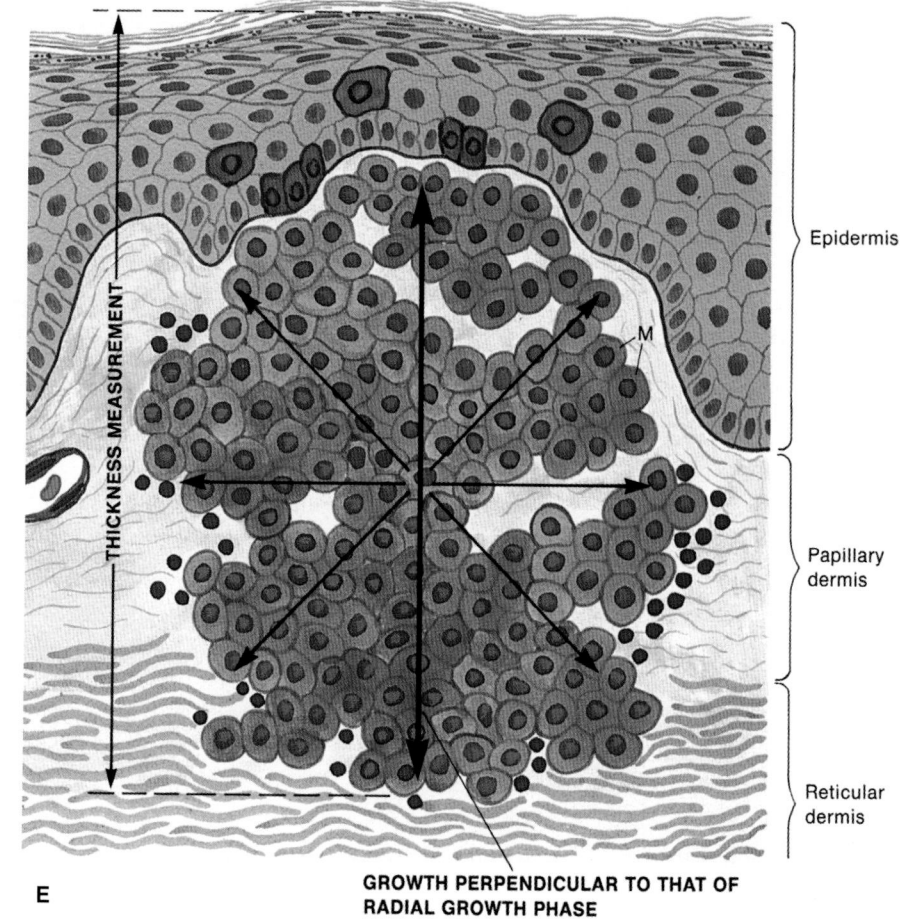

Figure 51.1 | E. Verticle growth phase.

HISTOGENESIS AND HISTOPATHOLOGY

Histogenesis

The melanocyte is a junctional cell usually located at the interface between the dermis and the epidermis. The integumentary system encompasses the entire skin surface, including its folds, openings, adnexae, derivatives, and appendages. In humans, it is the largest organ, and its derivatives include nails, hair, and sweat and sebaceous glands. The skin consists of two layers—the epidermis and the dermis (Fig. 51.2). The superficial epidermis is nonvascular and consists of a stratified squamous epithelium with distinct cell types and layers referred to as strata. The dermis is the vascular zone, and the epidermis is avascular. The majority of the dermis is a dense, irregular connective tissue, and below this is the hypodermis or subcutaneous tissue, which is mainly a mixture of connective tissue and fat that forms the fascial layers. The epidermis can be thick or thin in different regions of the body. Thick skin is largely keratinized and devoid of hair and glands, whereas thin skin contains hair and sweat and sebaceous glands and tends to be the sites for malignancy.

The dermis consists of a papillary and a reticular layer. The papillary layer is at the junction of epidermis and dermis and is irregular owing to projections of dermal papillae that interdigitate with epidermal ridges. This layer is loose connective tissue, which has capillary loops, fibroblasts, and macrophages. The reticular layer is thicker and denser; it has connective tissue without distinct boundaries. The hypodermis blends inferiorly and contains superficial fascia and fat tissues. This layer contains Pacinian corpuscles; Meissner's corpuscles are at the dermal papillary level. Both provide sensory receptors for skin. The skin appendages lie in the reticular layer, extend into the hypodermis, and include hair follicles, merocrine sweat glands, and apocrine sebaceous glands (Fig. 51.2A).

The layers that constitute the epidermis have germinal stem cells, stratum basale. The next layer is the stratum spinosum, which is four or five cells thick. The stratum granulosum is filled with granules of keratohyalin. When the cell loses its nucleus, it becomes the stratum lucidum. Finally, the piling of cells in the stratum corneum consists of flat, dead cells that provide the thickness to skin and account for desquamation.

Melanocytes are the key cell in determining skin color and are of neural crest origin, that is, dendrite cells. One melanocyte may supply more than 30 keratinocytes with dendrites and melanin granules via spider-like extensions. Melanosomes are the pigment granules in distinctive organelles synthesized on small filaments. Melanomas reflect visible light, resulting in different skin colors (Fig. 51.2B).

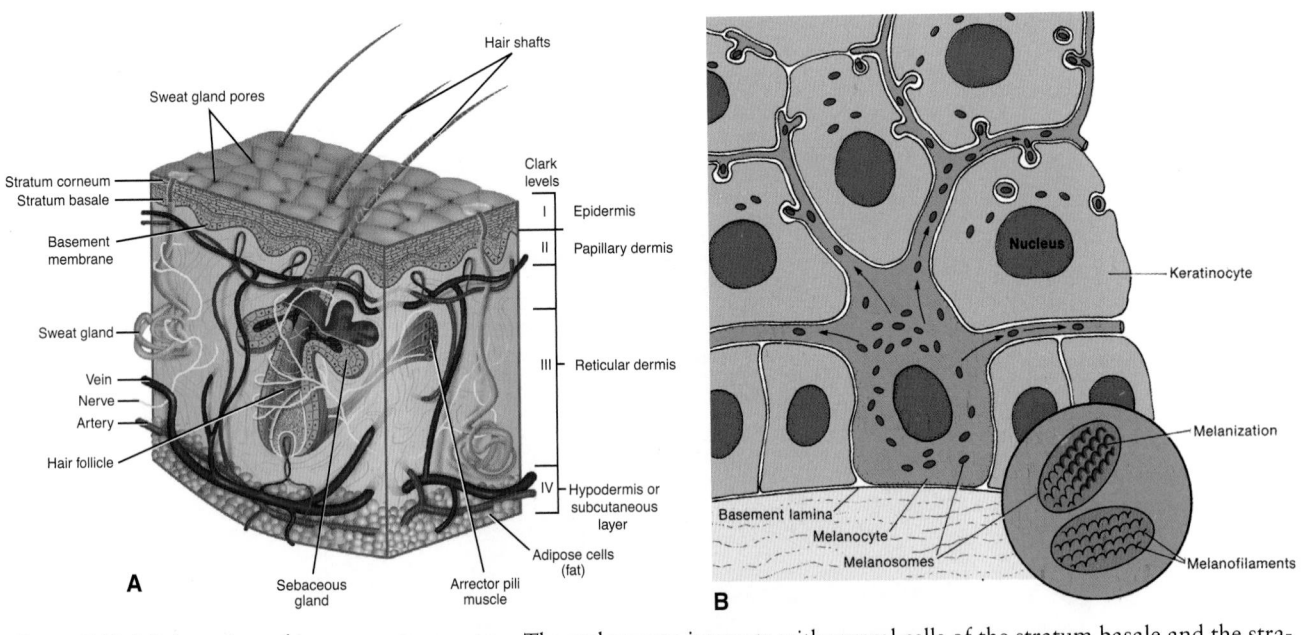

Figure 51.2 | Orientation of integumentary system. The melanocyte interacts with several cells of the stratum basale and the stratum spinosum. **A.** Epidermis showing Clark levels. I. Epidermis. II. Dermis papillary. III. Reticular dermis. IV. Hypodermis or subcutaneous layer. **B.** A melanocyte supplies more than 30 keratinocytes with melanin granules by way of complex dendritic cytoplasmic extensions. Melanin granules are transferred to keratinocytes and come to lie in a supranuclear cap, a site indicating their protective function. Pigment granules are actually formed in the melanocytes within distinctive organelles—the melanosomes. Pigment is synthesized on small filaments within this organelle (*inset*).

Histopathology

The melanoma develops and extends either in a horizontal or a vertical growth phase as illustrated previously (Fig. 51.2D, E).

The various histologic types of melanoma are listed in Table 51.2.

The dysplastic melanocyte may grow to become continuous streams bridging from rete to rete. Large atypical nuclei portend neoplasia.

- The superficial spreading type (in a radial growth phase), occurring at the dermal–epidermal junction (Fig. 51.3A).
- The superficial spreading types (in a vertical phase) (Fig. 51.3B).
- The lower half of the reticular layer.
- The nodular type, in which the invasive component extends into the dermis (Fig. 51.3C).
- The acral lentiginous type (Fig. 51.3D).

TABLE 51.2	Histopathologic Type: Common Melanomas of the Skin
Type	
Melanoma in situ	Desmoplastic melanoma
Malignant melanoma, NOS	Epithelioid cell melanoma
Superficial spreading melanoma	Spindle cell melanoma
Nodular melanoma	Balloon cell melanoma
Lentigo maligna melanoma	Blue nevus, malignant
Acral lentiginous melanoma	Malignant melanoma in giant pigmented nevus

NOS, not otherwise specified.
Modified from Edge SB, Byrd DR, Compton CC, et al., *AJCC Cancer Staging Manual. 7th ed.* New York: Springer; 2010:336.

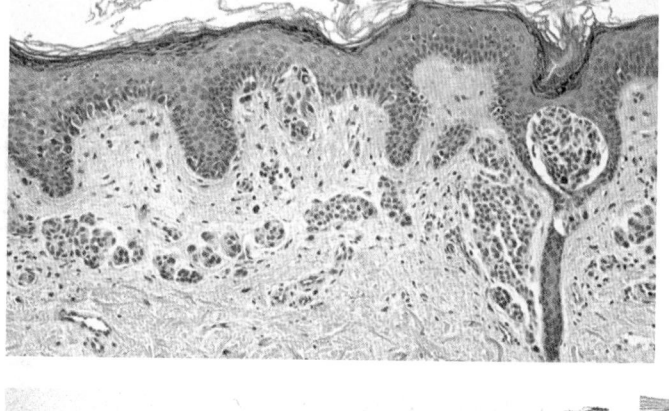

A

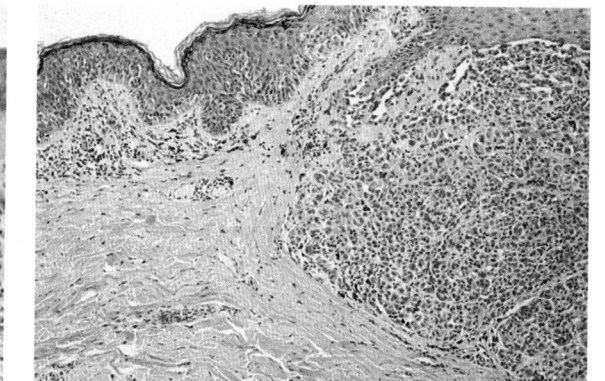

B

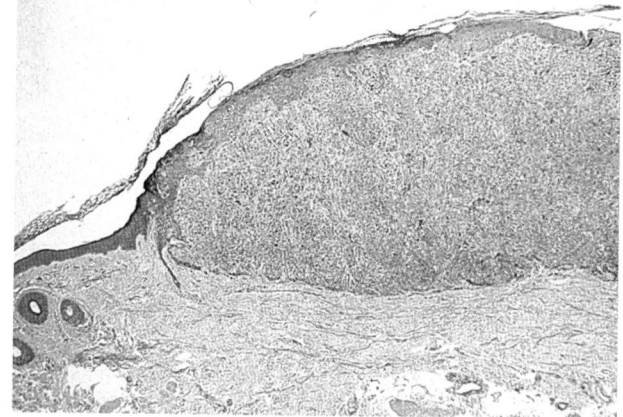

C

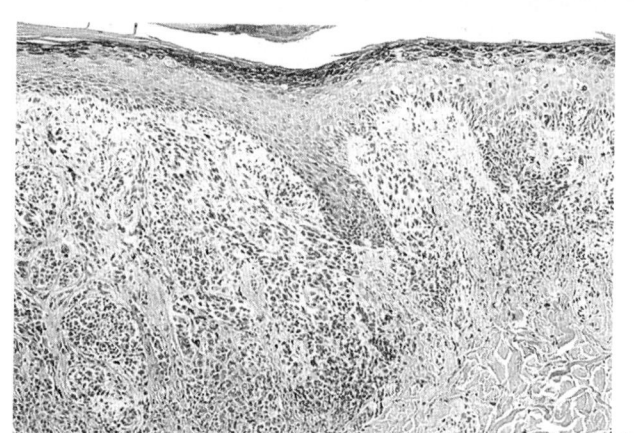

D

Figure 51.3 | A. Compound nevus with melanocytic dysplasia. On the right, a compound nevus is apparent with both intraepidermal and dermal components. To the left, within the epidermis are single atypical melanocytes within the basal unit, as well as incipient lamellar fibroplasia. Dermal melanocytes are present below. **B. Malignant melanoma, superficial spreading type, vertical growth phase.** Vertical growth is manifested by the distinct spheroid tumor nodule to the right. A focus of melanocytes clearly has a growth advantage (larger size) over other nests in the radial growth phase (left). The nodule distorts the papillary dermal–reticular dermal junction and therefore is level III. **C. Malignant melanoma, nodular type.** Intraepidermal growth is essentially absent. There is no radial growth lateral to the nodule. This tumor expands the papillary dermis and distorts the reticular dermal junction; it is therefore level III. **D. Malignant melanoma, acral lentiginous type, vertical growth phase.** On the left is confluent growth of atypical dermal melanocytes filling and expanding the papillary dermis.

TNM STAGING CRITERIA

TNM STAGING CRITERIA

The origin of melanoma can be as de novo lesions versus arising from nevi. It is due to the melanocyte, an ectodermal junctional cell located between the epidermal basale stratum and the dermal papillary zone. A completely revised melanoma staging system is described in the seventh edition of the *AJCC Cancer Staging Manual*, based on a major data analyses of numerous prognostic factors derived from a 17,000-patient database from 13 centers. The major differences between the new version and the previous criteria are given later in Table 51.4.

The biologic aggressiveness is noted in the change of only 1 mm in size, which singles this malignancy out. Rather than measuring the cancer in centimeters, the stage and/or substage in melanomas advances by 1 mm. The T categories of melanoma are currently defined in whole integers: T1, 1 mm; T2, 2 mm; and T3, 4 mm. Subcategories such as ulceration or loss of overlying epidermis, assessed by histopathology, advances the stage. Regional nodes (N) are defined by radioisotope injection at the site and dissection of the radioactive sentinel node. The number of nodes involved defines the N category. Stage grouping has many gradations of both primary and nodes. Collectively the current staging system is subcategorized into 20 subgroupings. The scientific survival data analysis is exemplary and perhaps one of the most thorough in the *Manual* to justify the new subgroups.

SUMMARY OF CHANGES SEVENTH EDITION AJCC

- Mitotic rate (histologically defined as mitoses/mm^2, not mitoses/10 HPF) is an important primary tumor prognostic factor. A mitotic rate equal to or greater than 1/mm^2 denotes a melanoma at higher risk for metastases. It should now be used as one defined criteria of T1b melanomas. (Fig. 51.4; Table 51.1B)

- Melanoma thickness and tumor ulceration continue to be used in defining strata in the T category. For T1 melanomas, in addition to tumor ulceration, mitotic rate replaces level of invasion as a primary criterion for defining the subcategory of T1b.

- The presence of nodal micrometastases can be defined using either H&E or immunohistochemical staining (previously, only the H&E could be used).

- There is no lower threshold of tumor burden defining the presence of regional nodal metastasis. Specifically, nodal tumor deposits less than 0.2 mm in diameter (previously used as the threshold for defining nodal metastasis) are included in the staging of nodal disease as a result of the consensus that smaller volumes of metastatic tumor are still clinically significant. A lower threshold of clinically insignificant nodal metastases has not been defined on evidence.

- The site of distant metastases [nonvisceral (i.e., skin/soft tissue/distant nodal) vs. lung vs. all other visceral metastatic sites] continues to represent the primary component of categorizing the M category.

- Survival estimates for patients with intralymphatic regional metastases (i.e., satellites and in transit metastasis) are somewhat better than for the remaining cohort of Stage IIIB patients. Nevertheless, Stage IIIB still represents the closest statistical fit for this group, so the current staging definition for intralymphatic regional metastasis has been retained.

- The prognostic significance of microsatellites has been established less broadly. The Melanoma Task Force recommended that this uncommon feature be retained in the N2c category, largely because the published literature is insufficient to substantiate revision of the definitions used in the Sixth Edition Staging Manual.

- The staging definitions of metastatic melanoma from an unknown primary site was clarified, such that isolated metastases arising in lymph nodes, skin, and subcutaneous tissues are to be categorized as Stage III rather than Stage IV.

- The definitions of tumor ulceration, mitotic rate, and microsatellites were clarified.

- Lymphoscintigraphy followed by lymphatic mapping and sentinel lymph node biopsy (sentinel lymphadenectomy) remain important components of melanoma staging and should be used (or discussed with the patient) in defining occult Stage III disease among patients who present with clinical Stage IB or II melanoma.

IMPORTANT DETAILS FOR STAGING

- *Tumor thickness* is the strongest prognostic factor and is measured from the most superficial aspect of stratum granulosum to the deepest margin in the dermis.

- *Dermal mitotic rate* predicts poorer survival with increase in mitotic activity, and it is recommended to find "hot spots" with the most mitotic cells and view areas equal to 1 mm^2. Lower rates are expressed as mitoses/mm^2.

- *Ulceration* is associated with poorer survival and upstages melanomas of the same thickness for T stage *a* to *b*.

- *Lymphocytic response* refers to tumor infiltrating lymphocytes (TILs) and improves prognosis if present "location" head and neck are worse than trunk, with extremities being best.

- *"Lymphatic spread"* satellite lesions are "in-transit" metastases and portend a poor prognosis; however, microsatellites are less reliable predictors. Immunohistochemical staining (IHS) is now advised.

- *"Node metastases"* are ominous and decrease survival. These are determined in sentinel nodes. N1, one node; N2, two or three nodes; N3, four or more nodes and update T lesions to stage III.

SKIN INTEGUMENTARY SYSTEM—MELANOMA

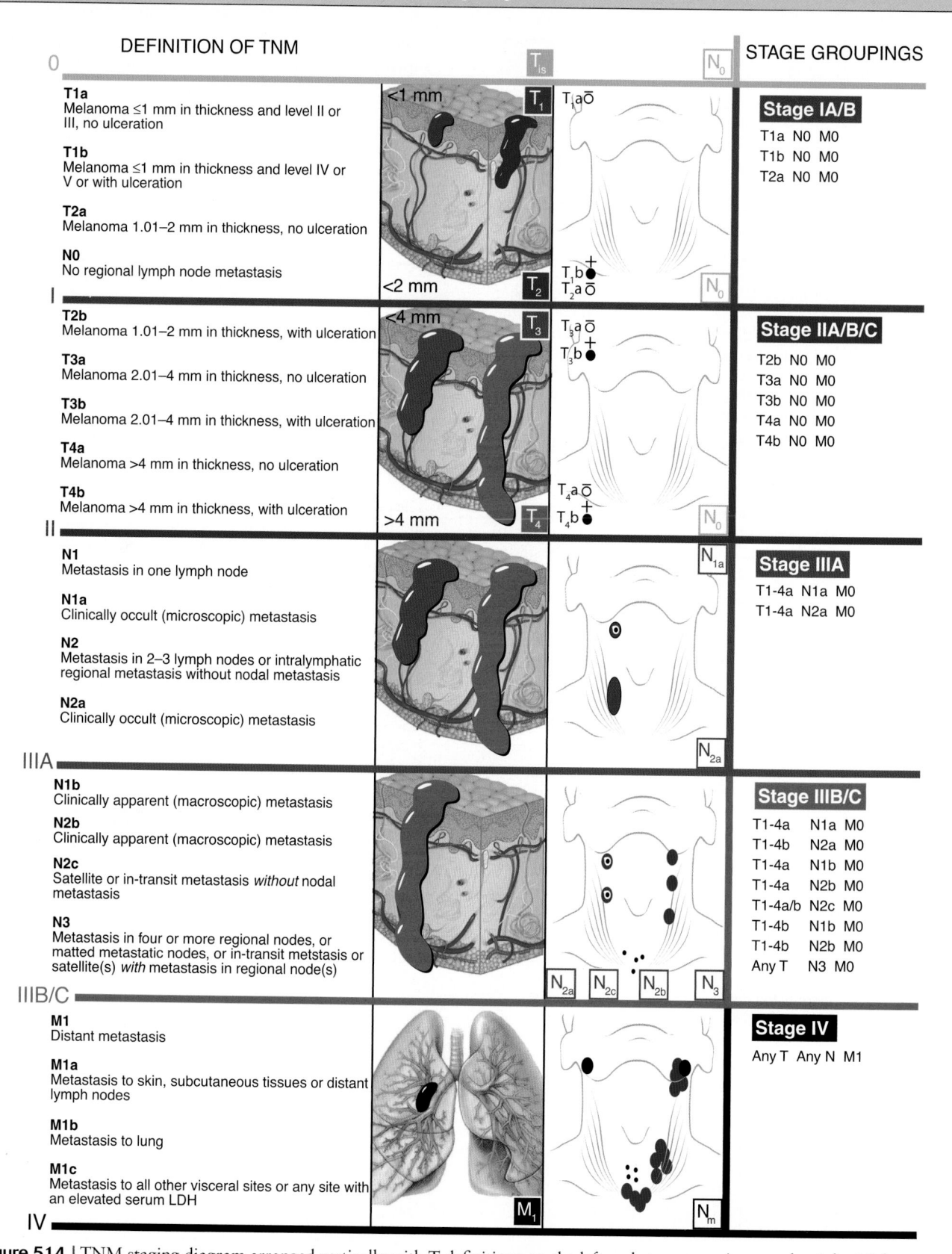

| DEFINITION OF TNM | | | STAGE GROUPINGS |

T1a
Melanoma ≤1 mm in thickness and level II or III, no ulceration

T1b
Melanoma ≤1 mm in thickness and level IV or V or with ulceration

T2a
Melanoma 1.01–2 mm in thickness, no ulceration

N0
No regional lymph node metastasis

Stage IA/B
T1a N0 M0
T1b N0 M0
T2a N0 M0

T2b
Melanoma 1.01–2 mm in thickness, with ulceration

T3a
Melanoma 2.01–4 mm in thickness, no ulceration

T3b
Melanoma 2.01–4 mm in thickness, with ulceration

T4a
Melanoma >4 mm in thickness, no ulceration

T4b
Melanoma >4 mm in thickness, with ulceration

Stage IIA/B/C
T2b N0 M0
T3a N0 M0
T3b N0 M0
T4a N0 M0
T4b N0 M0

N1
Metastasis in one lymph node

N1a
Clinically occult (microscopic) metastasis

N2
Metastasis in 2–3 lymph nodes or intralymphatic regional metastasis without nodal metastasis

N2a
Clinically occult (microscopic) metastasis

Stage IIIA
T1-4a N1a M0
T1-4a N2a M0

N1b
Clinically apparent (macroscopic) metastasis

N2b
Clinically apparent (macroscopic) metastasis

N2c
Satellite or in-transit metastasis *without* nodal metastasis

N3
Metastasis in four or more regional nodes, or matted metastatic nodes, or in-transit metstasis or satellite(s) *with* metastasis in regional node(s)

Stage IIIB/C
T1-4a   N1a   M0
T1-4b   N2a   M0
T1-4a   N1b   M0
T1-4a   N2b   M0
T1-4a/b N2c   M0
T1-4b   N1b   M0
T1-4b   N2b   M0
Any T   N3   M0

M1
Distant metastasis

M1a
Metastasis to skin, subcutaneous tissues or distant lymph nodes

M1b
Metastasis to lung

M1c
Metastasis to all other visceral sites or any site with an elevated serum LDH

Stage IV
Any T Any N M1

Figure 51.4 | TNM staging diagram arranged vertically with T definitions on the left and stage groupings on the right. Melanoma with regard to size is one of the most virulent malignancies and spreads insidiously into lymph nodes. Ulcerations of a primary lesion (symbolically without [open dot with minus sign above] or with [solid dot with plus sign above]) and in-transit metastases [cluster of points] are ominous signs prognostically. Occult lymph nodes are microscopically positive ones. Color bars are coded for stage: stage 0, yellow; I, green; II, blue; IIIA, purple; IIIB/C, red; and IV, metastatic disease to viscera and nodes, black.

T-ONCOANATOMY, N-ONCOANATOMY, AND M-ONCOANATOMY

T-ONCOANATOMY

The skin can be divided into its surface sectors and the lymph node region that drains a sector. The incidence of melanoma, according to body sectors, with emphasis on gender related differences is presented in Fig. 51.5A. This can be age related distribution of melanoma peaks between 25 and 70 years. 66% of all patients are between 25 and 64 years. Only 22% of cases are less than 40 years of age (Fig. 51.5B).

- The head and neck includes the face and scalp. It is the face and scalp that demand careful attention clinically because of the complex functions, cosmesis, and special senses that all need to be preserved. The lymph node drainage of the integumentary surface differs from the upper aerorespiratory and digestive passages. The first station or echelon draining the skin of the face and scalp is a ring of superficial nodes: submental, submaxillary, facial, preauricular, parotid, mastoid, and occipital.

- Anterior chest wall from the clavicles to the navel in males tends to be hirsute. Lesions on the anterior thoracic wall skin drain to the anterior axillary nodes.

- Posterior chest wall to the same level tends to be less hirsute, is exposed more often to the sun, and is subject to forming cancers. The regional nodes are along the posterior wall of the axilla, although all axillary nodes are at risk.

- The upper extremity is an infrequent sector involved with skin cancer but can be a site for burn and chronic inflammation. It is notorious for radiation-induced cancer in dentists who finger-held dental films during their practice. Serial resections occur with loss of fingers, then the hand, and then the forearm. Involvement of epitrochlear node, then axillary nodes, invariably leads to the patient's death from pulmonary metastases.

- The anterior abdominal wall draws into the femoral and inguinal nodes, but this sector of skin is rarely involved with skin cancers.

- The posterior abdominal wall or skin of the lower back is an infrequent site of malignancy and drains to femoral and inguinal nodes.

- The lower extremity is not a common site for skin cancers. Burns or chronic inflammation may cause lesions to evolve from hyperplasia to dysplasia and on to neoplasia. Popliteal nodes drain the foot and leg and ultimately drain into superficial femoral lymph nodes, which also drain the thigh.

Gender differences according to body locations differ for men and women. Males tend to have more lesions on the trunk and then the head and neck loci than do women. Females have more lesions on the lower and upper limbs than do men (Fig. 51.5A).

The vast majority of melanomas (66%) occur between 25 and 65 years of age, with a median age of 53 years, and peak between 65 and 70 years (Fig. 51.5B).

N-ONCOANATOMY

N-oncoanatomy of the skin surfaces emphasizes the anterior location for most if not all lymph node stations (see Fig. 51.6A, B, C).

- The concept of the sentinel lymph node began by injecting vital blue dye intradermally and then adding lymphoscintigraphy with 99mTc, draining lymph nodes were trapped and dissected. This is proved detection of sentinel nodes to 99% vs 83% for dye alone (Fig. 51.6C).

- The face and scalp drain into the superficial ring of nodes at the junction of the mandible and neck: submental, submandibular, preauricular, mastoid, and occipital nodes. Once involved, the rest of the deep lymph nodes in the neck along the carotid sheath and internal jugular vein are at risk.

- The axillary nodes are the recipient of lymphatics of the upper extremity and upper half body, both anterior and posterior skin surfaces.

- The femoral and inguinal nodes drain the lower extremity and the lower half of the body, both the anterior and posterior skin surfaces. The only exceptions are the popliteal lymph nodes that are posterior to knee joint, which drain the foot and leg.

M-ONCOANATOMY

There is a rich network of venous channels beneath all skin surfaces that allows for venous hematogenous spread once the dermal and hypodermal layers are penetrated by invading cancers. These venous collateral channels and plexus are rich and appear once obstruction occurs. (Fig. 51.6A, B).

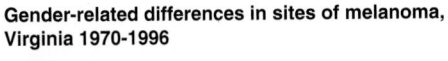

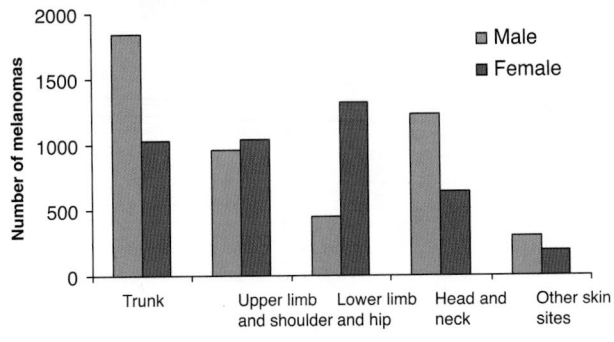

A Trunk M:F=1.8; lower limb M:F =1/3; head and neck M:F =1.9

Figure 51.5A | Incidence of melanoma in Virginia, 1970 to 1996, by gender. (From Virginia Cancer Registry, 1999.)

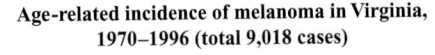

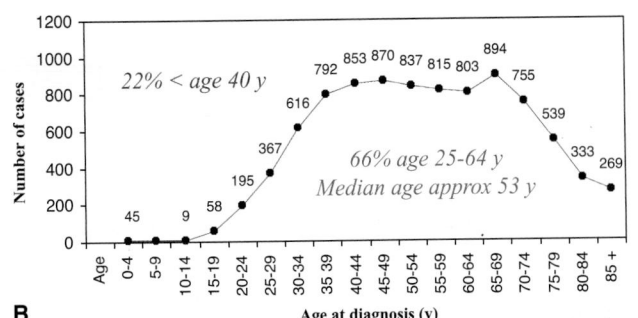

B

Figure 51.5B | Age related incidence of melanoma in Virginia, USA, 1970–1999. (From Virginia Cancer Registry, 1999.)

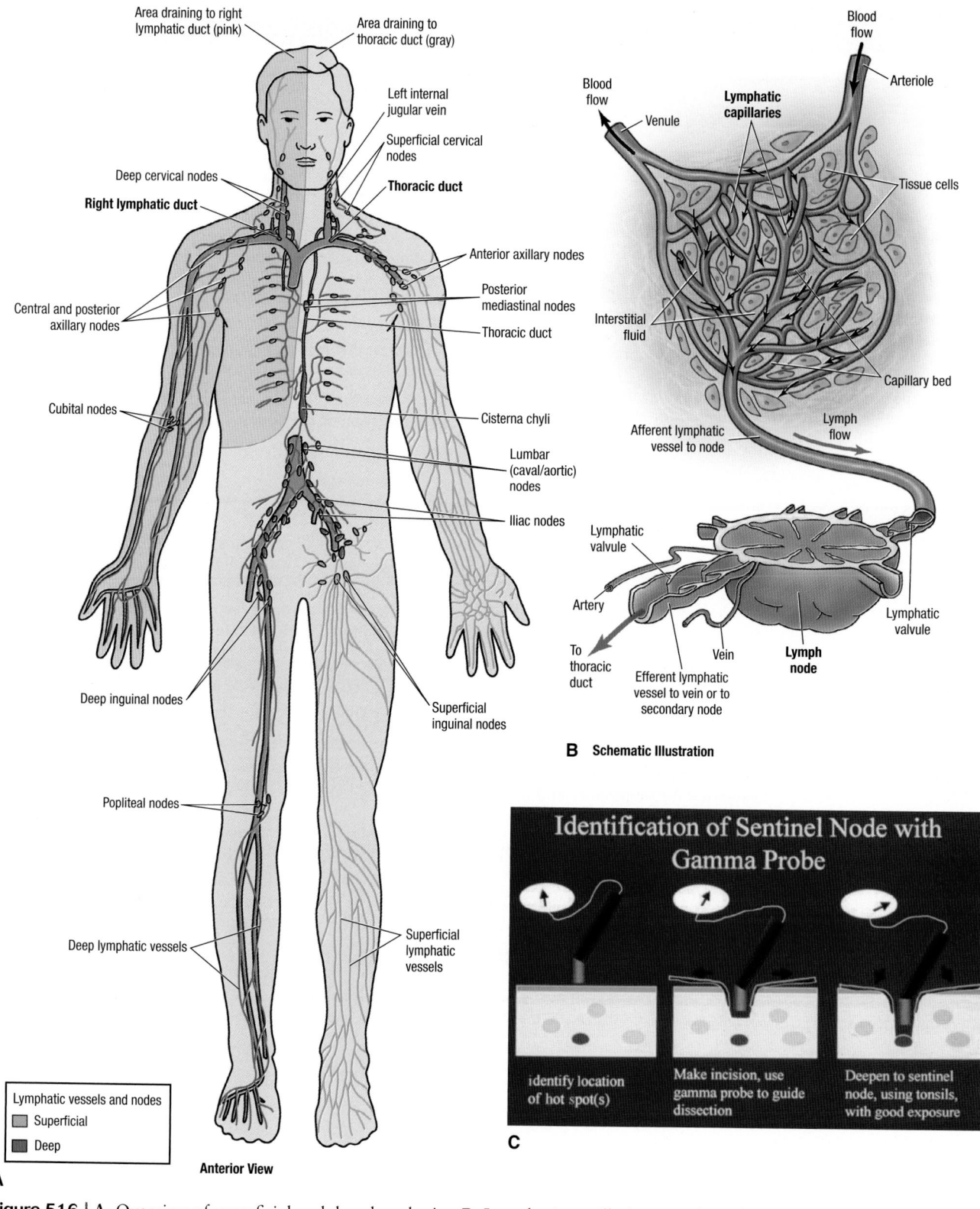

Figure 51.6 | **A.** Overview of superficial and deep lymphatics. **B.** Lymphatic capillaries, vessels, and nodes. Black arrows indicate the flow (leaking of interstitial fluid out of blood vessels and absorption) into the lymphatic capillaries. **C.** Schematic of the method to identify using lymphoscintigraphy with Tc99m. The draining sentinel node using a handheld gamma camera.

STAGING WORKUP

RULES OF CLASSIFICATION AND STAGING

The clinical and pathologic classifications are identified. Clinical staging is based on physical examination, inspection, and palpation of primary sites and draining regional nodes. Imaging with regular radiographs is adequate and includes skull films, facial bones, and mandible for deeply invading or fixed tumors beyond T1 in size. Computed tomography may be desirable for deeper invasion. Because of the high proclivity to metastasize, all advanced-stage melanoma must be thoroughly assessed with enhanced computed tomography and magnetic resonance imaging, especially if symptomatic (Table 51.3A).

It is important to compare the changes in the sixth versus the seventh edition of the *AJCC Manual* for accuracy in staging (Table 51.1B).

Pathologic Staging

Complete resection of the entire site is often performed with wide margins and the need to determine if there is any residuum. Skin grafting may be required to close the defect. Orientation of the section is critical to be sure the microsection is at a right angle to the skin surface. Any obliquity may increase the size of the melanoma depth of invasion. Ulceration advances the stage and must be determined on histopathology.

Sentinel lymph node biopsy is recommended for all T stages: T1b, T2, T3, and T4.

- Clinical assessment of regional lymph nodes is done after excision of the primary tumor.
- Complete staging of regional lymph nodes is done after surgical resection of the nodes.

TABLE 51.3	Imaging Modalities for Staging Skin Melanoma	
Method	Diagnosis and Staging Capability	Recommended for Use
Primary (T) Staging		
STUS	Mainly useful for recurrent, deeply invading melanomas	No, unless advanced
Nodal (N) Staging		
CT	Searching for adenopathy in regional lymph node station	Yes, for recurrent disease
Metastases (M) Staging		
CT-Ch	Evaluation for pulmonary and mediastinal disease	Yes, for advanced T3, T4 invasive disease
CT-Abd	Evaluation of liver for defects compatible with metastases	Yes, for advanced T3, T4 invasive disease
Bone scan Tc	Assessment of bone for activity followed by regular radiographs if positive	Yes, for advanced T3, T4 invasive disease or symptomatics
PET	Ability to find occult foci in total body scan, especially with CT	No, investigational mainly

CT, computed tomography; CT-Abd, abdominal CT; CT-Ch, chest CT; PET, positron emission tomography; STUS, soft tissue ultrasound.

PROGNOSIS AND CANCER SURVIVAL

PROGNOSIS

The limited number of prognostic factors are listed in Table 51.4.

Cox regression analysis of prognostic factors in 10,233 patients with localized cutaneous melanoma (stage I and II) is given in Table 51.5.

TABLE 51.4	Prognostic Factors
Clinically significant	Measured thickness
	Ulceration
	Serum lactate dehydrogenase (LDH)
	Mitotic rate
	Tumor-infiltrating lymphocytes (TIL)
	Level of invasion
	Vertical growth phase
	Regression

Data from Edge SB, Byrd DR, Compton CC, et al., *AJCC Cancer Staging Manual, 7th edition*, New York, Springer, 2010, p. 342.

TABLE 51.5	Analysis of Prognostic Factors in Localized Cutaneous Melanoma Stage I and II
Variable	**Chi-Square Value (1 d.f.)**
Tumor thickness	84.6
Mitotic rate	79.1
Ulceration	47.2
Age	40.8
Gender	32.4
Site	29.1
Clark's level	8.2

Edge SB, Byrd DR, Compton CC, et al., *AJCC Cancer Staging Manual, 7th edition*, New York, Springer, 2010, p. 330. Table 31.6.

CANCER STATISTICS AND SURVIVAL

Without exception, the cancer facts, findings, and statistics have been meticulously compiled (Fig. 51.7). The analysis of data on melanoma in the sixth edition of the *AJCC Manual* is very detailed and supports splitting four stages into 20 subgroupings as to outcomes. There are 63,130 new cases annually, 8,700 of whom will die. The 5-year survival rates of pathologically staged patients by Balch et al. demonstrate that ulceration and nodal involvement decrease survival. The differences in 15-year survival by stage are shown for localized stages IA and IB (>50%) versus stage III (30%) for nodal involvement and <10% survival at 5 years for stage IV metastasis based on the AJCC database of 17,000 patients with complete clinical and pathologic data.

Tumor Thickness as sole predictor of ten year survival after definitive therapy of primary melanoma Table 51.6. According to the recent American Cancer Society Figures and Facts 2010, the five year survival, according to stage, is:

- All stage 91%
- Localized 98%
- Regional 62%
- Metastatic 32%

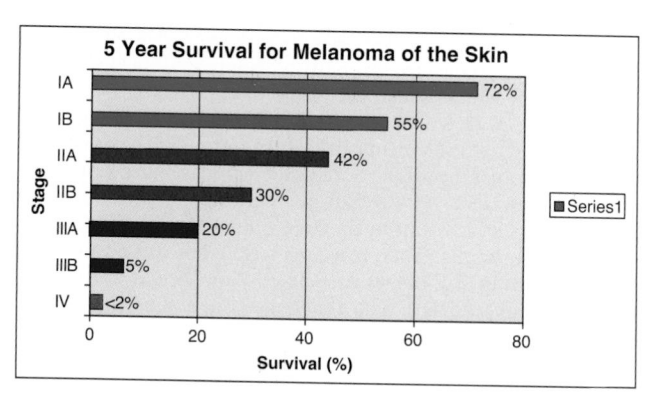

Figure 51.7 | Survival curves based on melanoma staging according to AJCC melanoma staging database. (Data from Edge SB, Byrd DR, Compton CC, et al., *AJCC Cancer Staging Manual, 7th edition*, New York, Springer, 2010, p. 329, Table 31.3.)

TABLE 51.6	Tumor Thickness as Sole Predictor of Outcome 10 years after Definitive Therapy of Primary Melanoma
Thickness (mm)	**Survival (%)**
≤1	83–88
1.01–2	64–79
2.01–4	51–64
>4	32–54

MMP: matrix metalloproteinase.
ADAM: proteins with A Disintegrin and A Metalloproteinase domain.
From Edge SB, Byrd DR, Compton CC, et al., *AJCC Cancer Staging Manual, 7th edition*, New York, Springer, 2010, p. 328. Table 31.3.

Musculoskeletal Soft Tissue Sarcoma

PERSPECTIVE, PATTERNS OF SPREAD, AND PATHOLOGY

Gauging the anatomic extent of soft tissue sarcoma requires an understanding of compartmental anatomy by investing fascia, which applies mainly but not exclusively to limbs.

PERSPECTIVE AND PATTERNS OF SPREAD

Soft tissues sarcomas are thought to originate exclusively from mesenchyme, which is also the origin of connective tissue. The mesenchyme is an embryonic stem cell that can have a variety of connective tissue elements, any and all of which can undergo malignant transformation. Soft tissue sarcomas are not common and represent <1% of all malignancies. Because of their rarity and their slow onset, they are often identified secondary to incidental trauma. Therefore, any suspicious soft tissue mass that increases in size or has associated pain should not be dismissed but investigated. The challenge is to achieve local control without sacrifice of a limb or vital axial part and yet early enough to avoid metastatic dissemination. Exciting advances in understanding the genetic determinants of this disease have allowed for new insights in its management. The incidence of musculoskeletal tumors is estimated at <10,000 new patients annually; only 25% occur in bone (2,500 cases). For every malignant soft tissue sarcoma, there are 100 benign neoplasms. The ratio is slightly higher in males than in females. By far, the most common sites are in lower and upper extremities, followed by axial and head and neck locations, with other sites such as retroperitoneum and pelvis being least common.

Patterns of spread tend to invade the compartment in which they arise. Superficial soft tissue sarcomas, that is, fibrosarcomas and liposarcomas, that arise in subcutaneous tissues spread along sagittal planes before invading underlying muscle. New muscle sarcomas invade within their muscle compartments initially, then the adjacent neurovascular bundles as they advance, and eventually bone (Fig. 52.1; Table 52.1).

The histopathologic types are highly varied and include malignant fibrous histiocytoma (40%), liposarcoma, synovial sarcoma, and neurofibrosarcoma as common types (each >10%); other varieties are infrequent (each <10%). Accurate assignment of histopathologic grade is the central component in staging of the patient's sarcoma. The essential features of establishing grade are nuclear and cellular morphology and pleomorphism. The number of mitoses per high-powered field,

the presence of necrosis, and the degree of cellularity all affect establishing grade by a pathologist with familiarity of soft tissue sarcomas. With modern molecular biology technology, cytogenetics and molecular genetics have been added to cytochemistry, immunohistochemistry, electron microscopy, and flow cytometry, supplementing routine hematoxylin and eosin staining microscopy. Grade has typically been assigned in terms of four grades, and the American Joint Committee on Cancer (AJCC) recommendation is into two tiers: low and high grade. From perusing the stage grouping it is evident that pathologic grade dominates the anatomic extent.

ETIOLOGY

Most soft tissue sarcomas occur sporadically. Their etiology is undefined, although, in rare cases, there is an association with familial disease syndromes:

- Desmoid tumors among patients with *familial polyposis.*

- Sarcomas of soft tissue and bone in patients with *hereditary or bilateral retinoblastoma.*

- *Neurofibromatosis type 1,* in which benign neurofibromas and malignant neurofibrosarcomas are seen.

- Bone and soft tissue sarcomas in patients with *Li–Fraumeni syndrome.*

In addition to genetic causes, soft tissue sarcomas are occasionally associated with exposure to carcinogens.

For example, radiation therapy has been linked to the development of bone and soft tissue sarcomas, although this occurrence is uncommon, and cohort studies of this phenomenon are rare. The frequency of radiation-induced sarcoma is higher following treatment in children, particularly those with Ewing's sarcoma and retinoblastoma. In addition to radiation, exposure to chemicals, such as chemotherapeutic agents, phenoxyacetic acid, chlorophenols, and vinyl chloride, is similarly related to the development of sarcomas.

An interesting feature of soft tissue sarcomas is that some of these tumors display stable chromosomal translocations; these translocations eventually may serve as diagnostic criteria. For example, a study in the Netherlands found patterns of structural and numeric imbalances in a series of malignant fibrous histiocytomas, the most common subtype of malignant

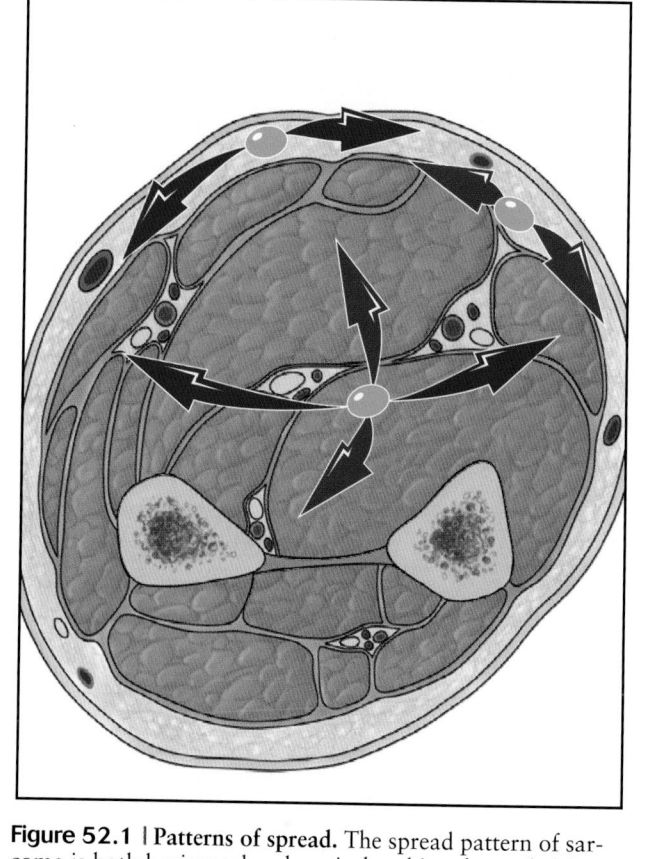

Figure 52.1 | Patterns of spread. The spread pattern of sarcoma is both horizontal and vertical and is color coded for stage: T0, yellow; T1, green; T2, blue; T3, purple; and T4, red. The concept of visualizing patterns of spread to appreciate the surrounding anatomy is well demonstrated by the six-directional pattern (SIMLAP, Table 52.1).

TABLE 52.1	SIMLAP
Musculoskeletal: Soft Tissue Sarcoma in Upper Extremity	
S	Axillary artery, vein, nerves, nodes
I	Epitrochlear nodes
M	Humerus
L	Dermis, skin
A	Anterior compartment
P	Posterior compartment, intermuscular septum

The six vectors of invasion are Superior, Inferior, Medial, Lateral, Anterior, and Posterior. The color-coded dots correlate the T stage with the specific anatomic structure involved.

- Synovial cell sarcomas are characterized by the translocation t(X;18)(p11.2;q11.2), which has been cloned and has led to the identification of two novel genes, *SYT* and *SSX*.

- Alveolar rhabdomyosarcomas show a translocation at t(2;13)(q35;q14). This chimeric gene has also been cloned and has been termed *PAX3-FKHR*. Molecular determination of minimal residual disease in alveolar rhabdomyosarcoma is possible with this gene, but the clinical significance of this finding is uncertain.

- Clear cell sarcomas often exhibit a t(12;22)(q13-14;q12) translocation. This entity is sometimes referred to as malignant melanoma of soft parts, although it should be noted that the t(12;22)(q13-14;q12) translocation is not seen in cutaneous malignant melanoma.

- Alterations of the retinoblastoma gene (*RB*) are a common finding in the sporadic development of soft tissue sarcomas. Loss of *RB* immunoreactivity and *RB* loss of heterozygosity have been correlated with a poorer outcome.

- Somatic alterations of the *TP53* gene are also common in soft tissue sarcomas. It is now well recognized that the high cancer incidence in patients with Li–Fraumeni syndrome, in which soft tissue and bone sarcomas are prominent, is the consequence of germline mutations on the *TP53* gene.

- The *MDM2* gene, located at 12q13-14, was observed to be frequently amplified in soft tissue sarcomas. *SAS*, another gene located at 12q13-14, was similarly amplified in soft tissue sarcomas.

Molecular characterizations of these chromosomal abnormalities serve as diagnostic criteria for soft tissue sarcomas. It is expected that diagnosis will be made on the basis of histology, immunohistochemistry, cytogenetics, and molecular biology in the near future. Indeed, genetic evaluation already is proving to be a useful complement to histopathologic assessment.

soft tissue sarcomas. Through the use of comparative genomic hybridization and conventional cytogenetic and Southern blot analyses, researchers have found increases in 1q21-q22 (69%) and 20q (66%), and decreases in 9p21-pter (55%) and 11q23-qter (55%), along with loss of *TP53* and amplification of *MDM2* genes.

Many of these chromosomal abnormalities have been characterized at the molecular level, and chimeric genes that are associated with these cytogenetic changes have been cloned. Some of these developments are providing clues to the molecular alterations that are fundamental to the development of soft tissue sarcomas:

- Myxoid liposarcoma displays a t(12;16)(q13;p11) translocation. The fusion gene, known as *TLS/FUS-CHOP*, fails to induce G_1/S arrest, whereas the nononcogenic form of *CHOP* induces a normal G_1/S arrest.

OVERVIEW OF HISTOGENESIS AND HISTOPATHOLOGY

The connective tissues are the derivatives of the mesenchymal stem cell. The derivative normal cells that can become malignant and give rise to a large variety of soft tissue sarcomas are given in Table 52.2. The composite illustration of loose connective tissue (LCT; Fig. 52.2) vividly illustrates the rich variety of cells and types of connective tissue fibers. LCT is constituted by the fibroblast, the fibrocyte, fat cells, mast cells, and macrophages in a rich matrix of extracellular materials such as collagen bundles, reticular fibers, and elastic fibers, along with abundant ground substance. This LCT constitutes the hypodermis and is the intermediate layer between the skin epidermis and dermis and the investing fascia, which is the initial tight wrapping around the musculature and neurovascular bundle and bone. This investing fascia is the dense connective tissue, which has more collagen bundles packed together with fewer cells and less ground substance. The "dense irregular connective tissue" defines the deep muscle compartment of limbs, the head and neck, and the trunk. The "dense regular connective tissue" constitutes the ligaments of muscles and joints. In dense connective tissue, fibroblasts and fibrocytes are the dominant cells.

The fusiform-shaped fibroblast synthesizes collagen fiber and ground substance. The fibrocyte is a resting cell, and the presence or absence of adipose cells determines whether the connective tissue is loose or dense, respectively. Macrophages and histiocytes are numerous in LCTs but are difficult to distinguish from fibrocytes unless they are phagocytic. It is for this reason that the malignant fibrous histiocytoma is the dominant soft tissue sarcoma. Mast cells, plasma cells, and lymphocytes permeate LCTs and occasional leukocytes owing to the rich network of capillaries and small vessels in the hypodermis. The collagen fibers are tough, thick proteinaceous bundles; the elastic fibers are fine, resilient, and, when stretched, return to their initial position; reticular fibers form delicate, netlike meshworks.

Collagen is abundant in soft tissues, muscle compartments, and fascial layer tendons. Elastic fibers are abundant in blood vessels, especially arteries, lungs, urinary bladder, and Cooper's ligaments in breasts. They enable return to the original shape after stretching. Reticular fibers are the network mesh in liver, lymph nodes, spleen, bone marrow, and generally in lymphatic and hematopoietic organs (Table 52.2; Fig. 52.2A, C).

To complete the story of soft tissues, the largest bulk of soft tissue—muscle mass—needs to be presented. There are three types of muscle tissues: skeletal, striated muscle, and, to a lesser degree, smooth, nonstriated muscle, and cardiac muscle. Muscle cells are inactive mitotically, largely consisting of sarcoplasm, surrounded by sarcolemma membrane. Muscle contains numerous myofibrils, which contain two types of contractile proteins—actin and myosin. Skeletal muscle fibers are multinucleated cells with cross-striations. They tend to hypertrophy rather than undergo hyperplasia to increase muscle mass, which may account for the rarity of adult rhabdomyosarcoma. In children, embryonal rhabdomyosarcoma is more common. The smooth muscle layer lines the wall of hollow viscera such as the digestive organ, ureter, urinary bladder, and blood vessels. They tend to form benign leiomyomas more than leiomyosarcomas. Cardiac myocytes rarely give rise to any tumefaction and, in blood vessels, proliferation of myofibroblasts cause restenosis rather than angiosarcomas, which account for <1% of all soft tissue sarcomas (Table 52.2; Fig. 52.2B, D).

The last soft tissue element is nerve fibers of the peripheral nervous system, which consists of neurons, nerves, and axons. The peripheral nervous system is composed of various sizes of axons, surrounded by layers of connective tissue that partition several nerve bundles (axons) into fascicles. The epineurium is the thicker outer layer, whereas the perineurium is the thinner inner layer of nerve fibers. The supportive cell is the myelin-forming neurolemmocyte (Schwann cells) and satellite cells surround the neuronal cells in paravertebral and peripheral ganglia. Neurofibrosarcoma are among the more common soft tissue malignancies and constitute 12% of soft tissue sarcomas (Table 52.2).

TABLE 52.2	Histopathologic Types of Soft Tissue Sarcomas
Type	**Derivative Normal Cell**
Alveolar soft-part sarcoma	Neuromyogenic cell
Desmoplastic small round-cell tumor	Epithelioid endothelial
Epithelioid sarcoma	Fascial tendon fibrocyte
Clear cell sarcoma	Primitive mesenchymal
Chondrosarcoma, extraskeletal	Chondroblast
Osteosarcoma, extraskeletal	Osteoblast
Gastrointestinal stromal tumor	Leiomyoblast
Ewing's sarcoma/primitive neuroectodermal tumor	Primitive mesenchymal
Fibrosarcoma	Fibroblast
Leiomyosarcoma	Smooth myocyte
Liposarcoma	Adipolyte
Malignant fibrous histiocytoma	Fibroblast/histiocyte
Malignant hemangiopericytoma	Pericytes
Malignant peripheral nerve sheath tumor	Neurilemma (Schwann)
Rhabdomyosarcoma	Myofibroblast
Synovial sarcoma	Biphasic synovial epithelial cell
Sarcoma, not otherwise specified	Mesenchymal cell

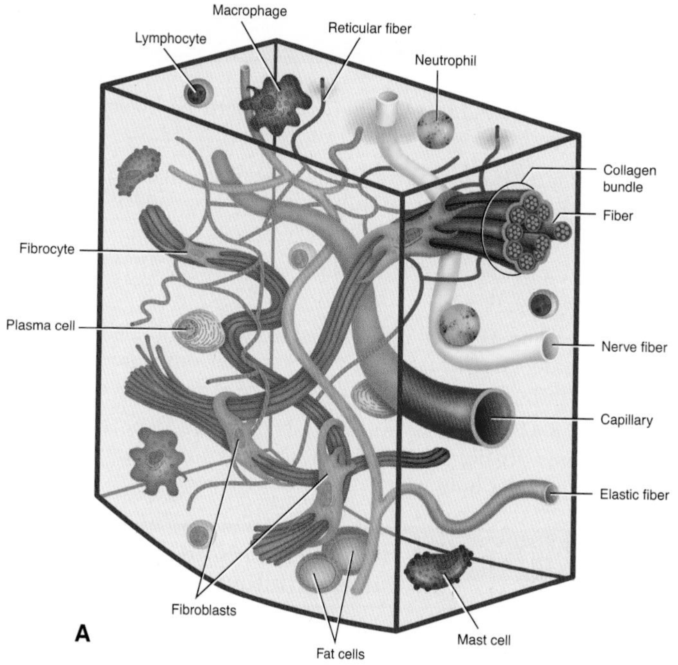

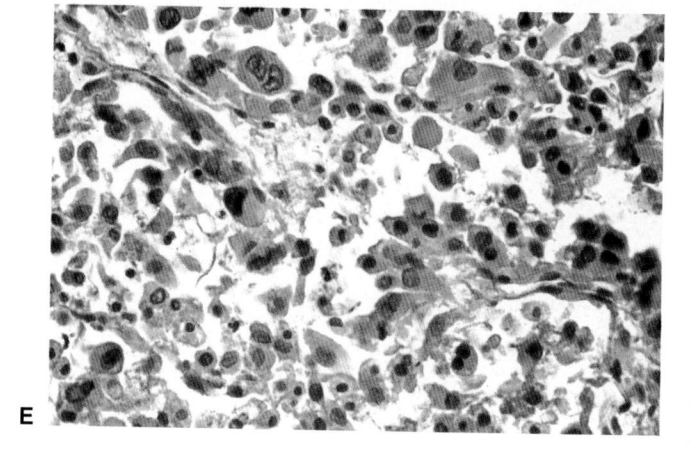

A. Macrophage, Reticular fiber, Neutrophil, Lymphocyte, Collagen bundle, Fiber, Fibrocyte, Plasma cell, Nerve fiber, Capillary, Elastic fiber, Fibroblasts, Fat cells, Mast cell

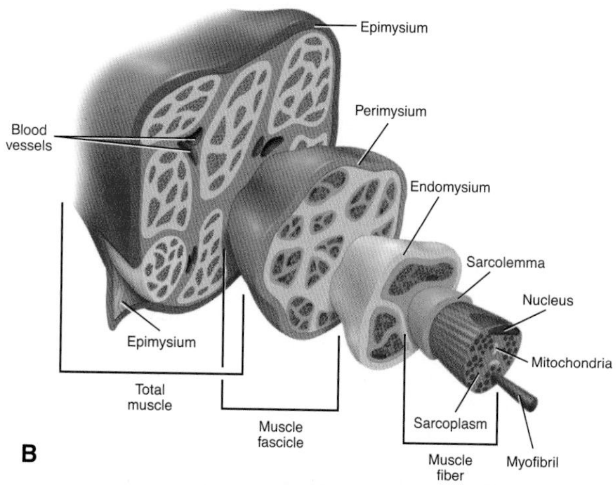

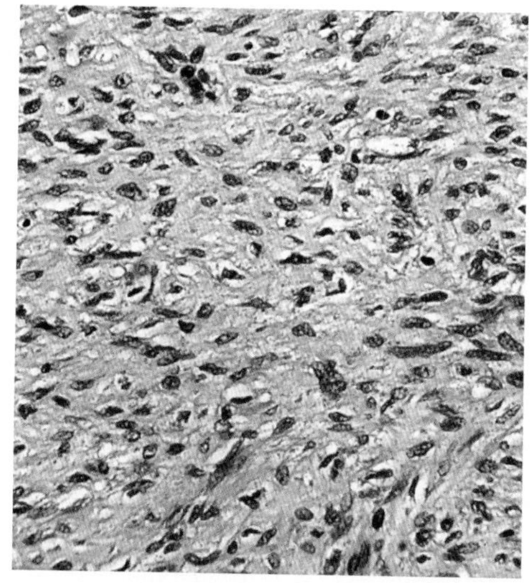

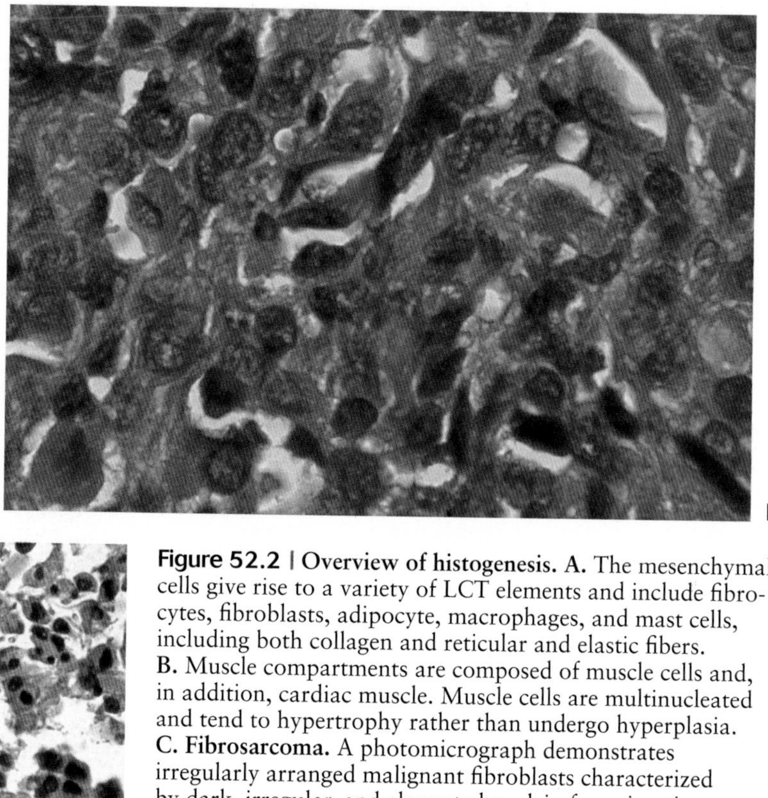

B. Epimysium, Perimysium, Endomysium, Sarcolemma, Nucleus, Mitochondria, Blood vessels, Epimysium, Total muscle, Muscle fascicle, Muscle fiber, Sarcoplasm, Myofibril

Figure 52.2 | Overview of histogenesis. A. The mesenchymal cells give rise to a variety of LCT elements and include fibrocytes, fibroblasts, adipocyte, macrophages, and mast cells, including both collagen and reticular and elastic fibers. **B.** Muscle compartments are composed of muscle cells and, in addition, cardiac muscle. Muscle cells are multinucleated and tend to hypertrophy rather than undergo hyperplasia. **C. Fibrosarcoma.** A photomicrograph demonstrates irregularly arranged malignant fibroblasts characterized by dark, irregular, and elongated nuclei of varying sizes. **D. Rhabdomyosarcoma.** The tumor contains polyhedral and spindle-shaped tumor cells with enlarged, hyperchromatic nuclei and deeply eosinophilic cytoplasm. A few cells have clearly visible cross-striations. **E. Alveolar rhabdomyosarcoma.** The neoplastic cells are arranged in clusters that display an alveolar pattern.

TNM STAGING CRITERIA

TNM STAGING CRITERIA

Gauging the anatomic extent of soft tissue sarcoma requires an understanding of compartmental anatomy, which applies mainly, but not exclusively, to the limbs. The depth of invasion of soft tissue sarcomas in limbs and the trunk is more important than size. The hypodermis is deep to the dermis and is the common location. The term "superficial" is defined as lack of involvement of the investing fascia, whereas "deep" implies deep to or involving the investing fascia. The relationship of the investing fascia is readily apparent in limbs. All intraperitoneal, retroperitoneal, intrathoracic truncal soft tissue sarcomas are considered deep. Head and neck tumors may be designated superficial or deep. There are two T stages based on size: T1, <5 cm; and T2, >5 cm. Each can be superficial (T1A or T2A) or deep (T1B or T2B) related to investing fascia. Grades I and II are low, and grades III and IV are high. Nodal invasion is less common than hematogenous spread, and N1 is equivalent to M1 or stage IV.

Grade is a very important criterion and has been extensively revised from a two-grade system to three tiers based on the National Institutes of Health and the French systems. The grade is determined by three parameters that are scored (Table 52.3A, B):

- Differentiation (1–3)
- Mitotic Activity (1–3)
- Necrosis (0–2)

SUMMARY OF CHANGES SEVENTH EDITION AJCC

- Gastrointestinal stromal tumor (GIST) is now included in Chapter 16; fibromatosis (desmoids tumor), Kaposi's

sarcoma, and infantile fibrosarcoma are no longer included in the histological types for this site (Fig. 52.3).

- Angiosarcoma, extraskeletal Ewing's sarcoma, and dermatofibrosarcoma protuberans have been added to the list of histologic types for this site.

- N1 disease has been reclassified as Stage III rather than Stage IV disease.

- Grading has been reformatted from a four grade to a three-grade system as per the criteria recommended by the College of American Pathologists.

- Kaposi's sarcoma, fibromatosis (desmoid tumor), and sarcoma arising from the dura mater, brain, parenchymatous organs, or hollow viscera are not included.

TABLE 52.3B	Histology-specific Tumor Differentiation Score

Histologic Type	Score
Atypical lipomatous tumor/well-differentiated liposarcoma	1
Myxoid liposarcoma	2
Round cell liposarcoma	3
Pleomorphic liposarcoma	3
Dedifferentiated liposarcoma	3
Fibrosarcoma	2
Myxofibrosarcoma [myxoid malignant fibrous histiocytoma (MFH)]	2
Typical storiform MFH (sarcoma, not otherwise specified)	2
MFH, pleomorphic type (patternless pleomorphic sarcoma)	3
Giant cell and inflammatory MFH (pleomorphic sarcoma, NOS with giant cells or inflammatory cells)	3
Well-differentiated leiomyosarcoma	1
Conventional leiomyosarcoma	2
Poorly differentiated/pleomorphic/epithelioid leiomyosarcoma	3
Biphasic/monophasic synovial sarcoma	3
Poorly differentiated synovial sarcoma	3
Pleomorphic rhabdomyosarcoma	3
Mesenchymal chondrosarcoma	3
Extraskeletal osteosarcoma	3
Ewing's sarcoma/primitive neuroectodermal tumor	3
Malignant rhabdoid tumor	3
Undifferentiated sarcoma	3

TABLE 52.3A	Scores Are Summed to Designate Tumor Grade

Score	Differentiation	Mitotic Count	Tumor Necrosis
1	Sarcomas closely resembling normal, mature mesenchymal tissue	0–9 mitoses per 10 HPFs	No tumor necrosis
2	Sarcomas of definite histologic type	10–19 mitoses per 10 HPFs	Less than or equal to ≤50% tumor necrosis
3	Synovial sarcomas, embryonal sarcomas, undifferentiated sarcomas, and sarcomas of unknown/doubtful tumor type	20 or more mitoses per 10 HPFs	>50% tumor necrosis

HPF, high-power field.
Used with the permission of the American Joint Committee on Cancer (AJCC) Chicago, Illinois. The original source for this material is the *AJCC Cancer Staging Manual*, Seventh edition (2010) published by Springer SBM, LLC, p 294.

Used with the permission of the American Joint Committee on Cancer (AJCC) Chicago, Illinois. The original source for this material is the *AJCC Cancer Staging Manual*, Seventh edition (2010) published by Springer SBM, LLC, p 294.

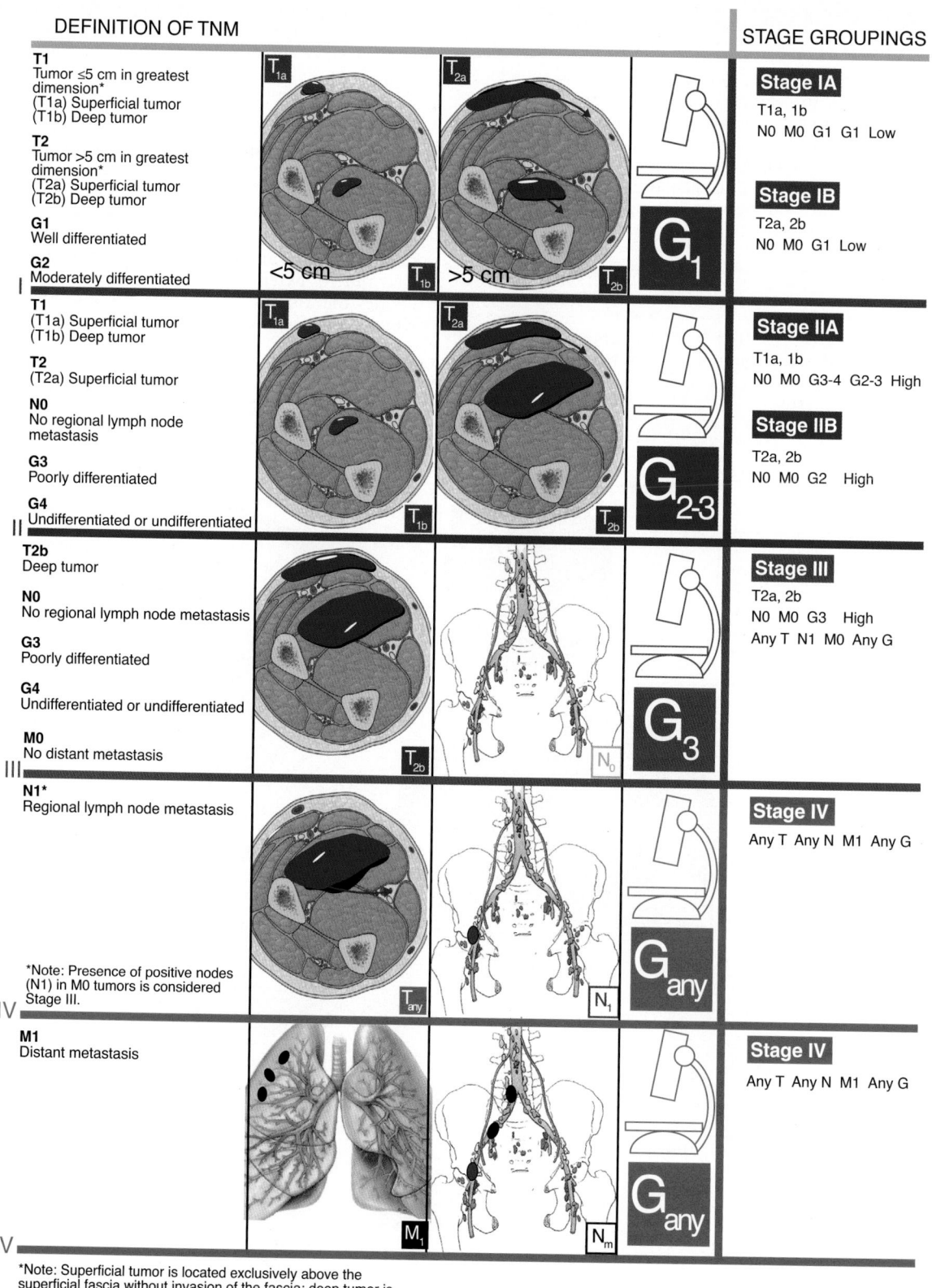

Figure 52.3 | TNM staging diagram. Soft tissue sarcomas are resected with the goal of limb preservation and are defined by compartmental anatomy. There are four stages when histologic grade is added to the T stage. N1 is equivalent to distant metastases. Color bars are coded for stage: stage I, green; II, blue; III, purple; IV, red; and metastatic disease to viscera and nodes, black. Note the importance of tumor grade in addition to anatomic extent.

T-ONCOANATOMY

ORIENTATION OF T-ONCOANATOMY

The ubiquitous distribution of connective tissue and muscle presents a challenge to defining this compartment anatomically. The major anatomic sectors are explored as functions of the frequency of soft tissue malignancies. The logical emphasis in oncoanatomy is on the limbs.

The three-dimensional and three-planar oncoanatomies are presented for each site, starting with the superficial investing fascia located deep to the skin in the hypodermis.

THREE-PLANAR ANATOMY

The upper limbs are presented in this chapter although the frequency of soft tissue sarcomas are in the lower limb.

Because compartmental anatomy is the key concept, the axial or transverse planes of limbs are the focus of the primary-site anatomy more than coronal or sagittal planes.

- *Upper limb* (Fig. 52.4ABC): The investing fascia is the superficial fascia and consists of the brachial fascia in the arm and the antebrachial fascia in the forearm. The brachial fascia is also the deep fascia of the arm and divides the muscle compartments into anterior (biceps) and posterior (triceps) compartments by its extensions, namely, the lateral and medial intermuscular septa. In the forearm, the antebrachial fascia is the superficial fascia, and its extension in the interosseous membrane divides the anterior from the posterior compartments, which is the deep aspect of the staging system for soft tissue sarcoma.

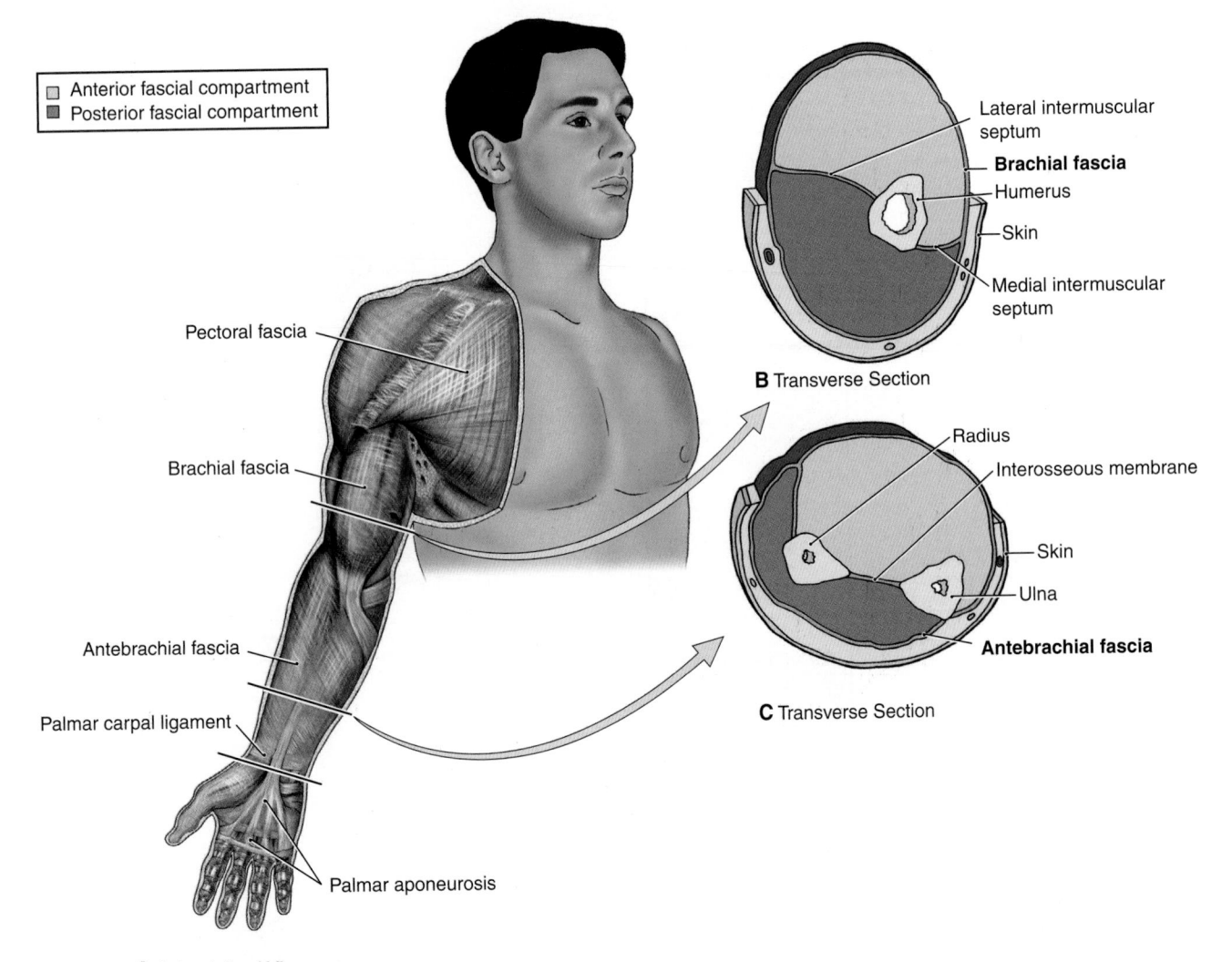

Figure 52.4 | Orientation of T-oncoanatomy of the upper limb. A. Anterior view of investing fascia. **B.** Transverse through arm. **C.** Transverse through forearm.

The anatomic and age distribution by pathology of soft tissue sarcomas is essential to understanding the challenges in diagnosis and treatment of these sarcomas which can occur in any site throughout the body. The majority are located in the extremities (41%), with 29% of all lesions occurring most commonly in the thigh of the lower limb; the intradominal location accounts for a third of the sarcomas and they are equally divided between visceral (21%) and retroperitoneal (15%) locations. Another 10%

are truncal and 5% are in the head and neck region (Fig. 52.4D). Soft tissue sarcomas, as are most cancers, are most common with increasing age; the median age at diagnosis is 65 years.

However, median age varies by histologic type and subtype. Alveolar rhabdomyosarcoma and desmoplastic small round cell sarcomas occur in young adults, whereas leiomyosarcomas, liposarcomas, and angiosarcomas occur most commonly in the 50–60 year old age group (Fig. 52.4E).

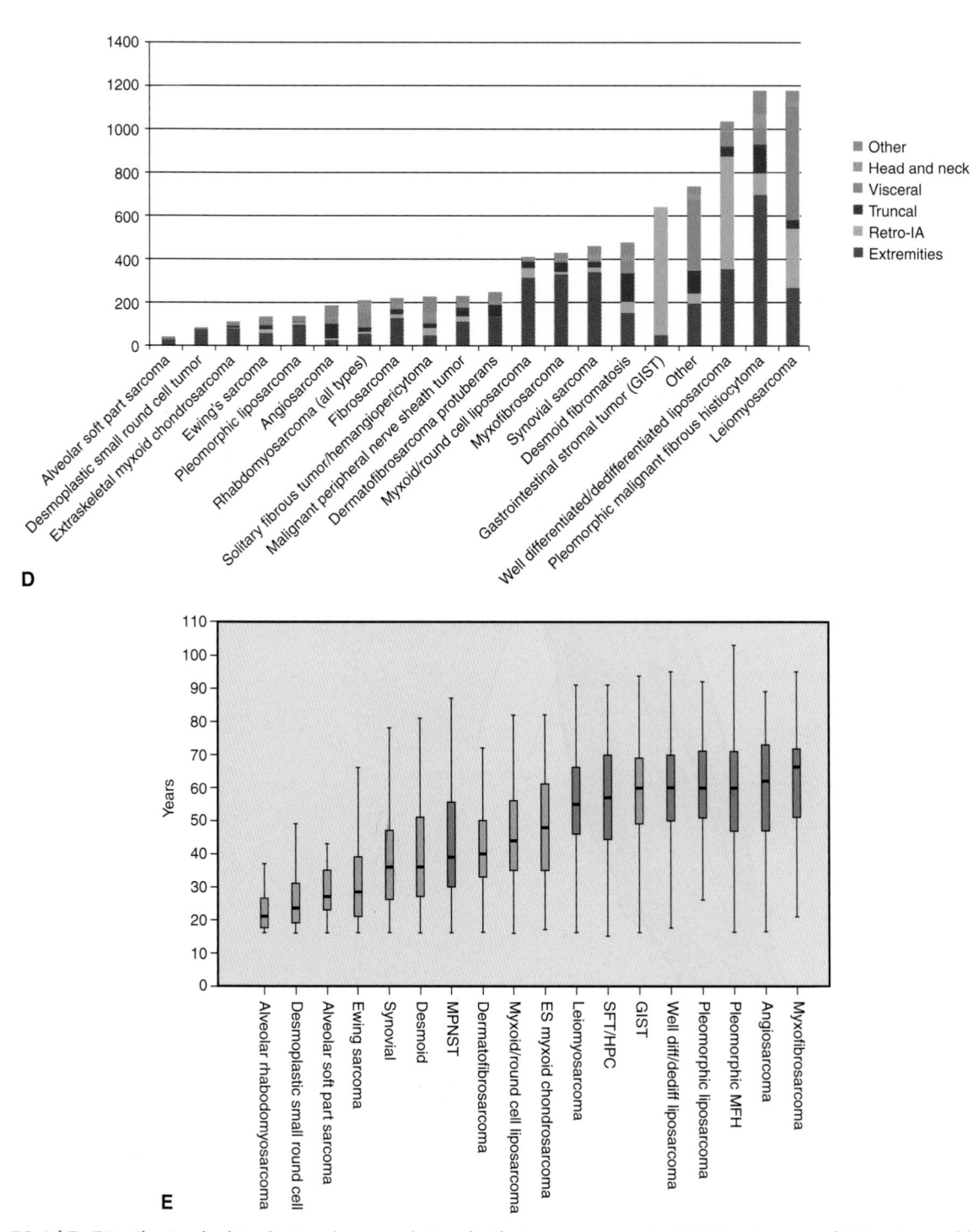

Figure 52.4 | D. Distribution by histologic subtype and site of soft tissue sarcomas in 8,328 patients aged 16 years or older admitted to the Memorial Sloan-Kettering Cancer Center from 1982 to 2009. The retroperitoneal/abdominal category excludes visceral sarcomas. **E.** Age at diagnosis for sarcoma subtypes. The boxes show median and interquartile range and the whiskers show range (with outliers excluded) for 7,212 patients aged 16 years or older admitted to Memorial Sloan-Kettering Cancer Center from 1982 through 2009. Sarcoma subtypes with simple genotypes, shown in red, are associated with younger median age at diagnosis than those with complex genotypes, shown in blue.

N-ONCOANATOMY AND M-ONCOANATOMY

N-ONCOANATOMY

N-oncoanatomy of the soft tissues beneath the skin surfaces emphasizes the anterior location for most if not all lymph node stations (Fig. 52.5).

- The axillary nodes are the recipients for lymphatics of the upper extremity and upper half body, including both anterior and posterior thoracic abdominal walls.

- The femoral and inguinal nodes drain the lower extremity and the lower half of the body on their anterior and posterior surfaces.

- The face and scalp drain into the superficial ring of nodes at the junction of the mandible and neck: submental, submandibular, preauricular, mastoid, and occipital nodes. Once involved, the rest of the lymph nodes in the neck along the carotid arterial sheath and internal jugular vein are at risk.

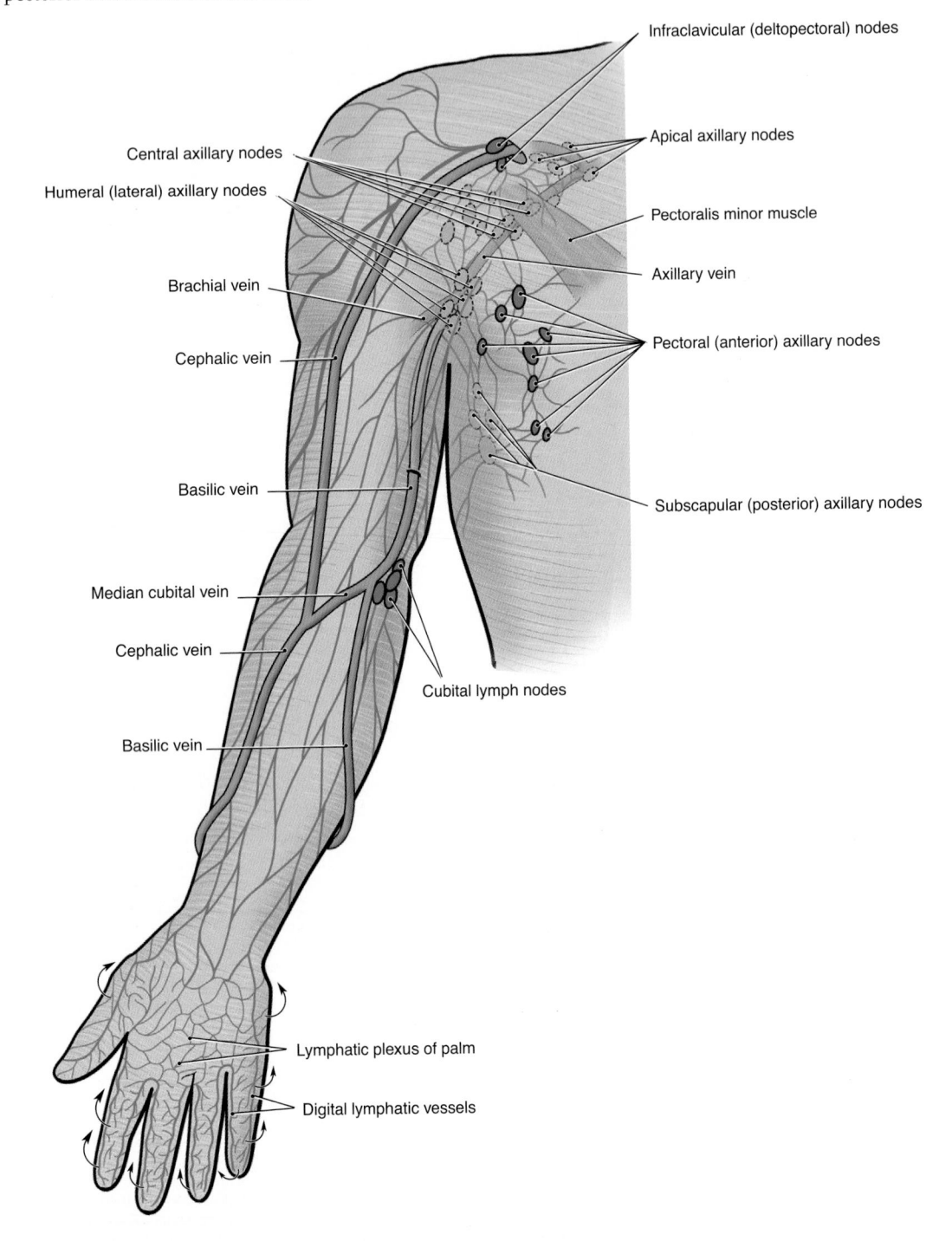

Anterior View

Figure 52.5 | N-oncoanatomy of the upper limb.

M-ONCOANATOMY

There is a rich network of venous channels in the hypodermis of all skin surfaces that allows for hematogenous spread once the dermal and hypodermal layers are invaded by soft tissue sarcoma. Collateral venous channels and plexus are rich and rapidly appear once obstruction occurs (Fig. 52.6). Pulmonary metastases are the most common site.

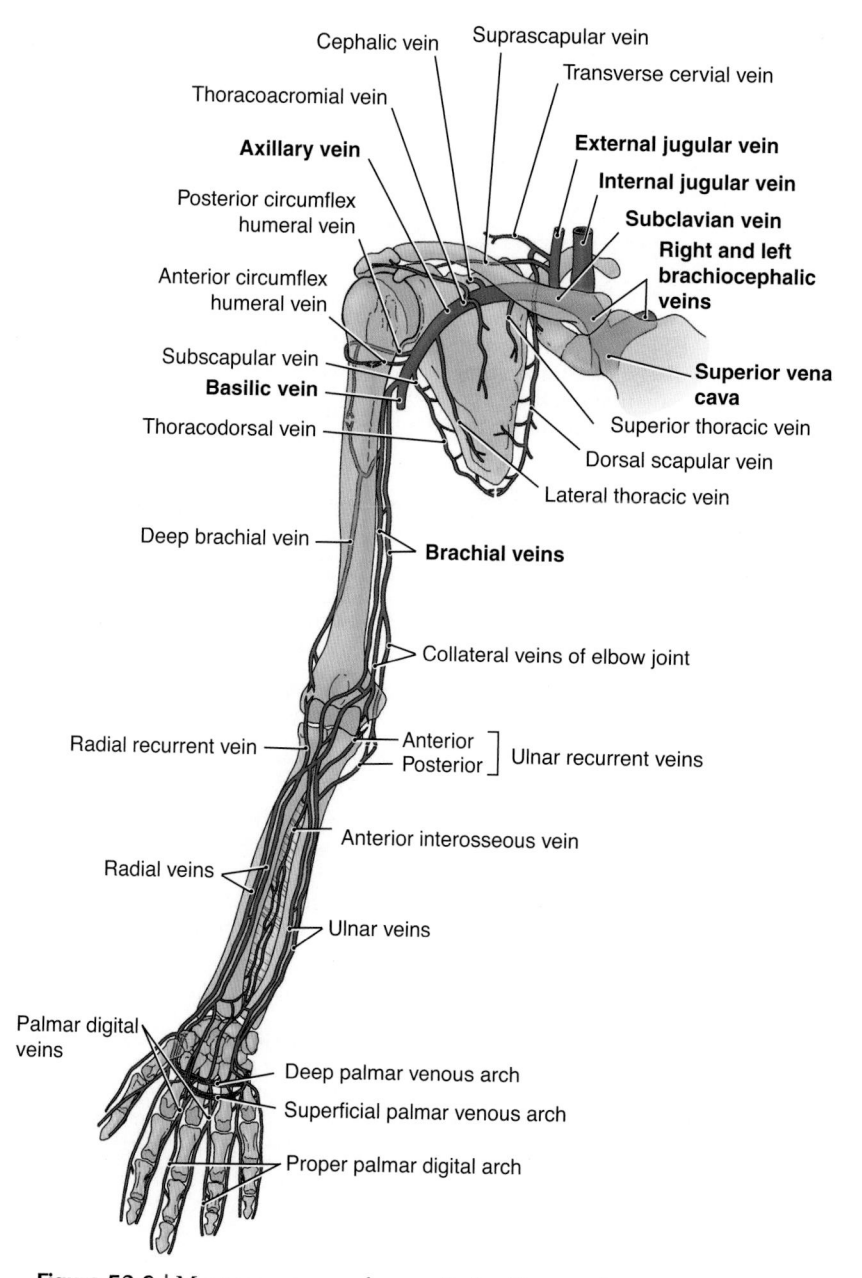

Figure 52.6 | M-oncoanatomy of upper limbs. Venous plexus and drainage.

STAGING WORKUP

RULES OF CLASSIFICATION AND STAGING

Clinical Staging and Imaging

Whenever feasible, physical examination in conjunction with imaging should establish size of the tumor: T1, <5 cm; or T2, >5 cm. Modern cross-sectional imaging is essential, and spiral computed tomography (CT) and magnetic resonance imaging (MRI) are of value and are complementary (Fig. 52.7; Table 52.4).

Pathologic Staging

Pathologic staging is an essential aspect of staging; histopathologic grading is critical. Imaging is valuable for orientation of surgical margins (ink markings), particularly for conservation surgery with reliance on postoperative radiation to ablate any residuum of tumor. Immunohistochemical staining and cytogenetics may be helpful for subtyping tumors.

- *Accurate measurement of tumor size* is important because it is regarded as a continuous variable, with 5 cm as an arbitrary dividing line between T1 and T2. Radiologic imaging can be used when resected specimens are difficult to interpret.

- *Depth* is very important to staging; superficial is designated A, and deep is designated B for each T category and stage. Superficial soft tissue sarcomas are in the hypodermis and do not involve the superficial investing fascia, which is the dividing line between the hypodermis and the deep muscle compartments. Note that all visceral soft tissue sarcomas are considered deep, as are retroperitoneal or intraperitoneal soft tissue sarcomas.

- *Grade* is critical to stage and is referred to as low or high. Low refers to grades I and II. High refers to grades III and IV.

- *Recurrent* soft tissue sarcomas are restaged following the same rules as the primary soft tissue sarcoma.

- *Nodes,* when enlarged, need histopathologic confirmation because they are so uncommon.

Oncoimaging Annotations

- Ultrasonography cannot discriminate between benign and malignant soft tissue tumors and is not recommended for their classification.

- Ultrasonography is useful in guiding percutaneous biopsy and may be useful in answering specific concerns in post-treatment follow-up.

- CT tends not to add value to the workup of the primary soft tissue tumor site compared with MRI.

- MRI is the primary modality in the pretreatment assessment of these tumors. Surface coils are necessary, and axial images are required. The utility of gadolinium enhancement is controversial.

- Hemorrhage, hematoma, and inflammatory changes can be confused with tumor on MRI.

- MRI has disappointing accuracy in assigning benign or malignant tumor status and even less reliability in predicting histology in most cases.

- MRI is the dominant imaging modality for determining intracompartmental and extracompartmental extent of a soft tissue sarcoma and its relationship to critical neurovascular structures.

- Sarcomas treated before limb salvage surgery with chemotherapy should be restaged with MRI before operation.

- The role of positron emission tomography in evaluating tumor response to neoadjuvant chemotherapy is still being explored.

- Systemic metastatic disease, usually to the lungs, and local recurrence have their maximum hazard rates within the first 2 years, defining the most frequent follow-up intervals for the first 2 years and tapering over a total of 5 years for osseous sarcomas.

TABLE 52.4	Imaging Modalities for Staging Soft Tissue Sarcomas	
Method	Diagnosis and Staging Capability	Recommended for Use
Primary (T) Staging		
MRI	MRI provides optimal cross-sectional three-planar views of both axial and appendicular anatomy	Yes, superior for soft tissue extensions
CT$_e$	CT preferably helical is complementary since it is superior in showing bony erosion and destruction by soft tissue sarcoma	Yes, advantage if bone is invaded
US	US may be of value in initial localizing of a mass or for guiding needle biopsies of primary sites or nodes	No, not detailed
Nodal (N) Staging and Metastases (M) Staging		
PET	Used with FDG as a total body scan, searching for disseminated disease	No, unless metastases are highly suspected

CT$_e$, computed tomography enhanced with intravenous contrast; FDG, fluorodeoxyglucose; MRI, magnetic resonance imaging; PET, positron emission tomography; US, ultrasound.

PROGNOSTIC FACTORS AND CANCER SURVIVAL

PROGNOSTIC FACTORS

Required for staging:
- grade

Clinically significant:
- neurovascular invasion as determined by pathology.
- Bone invasion as determined by imaging. If pM1, source of pathologic metastatic specimen.*

Anatomic extent and histologic grade determine the stage.

The TNM staging matrix is color coded for identification of stage group once T and N stages are determined (Table 52.6).

*Preceding passage from Edge SB, Byrd DR, and Compton CC, et al, *AJCC Cancer Staging Manual, 7th edition*. New York: Springer, 2010, p. 298.

TABLE 52.5 Five-Year Survival Rates in Extremity Soft Tissue Sarcoma

Stage	N	Freedom from Local Recurrence (%)	Disease-free Survival (%)	Overall Survival (%)
I	137	88.04	86.13	90.00
II	491	81.97	71.68	80.89
III	469	83.44	51.77	56.29

Data from Memorial Sloan-Kettering Cancer Center (MSKCC) for the time period of July 1, 1982, to June 30, 2000.
Used with the permission of the American Joint Committee on Cancer (AJCC) Chicago, Illinois. The original source for this material is the *AJCC Cancer Staging Manual,* Seventh edition (2010) published by Springer SBM, LLC, p 295.

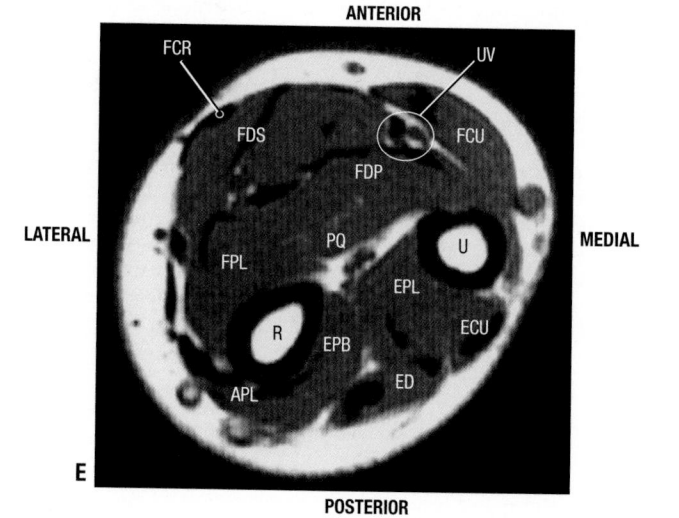

Figure 52.7 | Transverse MRI through the distal forearm.

CANCER STATISTICS AND SURVIVAL

Soft tissue sarcomas account for 10,520 cases annually (male, 5,680; female, 4,840). The number of deaths is <10% of these (1,460 annually). When compared with primary cancer sites, the current gains in survival over five decades dramatize the reversal of incurability of musculoskeletal sarcomas (<10%) in the 1940s and 1950s to its present 60% to 70% survival. This is a 700% increase in survival with limb preservation. The majority of these patients are pediatric and adolescent patients (Fig. 52.8; Table 52.5).

TABLE 52.6 Stage Summary Matrix

	N0	N0	N0	N1	M1
T1a	IA	IIA	IIA	III	IV
T1b	IA	IIA	IIA	III	IV
T2a	IB	IIB	III	III	IV
T2b	IB	IIB	III	III	IV

The T stage progression is modified by pathologic grade determines initial stage group progression. Then nodal progression determines stage progression.
- T1a, T1b, T2a, T2b = IA, IB, IIA, IIB
- N1 = III
- M1 = IV

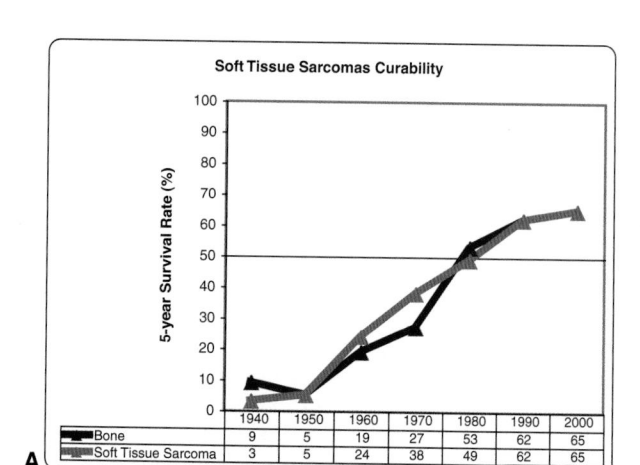

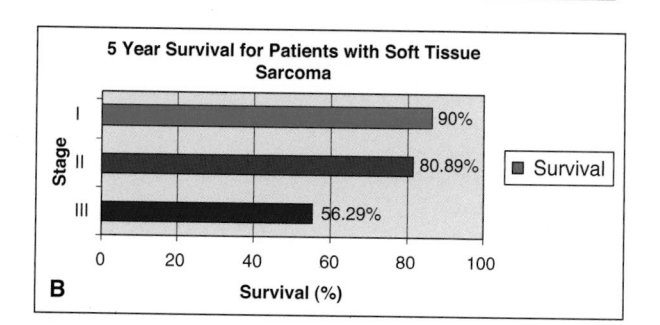

Figure 52.8 | **A.** Trajectory of soft tissue sarcoma curability. **B.** Five-year survival for patients with soft tissue sarcoma. Data taken from Table 56.6. (Data from Edge SB, Byrd DR, and Compton CC, et al, *AJCC Cancer Staging Manual, 7th edition*. New York, Springer, 2010, p. 295, Table 28.2.)

53

Osseous Skeletal System

PERSPECTIVE, PATTERNS OF SPREAD, AND PATHOLOGY

Knowledge of the relationship of the bone growth, its polarity, and amplification, particularly the amplification at each physis growth plate, and the modeling process is essential to understanding the classification and behavior of bone tumors.

PERSPECTIVE AND PATTERNS OF SPREAD

Primary malignant tumors of bone have been challenging for the multidisciplinary American Joint Committee on Cancer (AJCC)/International Union Against Cancer committees to develop a coherent classification and staging system. Although bone cancer is not common, it peaks in incidence in children, particularly in adolescence at the time of growth spurts. Because of the therapeutic specter of amputation, there is an emotional aspect in the management of both the patient, most often pediatric, and her or his family. There are approximately 2,500 new malignant bone and joint tumors annually in the United States. Although a virtual death warrant for most children afflicted in the 1950s and 1960s, bone cancers have with the multidisciplinary approach become curable with limb preservation. Despite the high incidence in teenagers, bone malignancies are only 5% to 6% of pediatric tumors.

From the first edition of the AJCC staging manual, the focus has been on histopathologic typing and grade. The determination traditionally of the bone tumor type has allowed for bone imaging to be an intrinsic part of bone tumor pathology analysis. The relationship of the bone growth and the modeling process to the classification of bone tumors had been advo-

cated by pathologists. The histopathologic types are tabulated in Fig. 53.1B as a function of bone growth and modeling, providing their site of origin and location. Cytogenetic alterations and aberrations are being uncovered but have not been formally included in staging. However, bone sarcoma grade, as in soft tissue sarcomas, plays an important part in staging and substaging.

Clinical detection is usually stimulated by persistence of bone pain in the area of the lesion, often initially being attributed to trauma from playing sports. Swelling and mass are signs of tumor progression, as are pathologic fractures. If the lesion is near a joint, unexplained sympathetic effusions and stiffness may be a presenting sign.

The initial staging criteria were influenced by tumor location and whether the osseous mass on film was confined to bone, within its cortex, or extended beyond the cortex. Tumefaction size has recently been added. Location in epiphysis, physis, metaphysis, or diaphysis is as noted earlier. **Patterns of spread** are within bone or beyond into soft tissues. The major concern is whether the neurovascular bundle is compromised in the lower extremity as the femoral artery wraps around the femoral shaft. Sites of rapid growth, such as the distal end of the femur and the proximal end of the tibia and humerus, are common sites of malignancies (Fig. 53.1A; Table 53.1).

With regard to bone tumors, oncogene overexpression or deletion is at the maximal growth, which is in the first 5 to 6 years of life, when skeletal growth is persistent, and then slows over the next 5 to 6 years. With puberty, there is a maximal growth spurt over the next 5 to 6 years. Malignancy in bone appears at those sites that grow the most, namely, the distal femur and proximal tibia and proximal humeri in adolescence.

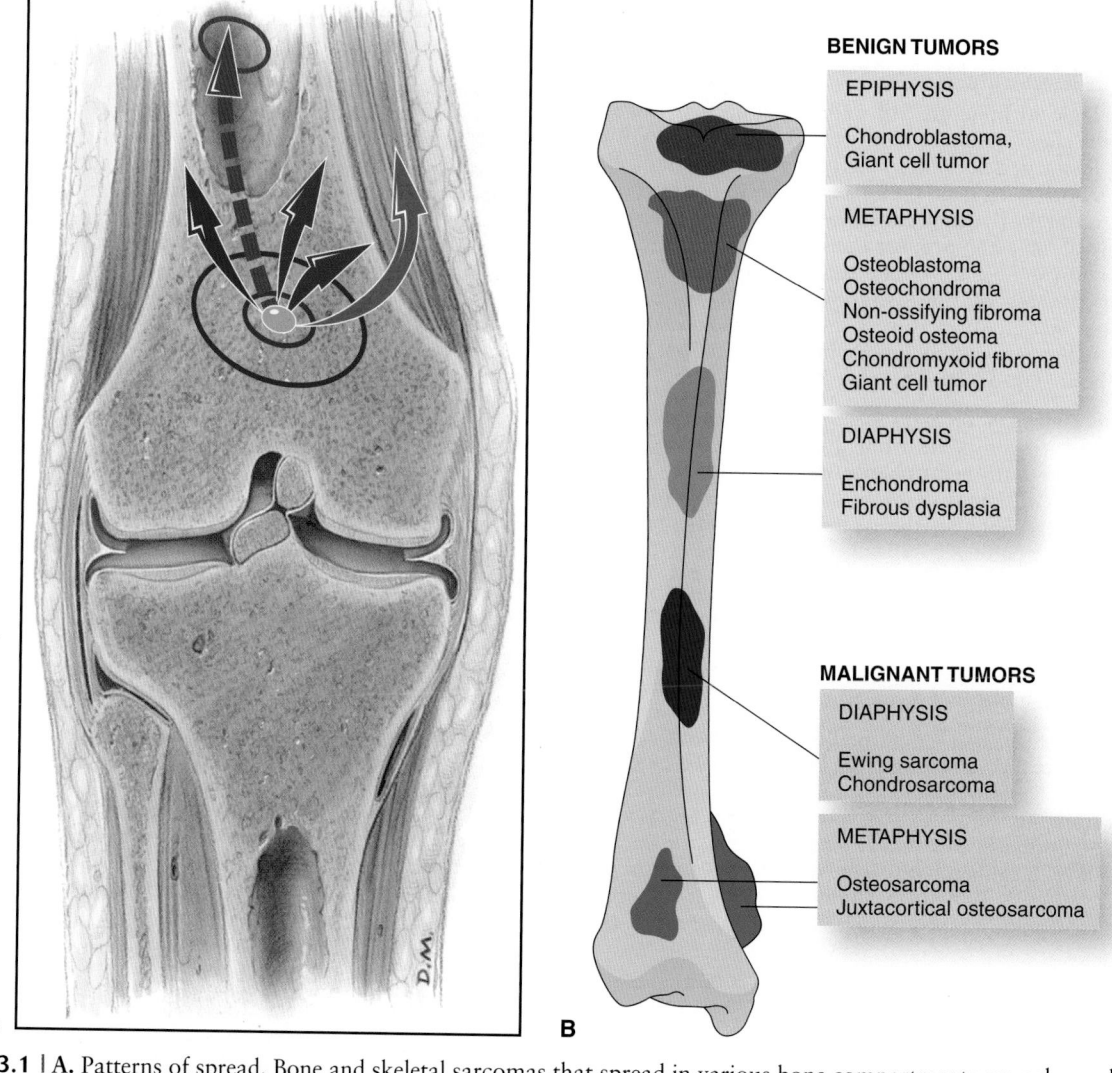

Figure 53.1 | **A.** Patterns of spread. Bone and skeletal sarcomas that spread in various bone compartments are color coded: T0,yellow; T1, green; T2, blue; T3, purple; and T4, red (into soft tissue). **B.** Location of primary bone tumors in long tubular bones. The concept of visualizing patterns of spread to appreciate the surrounding anatomy is well demonstrated by the six-directional pattern (SIMLAP, Table 53.1). Assuming origin in the distal metastasis of the femur.

TABLE 53.1	SIMLAP
Bone (Alternate) (Orientation Cross Section)	
T stage does not apply	
S	Diaphysis
I	Epiphysis
M	Metaphysis of femur (origin of tumor)
L	Cortex
A	Cortex-Anterior compartment
P	Cortex-Posterior compartment

The six vectors of invasion are Superior, Inferior, Medial, Lateral, Anterior, and Posterior. The T stage is more dependent on tumor size than with the specific anatomic structure involved.

OVERVIEW OF HISTOGENESIS AND HISTOPATHOLOGY

There is a logic to bone growth and modeling that can be applied to the classification of bone tumors. Skeletal growth is the critical factor in determining the probable location of the bone tumor. Borrowing from the concepts that were developed from research on the dynamic classification of bone dysplasias, the anatomy of bone and proposed terminology are presented to provide a broader basis for understanding the modeling and remodeling process of bone shaping in skeletal growth. Anatomic physiologic correlation is shown histologically with the vectors of bone growth and modeling in an idealized growing end of bone (Fig. 53.2A–D; Table 53.2).

- *Epiphyseal segment or epiphysis:* The epiphysis grows in the form of a hemisphere from the subarticular cartilage zone; thus the term hemispherization is used. It is recognized that the ultimate shape of any epiphysis is rarely a true hemisphere, but nevertheless the term allows us to visualize its growth pattern.

- *Physeal segment or growth plate:* By cellular division, the cartilage disk increases its length interstitially and increases in diameter by apposition. Thus, the normal tendency is toward expansion in this segment. The simplest and most appropriate term for this segment is growth.

- *Metaphyseal segment:* The normal tendency in this zone is toward a reduction in shaft caliber by internal and external absorption. The term "constriction" is deeply entrenched in the literature but is not descriptively accurate. The vascular erosion and osteoclastic absorption are not constrictive but are reductive in caliber. If one were to select a new term for these processes, it would be "funnelization." It preserves the image of these absorptive activities at the ends of the shaft, which allow for progressive narrowing of caliber and the resultant concave shape of the metaphysis as one passes from the end toward the middle of the shaft.

- *Diaphyseal segment:* There is a tendency in the middle of the shaft to maintain a certain structural balance between the flaring, growing ends. To maintain this balance, the diameter of the diaphysis increases in width as the tubular bone grows in length. Proliferation of osteoblasts on the periosteal surface exceeds osteoclastic endosteal absorption, in that the cortex thickens and the marrow cavity widens as the tubular bone matures.

The term "cylindrization" is applied to the vectors of the diaphyseal growth, which are such as to ensure a cylindrical shape to the shaft. The concept of the periosteum acting as a shaping force to narrow diaphyseal caliber has no functional basis. Similarly, a lax periosteum does not lead to widening of the shaft.

- *Hemispherization:* Growth in the epiphysis at first extends in all directions, but for most of its development the epiphysis grows as a hemisphere from the subarticular zone.

- *Growth:* The zone of resting cartilage grows by apposition, increasing the transverse diameter at the shaft.

- *Funnelization:* The metaphysis is shaped like a funnel, the shape being due to active bone resorption by osteoclasis, which results in a progressive reduction in shaft caliber.

- *Cylindrization:* The shaft of the bone increases in diameter by thickening of the cortex and expansion of the marrow by appositional periosteal growth.

The large variety of histopathology in bone is a function of the numerous derivative normal cells (Table 53.2). The histopathology of some of the common bone tumors is shown in Fig. 53.2E–G.

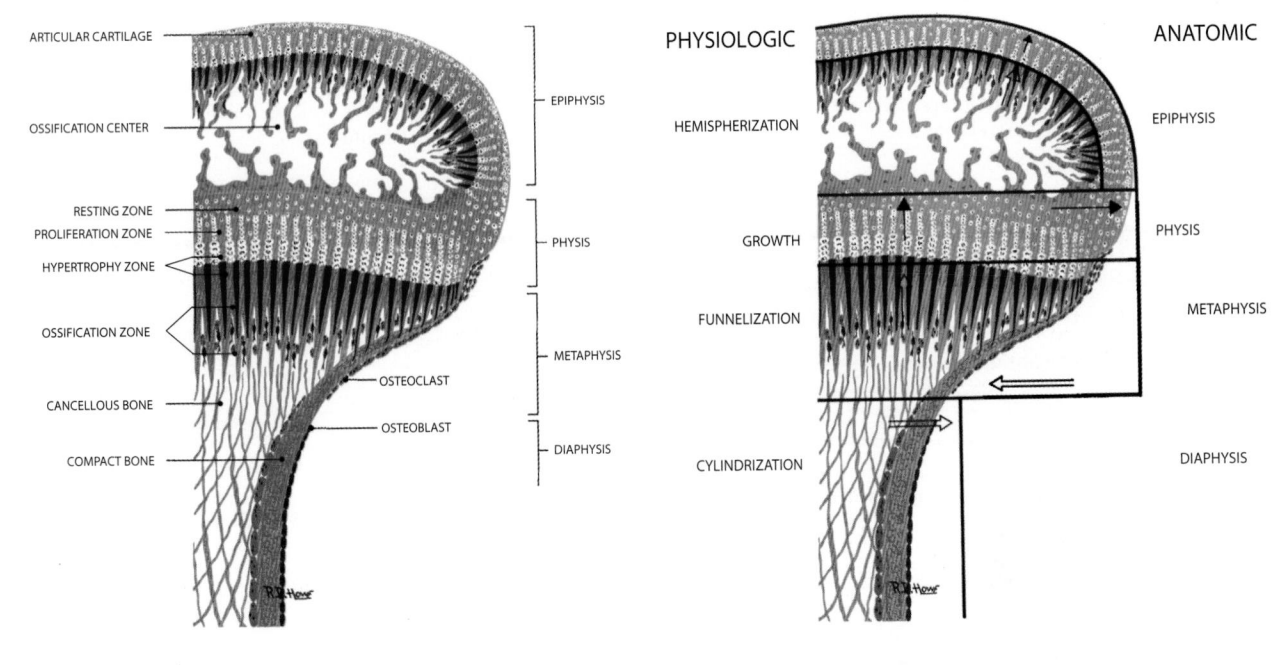

A Anatomic – Histologic correlation

B Anatomic – Physiologic correlation

Figure 53.2 | Overview of oncoanatomy. A. Anatomic–histologic correlation of the end of a growing long bone: epiphysis, physis, metaphysis, and diaphysis. **B.** Bone modeling at the same end of a growing long bone.

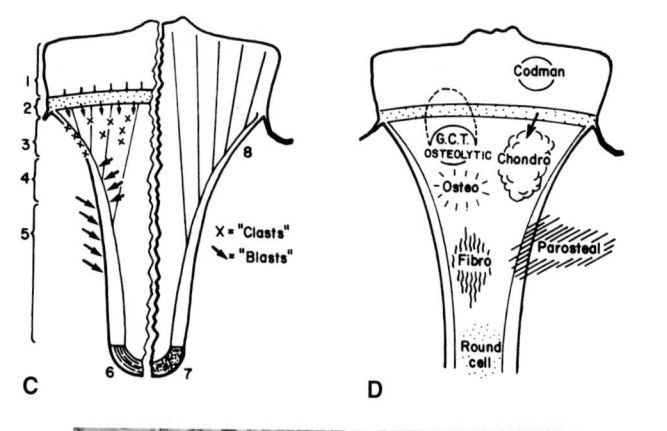

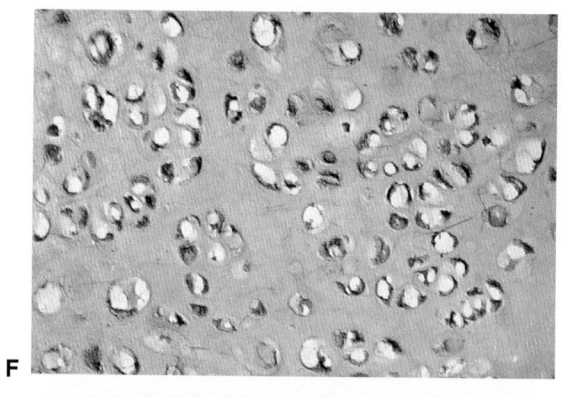

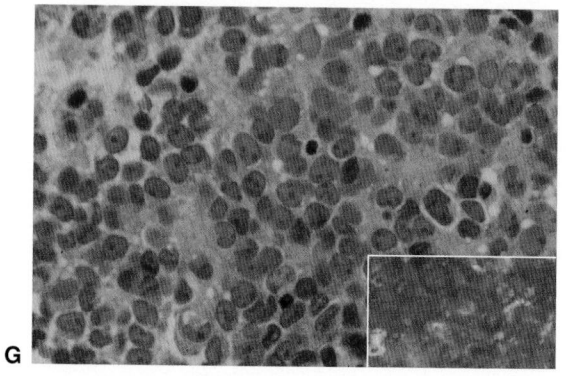

TABLE 53.2 | **Histopathologic Types of Bone Tumors**

I. Osteosarcoma (Fig. 53.2E)
  A. Intramedullary high grade
    1. Osteoblastic
    2. Chondroblastic
    3. Fibroblastic
    4. Mixed
    5. Small cell
    6. Other (telangiectactic, epithelioid, chondromyxoid fibroma–like, chodroblastoma-like, osteoblastoma-like, giant cell rich)
  B. Intramedullary low grade
  C. Juxtacortical high grade (high-grade surface osteosarcoma)
  D. Juxtacortical intermediate-grade chondroblastic (periosteal osteosarcoma)
  E. Juxtacortical low grade (parosteal osteosarcoma)
II. Chondrosarcoma (Fig. 53.2F)
  A. Intramedullary
    1. Conventional (hyaline/myxoid)
    2. Clear cell
    3. Dedifferentiated
    4. Mesenchymal
  B. Juxtacortical
III. Primitive neuroectodermal tumor/Ewing's sarcoma (Fig. 53.2G)
IV. Angiosarcoma
  A. Conventional
  B. Epithelioid hemangioendothelioma
V. Fibrosarcoma/malignant fibrous histiocytoma
VI. Chordoma
  A. Conventional
  B. Dedifferentiated
VII. Adamantinoma
  A. Conventional
  B. Well-differentiated osteofibrous dysplasia–like
VIII. Other
  A. Liposarcoma
  B. Leiomyosarcoma
  C. Malignant peripheral nerve sheath tumor
  D. Rhabdomyosarcoma
  E. Malignant mesenchymoma
  F. Malignant hemangiopericytoma
  G. Sarcoma, not otherwise specified; primary malignant lymphoma; and multiple myeloma are not included

Reprinted from Edge SB, Byrd DR, and Compton CC, et al, *AJCC Cancer Staging Manual. 7th ed.* New York, Springer, 2010, pp. 284–285.

Figure 53.2 | **C, D.** The relationship of modeling processes to bone tumors. **E. Osteosarcoma.** A photomicrograph reveals pleomorphic malignant cells, tumor giant cells, and mitoses. The tumor produces woven bone that is focally calcified. **F. Chondrosarcoma.** A photomicrograph of a chondrosarcoma shows malignant chondrocytes with pronounced atypia. **G. Ewing's sarcoma** A biopsy specimen shows fairly uniform small cells with round, dark-blue nuclei, paucity of mitotic activity, and poorly defined cytoplasm. A periodic acid–Schiff (PAS) stain demonstrates abundant intracellular glycogen (*inset*).

TNM STAGING CRITERIA

TNM STAGING CRITERIA

The staging criteria have remained simple, with a major modification in the sixth edition of the AJCC manual. T1 changed from confined within cortex and T2 beyond the cortex to tumors that are T1 (<8 cm) and T2 (>8 cm). T3 was added as a discontinuous primary tumor, that is, two separate anatomic sites in the same bone as metaphysis and diaphysis of the shaft. Stage III, previously undefined, is currently T3. Curiously, MIa lung metastases are regarded as more favorable than regional nodes N1, translating into stages IVA and IVB, respectively. Pathologic grade impacts the TNM anatomic stage, depending on whether the tumor grade is I or II (low grade) or III or IV (high grade). The substage designation of A or B depends on low or high grade, respectively, for stages I and II.

SUMMARY OF CHANGES SEVENTH EDITION AJCC

- Stage III is reserved for G3, G4 (Fig. 53.3)

The TNM staging matrix is color coded for identification of stage group once T and N stages are determined (Table 53.3).

TABLE 53.3 Stage Summary Matrix

	N0	N0	M1a	N1	M1b
T1	IA	IIA	IVA	IVB	IVB
T2	IB	IIB	IVA	IVB	IVB
T3	IB	III	IVA	IVB	IVB

The T stage progression as modified by pathologic grade determines initial stage group progression. Then nodal progression determines stage progression.

- T1, T2, T3 = IA, IB, IIA, B, and III, respectively modified by pathologic grade.
- N1 is stage IVB; also, Nx reflects rarity of node involvement.
- M1a is stage IVA (pulmonary), and is better than N1 or M1b (other sites).

BONE

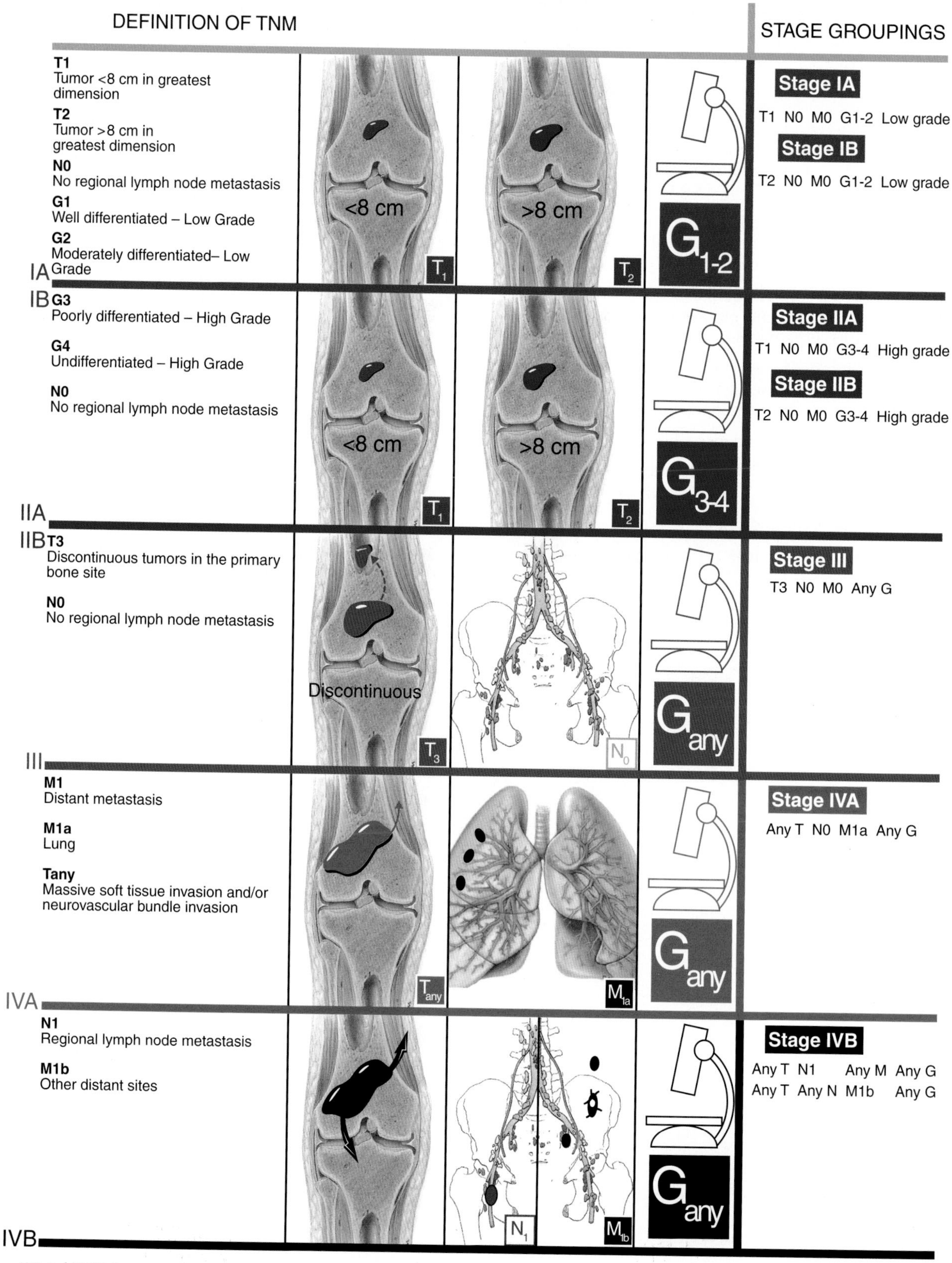

DEFINITION OF TNM

T1
Tumor <8 cm in greatest dimension

T2
Tumor >8 cm in greatest dimension

N0
No regional lymph node metastasis

G1
Well differentiated – Low Grade

G2
Moderately differentiated– Low Grade

IA

IB **G3**
Poorly differentiated – High Grade

G4
Undifferentiated – High Grade

N0
No regional lymph node metastasis

IIA

IIB **T3**
Discontinuous tumors in the primary bone site

N0
No regional lymph node metastasis

III

M1
Distant metastasis

M1a
Lung

Tany
Massive soft tissue invasion and/or neurovascular bundle invasion

IVA

N1
Regional lymph node metastasis

M1b
Other distant sites

IVB

<8 cm — T₁

>8 cm — T₂

G₁₋₂

<8 cm — T₁

>8 cm — T₂

G₃₋₄

Discontinuous — T₃

N₀

G_any

T_any

M₁ₐ

G_any

N₁

M₁ᵦ

G_any

STAGE GROUPINGS

Stage IA

T1 N0 M0 G1-2 Low grade

Stage IB

T2 N0 M0 G1-2 Low grade

Stage IIA

T1 N0 M0 G3-4 High grade

Stage IIB

T2 N0 M0 G3-4 High grade

Stage III

T3 N0 M0 Any G

Stage IVA

Any T N0 M1a Any G

Stage IVB

Any T N1   Any M Any G
Any T Any N M1b   Any G

Figure 53.3 | TNM stage criteria are color-coded bars. Note the importance of tumor grade in addition to anatomic extent. Bone sarcomas are characterized by early invasion of bone marrow sinuses in cancellous bone with rapid dissemination hematogenously to lung. Early detection of M1 lung nodules can be resected with long-term survival. Note that lymph node metastasis (N1) carries a poorer prognosis and worse stage than lung metastasis (M1). Stage I, green; II, blue; III, purple; IV, red; and metastatic, black.

T-ONCOANATOMY: POLARITY AND AMPLIFICATION OF SKELETAL GROWTH AND MODELING

To more fully understand normal skeletal growth, there are three basic considerations: (i) amplification or actual increases in size of bone, (ii) polarity or direction of growth, and (iii) time or scale of measurement (Fig. 53.4A).

- *Amplification* is the concept that the bone showing the greatest growth potential shows the greatest change because it magnifies the same defect to a greater degree.

- *Polarity* is the concept that tubular bones grow in a differential pattern, with one end predominating over the other. The maximal direction of longitudinal growth is its polarity

Traditionally, in classifying skeletal bone anatomy the orientation is regional. There are eight regions—head, neck, thorax, abdomen, back, pelvis, and upper and lower extremities.

- *Head*: skull, facial bones, and mandible

- *Neck*: cervical vertebrae (C1–C7), hyoid bone, and clavicle

- *Thorax*: ribs, thoracic vertebrae (T1–T12), sternum manubrium, and pectoral girdle

- *Abdomen*: lumbar vertebrae (L1–L5) and pelvic girdle (false pelvis)

- *Back*: vertebrae composing the spine—cervical (C4–C7), thoracic (T1–T12), lumbar (L1–L5), and sacral (S5–S1)

- *Pelvis*: sacrum (S1–S5), coccyx, and true pelvis

- *Upper limb*: pectoral girdle, arm, forearm, and hand

- *Lower limb*: pelvic girdle, thigh, leg, and foot

Bone typing (Fig. 53.4B–E) is based on size, shape, and modeling, and provides an insight into normal growth, which is a dynamic balance between appositional growth of endochondral bone and the resorption and regeneration of intramembranous bone. Each bone grows and models differently. Tumefactions are the sites of most active growth and resorption activities. The five types of bone shapes are long, short, irregular, flat, and special bones.

- *Long*: upper—humerus, radius, ulna; lower—femur, tibia, fibula

- *Short*: metacarpal, metatarsal, and phalanges

- *Irregular*: vertebrae

- *Flat*: ribs, scapula, and pelvis

- *Special*: skull, face, and mandible

The skeletal anatomic sites can be divided into five basic bone types for the purposes of presentation. Each site is presented diagrammatically to indicate sites of maximal bone growth and modeling as a correlate as to the most likely sites for bone tumors.

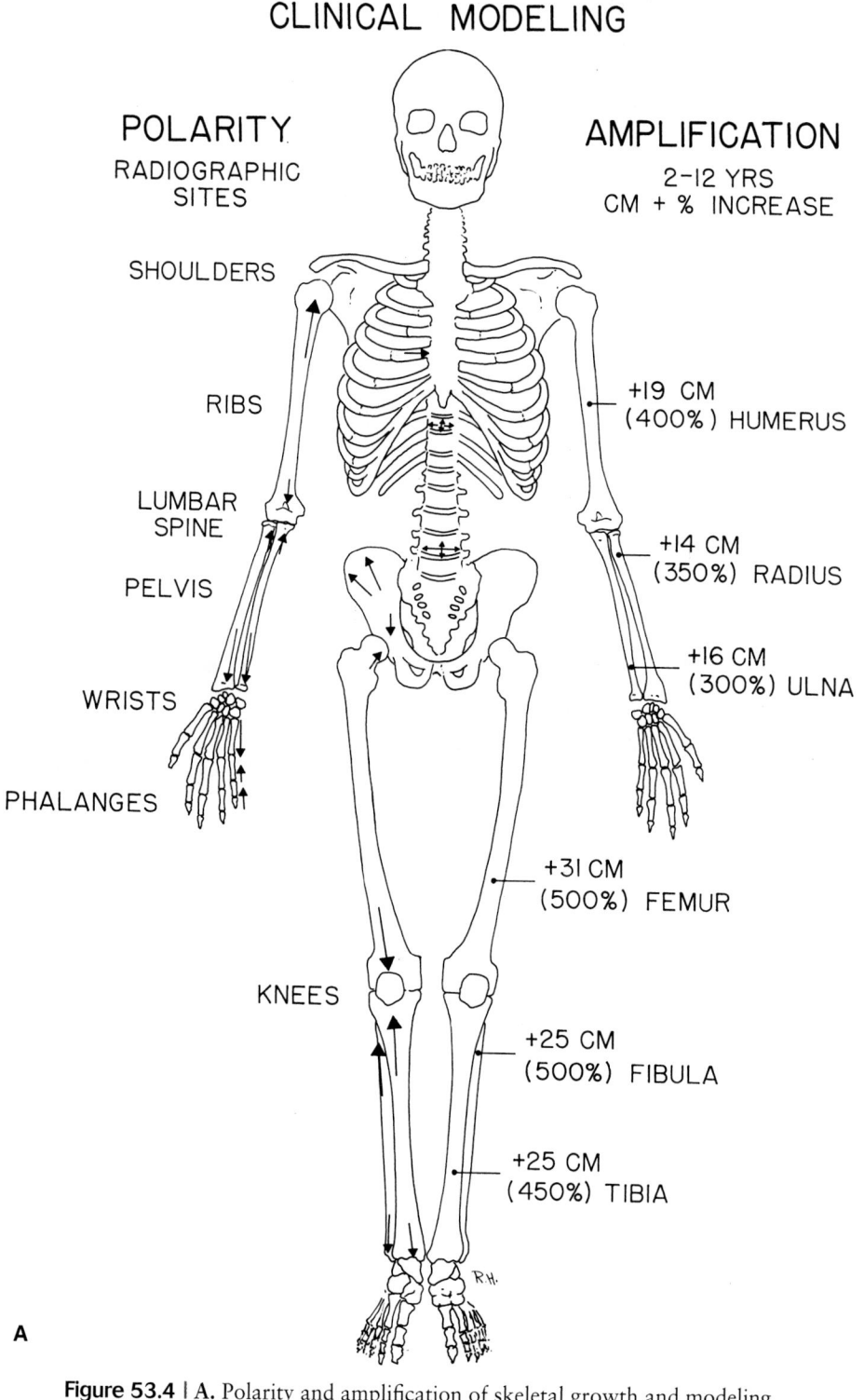

Figure 53.4 | A. Polarity and amplification of skeletal growth and modeling.

T-ONCOANATOMY

In osseous sarcomas, the anatomy of lower extremity is emphasized since this is the most common site for bone malignancies and as noted, the distal femoral physis and proximal tibial physis by virtue of their growth potential are the most prone sites.

- *Lower limb*: The basic design of muscle compartments is related to limb motion: anterior (flexion), posterior (extension), medial (adduction), and lateral (abduction). All of the compartments are not present in all parts of the limb, being

more common proximally than distally, where rotation becomes more important.

- *Knee*: The distal femoral physis and proximal tibia physis are most readily visualized on the MRI coronal section and are highlighted by the arrow head (>) in Fig. 53.4D,E. The number and letters of anatomy are correlated in the MRI with labels in the coronal section. In the sagittal view of the knee, the surrounding soft tissue anatomy is more readily appreciated (Fig. 53.4F,G).

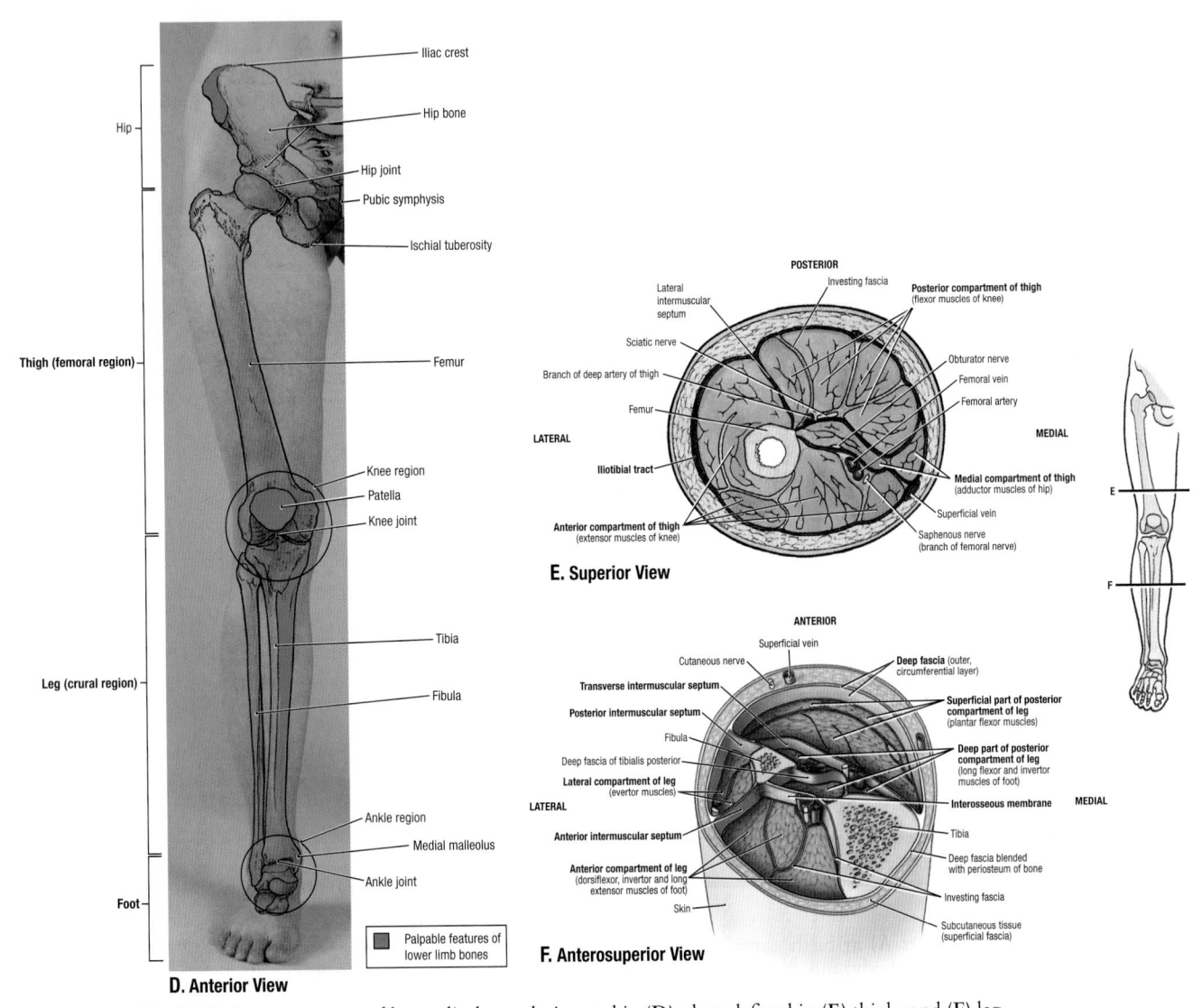

D. Anterior View

E. Superior View

F. Anterosuperior View

Figure 53.4 | D, E, F: Compartments of lower limb are designated in (D), then defined in (E) thigh, and (F) leg.

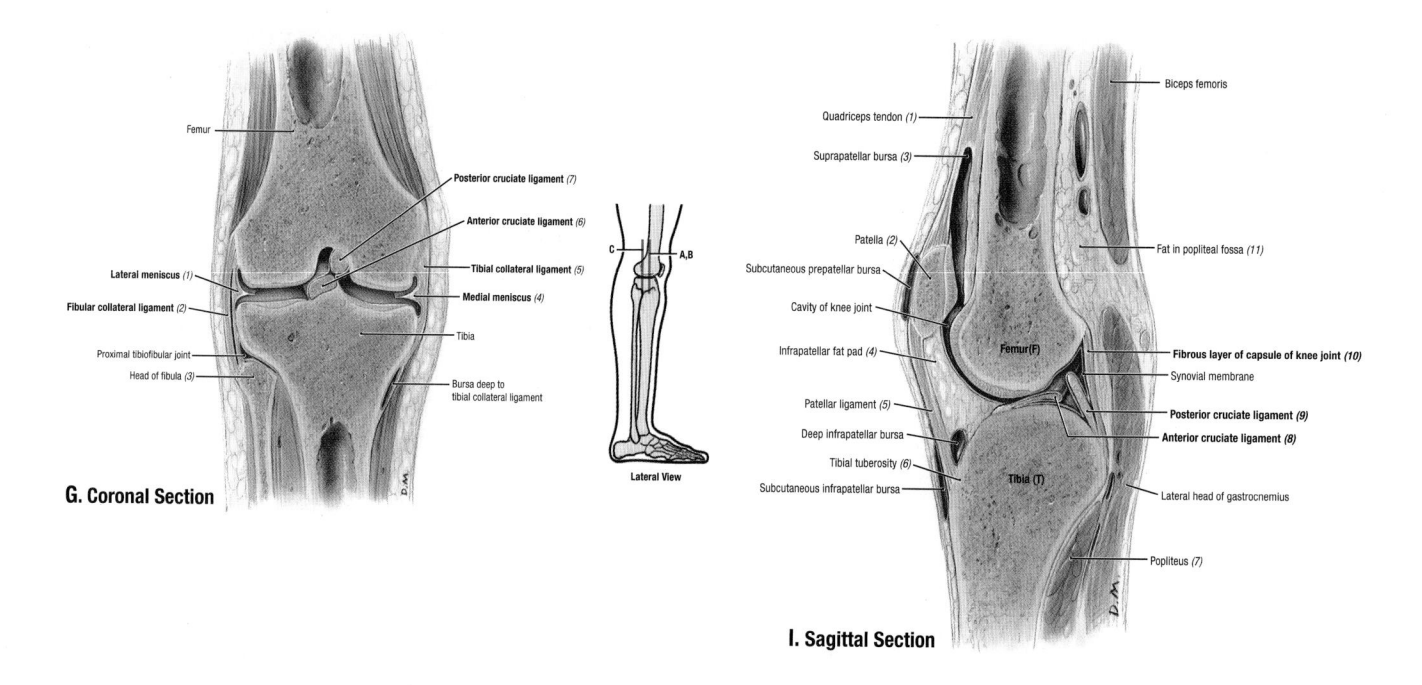

G. Coronal Section

Femur

Posterior cruciate ligament (7)

Anterior cruciate ligament (6)

Tibial collateral ligament (5)

Medial meniscus (4)

Lateral meniscus (1)

Fibular collateral ligament (2)

Tibia

Proximal tibiofibular joint

Head of fibula (3)

Bursa deep to tibial collateral ligament

Lateral View

I. Sagittal Section

Biceps femoris

Quadriceps tendon (1)

Suprapatellar bursa (3)

Fat in popliteal fossa (11)

Patella (2)

Subcutaneous prepatellar bursa

Cavity of knee joint

Femur(F)

Fibrous layer of capsule of knee joint (10)

Infrapatellar fat pad (4)

Synovial membrane

Patellar ligament (5)

Posterior cruciate ligament (9)

Deep infrapatellar bursa

Anterior cruciate ligament (8)

Tibial tuberosity (6)

Tibia (T)

Subcutaneous infrapatellar bursa

Lateral head of gastrocnemius

Popliteus (7)

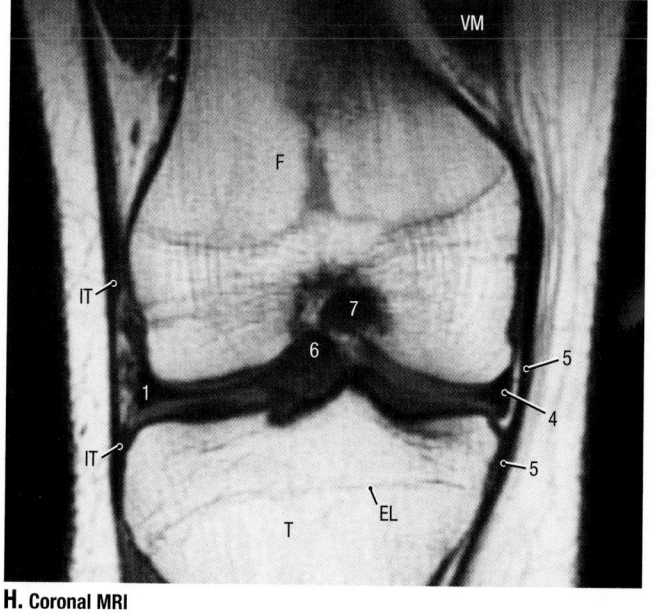

H. Coronal MRI

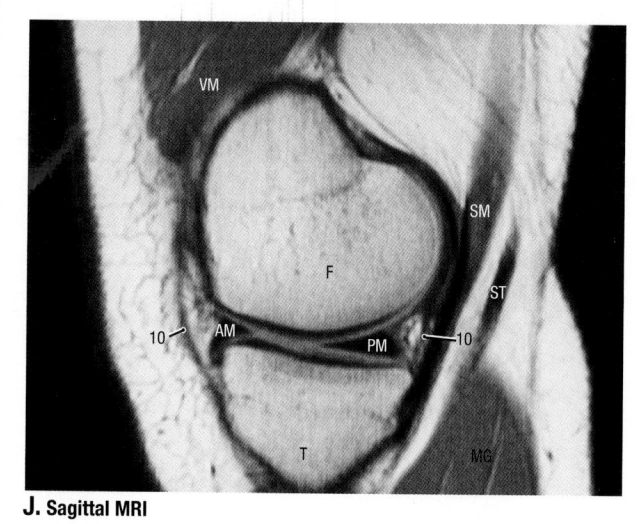

J. Sagittal MRI

Figure 53.4 | G, H, I, J. Anatomy of the two most active sites of bone growth: distal femur and proximal tibia are correlated in (**H**) coronal and (**J**) sagittal MRIs. Letters and numbers define specific structures which are noted in (#) anatomy illustrations (G/I).

N-ONCOANATOMY AND M-ONCOANATOMY

N-ONCOANATOMY

Bone and bone marrow are richly supplied with blood and lymphatics are intimately related to regional veins that also drain surrounding soft tissue, which so often are invaded owing to penetration of cortex. Only the major regional nodes are listed here, and only the lower extremity regional nodes are shown in Fig. 53.5A–D.

- *Femoral nodes*: lower limb and lower half of the truncal skeleton
- *Axillary*: upper limb and upper half of the truncal skeleton
- *Neck nodes*: skull and facial bones

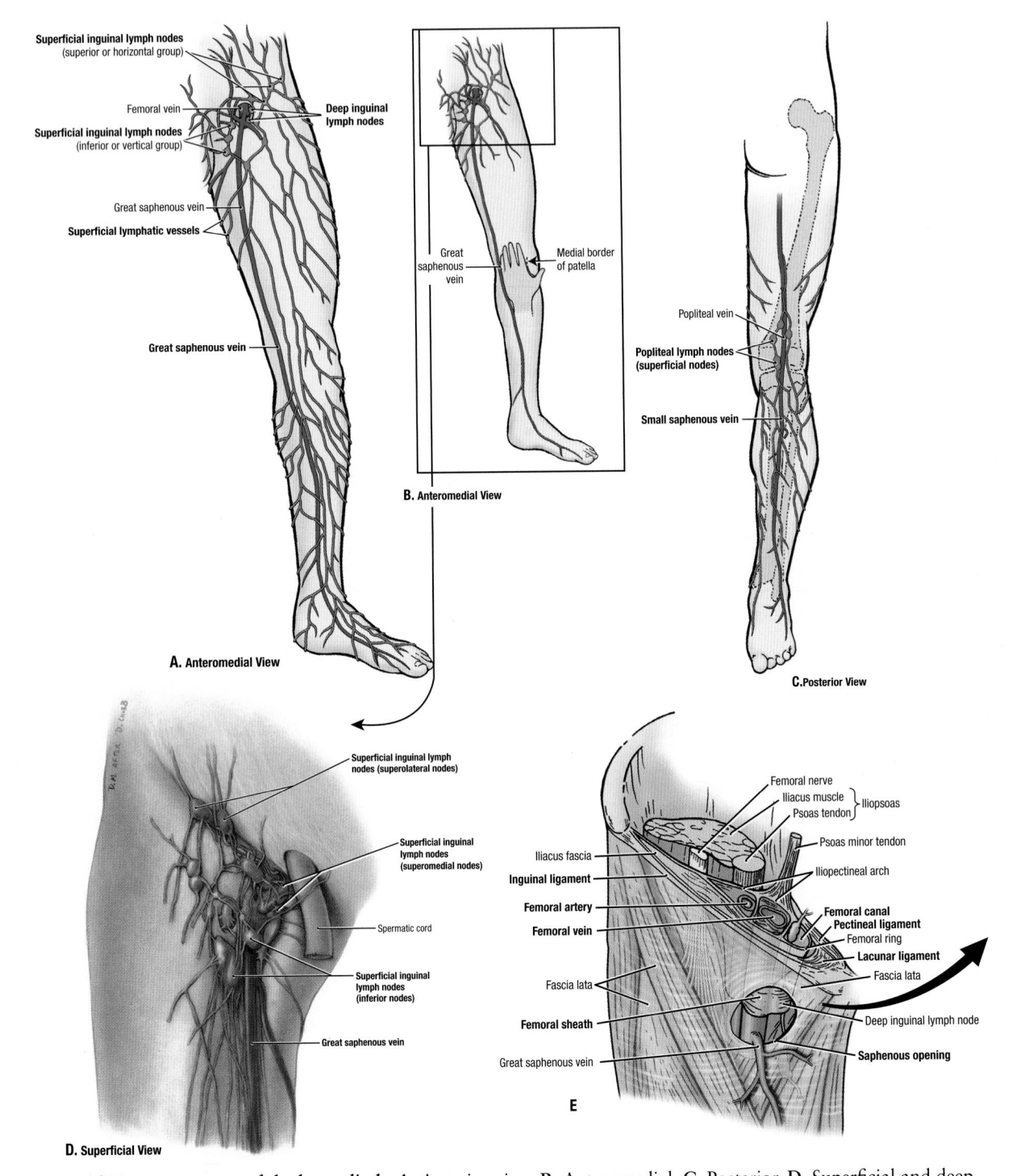

Figure 53.5 | N-oncoanatomy of the lower limb. **A.** Anterior view. **B.** Anteromedial. **C.** Posterior. **D.** Superficial and deep inguinal nodes and superficial veins. **E.** Dissected femoral triangle presents the order of neurovascular bundle and lymph nodes – Nerve, Artery, Vein, Lymph Node (NAVEL), from lateral to medial.

M-ONCOANATOMY

The venous drainage surrounding the skeletal anatomy is a rich network and accounts for both skip lesions in the same bone and the propensity of bone tumors to metastasize to other bones (Fig. 53.6A). The rich axial intervertebral venous network readily explains why once one vertebra is involved, others are at risk.

To complete the picture, the neurovascular bundle is presented in Fig. 53.6B (popliteal fossa with nerve, artery, vein) and lymph nodes (not shown but are medial in location similar to NAVEL of femoral triangle).

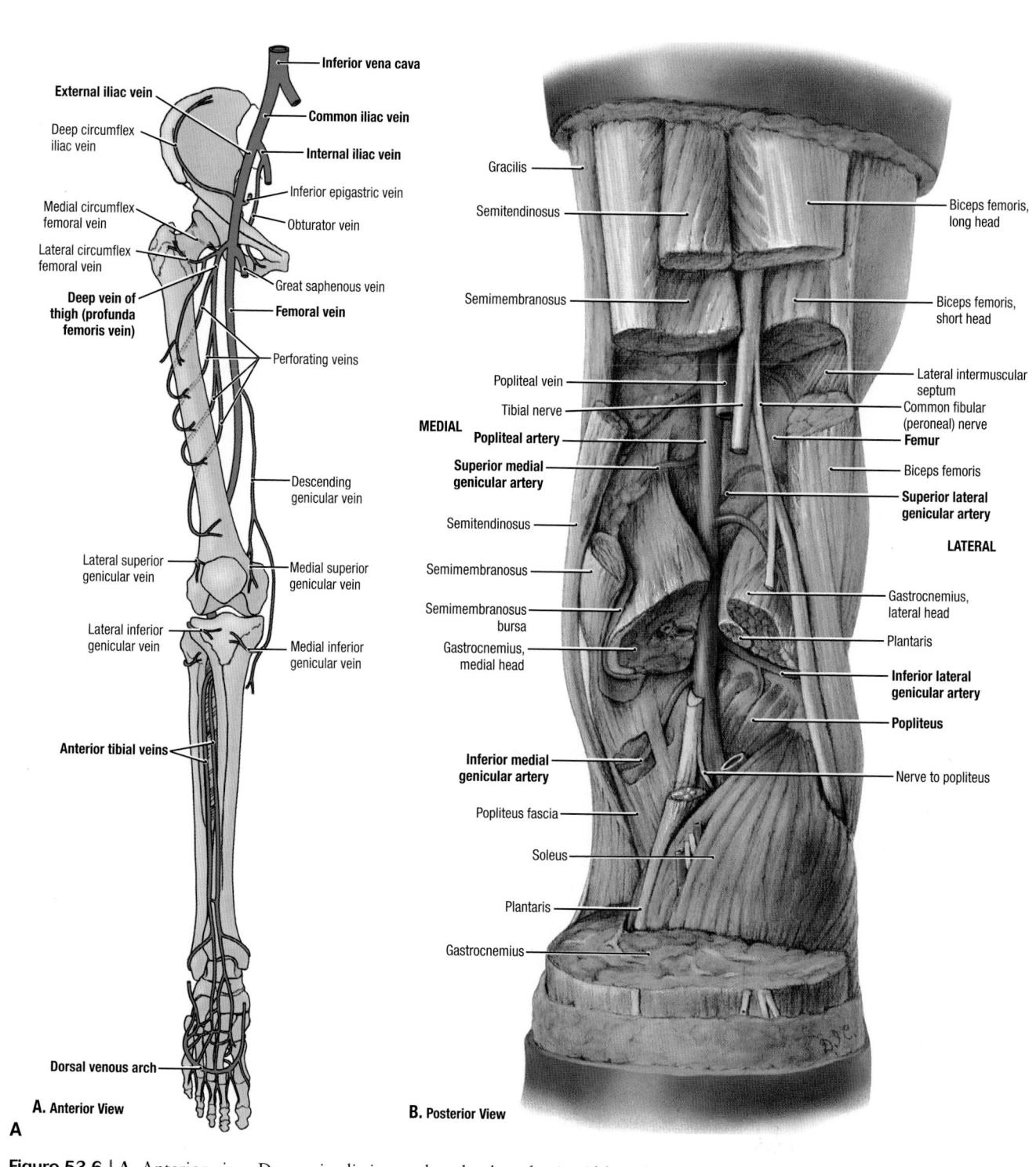

Figure 53.6 | A. Anterior view. Deep veins lie internal to the deep fascia. Although only the anterior and posterior tibial veins are depicted as paired structures in this schematic illustration, typically in the limbs deep veins occur as paired, continually interanastomosing accompanying veins surrounding and sharing the name of the artery they accompany. **B.** Posterior view. Neurovascular bundle and lymph nodes maintain NAVEL, i.e., tibial nerve, popliteal artery, vein, and lymph nodes are lateral to medial.

STAGING WORKUP

RULES OF CLASSIFICATION AND STAGING

Clinical Staging and Imaging

Clinical staging and imaging includes physical examination, modern cross-sectional imaging, and image-guided biopsies. Standard bone radiographs identify the osseous malignancy but need to be supplemented with magnetic resonance imaging (MRI) and enhanced computed tomography (CT). MRI is superior for soft tissue and bone marrow invasion and enhanced CT for bone cortex erosion. Tumor size is estimated for staging: <8 cm or >8 cm. The entire skeleton deserves to be overviewed for metastases using ^{99m}Tc colloid. Chest CT is essential for surveying lungs for pulmonary metastases.

Image-guided biopsy is essential, but a note of caution is warranted. The biopsy site needs to be carefully planned to allow for eventual en bloc resection of the entire biopsy tract with excision of the malignant bone tumor (Table 53.4).

Pathologic Staging

Pathologic staging incorporates the clinical findings, the complete imaging file, and the completely resected specimen. Histopathologic analyses for sarcoma grade affect cancer staging more than tumor type. Resected regional lymph nodes need to be included. Suspicious metastatic lesions in long or other bones should be needled and confirmed by histopathology.

Oncoimaging Annotations

- MRI is the dominant imaging modality for determining intracompartmental and extracompartmental extent of an intraosseous tumor and its relationship to critical neurovascular structures.
- CT allows accurate determination of intraosseous and extraosseous extension and invasion of tumor.

- The routine radiograph remains the most reliable predictor of the histologic nature of a bone lesion.
- Metastases account for 65% of all malignant bone tumors in adults.
- All suspected sarcomas of bone should be staged with MRI before rather than after biopsy. As a consequence of post-biopsy edema and hemorrhage, MRI often overestimates the size and extent of tumor.
- With osteosarcoma and Ewing's sarcoma, which are known to produce skip lesions, it is important to examine the entire long bone with MRI.
- Systemic metastatic disease, usually to the lungs, and local recurrence have their maximum hazard rates within the first 2 years, defining the most frequent follow-up intervals for the first 2 years and tapering over a total of 5 years for osseous sarcomas.
- Geographic lesions are well circumscribed, and they frequently have a well-defined, sclerotic border. There is typically no extension of the tumor beyond the radiographically evident lesion border, implying a slow growth rate. This, typically, is seen in benign tumors, such as osteoblastomas, giant cell tumors, or nonossifying fibromas. This pattern also can be observed in low-grade malignant lesions, such as a low-grade chondrosaroma.
- A so-called moth-eaten pattern suggests an aggressive tumor, with multiple lytic areas and, frequently, cortical destruction. The tumor extends within the bone beyond the radiographically evident lytic areas and suggests an intermediate rate of growth.
- A permeative pattern implies extremely rapid and infiltrative growth, with diffuse areas of lytic destruction invading the bone. Permeative lesions are often associated with cortical disruption and extraosseous soft tissue mass, and they are characteristic of high-grade lesions. However, acute infection also can have this appearance, as well as, occasionally, benign tumors, such as eosinophilic granulomas. This overlap underscores the necessity for accurate diagnostic biopsy.

TABLE 53.4	Imaging Modalities for Staging Bone Cancer	
Method	Diagnosis and Staging Capability	Recommended for Use
Primary (T) Staging		
MRI	MRI provides optimal cross-sectional three-planar views of both axial and appendicular anatomy	Yes, superior for soft tissue extensions and neurovascular invasion
CT$_e$	CT (preferably helical) is complementary; it is superior in showing bony erosion and destruction by osseous sarcoma	Yes, advantage if bone is invaded
US	US may be of value in initial localizing of a mass or for guiding needle biopsies of primary sites or nodes	No, not detailed
Nodal (N) and Metastases (M) Staging		
Tc 99m scan	Yes, for evaluating entire skeleton for multiple bone lesions.	
PET	Used with FDG as a total body scan, searching for disseminated disease	No, unless metastases are highly suspected on the Tc scan

CT$_e$, computed tomography enhanced with intravenous contrast; FDG, fluorodeoxyglucose; MRI, magnetic resonance imaging; PET, positron emission tomography; US, ultrasound.

PROGNOSIS AND CANCER SURVIVAL

- Periosteal reactions can be of several types. A so-called sunburst periosteal reaction implies very proliferative malignant bone formation, and it is characteristic of an aggressive tumor, such as osteosarcoma or Ewing's sarcoma.

- Codman's triangle refers to the raised, normal periosteum at the margin of a bone tumor associated with reactive periosteal new bone formation; it can be seen with a variety of malignant bone tumors. A lamellar periosteal reaction (onion skin) implies rapid cyclic tumor growth, and it is most classically associated with Ewing's sarcoma, although it is not specific for this tumor. Spiculated periosteal reactions also occur in aggressive, rapidly growing tumors such as Ewing's sarcoma, and they represent reactive periosteal bone being deposited along periosteal vessels, as the expanding tumor stretches the periosteum.

PROGNOSTIC FACTORS

Clinically significant:

- Three dimensions of tumor size

- Percentage necrosis post neoadjuvant systemic therapy from pathology report

- Number of resected pulmonary metastases from pathology report*

From Edge SB, Byrd DR, and Compton CC, et al, *AJCC Cancer Staging Manual, 7th edition.* New York, Springer, 2010, p. 289.

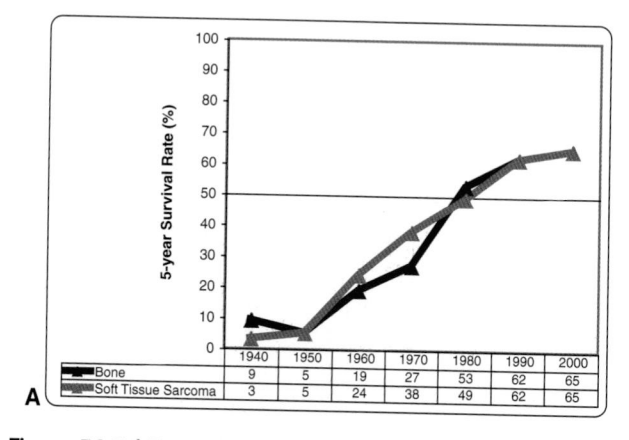

Figure 53.7 | Trajectory of bone sarcoma curability.

In addition to known prognostic factors of tumor size, histopathology, and grade, the following factors are incorporated in the staging system:

- Lung metastases do better than bony or hepatic metastases.

- Histologic response to chemotherapy is good, >90% tumor necrosis.

- Pathologic fractures are a poor response if now healing after chemotherapy.

- Molecular aberrations and fusion genes are under investigation in different bone sarcomas.

- Ewing's Sarcoma: EWS-FLI1 type 1 fusion gene predicts for longer relapse free survival. Aberrant P53, p16 INK4A and p14ARF are associated with more aggressive behavior and metastases, p27 correlates with improved survival.

- Osteosarcoma: P-glycoprotein predicts 9× increase of death and 5× increase in metastases. HER2/erbB-2 expression is associated with increased risk of metastases but correlates with response to chemotherapy. KI-67 is a marker for pulmonary metastases and HSP27 is associated with a negative prognosis.

- Chondrosarcoma: Decreased Hedgehog signaling and loss of INK 4A/p16 correlates with tumor progression in peripheral tumors.

CANCER STATISTICS AND SURVIVAL

Soft tissue sarcomas account for 10,520 cases annually, whereas bone sarcomas occur in only 2,650 patients. Together, musculoskeletal tumors reached an incidence of 13,170 patients; <50% will die. When compared with primary cancer sites, the current gains in survival over five decades dramatize the reversal of incurability of musculoskeletal sarcomas (<10%) in the 1940s and 1950s to its 60% to 70% survival rate. This is a 700% increase in survival with limb preservation (see Fig. 53.6). There are 2,650 new cases of bone sarcoma in the United States, slightly more in males 1,530 than in females 1120. Approximately 40% become long-term survivors, with deaths resulting in 60% of this population. In children, the most common tumors form a very small percentage of pediatric malignancies, that is, osteosarcomas (2.5%) and Ewing's tumor (1.6%).

54

Lymphoid Neoplasms: Hodgkin's Lymphoma and Non-Hodgkin's Lymphoma

PERSPECTIVE, PATTERNS OF SPREAD, AND PATHOLOGY

The lymphoid neoplasms include an ever-increasing spectrum of disorders defined by a combination of morphologic, immunophenotypic, and genetic features.

PERSPECTIVE AND PATTERNS OF SPREAD

Hodgkin's Lymphoma

The first case described by Thomas Hodgkin, entitled "On some morbid appearances of the absorbent glands and spleen," dramatically demonstrates the concept of contiguous spread of this lymphoid disorder (Fig. 54.1). This concept of "contiguous spread" was promulgated by Kaplan, who argued for a unicentric origin, along with other pioneer radiation oncologists who advocated for prophylactically treating the uninvolved contiguous nodal regions. Hodgkin's lymphoma (HL), which usually starts in a cervical lymph node, is believed to spread in an orderly fashion. Each contiguous nodal area is believed to be the next most likely site to be involved.

Each node, depending on its location, would involve the juxtaposed neighboring site (Fig. 54.2).

Three illustrations of cervical node involvement portray advancing stages: stage I, high cervical node (Fig. 54.2A); stage II, cervical node with mediastinal mass (Fig. 54.2B); and stage III, supraclavicular node with para-aortic node spread via thoracic duct (Fig. 54.2C). For the clinician, the patterns of spread of HL highlight the regional node-bearing areas and emphasize the need to know the location of the lymph nodes. HL can originate in any one of the different lymph node regions in the body and spread through adjacent normal lymphatic pathways. The more likely contiguous site of involvement is the one that is "upstream," because lymph flows in prograde and centrifugal fashion from the peripheral limbs to the central core.

Lymphatic trunks gather the lymph and allow flow from different viscera and anatomic sites into lymph nodes. Once obstruction occurs, retrograde flow takes place in lymphatics, and contiguous sites may be the "downstream" lymph nodes.

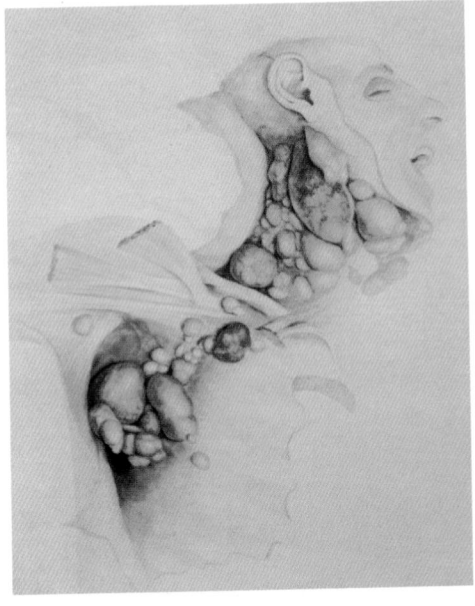

Figure 54.1 | Water color painting by Robert Carswell (1793–1857) of a patient seen by him at postmortem examination in 1828; this case was the seventh described in Hodgkin's paper. Carswell's five magnificent water color paintings are the property of University College Medical School, University of London, and were rediscovered by Dr. Peter J. Dawson, who published three of them in an article in the *Archives of Internal Medicine* (1968;121:288–290).

PATTERNS OF SPREAD

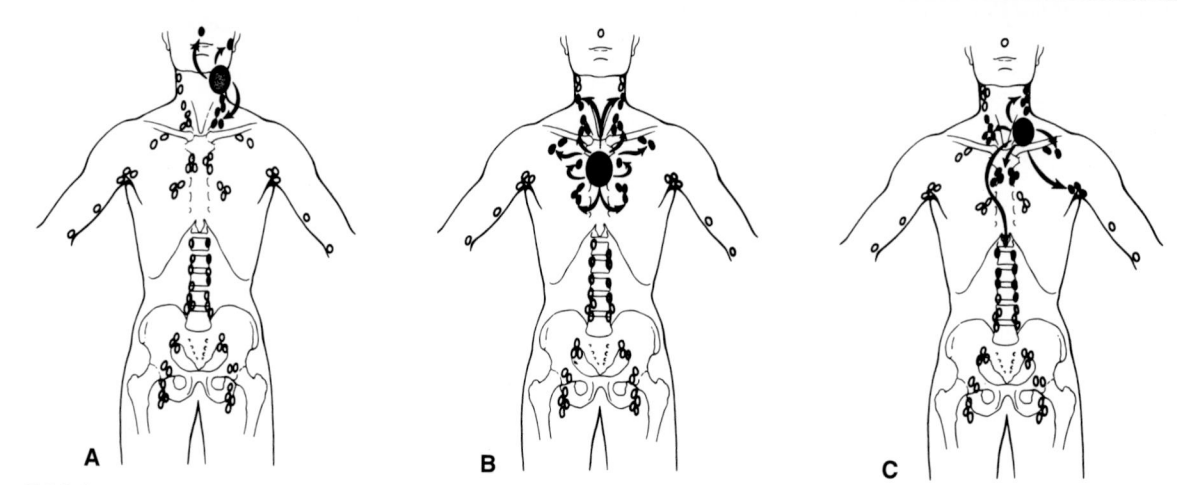

Figure 54.2 | Patterns of spread in Hodgkin's lymphoma are due to contiguous involvement of adjacent node-bearing regions. **A.** High cervical nodes could retrograde to involve the parotid lymph node or Waldeyer's ring or prograde to the supraclavicular area. **B.** Mediastinal lymph nodes could spread to supraclavicular, infraclavicular, or cervical lymph nodes or involve hilar nodes as a gateway to pulmonary infiltration. **C.** Supraclavicular node retrograde can spread to epigastric and celiac para-aortic lymph nodes, as well as to ipsilateral axillary, cervical nodes, and contralateral supraclavicular nodes.

The common presentation of Hodgkin's disease is a unifocal painless enlargement of a lymph node (90%). Most often the nodal involvement is supradiaphragmatic: cervical and supraclavicular nodes can be involved in 60–80%. Primary mediastinal presentations are not very common despite mediastinal involvement often being present after staging work-up. Subdiaphragmatic involvement occurs in only 3–10% of clinical cases initially. The initial anatomic distribution of disease provides an overview of nodal vs. extranodal disease. The dissemination of HL is usually a late manifestation if the disease recurs (Fig. 54.2ABC).

In this illustration of the SIMLAP, construction of multidirectional spread, the presenting site of involvement is the anterior mediastinum (Fig. 54.2D).

The stage assumes the origin of the lymphoma in the anterior mediastinum.

To illustrate the SIMLAP construct of multidirectional spread, the presenting **site of involvement is the anterior mediastinum** (Table 54.2).

The concept of visualizing patterns of spread to appreciate the surrounding anatomy is well demonstrated by the six-directional pattern (SIMLAP, Table 54.2).

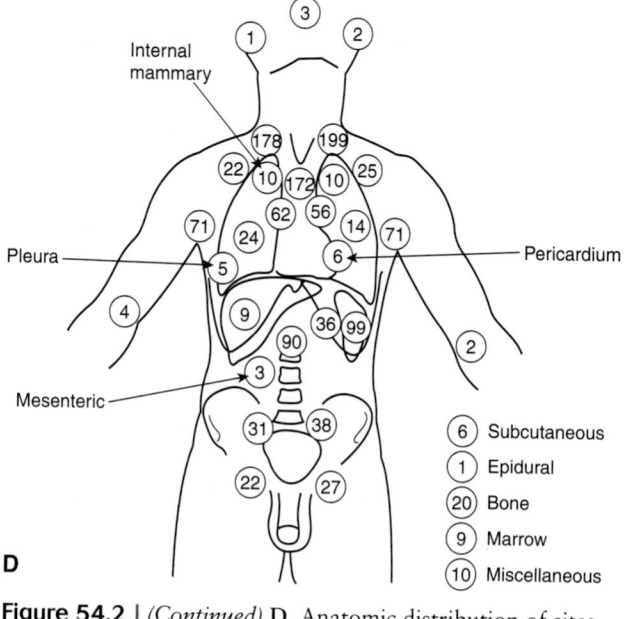

Figure 54.2 | *(Continued)* **D.** Anatomic distribution of sites of involvement. (From Kaplan HS, Dorfman RF, Nelson TS, et al: Staging laparotomy and splenectomy in Hodgkin's disease: analysis of indication and patterns of involvement in 285 consecutive cases, unselected patients. NCI Monograph 1973:36:291.)

TABLE 54.1	SIMLAP	
Lymphoid/Lymph Node Regions (Carinal Lymph Node)		
Subcarinal		
S	Waldeyer's	II E •
	Cervical/supraclavicular	II •
I	Inguinal femoral	III •
	Popliteal	III •
M	Mediastinal	I •
	Hilar	II •
L	Infraclavicular	II •
	Axillary, pectoral	II •
	Epitrochlear	II •
A	Thymus	II E •
	Anterior mediastinum	I •
P	Posterior mediastinum	II •
	Para-aortic	III •

The six vectors of invasion are <u>S</u>uperior, <u>I</u>nferior, <u>M</u>edial, <u>L</u>ateral, <u>A</u>nterior, and <u>P</u>osterior. The color-coded dots correlate the T stage with the specific anatomic structure involved.

Non-Hodgkin's Lymphoma (NHL)

Diffuse large B cell lymphoma and follicular lymphomas are most prevalent, accounting for 50% of all cases. A large variety of associated disorders are noted that have an altered state of immunity—that is, autoimmune, immune suppression, or viral infections—and predispose the host to developing a secondary malignant lymphoma (Table 54.2A).

Understanding how lymphomas spread and advance in stage requires understanding the intricate structure of a lymph node. Lymph nodes consist of collections of lymphoid tissues, draining lymphatic vessels, typically lima bean shaped ovoids, normally ≤ 1.0 cm in size. The interstital fluid (lymph) enters via afferent channels in the convex cortex and exits via an efferent lymphatic at the hilus. This contains B and T cell domains and circulating lymphocytic cells enter via post capillary venules.

Although the cause of NHL is unknown, there are several genetic diseases and infectious agents that are believed to increase the risk. For example, some rare immunodeficiency states can result in 25% developing lymphomas. In Sjogren's syndrome there is a 30–40 times increase risk of developing lymphomas, usually in salivary glands as marginal zone NHL. In contrast T cell lymphomas are associated with celiac sprue disease (Table 54.2A).

Understanding how lymphomas spread and advance in stage requires an intimate knowledge of the intricate structures of lymph nodes and the function served by T cells and B cells.

- **T cells remain in paracortex:** T cells migrate to the thymus, where in T cell receptors, each recognize a single antigen and in their diversity, T cell receptors acquire CD_3 and CD_2 antigens define these lymphocytes as T cells. As other antigens appear, such as CD_4 – defines helper cells and CD_8 suppressor cells. The cells migrate from the thymus gland to lymph nodes. Once exposed to antigens specific for receptors, CD_4 (helper) cells become activated. T lymphocytes once activated by antigen peptides become "killer cells", eliminating viruses and foreign cells. A subpopulation of natural killer cells (NK cells) do not require antigenic recognition for their cytotoxic activity.

- **B cells home to germinal centers:** B cells acquire and collect cytoplasmic and cell surface antigens in the bone marrow i.e., CD_{19}, CALLA, CD_{10}, and a nuclear antigen TdT and mature expressing additional surface antigens CD_{22}, plus lg heavy and light chains. Terminally differentiated B lymphocytes are plasma cells.

The numerous B and T/NK cell lymphomas are tabulated as to their incidence in Table 54.2B.

TABLE 54.2A — Disorders with Increased Risk of Secondary Malignant Lymphoma

Sjögren's syndrome

Hashimoto thyroiditis

Renal and cardiac transplant recipients

Acquired immunodeficiency syndrome (AIDS)

Epstein–Barr virus infection

Human herpes virus 8 infection

Helicobacter pylori–positive gastritis

Hepatitis C

Congenital immune deficiency syndromes

Chédiak–Higashi

Wiskott–Aldrich

Ataxia telangiectasia

Immunoglobulin A deficiency

Severe combined immune deficiency

α Heavy-chain disease

Celiac disease

Hodgkin's lymphoma (posttreatment)

TABLE 54.2B — Frequency of B and T/NK Cell Lymphomas

Diagnosis	Percent of Total Cases
Diffuse large B cell lymphoma	30.6
Follicular lymphoma	22.1
MALT lymphoma	7.6
Mature T cell lymphomas (except ALCL)	7.6
Chronic lymphocytic leukemia/small-cell lymphocytic lymphoma	6.7
Mantle cell lymphoma	6.0
Mediastinal large B cell lymphoma	2.4
Anaplastic large cell lymphoma	2.4
Burkitt's lymphoma	2.5
Nodal marginal zone lymphoma	1.8
Precursor T lymphoblastic lymphoma	1.7
Lymphoplasmacytic lymphoma	1.2
Other types	7.4

ALCL, anaplastic large cell lymphoma; MALT, mucosa-associated lymphoid tissue; NK, natural killer.

OVERVIEW OF LYMPHOID SYSTEM

The lymphoid system is represented diagrammatically in Table 54.3; Fig. 54.5 shows more explicit anatomic identification of lymph node stations and sites.

The term "variant lymphocytes" covers atypical lymphocytes and large granular lymphocytes. Atypical lymphocytes are large and exhibit deep blue to pale gray cytoplasm; they are seen in benign reactive processes. Large granular lymphocytes are medium-to-large lymphoid cells with some pink cytoplasmic granules. They are suppressor T lymphocytes, some with natural killer (NK) function, and may be increased in benign or malignant disorders. Plasmacytoid lymphocytes have abundant blue cytoplasm and are seen in some reactive disorders.

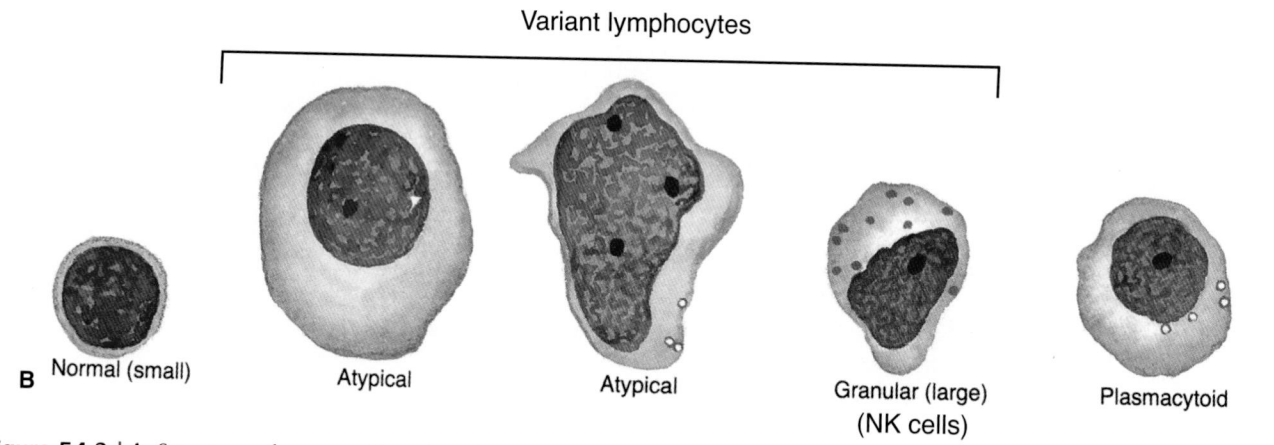

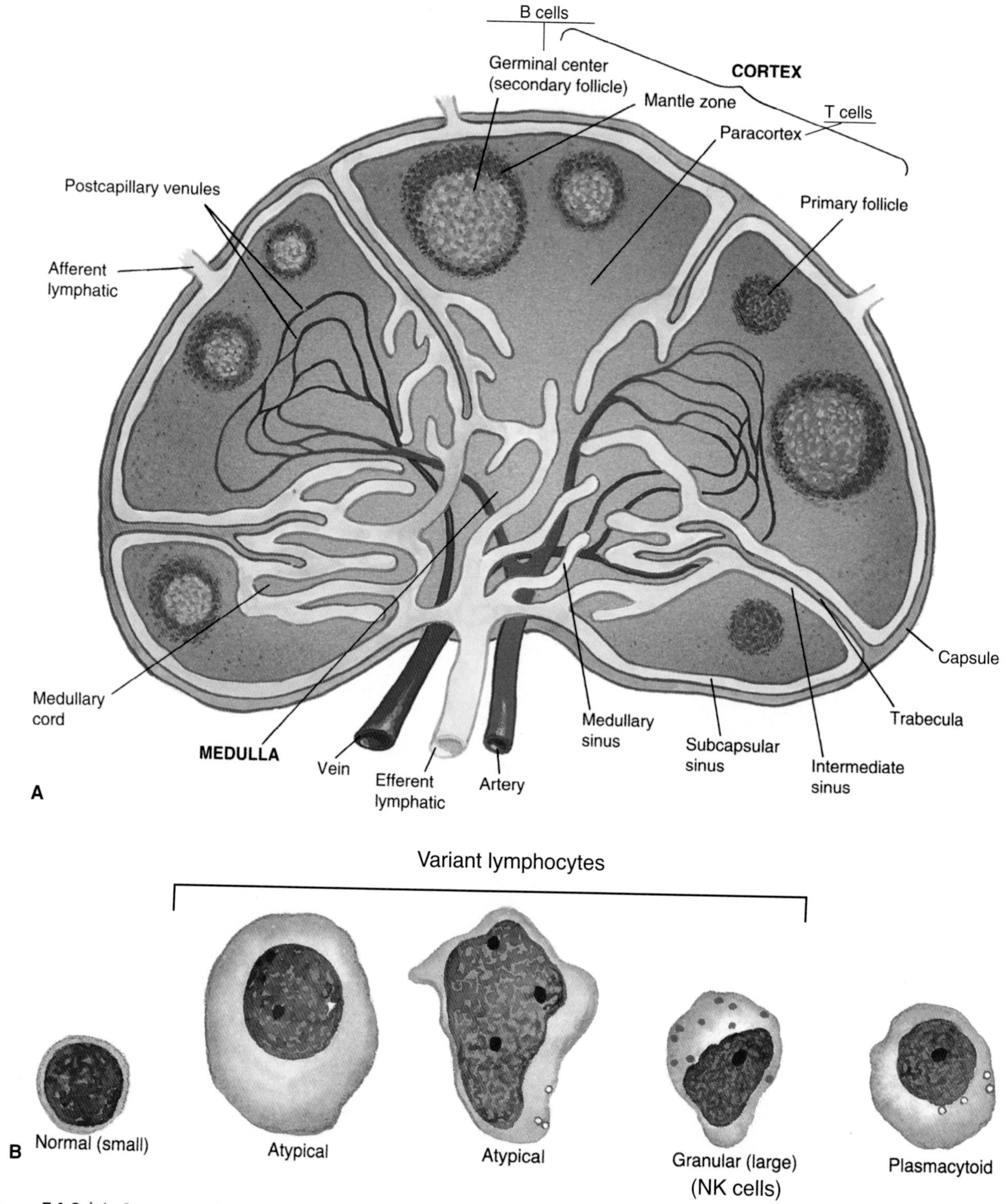

Figure 54.3 | A. Structure of a normal lymph node. **B. Lymphocyte morphology.** The term "variant lymphocytes" covers atypical lymphocytes and large granular lymphocytes. *Atypical lymphocytes* are large and exhibit deep blue to pale gray cytoplasm; they are seen in benign reactive processes. *Large granular lymphocytes* are medium-to-large lymphoid cells with some pink cytoplasmic granules. They are suppressor T lymphocytes, some with natural killer (NK) function, and may be increased in benign or malignant disorders. *Plasmacytoid lymphocytes* have abundant blue cytoplasm and are seen in some reactive disorders.

OVERVIEW OF HISTOGENESIS

Anatomically, the lymphoid system is ubiquitous in design and provides the immunologic function throughout the body, consisting of lymphatic channels, lymph node stations, and lymphoid extranodal sites. Lymphocytes can circulate in blood and lymphoid tissues and are characterized by preferentially homing to and from lymph nodes (Fig. 54.4A). Each lymph node has an outer cortex and inner medulla, as well as aggregations of lymphocytes in lymphoid nodules, which exhibit a lighter central area, called the germinal center. The medulla consists of cords and sinuses that are filled with lymphocytes, plasma cells, and macrophages. Lymph enters from afferent channels through the medullary sinuses in the node and exits from the hilus with the arteriole and vein into efferent channels (Fig. 54.4B). Lymphatic tissue in extranodal sites is part of other organs such as:

- GALT: gut-associated lymphoid tissue in small intestine, appendix (Fig. 54.4E)

- BALT: bronchus-associated lymphoid tissue in the respiratory system
- MALT: Mucosal-associated lymphoid tissue in mucous membranes of digestive septa or tonsil (Fig. 54.4C)

In the embryo and newborn, lymphocytes are generated as T cells in the thymus gland (Fig. 54.4D) and B cells in the bursa of Fabricius (as in the appendix; Fig. 54.4E), which populate bone marrow and peripheral nodal sites. The spleen can be viewed as a large node or an extranodal site with a more elaborate vascular supply (Fig. 54.4F). A connective tissue capsule with its fibrous septa divides the interior into incomplete compartments, that is, white and red pulp. The red pulp consists of splenic cords and sinuses, which interconnect, and eventually these blood channels exit via its vein. Perhaps the largest accumulation of lymphocytes is in peripheral lymph nodes and the central bone marrow, with rapid exchange among lymphoid sites.

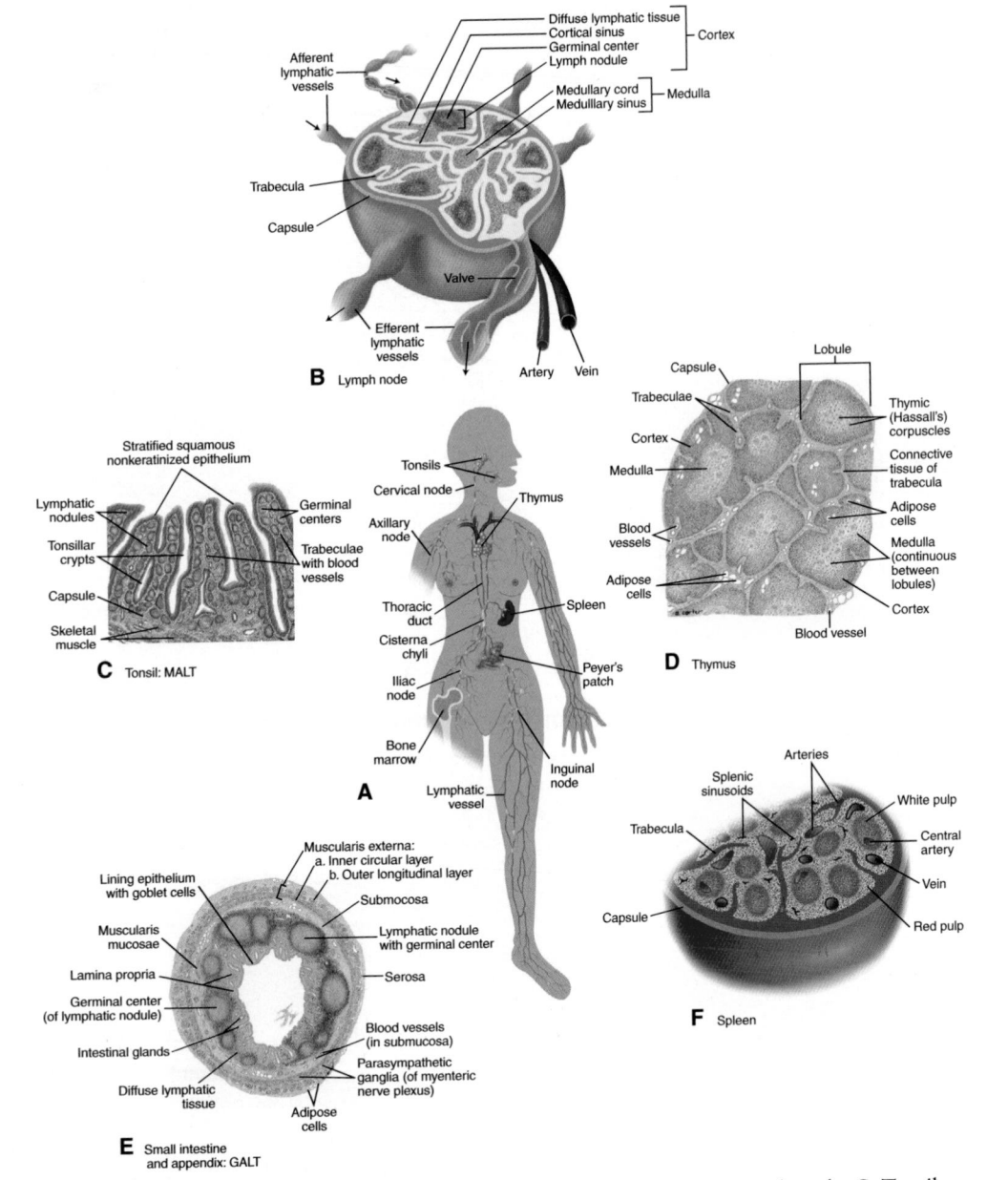

Figure 54.4A | Overview of lymphoid system histogenesis. A. Total lymphoid system. **B.** Lymph node. **C.** Tonsil: mucosa-associated lymphoid tissue (MALT). **D.** Thymus. **E.** Small intestine and appendix: gut-associated lymphoid tissue. **F.** Spleen.

HISTOPATHOLOGY

To provide a basis for the classification of lymphomas, the histologic and physiologic elements of the structure of lymph node with its T cell and B cell lymphocyte domains are important. Lymphocytes mature in the thymus by virtue of developing CD_3 antigen receptors. The large diversity in T cell receptors reflects the fact that each T cell recognizes a single antigen. Other key antigens are CD_4 (helper) and CD_8 (suppressor) lymphocytes.

- B lymphocytes mature in the bone marrow and express surface antigens CD_{19}, CD_{20}, and CD_{22}, plus light and heavy immunoglobulin (Ig) chains.

- The cortex of a lymph node contains the T cell and B cell domains, and, circulating, they enter via the paracortex. T lymphocytes remain in paracortex; B cells migrate to the germinal centers (Fig. 54.3A).

Many different classifications of lymphomas have evolved over time. Currently, the revised European–American Classification of Lymphoid Neoplasms (REAL) has been adopted by the World Health Organization (WHO) and is standard for clinical trials. The list in Table 54.3 is defined by a combination of morphologic, immunophenotypic, and genetic aspects that have distinct clinical features. However, morphology is the most reliable and basic approach for classification, with immunotyping reserved for difficult cases. Some of the more common histopathologies are presented in Fig. 54.4A–E.

TABLE 54.3	Revised European–American Classification of Lymphoid Neoplasms (REAL)
B Cell Neoplasms	**T Cell and NK Cell Neoplasms**
Precursor B cell neoplasm	**Precursor T cell neoplasm**
Precursor B lymphoblastic leukemia/lymphoma (precursor B cell acute lymphoblastic leukemia)	Precursor T lymphoblastic lymphoma/leukemia (precursor T cell acute lymphoblastic leukemia)
Mature (peripheral) B cell neoplasms	**Mature (peripheral) T/NK cell neoplasms**
Chronic lymphocytic leukemia/small lymphocytic lymphoma	T cell prolymphocytic leukemia
B cell prolymphocytic leukemia	T cell granular lymphocytic leukemia
Lymphoplasmacytic lymphoma	Aggressive NK cell leukemia
Splenic marginal zone B cell lymphoma of MALT type	Systemic EBV-positive T cell lymphoproliferative disease of childhood (associated with chronic active EBV infection)
Hairy cell leukemia	Hydroa vacciniforme–like lymphoma
Splenic lymphoma/leukemia, unclassifiable	Adult T-cell lymphoma/leukemia (HTLV 1+)
Plasma cell myeloma/plasmacytoma	Extranodal NK/T cell lymphoma, nasal type
Heavy chain diseases	Enteropathy-type T cell lymphoma
Extranodal marginal zone B cell lymphoma of MALT type	Hepatosplenic γδ T cell lymphoma
Nodal marginal zone B cell lymphoma (with or without monocytoid B cells)	Subcutaneous panniculitis-like T cell lymphoma
Follicular lymphoma	Mycosis fungoides/Sézary syndrome
Primary cutaneous follicle center lymphoma	Primary cutaneous anaplastic large-cell lymphoma
Mantle cell lymphoma	Primary cutaneous γδ T-cell lymphoma
Diffuse large B cell lymphoma (DLBCL)	Primary cutaneous small/medium CD4-positive T cell lymphoma
DLBCL, not otherwise specified	Peripheral T cell lymphoma, not otherwise characterized
T cell/histiocyte–rich large B cell lymphoma	Angioimmunoblastic T-cell lymphoma
DLBCL associated with chronic inflammation	Anaplastic large-cell lymphoma, ALK-positive
EBV-positive DLBCL of the elderly	Anaplastic large-cell lymphoma, ALK-negative
Lymphomatoid granulomatosis	
Primary mediastinal (thymic) large B cell lymphoma	
Intravascular large B cell lymphoma	
Primary cutaneous DLBCL, let type	
ALK-positive DLBCL	
Plasmablastic lymphoma	
Primary effusion lymphoma	
Large B cell lymphoma arising in HHV-8–associated multicentric Castleman's disease	
Burkitt's lymphoma/Burkitt's cell leukemia	
B cell lymphoma, unclassifiable, with features intermediate between those of diffuse large B cell lymphoma and Burkitt's lymphoma	
B cell lymphoma, unclassifiable, with features intermediate between those of diffuse large B cell lymphoma and classic Hodgkin's lymphoma	

ALK, anaplastic lymphoma kinase; EBV, Epstein–Barr virus; HTLV 1, human T-cell leukemia virus type 1; MALT, mucosa-associated lymphoid tissue. From Swerdlow SH, Campo E, Harris NL, et al. *WHO Classification of Tumours of Haematopoietic and Lymphoid Tissues.* 4th ed. Lyon, France: IARC, 2008, with permission. Used with the permission of the American Joint Committee on Cancer (AJCC) Chicago, Illinois. The original source for this material is the *AJCC Cancer Staging Manual,* Seventh edition (2010) published by Springer SBM, LLC, p 602.

LYMPHOMAS

Malignant lymphomas are a very heterogeneous group derived from B cells and T cells. The REAL classification has been adopted by the WHO, which distinguishes between non-Hodgkin's lymphoma (NHL) and Hodgkin's lymphomas. The more common histopathologic types are illustrated, as well as some less frequent types, to provide an overview of the spectrum of the lymphomas. The incidence is noted (%) for each group of lymphomas.

- (30%) Diffuse large B cell lymphomas (DLBCLs) are a heterogeneous group of aggressive, potentially curable B cell neoplasms.

- (22%) Follicular lymphoma (FL) is the malignant counterpart of lymphocytes derived from follicle centers. Unlike any other type of lymphoma, FL mimics an entire functional unit of lymphocytes, including their ancillary cells. The opposite of FL is diffuse lymphoma.

- (7.6%) MALT lymphomas are indolent, malignant T lymphocyte proliferations of small to medium-sized lymphocytes, with frequent monocytoid features and variable admixtures of plasma cells.

- (6%) Mantle cell lymphoma is a B cell neoplasm of small to medium-sized lymphocytes with irregular nuclear features.

- (6.1%) Small-cell lymphoma is a malignant B cell proliferation of small, mature-appearing lymphocytes and a variable number of larger cells (prolymphocytes and paraimmunoblasts).

- (2.5%) Burkitt's lymphoma is one of the most rapidly growing malignancies.

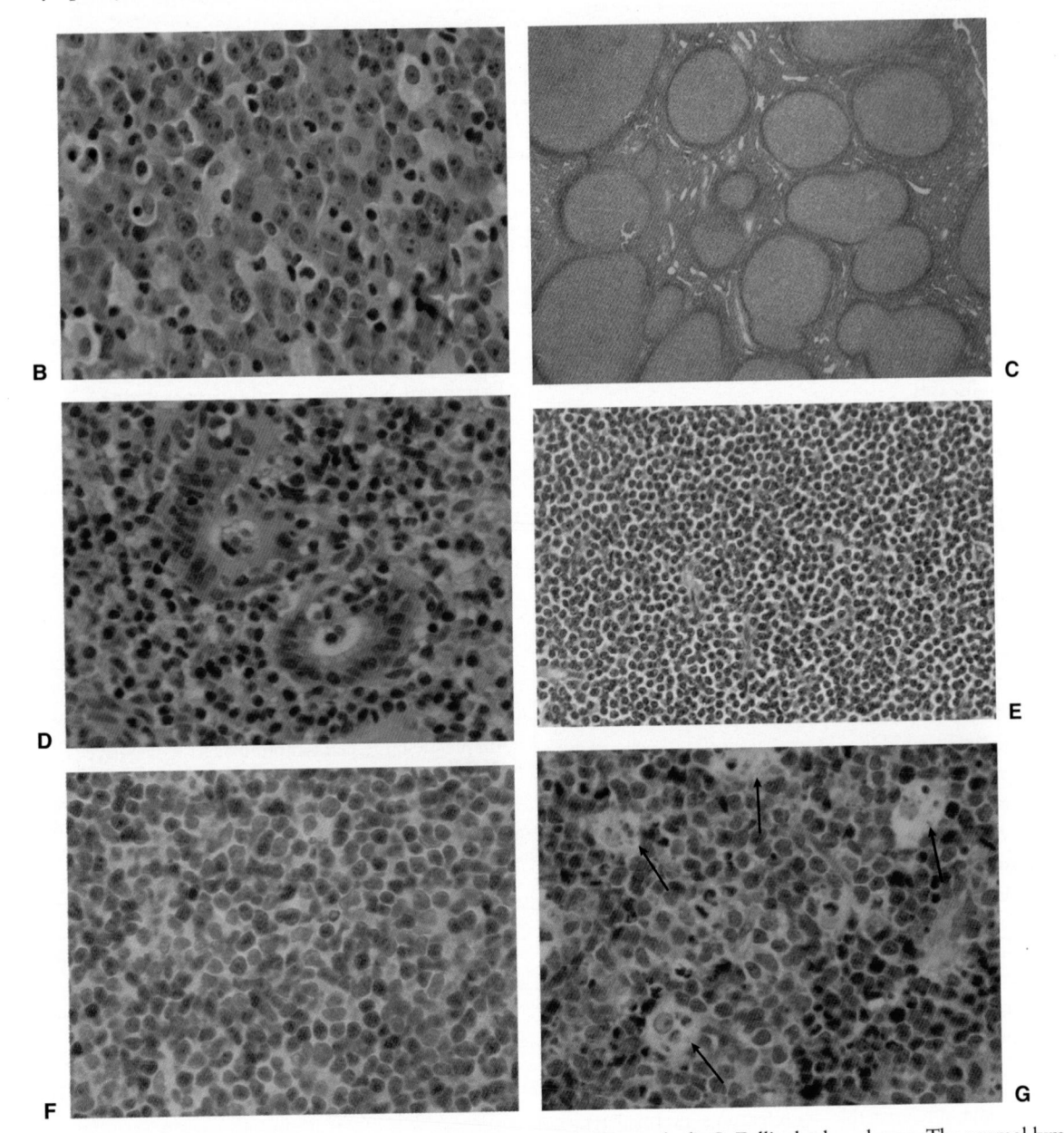

Figure 54.4 | B. Diffuse large B cell lymphoma. Tumor cells show prominent nucleoli. C. Follicular lymphoma. The normal lymph node architecture is replaced by malignant lymph follicles. D. Mucosa-associated lymphoid tissue (MALT) lymphoma. Lymphoepithelial lesions of the stomach are present. E. Small lymphocytic lymphoma/leukemia. On microscopic examination, the lymph nodal architecture is replaced by a diffuse infiltration of normal-appearing small lymphocytes. F. Mantle cell lymphoma. A nuclear stain for BCL-1 is positive. G. Burkitt's lymphoma. Lymph node is effaced by neoplastic lymphocytes with several starry-sky macrophages (*arrows*).

HODGKIN'S DISEASE

Classic Hodgkin's disease is identified by the clonal proliferation of mononuclear cells that are multinucleated and express CD_{30}; they were described by Reed and Sternberg and referred to by their names (Fig. 54.4H, I).

There are histopathologic varieties:

- Nodular lymphocyte-predominant Hodgkin's lymphoma (NLPHL) features Reed–Sternberg cell variants called "popcorn" of lymphohistocytic (LH) cells (Fig. 54.4I).

- Nodular sclerosis Hodgkin's lymphoma (NSHL) features a nodular architecture creating islands of lymphoid tissue surrounded by fibrosis (Fig. 54.4J).

- Mixed cellularity Hodgkin's lymphoma (MCHL) contains Hodgkin and RS cells against a mixed inflammatory background of eosinophils, neutrophils, macrophages, and plasma cells (Fig. 54.4K).

- Lymphocyte depleted HL shows a predominance of Reed–Sternberg cells with relatively low number of lymphocytes (Fig. 54.4L).

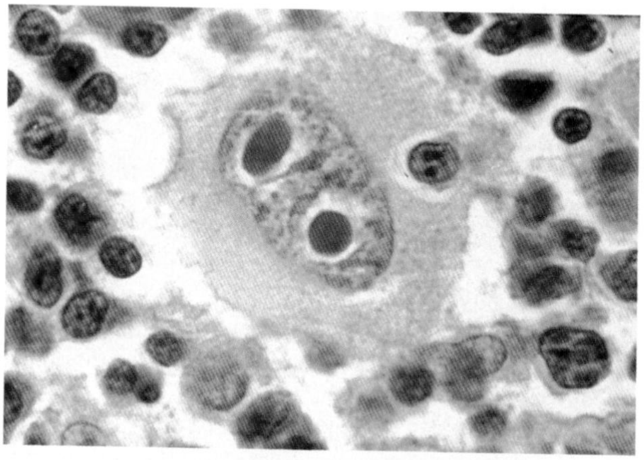

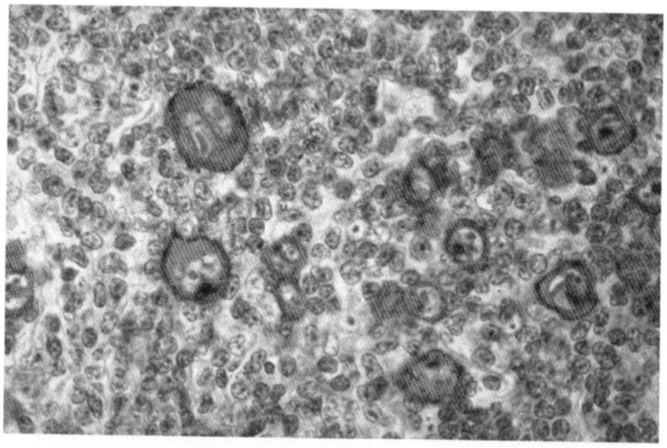

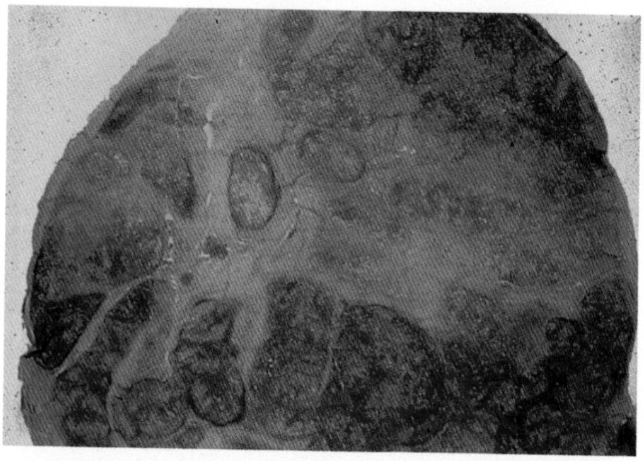

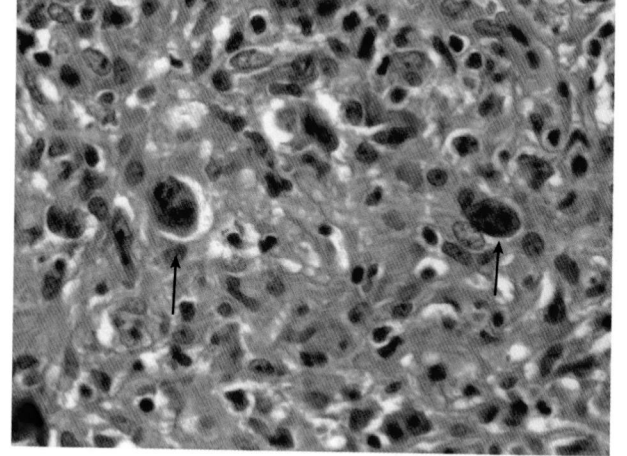

Figure 54.4 | H. Classic Reed–Sternberg cell. Mirror-image nuclei contain large eosinophilic nucleoli. **I.** Reed–Sternberg and Hodgkin cells. The cells are positive for CD30 (immunohistochemistry). **J.** Hodgkin's lymphoma; nodular sclerosis. A low-power photomicrograph demonstrates broad bands of fibrosis. **K.** Hodgkin's lymphoma; mixed cellularity. A photomicrograph of a lymph node shows classic, binucleated, and mononuclear Reed–Sternberg cells; lymphocytes; and mild diffuse fibrosis. **L.** Hodgkin's lymphoma; lymphocyte-depleted type. Two tumor cells are seen (*arrows*). The number of reactive lymphocytes in the fibrotic background is markedly reduced.

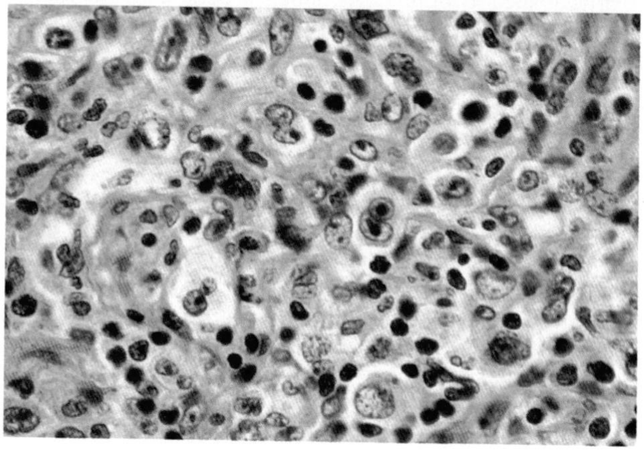

ANATOMIC STAGING SYSTEM—LYMPHOMAS

In 1971, the Ann Arbor staging system was introduced; it was internationally adopted with minor modification in Cotswold, England, in the earliest joint editions of the American Joint Committee on Cancer/International Union Against Cancer (Fig. 54.5). This classification has remained stable with minor modifications and is applicable to both HL and non-Hodgkin's lymphoma (NHL). Most classifications rate an extranodal site as "localized," which deserves an "E" designation as part of the staging process. Briefly, stage I is one node-bearing region; stage II is two or more node-bearing regions on one side of the diaphragm; stage III is a node-bearing region on both sides of the diaphragm; and stage IV is dissemination to extranodal visceral sites. This anatomic classification was based on two new definitions: (1) a node-bearing region and (2) an extranodal site of involvement.

- Node-bearing regions: There are six major and five minor regions, but they do not have a foundation anatomically and have been assigned by consensus.

- The diaphragm is a critical landmark in the staging process, and supradiaphragmatic presentations carry a better prognosis than infradiaphragmatic ones. The diaphragm again is an anatomic but not a physiologic divide of the lymphoid system.

- Extranodal sites include Waldeyer's ring of pharyngeal lymphoid tissue, the spleen, Peyer's patches in the intestine, and bone. In immunosuppressed patients, when visceral sites are involved, such as brain, liver, lung, or bone marrow, these are considered to be disseminated sites similar to metastases.

For lymphomas, the TNM system could be visualized (similar to cancer) if "extranodal (E) sites" were the origin of the malignant lymphoid process and then spread to regional nodes. However, this parallel is not a common occurrence. Noncontiguous spread, which is less predictable and less orderly, occurs in NHL. The malignant lymphocyte is like the normal lymphocyte; it tends to enter the general circulation but homes back to lymphoid tissue and accounts for the random general spread pattern of lymphomas. The normal cellular migration streams have been diagrammed by Yoffey and are referred to as "the fourth circulation." The therapeutic and diagnostic implications in treating lymphomas require a thorough evaluation of all lymphoid sites.

The lymphocyte is a highly mobile cell both when healthy and diseased. It can enter rapidly into the general circulation in the lymph nodes, which have rich beds of postcapillary venules, or move in a more orderly fashion from one nodal station to the next through lymphatic channels, eventually returning to the blood via the thoracic duct. Patterns of spread in lymphomas and HL are as follows.

- An early phase involves only lymphoid tissue and lymph nodes.

- In HL, the spread is more predictable, using lymphatic channels between contiguous sites.

- In lymphomas, the spread is random, confined to nodal and extranodal lymphoid tissues and organs.

- Virtually all lymphoid tissues can be involved and are at risk.

- Dissemination via hematogenous channels often is a late event, and transformation of lymphoma into a leukemic phase can be the terminal event.

Some clarification regarding extranodal sites:

- Spleen involvement is established if there is splenomegaly along with imaging of multiple focal defects.

- Liver involvement is due to hepatomegaly with multiple focal defects.

- Lung and bone involvement can be found as single infiltrates or multiple lesions. Both can be considered extranodal sites (E) if they are contiguous to a node. They need to be the only anatomic site involved to be considered focal extranodal (E) sites. If both or more sites are involved, the patient is stage IV.

- Neurologic involvement is considered disseminated disease and is common in advanced stages and/or immunosuppressed patients.

- Bone marrow involvement is distinguished from bone involvement and is always considered to be disseminated disease (stage IV).

- For the purposes of staging, some extranodal sites are considered as nodal sites—Waldeyer's ring, thymus, and spleen. NHL in 25% of presentations is an extranodal site.

SUMMARY OF CHANGES SEVENTH EDITION AJCC

There are no changes to the stage groups in the seventh edition for Hodgkin's lymphoma and non-Hodgkin's lymphoma.

Primary cutaneous T cell lymphoma (CTLC): Mycoses Fundoides and Sezary Syndrome. Although there are no major changes in the staging of Mycosis Fungoides, when comparing the 6th vs. 7th edition of AJCC Manuals, there are more refinements in substages and peripheral blood involvement has been added and emphasized as a new feature. Erythematous patches progress to plaques, then tumors. Sezary syndrome is the aggressive leukemic and erythrodermic form of CTLC with circulating atypical malignant T lymphocytes with cerebriform nuclei (Sezary cells).

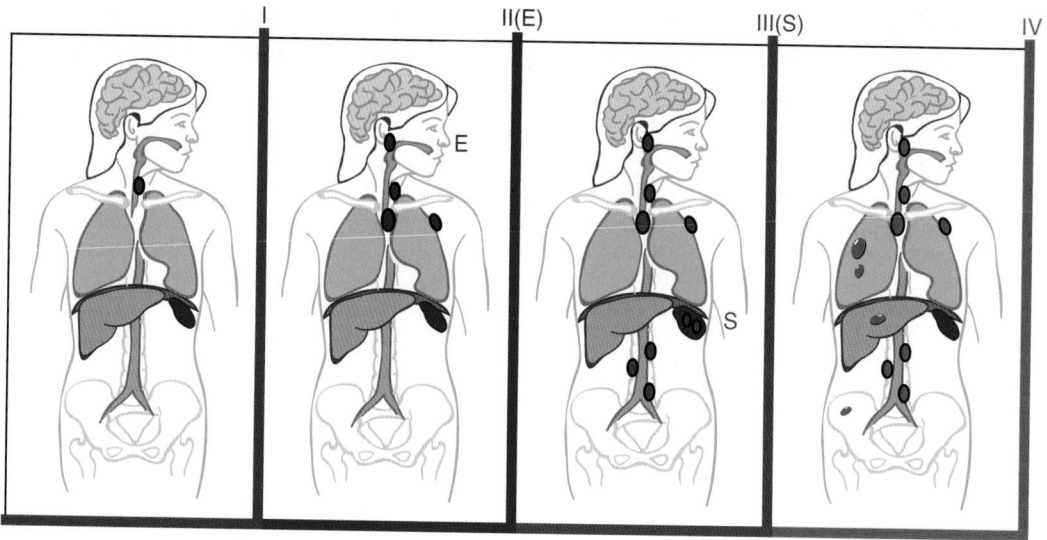

Figure 54.5 | ENM anatomic staging. Bars are color coded: stage I, green; II, blue; III, purple; and IV, red.

- Stage I: involvement of a single lymphatic site (i.e., nodal region, Waldeyer's ring, thymus, or spleen) (I), or localized involvement of a single extralymphatic organ or site in the absence of any lymph node involvement (IE) (rare in Hodgkin's lymphoma).

- Stage II: involvement of two or more lymph node regions on the same side of the diaphragm (II), or localized involvement of a single extralymphatic organ or site in association with regional lymph node involvement with or without involvement of other lymph node regions on the same side of the diaphragm (IIE). The number of regions involved may be indicated by a subscript.

- Stage III: involvement of lymph node regions on both sides of the diaphragm (III), which also may be accompanied by extralymphatic extension in association with adjacent lymph node involvement (IIIE) or by involvement of the spleen (IIIS) or both (IIIE, S). Splenic involvement is designated by the letter S.

- Stage IV: diffuse or disseminated involvement of one or more extralymphatic organs, with or without associated lymph node involvement, or isolated extralymphatic organ involvement in the absence of adjacent regional lymph node involvement, but in conjunction with disease in distant site(s). Stage IV includes any involvement of the liver or bone marrow, lungs (other than by direct extension from another site), or cerebrospinal fluid.

TABLE 54.4	TNM Classification for Mycosis Fungoides	
T1	Limited patch/plaque	(<10% of skin surface involved)
T2	Generalized patch/plaque	(≥10% of skin surface involved)
T3	Cutaneous tumors	(one or more)
T4	Generalized erythroderma	(with or without patches, plaques, or tumors)
N0		Lymph nodes clinically uninvolved
N1		Lymph nodes clinically enlarged, histologically uninvolved
N2		Lymph nodes clinically enlarged, histologically involved
N3		Lymph nodes enlarged and histologically involved
M0		No visceral disease
M1		Visceral disease present
B0		No circulating atypical cells (<1,000 Sezary cells [CD4 + CD7 −]/ml)
B1		Low circulating atypical cells (<1,000 Sezary cells [CD4 + CD7 −]/ml)
B2		High circulating atypical cells (≥1,000 Sezary cells [CD4 + CD7 −]/ml)

Stage Classification of Mycosis Fungoides

IA	T1	N0	M0	0,1
IB	T2	N0	M0	0,1
IIA	T1–2	N1	M0	0,1
IIB	T3	N0–1	M0	0,1
IIIA	T4	N0	M0	0
IIIB	T4	N0	M0	1
IVA	T1–4	N2–3	M0	0,2
IVB	T1–4	N0–3	M1	0,−2

Original table from Greene FL, Page DL, Fleming ID, et al, eds. *AJCC Cancer Staging Manual. 6th edition.* New York: Springer, 2002, p. 397. Updated with data from Edge SB, Byrd DR, and Compton CC, et al, *AJCC Cancer Staging Manual, 7th edition.* New York, Springer, 2010, p. 615.

N-ONCOANATOMY

OVERVIEW OF LYMPHOID N-ONCOANATOMY

For staging, lymph node regions are defined in Fig. 54.6A based on general agreement at the Rye, New York, and Ann Arbor, Michigan, meetings rather than any anatomic–physiologic principles. A more comprehensive overview is presented from an anatomic physiologic viewpoint (Fig. 54.6B).

The lymphoid and lymphatic system is diverse. The organization of this system is akin to a separate circulation, which allows lymphocytes, interstitial fluid, and plasma proteins from every tissue and organ system to be collected through lymphatic channels, at regional lymph node stations. Depending on the anatomic location of the organ, the collected lymph then passes through an array of distant lymph nodes and channels, coalescing first into the cisterna chyli below the diaphragm, into the thoracic duct, and finally into the bloodstream. Malignant lymphocytes follow the pathway of normal lymphocytes. An understanding of this normal pathway makes the concepts of both contiguous spread and random spread of lymphoid malignancies more readily appreciated.

The classic book on the anatomy of the lymphoid system is *Anatomy of Human Lymphatics* by H. Rouviere (1832). The drawings have been modified largely from his renderings of lymphatics and lymph nodes for each site. The lymphoid system has been of interest to many other anatomists and pathologists. Such sources as Cruikshank's *The Anatomy of the Absorbing Vessels of the Human Body* (1786), Kampmeier's *Developmental Anatomy* (1919), and Yoffey's *Lymphatics, Lymph and Lymphomyeloid Complex* (1970) are excellent historical references, which still apply today. Excellent renderings of regional node-bearing areas and anatomy exist in surgical dissection and resection diagrams for cancers of specific organs. The classic "en bloc" or "radical" operation of cancer surgery is the removal of first station or regional lymph nodes with the primary tumor. For example, a radical mastectomy is the removal of primary breast cancer, the breast, and axillary lymph nodes, as compared with a simple mastectomy, which usually does not remove lymph nodes. Simple hysterectomy versus radical hysterectomy emphasizes the removal of lymph nodes in addition to the cervix and uterus in the latter operation. Some key anatomic factors are summarized as follows.

- There are 12 so-called "lymph node bearing regions" as defined based on general agreement (Fig. 54.6A). However, if all specific lymph node stations are counted, there are 36 lymph node stations (Fig. 35.6B).

- Specific major lymphatic trunks drain each structure, site, and viscera, and generally coalesce in two major sites on either side of the diaphragm—the cisterna chyli or the thoracic duct. The cisterna chyli drains the abdomen and pelvis and empties into the thoracic duct, which drains the lungs, mediastinum, heart, breast, and head and neck.

- The first station (echelon) of lymph nodes comprises the "regional" lymph nodes that first receive the lymph from the major lymphatic trunks draining a structure, site, or viscera.

- The second station (echelon) of lymph nodes is referred to as "juxtaregional." It is the next region to receive lymph from first-station nodes.

- Although bypass mechanisms and collateral channels exist, lymph generally flows from organs in a prograde fashion to their first-station regional nodes.

- The thoracic duct drains into the junction of the left subclavian vein and the internal jugular vein.

- The diaphragm is rich in lymphatics and drains the peritoneal cavity. The lymphatics, located on its undersurface, are greater on the right than on the left.

Lymph from the right side of the head, right upper extremities, and right upper thorax drain into the right subclavian duct, which empties into the venous circulation at the junction of the right subclavian and internal jugular veins. Lymph from the rest of the body drains alternately to the thoracic duct, which empties on the left side at the junction of left subclavian and internal jugular vein.

The staging of HL depends on biopsy of major lymph nodal sites below the diaphragm. One needs to identify the sites that commonly are sampled. These include any enlarged para-aortic or pelvic lymph nodes and the splenic hilar nodes and spleen (which are removed). The liver and the bone marrow are biopsied, the porta hepatis is explored, and the mesentery is biopsied, particularly in NHL.

Extranodal or extralymphatic sites (ENM) include the bone marrow, the gastrointestinal tract, skin, bone, central nervous system, lung, gonads, ocular adnexae (conjunctiva, lacrimal glands, and orbital soft tissue), liver, kidneys, uterus, etc. Hodgkin's lymphoma rarely presents in an extranodal site alone, but about 25% of non-Hodgkin's lymphomas are extranodal at presentation. The frequency of extranodal presentation varies dramatically among different lymphomas, however, with some (mycosis fungoides and MALT lymphomas) being virtually always extranodal, except in advanced stages of the diseases, and some (follicular lymphoma, B-cell small lymphocytic lymphoma) seldom being extranodal, except for bone marrow involvement. For the purpose of coding and staging, lymph nodes, Waldeyer's ring, thymus, and spleen are considered *nodal* or *lymphatic sites*.

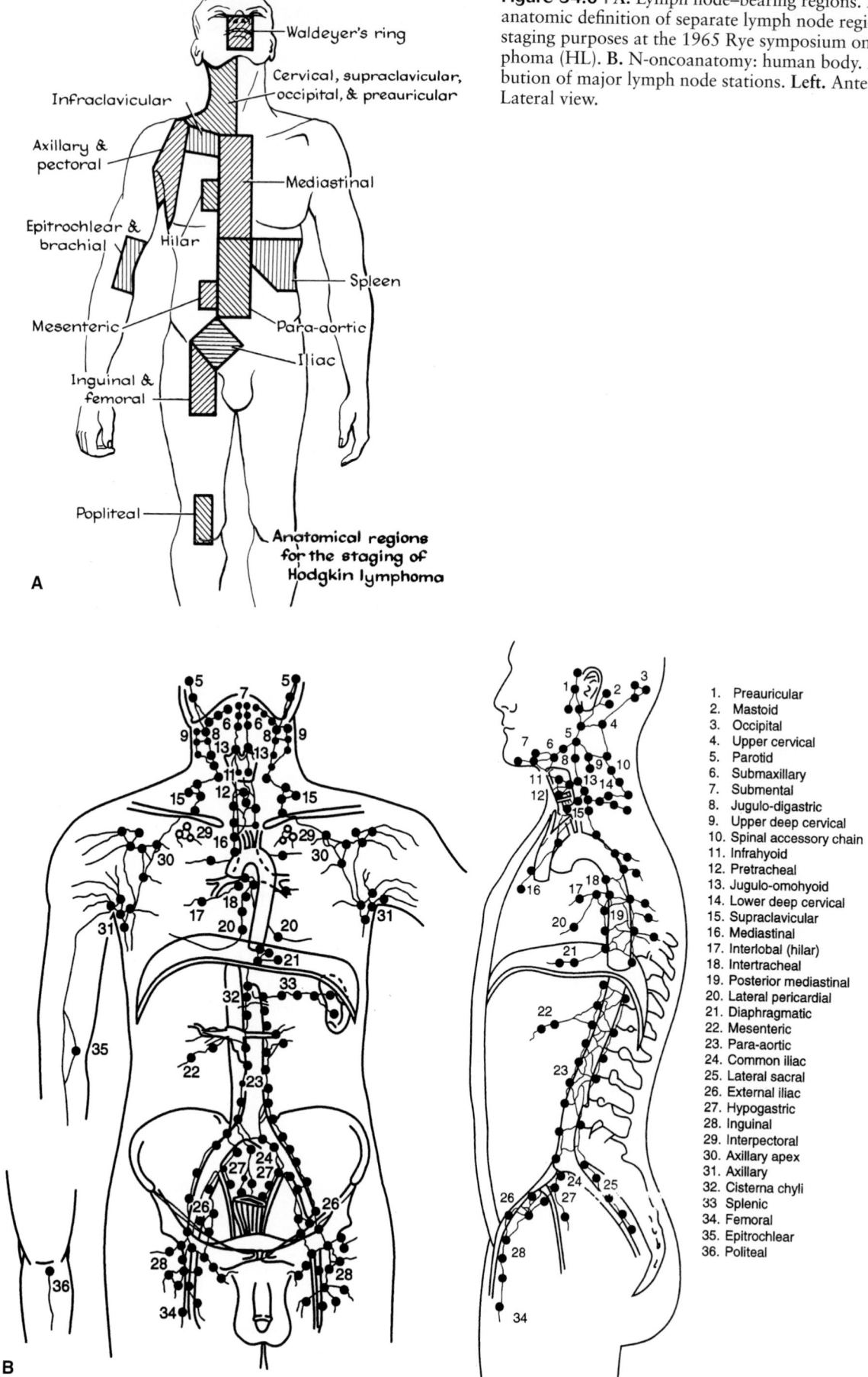

Figure 54.6 | A. Lymph node–bearing regions. Diagram of the anatomic definition of separate lymph node regions adopted for staging purposes at the 1965 Rye symposium on Hodgkin's lymphoma (HL). **B.** N-oncoanatomy: human body. Anatomic distribution of major lymph node stations. **Left.** Anterior view. **Right.** Lateral view.

Waldeyer's ring

Cervical, supraclavicular, occipital, & preauricular

Infraclavicular

Axillary & pectoral

Mediastinal

Epitrochlear & brachial

Hilar

Spleen

Mesenteric

Para-aortic

Iliac

Inguinal & femoral

Popliteal

Anatomical regions for the staging of Hodgkin lymphoma

A

1. Preauricular
2. Mastoid
3. Occipital
4. Upper cervical
5. Parotid
6. Submaxillary
7. Submental
8. Jugulo-digastric
9. Upper deep cervical
10. Spinal accessory chain
11. Infrahyoid
12. Pretracheal
13. Jugulo-omohyoid
14. Lower deep cervical
15. Supraclavicular
16. Mediastinal
17. Interlobal (hilar)
18. Intertracheal
19. Posterior mediastinal
20. Lateral pericardial
21. Diaphragmatic
22. Mesenteric
23. Para-aortic
24. Common iliac
25. Lateral sacral
26. External iliac
27. Hypogastric
28. Inguinal
29. Interpectoral
30. Axillary apex
31. Axillary
32. Cisterna chyli
33 Splenic
34. Femoral
35. Epitrochlear
36. Politeal

B

STAGING WORKUP

RULES FOR CLASSIFICATION AND STAGING

Histopathology

The lymphoid neoplasms include an ever-increasing spectrum of disorders. The large variety of sites affected and the systemic distribution of lymphomas reflects the ubiquitous distribution of the lymphocyte. The array of lymphomas and lymphoproliferative conditions has undergone a metamorphosis over the last five decades and has made their classification more accurate and perhaps more confusing. Morphologic criteria based on both the macropathology and micropathology of the lymph node have been supplemented by immunotyping and genetic features of the lymphocyte. These lymphoid neoplasms have a common ancestry with either B cells, T cells, or natural killer cells. Accordingly, the NHLs collectively include the neoplastic versions of these cells and in addition include HL and lymphoid leukemias. Currently, the Revised European–American Classification of Lymphoid Neoplasms (REAL) has incorporated the histopathology of the original Working Formulation of the International Lymphoma Study Group with the newer immunomolecular markers to define 50 different categories of lymphoid neoplasms in NHL (Table 54.3) whereas in HL there are 4 varieties histopathologically (Fig. 54.4H,I,J,K,L).

Clinical Staging and Imaging

Careful inspection and clinical palpation of all peripheral sites is mandatory: head and neck, upper limb (epitrochlear node) and axilla, inguinal/femoral area, and lower limb (popliteal and femoral nodes). Thoracic and abdominal nodes require imaging. Liver and spleen should be palpable if enlarged. Spiral computed tomography (CT) and magnetic resonance imaging (MRI) can provide cross-sectional anatomy. Suspicious nodes are defined with different size thresholds. Most nodes ≥1 cm and certainly 1.5- to 2-cm rounded nodes are considered positive and, if possible, deserve needle aspiration or excisional biopsy to confirm. Retrocrural nodes >0.5 cm are considered highly suspicious. Imaging can establish organ invasion of liver, spleen, lung, bone, and central nervous system. MRI is excellent to show bone marrow invasion, but aspiration biopsy is advised for confirmation (Table 54.4).

Pathologic Staging

Laparotomy, once routine in HL, allowed for histopathologic verification of lymphomatous invasion of liver, spleen, bowel, mesentery, omentum, accessible bone, and bone marrow.

TABLE 54.5A   **Recommendation for the Diagnostic Evaluation of Patients with Lymphoma**

A. Mandatory procedures
1. Biopsy (preferably excisional), with interpretation by a qualified pathologist
2. History, with special attention to the presence and duration of fever, night sweats, and unexplained loss of 10% or more of body weight in the previous 6 months
3. Physical examination
4. Lab tests
    a. Complete blood cell count and platelet count
    b. Erythrocyte sedimentation rate or C-reactive protein (Hodgkin's lymphoma patients)
    c. Chemistry panel (electrolytes, blood urea nitrogen, creatinine, calcium, phosphorus, uric acid, aspartate aminotransferase, alanine aminotransferase, bilirubin, lactase dehydrogenase, and alkaline phosphatase)
5. Radiographic examination
    a. Chest X-ray
    b. Computed tomography of neck, chest, abdomen, and pelvis
    c. Metabolic imaging (deoxyfluoroglucose-positron emission tomography) in appropriate indications
6. Bone marrow examination*
7. HIV testing in patients with an aggressive histology
8. Hepatitis B serology in patients being considered for rituximab

B. Ancillary procedures
1. Radioisotopic bone scans, in selected patients with bone pain
2. Gastroscopy and/or gastrointestinal series in patients with gastrointestinal presentations
3. Magnetic resonance imaging (MRI) of the spine in patients with suspected spinal cord involvement
4. MRI of the brain in patients with cranial nerve palsy or suspected primary central nervous system lymphoma
5. MRI of bone if nuclear imaging abnormality is identified
6. Cerebrospinal fluid cytology in patients with stage IV disease and bone marrow involvement, testis involvement, or parameningeal involvement and in all children and all adults with lymphoblastic and Burkitt's lymphoma. Flow cytometric analysis may be more sensitive than cytologic assessment.

---

*May include unilateral/bilateral bone marrow aspiration and biopsy in adults and children with non-Hodgkin's lymphoma and unilateral/bilateral biopsies in children with Hodgkin's lymphoma who present with B symptoms or advanced stage disease (III/IV).
Used with the permission of the American Joint Committee on Cancer (AJCC) Chicago, Illinois. The original source for this material is the *AJCC Cancer Staging Manual*, Seventh edition (2010) published by Springer SBM, LLC, p 609.

Currently, imaging and selected image-guided biopsy of suspicious areas can provide histopathologic verification for more accurate staging. Needle biopsy is limited in HL because aspiration of a Reed–Sternberg cell is essential for the diagnosis. An excisional biopsy of an enlarged node is preferred.

ONCOIMAGING ANNOTATIONS

Hodgkin's Lymphoma

- Generally, tumor is detected in cervical nodes when they are enlarged (≤10 mm), become more round, or increase in number.

- Lymphomas usually show homogeneous nodal enhancement. Central nodal necrosis is exceedingly rare.

- In the patient with low mediastinal or hilar abnormalities, CT is critical in verifying disease and better in defining the contiguous lung parenchyma for unsuspected involvement.

- Nodal size criterion is reduced to 6 mm for prevascular, internal mammary, posterior mediastinal, and anterior diaphragmatic nodes.

- HL primarily involves the upper abdominal and retroperitoneal nodes, whereas NHL may involve any of the nodes, including the mesenteric nodes. Retroperitoneal lymph nodes involved with HL rarely become grossly enlarged, detracting from the accuracy of CT.

Non-Hodgkin's Lymphoma

- On both ultrasonography and CT, a relatively specific finding of mesenteric NHL is the "sandwich" sign, in which tumor infiltrating the mesenteric leaves or nodes encase the mesenteric vessels.

- Waldeyer's ring is the most common head and neck site for extranodal NHL.

- Single or multiple submucosal nodules or masses are common in bowel lymphoma, and as the lesion outgrows its blood supply, mucosal necrosis may occur, leading to ulceration and cavitation.

- Diffuse infiltration of the submucosa causes wall thickening and enlargement of the folds.

- One of the unusual features of small-bowel lymphoma occurs after transmural extension of the lymphoma, resulting in aneurysmal dilation of the involved bowel.

- Lymphomatous involvement of the spleen occurs in three patterns: diffuse infiltration, small nodules <1 cm in diameter, and macronodules. Imaging typically detects only the macronodular form.

- Lymphomatous renal masses are frequently bilateral and often significant retroperitoneal lymphadenopathy is absent.

- MRI is exquisitely sensitive to bone marrow involvement, and in select patients, it may serve to guide biopsies.

TABLE 54.5B	Prognostic Systems in Common Use for Patients with Lymphoma
Non-Hodgkin's lymphoma: risk factors in the International Prognostic Index (IPI) for non-Hodgkin's lymphoma	Age ≥60 years
	Reduced performance status (such as ECOG ≥2)
	Elevated LDH
	≥2 extranodal sites of disease
	Ann Arbor stage III or IV
Follicular lymphoma: risk factors in the Follicular Lymphoma Prognostic Index (FLIPI)	Number of nodal sites ≥5
	Elevated LDH
	Age ≥60 years
	Ann Arbor Stage III or IV
	Hemoglobin (<12 g/dL)
Hodgkin's lymphoma: risk factors in the International Prognostic Score (IPS)	Serum albumin <4 g/dL
	Hemoglobin <10.5 g/dL
	Age ≥45 years
	Male sex
	Ann Arbor stage IV
	White blood cell count ≥15 × 10^9/L
	Lymphocytopenia <0.6 × 10^9/L or <8%

ECOG, Eastern Cooperative Oncology Group; LDH, lactase dehydrogenase.
Used with the permission of the American Joint Committee on Cancer (AJCC) Chicago, Illinois. The original source for this material is the *AJCC Cancer Staging Manual,* Seventh edition (2010) published by Springer SBM, LLC, p 611.

Introduction and Orientation

PERSPECTIVE AND PATTERNS OF SPREAD

The eye is a palindrome of three letters, and its oncoanatomy is characterized by being a trilogy anatomically, reflecting its embryonic origin.

PERSPECTIVE AND PATTERNS OF SPREAD

Blindness is a major concern at any age, and any form of tumefaction is a challenge to the preservation of vision. The tissues of the eye in their embryogenic development are derived from neuroectoderm, surface ectoderm, and mesoderm. There are many different tumors that can arise around the orbit and in the eye due to the large variety of tissues that constitute this sensory organ and its anatomic environment (Table 55.1).

The eye is composed of three different layers, each with its unique structures. The neoplasms are different for adults and children. Each structure gives rise to a characteristic tumor that can only occur in that layer; that is, in the retina, retinoblastomas; in the pigmented choroids, the pigmented melanoma; or the sclera and conjunctiva squamous cell cancers. Each tumor

spreads in a specific pattern depending on the layers involved; however, each can advance and invade into other layers and structures of the eye and orbit (Fig. 55.1; Table 55.2).

An exact understanding of three-dimensional anatomy is essential in radiation oncology, where precision proton beams with sharp and limited Bragg peaks or strategically placed radioisotopic plaques have successfully eradicated choroidal melanomas and preserved vision. In a similar fashion, carefully shaped photon beams with appropriate shielding can save an eye in children with retinoblastomas and embryonal rhabdomyosarcomas.

Preservation of vision with tumor ablation is the essential goal for both the ophthalmologic surgeon and the radiation oncologist. Precise surgical ablative procedures match accurate proton beams and have allowed for high cure rates with eye and vision conservation. Enucleation and exenteration are reserved for very advanced and recurrent sarcomas and cancers.

The patterns of spread are presented to provide an overview of how neoplasms at each site of origin ultimately invade the eye globe from extraocular sites in contrast to intraocular sites. The accompanying SIMLAP tables provide the malignant gradient based on six patterns or vectors of invasion that determine stage advancement.

TABLE 55.1	Most Common Tumors of the Eye					
	Adult			**Child**		
Site	**Tumor Type**	**Sign**	**Visual Loss**	**Tumor Type**	**Sign**	**Visual Loss**
Lid	Basal cell carcinoma	Scabbing ulcer	None	Hemangioma	Red strawberry mass	Closed eyelid
Conjunctiva	Squamous cell carcinoma	Fleshy lesion	None	Leukemia	Raised, infiltrative mass	None
Intraocular	Melanoma	Black-to-brownish elevated area in choroids	Scotoma	Retinoblastoma	White reflex	Blindness
Intraorbital	Lymphoma	Mass, displacement of globe	Diplopia	Embryonal rhabdomyosarcoma	Mass, displacement of globe	Diplopia
Metastatic	Breast (lung)	Raised area in retina	Scotoma	Neuroblastoma	Proptosis, ecchymosis, pain, orbit mass	Diplopia

Used with permission from Rubin P. *Clinical Oncology*. 7th ed. Philadelphia: WB Saunders; 1993:300.

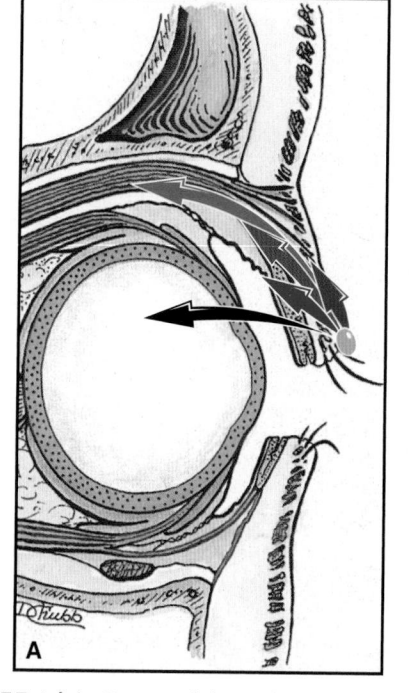 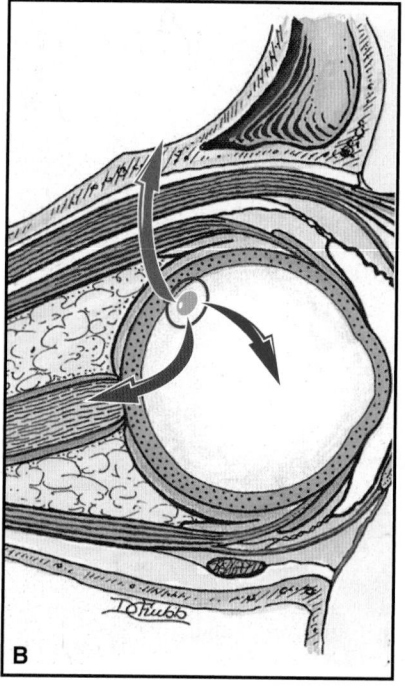 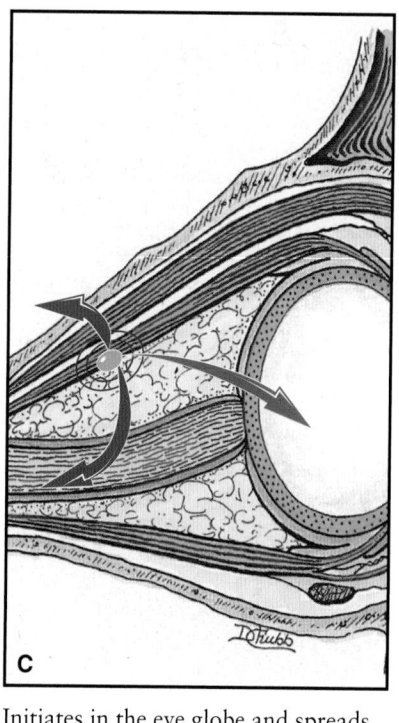

Figure 55.1 | A. Cancer of the eyelid. Invasion of globe is a late stage. **B.** Retinoblastoma. Initiates in the eye globe and spreads in an extraocular fashion. **C.** Orbital sarcomas begin in the orbit soft tissue/muscle and can invade into the eye globe as the tumor advances.

TABLE 55.2A–C	SIMLAP		

Cancer of Eyelid		**Retinoblastoma**		**Sarcoma**	
Upper Eyelid					
S Conjunctiva fornix, eyelash	• T3	Macula	• T1	**S** Orbit, extraocular muscles	• T1
Lacrimal gland, orbit bone	• T4b	**S** Orbit, extraocular muscles	• T4	Extraocular muscles	• T2
I Conjunctival fornix, eyelash margin	• T1			Bone orbit	• T3
		I Orbit, extraocular muscles	• T4	Frontal sinus	• T4
Sebaceous gland, sweat gland	• T2			**I** Soft tissue orbit	• T3
M Canaliculi, nasolacrimal duct	• T4a	**M** Retina	• T1	Maxillary sinus	• T4
Nasal cavity, paranasal sinus	• T4c	Choroid focal	• T2b	Soft tissue orbit	• T3
L		**L** Retina	• T1	**M** Orbit extraocular muscles, fat	• T3
A Epidermis, orbicularis oculi	• T1 • T3	Choroid focal	• T2b	Nasal cavity, ethmoid paranasal sinus	• T4
P Bulbar conjunctiva	• T4	**A** Vitreous seeding	• T2	**L** Nasal cavity, ethmoid paranasal sinus	• T4
Palpebral conjunctiva	• T3	Orbit	• T4		
Cornea, uvea	• T4	**P** Optic nerve disc	• T2a	**A** Globe	• T4
Globe of eye	• T4	Optic coats	• T3	Eyelids	• T4
Tarsal plate	• T2	Retro-orbital space	• T4	**P** Temporal fossa	• T4
Sclera	• T4	Choroid focal	• T2b	Central nervous system	• T4
Central nervous system	• T4d	Choroid massive	• T3c		
Orbit soft tissues	• T4d	Optic nerve	• T3a		
Bone orbit	• T4d	Chiasm	• T4		
		Orbit	• T4		
		Subarachnoid space	• T4		
		Apex orbit	• T4		
		Brain	• T4		

The six vectors of invasion are <u>S</u>uperior, <u>I</u>nferior, <u>M</u>edial, <u>L</u>ateral, <u>A</u>nterior, and <u>P</u>osterior. The color-coded dots correlate the T stage with the specific anatomic structure involved.

OVERVIEW OF EMBRYOGENESIS

Embryogenesis determines the histogenesis and offers insights into the variety of malignancies that form from birth to infants to children in rapid growth and adults (Table 55.3). Knowing specific normal tissue derivation in the eye provides an understanding of the carcinogenesis to sarcomagenesis (Fig. 55.2). The eye is uniquely designed for perceiving of light and color and distinguishing different forms.

Table 55.3 provides a concise list of the trigermal origin of specific tissues of the eye.

- *The optic cup* is a neuroectodermal outpouching that forms retina and optic nerve; therefore, primitive retinoblastomas are derived in this layer and spread into the optic nerve and disseminate into the central nervous system.

- *Surface ectoderm* forms the eyelid epidermis and its epithelial extensions, which become the conjunctival cover inside the eyelid and cover the eye globe. As in skin, epithelial skin cells give rise to basal cell and squamous cell cancers; more rare are melanomas.

- *Glandular appendages* in the eyelid and the lacrimal gland can give rise to adenocarcinomas, which are ectodermal derivatives.

- *Mesoderm* forms the connective tissue and mesenchyme of eye and includes the sclera of the eye, the vasculature in retina and choroid, and its arterial and venous drainage. The extraocular muscles can transform into embryonal *rhabdomyosarcomas*.

The choroid of the eye is the portion of the retina that lies next to the retina and consists of a choriocapillary layer, which consists of branching lamellae that have large, flat melanocytes scattered between connective tissue elements. As in the skin, the melanin protects against the damaging effects of non-ionizing ultraviolet light as it reaches the retina. *Melanomas of the iris,*

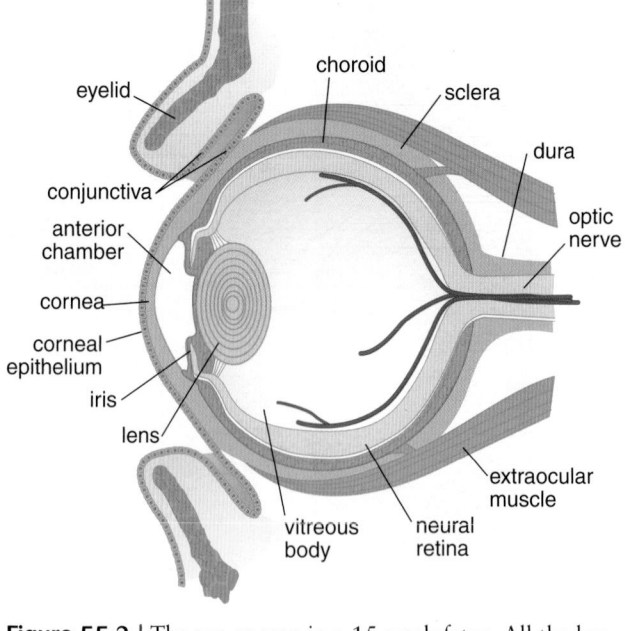

Figure 55.2 | The eye as seen in a 15-week fetus. All the layers of the eye are established, and the hyaloid artery traverses the vitreous body from the optic disc to the posterior surface of the lens.

uvea, and choroid can be aggressive, and their access to the loose vascular tissue in choroid allows for their metastatic spread. The iris is the anterior part of the vascular coat. The retina is neural ectoderm and can transform into retinoblastomas and invade via the optic nerve into the CNS.

Each source is a derivative of specific structural sites and in turn can lead to tumefactions that are unique.

TABLE 55.3	Embryonic Origins of the Individual Structures of the Eye
Source	**Derivative**
Surface ectoderm	Epithelium of the cornea, conjunctiva, and lacrimal gland and its drainage system
	Lens
Neural ectoderm	Epithelium of the retina, iris, and ciliary body
	Sphincter pupillae and dilator pupillae muscles
	Vitreous body (derived partly from neural ectoderm of the optic cup and partly from mesenchyme)
	Optic nerve
Mesoderm	Eyelids (except epithelium and conjunctiva)
	Stroma of the cornea, ciliary body, iris, and choroid
	Sclera
	Extraocular muscles
	Hyaloid system (most of which degenerates before birth)
	Coverings of the optic nerve
	Connective tissue and blood vessels of the eye, bony orbit, and vitreous body

Anterior to Posterior order.

OVERVIEW OF HISTOGENESIS OF EYE PRIMARY SITES

- The overview begins with the sagittal section of the *eye*, which provides a framework for presenting the derivative normal cells and consequential tumors that arise from them (Table 55.4; Fig. 55.3).

- The *eyelid* forms the external covers of the eye, which are composed of epidermis and dermal glandular appendages that are special and specific to this site. Basal cell cancers are most common, squamous cell cancers are less common, and adenocarcinomas arising from meibomian, sebaceous (Zeis), or apocrine (Moll) glands are rare.

- Squamous cell cancers of the *conjunctiva* arise from stratified squamous epithelium.

- Adenocarcinomas of the *lacrimal gland* parallel salivary gland neoplasms histopathologically, and both tend to be involved by lymphoma, which can be present in the conjunctiva and/or orbit, often as isolated sites of disease.

- Melanomas can arise from the pigmented uveal or *choroid* layer of the eye globe, very uncommonly on the iris, and even less so in the conjunctiva.

- The common pediatric tumors arising from the *retina* are retinoblastomas.

- Embryonal cancers arise from the *orbital recti muscles*.

- Sarcomas (not cancers).

TABLE 55.4	Histogenesis of Eye Primary Sites and Derivative Tumors	
Normal Structure	**Derivative Cell**	**Malignancy**
Eyelid, skin, glands	Germinal basal keratinocyte Simple columnar cells	Basal cell cancers Adenocarcinomas
Conjunctiva	Stratified squamous cell	Squamous cell cancer
Uvea, choroids	Melanocyte in pigmented epithelial layer	Melanomas of choroid, uvea
Retina	Retinoblast, precursor cell to inner and outer nuclear cells	Retinoblastoma
Lacrimal gland	Columnar cell	Adenocarcinoma
Recti muscles	Striated muscle cell Lymphocyte	Embryonal rhabdomyosarcoma Lymphoma

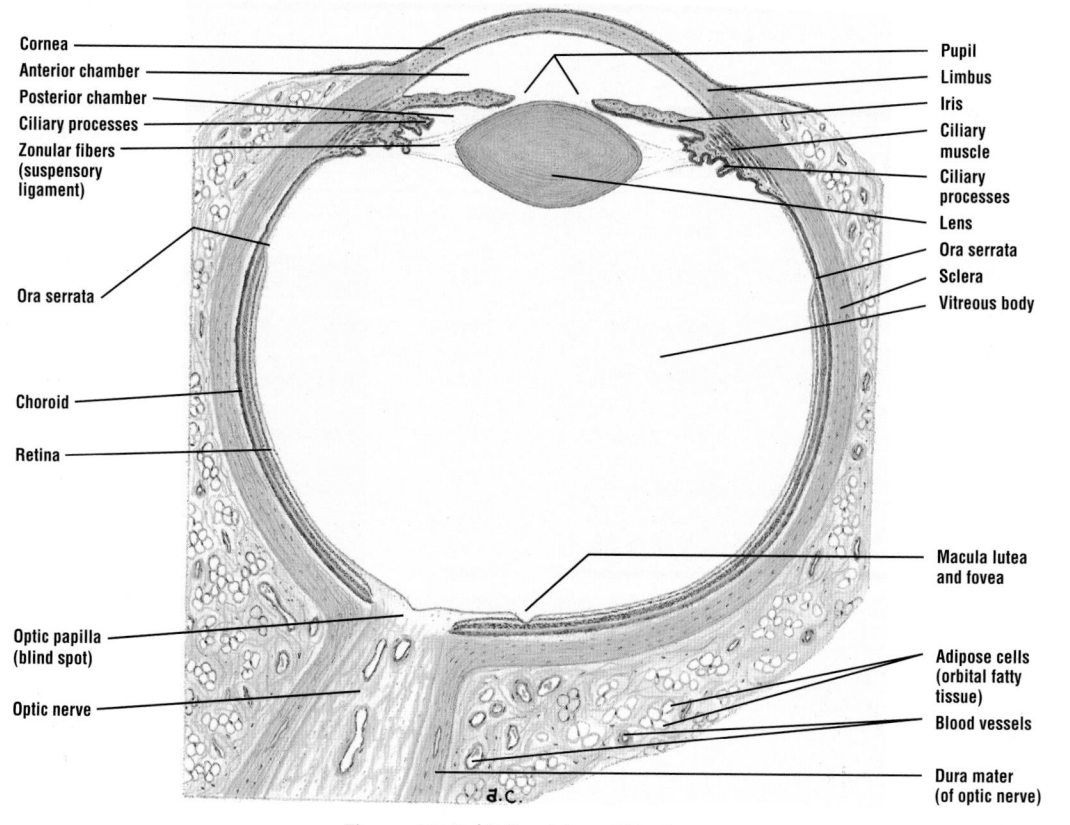

Figure 55.3 | Sclera/choroid/retina.

TNM STAGING CRITERIA

TNM STAGING CRITERIA

For all intents and purposes, the T category determines the stage. The TNM stage grouping is not used to stage eye malignancies, with the exception of uveal melanomas. Usually, malignancies of the eye are diagnosed and staged when they are millimeters in size rather than centimeters (Table 55.5A). Most often, T1 to T3 in all sites are measured in millimeters, not centimeters, for tumor progression. Careful mapping of tumor depth or height by width is often used. T4 lesions that invade into the orbit soft tissues tend to spread to preauricular, submandibular, and cervical nodes. The globe of the eye is immunologically privileged and without a lymphatic system. N1 is noted, but does not affect stage grouping. M1 is noted, but does not affect or modify stage IV.

The staging of different primary cancers depends on their origin (Fig. 55.4).

A. Eyelid cancers advance by invading the conjunctiva and eye globe.

B. Uvea melanoma of iris and ciliary body invade into canal of Schlemm, cause glaucoma, and extend into choroid and sclera.

C. Retinoblastoma invades globe and optic nerve.

D. Embryonal sarcomas invade orbit and advance, invading eye globe and into the base of the skull.

Stage grouping is new in the seventh edition of AJCC and applies only to eyelid and conjunctiva (Table 55.5B) and Uvea (Table 55.5C).

TABLE 55.5A T Size Staging Criteria for the Eye

	T1	T2	T3	N
Eyelid*	<5 mm	>5–10 mm	>10 mm	
Conjunctiva	≤5 mm	>5 mm		
Conjunctival melanoma	—	≤0.8 mm	>0.8 mm	N1
Melanoma uvea*	—	<10 mm	>10–16 mm	N1
Retinoblastoma	—	≤3 mm		
Lacrimal gland	≤2.5 mm	25–50 mm	>50 mm	N1
Sarcoma orbit	<15 mm	>15 mm		N1

*Stage grouping recommended for eyelid and uveal melanomas of choroids.

TABLE 55.5B Stage Summary Matrix for Eyelid and Conjunctiva

	N0	N1	M1
T1	IA	IIIB	IV
T2a	IB	IIIB	IV
T2b	IC	IIIB	IV
T3a	II	IIIB	IV
T3b	IIIA	IIIB	IV
T4	IIIC	IIIC	IV

The T stage determines stage group.
T3 = N1

TABLE 55.5C Stage Summary Matrix for Uvea

	N0	M0	N1	M1a-c
T1a	I	I	IV	IV
T1b-d	IIA	IIA	IV	IV
T2a	IIA	IIA	IV	IV
T2b	IIB	IIB	IV	IV
T3a	IIB	IIB	IV	IV
T2c-d	IIIA	IIIA	IV	IV
T3b-c	IIIA	IIIA	IV	IV
T4a	IIIA	IIIA	IV	IV
T3d	IIIB	IIIB	IV	IV
T4b-c	IIIB	IIIB	IV	IV
T4d-e	IIIC	IIIC	IV	IV

The T stage determines stage group.

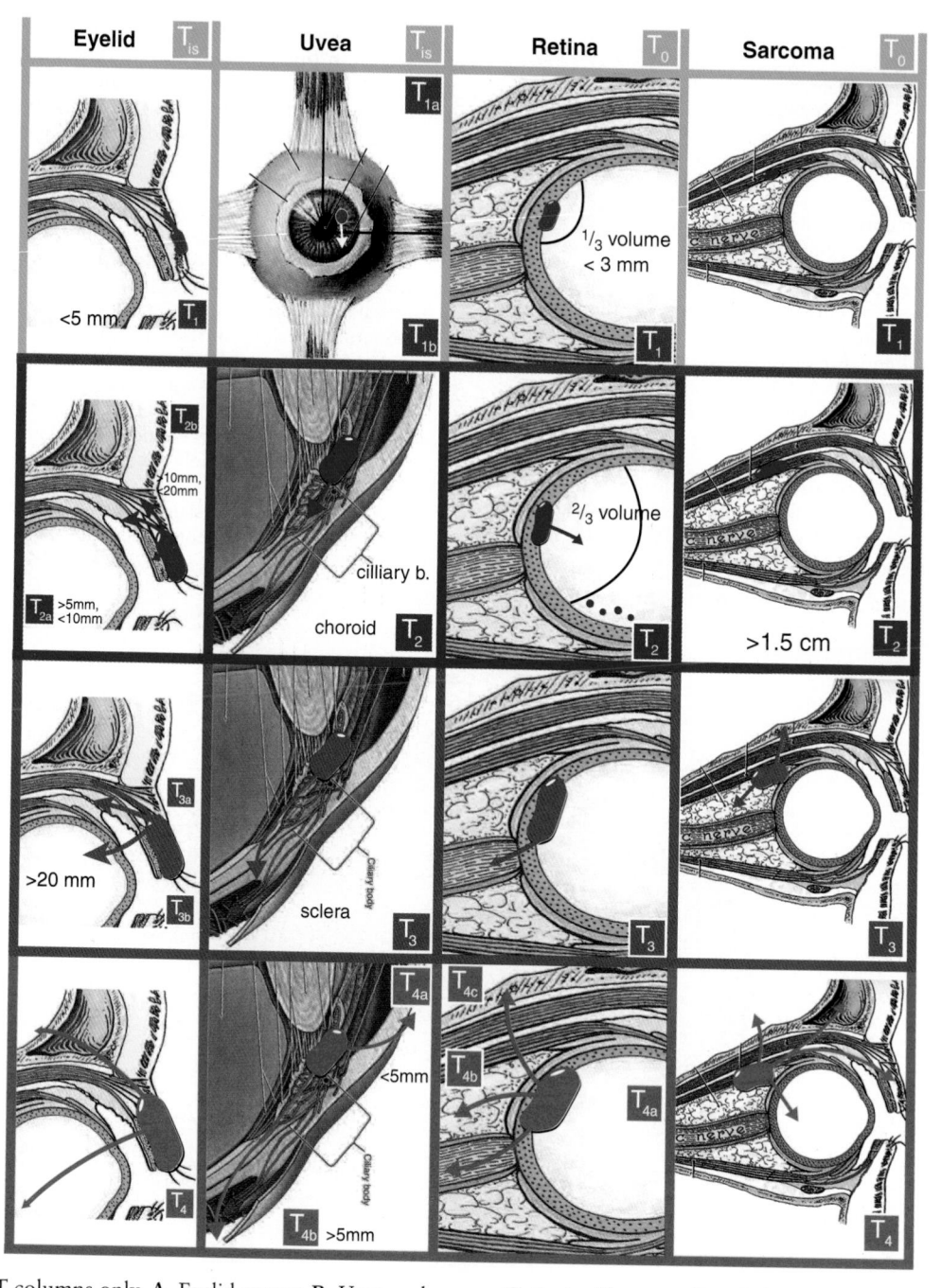

Figure 55.4 | T columns only. **A.** Eyelid cancer. **B.** Uvea melanoma. **C.** Retinoblastoma. **D.** Rhabdomyosarcoma. TNM staging criteria are color-coded bars for T advancement: Tis, yellow; T1, green; T2, blue; T3, purple; T4, red.

Orientation of Primary T-oncoanatomy

To appreciate the eye oncoanatomy, one needs to be aware of the trilogy segmentation, beginning with the globe of the eye (Fig. 55.5). A brief description of primary sites follows:

- *Globe layers* (Fig. 55.5A) are organized in three concentric coats: (i) Outer corneoscleral, (ii) middle vascular uvea/choroid, and (iii) inner photosensitive retina.

- *Chambers of the eye* (Fig. 55.5B) consist of (i) the anterior chamber, between the cornea and the iris; (ii) the posterior chamber, between the posterior surface of the iris and anterior surface and equator of the lens; and (iii) the vitreous chamber—the space between the lens and retina. The vitreous is filled with a gelatinous substance.

From anterior to posterior.

- *Eyelid of the eye* (Fig. 55.6A) consists of three layers: (i) skin with eyelashes; (ii) meibomian glands, sebaceous glands of Zeis, and apocrine glands of Moll; and (iii) tarsal muscle and conjunctiva cover.

- *Lacrimal apparatus* (Fig. 55.6B) consists of three parts, as do the tears: (i) the lacrimal gland secretions are watery;

the glands of the tarsal plate provide a waxy sebaceous secretion (meibomian) and an oily film (Zeis and Moll), which is collected by (ii) canaliculi at the inner canthus into a lacrimal sac; and (iii) a lacrimal canal that vertically descends into the nares below the inferior turbinate.

- *Uvea* (Fig. 55.6C) includes the iris, the ciliary body, and choroid.

- *Orbit* (Fig. 55.6D) contains the globe and consists of three compartments, each of which gives rise to retro-orbital tumors, that is, by adipose tissue in which the recti muscles (medial, lateral, superior, and inferior) and oblique (superior and inferior) muscles are innervated by three cranial nerves (III, IV, and VI), and surrounded by the bony orbit. The bony orbits are like inverted pyramids tipped medially, with four walls, an apex where the optic nerve enters, and the orbital opening surrounded by the eyelids that forms the base. It is approximately 4 cm at its base and 5 cm on its axis. The optic canal is less than 1 cm long. The superior and inferior orbital fissure and foramen allow for nerves, arteries, and veins to enter and exit.

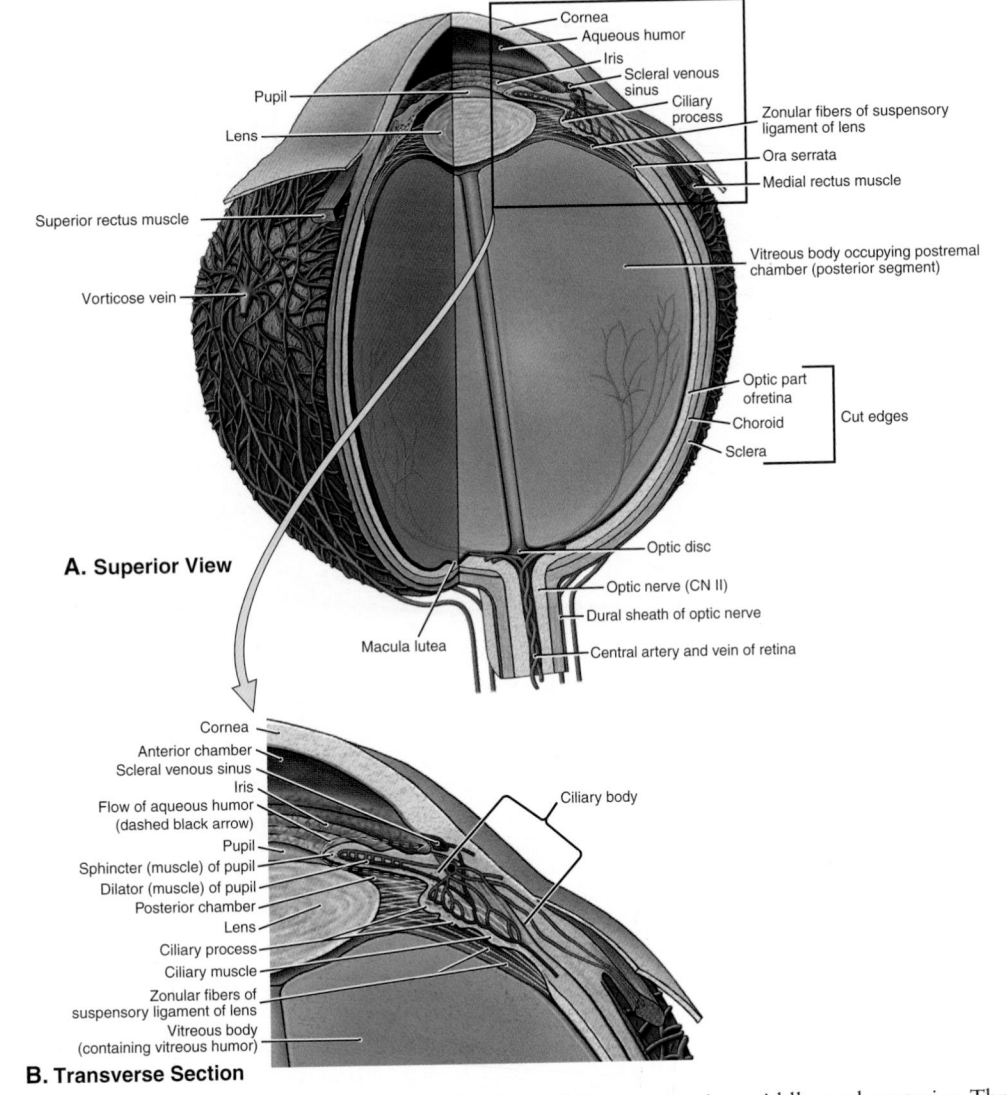

Figure 55.5 | Overview of T-oncoanatomy trilogy: Three chambers of the eye, anterior, middle, and posterior. Three layers: sclera, choroid, and retina.

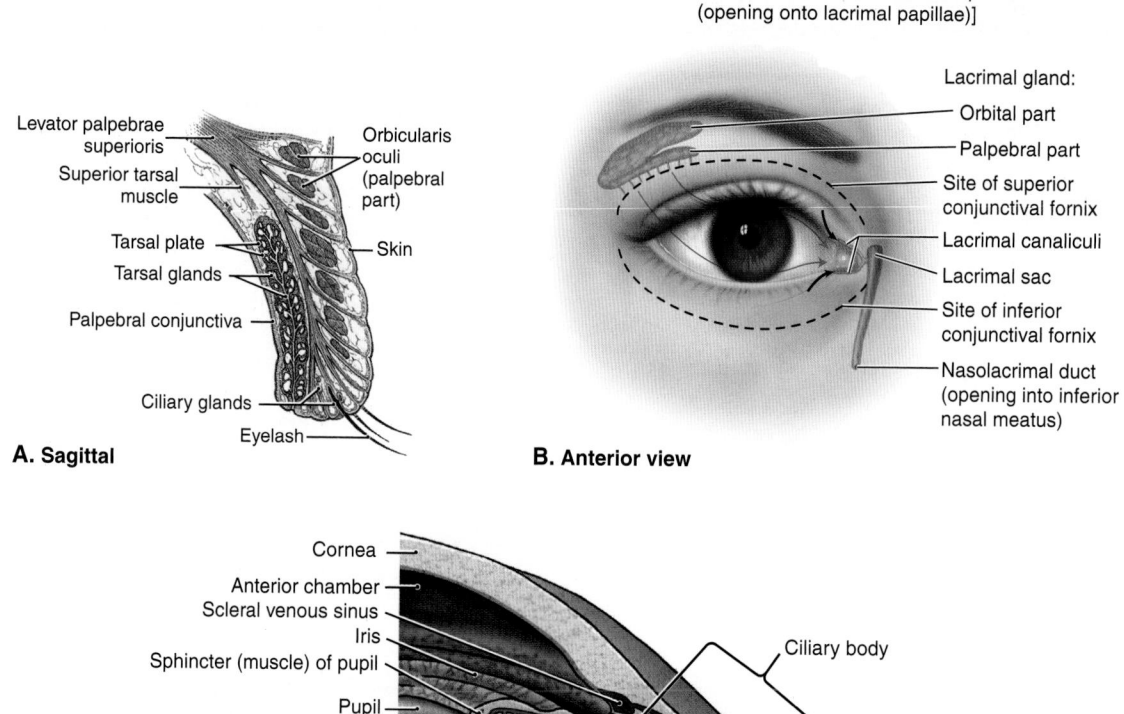

[*Black arrows* indicate lacrimal punctae (opening onto lacrimal papillae)]

A. Sagittal

Levator palpebrae superioris
Superior tarsal muscle
Tarsal plate
Tarsal glands
Palpebral conjunctiva
Ciliary glands
Eyelash
Orbicularis oculi (palpebral part)
Skin

B. Anterior view

Lacrimal gland:
Orbital part
Palpebral part
Site of superior conjunctival fornix
Lacrimal canaliculi
Lacrimal sac
Site of inferior conjunctival fornix
Nasolacrimal duct (opening into inferior nasal meatus)

Cornea
Anterior chamber
Scleral venous sinus
Iris
Sphincter (muscle) of pupil
Pupil
Dilator (muscle) of pupil
Posterior chamber
Lens
Ciliary process
Ciliary muscle
Zonular fibers of suspensory ligament of lens
Vitreous body (containing vitreous humor)
Ciliary body

C

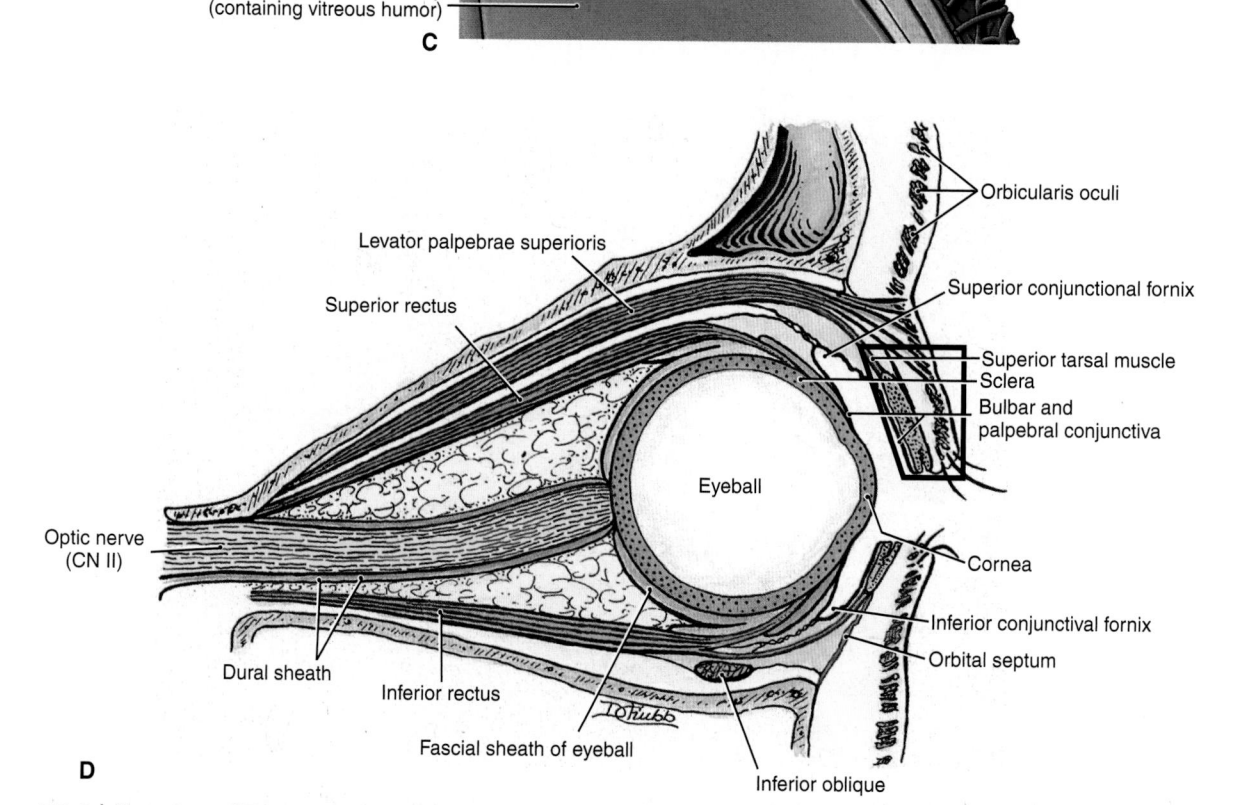

Orbicularis oculi
Levator palpebrae superioris
Superior rectus
Superior conjunctional fornix
Superior tarsal muscle
Sclera
Bulbar and palpebral conjunctiva
Eyeball
Optic nerve (CN II)
Cornea
Inferior conjunctival fornix
Orbital septum
Dural sheath
Inferior rectus
Fascial sheath of eyeball
Inferior oblique

D

Figure 55.6 | Overview of T-oncoanatomy Tripartite. A. Eyelid: skin, glands, conjunctiva. **B.** Lacrimal apparatus: gland, sac, duct. **C.** Uvea: Iris, ciliary body, choroid. **D.** Orbit: fat, extraocular muscles, optic nerve.

N-ONCOANATOMY AND M-ONCOANATOMY

N-ONCOANATOMY

The eye globe is immunologically privileged, in that it is free of lymphatics and is similar to the central nervous system. However, the eyelids and orbital contents can be involved with infiltrations of inflammatory lymphocytes, pseudolymphomas, and true lymphomas. A unique feature is the presence of direct lymphatic channels between lacrimal and parotid glands. The orbit and eyelids drain to preauricular or parotid nodes. Lesions at the inner canthus and lacrimal apparatus drain to facial and submandibular nodes (Fig. 55.7A, B; Table 55.6).

TABLE 55.6	Specific Site of Malignancy: Sentinel and Regional Lymph Nodes	
	Sentinel	**Regional**
Eyelid	Preauricular Facial node	Superficial cervical Parotid gland nodes
Conjunctiva	Preauricular Facial node	Superficial cervical Parotid gland nodes
Lacrimal gland	Preauricular Facial node	Submandibular Superficial cervical Preauricular
Sarcoma orbit	Preauricular Facial node	Superficial cervical Deep cervical
Uvea	Preauricular Facial node	Superficial cervical Parotid gland nodes
Lymphoma	Preauricular Facial node Rouvière's	Superficial cervical Parotid gland nodes Deep cervical

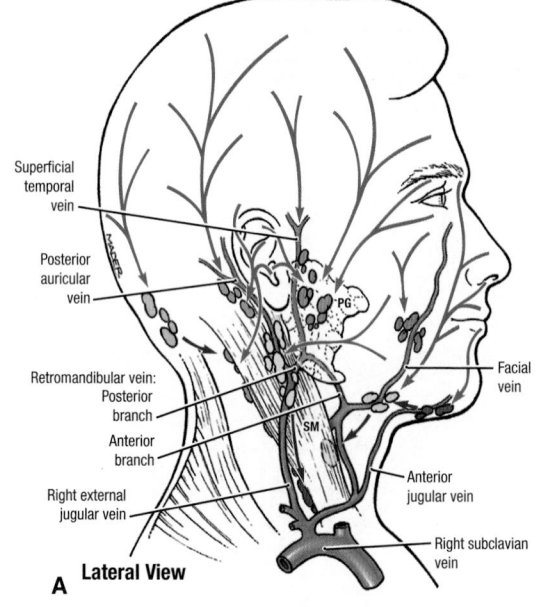

A Lateral View

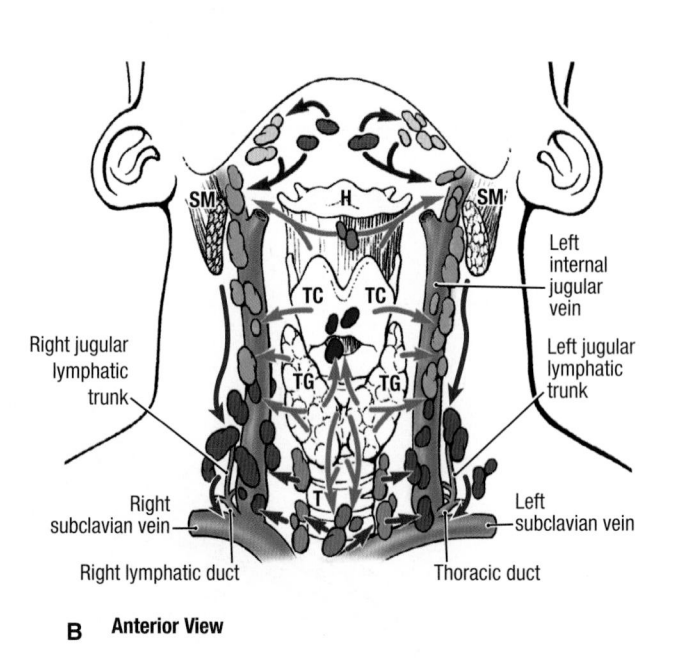

B Anterior View

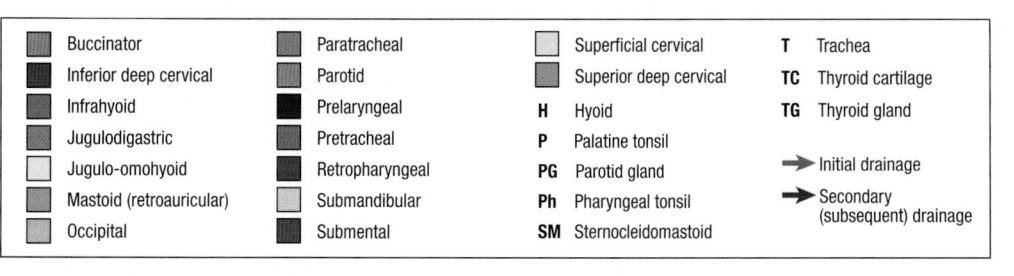

▉ Buccinator	▉ Paratracheal	▉ Superficial cervical	**T** Trachea
▉ Inferior deep cervical	▉ Parotid	▉ Superior deep cervical	**TC** Thyroid cartilage
▉ Infrahyoid	▉ Prelaryngeal	**H** Hyoid	**TG** Thyroid gland
▉ Jugulodigastric	▉ Pretracheal	**P** Palatine tonsil	
▉ Jugulo-omohyoid	▉ Retropharyngeal	**PG** Parotid gland	➡ Initial drainage
▉ Mastoid (retroauricular)	▉ Submandibular	**Ph** Pharyngeal tonsil	➡ Secondary (subsequent) drainage
▉ Occipital	▉ Submental	**SM** Sternocleidomastoid	

Figure 55.7 | N-oncoanatomy. A. Superficial drainage. **B.** Drainage of the trachea, thyroid gland, larynx, and floor of the mouth. *(continued)*

M-ONCOANATOMY

The venous supply is the pathway for metastatic spread of cancers and/or sarcomas that occur with relative frequency in the orbit and the globe of the eye in both children and adults (Fig. 55.7C, D).

- *Orbital:* Neuroblastoma metastasis in children produces proptosis and ecchymosis (Hutchinson syndrome), whereas lymphomas and pseudolymphomas are more common in adults.

- *Global:* Metastatic choroidal deposits from the common adult cancers of the lung and the eye cause scotomas.

The venous drainage of the eye and orbit are more the recipient of metastatic cancer than viaducts for dissemination. The eye is relatively avascular, except for the choroidal layer, which has a rich venous network. The optic nerve is surrounded by all of the meningeal layers of the brain; the optic disc is a direct window into the central nervous system. Once the optic nerve is invaded by malignancy, a tumor can disseminate in the central nervous system via the subarachnoid space.

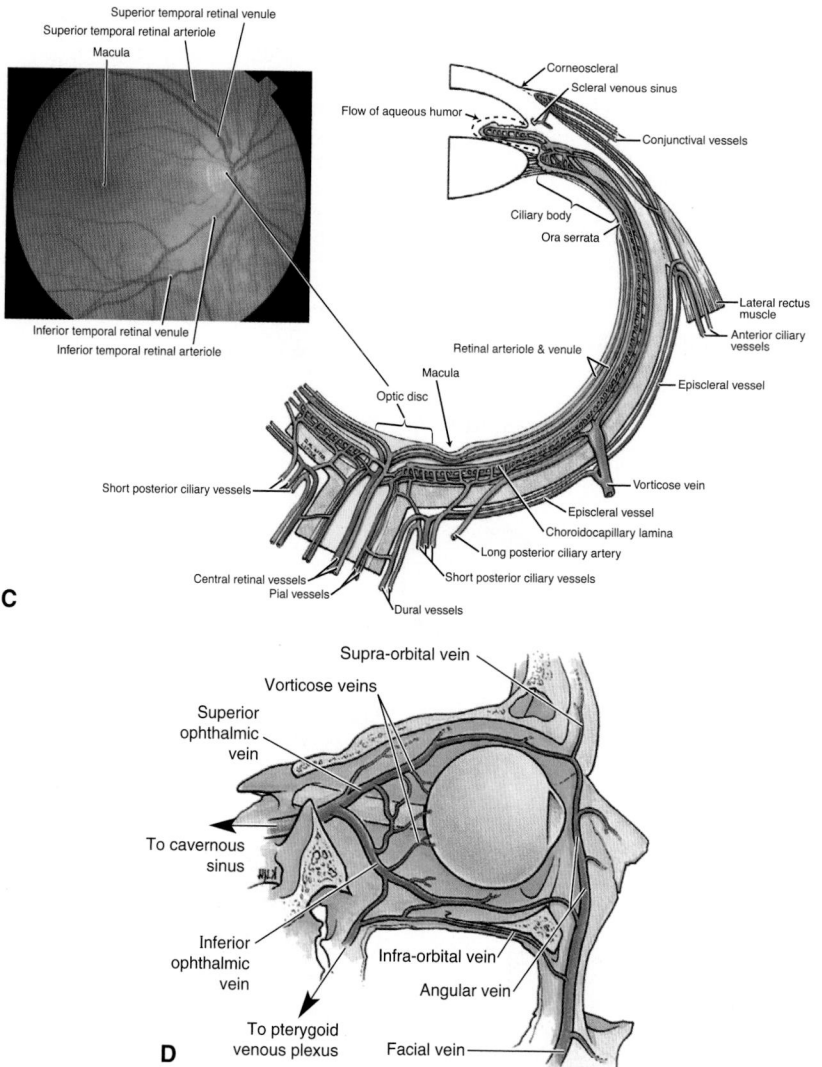

Figure 55.7 | *(Continued)* **M-oncoanatomy. C.** Right ocular fundus, ophthalmoscopic view. Retinal venules (wider) and retinal arterioles (narrower) radiate from the center of the oval optic disc, formed in relation to the entry of the optic nerve into the eyeball. The round, dark area lateral to the disc is the macula; branches of vessels extend to this area, but do not reach its center—the fovea centralis, a depressed spot that is the area of most acute vision. It is avascular but, like the rest of the outermost (cones and rods) layer of the retina, is nourished by the adjacent choriocapillaris. An increase in cerebrospinal fluid pressure slows venous return from the retina, causing edema of the retina (fluid accumulation). The edema is viewed during ophthalmoscopy as swelling of the optic disc, a condition called papilledema. **D.** Blood supply to the eyeball. The eyeball has three layers: (a) the external, fibrous layer is the sclera and cornea; (b) the middle, vascular layer is the choroid, ciliary body, and iris; and (c) the internal, neural layer or retina consists of a pigment cell layer and a neural layer. The central artery of the retina—a branch of the ophthalmic artery—is an end artery. Of the eight posterior ciliary arteries, six are short posterior ciliary arteries and supply the choroid, which in turn nourishes the outer, nonvascular layer of the retina. Two long posterior ciliary arteries, one on each side of the eyeball, run between the sclera and choroid to anastomose with the anterior ciliary arteries, which are derived from muscular branches. The choroid is drained by posterior ciliary veins, and four to five vorticose veins drain into the ophthalmic veins. The superior and inferior ophthalmic veins receive the vorticose veins from the eyeball and drain into the cavernous sinus posteriorly and the pterygoid plexus inferiorly. They communicate with the facial and supraorbital veins anteriorly.

Cranial Nerve Oncoanatomy

A diagrammatic presentation of the innovation of the eye: Cranial nerves (CN) II, III, IV, V sensory, and VI (Fig. 55.8A).

- The superior division of the oculomotor nerve (CN III) supplies the superior rectus and levator palpebrae muscles, the optic nerve CNII and optic nerve, chiasm, and tracts (Fig. 55.8B).

- The trochlear nerve (CN IV) lies on the medial side of the superior oblique muscle, and the abducent nerve (CN VI) lies on the medial side of the lateral rectus muscle.

- The lacrimal nerve runs superior to the lateral rectus muscle, supplying sensory fibers to the conjunctiva and skin of the superior eyelid; it receives a communicating branch of the zygomaticotemporal nerve carrying secretory motor fibers from the pterygopalatine ganglion to the lacrimal gland.

- The parasympathetic ciliary ganglion, placed between the lateral rectus muscle and the optic nerve (CN II), gives rise to many short ciliary nerves; the nasociliary nerve gives rise to two long ciliary nerves that anastomose with each other and the short ciliary nerves.

Superficial dissection is shown in Fig. 55.8C.

- The orbital plate of the frontal bone is removed.

- The levator palpebrae superioris muscle lies superficial to the superior rectus muscle.

- The trochlear, frontal, and lacrimal nerves lie immediately inferior to the roof of the orbital cavity.

Figure 55.8D shows deep dissection before (right side) and after (left side) section of the optic nerve (CN II).

- The eyeball occupies the anterior half of the orbital cavity.

- Nerves supplying the four recti (superior, medial, inferior, lateral) enter their ocular surfaces (the superior rectus is not shown).

- The parasympathetic ciliary ganglion lies posteriorly between the lateral rectus muscle and the sheath of the optic nerve.

- The nasociliary nerve (CN V^1) sends a branch to the ciliary ganglion and crosses the optic nerve (CN II), where it gives off two long ciliary nerves (sensory to the eyeball and cornea) and the posterior ethmoidal nerve (to the sphenoidal sinus and posterior ethmoidal cells). The nasociliary nerve then divides into the anterior ethmoidal and infratrochlear nerves.

Figure 55.8E is a cross section of the optic nerve with three meningeal surrounding layers.

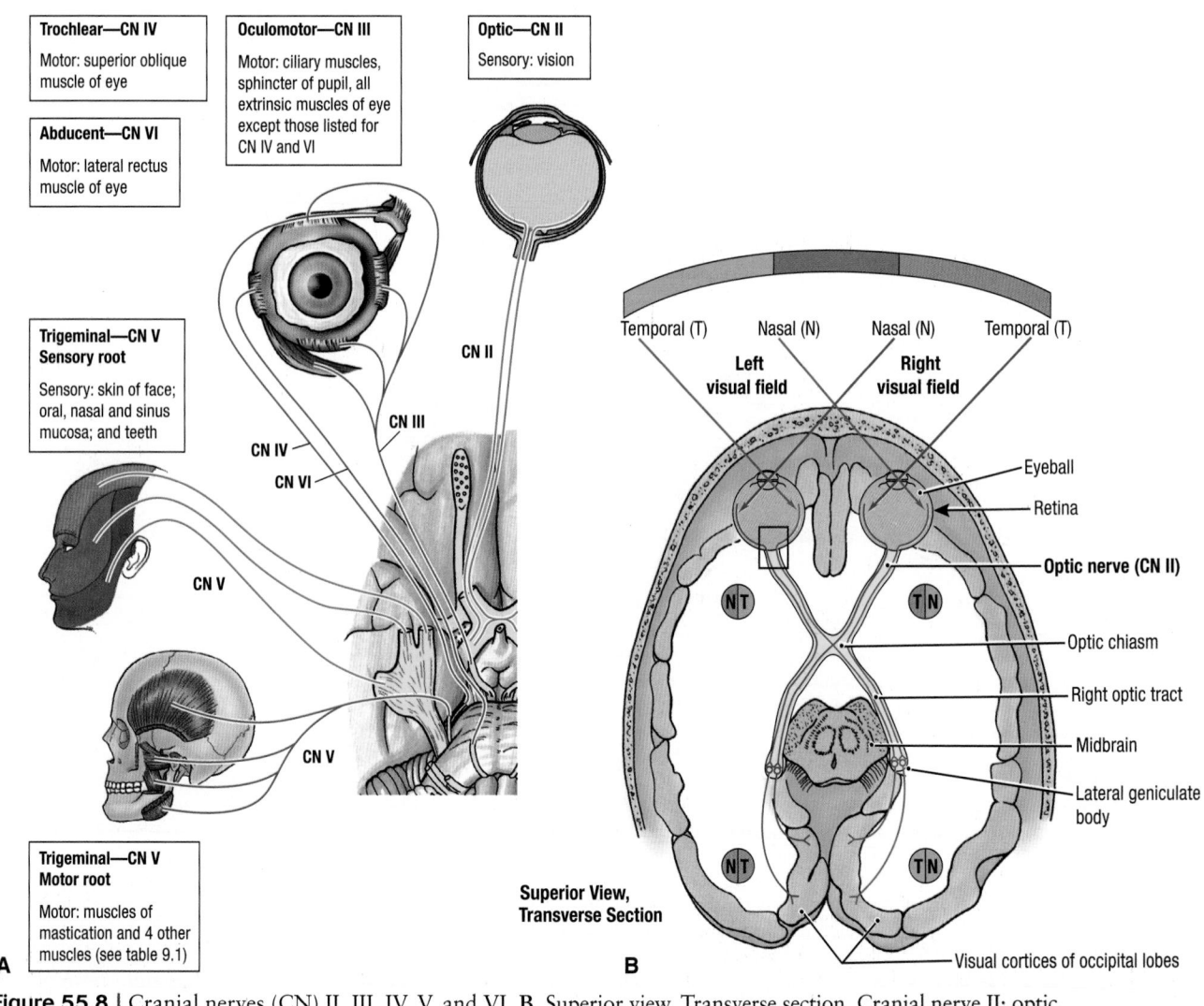

Figure 55.8 | Cranial nerves (CN) II, III, IV, V, and VI. **B.** Superior view, Transverse section, Cranial nerve II: optic.

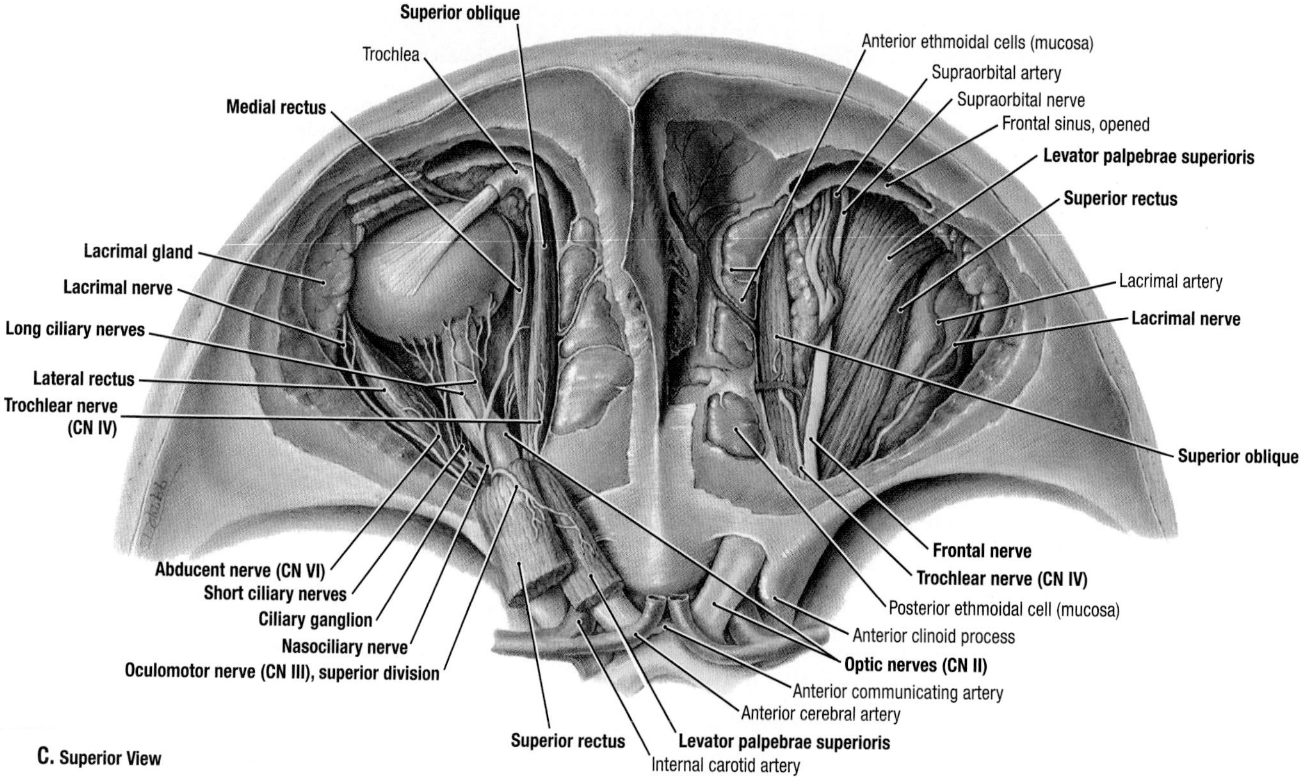

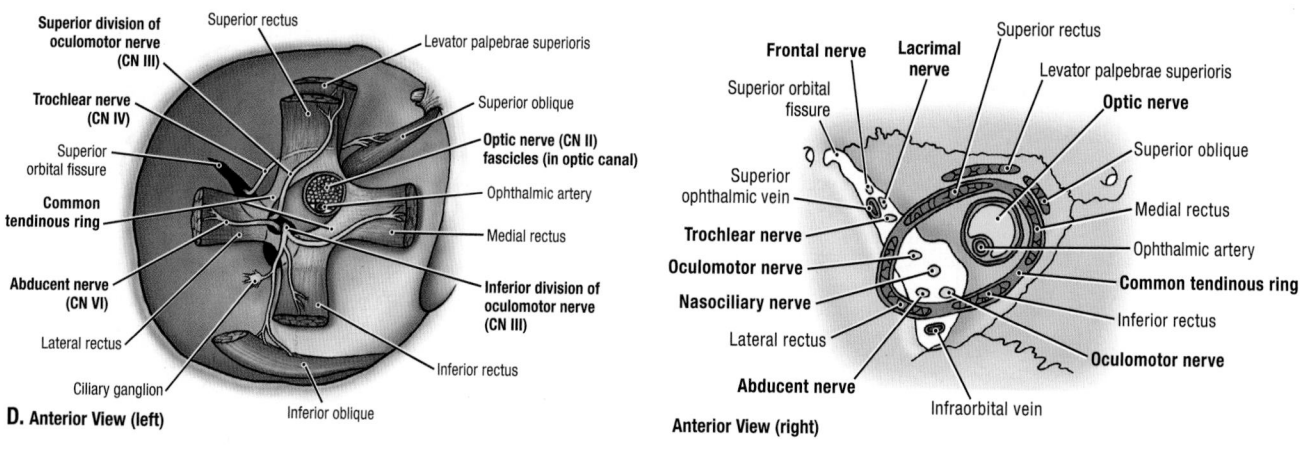

Superior oblique

Trochlea

Medial rectus

Lacrimal gland

Lacrimal nerve

Long ciliary nerves

Lateral rectus

Trochlear nerve
(CN IV)

Abducent nerve (CN VI)
Short ciliary nerves
Ciliary ganglion
Nasociliary nerve
Oculomotor nerve (CN III), superior division

Anterior ethmoidal cells (mucosa)
Supraorbital artery
Supraorbital nerve
Frontal sinus, opened
Levator palpebrae superioris
Superior rectus

Lacrimal artery
Lacrimal nerve

Superior oblique

Frontal nerve
Trochlear nerve (CN IV)
Posterior ethmoidal cell (mucosa)
Anterior clinoid process
Optic nerves (CN II)
Anterior communicating artery
Anterior cerebral artery

Superior rectus   **Levator palpebrae superioris**
Internal carotid artery

C. Superior View

Superior division of oculomotor nerve (CN III)
Trochlear nerve (CN IV)
Superior orbital fissure
Common tendinous ring
Abducent nerve (CN VI)
Lateral rectus
Ciliary ganglion

Superior rectus
Levator palpebrae superioris
Superior oblique
Optic nerve (CN II) fascicles (in optic canal)
Ophthalmic artery
Medial rectus
Inferior division of oculomotor nerve (CN III)
Inferior rectus
Inferior oblique

D. Anterior View (left)

Frontal nerve   **Lacrimal nerve**
Superior orbital fissure
Superior ophthalmic vein
Trochlear nerve
Oculomotor nerve
Nasociliary nerve
Lateral rectus
Abducent nerve

Superior rectus
Levator palpebrae superioris
Optic nerve
Superior oblique
Medial rectus
Ophthalmic artery
Common tendinous ring
Inferior rectus
Oculomotor nerve
Infraorbital vein

Anterior View (right)

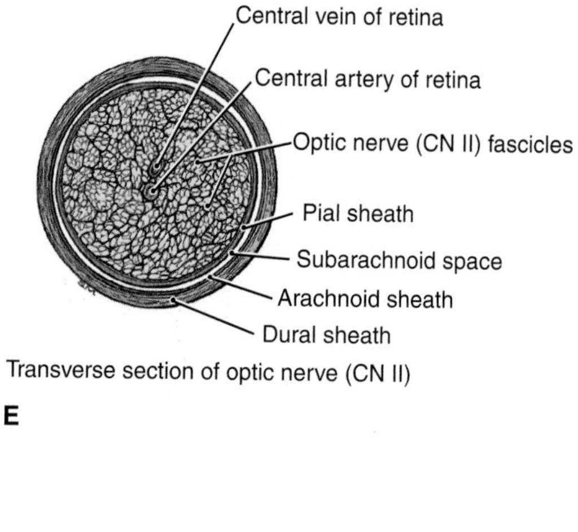

Central vein of retina
Central artery of retina
Optic nerve (CN II) fascicles
Pial sheath
Subarachnoid space
Arachnoid sheath
Dural sheath

Transverse section of optic nerve (CN II)

E

Figure 55.8C–E | C. Orbital cavity, superior view. D. Nerves of the orbit in relation to the orbital fissures and the common tendinous ring. The common tendinous ring is formed by the origin of the four recti and encircles the dural sheath of the optic nerve, CN VI, and the superior and inferior branches of CN III; the nasociliary nerve (CN V^1) also passes through this cuff. E. Optic nerve with three meningeal surrounding layers.

STAGING WORKUP

RULES FOR CLASSIFICATION AND STAGING

In general, clinical and pathologic assessment is essential to diagnosis and to staging with surgical resection or biopsy to establish the histopathology of the lesion. Imaging plays an important role in the evaluation.

Clinical Staging

The assessment of the tumor is based on physical examination, including careful inspection and palpation of eyelids and conjunctiva, followed by slit-lamp examination and direct and indirect ophthalmoscopy. Additional imaging techniques, such as ultrasonography, computed tomography (CT), MRI, fluorescein angiography, and isotopic studies may be indicated (Table 55.7). The three planar views of the eye, globe, and orbit are shown in Fig. 55.9. **A.** CT coronal, **B.** MRI sagittal, **C.** MRI transverse.

Pathologic Staging

Resection of primary site and careful assessment of tumor size, extent, and both dimensions—height or depth plus width—is important. Margins of the resected specimen are noted when wedge resection or enucleation of the globe is done. Histopathologic type and tumor grade apply to all sites; R1 is for microscopic and R2 is for macroscopic residual tumor. Venous invasion V1 microscopic and V2 macroscopic also should be noted.

TABLE 55.7	Imaging Modalities of the Eye and Orbit	
Method	**Diagnosis and Staging Capability**	**Recommended for Use**
CT	Provides excellent anatomic detail of globe, orbital content, and bony orbit; can distinguish smooth, round cysts from infiltrative tumors versus pseudotumors and detect bone destruction and sinus invasion	Yes
Primary tumor ultrasonography and fine needle aspiration biopsy	A scan and B scan can be used to screen intraocular and orbital tumors and cysts, especially melanomas	No
MRI	Provides excellent three-dimensional view, orbital fat hyperintense and vitreous hypointense in tumor (T1) and reverse in T2; can detect tumors versus pseudotumors and cysts; may be superior for diagnosis of vascular lesions, demyelinating disease	Yes
Endoscopy	Orbital endoscopy with fiber-optic lights is used in conjunction with CT and/or MRI for obtaining core biopsy	Yes, when indicated
Standard orbital view	Useful for assessing optic nerve foramen and supraorbital fissure, but supplanted by CT; can detect intraocular calcification	No
Orbital phlebography	Venography particularly useful for detecting orbital varices, but is less efficient and more invasive than CT	No
Carotid angiography	Useful in diagnosis of vascularized tumors and aneurysms, but replaced by CT, MRI	No
Fluorescein angiography	Sometimes used in diagnosis of ocular melanoma	No
Biopsy	Usually an incisional or excisional biopsy is indicated to confirm malignant versus pseudotumors; directed stereotactically by CT/MRI; contraindicated for melanomas due to high risk of seeding.	Yes, if indicated

CT, computed tomography; MRI, magnetic resonance imaging.
Used with permission from Rubin P. *Clinical Oncology.* 7th ed. Philadelphia: WB Saunders; 1993:300.

PROGNOSIS AND CANCER SURVIVAL

CANCER STATISTICS AND SURVIVAL

The eye and orbit only account for 2,090 new diagnoses, excluding carcinomas of the eyelids. Deaths attributed to ocular malignancy are less than 10% of the entire group (fewer than 200 patients per year). Some of the most elegant proton and three-dimensional conformal radiation stereotactic techniques allow for cure of choroidal melanomas and retinoblastoma with preservation of vision.

Survival results are impressive. Virtually all eye tumor patients, when properly treated, reach 90% long-term survival.

- Basal cell cancers of the eyelids are greater than 95% curable.

- Radiation isotopic plaque and enucleation were found to be comparable in treating posterior uveal/choroidal melanomas in the Collaborative Ocular Melanoma Study group, consist-

ing of 1,300 patients over 11.5 years. Recurrence rates with radiation range from about 15% to less than 5% with surgery. Cure rates range from 85% to 95%.

- Retinoblastomas are highly curable, with radiation yielding greater than 90% local tumor control, most often with vision conservation. Those patients who relapse can still be cured by enucleation.

- Optic nerve gliomas are extremely curable by stereotactic radiation therapy. The University of Pittsburgh group reports 96%, 90%, and 90% survival at 5, 10, and 15 years, respectively, with 86% retaining vision.

- Orbital and conjunctival lymphomas, when isolated, are 100% locally controlled with chemoradiation, and virtually all patients are long-term survivors.

- Embryonal rhabdomyosarcomas have the highest survivorship compared with all other sites, with up to greater than 90% long-term outcomes.

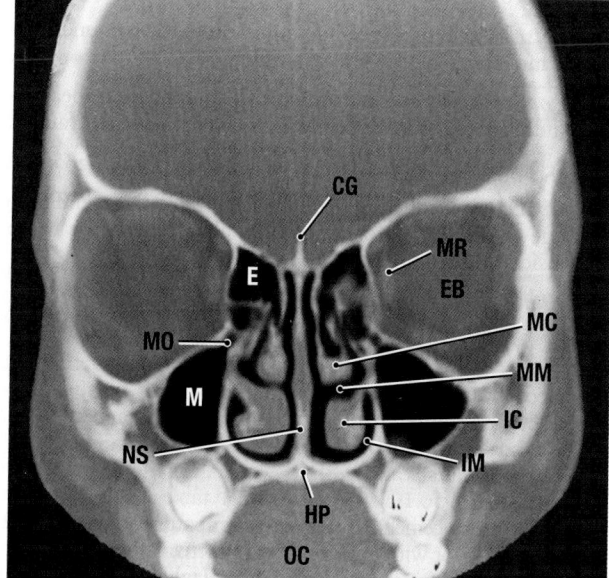

A

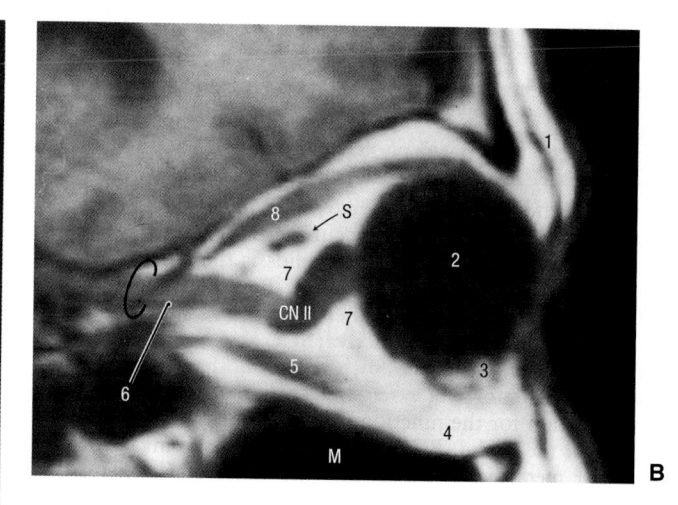

B

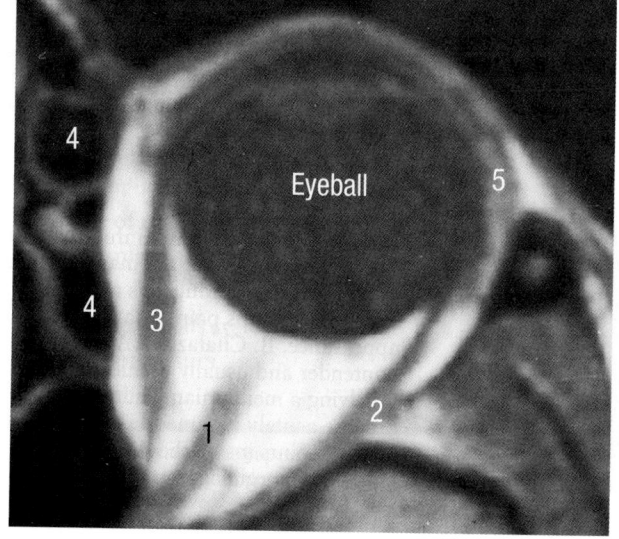

C

Figure 55.9 | Orbit, eye globe, and eyelid. **A.** Coronal view. Note the relationship of the orbit to paranasal sinuses: ethmoid, maxillary, and frontal. E. Ethmoid, CG. Crista Galli, EB. Eyeball, C. Inferior Concha, M. Maxillary Sinus, HP. Hard Palate, OC. Oral Cavity, IM. Inferior Meatus, NS. Nasal Septum, MR. Medial Rectus Muscle, MC. Air cell in middle concha, MM. Middle Meatus, MO. Opening of Maxillary Sinus. **B.** Sagittal view. Note the relationship of the eye globe and orbit to the cranial cavity and brain and the optic nerve chiasm. 1. Orbicularis oculi, 2. Eyeball, 3. Inferior Oblique Muscle, 4. Extracoronal Fat, 5. Inferior Rectus Muscle, 6. Dural and Arachnoid Sheath, 7. Retrobulbar Fat, 8. Superior Rectus Muscle, M. Maxillary Sinus. **C.** Axial transverse view. Note the relationship of the extraocular muscles in the orbit. 1. Optic Nerve, 2. The Lateral Rectus Muscle, 3. The Medial Rectus Muscle, 4. The Ethmoid Sinus, 5. Lacrimal Gland.

OVERVIEW OF HISTOGENESIS AND HISTOPATHOLOGY

Overview of Eyelid

The eyelids are essential to protect the eye from pollutions—dust and debris—with skin on the outer surface and conjunctiva the inner surface. Between these two epithelial layers is a variety of glandular adnexa—sebaceous glands (Zeis), apocrine glands (Moll), and eccrine glands (meibomian)—each of which can transform into adenocarcinomas. Accessory lacrimal gland (Krause) and lacrimal gland form an inferior border in the upper eyelid. Eyelashes are hair follicles and are of importance in cosmesis. Table 56.2A lists the various cancers. The eyelid of the eye (Fig. 56.2A) consists of three layers: (i) skin with eyelashes; (ii) meibomian glands, sebaceous glands of Zeis, and apocrine glands of Moll; and (iii) tarsal muscle and conjunctiva cover. Tears consist of three elements: (i) The lacrimal gland secretions are watery, and the glands of the tarsal plate provide (ii) a waxy sebaceous secretion (meibomian) and (iii) an oily film (Zeis and Moll).

The conjunctiva consists of stratified columnar epithelium containing numerous goblet cells whose secretion bathes the eye. Tears drain from the eye through lacrimal puncta canaliculi located at a medial angle into a lacrimal sac lined by pseudostratified epithelium, as is the nasolacrimal duct. The conjunctiva has another list of histopathologic types (Table 56.2B; Fig. 56.2B). Note that conjunctiva can occur although this is the least common site.

Embryogenesis is an indication of histogenesis. The eyelid and conjunctiva are ectodermal structures giving rise to a variety of carcinomas.

TABLE 56.2A	Eyelid Histopathologic Type

The primary eyelid carcinoma tumors include the following group and list of histologies:

- Basal cell carcinoma
- Squamous cell carcinoma
- Mucoepidermoid carcinoma
- Sebaceous carcinoma
- Primary eccrine adenocarcinoma
- Primary apocrine adenocarcinoma
- Adenoid cystic carcinoma
- Merkel cell carcinoma

From Edge SB, Byrd DR, and Compton CC, et al, AJCC Cancer Staging Manual, 7th edition. New York, Springer, 2010, p. 528.

TABLE 56.2B	Conjunctiva Histopathologic Type

The classification applies only to carcinoma of the conjunctiva.

Conjunctival intraepithelial neoplasia (CIN), including in situ squamous cell carcinoma

- Squamous cell carcinoma
- Mucoepidermoid carcinoma
- Spindle cell carcinoma
- Sebaceous gland carcinoma including pagetoid (conjunctival) spread
- Basal cell carcinoma
- Melanoma

From Edge SB, Byrd DR, and Compton CC, et al, AJCC Cancer Staging Manual, 7th edition. New York, Springer, 2010, p. 532.

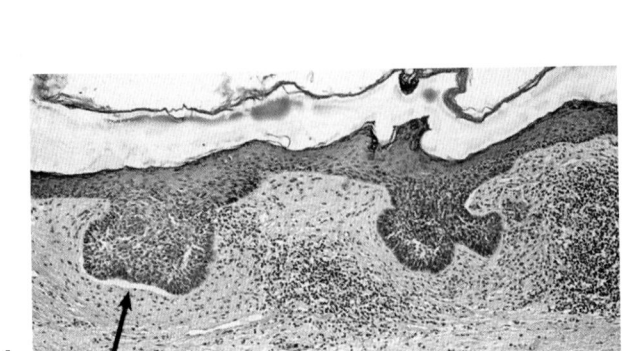
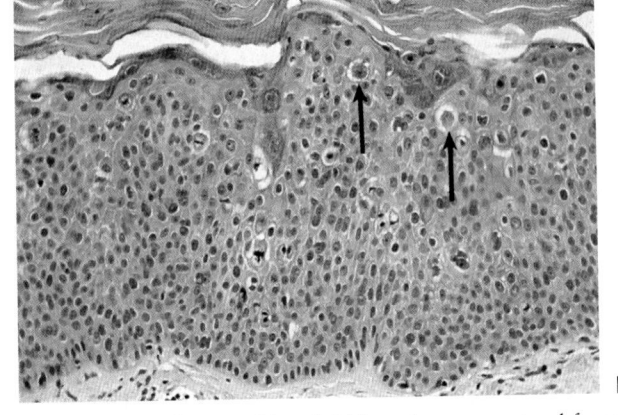

Figure 56.2 | Eyelid histopath overview. A. Basal cell carcinoma, (eyelid). Buds of atypical basaloid keratinocytes extend from the overlying epidermis into the papillary dermis. The peripheral keratinocytes mimic the stratum basalis by palisading. The separation artifact (*arrow*) is present because of poorly formed basement membrane components and the hyaluronic acid–rich stroma that contains collagenase. **B. Squamous cell carcinoma (conjunctiva).** A microscopic view of the periphery of the lesion shows squamous cell carcinoma in situ. The entire epidermis is replaced by atypical keratinocytes. Mitoses and multinucleation of keratinocytes are apparent, as is apoptosis (*straight arrows*).

EYELID BASAL CELL SQUAMOUS CELL CANCER

SUMMARY OF CHANGES SEVENTH EDITION AJCC

Carcinoma of the Eyelid

- A section on Lymph Node Staging was added (Fig. 56.3A).
- T3 was redefined, and the lesions have been divided into T3a and T3b.

- T4 has been redefined.
- N0 was redefined and divided into cN0 (no regional lymph node metastasis, based upon clinical evaluation or imaging) and pN0 (no regional lymph node metastasis, based upon lymph node biopsy).
- Stage groupings have been defined and added.

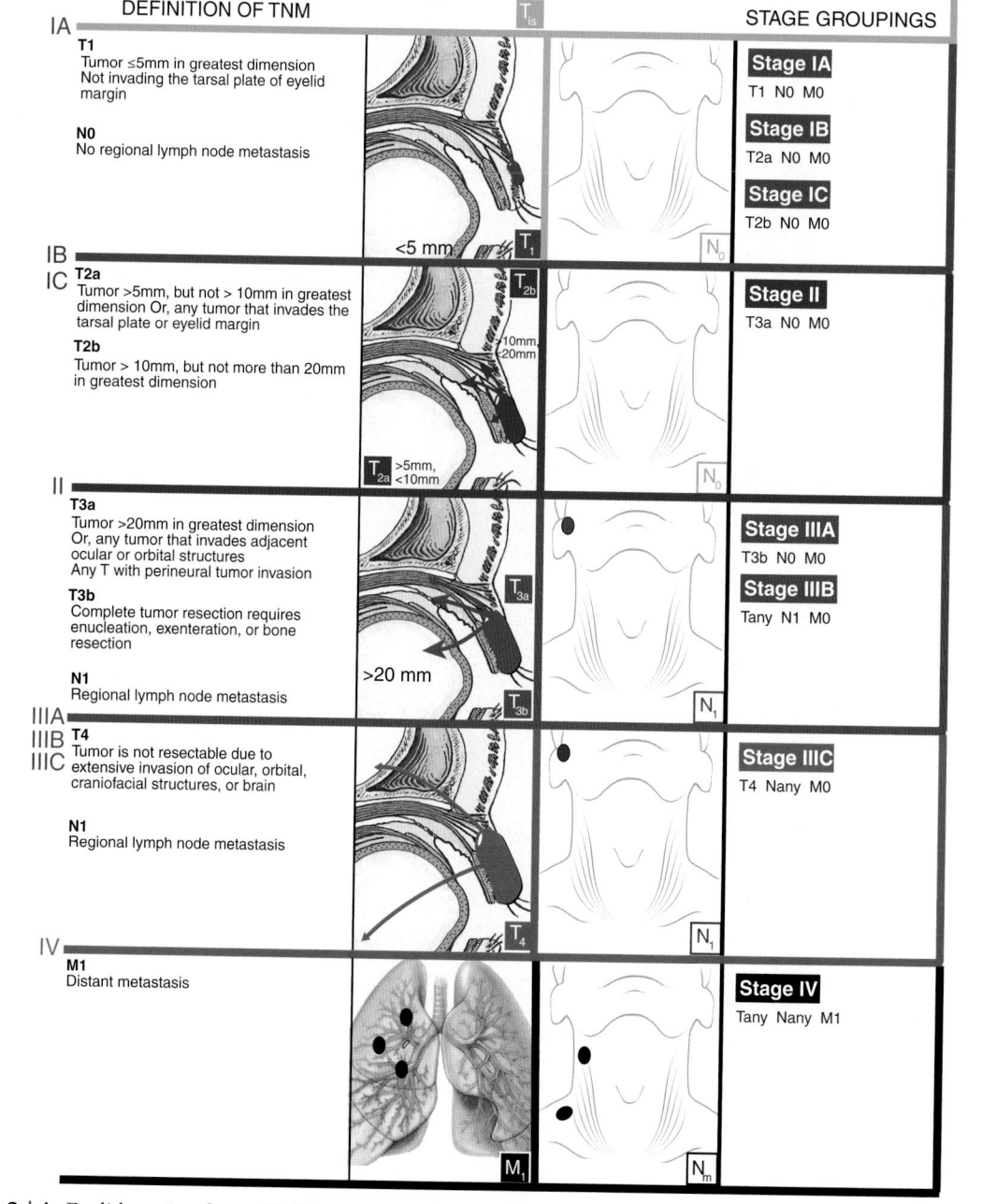

Figure 56.3 | A. Eyelid staging figure. TNM staging criteria are color coded bars for T advancement: Tis, yellow; T1, green; T2, blue; T3, purple; T4, red. *(continued)*

TNM STAGING CRITERIA

TNM STAGING CRITERIA

Because of the fineness and thin character of the layers of the eyelid, conjunctiva size is the key criterion for localized stages, measured in millimeters (Fig. 56.3B).

- Skin cancer of the eyelid: T1, <5 mm; T2, >5 to <10 mm; T3, >10 mm.
- Conjunctival carcinoma: T1, >5 mm; T2, >5 mm.

SUMMARY OF CHANGES SEVENTH EDITION AJCC

Carcinoma of Conjunctiva

- A listing of site-specific categories is included in T3.
- Sebaceous gland carcinoma with pagetoid conjunctival spread was added under histopathologic type.

The TNM staging matrix allows for identification of stage group once T and N stages are determined (Table 56.3).

CONJUNCTIVA CANCER

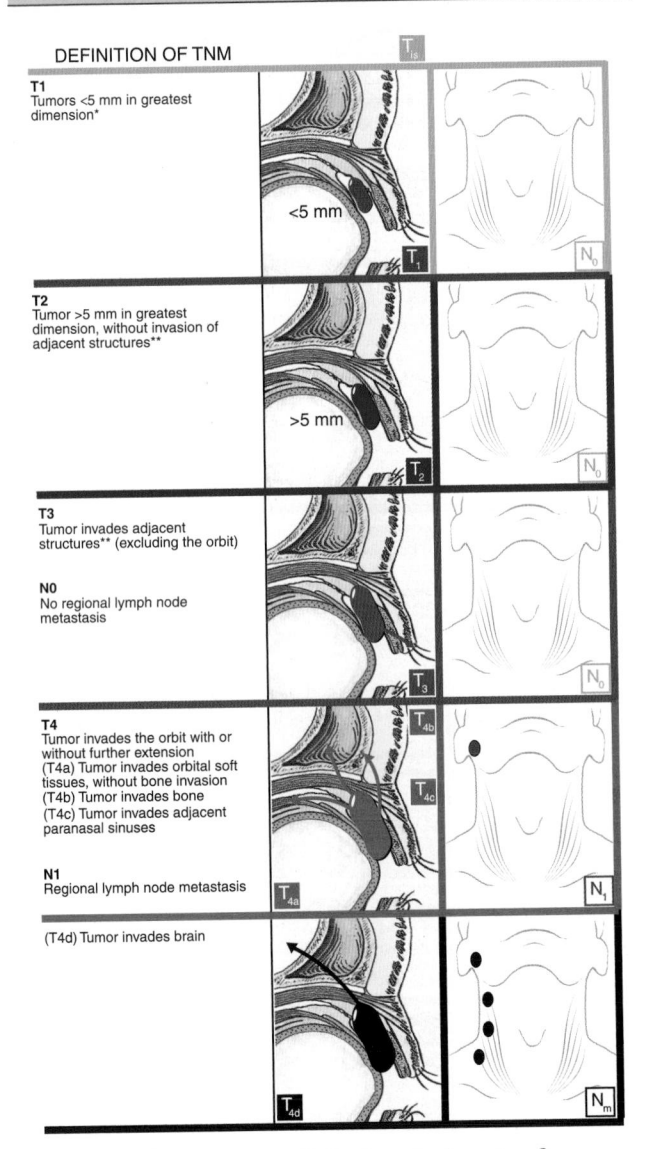

DEFINITION OF TNM

T1
Tumors <5 mm in greatest dimension*

T2
Tumor >5 mm in greatest dimension, without invasion of adjacent structures**

T3
Tumor invades adjacent structures** (excluding the orbit)

N0
No regional lymph node metastasis

T4
Tumor invades the orbit with or without further extension
(T4a) Tumor invades orbital soft tissues, without bone invasion
(T4b) Tumor invades bone
(T4c) Tumor invades adjacent paranasal sinuses

N1
Regional lymph node metastasis

(T4d) Tumor invades brain

Figure 56.3 | B. (*Continued*) Conjunctival staging figure. TNM staging criteria are color coded bars for T advancement: Tis, yellow; T1, green; T2, blue; T3, purple; T4, red. (*continued*)

TABLE 56.3 **Stage Summary Matrix for Eyelid and Conjunctiva**

	N0	N1	M1
T1	IA	IIIB	IV
T2a	IB	IIIB	IV
T2b	IC	IIIB	IV
T3a	II	IIIB	IV
T3b	IIIA	IIIB	IV
T4	IIIC	IIIC	IV

T stage determines stage group.

Malignant Melanoma of the Conjunctiva

- Definitions of T classification have changed to describe location (bulbar, noncaruncular, caruncular) (Fig. 56.3C).

- Definitions of N category have changed to describe whether a biopsy was performed.

- Definitions of pT status have changed to describe local invasion and tumor thickness.

- Definition of T(is) or melanoma in situ when tumor is limited to the epithelium.

- Definitions of "Histologic Grade" were changed to describe cases of synchronous PAM with atypia and conjunctival melanoma (G3 and G4).

CONJUNCTIVA MELANOMA

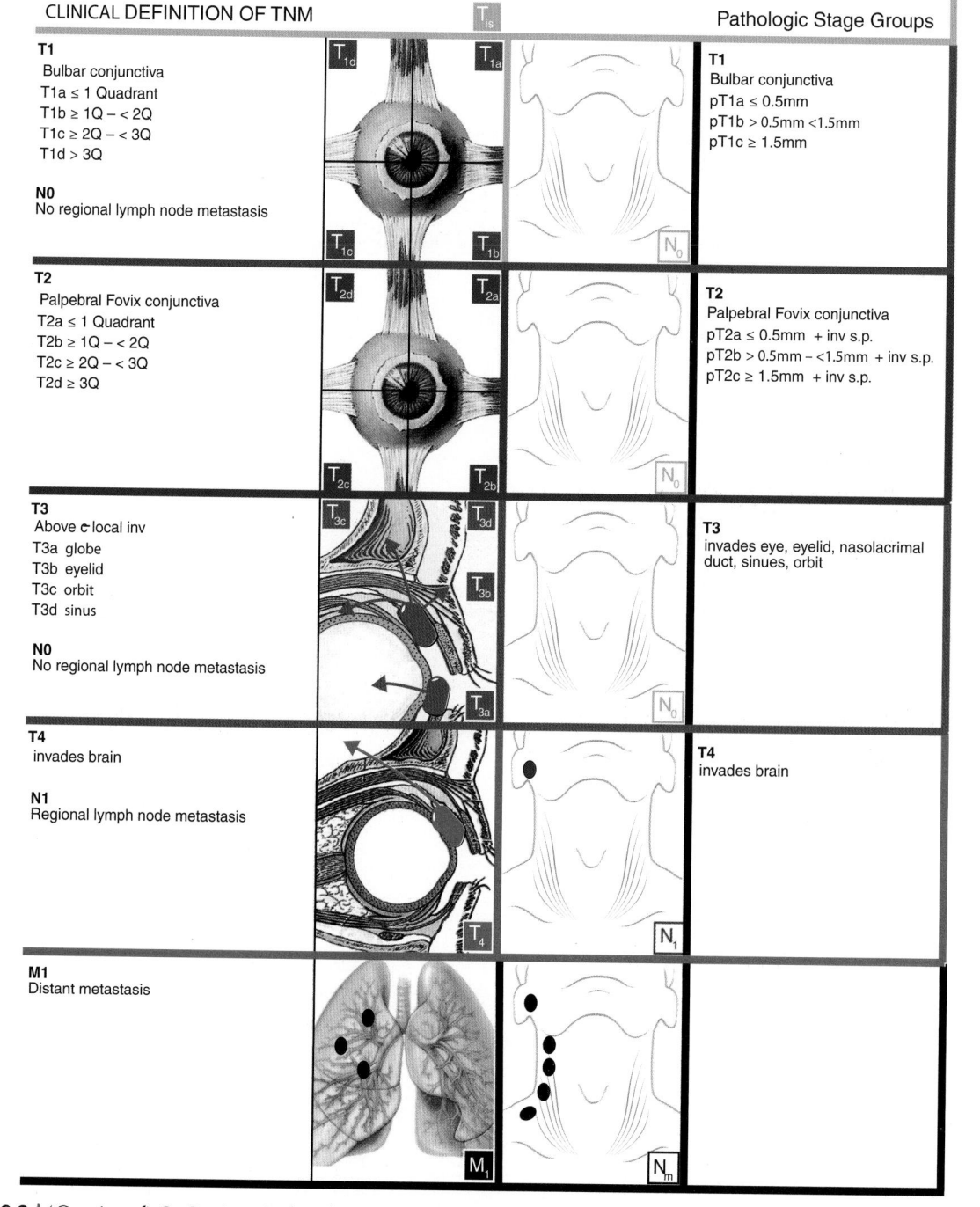

Figure 56.3 | (*Continued*) **C.** Conjunctival melanoma staging figure. TNM staging criteria are color coded bars for T advancement: Tis, yellow; T1, green; T2, blue; T3, purple; T4, red.

TNM STAGING

T-ONCOANATOMY

The eyelid is the anterior protective layer of skin and mucosa and can rapidly close when needed to avoid harm to the globe. The intricate anatomy is rarely appreciated until tumefaction occurs and benign conditions need to be distinguished from cancers. The three-planar views are most revealing if the oncoanatomy is related to specific tumors (Fig. 56.4).

- *Coronal (Fig. 56.4A):* The important features to note are at the inner canthus of the eye, where two fine lacrimal puncta and canaliculi drain into a hidden sac, which drains into the lacrimal duct and into the inferior meatus of the nose.

- *Sagittal (Fig. 56.4B):* The true complexity and the rich variety of tissues are noted as to lesion formation. The infected eyelash can give rise to a *sty* or *hordeolum* (a plugged tarsal gland to a *chalazion*), not to be confused with the variety of cancers that occur as adenocarcinomas of tarsal glands of Zeis or ciliary glands at the edge of the lids and squamous cell cancer of the conjunctiva. The magnified sagittal view provides the intricate organization of layers. Note the insertion of the levator palpebrae muscle in the upper lid. The conjunctiva covers the globe and lid, meeting at the fornix.

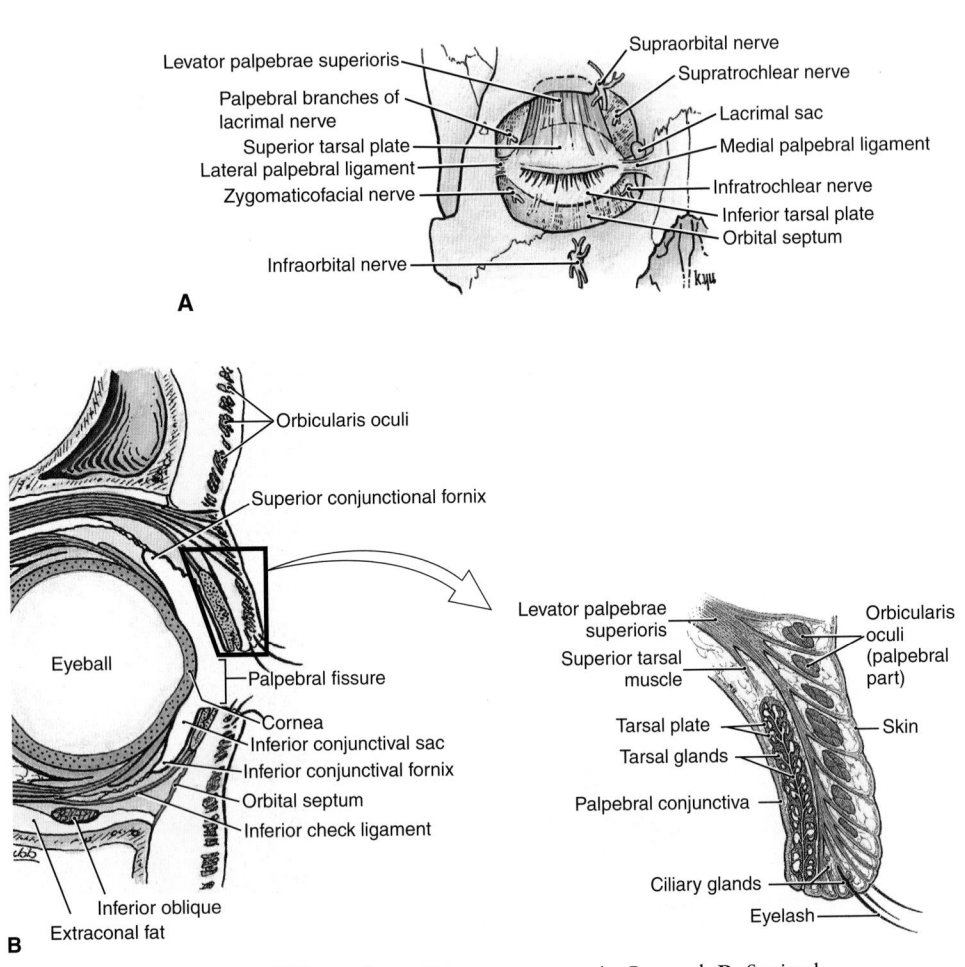

Figure 56.4 | Three-planar T-oncoanatomy. A. Coronal. **B.** Sagittal.

N-ONCOANATOMY AND M-ONCOANATOMY

N-ONCOANATOMY

The eyelids and conjunctiva drain predominantly into the preauricular nodes except for its medial margin, which follows medial lymphatics into the submandibular nodes (Figs. 56.5A, 56.5B; Table 56.4).

M-ONCOANATOMY

The pterygoid plexus of veins drains the fine veins of the eyelids into the internal jugular vein (Fig. 56.5C). Pulmonary metastases are the most common site of dissemination.

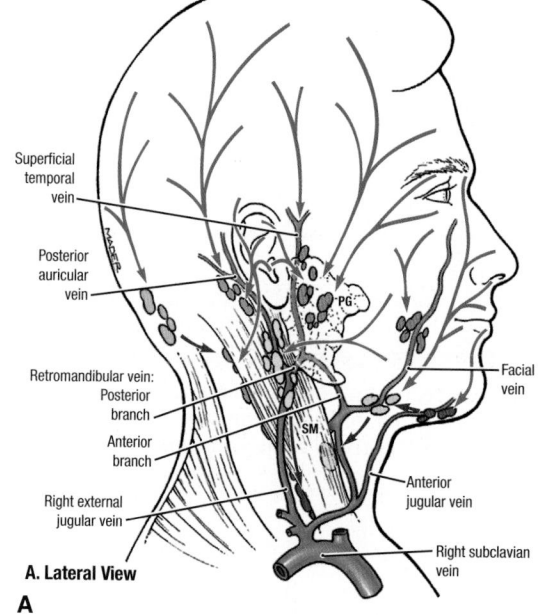

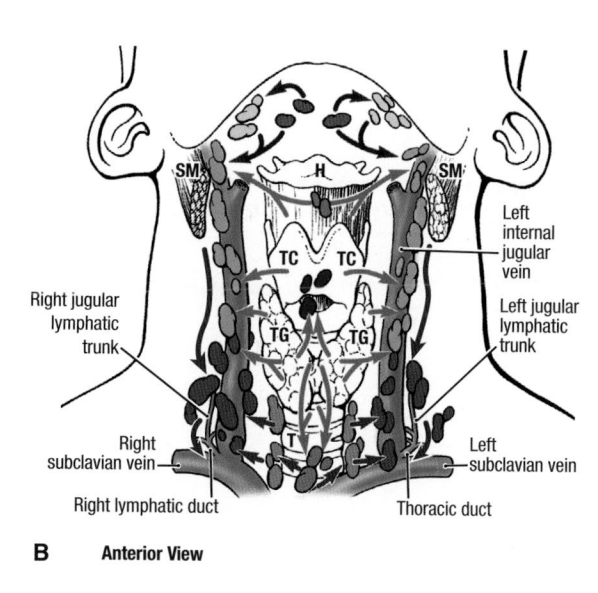

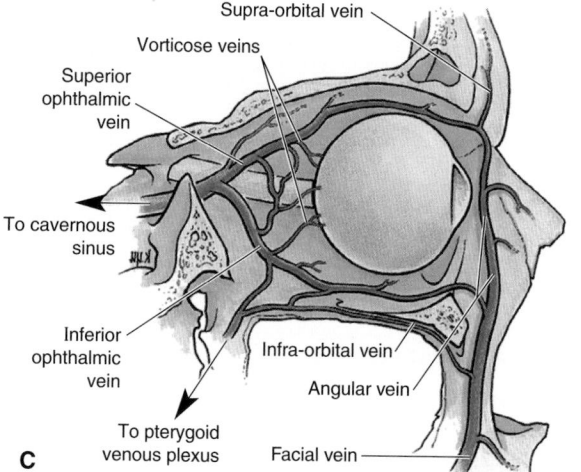

Figure 56.5 | A,B. N-oncoanatomy. Lateral view. The sentinel node is the preauricular node. **C. M-oncoanatomy of the eye.** Venous drainage of the eyelid. Retinal arteries and veins.

TABLE 56.4	Eyelid-Lymph Node Drainage	
	Sentinel	Regional
Eyelid	Preauricular Facial node	Superficial cervical Parotid gland nodes
Conjunctiva	Preauricular Facial node	Superficial cervical Parotid gland nodes

STAGING WORKUP

RULES FOR CLASSIFICATION AND STAGING

Clinical Staging

Clinical staging begins with histopathologic identification of cancer type and grade and then involves careful inspection, palpation, and slit-lamp biomicroscopy. The entire conjunctival surface needs viewing with upper-lid eversion. If the cancer is deeply invading T3, T4, imaging procedures are highly recommended to determine anatomic extent. Conjunctival melanoma needs to be distinguished from acquired melanosis, junctional and compound nevi, and melanoma in situ (Table 56.5; Fig. 55.6).

Pathologic Staging

Pathologic staging is appropriate for total excision of cancers and exenterations. Deeply invading malignancies require notation of margins of conjunctiva and, if globe is included, optic nerves. Depth of lesions suspected as melanomas need to be perpendicular to the skin. Sentinel node biopsy is encouraged using 99m-technicium.

For lacrimal gland cancer resections, the complete specimen should be studied for margins. Perineural and sentinel preauricular/parotid node evaluation needs to be recorded if positive.

TABLE 56.5	Imaging Modalities: Eye and Orbit	
Method	**Diagnosis and Staging Capability**	**Recommended for Use**
CT	Provides excellent anatomic detail of globe, orbital content, and bony orbit; can distinguish smooth, round cysts from infiltrative tumors versus pseudotumors and detect bone destruction and sinus invasion	Yes
Primary tumor ultrasonography and fine-needle aspiration biopsy	A scan and B scan can be used to screen intraocular and orbital tumors and cysts, especially melanomas	No
MRI	Provides excellent three-dimensional view, orbital fat hyperintense and vitreous hypointense in tumor (T1) and reverse in T2; can detect tumors versus pseudotumors and cysts; may be superior for diagnosis of vascular lesions, demyelinating disease	Yes
Endoscopy	Orbital endoscopy with fiber-optic lights is used in conjunction with CT and/or MRI for obtaining core biopsy	Yes, when indicated
Standard orbital view	Useful for assessing optic nerve foramen and supraorbital fissure, but supplanted by CT; can detect intraocular calcification	No
Orbital phlebography	Venography is particularly useful for detecting orbital varices but is less efficient and more invasive than CT	No
Carotid angiography	Useful in diagnosis of vascularized tumors and aneurysms, but replaced by CT/MRI	No
Fluorescein angiography	Sometimes used in diagnosis of ocular melanoma	No
Biopsy	Usually an incisional or excisional biopsy is indicated to confirm malignant versus pseudotumors; directed stereotactically by CT/MRI; contraindicated for melanomas owing to high risk of seeding	Yes, if indicated

CT, computed tomography; MRI, magnetic resonance imaging.
Used with permission from Rubin P. *Clinical Oncology*. 7th ed. Philadelphia: WB Saunders; 1993:300.

PROGNOSIS AND CANCER SURVIVAL

PROGNOSTIC FACTORS

See Table 56.6.

TABLE 56.6 | Prognostic Factors

*Eyelid**

Clinically significant:

Sentinel lymph node biopsy (SLNB) results

Regional nodes identified on clinical or radiographic examination

Perineural invasion

Tumor necrosis

Pagetoid spread

More than 3 Mohs micrographic surgical layers required

Immunosuppression—patient has HIV disease

Immunosuppression—history of solid-organ transplant or leukemia

Prior radiation to the tumor field

Excluding skin cancer, patient has history of two or more carcinomas

Patient has Muir–Torre syndrome

Patient has xeroderma pigmentosa

Required for staging:

Tumor thickness (in mm)

Clark's level

Presence/absence of perineural invasion

Primary site location on ear or hair-bearing lip

Histologic grade

Size of largest lymph node metastasis

Conjunctiva

Clinically Significant:

Ki-67 growth fraction

AIDS

Immunosuppression

Neurodermatitis

Ultraviolet radiation excess

Papilloma virus 16/18

*For eyelid cutaneous squamous cell carcinoma only.
Edge SB, Byrd DR, Compton CC, et al., *AJCC Cancer Staging Manual, 7th edition.* New York, Springer, 2010, p. 528.

CANCER STATISTICS AND SURVIVAL

The eye and orbit only account for 2,750 new diagnoses, excluding carcinomas of the eyelids. Deaths attributed to ocular malignancy are less than 10% of the entire group (240). Some of the most elegant proton and three-dimensional conformal radiation stereotactic techniques allow for the cure of choroidal melanomas and retinoblastoma with preservation of vision.

Survival remains impressive; 90% survive long term. Most skin cancers about the eyelids are detected early and are readily controlled by excision and/or radiation. Only recurrent cancers that deeply invade can lead to deformity, loss of eye, and death.

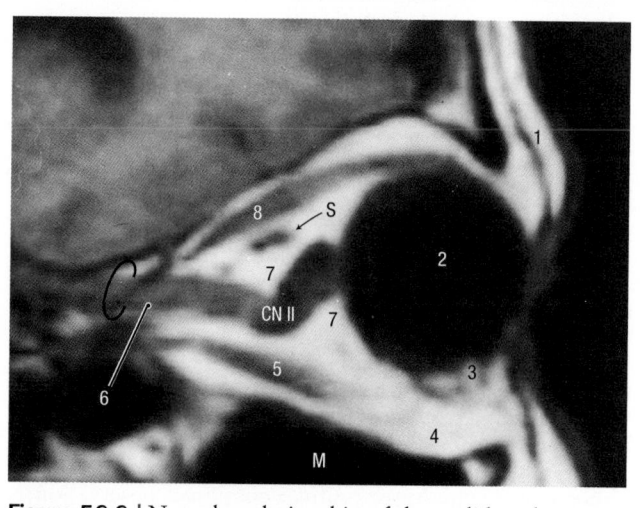

Figure 56.6 | Note the relationship of the eyelid to the eye globe and skull base. Correlates with Fig. 56.4B Sagittal View T-oncoanatomy. 1. Orbicularis oculi, 2. Eyeball, 3. Inferior Oblique Muscle, 4. Extracoronal Fat, 5. Interior Rectus Muscle, 6. Dural and Arachnoid Sheath, 7. Retrobulbar Fat, 8. Superior Rectus Muscle, M. Maxillary Sinus.

57

Uvea (Malignant Melanoma)

PERSPECTIVE, PATTERNS OF SPREAD, AND PATHOLOGY

The uveal layer consists of three parts: the iris, ciliary body, and choroid.

PERSPECTIVE AND PATTERNS OF SPREAD

A nevus of the uveal tract may occur in the iris, ciliary body, or choroids (Fig. 57.1; Table 57.1). It can be recognized by its clinical appearance and course. The principal concern about a nevus of the eye is that it must be distinguished from a melanoma. This usually is possible because of its unchanging size, the absence of much elevation, and the fact that it interferes little with the function of the overlying retina when it occurs in the choroidal layer. However, differentiation of a large nevus from a small, dormant melanoma can be virtually impossible. In this case, routine, continued observation is mandatory. Hemangiomas of the uveal tract can be more troublesome and can show some signs of growth over a period of many years. It is usually possible to identify these tumors by the use of intravenous fluorescein combined with examination of the fundus with cobalt blue light. Under these circumstances, hemangiomas fluoresce brightly.

Intraocular malignant melanoma is estimated to occur in about 0.05% of the eye-patient population. It is a tumor of adults; the average age is 50 years. It is rare in blacks.

Intraocular melanoma is the most common primary intraocular malignancy in countries with mainly white populations. Metastatic disease is the most common intraocular malignancy. There is no difference in distribution between the genders, nor is there any significant genetic relationship, except for the tumor's predilection for whites. It is rarely associated with other melanomas, such as those of the skin. Conversely, cutaneous malignant melanomas do not commonly metastasize to the eye.

The derivation of melanomas of the uvea has been the subject of a great deal of study and theory. It is possible that the stromal melanocytes of the uvea are the precursors of malignant melanoma. The pigmented epithelium of the retina (or of other neural crest–derived cells) is also implicated by some observers. Another hypothesis is that most melanomas arise in preexisting nevi.

Typical presentation depends on ophthalmoscopic examination. However, the term "intraocular melanoma" may refer to a tumor appearing in any part of the uveal tract; this may include the iris, in which case the tumor may be visible on direct inspection. Iris melanomas may be diffuse rather than discrete nodules, presenting as heterochromia, or darkening of the iris. Acquired heterochromia in the presence of elevated intraocular pressure is particularly suspicious.

When it occurs in the choroid, the tumor most characteristically appears in an equatorial position within the eye. It is possible for the tumor to reach a relatively large size before it produces symptoms, such as loss of side vision or a sensation

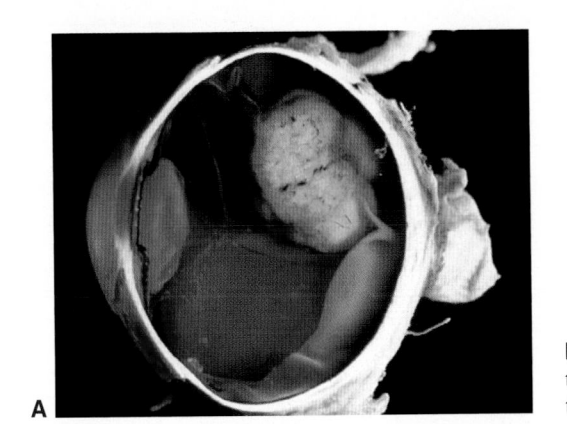

A

Figure 57.1 | Malignant Melanoma. A. A mushroom-shaped melanoma of the choroid is present in this eye. Choroidal melanomas commonly invade through Bruch's membrane and result in this appearance. *(continued)*

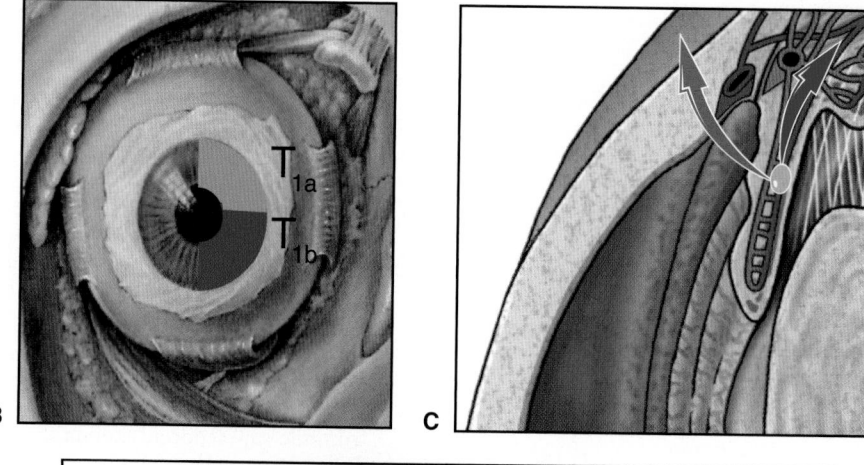

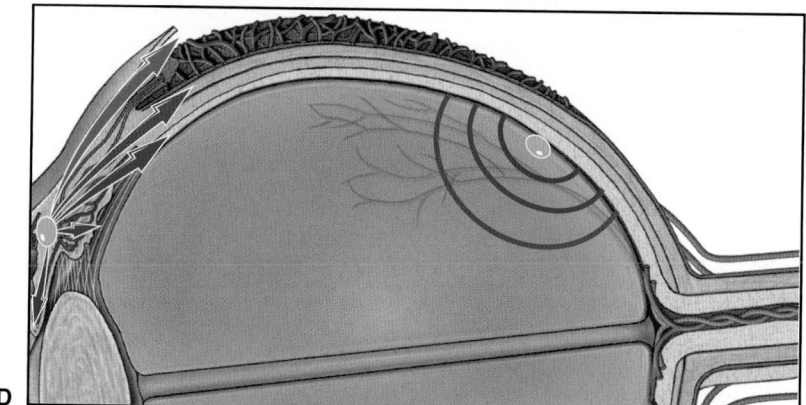

Figure 57.1 | *(Continued)* **Patterns of spread.** Primary melanomas of the uvea include iris and choroid. Cancers are color coded for progression: Tis, yellow; T1, green; T2, blue; T3, purple; T4, red. **B.** Iris. **C.** Ciliary body. **D.** Choroid. The concept of visualizing patterns of spread to appreciate the surrounding anatomy is well demonstrated by the six-directional pattern (SIMLAP; Table 57.1).

of floating spots. Therefore, the investigation of minor visual symptoms may be important. Tumor growth produces deterioration of vision as the retina overlying the tumor loses its function. The tumor frequently produces secondary changes within the eye, such as the induction of cataract, secondary glaucoma, iridocyclitis, and retinal detachment.

Primary acquired melanosis can be particularly difficult to manage because of its widespread involvement of the conjunctiva and eyelids. Because histopathologic examination of the involved tissue can differentiate melanosis from melanomas of low malignant potential, repeat biopsy of suspicious areas is indicated.

TABLE 57.1	SIMLAP (Primary in the Iris)	
Uvea Melanoma		
S	Ciliary body	• T2
	Choroid	• T2
I	Ciliary body	• T2
	Choroid	• T2
M	Iris <3 o'clock	• T1a
	Iris >3 o'clock	• T1b
L		
A	Scleral external	• T3
	Canal of Schlemm	• T3
P	Extraocular	• T4

Choroid melanoma is size related.
The six vectors of invasion are <u>S</u>uperior, <u>I</u>nferior, <u>M</u>edial, <u>L</u>ateral, <u>A</u>nterior, and <u>P</u>osterior. The color-coded dots correlate the T stage with the specific anatomic structure involved.

HISTOGENESIS AND HISTOPATHOLOGY

Melanocyte loci determine melanoma sites. Histopathology has relied on Callender's classification (Table 57.2, Fig. 57.2): Small, spindle-shaped cells with small condensed nuclei, referred to as spindle A, are the most benign. The 5-year mortality rate is less than 5%. Spindle melanoma type B is characterized by larger, more loosely packed spindle cells with prominent nucleoli. It is also relatively benign and has a 14% 5-year mortality rate. The pure epithelioid cell type occurs least commonly. This type is large and polygonal and has round nuclei and prominent cytoplasm and resembles epithelial tumors. The mortality rate is 69%. Half of the melanomas of the eye have a mixture of cell types. The dangerous epithelioid cell types exhibit a 51% 5-year mortality rate.

Necrosis is rare in melanomas and occurs in only 7% of tumors. When it occurs, it may create severe inflammatory signs and secondary glaucoma. Pigmentation of the tumor varies from intense to amelanotic. The degree of pigmentation correlates only slightly with the degree of malignancy. Reticulin fibers are frequent and heavy in some tumors and light in others. Reticulin content is only slightly correlated with prognosis. Newer prognostic parameters include number of mitotic figures per high-power field and inverse standard deviation of tumor cell nucleolar area.

- *Conjunctiva*: It is important to differentiate melanosis from melanoma of low grade potential (Fig. 57.2B).

- The *iris* has melanocytes and fibroblasts in loose connective tissue resting on pupil dilator muscle, then myoepithelial cells and a layer of epithelial cells. The color of the iris depends on the number of stromal melanocytes scattered in the connective tissue (Fig. 57.2B).

- The *ciliary body epithelium* consists of two layers—the outer pigmental layer with its melanocytes, and the inner nonpigment epithelium. The ciliary body contains the ciliary muscle and vascular connective tissue, with the ciliary epithelium producing the aqueous humor. The scleral venous sinus (canal of Schlemm) in close proximity to the iridocorneal angle drains the aqueous humor and regulates intraocular pressure. If it is invaded by the melanoma, glaucoma occurs (Fig. 57.2B).

- The *choroid layer* is between the retina and sclera and is the dominant vascular coat of the eye. It is a dark brown layer and is traversed by lamellae strands that originate from the suprachoroid lamina (lamina fusca) and consists of flat, large melanocytes between connective tissue. *This is the largest collection of melanocytes in the eye and receives the most ultraviolet radiation.* Therefore this is the most common site in the eye to transform into malignant melanomas (Fig. 57.2C).

- *Retinal pigment epithelium* (RPE) has pigmented cells that are the bottom layer of 10 layers that constitute the retina; some postulate that these also may give rise to melanomas (Fig. 57.2C).

The embryogenesis of neural ectoderm determines the epithelium of the iris, ciliary body, and choroid.

TABLE 57.2	Histopathologic Type for Uvea

The histopathologic types are as follows:

Spindle cell melanoma (>90% spindle cells)

Mixed cell melanoma (>10% epithelioid cell and <90% spindle cells)

Epithelioid cell melanoma (>90% epithelioid cells)

Histopathologic Grade

GX: Grade cannot be assessed

G1: Spindle cell melanoma

G2: Mixed cell melanoma

G3: Epithelioid cell melanoma

(Edge SB, Byrd DR, Compton CC, et al., *AJCC Cancer Staging Manual, 7th ed.* New York: Springer, 2010, p. 552).

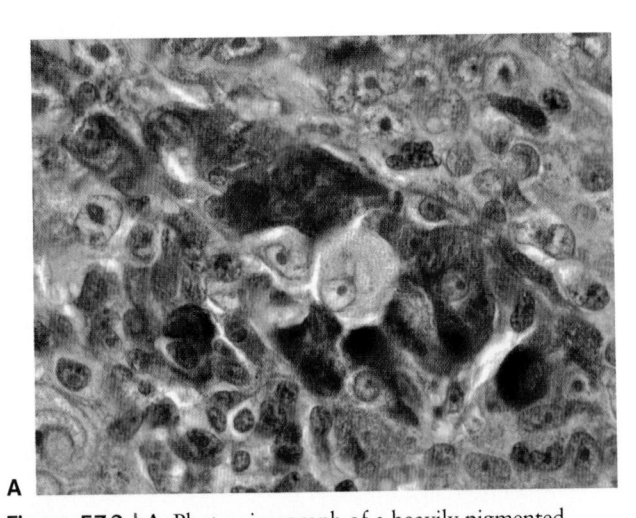

A

Figure 57.2 | A. Photomicrograph of a heavily pigmented melanoma of the choroid depicting epithelioid tumor cells with prominent nucleoli. *(continued)*

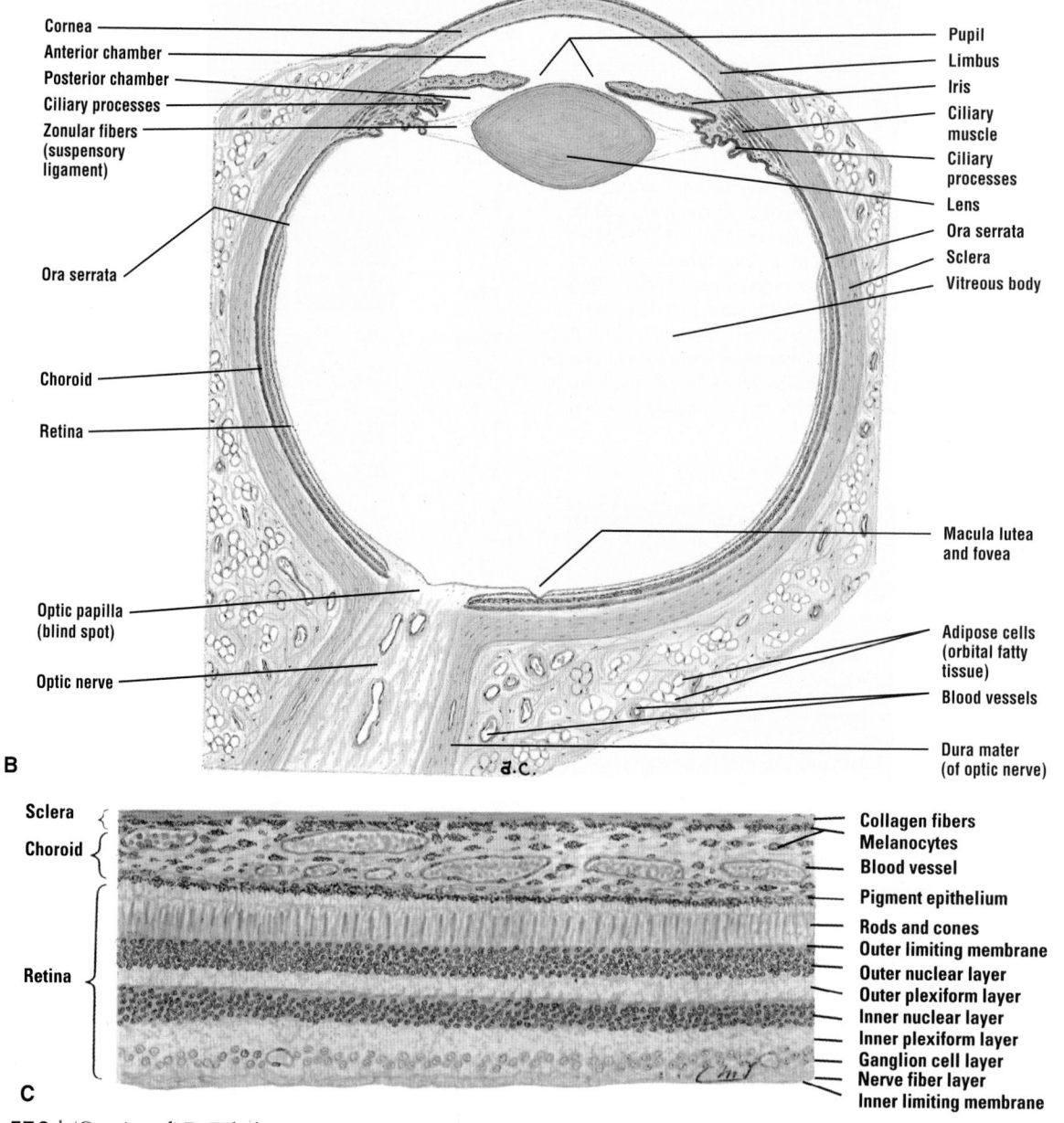

Figure 57.2 | *(Continued)* **B.** Whole eye (sagittal section). Stain: hematoxylin and eosin. Low magnification. **C.** Retina, choroid, and sclera (panoramic view). Stain: hematoxylin and eosin. Medium magnification.

TNM STAGING CRITERIA

According to Reese, the distribution of melanomas is predominantly in the choroid (78%), then the iris (12%) and the ciliary body (10%). It is for this reason that choroidal melanoma will be emphasized and illustrated first. Other loci of origin will be presented more concisely because each has special anatomic features. The most common patterns of spread are intraocular via the choroidal venous network and then through the sclera extraocularly into the orbit. Distant spread is possible because melanomas of the choroid exit via retinal veins into the internal jugular vein. Remarkably, liver is the target organ rather than lung. In fact, severe hepatomegaly due to extensive metastatic disease without an obvious gastrointestinal tract cancer should suggest a search for an intraocular choroidal melanoma. The classic professorial diagnosis of choroid melanoma is made on rounds in which a patient with palpable hepatomegaly is noted to have a glass eye.

SUMMARY OF CHANGES SEVENTH EDITION AJCC

Major changes with numerous prognostic factors and size: Thickness and diameter are important for both choroid uveal and ciliary body (Fig. 57.3). The Stage Summary Matrix for Uvea Iris, and Ciliary body is shown in Table 57.3. Uvea choroid melanomas are compared by 3 criteria: Ciliary Body (CB), Extraocular extensions (EOE), and size (Fig. 57.4A), uvea iris melanomas (Fig. 57.4B), and conjunctiva (Fig. 57.5C).

Ciliary Body and Choroid

- The definitions of T1-T4 lesions have been modified.
- The definitions of T1a-c, T2a-c, and T3a have been modified, and T1-T3 has been divided into T1a-d, T2a-d, and T3a-d.
- *T4 has been divided into T4a-e.*
- T1 through T4 are defined as tumors representing tabulated combinations of largest basal tumor diameter and tumor thickness (height).
- T1a, T2a, T3a, T4a are defined as tumors without ciliary body involvement and without extrascleral extension.
- T1b, T2b, T4b, T4b are defined as tumors with ciliary body involvement but without extrascleral extension.
- T1c, T2c, T3c, T4c are defined as tumors with ciliary body involvement but with extrascleral extension equal to or less than 5 mm.

TABLE 57.3 Stage Summary Matrix for Uvea

	N0	M0	N1	M1a-c
T1a	I	I	IV	IV
T1b-d	IIA	IIA	IV	IV
T2a	IIA	IIA	IV	IV
T2b	IIB	IIB	IV	IV
T3a	IIB	IIB	IV	IV
T2c-d	IIIA	IIIA	IV	IV
T3b-c	IIIA	IIIA	IV	IV
T4a	IIIA	IIIA	IV	IV
T3d	IIIB	IIIB	IV	IV
T4b-c	IIIB	IIIB	IV	IV
T4d-e	IIIC	IIIC	IV	IV

The T stage determines stage group.

- T1d, T2d, T3d, and T4d are defined as tumors with ciliary body involvement and with extrascleral extension equal to or less than 5 mm.
- T4e is defined as tumor of any size with an extrascleral extension greater than 5 mm in diameter.

Malignant Melanoma of Uvea-Iris

In clinical practice, the largest tumor basal diameter may be estimated in optic diameters (dd, average: 1 dd = 1.5 mm). Tumor thickness may be estimated in diopters (average: 2.5 dd = 1 mm). However techniques such as ultrasonography and fundus photography are used to provide more accurate measurements. Ciliary body involvement can be evaluated by the slit-lamp, ophthalmoscopy, gonioscopy, and transillumination. However, high frequency ultrasonography (ultrasound biomicroscopy) is used for more accurate assessment. Extension through the sclera is evaluated visually before and during surgery and with ultrasound, computed tomography or magnetic resonance imaging.

Thickness (mm)	≤3.0	3.1-6.0	6.1-9.0	9.1-12.0	12.1-15.0	15.1-18.0	>18.0
>15.0					4	4	4
12.1-15.0				3	3	4	4
9.1-12.0		3	3	3	3	3	4
6.1-9.0	2	2	2	2	3	3	4
3.1-6.0	1	1	1	2	2	3	4
≤3.0	1	1	1	1	2	2	4

Largest basal diameter (mm)

Figure 57.3 | Classification for ciliary body and choroid uveal melanoma based on thickness and diameter. (From Edge SB, Byrd DR, Compton CC, et al., *AJCC Cancer Staging Manual, 7th edition*. New York, Springer, 2010, p. 556.)

UVEA CHOROID MELANOMA

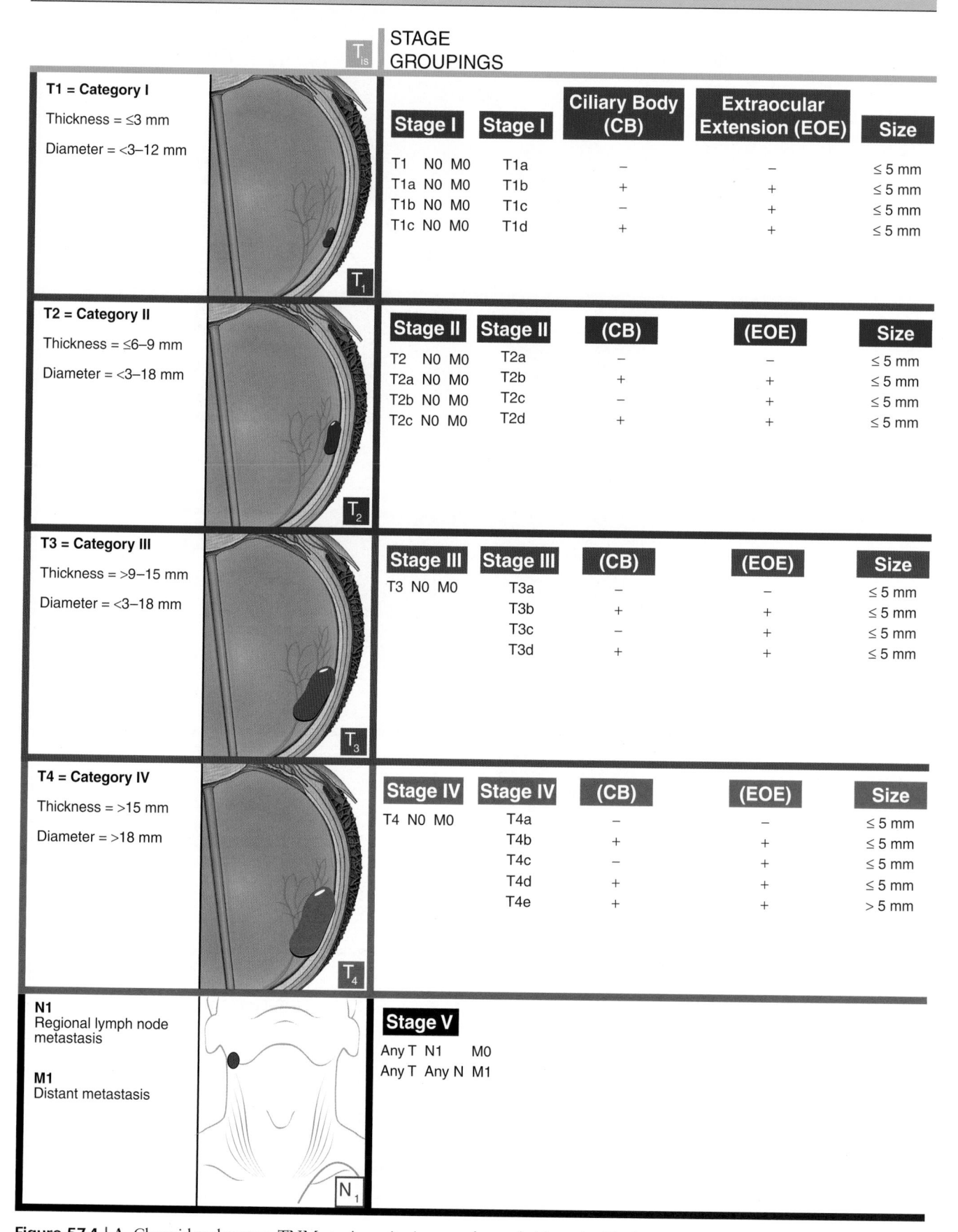

STAGE GROUPINGS

T1 = Category I

Thickness = ≤3 mm

Diameter = <3–12 mm

Stage I	Stage I	Ciliary Body (CB)	Extraocular Extension (EOE)	Size
T1 N0 M0	T1a	–	–	≤ 5 mm
T1a N0 M0	T1b	+	+	≤ 5 mm
T1b N0 M0	T1c	–	+	≤ 5 mm
T1c N0 M0	T1d	+	+	≤ 5 mm

T2 = Category II

Thickness = ≤6–9 mm

Diameter = <3–18 mm

Stage II	Stage II	(CB)	(EOE)	Size
T2 N0 M0	T2a	–	–	≤ 5 mm
T2a N0 M0	T2b	+	+	≤ 5 mm
T2b N0 M0	T2c	–	+	≤ 5 mm
T2c N0 M0	T2d	+	+	≤ 5 mm

T3 = Category III

Thickness = >9–15 mm

Diameter = <3–18 mm

Stage III	Stage III	(CB)	(EOE)	Size
T3 N0 M0	T3a	–	–	≤ 5 mm
	T3b	+	+	≤ 5 mm
	T3c	–	+	≤ 5 mm
	T3d	+	+	≤ 5 mm

T4 = Category IV

Thickness = >15 mm

Diameter = >18 mm

Stage IV	Stage IV	(CB)	(EOE)	Size
T4 N0 M0	T4a	–	–	≤ 5 mm
	T4b	+	+	≤ 5 mm
	T4c	–	+	≤ 5 mm
	T4d	+	+	≤ 5 mm
	T4e	+	+	> 5 mm

N1
Regional lymph node metastasis

M1
Distant metastasis

Stage V

Any T N1 M0
Any T Any N M1

Figure 57.4 | A. Choroid melanoma. TNM staging criteria are color coded bars for T advancement: Tis, yellow; T1, green; T2, blue; T3, purple; T4, red. *(continued)*

UVEA IRIS MELANOMA

DEFINITION OF TNM

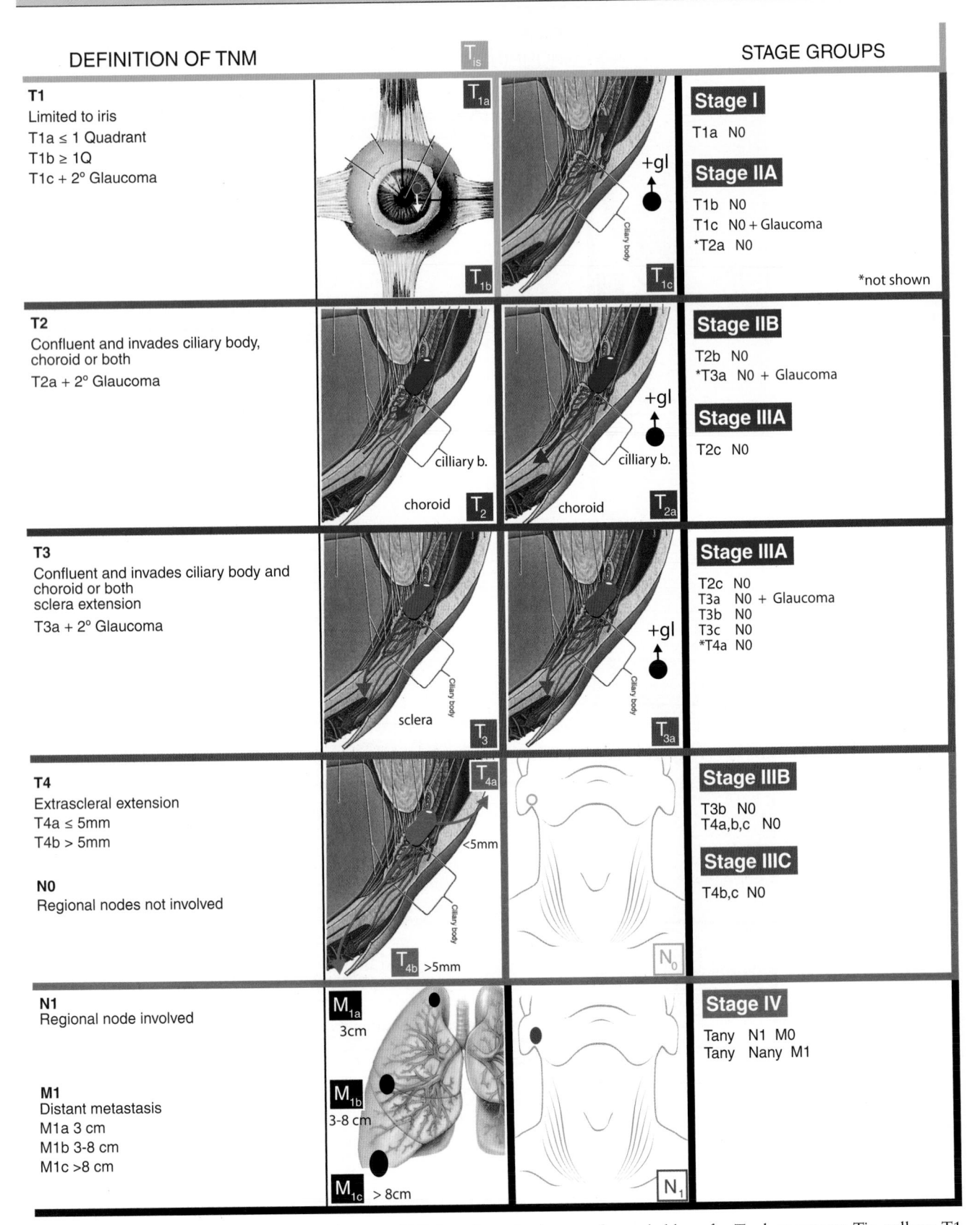

T1
Limited to iris
T1a ≤ 1 Quadrant
T1b ≥ 1Q
T1c + 2° Glaucoma

T2
Confluent and invades ciliary body, choroid or both
T2a + 2° Glaucoma

T3
Confluent and invades ciliary body and choroid or both
sclera extension
T3a + 2° Glaucoma

T4
Extrascleral extension
T4a ≤ 5mm
T4b > 5mm

N0
Regional nodes not involved

N1
Regional node involved

M1
Distant metastasis
M1a 3 cm
M1b 3-8 cm
M1c >8 cm

STAGE GROUPS

Stage I
T1a N0

Stage IIA
T1b N0
T1c N0 + Glaucoma
*T2a N0

*not shown

Stage IIB
T2b N0
*T3a N0 + Glaucoma

Stage IIIA
T2c N0

Stage IIIA
T2c N0
T3a N0 + Glaucoma
T3b N0
T3c N0
*T4a N0

Stage IIIB
T3b N0
T4a,b,c N0

Stage IIIC
T4b,c N0

Stage IV
Tany N1 M0
Tany Nany M1

Figure 57.4 | *(Continued)* **B.** Uvea iris melanoma. TNM staging criteria are color coded bars for T advancement: Tis, yellow; T1, green; T2, blue; T3, purple; T4, red. *(continued)*

CONJUNCTIVA MELANOMA

CLINICAL DEFINITION OF TNM

Pathologic Stage Groups

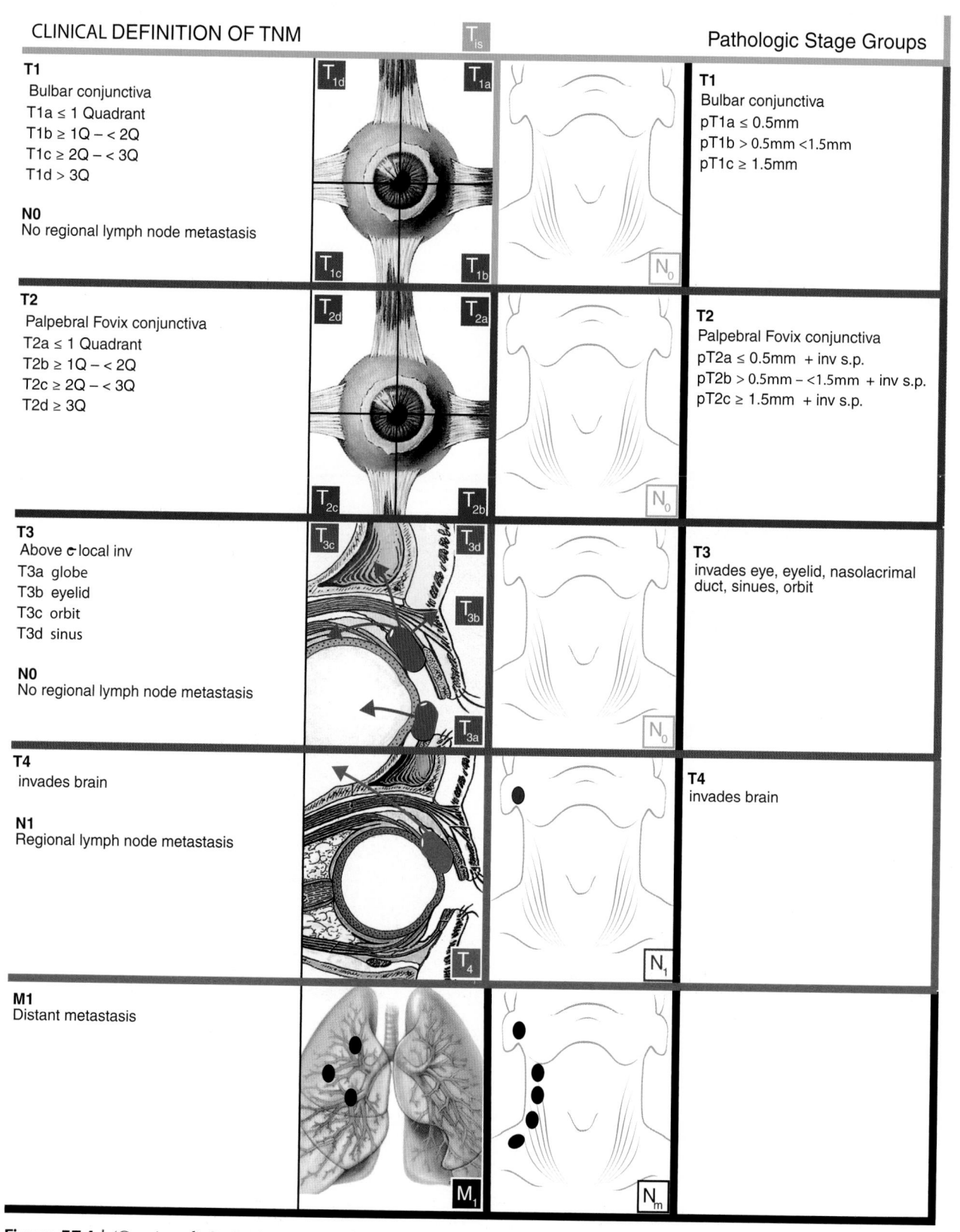

T1
 Bulbar conjunctiva
 T1a ≤ 1 Quadrant
 T1b ≥ 1Q – < 2Q
 T1c ≥ 2Q – < 3Q
 T1d > 3Q

N0
No regional lymph node metastasis

T2
 Palpebral Fovix conjunctiva
 T2a ≤ 1 Quadrant
 T2b ≥ 1Q – < 2Q
 T2c ≥ 2Q – < 3Q
 T2d ≥ 3Q

T3
 Above c local inv
 T3a globe
 T3b eyelid
 T3c orbit
 T3d sinus

N0
No regional lymph node metastasis

T4
 invades brain

N1
Regional lymph node metastasis

M1
Distant metastasis

T1
Bulbar conjunctiva
pT1a ≤ 0.5mm
pT1b > 0.5mm <1.5mm
pT1c ≥ 1.5mm

T2
Palpebral Fovix conjunctiva
pT2a ≤ 0.5mm + inv s.p.
pT2b > 0.5mm – <1.5mm + inv s.p.
pT2c ≥ 1.5mm + inv s.p.

T3
invades eye, eyelid, nasolacrimal
duct, sinuses, orbit

T4
invades brain

Figure 57.4 | *(Continued)* **C.** Conjunctiva Melanoma. TNM staging criteria are color coded bars for T advancement: Tis, yellow; T1, green; T2, blue; T3, purple; T4, red.

TNM STAGING CRITERIA

T-ONCOANATOMY

The middle layer of the globe is best appreciated in an axial view through the isocenter of the globe at the pupil of the eye through to the optic nerve. The uvea is the rich vascular layer of the eye.

- *Coronal:* Anterior view of Iris (Fig. 57.5A).

- *Sagittal:* The pupil is surrounded by the iris and is the window of the eye. It is under control of the sympathetic and oculomotor nerves. Horner's syndrome results in a small pupil and lid lag or ptosis. The pupil of the eye often can provide a major insight into numerous systemic disorders. Dilation of conjunctival capillaries is often benign and due to irritation, allergy, or infection. The presence of ciliary

injections as small capillaries surrounding a dilated pupil is an emergency suggesting glaucoma. The lens of the eye—the site of potential cataract formation—completes the middle layer of the eye and iris.

- *Axial:* As with most eye structures, this layer consists of three parts: (i) the iris (Fig. 57.5A), (ii) a ciliary body (pupil) (Fig. 57.5B), and (iii) the choroid (Fig. 57.5C). The eye also contains three chambers: (i) anterior between cornea and iris, (ii) posterior between the iris and lens, and (iii) the vitreous body, which fills the globe with a gelatinous substance between lens and retina. Because this layer is pigmented, it can give rise to melanoma at any site. The major anatomic feature is the extensive vascular mesh, and one can appreciate the access melanomas have to venous drainage via the vorticose vein.

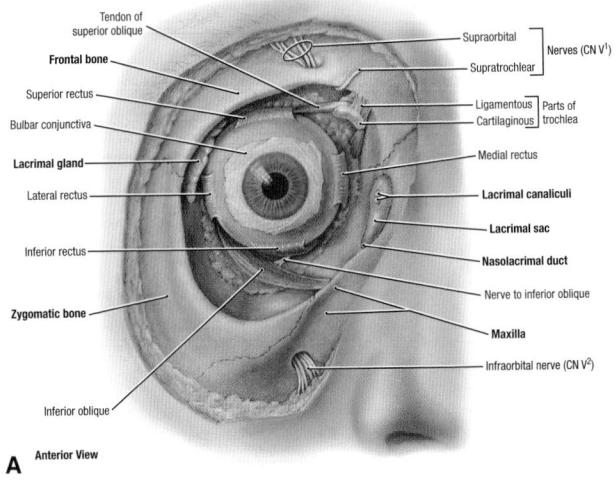

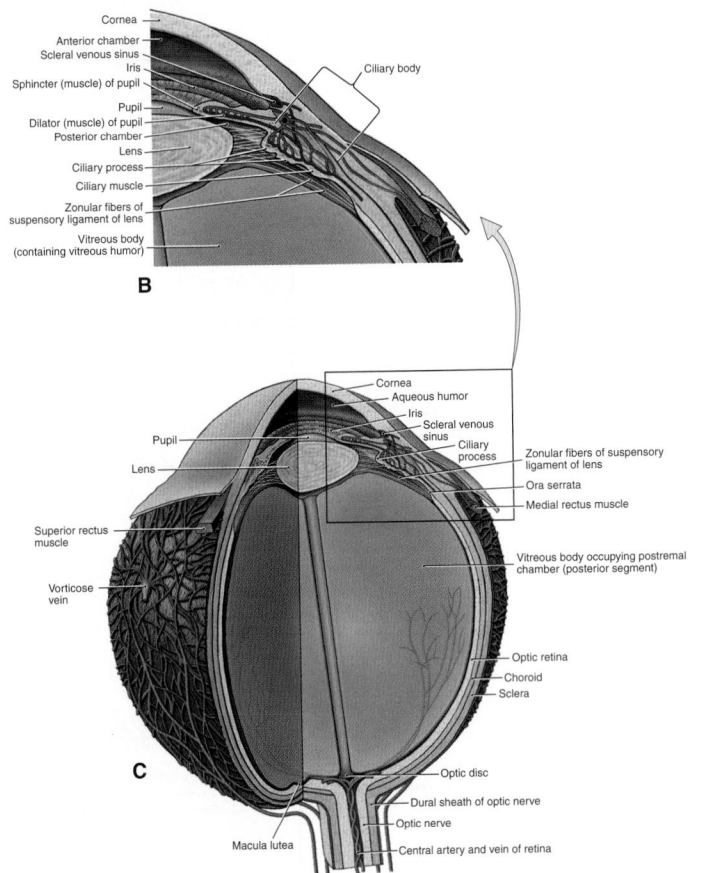

Figure 57.5 | A. Iris. Anterior dissection of the orbital cavity. The eyelids, orbital septum, levator palpebrae superioris, and some fat are removed. **Three-planar T-oncoanatomy. B.** Ciliary body; sagittal. **C.** Choroid; coronal and transverse.

N-ONCOANATOMY AND M-ONCOANATOMY

N-ONCOANATOMY

The eye globe is immunologically privileged and has no lymphatics or regional lymph nodes (Fig. 57.6A).

This applies to only uveal melanomas with extrascleral extension but applies to all conjunctival melanomas.

TABLE 57.4	Uvea-Regional Lymph Nodes	
	Sentinel	**Regional**
Uvea	Preauricular Facial node	Superficial cervical Parotid gland nodes

M-ONCOANATOMY

The pterygoid plexus of veins drains the fine veins of the eyelids into the internal jugular vein (Fig. 57.6B). Metastases occur most commonly to liver (90%) and can be massive. The astute clinical observation is "patient with glass eye" and hepatomegaly can offer the diagnosis of metastatic choroidal melanoma at the bedside. Other metastatic sites are lung, bone, brain, and subcutaneous.

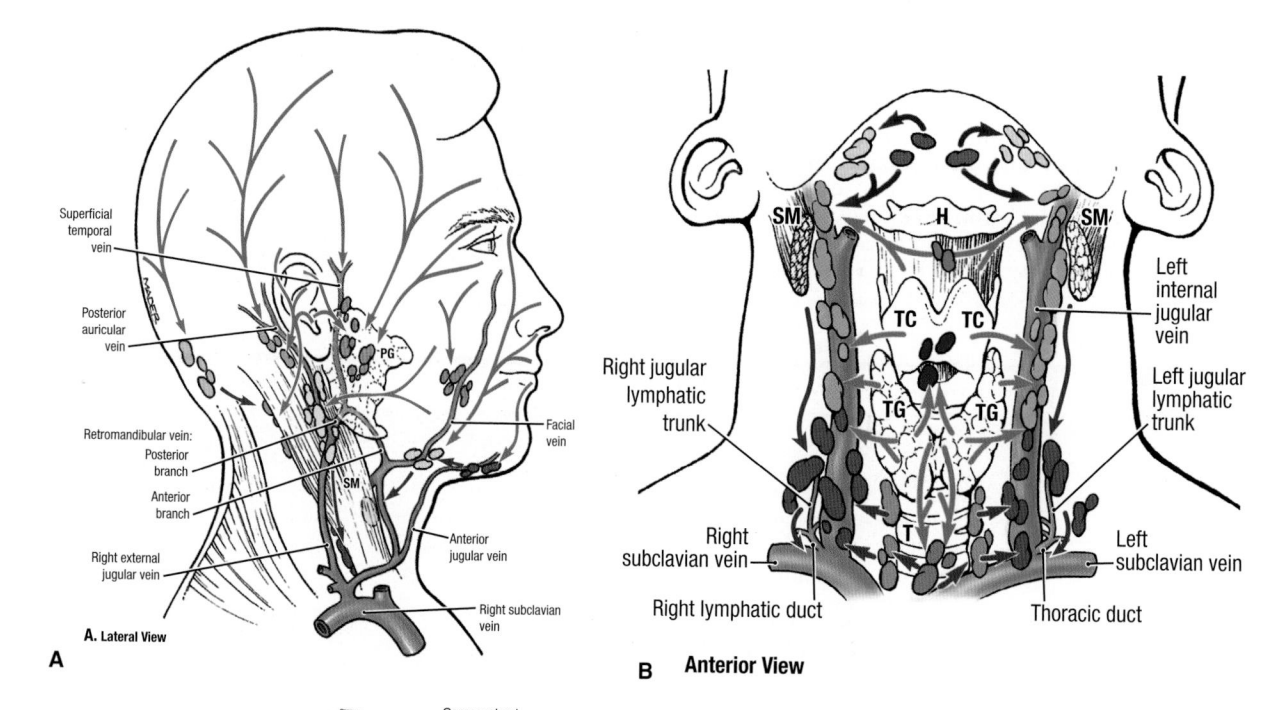

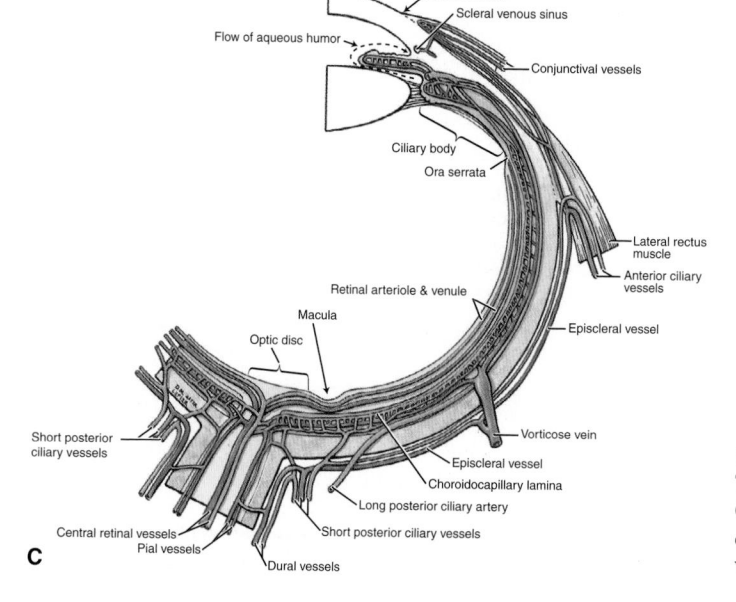

Figure 57.6 | A,B. N-oncoanatomy. Lateral view. The sentinel node is the preauricular node. **C. M-oncoanatomy of the eye.** The choroid is drained by posterior ciliary veins, and four to five vorticose veins drain into the ophthalmic veins.

STAGING WORKUP

RULES FOR CLASSIFICATION AND STAGING

Clinical Staging and Imaging

The clinical assessment requires inspection by slit-lamp examination and ophthalmoscopy. Imaging is highly desirable, especially computed tomography (CT) and fluorescein angiography (Table 57.5; Fig. 57.7). If retinal detachment raises suspicion of choroidal metastases, films or CT of chest should be considered. In women, mammography is worthwhile.

Clinical Staging

The assessment of cancer is based on inspection, slit-lamp examination, and palpation of the regional lymph nodes. All conjunctival surfaces are inspected and photographed with eversion of the upper eyelid. High-frequency ultrasound (UBM) imaging should be performed when the tumor is found to be affixed to the globe and when intraocular invasion is suspected. Low-frequency ultrasound may also be used to evaluate the sclera, eye, and orbit. Radiologic examinations (computed axial tomography, magnetic resonance imaging, and positron emission tomography [PET]/CT imaging) can be used to examine regional lymph nodes, paranasal sinuses, the orbit, brain, and chest. There are ongoing studies to clarify the role of sentinel lymph node involvement and sentinel lymph node biopsy.

Conjunctival carcinoma has been particularly associated with AIDS, neurodermatitis (atopic keratoconjunctivitis), other forms of immunosuppression (including iatrogenic), ultraviolet radiation, and human papillomavirus (HPV 16 and 18).

PATHOLOGIC STAGING

Complete resection of the primary site is indicated (if possible). Cryotherapy and/or topical chemotherapy (mitomycin, 5-fluorouracil, and/or interferon alpha-2b) may be considered as adjunctive therapies. Extensive tumor involvement of orbital soft tissues may require exenteration with or without adjuvant external beam radiation therapy. The specimen should be thoroughly sampled for histologic study of surgical margins, type of tumor, and grade of malignancy.

Resection of primary site with margins is essential and may include iridectomy to eye wall resection to enucleation of globe. Measurements should include size (height and depth) of choroidal lesion, measurements of iris uveal lesion in clock-hours of involvement, and margin of resection. Sentinel and/or palpable regional nodes include size and location.

TABLE 57.5	**Imaging Modalities: Eye and Orbit**	
Method	**Diagnosis and Staging Capability**	**Recommended for Use**
CT	Provides excellent anatomic detail of globe, orbital content, and bony orbit; can distinguish smooth, round cysts from infiltrative tumors versus pseudotumors and detect bone destruction and sinus invasion	Yes
Primary tumor ultrasonography and fine-needle aspiration biopsy	A scan and B scan can be used to screen intraocular and orbital tumors and cysts, especially melanomas	No
MRI	Provides excellent three-dimensional view, orbital fat hyperintense and vitreous hypointense in tumor (T1) and reverse in T2; can detect tumors versus pseudotumors and cysts; may be superior for the diagnosis of vascular lesions, demyelinating disease	Yes
Endoscopy	Orbital endoscopy with fiber-optic lights is used in conjunction with CT and/or MRI for obtaining core biopsy	Yes, when indicated
Standard orbital view	Useful for assessing optic nerve foramen and supraorbital fissure, but supplanted by CT; can detect intraocular calcification	No
Orbital phlebography	Venography is particularly useful for detecting orbital varices but is less efficient and more invasive than CT	No
Carotid angiography	Useful in diagnosis of vascularized tumors and aneurysms, but replaced by CT/MRI	No
Fluorescein angiography	Sometimes used in diagnosis of ocular melanoma	No
Biopsy	Usually an incisional or excisional biopsy is indicated to confirm malignant versus pseudotumors; directed stereotactically by CT/MRI; contraindicated for melanomas owing to high risk of seeding	Yes, if indicated

CT, computed tomography; MRI, magnetic resonance imaging.
Used with permission from Rubin P. *Clinical Oncology*. 7th ed. Philadelphia: WB Saunders; 1993:300.

PROGNOSIS AND CANCER SURVIVAL

PROGNOSTIC FACTORS

See Table 57.6.

TABLE 57.6 | Prognostic Factors

Uvea

Required for staging:
  Height
  Largest tumor diameter
Clinically significant:
  Measured thickness (height)
  Chromosomal alterations
  Gene expression profile
  Positron emission tomography/computed tomography
  Mitotic count per 40 high-power fields (HPF)
  Mean diameter of the 10 largest nucleoli (MLN)
  Presence of extravascular matrix patterns
  Microvascular density (MVD)

From Edge SB, Byrd DR, Compton CC, et al., *AJCC Cancer Staging Manual, 7th edition.* New York, Springer, 2010, p. 552.

CANCER STATISTICS AND SURVIVAL

The eye and orbit only account for 2,750 new diagnoses annually, excluding carcinomas of the eyelids. Deaths attributed to ocular malignancy are less than 10% of the entire group (240). Some of the most elegant proton and three-dimensional conformal radiation stereotactic techniques allow for cure of choroidal melanomas and retinoblastoma with preservation of vision.

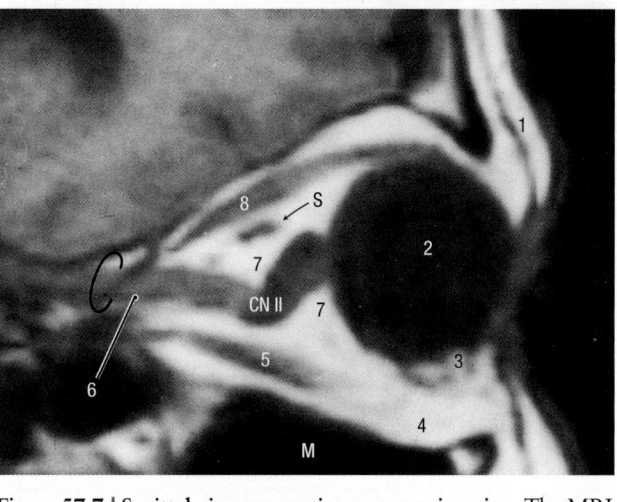

Figure 57.7 | Sagittal view magnetic resonance imaging. The MRI can be correlated with Fig. 57.5C. 1. Orbicularis oculi, 2. Eyeball, 3. Inferior Oblique Muscle, 4. Extracoronal Fat, 5. Interior Rectus Muscle, 6. Dural and Arachnoid Sheath, 7. Retrobulbar Fat, 8. Superior Rectus Muscle, M. Maxillary Sinus.

Results from ocular melanomas are presented in Fig. 57.8. Survival is impressive, with 90% long-term survival.

- Radiation isotopic plaque and enucleation were found to be comparable treatments in posterior uveal/choroidal melanomas in the Collaborative Ocular Melanoma Study group, consisting of 1,300 patients over 11.5 years. Recurrence rates with radiation range from about 15% to less than 5% with surgery.

- The probability of choroid melanoma control by Harvard proton beam control is 96.3%. The absolute local recurrence rate after helium ion therapy is less than 3%. Custom plaque irradiation appears to be an effective method for treating iris melanomas as well.

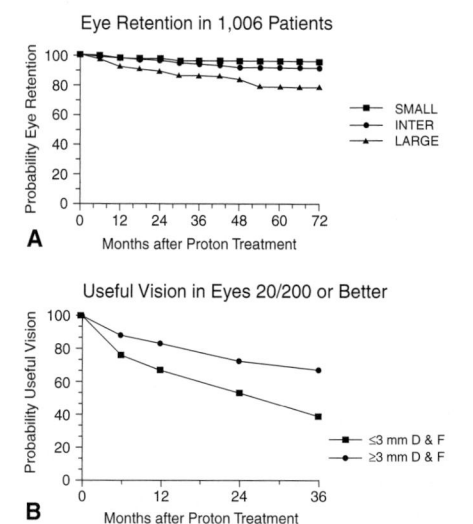

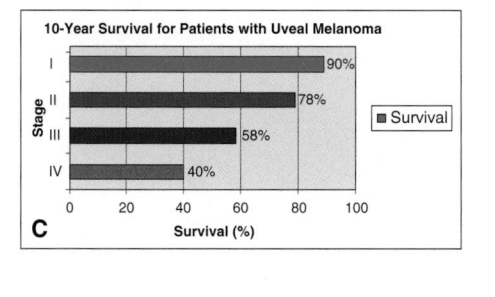

Figure 57.8 | Survival and eye retention probability. A. Kaplan–Meier plot of eye retention probability after proton therapy in 1,006 patients with small (<3 mm high and <10 mm in diameter), intermediate (3.1–8 mm high and/or 10.1–16 mm in diameter), and large (>8 mm high and >16 mm in diameter) uveal melanomas. **B.** Kaplan–Meier plot of the probability of retaining useful vision in patients with tumors 3 mm from the optic disc (D) and fovea (F) and >3 mm from the optic disc and/or fovea in 562 eyes with initial visual acuity 20/200 (6/60) or better. **C.** Ten-year survival for patients with uveal melanoma. (Data for part C from Edge SB, Byrd DR, Compton CC, et al., *AJCC Cancer Staging Manual. 7th edition.* New York, Springer, 2010.)

Retina

PERSPECTIVE, PATTERNS OF SPREAD, AND PATHOLOGY

Trilateral neuroblastoma occurs when both eyes are involved with retinoblastomas and there is a pinealblastoma in the pineal gland.

PERSPECTIVE AND PATTERNS OF SPREAD

Retinoblastoma is a hereditary malignancy and occurs in approximately 1 in 20,000 live births. There is no known difference in the incidence between whites and blacks, between males and females, or in children in various parts of the world (Fig. 58.1). Thirty percent of retinoblastomas are bilateral, and all bilateral tumors are germinal. Forty percent of all retinoblastomas are germinal (i.e., 25% of all unilateral tumors are germinal). In these cases, there is a 100% chance of an autosomal-dominant pattern of hereditary transmission to the next generation, as well as a lifelong significant risk of development of a second, nonocular malignancy (85%). More than 90% of retinoblastoma cases are diagnosed before age 5 years. The median age at diagnosis is 14 months for bilateral cases and 23 months for unilateral tumors. There is a 5% association with other congenital defects, of which mental retardation is the most common. In the syndrome designated Dq-1, half of the patients have retinoblastoma, as well as a high incidence of other defects, including psychomotor retardation, skeletal abnormalities, congenital heart disease, and other eye defects. Spontaneous regression occurs in 1% of all retinoblastoma

patients. This has been attributed to the tumor's outgrowing its vascular supply and becoming infarcted and necrotic.

Retinoblastoma has been documented to result from a genetic mutation. Retinoblastoma behaves like an autosomal-dominant syndrome with >90% penetrance, but the abnormal tumor-producing mutant allele is recessive. Seventy percent of retinoblastomas present as unilateral tumors. In all the bilateral and in 25% of the unilateral presentations, a germinal mutation affecting all cells in the body has occurred. Despite the high occurrence rate of germinal mutations (40% of cases), only 12% of patients have a positive family history; the other 88% represent the first germinal mutation in the family.

Retinoblastoma conforms to the two-hit Knudson hypothesis, in which two chromosomal mutational events are necessary to cause cancer. In the hereditary form, the mutational event affects a germ cell and thus all cells in the body, whereas in nongerminal cell cases, a single retinal cell is affected. The normal allele at the retinoblastoma locus is believed to act as a controller gene or suppressor of the malignant retinoblastoma growth. Thus, both alleles must be lost before malignant growth can ensue. In the hereditary cases, all cells have lost one normal allele, and the chance of several retinal cells losing the second allele is quite high, resulting in bilateral or multicentric tumor growth at an earlier age (median, 14 months). In the nonhereditary or somatic form, one retinal cell has lost one allele and must lose the second before a unicentric, unilateral tumor arises, usually at a later age (median, 23 months). Thus, in nongerminal cases, the chance of bilateral mutations (two hits) on two separate retinal cells is low, and the chance that a

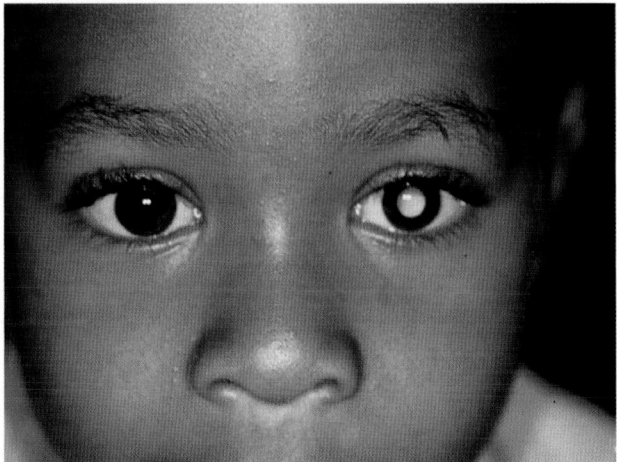
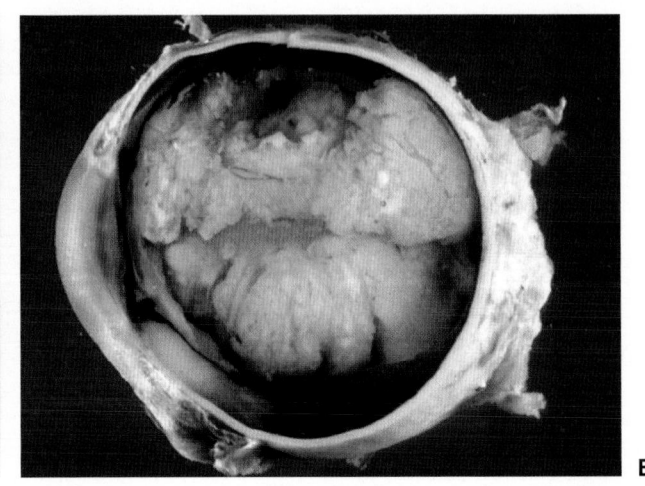

A   B

Figure 58.1 | Retinoblastoma. A. The white pupil (leukocoria) in the left eye is the result of an intraocular retinoblastoma. **B.** This surgically excised eye is almost filled by a cream-colored intraocular retinoblastoma with calcified flecks.

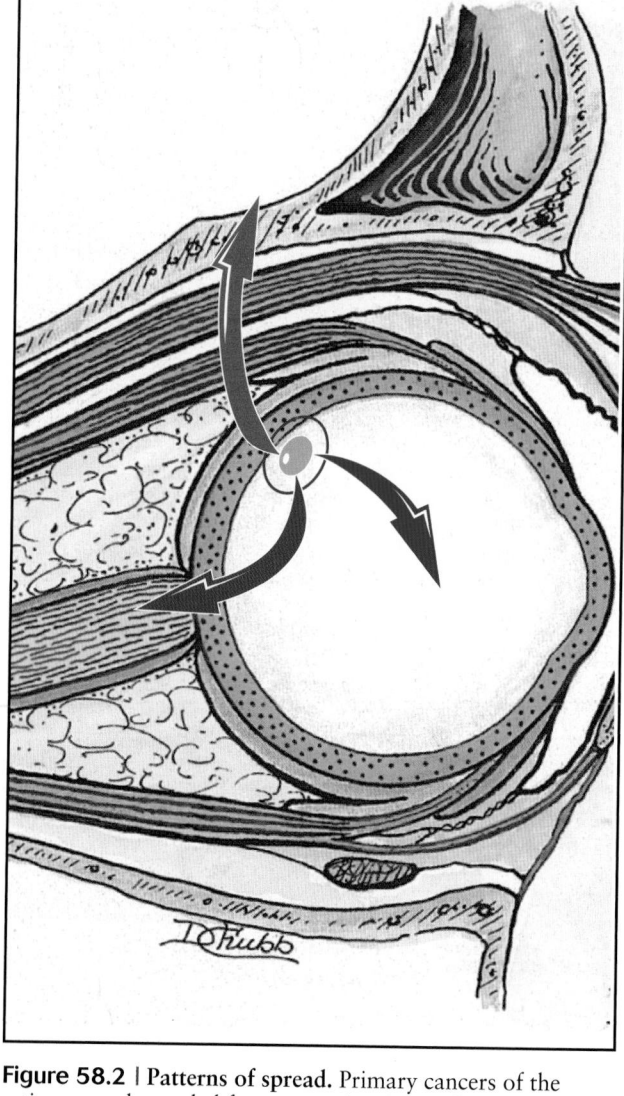

TABLE 58.1		SIMLAP

	Retinoblastoma	
	Macula	• T1
S	Orbit, extraocular muscles	• T4
I	Orbit, extraocular muscles	• T4
M	Retina	• T1
	Choroid focal	• T2b
L	Retina	• T1
	Choroid focal	• T2b
A	Vitreous seeding	• T2
	Orbit	• T4
P	Optic nerve disc	• T2a
	Optic coats	• T3
	Retro-orbital space	• T4
	Choroid focal	• T2b
	Choroid massive	• T3c
	Optic nerve	• T3a
	Chiasm	• T4
	Orbit	• T4
	Subarachnoid space	• T4
	Apex orbit	• T4
	Brain	• T4

The six vectors of invasion are Superior, Inferior, Medial, Lateral, Anterior, and Posterior. The color-coded dots correlate the T stage with the specific anatomic structure involved.

Figure 58.2 | Patterns of spread. Primary cancers of the retina are color coded for progression: T0, yellow; T1, green; T2, blue; T3, purple; T4, red. The concept of visualizing patterns of spread to appreciate the surrounding anatomy is well demonstrated by the six-directional pattern (SIMLAP, Table 58.1).

bilateral tumor would be nongerminal or somatic is equally low. Because 50% of the offspring of germinal retinoblastoma patients are affected, prenatal or presymptomatic diagnosis is crucial. A few laboratories have developed diagnostic tests to identify the retinoblastoma gene in this group of patients. Detection of the gene in the 15% of patients with unilateral disease that have the germinal mutation is also important because they carry a lifelong risk of secondary malignancies. Healthy parents who have a single affected child can expect an attack rate of 6% among their other offspring. An unaffected sibling of a child with sporadic retinoblastoma, like one of his parents, may be a carrier; however, the risk is extremely low (<1%). If retinoblastoma occurs more than once in a given pedigree, there is a 40% to 48% chance that the affected members of this pedigree will have offspring with retinoblastoma. The unaffected members have a chance of only 5% to 20%.

History of prematurity and oxygen therapy may predispose the infant, but the likely presenting sign is "leukoria" or recognition of "white reflex" in the pupil of the eye instead of red at angles of light or photographs. Binocular indirect ophthalmoscopy is an important diagnostic exam to verify the presence of a tumor with whitish color due to calcification (Fig. 58.1).

The tumor spreads readily within the eye (Fig. 58.2; Table 58.1). Trilateral retinoblastoma occurs when both eyes are involved and pineoblastoma occurs in the pineal gland. This rare but interesting combination illustrates that the pineal or third eye shares the same developmental anlage as the retina. This diagnosis must be considered in a patient with bilateral retinoblastoma who subsequently develops headache or lethargy.

Early recognition, especially in the hereditary form, allows for conservation of the eye using modern radiation techniques that conform to the tumor shape and size while sparing the eye. As the retinoblastoma advances and fills the eye globe and invades the optic nerve, the surgical enucleation of the eye globe and optic nerve leads to a pathologic staging that is most important.

Trilateral retinoblastomas are rare (2% to 5%): Bilateral retinoblastomas in addition to ectopic retinoblastomas of the pineal gland. This atypical presentation can begin as an increase in intracranial pressure with lethargy, vomiting, and ataxia.

OVERVIEW OF HISTOGENESIS AND HISTOPATHOLOGY

The embryogenesis of the eye has no endoderm and is tripartite: it is the neural ectoderm that is the focus for the epithelium of retina and optic nerve and partly of vitreous body that is our concern. The retina is the most complex tissue of the eye and consists of numerous cell layers (six) (Fig. 58.4B) and cell populations (10). It is similar in its organization to the cerebral cortex (Fig. 58.4A).

The analogy is essential to understanding the behavior of the retinoblastoma and its spread pattern into the optic nerve and ultimately into the subarachnoid space. The eye is unlike other cranial nerves, which are more akin to peripheral nerves. The optic nerve is more vulnerable to invasion of the central nervous system (CNS) than other forms of perineural invasion of cranial nerves. The optic nerve is a projection of the forebrain, and its fibrous covers are an extension of the meninges; its most innermost layer is the neural retina. The sclera is penetrated by the optic nerve that forms the optic disc and is the lamina cribrosa or cribriform plate, sometimes referred to as a blind spot. Thus, the importance in the TNM classification is to the distance to optic nerve because this is the gateway to CNS invasion and spread. Once the retinoblastoma crosses the lamina cribrosa, it has invaded the CNS. Retinoblastomas have three growth patterns: *endophytic* (into the vitreous), *exophytic* (between sensory and pigmented layer, which leads to retinal detachment), and *diffuse multicentric*—seeding and snowballing.

Retinoblastoma usually arises from the posterior portion of the retina and consists of small, closely packed, round or polygonal cells with dark-staining nucleus and scanty cytoplasm (Table 58.2, Fig. 58.3). In many cases, the tumor cells are arranged in rosettes, but their absence does not necessarily exclude this diagnosis. Histopathologic classification of retinoblastoma permits a certain amount of separation between more- and less-differentiated tumor varieties. The more-differentiated tumors show small rosettes that are believed to represent differentiated spongioblasts (neuroepitheliomas). The tumor often outgrows its blood supply. Areas of necrosis are common and are responsible for the formation of calcium deposits. Rarely, the tumor may become so necrotic as to destroy itself entirely, giving rise to the rare instance of spontaneous regression. The necrotizing tendency of the tumor is one of the factors responsible for the occasional intense ocular inflammation that may be highly misleading clinically.

Layers of the retina, including the interrelationships of the neurons and the supporting cells, are variously defined as many different types of neurons and multiple synapses but are classified in three categories: (i) photoreceptors—retinal rods and cones, (ii) conducting neurons—bipolar and ganglion cells, and (iii) association with other neurons—horizontal, centrifugal amacrine supporting cells. The ultrastructure of the rod and cone is an (i) inner fiber, (ii) an inner segment, and (iii) an outer segment (Fig. 58.4).

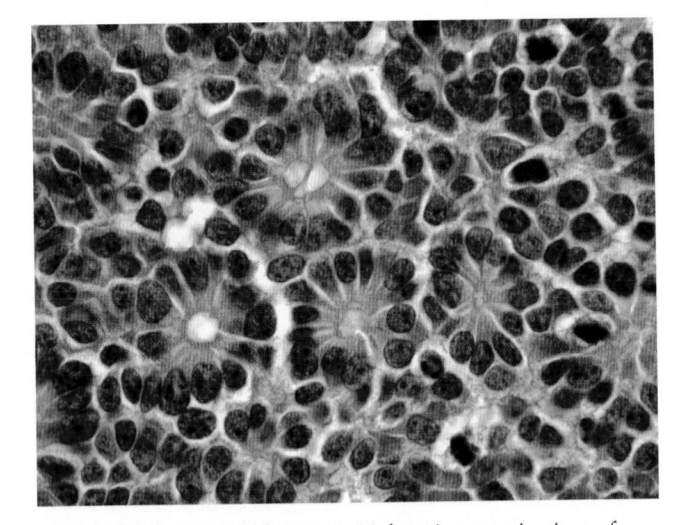

Figure 58.3 | Retinoblastoma. Light microscopic view of a retinoblastoma showing Flexner–Wintersteiner rosettes characterized by cells that are arranged around a central cavity.

TABLE 58.2	Histopathologic Types of Retinoblastomas
Retinoblastoma, not otherwise specified	
Retinoblastoma, differentiated	
Retinoblastoma, undifferentiated	
Retinoblastoma, diffuse	

Used with permission from Greene FL, Page DL, Fleming ID, et al., eds. *AJCC Cancer Staging Manual.* 7th ed. New York: Springer; 2002:373.

HISTOGENESIS

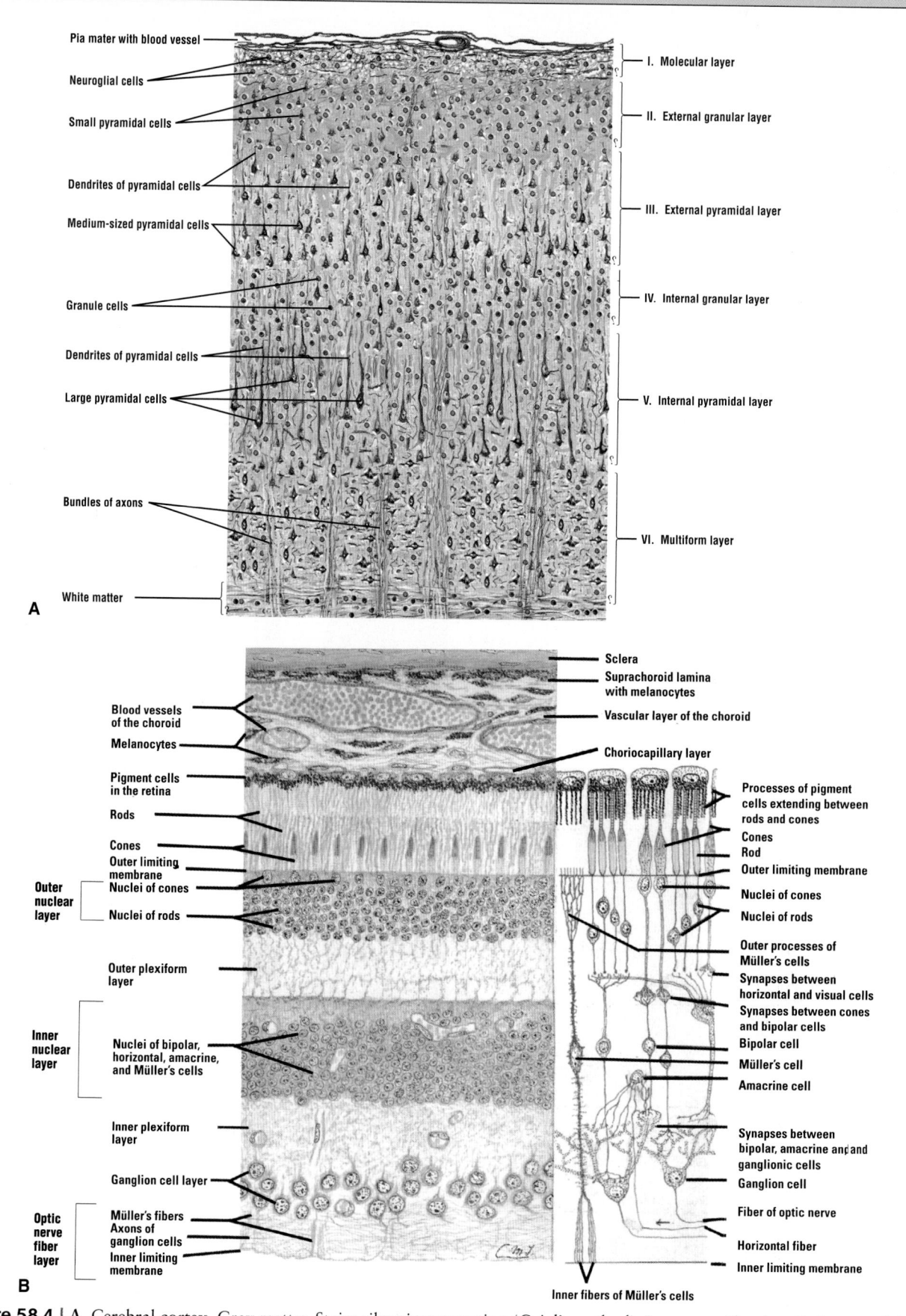

Pia mater with blood vessel

Neuroglial cells

Small pyramidal cells

Dendrites of pyramidal cells

Medium-sized pyramidal cells

Granule cells

Dendrites of pyramidal cells

Large pyramidal cells

Bundles of axons

White matter

A

I. Molecular layer

II. External granular layer

III. External pyramidal layer

IV. Internal granular layer

V. Internal pyramidal layer

VI. Multiform layer

Blood vessels of the choroid

Melanocytes

Pigment cells in the retina

Rods

Cones

Outer limiting membrane

Outer nuclear layer — **Nuclei of cones** / **Nuclei of rods**

Inner nuclear layer — **Outer plexiform layer** / **Nuclei of bipolar, horizontal, amacrine, and Müller's cells** / **Inner plexiform layer**

Ganglion cell layer

Optic nerve fiber layer — **Müller's fibers** / **Axons of ganglion cells** / **Inner limiting membrane**

B

Sclera

Suprachoroid lamina with melanocytes

Vascular layer of the choroid

Choriocapillary layer

Processes of pigment cells extending between rods and cones

Cones
Rod

Outer limiting membrane

Nuclei of cones

Nuclei of rods

Outer processes of Müller's cells

Synapses between horizontal and visual cells

Synapses between cones and bipolar cells

Bipolar cell

Müller's cell

Amacrine cell

Synapses between bipolar, amacrine and ganglionic cells

Ganglion cell

Fiber of optic nerve

Horizontal fiber

Inner limiting membrane

Inner fibers of Müller's cells

Figure 58.4 | A. Cerebral cortex. Gray matter. Stain: silver impregnation (Cajal's method). Low magnification. **B.** Layers of the choroid and retina (detail). Stain: hematoxylin and eosin. High magnification.

SUMMARY OF CHANGES SEVENTH EDITION AJCC

Clinical Classification (Fig. 58.5A; Table 58.3)

- The definitions of T1–T4 were modified.
- The definitions for M1 were modified.

	Clinical	Pathologic
T1	<2/3 globe, no seeding	Confined to eye No optic nerve/choroid invasion
T2	<2/3 globe with seeding	Minimal optic nerve/choroid invasion
T3	>2/3 Globe	Significant optic nerve/choroid invasion
T4	Extraocular	Invasion beyond nerve resection Massive choroidal invasion

TABLE 58.3 Comparing Clinical versus Pathologic Features/Descriptors

CLINICAL

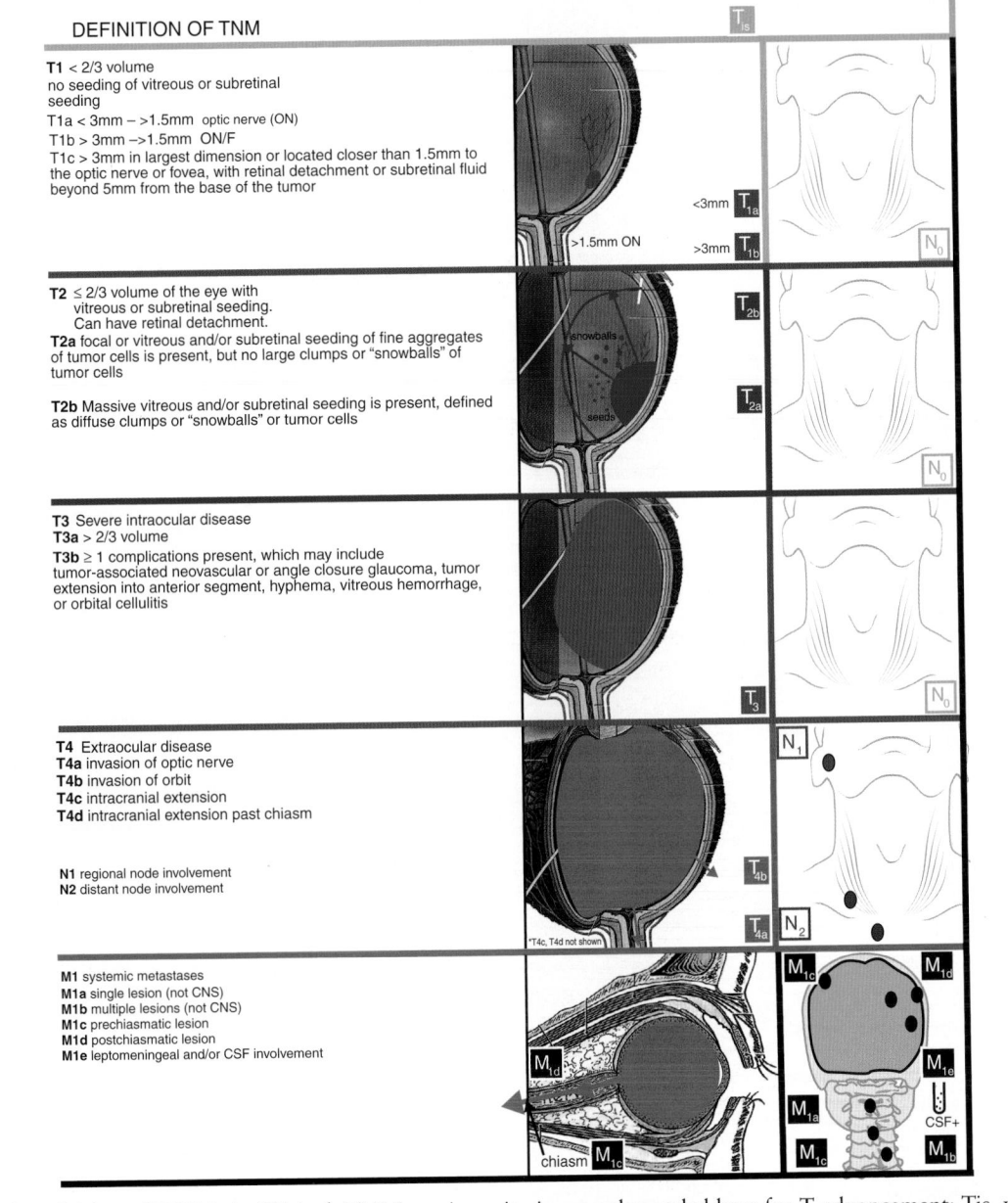

DEFINITION OF TNM

T1 < 2/3 volume
no seeding of vitreous or subretinal
seeding
T1a < 3mm – >1.5mm optic nerve (ON)
T1b > 3mm –>1.5mm ON/F
T1c > 3mm in largest dimension or located closer than 1.5mm to
the optic nerve or fovea, with retinal detachment or subretinal fluid
beyond 5mm from the base of the tumor

T2 ≤ 2/3 volume of the eye with
vitreous or subretinal seeding.
Can have retinal detachment.
T2a focal or vitreous and/or subretinal seeding of fine aggregates
of tumor cells is present, but no large clumps or "snowballs" of
tumor cells

T2b Massive vitreous and/or subretinal seeding is present, defined
as diffuse clumps or "snowballs" or tumor cells

T3 Severe intraocular disease
T3a > 2/3 volume
T3b ≥ 1 complications present, which may include
tumor-associated neovascular or angle closure glaucoma, tumor
extension into anterior segment, hyphema, vitreous hemorrhage,
or orbital cellulitis

T4 Extraocular disease
T4a invasion of optic nerve
T4b invasion of orbit
T4c intracranial extension
T4d intracranial extension past chiasm

N1 regional node involvement
N2 distant node involvement

M1 systemic metastases
M1a single lesion (not CNS)
M1b multiple lesions (not CNS)
M1c prechiasmatic lesion
M1d postchiasmatic lesion
M1e leptomeningeal and/or CSF involvement

Figure 58.5 | Definition of TNM. A. Clinical. TNM staging criteria are color coded bars for T advancement: Tis, yellow; T1, green; T2, blue; T3, purple; T4, red. (*continued*)

Pathologic Classification

- Minor modifications were made to the definitions for pT2–pT4 (Fig. 58.5B).
- The definitions for pM1 were modified.

Other

- A description of proper processing of the enucleated retinoblastoma globe for pathological examination was added.
- Definitions of the T stage progression can be described as:
  - Minimal T1 Focal
  - Moderate T2 Massive
- Severe T3 Massive
- Extraocular T4 Massive

There is variation in descriptors from the sixth to the seventh edition.

In pathologic staging, the following definitions have been added:

Artifactual invasion: cluster of tumor cells in open spaces between intraocular and extraocular spaces.

True invasion: one or more solid clusters fills/replaces choroid with pushing borders.

Focal choroidal: solid clusters ≤3 mm diameter.

Massive choroidal: solid clusters ≥3 mm diameter.

NB: There are numerous details to fixation sampling of the enucleated eye globe/optic nerve anterior-posterior in a "bread loaf" fashion.

PATHOLOGIC

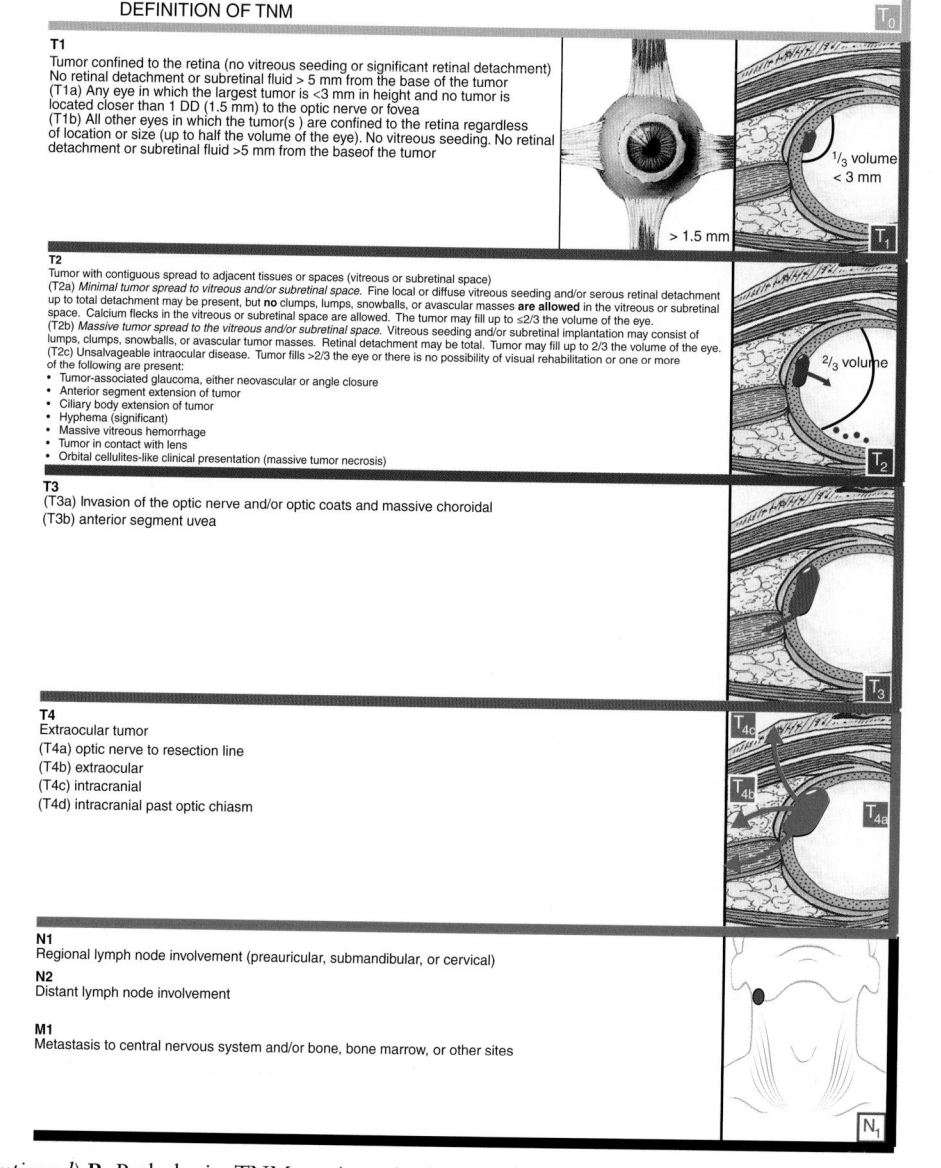

DEFINITION OF TNM

T1
Tumor confined to the retina (no vitreous seeding or significant retinal detachment)
No retinal detachment or subretinal fluid > 5 mm from the base of the tumor
(T1a) Any eye in which the largest tumor is <3 mm in height and no tumor is located closer than 1 DD (1.5 mm) to the optic nerve or fovea
(T1b) All other eyes in which the tumor(s) are confined to the retina regardless of location or size (up to half the volume of the eye). No vitreous seeding. No retinal detachment or subretinal fluid >5 mm from the baseof the tumor

T2
Tumor with contiguous spread to adjacent tissues or spaces (vitreous or subretinal space)
(T2a) *Minimal tumor spread to vitreous and/or subretinal space.* Fine local or diffuse vitreous seeding and/or serous retinal detachment up to total detachment may be present, but **no** clumps, lumps, snowballs, or avascular masses **are allowed** in the vitreous or subretinal space. Calcium flecks in the vitreous or subretinal space are allowed. The tumor may fill up to ≤2/3 the volume of the eye.
(T2b) *Massive tumor spread to the vitreous and/or subretinal space.* Vitreous seeding and/or subretinal implantation may consist of lumps, clumps, snowballs, or avascular tumor masses. Retinal detachment may be total. Tumor may fill up to 2/3 the volume of the eye.
(T2c) Unsalvageable intraocular disease. Tumor fills >2/3 the eye or there is no possibility of visual rehabilitation or one or more of the following are present:
- Tumor-associated glaucoma, either neovascular or angle closure
- Anterior segment extension of tumor
- Ciliary body extension of tumor
- Hyphema (significant)
- Massive vitreous hemorrhage
- Tumor in contact with lens
- Orbital cellulites-like clinical presentation (massive tumor necrosis)

T3
(T3a) Invasion of the optic nerve and/or optic coats and massive choroidal
(T3b) anterior segment uvea

T4
Extraocular tumor
(T4a) optic nerve to resection line
(T4b) extraocular
(T4c) intracranial
(T4d) intracranial past optic chiasm

N1
Regional lymph node involvement (preauricular, submandibular, or cervical)
N2
Distant lymph node involvement

M1
Metastasis to central nervous system and/or bone, bone marrow, or other sites

Figure 58.5 | (*Continued*) **B.** Pathologic. TNM staging criteria are color coded bars for T advancement: Tis, yellow; T1, green; T2, blue; T3, purple; T4, red.

TNM STAGING CRITERIA

T-ONCOANATOMY

The retina is the innermost layer of the eye, and its posterior (75%) portion is photosensitive and is stimulated by light. Anteriorly, it ends at the ora serrata. The photoreceptor cells are rods and cones. Leaving the retina are nerve fibers that form the optic disc and nerve and pass signals to the brain. There are sight strata of cells; in addition to the optic disc, there is the macula and an array of retinal arterioles and venules that characterize the eye grounds (Fig. 58.6).

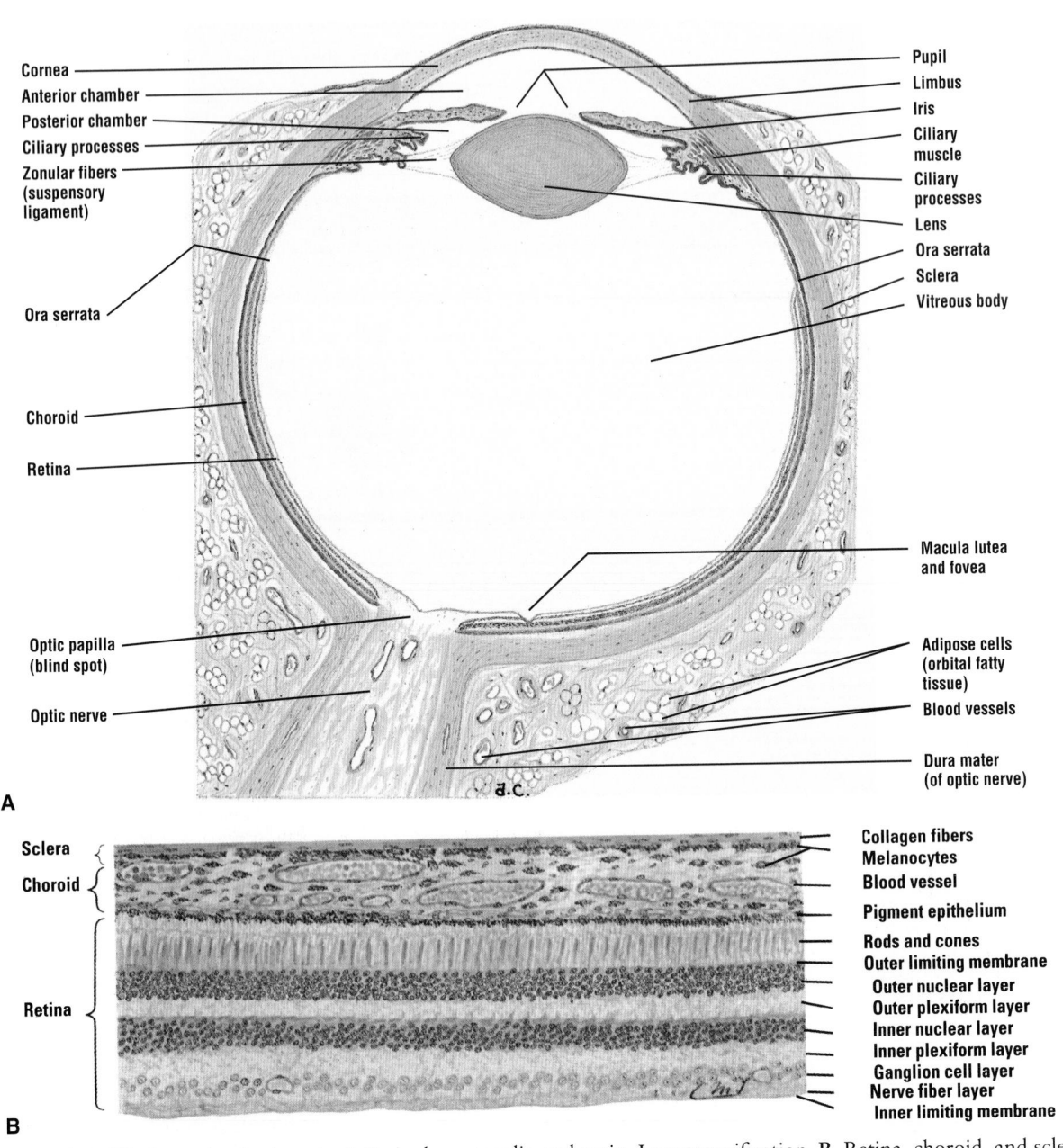

Figure 58.6 | A. Whole eye (sagittal section). Stain: hematoxylin and eosin. Low magnification. **B.** Retina, choroid, and sclera (panoramic view). Stain: hematoxylin and eosin. Medium magnification.

N-ONCOANATOMY AND M-ONCOANATOMY

N-ONCOANATOMY

The eye globe is immunologically privileged and has no lymphatics or regional lymph nodes.

M-ONCOANATOMY

The lesion can seed itself throughout the interior of the eye and include the iris and anterior chamber (Fig. 58.7). Distant spread of retinoblastoma commonly occurs along the optic nerve. Here the tumor can spread readily along the meningeal spaces of the optic sheath and soon reach the subarachnoid space and seed out into the cerebrospinal fluid. Distant spread can also occur though the bloodstream, most commonly to bone, lungs, and liver. The causes of death in this tumor are interesting. More than 90% of the patients have intracranial involvement; in almost 50% of all deaths, disease is confined to the cranial cavity and spinal cord; the remaining half have distant metastases. Distant metastasis occurs with equal incidence (~50%) of spread to lymph nodes, skull bones, distant bones, and viscera.

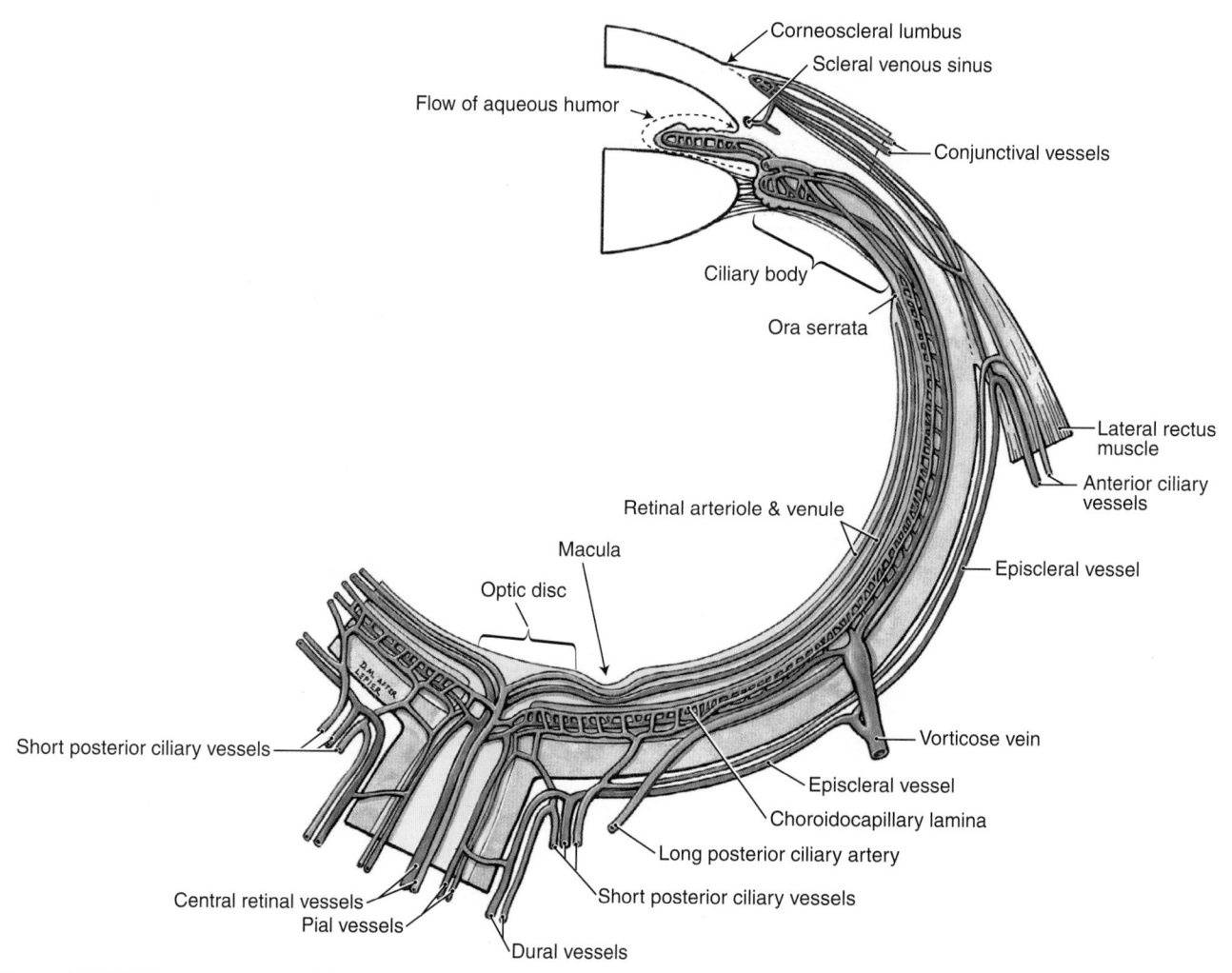

Figure 58.7 | **M-oncoanatomy of the eye.** The choroid is drained by posterior ciliary veins, and four to five vorticose veins drain into the ophthalmic veins.

STAGING WORKUP

RULES FOR CLASSIFICATION AND STAGING

Clinical Staging and Imaging

Examination under anesthesia is most desirable, and if simple orbital radiographs show calcification in the child's globe, it is pathognomonic for retinoblastoma (Table 58.4). Enhanced computed tomography is the preferred cross-sectional imaging, although magnetic resonance imaging is complementary for extraocular soft tissue extension and especially to assess for optic nerve invasion. With multiple lesions, ultrasound identification of their location is done with detailed retinal drawings. In bilateral cases, each eye should be staged separately. Distance of tumor from disc, fovea, and ora serrata should be noted in millimeters or estimated in terms of size of optic nerve disc (e.g., 1.5×1 or 2, etc.).

Pathologic Staging

If the eye is sacrificed and enucleated, tumor size, invasion of optic nerve, and margins, if there is extraocular spread, need notation.

TABLE 58.4	Imaging Modalities: Eye and Orbit	
Method	Diagnosis and Staging Capability	Recommended for Use
CT	Provides excellent anatomic detail of globe, orbital content, and bony orbit; can distinguish smooth, round cysts from infiltrative tumors versus pseudotumors and detect bone destruction and sinus invasion	Yes
Primary tumor ultrasonography and fine-needle aspiration biopsy	A and B scans can be used to screen intraocular and orbital tumors and cysts, especially melanomas	No
MRI	Provides excellent three-dimensional view, orbital fat hyperintense and vitreous hypointense in tumor (T1) and reverse in T2; can detect tumors versus pseudotumors and cysts; may be superior for diagnosis of vascular lesions, demyelinating disease; best for extraocular extension	Yes
Endoscopy	Orbital endoscopy with fiber-optic lights is used in conjunction with CT and/or MRI for obtaining core biopsy	Yes, when indicated
Standard orbital view	Useful for assessing optic nerve foramen and supraorbital fissure, but supplanted by CT; can detect intraocular calcification	No
Orbital phlebography	Venography particularly useful for detecting orbital varices, but is less efficient and more invasive than CT	No
Carotid angiography	Useful in diagnosis of vascularized tumors and aneurysms, but replaced by CT/MRI	No
Fluorescein angiography	Sometimes used in diagnosis of ocular melanoma	No
Biopsy	Usually an incisional or excisional biopsy is indicated to confirm malignant versus pseudotumors; directed stereotactically by CT/MRI; contraindicated for melanomas owing to high risk of seeding	Yes, if indicated

CT, computed tomography; MRI, magnetic resonance imaging.
Used with permission from Rubin P. *Clinical Oncology.* 7th ed. Philadelphia: WB Saunders; 1993:300.

PROGNOSIS AND CANCER SURVIVAL

PROGNOSTIC FACTORS

Clinically significant:

- Extension evaluated at enucleation
- RB gene mutation
- Positive family history of retinoblastoma
- Primary globe-sparing treatment failure
- Greatest linear extent of choroid involved by choroidal tumor invasion*

CANCER STATISTICS AND SURVIVAL

The eye and orbit only account for 2,750 new diagnoses, excluding carcinomas of the eyelids. Deaths attributed to

*Preceding passage from Edge SB, Byrd DR, Compton CC, et al., *AJCC Cancer Staging Manual, 7th edition*. New York, Springer, 2010, p. 566.

ocular malignancy are <10% of the entire group (240). Some of the most elegant proton and three-dimensional conformal radiation stereotactic techniques allow for cure of choroidal melanomas and retinoblastoma with preservation of vision, the majority with eye preservation (Table 58.5). Survival remains impressive; 90% achieve long-term survival.

- Retinoblastomas are highly curable; with radiation, >90% local tumor control is achieved with vision conservation. Those that relapse can still be cured by enucleation.

- In Africa and Asia, retinoblastoma is the most common primary intraocular malignancy.

TABLE 58.5 Visual Preservation Following External Beam Irradiation: Selected Series Reese-Ellsworth Group

Author	Year	I	II	III	IV	V
Cassady	1969	84%	67%	69%	30%	66%
Egbert	1978	88%	60%	67%	0%	33%
Schipper	1985	100%	100%	83%	79%	0%
Foote	1989	100%	100%	85%	50%	53%
Amendola	1990	100%	83%	100%	67%	50%
Buckley	1992	—	—	100%	100%	100%
Fontanesi	1995	100%	67%	67%	100%	57%
Fontanesi	1996	75%	100%	50%	100%	43%
Toma	1995	78%	67%	64%	100%	—
Blach	1996	67%	67%	67%	44%	44%
Pradhan	1997	86%	100%	50%	50%	54%
Scott	1999	—	—	—	—	54%
Merchant	2002	—	95%	—	66%	—

HISTOGENESIS AND HISTOPATHOLOGY

Orbital sarcomas are mesenchymal malignancies and can range from rhabdomyosarcomas, to fibrosarcomas, and to angiosarcomas. Rhabdomyosarcomas are malignant tumors with characteristics of striated muscle differentiation that occur in young adults and children (Fig. 59.3A, B). There are four subtypes: embryoid, alveolar, pleomorphic, and botryoid (Table 59.3A).

TABLE 59.3A	Histology-specific Sarcoma Differentiation Score

Histologic Type	Score
Atypical lipomatous tumor/ well-differentiated liposarcoma	1
Myxoid liposarcoma	2
Round cell liposarcoma	3
Pleomorphic liposarcoma	3
Dedifferentiated liposarcoma	3
Fibrosarcoma	2
Myxofibrosarcoma [myxoid malignant fibrous histiocytoma (MFH)]	2
Typical storiform MFH (sarcoma, NOS)	2
MFH, pleomorphic type (patternless pleomorphic sarcoma)	3
Giant cell and inflammatory MFH (pleomorphic sarcoma, NOS with giant cells or inflammatory cells)	3
Well-differentiated leiomyosarcoma	1
Conventional leiomyosarcoma	2
Poorly differentiated/pleomorphic/ epithelioid leiomyosarcoma	3
Poorly differentiated synovial sarcoma	3
Pleomorphic rhabdomyosarcoma	3
Mesenchymal chondrosarcoma	3
Extraskeletal osteosarcoma	3
Ewing sarcoma/primitive neuroectodermal tumor	3
Malignant rhabdoid tumor	3
Undifferentiated sarcoma	3

Grading of malignant peripheral nerve sheath tumor, embryonal and alveolar rhabdomyosarcoma, angiosarcoma, extraskeletal myxoid chondrosarcoma, alveolar soft part sarcoma, clear cell sarcoma, and epithelioid sarcoma is not recommended under this system.
(Edge SB, Byrd DR, Compton CC, et al., *AJCC Cancer Staging Manual*, *7th ed*. New York: Springer, 2010, Table 28.1, p. 24).
Modified from Guillou L, Coindre JM, Bonichon F, et al. Comparative study of the National Cancer Institute and French Federation of Cancer Centers Sarcoma Group grading systems in a population of 410 adult patients with soft tissue sarcoma. *J Clin Oncol*. 1997;15:350–362, with permission.

Non-Hodgkin's lymphomas are highly varied as well and refer to a spectrum of T and B cell lymphomas that can occur (Table 59.3B, Fig. 59.3C). Typically, ocular adnexal lymphomas (OALs) are mainly B cell lymphomas of mucosa-associated lymphatic tissue type and more rarely T/NK cell lymphomas.

The embryogenesis determines the histogenesis, and in the orbit there are mainly mesodermal mesenchymal-derived tissues, each of which can give rise to a wide spectrum of malignancies. Prominent in retro-orbital tissues are the extraocular muscles, adipose tissue, peripheral nerves, connective tissues, fascia, lymphatics and lymphoid cells, retinal artery, and veins.

The major sarcomas that can arise are soft tissue sarcomas (refer to Chapter 52).

The proposed TNM classification of OALs defines the anatomic extent of disease in greater detail. This has been considered a prognostic value in the literature. Similar to nodal lymphomas, the International Prognostic Index (IPI) should be applied to subdivide patients with primary diffuse large B cell lymphomas of the ocular adnexa according to prognosis, thereby enhancing individual patient care. Similarly, the Follicular Lymphoma International Prognostic Index (FLIPI), which includes age, Ann Arbor stage, number of nodal sites, serum lactate dehydrogenase level, and hemoglobin level to build a three-category index, should be applied in patients with primary ocular adnexal follicular lymphomas.

The major lymphomas that can occur are listed in Table 59.3B.

The major malignant primary epithelial tumors are shown in Table 59.C.

TABLE 59.3B	Histopathologic Type: Lymphomas

The lymphomas arising as primary tumors in the ocular adnexa are subtyped according to the World Health Organization lymphoma classification. The main ocular adnexal lymphoma subtypes include the following:

Extranodal marginal zone B cell lymphoma (MALT lymphoma)

Diffuse large B cell lymphoma

Follicular lymphoma

Mantle cell lymphoma

Lymphoplasmacytic lymphoma

Plasmacytoma

Burkitt lymphoma

Peripheral T cell lymphoma, unspecified

Mycosis fungoides

Extranodal NK/T cell lymphoma, nasal type

Anaplastic large-cell lymphoma

(Edge SB, Byrd DR, Compton CC, et al., *AJCC Cancer Staging Manual*, *7th ed*. New York: Springer, 2010, p. 585).

Alveolar Rhabdomyosarcoma

This neoplasm occurs less frequently than the embryonal type and principally affects persons between ages 10 and 25 years; rarely, it may be seen in elderly patients. It is most common in the upper and lower extremities, but it can also be distributed in the same sites as the embryonal type. Typically, club-shaped tumor cells are arranged in clumps that are outlined by fibrous septa. The loose arrangement of the cells in the center of the clusters leads to the "alveolar" pattern (see Fig. 59.3B). The tumor cells exhibit intense eosinophilia, and occasional multinucleated giant cells are identified. Malignant rhabdomyoblasts, recognizable by their cross-striations, occur less commonly in the alveolar variant than in embryonal rhabdomyosarcoma, being present in only 25% of cases. Most alveolar rhabdomyosarcomas express *PAX3–FKHR* or *PAX7–FKHR* gene fusions, resulting from t(2;13)(q35;q14) or t(1;13)(p36;q14) translocations, respectively. In patients with localized tumors, the type of fusion does not correlate with the clinical outcome. However, in the presence of metastatic disease, *PAX3–FKHR*-positive tumors have a worse prognosis than do *PAX7–FKHR*-positive ones.

Pleomorphic Rhabdomyosarcoma

The least common form of rhabdomyosarcoma is found in the skeletal muscles of older persons, often in the thigh. This tumor differs from the other types of rhabdomyosarcoma in the pleomorphism of its irregularly arranged cells and can be categorized as one type of adult pleomorphic spindle cell sarcoma. Large, granular, eosinophilic rhabdomyoblasts, together with multinucleated giant cells, are common. Cross-striations are virtually nonexistent.

The historically dismal prognosis associated with most rhabdomyosarcomas has improved in the last two decades as a result of the introduction of combined therapeutic modalities, including surgery, radiation therapy, and chemotherapy. Today, more than 80% of patients with localized or regional disease are cured. Factors indicating a worse prognosis include age older than 10 years, tumor size greater than 5 cm, alveolar and pleomorphic histologic subtypes, and advanced stage of disease.

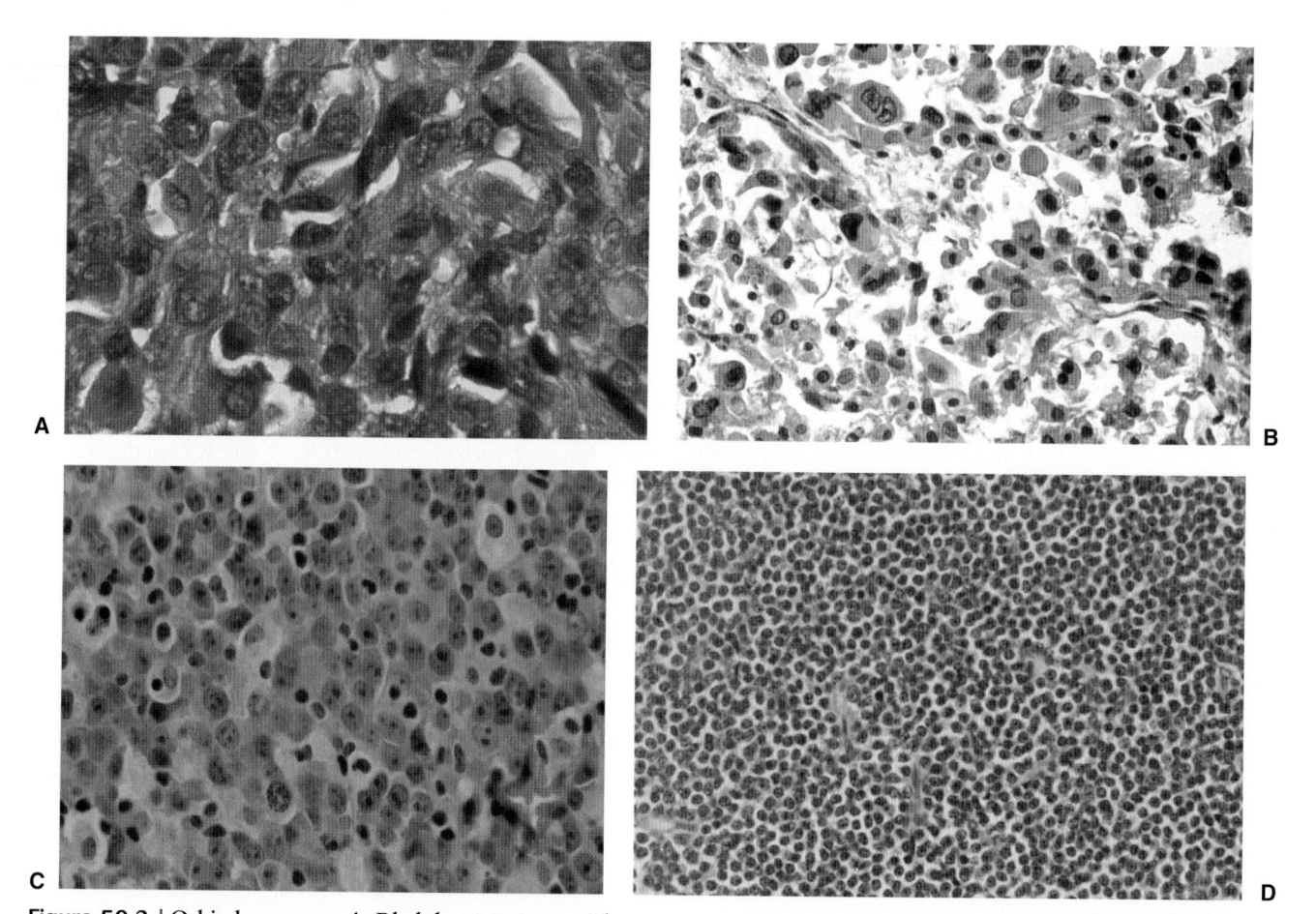

Figure 59.3 | Orbital sarcomas. A. Rhabdomyosarcoma. The tumor contains polyhedral and spindle-shaped tumor cells with enlarged, hyperchromatic nuclei and deeply eosinophilic cytoplasm. A few cells have clearly visible cross striations. **B. Alveolar rhabdomyosarcoma.** The neoplastic cells are arranged in clusters that display an alveolar pattern. **C. Diffuse large B cell lymphoma.** Tumor cells show prominent nucleoli. **D. Small lymphocytic lymphoma/leukemia.** On microscopic examination, the lymph nodal architecture is replaced by a diffuse infiltration of normal-appearing small lymphocytes. *(continued)*

TNM STAGING CRITERIA

TNM STAGING CRITERIA

Lacrimal gland cancers remain confined to the gland: T1, <2.5 cm; T2, <5 cm, but with extraglandular invasion; T3, in periosteum; and T4, into orbital soft tissues, optic nerve, globe, and brain (Table 59.3C).

Sarcomas of the orbit have minimal change in the seventh edition of the *AJCC Cancer Staging Manual* (Fig. 59.4A).

The embryonal RMS can invade the orbit and progress to involve the globe, optic nerve, and even bone (Fig. 59.4C). However, size is the dominant criterion in the staging system: early with T1, <15 mm; T2, >15 mm; T3, limited invasion of orbital tissue and bone wall; and T4, extensive invasion into the globe and periorbital tissues, central nervous system, and brain (Fig. 59.3C).

Lymphomas of the orbit are entirely new for the eye and are referred to as ocular adnexal lymphomas because they can arise in various regions of the eye and orbit—anteriorly in conjunctiva, lacrimal gland, and nasolacrimal duct or in the retro-orbital area behind the eye globe. OALs have a separate staging system as primary sites of origin, and this is not recommended for secondary adnexal involvement of the eye in a disseminated lymphoma. The basic features emphasize anterior–posterior origin and spread for T1 and T3 and juxtaorbital spread into adjacent structures for T4.

Lymphomas do not arise in the eye interior because the eye is immunologically a privileged site and has no lymphatic drainage (Fig. 59.4B).

SUMMARY OF CHANGES SEVENTH EDITION AJCC

- A listing of site-specific categories is now included in T4.
- The anatomy description was expanded.
- Regional lymph nodes were defined.

Carcinoma of the Lacrimal Gland

The staging system for lacrimal gland carcinomas has been made consistent with that for salivary gland carcinomas by:

- Proposing changes in the size cutoffs between T1, T2, and T3
- By subdividing T4
- By expanding the histologic categories to those used for salivary gland malignancies, since all of these have been reported in the lacrimal gland
- Lacrimal sac tumors have been removed from this section.

Although each of the tumors has T and N categories, none are stage grouped.

TABLE 59.3C	Histopathologic Type: Lacrimal Gland

Low Grade

Carcinomas ex pleomorphic adenoma [where the carcinoma is noninvasive or minimally invasive as defined by the World Health Organization (WHO) classification (extension <1.5 mm, beyond the capsule into surrounding tissue)]

Polymorphous low-grade carcinoma

Mucoepidermoid carcinoma, grades 1 and 2

Epithelial-myoepithelial carcinoma

Cystadenocarcinoma and papillary cystadenocarcinoma

Acinic cell carcinoma

Basal cell carcinoma

Mucinous adenocarcinoma

High Grade

Carcinoma ex pleomorphic adenoma (malignant mixed tumor) that includes adenocarcinoma and adenoid cystic carcinoma arising in a pleomorphic adenoma [where the carcinoma is invasive as defined by the WHO classification (extension >1.5 mm beyond the capsule, into surrounding tissue)]

Adenoid cystic carcinoma, not otherwise specified

Adenoidcarcinoma, not otherwise specified

Mucoepidermoid carcinoma, grade 3

Ductal adenocarcinoma

Squamous cell carcinoma

Sebaceous adenocarcinoma

Myoepithelial carcinoma

Lymphoepithelial carcinoma

Other Rare and Unclassifiable Carcinomas

(Edge SB, Byrd DR, Compton CC, et al., *AJCC Cancer Staging Manual, 7th ed.* New York: Springer, 2010, p. 571).

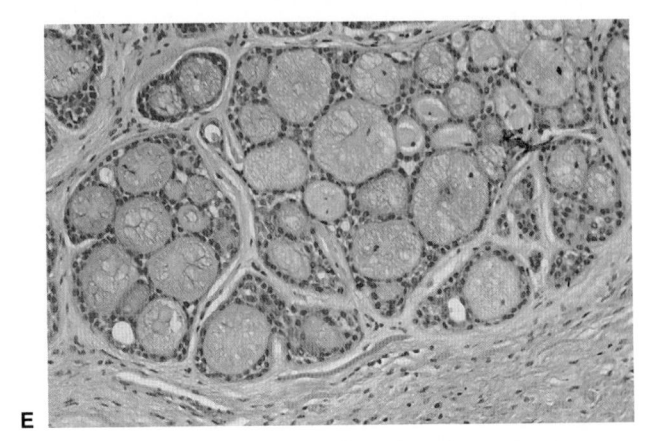

E

Figure 59.3 | *(Continued)* **E. Adenoid cystic carcinoma** showing cribriform growth in which cystlike spaces are filled with basophilic material. The cyst spaces are really pseudocysts surrounded by myoepithelial cells.

LACRIMAL GLAND ADENOCARCINOMA

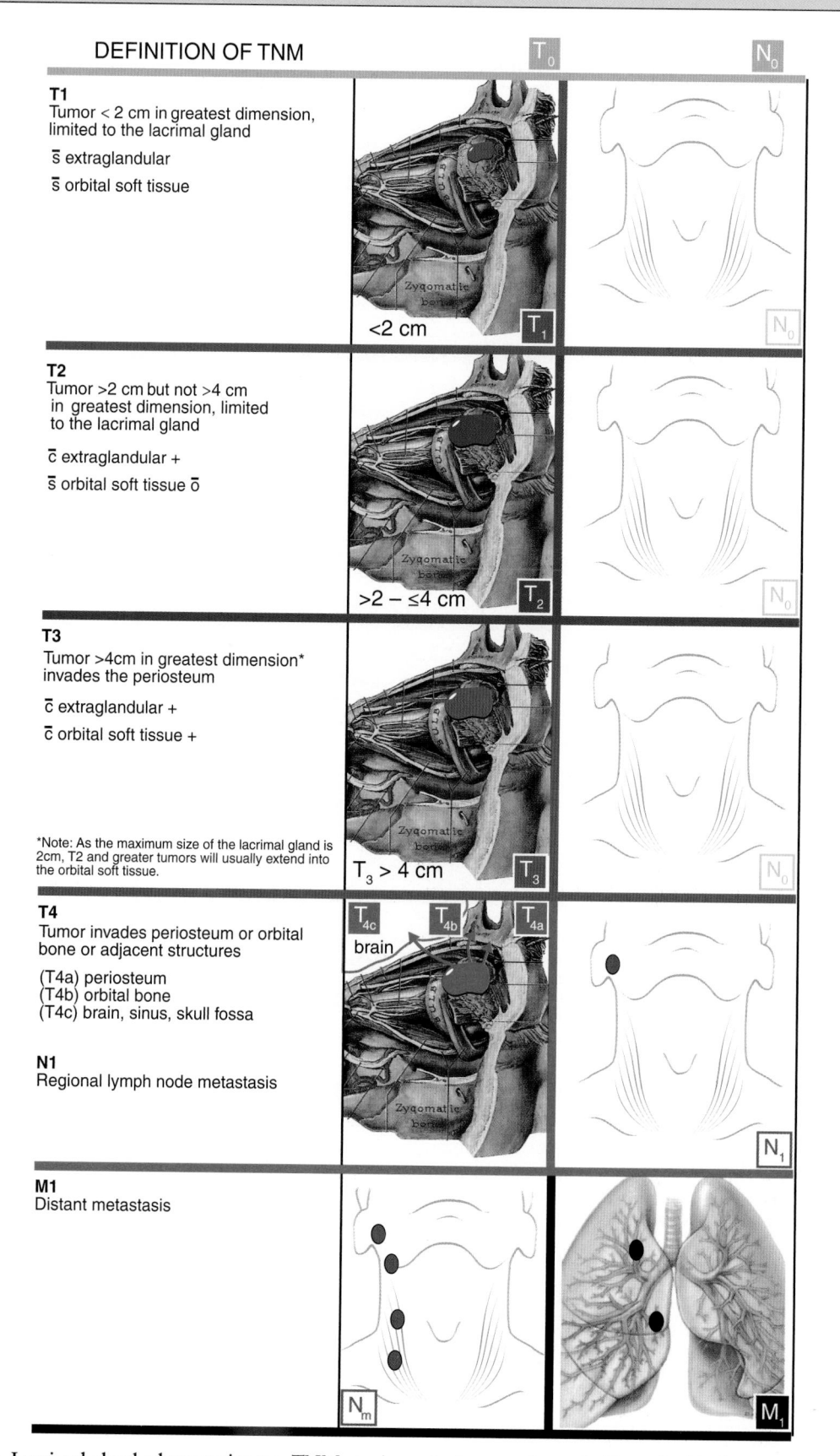

DEFINITION OF TNM

T1
Tumor < 2 cm in greatest dimension, limited to the lacrimal gland

s̄ extraglandular

s̄ orbital soft tissue

T2
Tumor >2 cm but not >4 cm in greatest dimension, limited to the lacrimal gland

c̄ extraglandular +

s̄ orbital soft tissue ō

T3
Tumor >4cm in greatest dimension* invades the periosteum

c̄ extraglandular +

c̄ orbital soft tissue +

*Note: As the maximum size of the lacrimal gland is 2cm, T2 and greater tumors will usually extend into the orbital soft tissue.

T4
Tumor invades periosteum or orbital bone or adjacent structures

(T4a) periosteum
(T4b) orbital bone
(T4c) brain, sinus, skull fossa

N1
Regional lymph node metastasis

M1
Distant metastasis

Figure 59.4 | A. Lacrimal gland adenocarcinoma. TNM staging criteria are color coded bars for T advancement: Tis, yellow; T1, green; T2, blue; T3, purple; T4, red. *(continued)*

ORBITAL SARCOMA

DEFINITION OF TNM

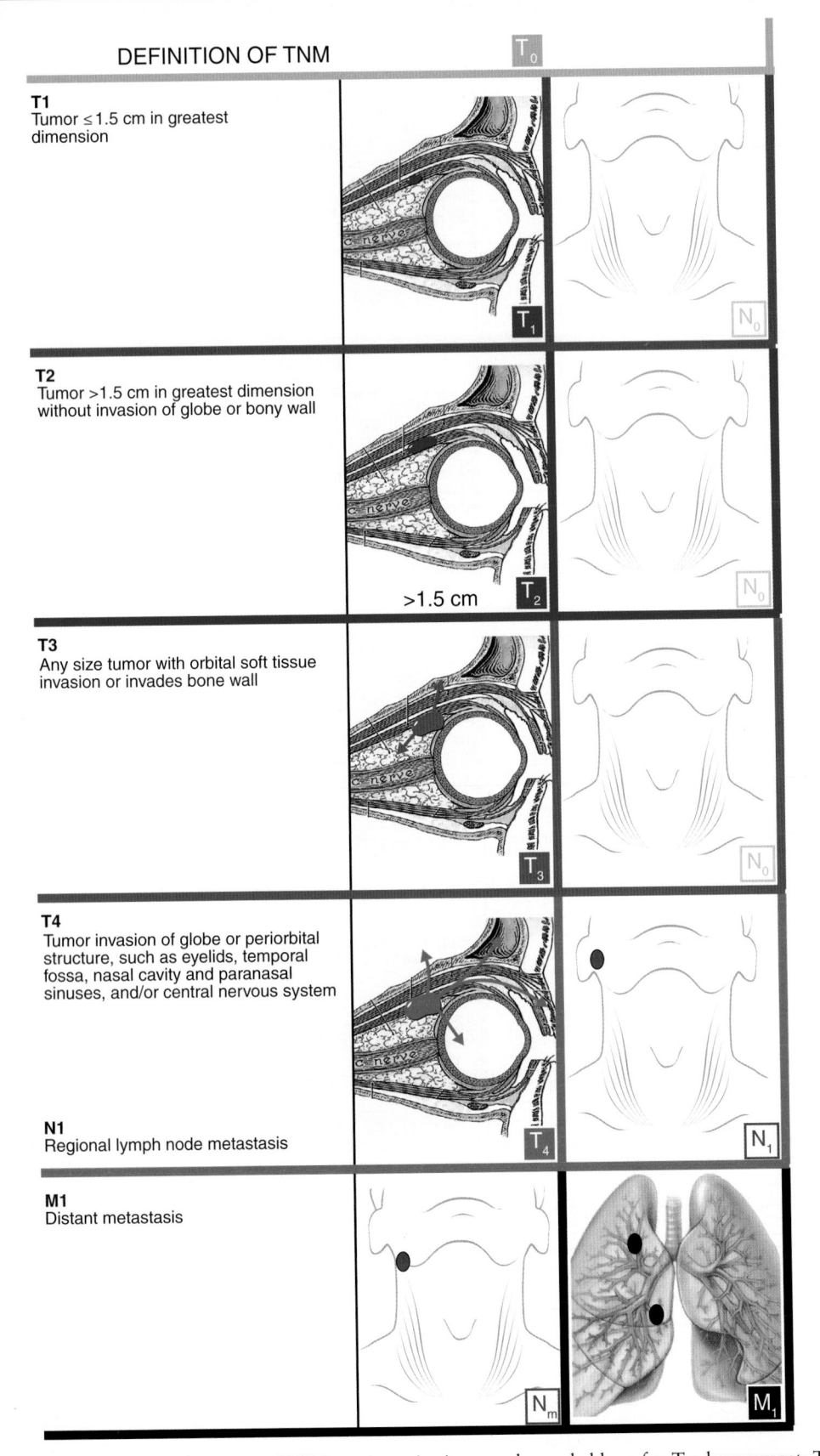

T1
Tumor ≤1.5 cm in greatest dimension

T2
Tumor >1.5 cm in greatest dimension without invasion of globe or bony wall

T3
Any size tumor with orbital soft tissue invasion or invades bone wall

T4
Tumor invasion of globe or periorbital structure, such as eyelids, temporal fossa, nasal cavity and paranasal sinuses, and/or central nervous system

N1
Regional lymph node metastasis

M1
Distant metastasis

Figure 59.4 | *(Continued)* **B. Orbital sarcoma.** TNM staging criteria are color coded bars for T advancement: Tis, yellow; T1, green; T2, blue; T3, purple; T4, red. *(continued)*

ORBITAL LYMPHOMA

DEFINITION OF TNM

T1 Conjunctiva

T1a Bulbar conjunctiva only

T1b Papebral conjunctiva
± fornix ± caruncle

T1c extensive conjunctival involvement

N0
No evidence of lymph node involvement

T2 Orbital ± conjunctiva

T2a anterior orbital ± conjunctiva

T2b anterior orbital ± conjunctiva
+ lacrimal gland

T2c posterior orbital ± conjunctiva
± anterior
± extraocular muscle

T2d + nasolacrimal drainage system
involvement ± conjunctiva

N1
Involvement of ipsilateral regional lymph
nodes*

T3

Lymphoma with preseptal eyelid
involvement (defined above)16
± orbital involvement ± any conjunctival
involvement

N2

Involvement of contra lateral or bilateral
regional lymph nodes*

T4
Orbital adnexal lymphoma extending
beyond orbit to adjacent structures such
as bone and brain
T4a Involvement of nasopharynx
T4b Osseous involvement (including
periosteum)
T4c Involvement of maxillofacial,
ethmoidal, and/or frontal sinuses
T4d Intracranial spread

N3
Involvement of peripheral lymph nodes
not draining ocular adnexal region

M1a
Noncontiguous involvement of tissues of
organs external to the ocular adnexa (e.g.,
parotid glands, submandibular gland, lung,
liver, spleen, kidney, breast, etc.)

M1b Lymphomatous involvement of the
bone marrow

M1c Both M1a and M1b involvement

N4
Involvement of central lymph nodes

*Note: The regional lymph nodes include
preauricular (parotid), submandibular, and
cervical.

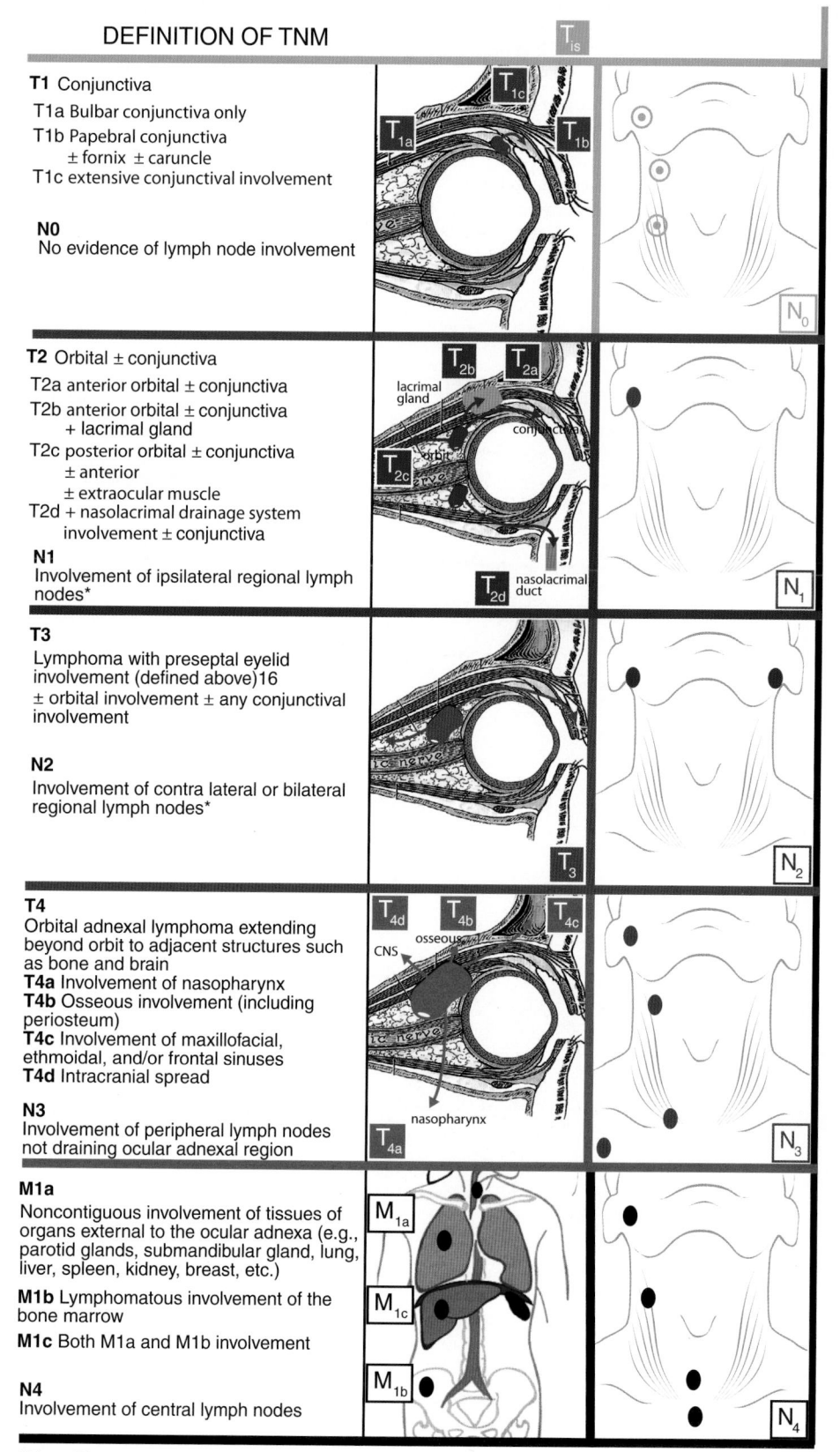

Figure 59.4 | *(Continued)* **C. Orbital lymphoma.** TNM staging criteria are color coded bars for T advancement: Tis, yellow; T1, green; T2, blue; T3, purple; T4, red.

TNM STAGING CRITERIA

T-ONCOANATOMY

The isocenter of the bony wall of the orbit, the eye socket, is through the optic nerve exiting at the optic foramen in its posterior wall. The orbital content anteriorly is the location of the lacrimal gland on its superior lateral wall.

- *Coronal*: The true content is posterior to the globe, with the extraocular muscles and their innervation by cranial nerves III, IV, and VI, which enter through the medially placed

optic nerve, as well as cranial nerve V and the nasociliary nerve (Fig. 59.5A).

- *Sagittal*: The extraocular muscles (EOM) and fat are appreciated in relation to the bony eye socket (Fig. 59.5B) and EOM function (Fig. 59.5D, Table 59.4).

- *Axial*: This provides the medial entry of cranial nerves, particularly the optic nerve, which offer access to the subarachnoid space and accounts of blurring of the optic disc when intracranial metastatic disease occurs. Note the lateral superior location of the lacrimal gland (Fig. 59.5C).

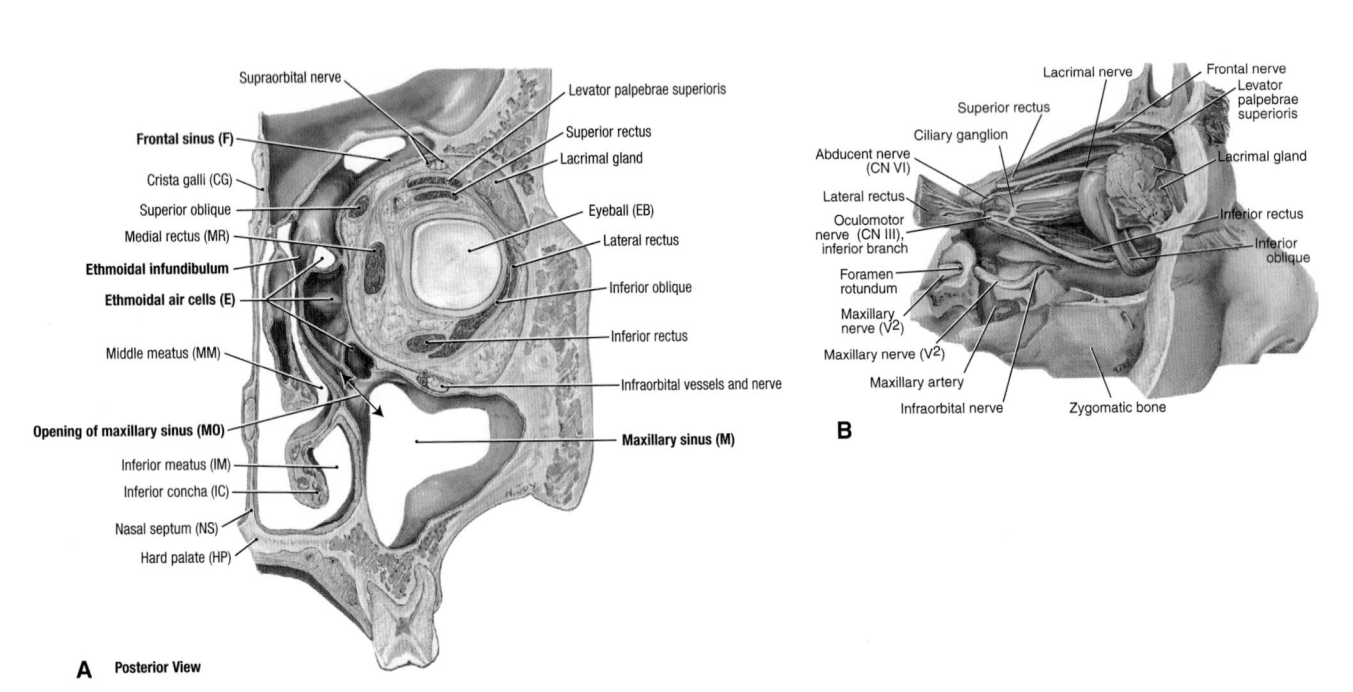

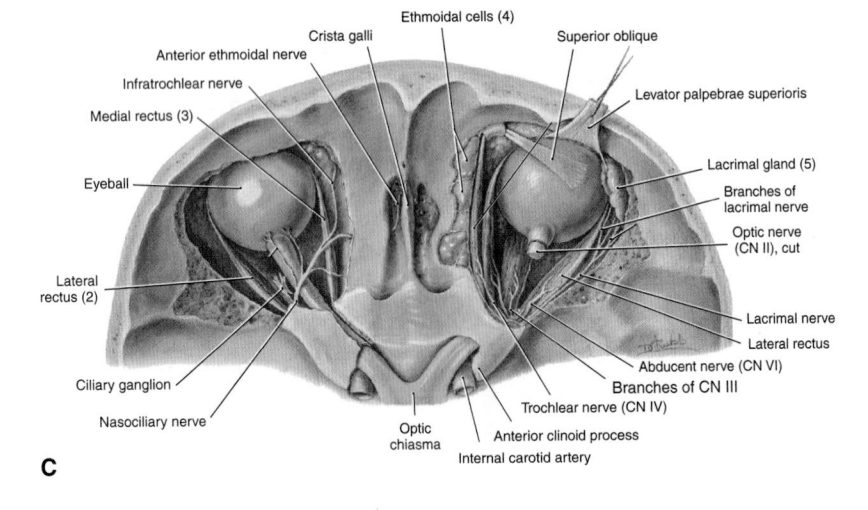

Figure 59.5 | T-oncoanatomy. A. Coronal. This coronal view shows the important relationships between the paranasal sinuses and the orbit. The frontal sinus is superior, the ethmoid sinus is medial, and the maxillary antrum is inferior and extends posteriorly. This is the most common site of sinus cancers, and, when invading superiorly, there is perineural invasion of infraorbital nerve. A focus of hypesthesia develops in the cheek below the eye. B. Sagittal. C. Axial.

- **Extraocular Muscles** are often impaired with orbital malignancies causing strabismus and proptosis.

Movement from the primary position always involves more than one muscle acting synergistically. When testing muscles, it is desirable to test actions produced by one muscle acting independently. Because the axes of the orbits diverge and do not correspond to the axis of gaze in the primary position, responsibility for elevation and depression changes with abduction and adduction. When the eye is adducted, the oblique muscles are solely responsible; when the eye is abducted, the rectus muscles are solely responsible.

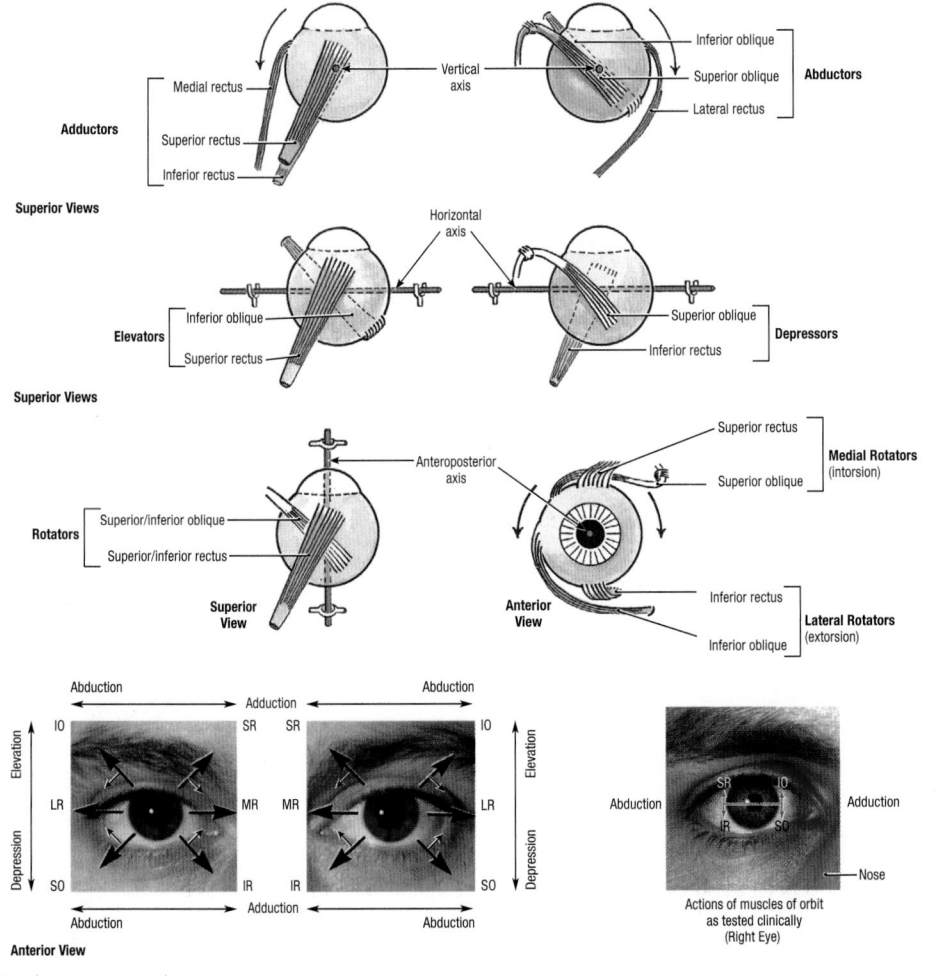

Figure 59.5D | Muscle groups and eye movement.

TABLE 59.4	Actions of Muscles of the Orbit Starting from Primary Position[a]		
	Main Action		
Muscle	**Vertical Axis (A)**	**Horizontal Axis (B)**	**Anteroposterior Axis (C)**
Superior rectus (SR)	Elevates	Adducts	Rotates medially (intorsion)
Inferior rectus (IR)	Depresses	Adducts	Rotates laterally (extorsion)
Superior oblique (SO)	Depresses	Abducts	Rotates medially (intorsion)
Inferior oblique (IO)	Elevates	Abducts	Rotates laterally (extorsion)
Medial rectus (MR)	N/A	Adducts	N/A
Lateral rectus (LR)	N/A	Abducts	N/A

[a]Primary position, gaze directed anteriorly.

N-ONCOANATOMY AND M-ONCOANATOMY

N-ONCOANATOMY

The orbit and lacrimal glands drain predominantly into the preauricular nodes, except for its medial margin, which follows medial lymphatics into the submandibular nodes (Fig. 59.6A, B; Table 59.5). The most likely sentinel node is the preauricular node and can be determined with ^{99m}Tc lymphoscintography. Once lymphatic spread occurs, the superficial ring of nodes is at risk, including occipital, mastoid, parotid, and submandibular nodes. When orbital tumors invading into paranasal sinuses are ethmoid or extending into nasopharynx, the retropharyngeal are at risk. This places the deep cervical jugular nodes at risk. The incidence of lymph node involvement for orbital rhabomyosarcomas compared to other head and neck sites, is 0–8%; for other body sites, the incidence ranges between 10–25%.

TABLE 59.5	Orbital Tumors: Sentinel and Regional Nodes	
	Sentinel	**Regional**
Sarcoma orbit	Preauricular Facial node	Superficial cervical Deep cervical
Lymphoma	Preauricular Facial node Rouvière's	Superficial cervical Parotid gland nodes Deep cervical
Lacrimal Gland	Preauricular Facial node	Submandibular Superficial cervical Preauricular

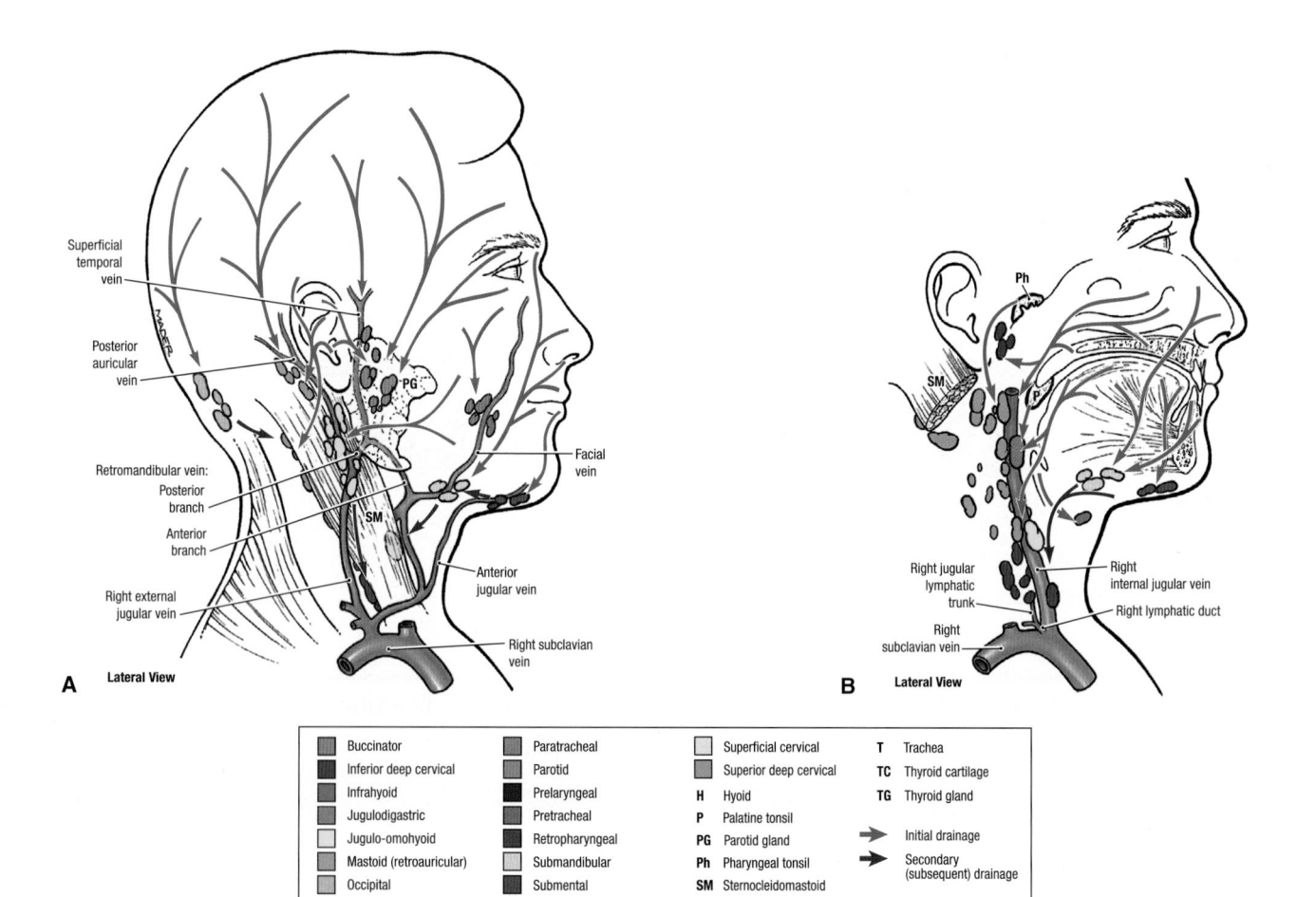

Buccinator	Paratracheal	Superficial cervical	**T** Trachea
Inferior deep cervical	Parotid	Superior deep cervical	**TC** Thyroid cartilage
Infrahyoid	Prelaryngeal	**H** Hyoid	**TG** Thyroid gland
Jugulodigastric	Pretracheal	**P** Palatine tonsil	
Jugulo-omohyoid	Retropharyngeal	**PG** Parotid gland	Initial drainage
Mastoid (retroauricular)	Submandibular	**Ph** Pharyngeal tonsil	Secondary (subsequent) drainage
Occipital	Submental	**SM** Sternocleidomastoid	

Figure 59.6 | A. Superficial cervical lymph node. B. Deep cervical lymph node. *(continued)*

M-ONCOANATOMY

The orbital plexus of veins drain into 3 different veins: (1) Lacrimal gland drains into the supra-orbital vein, then the facial vein (2) the orbit drains via the superior and inferior ophthalmic veins into the cavernous sinus and also (3) the pterygoid venous plexus into the internal jugular vein. Eventually the lung is the target organ for metastases (Fig. 59.6C).

CRANIAL NERVE ONCOANATOMY

The frequency of cranial nerve involvement in orbital malignancies supports the need to be aware of the cranial nerve oncoanatomy. Equally important are tumors that can invade the orbit from surrounding anatomic sites and present with neurologic impairments (Fig. 59.6D; Table 59.6). Nasopharyngeal carcinomas can invade cavernous sinus via foramen lacerum and involve CN VI, IV, and III in that order.

TABLE 59.6	Oculomotor (CN III), Trochlear (CN IV), and Abducent (CN VI) Nerves[a]			
Nerve	Functional Components	Cells of Origin/ Termination	Cranial Exit	Distribution and Functions
Oculomotor	Somatic motor	Oculomotor nucleus		Motor to superior, inferior, and medial recti, inferior oblique, and levator palpebrae superioris muscles; raises upper eyelid; rotates eyeball superiorly, inferiorly, and medially
	Visceral motor (parasympathetic)	Presynaptic: midbrain (Edinger-Westphal nucleus); Postsynaptic: ciliary ganglion	Superior orbital fissure	Motor to sphincter pupillae and ciliary muscle that constrict pupil and accommodate lens of eyeball
Trochlear	Somatic motor	Trochlear nucleus		Motor to superior oblique that assists in rotating eyeball inferolaterally
Abducent	Somatic motor	Abducent nucleus		Motor to lateral rectus that rotates eyeball laterally

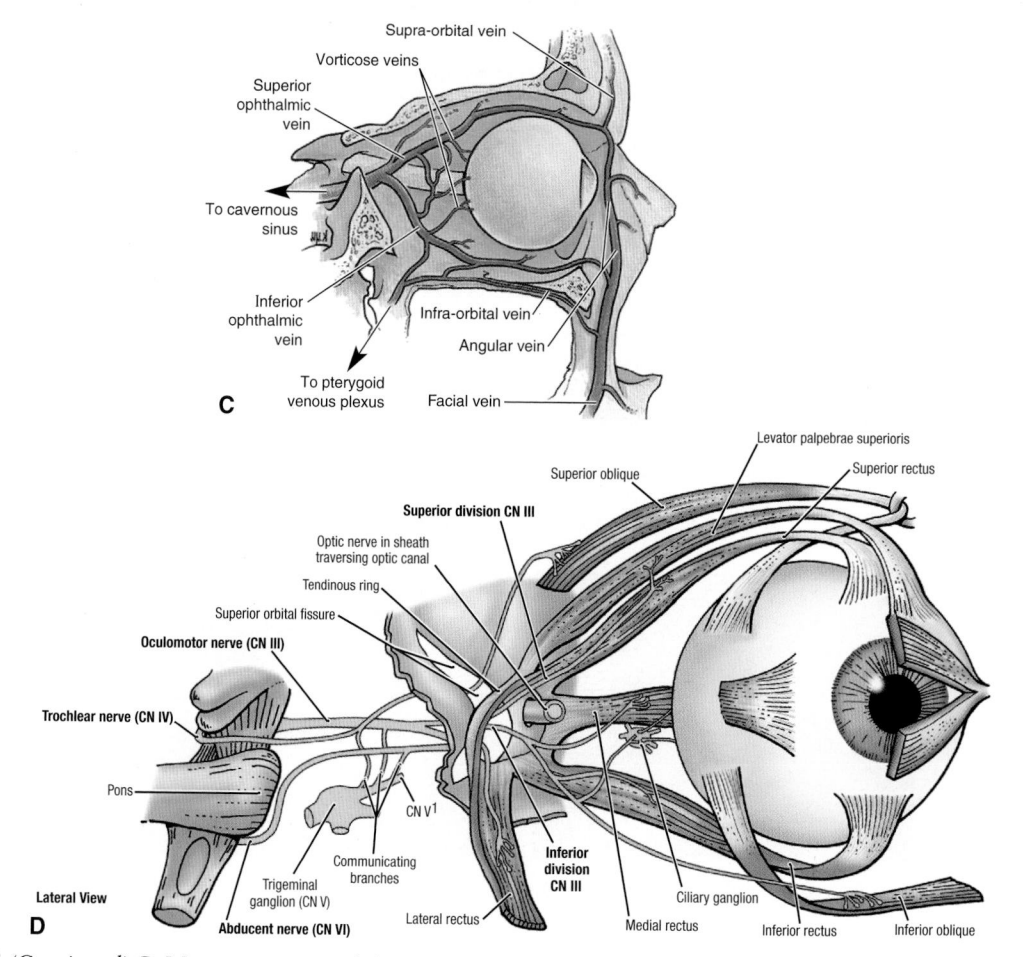

Figure 59.6 | *(Continued)* **C.** M-oncoanatomy of the eye. The orbital vein drains into the cavernous sinus posteriorly or the facial vein anteriorly. **D.** Major cranial nerves (CN) of eye and muscles CN activate.

STAGING WORKUP

RULES FOR CLASSIFICATION AND STAGING

Clinical Staging and Imaging

Careful examination is undertaken, preferably under anesthesia if deep in orbit. Imaging is essential to determine whether the orbital mass is primary or metastatic. Cross-sectional imaging such as enhanced computed tomography and magnetic resonance imaging is worthwhile (Fig. 59.7). Ultrasound-guided biopsy deserves consideration (Table 59.7; Fig. 59.7).

Pathologic Staging

For lacrimal gland cancer resections, complete specimen should be studied for margins. Perineural and sentinel preauricular/parotid node evaluation needs to be recorded if positive.

TABLE 59.7	Imaging Modalities: Eye and Orbit	
Method	Diagnosis and Staging Capability	Recommended for Use
CT	Provides excellent anatomic detail of globe, orbital content, and bony orbit; can distinguish smooth, round cysts from infiltrative tumors versus pseudotumors and detect bone destruction and sinus invasion	Yes
Primary tumor ultrasonography and fine-needle aspiration biopsy	A and B scans can be used to screen intraocular and orbital tumors and cysts, especially melanomas	No
MRI	Provides excellent three-dimensional view, orbital fat hyperintense and vitreous hypointense in tumor (T1) and reverse in T2; can detect tumors versus pseudotumors and cysts; may be superior for diagnosis of vascular lesions, demyelinating disease	Yes
Endoscopy	Orbital endoscopy with fiber-optic lights is used in conjunction with CT and/or MRI for obtaining core biopsy	Yes, when indicated
Standard orbital view	Useful for assessing optic nerve foramen and supraorbital fissure, but supplanted by CT; can detect intraocular calcification	No
Orbital phlebography	Venography particularly useful for detecting orbital varices, but is less efficient and more invasive than CT	No
Carotid angiography	Useful in diagnosis of vascularized tumors and aneurysms, but replaced by CT/MRI	No
Fluorescein angiography	Sometimes used in diagnosis of ocular melanoma	No
Biopsy	Usually an incisional or excisional biopsy is indicated to confirm malignant versus pseudotumors; directed stereotactically by CT/MRI; contraindicated for melanomas owing to high risk of seeding	Yes, if indicated

CT, computed tomography; MRI, magnetic resonance imaging.
Used with permission from Rubin P. *Clinical Oncology.* 7th ed. Philadelphia: WB Saunders; 1993:300.

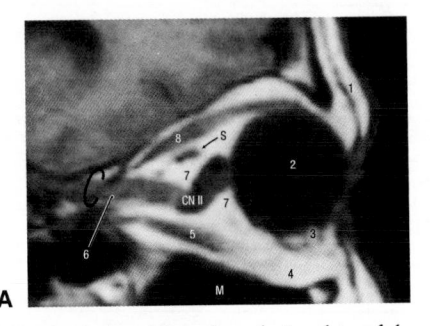 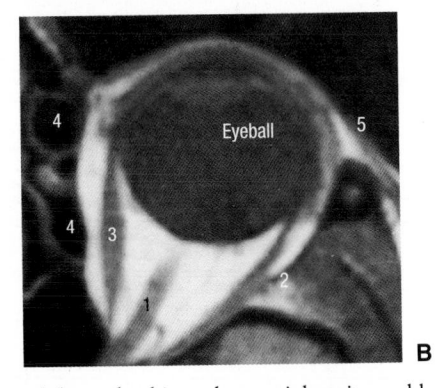

Figure 59.7 | Orbit A. Sagittal view. Note the relationship of the eye globe and orbit to the cranial cavity and brain and the optic nerve chiasm. 1. Orbicularis oculi, 2. Eyeball, 3. Inferior Oblique Muscle, 4. Extracoronal Fat, 5. Interior Rectus Muscle, 6. Dural and Arachnoid Sheath, 7. Retrobulbar Fat, 8. Superior Rectus Muscle, M. Maxillary Sinus. **B.** Axial transverse view. Note the relationship of extraocular muscles in the orbit. 1. Optic Nerve, 2. The Lateral Rectus Muscle, 3. The Medial Rectus Muscle, 4. The Ethmoid Sinus, 5. Lacrimal Gland.

PROGNOSIS AND CANCER SURVIVAL

PROGNOSTIC FACTORS

Lacrimal Gland Prognostic Factors

Required for staging: none.
Clinically significant:
Ki-67 growth fraction
Nuclear nm23 staining

Sarcomas

Required for staging: none.
Clinically significant: none.

Lymphomas

Clinically significant:
Tumor cell growth fraction (Ki-67, MIB-1)
Serum lactate dehydrogenase (LDH) at diagnosis
History of rheumatoid arthritis
History of Sjögren's syndrome
History of connective tissue disease
History of recurrent dry eyes syndrome (sicca syndrome)
Any evidence of a viral infection (e.g., hepatitis C or HIV)
Any evidence of a bacterial infection (e.g., *Helicobacter pylori*)
Any evidence of an infection caused by other microorganisms (e.g., *Chlamydia psittaci*).*

CANCER STATISTICS AND SURVIVAL

The eye and orbit only account for 2,090 new diagnoses, excluding carcinomas of the eyelids. Deaths attributed to ocular malignancy are <10% of the entire group (<200 patients/year). Some of the most elegant proton and three-dimensional conformational radiation stereotactic techniques allow for cure of choroidal melanomas and retinoblastoma with preservation of vision. Survival remains impressive; 90% achieve long-term survival (Fig. 59.8).

*Preceding passage from Edge SB, Byrd DR, Compton CC, et al., *AJCC Cancer Staging Manual, 7th ed.* New York: Springer, 2010, p. 573, 579, 588.

- Optic nerve gliomas are extremely curable by stereotactic radiation therapy. The University of Pittsburgh group reports 96%, 90%, and 90% survival at 5, 10, and 15 years, respectively; 86% retain vision.

- Orbital lymphomas and orbital rhabdomyosarcomas are 100% locally controlled with chemoradiation.

- The most recent IRS (IV) has achieved a 100% successful outcome, compared with 83% in IRS III.

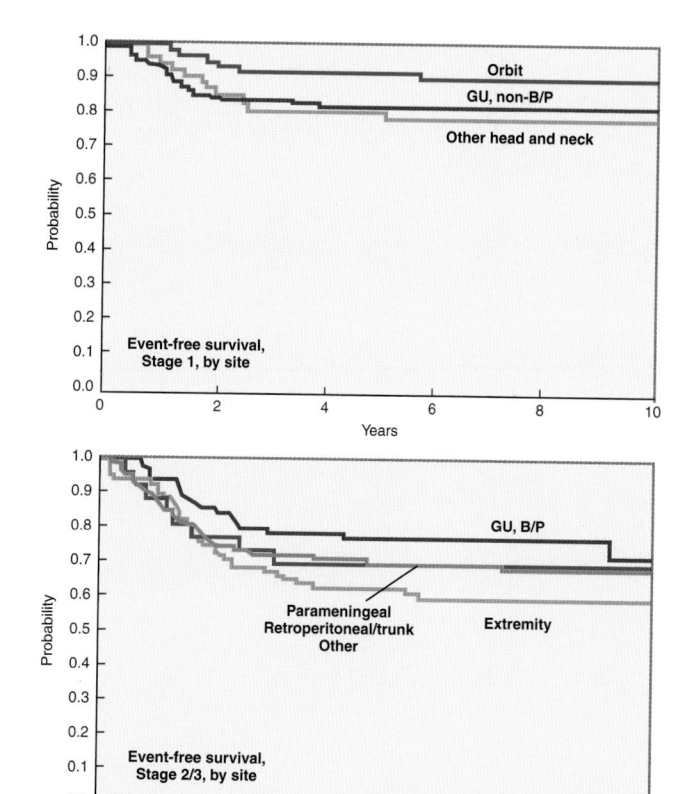

Figure 59.8 | Event-free survival of patients treated on Intergroup Rhabdomyosarcoma Study IV by stage and site. **A.** For patients with nonmetastatic favorable site tumors (stage 1), the best outcome was seen for orbital primary tumors. **B.** For patients with nonmetastatic unfavorable site tumors (stage 2 or 3), the best outcome was for those with genitourinary (bladder-prostate) tumors, whereas those with extremity tumors had an inferior outcome. GU B/P genitourinary tract (bladder or prostate); GU non B/P genitourinary tract (non-bladder, non-prostate).

Appendix A
Recommended Reading and References

The gains in survival and excellence in outcomes are due not only to improvements in each treatment modality, but to the multidisciplinary approach that has been adopted. Goals include eradication of the cancer and conservation of normal tissues, cosmesis with maintenance of physiologic function, and the need to achieve a socially acceptable result. Reference to multi-authored, multidisciplinary oncology textbooks presents the progress detailed in cooperative group clinical trials and the gains in practice due to evidence-based medicine over the past five decades. There are an equal number of single-or dual-authored monographs on upper aerorespiratory and digestive tract cancers.

Perspective and Patterns of Spread

Agur AMR, Dalley AF. *Grant's Atlas of Anatomy*, 12th ed. Philadelphia: Lippincott Williams & Wilkins; 2009.

Ross MH. Histology: A Text and Atlas with Cell and Molecular Biology. 5th ed. Philadelphia: Lippincott Williams & Wilkins; 2010.

American Cancer Society. *Cancer Facts & Figures*. Atlanta: Author; 2011.

Hedinger C. Histological typing of thyroid tumours. In: International Histological Classification of Tumors 2nd ed. New York: Springer; 1988.

Howlader N, Noone AM, Krapcho M, Neyman N, Aminou R, Waldron W, Altekruse SF, Kosary CL, Ruhl J, Tatalovich Z, Cho H, Mariotto A, Eisner MP, Lewis DR, Chen HS, Feuer EJ, Cronin KA, Edwards BK (eds). SEER Cancer Statistics Review, 1975–2008, National Cancer Institute. Bethesda, MD, http://seer.cancer.gov/csr/1975_2008/, based on November 2010 SEER data submission, posted to the SEER web site, 2011.

Histogenesis and Histology

Eroschenko VP. *diFiore's Atlas of Histology with Functional Correlations*. 11th ed. Philadelphia: Lippincott Williams & Wilkins; 2008.

Rubin R, Strayer DS. *Rubin's Pathology: Clinicopathologic Foundations of Medicine*. 5th ed. Philadelphia: Lippincott Williams & Wilkins; 2008.

TNM Staging Criteria

Edge SB, Byrd DR, Compton CC, et al (eds). American Joint Committee on Cancer (AJCC). AJCC Cancer Staging Manual 7th ed. New York: Springer; 2010.

International Union against Cancer (UICC). *TNM Classification of Malignant Tumours*, 7th ed. New York: Wiley-Liss; 2009.

Sobotta. *Atlas of Human Anatomy, Head, Neck, and Upper Limb*. Vol. 1. 14th ed. Philadelphia: Lippincott Williams & Wilkins; 2008.

Tobias MJ. Anatomy of the Human Lymphatic System: A Compendium Translated From the Original "Anatomie des Lymphatiques del' Homme" by H. Rouviere Rearranged for the Use of Students and Practitioners. Ann Arbor: Edward Bros; 1938.

Rules for Classification and Staging (Imaging)

Edge SB, Byrd DR, Compton CC, et al (eds). American Joint Committee on Cancer (AJCC). AJCC Cancer Staging Manual 7th ed. New York: Springer; 2010.

Bragg DG, Rubin P, Hricak H. Oncologic Imaging 2nd ed. Philadelphia: W B Saunders; 2002.

Husband JES, Reznek RH. *Imaging in Oncology* 3rd ed. Informa Healthcare; 2009.

International Union against Cancer (UICC). *TNM Classification of Malignant Tumours*. 7th ed. New York: Wiley-Liss; 2009.

Cancer Statistics and Survival

American Cancer Society: *Cancer Facts & Figures*. Atlanta: Author; 2011.

Berek JS, Hacker NF. *Gynecologic Oncology*. 5th ed. Philadelphia: Lippincott Williams & Wilkins; 2010.

Lin EH, Lozano R. *Cancer-Matrix Manual*. 5th ed. USA: Advanced Medical Publishing, Inc.; 2010.

Aisner J, Arrigada R, Green MR, eds. *Comprehensive Textbook of Thoracic Oncology*. Baltimore: Williams and Wilkins; 1996.

American Cancer Society (ACS). *Cancer Facts & Figures*. Atlanta: Author; 2011.

Ang KK, Garden AS. *Radiotherapy for Head and Neck Cancers: Indications and Techniques*, 4th ed. Philadelphia: Lippincott Williams & Wilkins; 2012.

Bartlett D, Ramanathan R, Deutsch M, Cancer of the Biliary Tree. In DeVita, Jr, VT, Hellman S, Rosenberg SE [eds]: Cancer: Principles and Practice of Oncology. 9th ed. Philadelphia: Lippincott Williams & Wilkins; 2011.

Harris JR, Lippman ME, Osborne KC, Morrow M (eds). *Diseases of the Breast*, 4th ed. Philadelphia: Lippincott Williams & Wilkins; 2009.

HHS/HRSA/OSP/DOT and UNOS. 2009 Annual Report of the U.S. Scientific Registry Transplant Recipients and the Organ Procurement and Transplantation Network: Transplant Data: 1999–2008, 2009. Rockville, MD and Richmond, VA.

Libutti S, Saltz L, Rustgi A, Tepper J. Cancer of the Colon. In DeVita V, Hellman S, Rosenberg SE [eds]: Cancer Principles and Practice of Oncology. 9th ed. Philadelphia: Lippincott Williams & Wilkins; 2011.

Libutti S, Tepper J, Saltz L, Rustgi A. Cancer of the Rectum. In DeVita V, Hellman S, Rosenberg SE[eds]: Cancer

Principles and Practice of Oncology. 9th ed. Philadelphia: Lippincott Williams & Wilkins; 2011.

Pass HI, Carbone DP, Johnson, DH, Minna JD, Scagliotti GV, Turrisi III, AT (eds). Principles and Practice of Lung Cancer: The Official Reference Text of the International Association for the Study of Lung Cancer (IASLC) 4th ed. Philadelphia: Lippincott Williams & Wilkins; 2010.

Halperin EC, Perez CA, Brady LW. *Principles and Practice of Radiation Oncology*, 5th ed. Philadelphia: Lippincott Williams & Wilkins; 2008.

Rubin P. *Clinical Oncology*, 8th ed. New York: Elsevier; 2001.

Wang CC. Radiation Therapy for Head and Neck Neoplasms. 3rd ed. New York, John Wiley, 1996.

Imaging

Atlas SW, Kaplan RT. Pocket Atlas of Cranial Magnetic Resonance Imaging. 2nd ed. Philadelphia: Lippincott Williams & Wilkins; 2001.

Halperin EC, Constine LS, Tarbell NJ, Kun LE. Pediatric Radiation Oncology. 5th ed. Philadelphia: Lippincott Williams & Wilkins; 2011.

Smith MM, Smith TL. *Pocket Atlas of Normal CT Anatomy of the Head and Brain*. 2nd ed. Philadelphia: Lippincott Williams & Wilkins; 2001.

Webb WR, Gotway MB. *Pocket Atlas of Body CT Anatomy*. 2nd ed. Philadelphia: Lippincott Williams & Wilkins; 2002.

Appendix B
Figure and Table Credits

Section 1 (Chapters 1–11)

Modified from

Agur AMR, Dalley AF, eds. *Grant's Atlas of Anatomy*, 12th edition. Philadelphia: Lippincott Williams & Wilkins: 2009. **Figures 1.1, 1.2A, 1.4, 1.5, 1.6, 1.7AB, 1.8, 2.2, 2.4, 2.5, 2.7C, 3.2, 3.3, 3.4, 3.5, 3.6, 3.7C, 3.8, 4.2, 4.3, 4.4, 4.5, 4.6, 4.8, 5.2, 5.3, 5.4, 5.5, 5.6, 6.2, 6.4, 6.5, 6.6, 6.7B, 7.2, 7.3, 7.4, 7.5, 7.6, 8.2, 8.3, 8.4, 8.5, 8.6, 9.2, 9.3, 9.4, 9.5, 9.6, 10.2, 10.3, 10.4, 10.5, 10.6, 11.2, 11.3, 11.4, 11.5, 11.6**

Edge SB, Byrd DR, Compton CC, et al, eds. *AJCC Cancer Staging Manual*, 7th edition. New York: Springer Science and Business Media, LLC. Publishers. Copyright American Joint Committee on Cancer, 2010.
Summary of changes text pages *(page in AJCC 7th edition)* 6 *(21)*, 22 *(69)*, 34 *(69)*, 44 *(41)*, 54 *(29)*, 64 *(79)*, 74 *(41)*, 84 *(41)*, 94 *(57)*, 104 *(57)*, 116 *(87)*

Modified from

Eroschenko VP, ed. *di Fiore's Atlas of Histology with Functional Correlations*, 10th ed. Philadelphia: Lippincott Williams & Wilkins; 2005. **Figure 1.2B-G**

Data from Halperin EC, Perez, CA, Brady, LW, eds: *Perez & Brady's Principles and Practice of Radiation Oncology*, 5th edition. Philadelphia: Lippincott Williams & Wilkins, 2008. **Table 42.3, Figure 1.7C**

Based on Lin EH and Lozano R, *Cancer Matrix Manual*. Madison, WI: Advanced Medical Pub Inc; 5th edition (2010) p. 180, **Table 4.3**

Lufkin: Pocket Alas of Head and Neck MRI Anatomy, Philadelphia: Lippincott Williams & Wilkins, 2000. **Figure 2.8**

Adapted from

Rubin P. *Clinical Oncology: A Multidisciplinary Approach for Physicians and Students*, 8th edition. Philadelphia: W.B. Saunders, 2001:408. **Tables 2.1, 3.1**

Rubin R and Strayer DS: *Rubin's Pathology: Clinicopathologic Foundations of Medicine*, 5th edition. Philadelphia: Lippincott Williams & Wilkins, 2008. **Figures 1.3, 2.1, 2.3B. 3.1, 4.1, 5.1, 6.1, 7.1, 8.1, 9.1, 10.1, 11.1**

Webb WR and Gotway MB. *Pocket Atlas of Body CT Anatomy*, 2nd edition. Philadelphia: Lippincott Williams & Wilkins, 2002. **Figures 1.9, 5.8, 7.8, 8.8, 9.8, 10.8, 11.8**

Section 2 (Chapters 12–21)

Modified from

Agur AMR, Dalley AF, eds. *Grant's Atlas of Anatomy*, 12th edition. Philadelphia: Lippincott Williams & Wilkins: 2009. **Figures 12.1, 12.2, 12.3A, 12.4, 12.5A, 12.6A, 13.2, 13.4, 13.5, 13.6A, 14.2, 14.3, 14.4, 14.5, 15.2, 15.3, 15.4, 15.5, 16.2, 16.3, 16.4, 16.5, 17.2, 17.3, 17.4, 17.5, 18.2, 18.3, 18.4, 18.5, 19.2, 19.3, 19.4, 19.5D, 19.7, 20.2, 20.3, 20.4, 20.5, 20.6, 20.7, 21.2, 21.3, 21.4, 21.5, 21.6A**

With kind permission of
Springer Science and Business Media from Bates M, ed. *Bronchial Carcinoma. An Integrated Approach to Diagnosis and Management*. Berlin: Springer-Verlag; 1984. **Figure 12.7**

Used with permission from
Constine LS, Rubin P, Qazi R. Malignant lymphomas. In Rubin P, ed. *Clinical Oncology*, 7th ed. Philadelphia: WB Saunders; 1993:217–250. **Figure 12.3C**

Edge SB, Byrd DR, Compton CC, et al, eds. *AJCC Cancer Staging Manual*, 7th edition. New York: Springer Science and Business Media, LLC. Publishers. Copyright American Joint Committee on Cancer, 2010.
Summary of changes text pages *(page in AJCC 7th edition)* 128 *(253)*, 144 *(253)*, 154 *(253)*, 164 *(253)*, 174 *(253)*, 184 *(253)*, 194 *(253)*, 204 *(253)*, 214 *(347-348)*, 216 *(347-348)*, 228 *(103)*

From Gartner LP, and Hiatt JL: *Color Atlas of Histology*, 11th edition. Philadelphia: Lippincott Williams & Wilkins, 2009. **Figure 12.3B**

Used with permission of
the American Joint Committee on Cancer (AJCC), Chicago, Illinois. The original source for this material is the *AJCC Cancer Staging Manual*, 6th edition. New York: Springer-Verlag; 2002. **Figure 12.5D**

From Halperin EC, Perez CA, Brady LW, eds. *Perez & Brady's Principles and Practice of Radiation Oncology*, 5th edition. Philadelphia: Lippincott Williams & Wilkins, 2008. **Figure 12.3C**

From Harris JR, Lippman ME, Osborne KC, Morrow M: *Diseases of the Breast*, 4e. Philadelphia: Lippincott Williams & Wilkins, 2009. **Figure 20.3B**

Used with permission of
the Mayo Foundation for Medical Education and Research. Lymph node classification adapted from Mountain CF, Dresler CM. Regional lymph node classification for lung cancer staging. *Chest* 1977;111:1718–1723. **Figures 12.5B, 13.6B, 15.6B, 16.6B, 17.6B, 18.6B, 19.6B**

From Rubin R and Strayer DS: *Rubin's Pathology: Clinicopathologic Foundations of Medicine*, 5th edition. Philadelphia: Lippincott Williams & Wilkins, 2008. **Figures 13.1, 14.1, 15.1, 16.1, 17.1, 18.1, 19.1, 20.1, 21.1**

Stelow EB, Mills SE: *Biopsy Interpretation of the Upper Aerodigestive Tract and Ear*. Philadelphia, Lippincott Williams & Wilkins, 2008. **Figure 21.1**

Webb WR and Gotway MB. *Pocket Atlas of Body CT Anatomy*, 2nd edition. Philadelphia: Lippincott Williams & Wilkins, 2002. **Figures 13.8, 14.8, 15.8, 16.8, 17.8, 18.8, 19.8, 20.8, 21.7**

Section 3 (Chapters 22–33)

Modified from
Agur AMR, Dalley AF, eds. *Grant's Atlas of Anatomy*, 12th edition. Philadelphia: Lippincott Williams & Wilkins: 2009. **Figures 22.2, 22.3, 22.4A, 22.5, 22.6, 22.7, 23.2, 23.3, 23.4, 23.5, 23.6BC, 24.2, 24.3, 24.4, 24.5, 24.6, 25.2, 25.3, 25.4, 25.5, 25.6, 26.2, 26.3, 26.4, 26.5, 26.6, 27.2, 27.3, 27.4, 27.5, 27.6, 28.1, 28.3, 28.4, 28.5, 28.6, 29.2, 29.3, 29.4, 29.5, 29.6, 30.2, 30.3, 30.4, 30.5, 30.6, 31.2, 31.3, 31.5, 31.6, 32.2, 32.3, 32.4, 32.5, 32.6, 33.1, 33.2, 33.3, 33.4, 33.5**

Adapted from
Culver KW. *Gene Therapy: A Primer for Physicians*, 2nd edition. Larchmont: Mary Ann Liebert, Inc., 1996. **Figure 22.1**

Edge SB, Byrd DR, Compton CC, et al, eds. *AJCC Cancer Staging Manual*, 7th edition. New York: Springer Science and Business Media, LLC. Publishers. Copyright American Joint Committee on Cancer, 2010. Summary of changes text pages (*page in AJCC 7e*) 256 (*103*), 266 (*117*), 278 (*191*), 278 (*201*), 290 (*227*), 292 (*227*), 302 (*211*), 314 (*241*), 326 (*143*), 336 (*127*), 346, 347 (*133*), 354 (*143*), 364 (*165*)

From Eroschenko VP, ed. *di Fiore's Atlas of Histology with Functional Correlations*, 11th ed. Philadelphia: Lippincott Williams & Wilkins; 2008. **Figure 23.4B-G**

Halperin EC, Perez, CA, Brady, LW, eds: *Perez & Brady's Principles and Practice of Radiation Oncology*, 5th edition. Philadelphia: Lippincott Williams & Wilkins, 2008. **Figure 23.6A**

Kadish SL, Kochman ML. *Oncology* 1995;9(10):967–983. **Figure 22.8**

Rubin R and Strayer DS: *Rubin's Pathology: Clinicopathologic Foundations of Medicine*, 5th edition. Philadelphia: Lippincott Williams & Wilkins, 2008. **Figures 23.1, 24.1, 25.1, 26.1, 27.1, 28.2, 29.1, 30.1, 31.1, 32.1**

Webb WR and Gotway MB. *Pocket Atlas of Body CT Anatomy*, 2nd edition. Philadelphia: Lippincott Williams & Wilkins, 2002. **Figures 22.9, 23.7, 24.7, 25.7, 26.7, 27.7, 28.7, 29.7, 30.7, 31.7, 32.7, 33.6**

Section 4 (Chapters 34–41)

Modified from
Agur AMR, Dalley AF, eds. *Grant's Atlas of Anatomy*, 12th edition. Philadelphia: Lippincott Williams & Wilkins: 2009. **Figures 34.1, 34.2, 34.3A, 34.4, 34.5, 34.6, 34.7, 35.2, 35.3, 35.5, 35.6, 35.7, 36.2, 36.3, 36.4, 36.5, 36.6, 37.2, 37.3, 37.4, 37.5, 37.6, 38.2, 38.3, 38.4, 38.5B-D, 38.6, 39.2, 39.3, 39.4, 39.5, 39.6BC, 40.2, 40.3, 40.4, 40.5, 40.6, 41.2, 41.3, 41.4, 41.5, 41.6**

Edge SB, Byrd DR, Compton CC, et al, eds. *AJCC Cancer Staging Manual*, 7th edition. New York: Springer Science and Business Media, LLC. Publishers. Copyright American Joint Committee on Cancer, 2010. Summary of changes text page (*page in AJCC 7e*): 392 (*479*), 404 (*491*), 414 (*497*), 424 (*457*), 436 (*447*), 446 (*507*)

DeVita V, Lawrence TS, Rosenberg SA: *DeVita, Hellman and Rosenberg's Cancer: Principles and Practice of Oncology*,

9th edition. Philadelphia, Lippincott Williams & Wilkins, 2011. **Figure 38.8**

DeVita VT, Lawrence TS, Rosenberg SA, et al., eds., *DeVita, Hellman, and Rosenberg's Cancer: Principles and Practice of Oncology*, 8th ed. Philadelphia: Lippincott Williams & Wilkins, 2008:1459, 1460. **Figures 35.1, 39.6A, 39.8, 41.8**

Eroschenko VP: *diFiore's Atlas of Histology with Functional Correlations*, 11th edition. Philadelphia, Lippincott Williams & Wilkins, 2008. **Figure 34.3F**

Gartner LP, and Hiatt JL: *Color Atlas of Histology*, 11th edition. Philadelphia: Lippincott Williams & Wilkins, 2009. **Figure 34.3BCDE**

Higgins CB, Hricak H, Helms CA. *Magnetic Resonance Imaging of the Body*, 3rd edition. Philadelphia, Lippincott Williams & Wilkins, 1996. **Figures 34.8, 40.7**

Rubin R and Strayer DS: *Rubin's Pathology: Clinicopathologic Foundations of Medicine*, 5th edition. Philadelphia: Lippincott Williams & Wilkins, 2008. **Figures 35.1, 35.4BC, 36.1, 37.1, 38.1, 39.1, 40.1, 41.1**

Webb WR and Gotway MB. *Pocket Atlas of Body CT Anatomy*, 2nd edition. Philadelphia: Lippincott Williams & Wilkins, 2002. **Figures 35.8, 36.7, 37.7, 38.7, 39.7**

Section 5 (Chapters 42–48)

Modified from
Agur AMR, Dalley AF, eds. *Grant's Atlas of Anatomy*, 12th edition. Philadelphia: Lippincott Williams & Wilkins: 2009. **Figures 42.1, 42.2, 42.3A, 42.4, 42.5, 42.6, 43.1, 43.3, 43.4, 43.5, 43.6, 44.2, , 44.3, 44.4, 44.5, 44.6, 45.2, 45.3, 45.4, 45.5, 45.6, 46.2, 46.3, 46.4, 46.5, 46.6, 47.2, 47.3, 47.4, 47.5, 47.6, 48.2, 48.3, 48.4, 48.5, 48.6**

Berek JS, Friedlander M, Hacker NF. *Epithelial Ovarian, Fallopian Tube, and Peritoneal Cancer*. Berek JS and Hacker NF, eds. *Berek and Hacker's Gynecologic Oncology*, 2010. **Table 43.4B**

Campos Z, Narumi Y, Hricak H. *Pocket Atlas of MRI of the Pelvis*. New York: Raven Press, 1993. **Figure 42.7B**

Edge SB, Byrd DR, Compton CC, et al, eds. *AJCC Cancer Staging Manual*, 7th edition. New York: Springer Science and Business Media, LLC. Publishers. Copyright American Joint Committee on Cancer, 2010. Summary of changes text page (*page in AJCC 7e*): 486 (*419*), 498 (*403*), 500 (*403*), 502 (*403*), 512 (*437*), 524 (*395*), 534 (*387*), 544 (*379*)

Eroschenko VP: *diFiore's Atlas of Histology with Functional Correlations*, 11th edition. Philadelphia, Lippincott Williams & Wilkins, 2008. **Figure 42.3G**

Gartner LP, and Hiatt JL: *Color Atlas of Histology*, 11th edition. Philadelphia: Lippincott Williams & Wilkins, 2009. **Figure 42.3BCDEF**

Halperin EC, Perez CA, Brady LW, eds. *Perez & Brady's Principles and Practice of Radiation Oncology*, 5th edition. Philadelphia: Lippincott Williams & Wilkins, 2008. **Table 37.4B, Figure 38.5A**

Rubin R and Strayer DS: *Rubin's Pathology: Clinicopathologic Foundations of Medicine*, 5th edition. Philadelphia: Lippincott Williams & Wilkins, 2008. **Figures 43.2, 44.1, 45.1, 46.1, 47.1, 48.1**

Webb WR and Gotway MB. *Pocket Atlas of Body CT Anatomy*, 2nd edition. Philadelphia: Lippincott Williams & Wilkins, 2002. **Figures 42.7A, 43.7, 44.7, 45.7, 46.8, 47.7, 48.7**

Section 6 (Chapters 49–54)

Modified from
Agur AMR, Dalley AF, eds. *Grant's Atlas of Anatomy*, 12th edition. Philadelphia: Lippincott Williams & Wilkins: 2009. **Figures 50.1B, 50.2A, 50.3, 50.4, 50.5, 50.6BC, 51.4, 52.3, 52.5, 52.6, 53.1A, 53.3, 53.4DEFGHIJ, 53.5, 53.6, 54.3A**

Bragg DG, Rubin P, Hricak H, eds. *Oncologic Imaging*, 2nd ed. Philadelphia: W.B. Saunders, 2002. **Figure 54.6B**

Edge SB, Byrd DR, Compton CC, et al, eds. *AJCC Cancer Staging Manual*, 7th edition. New York: Springer Science and Business Media, LLC. Publishers. Copyright American Joint Committee on Cancer, 2010.
Summary of changes text page (*page in AJCC 7e*): 572 *(301)*, 588 *(325)*, 598 *(291)*, 610 *(281)*

DeVita V, Lawrence TS, Rosenberg SA: *DeVita, Hellman and Rosenberg's Cancer: Principles and Practice of Oncology*, 9th edition. Philadelphia, Lippincott Williams & Wilkins, 2011. **Figures 51.1BC, 51.5, 51.6C, 52.4DE.**

Modified from
Eroschenko VP: *diFiore's Atlas of Histology with Functional Correlations*, 10th edition. Philadelphia, Lippincott Williams & Wilkins, 2005. **Figures 49.2, 49.6B, 49.7, 50.2B, 50.3, 50.4A, 51.1A, 51.2A, 51.4, 52.2AB, 52.3, 54.4A (parts A-F).**

Gartner LP, and Hiatt JL: *Color Atlas of Histology*, 11th edition. Philadelphia: Lippincott Williams & Wilkins, 2009. **Figures 50.2C, 51.6AB**

Kaplan HS. *Hodgkin's Disease*, 2nd edition. Cambridge: Harvard University Press; 1980. **Figure 54.6A**

Rubin P. *Dynamic Classification of Bone Dysplasia*. Chicago: Yearbook Medical Publishers; 1964. **Figures 53.2AB, 53.4ABC**

Rubin P, Williams J, eds. *Clinical Oncology: A Multidisciplinary Approach for Physicians and Students*, 8th ed. Philadelphia: Elsevier; 2001. **Figures 49.1, 49.3, 49.4, 49.5**

Rubin R and Strayer DS: *Rubin's Pathology: Clinicopathologic Foundations of Medicine*, 5th edition. Philadelphia: Lippincott Williams & Wilkins, 2008. **Figures 50.2DE, 50.4B, 51.1DE, 51.3, 53.2EFG, 54.3B, 54.4B-L**

Section 7 (Chapters 55–59)

Modified from
Agur AMR, Dalley AF, eds. *Grant's Atlas of Anatomy*, 12th edition. Philadelphia: Lippincott Williams & Wilkins: 2009. **Figures 55.1, 55.4, 55.6D, 55.7, 55.8, 56.1CD, 56.3, 56.4, 56.5, 56.6, 57.1CD, 57.4, 57.5, 57.6, 57.7, 58.2, 58.5, 58.7, 59.1, 59.2, 59.4, 59.5, 59.6,59.7**

Bragg DG, Rubin P, Hricak H, eds. *Oncologic Imaging*, 2nd ed. Philadelphia: W.B. Saunders, 2002. **Figure 54.6B**

Edge SB, Byrd DR, Compton CC, et al, eds. *AJCC Cancer Staging Manual*, 7th edition. New York: Springer Science and Business Media, LLC. Publishers. Copyright American Joint Committee on Cancer, 2010. Figure 57.3 *(p. 556)*
Summary of changes text page (*page in AJCC 7e*): 657 *(523)*, 658 *(531)*, 659 *(539)*, 668 *(547)*, 680-681 *(561)*, 690 *(577)*

Modified from
Eroschenko VP: *diFiore's Atlas of Histology with Functional Correlations*, 10th edition. Philadelphia, Lippincott Williams & Wilkins, 2005. **Figures 55.3, 55.6A, 57.1B, 57.2B, 58.4, 58.6A**

Gartner LP, and Hiatt JL: *Color Atlas of Histology*, 11th edition. Philadelphia: Lippincott Williams & Wilkins, 2009. **Figure 55.6B**

Moore KL, Dalley AF, Agur AMR. *Clinically Oriented Anatomy*, 6th edition. Philadelphia, Lippincott Williams & Wilkins, 2010. **Figures 55.5AB, 55.6C, 55.7BCD**

Rubin R and Strayer DS: *Rubin's Pathology: Clinicopathologic Foundations of Medicine*, 5th edition. Philadelphia: Lippincott Williams & Wilkins, 2008. **Figures 56.2AB, 57.1A, 57.2A, 58.1, 58.3, 59.3**

Index

Note: Page numbers followed by f denote figures, and page numbers followed by t denote tables.